EIGHTH EDITION

MOSBY'S FUNDAMENTALS of Therapeutic Massage

Sandy Fritz, MS, BCTMB, CMBE
Founder, Owner, Director, and Head Instructor
Health Enrichment Center
School of Therapeutic Massage and Bodywork
Lapeer, Michigan

Luke Allen Fritz, BAS (Massage Therapy), LMT
Instructor
Health Enrichment Center
School of Therapeutic Massage and Bodywork
Lapeer, Michigan

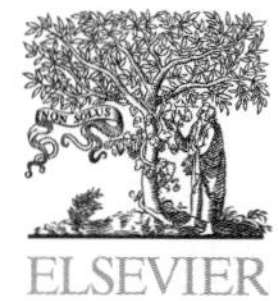

ELSEVIER
3251 Riverport Lane
St. Louis, Missouri 63043

MOSBY'S FUNDAMENTALS OF THERAPEUTIC MASSAGE, EIGHTH EDITION ISBN: 978-0-443-11720-6

Publishing Director: Kristin Wilhelm
Content Strategist: Melissa Rawe
Senior Content Development Manager: Lisa Newton
Senior Content Development Specialist: Laura Goodrich
Publishing Services Manager: Deepthi Unni
Senior Project Manager: Kamatchi Madhavan
Book Designer: Maggie Reid

Printed in India
Last digit is the print number: 9 8 7 6 5 4 3 2 1

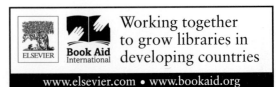

MOSBY'S

FUNDAMENTALS

of Therapeutic Massage

Reviewers

Damien A. Archambeau, LMT, BCTMB, A.A.S in Massage Therapy, CLT-ALM, Instructor and Approved Continuing Education Provider
Corporate Controller
TruMantra Education Group
New York, New York

Kevin Pierce, FL Massage License, MBA
Neuromuscular Massage Therapy Certification
Faculty at Sarasota School of Massage Therapy
Owner of Focus Massage & Bodywork
Florida Massage CEU Provider
Sarasota School of Massage Therapy
Sarasota, Florida

CONTRIBUTORS AND REVIEWERS TO PREVIOUS EDITIONS

Wayne J. Albert, PhD, CK, FCSB
Robin B. Anderson, MEd, BA, LMT, BCTMB, CEAS
Sandra K. Anderson, BA, LMT, ABT, NCTMB
Damien A. Archambeau, LMT, BCTMB, ERYT, YACEP
Lurana S. Bain, LMT, BCTMB
Carla M. Banshaw, BA, LMT
Patricia J. Benjamin, PhD
Paul V. Berry Jr., BSHA, LMT, NCTMB, PTA, NCMA
Leon K. Chaitow, ND, DO
Kelly Challis
Whitney Christiano, LMT, RYT, CPT, BA
Emily Edith Safrona Cowall, Reg MT
Karen Craig, LMT, NCTMB
Neal Delaporta, LMT, NCTMB, CPT
Robin Devine, RMT, CLT
Marjorie Foley, LMT Certified Paralegal
Luke Allen Fritz, LMT
Michael Garcia, RN, LMT
Jimmy Gialelis, LMT, BCTMB
Peter A. Goldberg, DIPL AC (NCCA), LMT
MaryAnne Hochadel, PharmD, BCPS
Cher Hunter, MA, LMT, NCTMB
Christopher V. Jones, CMT, NCTMB
Don Kelley, LMT, NCBTMB
Megan Lavery, LAPC, LMT, BCTMB, CZB, CPA
Kathy Lee, LMT, BS Business Administration
Lucy Liben, MS, LMT
Jean E. Loving, BA, LMT
Edward G. Mohr, MSIE, CPE, CSP, NCTM
Karen B. Napolitano, MS
Kathleen Maison Paholsky, MS, PhD
Kevin Pierce, MBA, NCBTMB
Monica J. Reno, AAS, LMT
Diana M. Reeder, BSHA, CCMA, CBCS
Shannon Saunders, LMT AAS Therapeutic Massage
Richard Schekter, MS, LMT
Jeffrey A. Simancek, BS, CMT, NCBTMB
Cherie Marilyn Sohnen-Moe, BA
Rebecca Steele, RMT
Diana L. Thompson, BA, LMP
Mary Margaret Tuchscherer, DC, PhD
Richard van Why
Sherri Williamson, LMT
Ed Wilson, PhD, LMT
Jeffrey B. Wood, LMT, COTA/L, BS

Preface

More than 45 years ago, when I was exploring a career in therapeutic massage, there were few schools. Because none of them were readily accessible to me, I taught myself. I took a course of less than 100 hours, which at least provided basic skills. The rest of my massage therapy training has come from reading a multitude of books and research papers; attending hundreds of hours of workshops; undergoing apprenticeship training; taking college courses in related subjects; teaching more than 7000 beginning students and approximately 1500 advanced students at my school, the Health Enrichment Center School of Therapeutic Massage and Bodywork; and providing more than 50,000 massage sessions. Since the publication of the first edition, I completed my bachelor's degree at Central Michigan University and master's degree at Thomas Edison State University. Becoming a student again in the university environment had a great influence on my perspective about education, as well as on my professional development.

I am still learning the importance of the fundamental concepts upon which all manual therapy approaches are based. I learn more about the elegant simplicity of massage each time I teach or do massage, and I have learned a great deal through researching and writing textbooks as well. More than ever, I am convinced that a strong understanding of the fundamental concepts of therapeutic massage and the ability to reason effectively through a decision-making process are essential for proficient professional practice. In the more than four decades of my massage career, I have experienced an evolution of massage therapy, from a fringe alternative method to the integration of massage into the maturity of evidence-based and informed practice. When I compare the first edition of this textbook to this eighth edition, it is apparent that the knowledge necessary to begin a massage therapy career has increased, yet the underlying fundamental principle remains—compassionate, beneficial application of touch to help people feel better.

A CO-AUTHOR FOR THE TEXTBOOKS

I am proud of my co-author, Luke Fritz. Luke has 20 years of massage experience in multiple settings but primarily with professional sports teams. He has his BAS in massage therapy and is teaching in both entry- and advanced-level education. Luke brings a contemporary view of massage practice for those 35 years old and younger. Yes, Luke is my son, and his input and perspective are an added value to the textbook content and design.

WHO WILL BENEFIT FROM THIS BOOK?

The eighth edition of *Mosby's Fundamentals of Therapeutic Massage* is intended to be used by skilled therapeutic massage educators and beginning and advanced students in the classroom setting. It will also be used as a continuing education resource by practitioners and as a reference text for health professionals and massage and bodywork practitioners.

WHY IS THIS BOOK IMPORTANT TO THE PROFESSION OF MASSAGE THERAPY?

The changes and additions to the eighth edition reflect how much therapeutic massage has evolved as a profession over the past few years. Today, therapeutic massage is in the process of standardizing and organizing. Projects such as the Entry-Level Analysis Program (elapmassage.org) and the Massage Therapy Body of Knowledge (MTBOK.org) have been an effort to unify the practice and terminology of massage and its various modalities, attesting to the growing awareness among massage professionals that their success depends on clarity and an agreed-upon base of knowledge, as in other skilled fields. It is an exciting time in massage therapy, as we see more and more people turning to massage as a reliable and practical form of self-care. A curriculum that is mindful of all these points is a curriculum that aims high.

A well-rounded education in massage therapy includes learning all of the following: how to perform massage manipulations and techniques; understanding the anatomical and physiological underpinnings for why the methods work based on research and a biologically plausible and logical framework; and the importance of structure, intent, and purpose of touch. It is as important to touch the whole person as it is to skillfully apply techniques. The massage professional must do both. In addition, the learner needs to understand the importance of sanitation, hygiene, body mechanics, research literacy, business practices, and ethics, and then apply this knowledge through effective decision making to build a well-balanced, professional massage career. To justify the cost and time spent, massage therapy needs to be beneficial and meet the outcomes and results desired by the clients served. Massage therapists need to be able to adapt to the individual client to be successful.

The fundamentals of massage methods remain relatively simple. Fundamentally, massage methods are mechanical force push and pull applications. Certainly then there must be more to massage therapy than just being able to give a massage. A well-planned school curriculum, as developed in this textbook and its instructor resources (TEACH Lesson Plan Manual and instructor resources), combined with a comprehensive science curriculum as presented in *Mosby's Essential Sciences for Therapeutic Massage* and its various ancillaries provide a foundation for massage educational programs and present information necessary for entry-level licensing. With in-depth study, these textbooks also provide the information and skill foundation for the advanced credential, the Board Certification Exam from the National Certification Board for Therapeutic Massage and Bodywork.

Massage education should be competency based, meaning all information in the educational setting is relevant to the actual professional practice of therapeutic massage. The design of this textbook, combined with the Evolve website, also supports various types of Web-enhanced education.

The level of knowledge in this eighth edition has been increased to reflect the skills necessary to work effectively in the medical care world with supervision. Although my personal love for this profession lies in humble service to the general public in the support of their wellness, and compassion and help for the daily aches and pains of life, I recognize the importance of being able to also work within the medical care and sport and fitness systems. My work over the past several years with a clinical physiologist, numerous physicians, athletic trainers, and physical therapists supports this observation. Because of the development of comprehensive textbooks, more schools will be better able to expand their curricula for those who wish to pursue therapeutic massage applications in health/medical care.

The foundation for therapeutic massage was laid centuries ago and will not change, provided human physiology remains constant. It is virtually impossible to acknowledge all those who have contributed to the knowledge base of this field. Our observations of the natural world are a good starting point for this basic knowledge. For example, animals know the value of rhythmic touch. Just watch a litter of puppies or kittens and observe the structured application of touch. The base of information goes beyond us to an innate need to rub an area that is hurting and to touch others to provide comfort, pleasure, and bonding.

TEXTBOOK THEMES

These major themes guide the structure of this textbook.

- Massage therapy is an outcome-based approach targeting the four main outcomes of relaxation and well-being, stress management, pain management, and functional mobility.
- Massage is based on four main approaches to care: palliative, restorative, condition management, and therapeutic change.
- Massage is uniquely adapted to every client based on goals, assessment, special circumstances, client-centered intention, and compassion and nurturance.
- Massage is uniquely designed for each client based on critical thinking, clinical reasoning, and evidence-informed practice.
- Massage is an evidence-informed and biologically plausible system based on applied mechanical forces modified in multiple ways to both assess the client and provide appropriate intervention to achieve client goals.
- Massage is a professional health service provided in multiple environments and is dependent on the therapeutic relationship between the massage therapist and the client.

TEXTBOOK ORGANIZATION

The textbook is divided into four units based on related content.

Unit I: Professional Practice

1 Therapeutic Massage as a Profession
2 Ethics, Professionalism, and Legal Issues
3 Business Considerations for a Career in Therapeutic Massage
4 Massage and Medical Terminology for Professional Record Keeping

The chapters focus on building a solid basis for professionalism and decision-making skills before moving into the actual physical and mental work of practicing massage. Chapter 1 begins with an exploration of touch and reveals its historical foundations. Chapter 2 introduces the clinical-reasoning, problem-solving model for ethical decision making and also explains what it means to be a professional, including awareness of laws and regulations. Chapter 3 provides a newly expanded look at the business of massage, job-seeking skills, and the options of creating a career as a business owner or as an employee. Chapter 4 presents appropriate medical and massage therapy terminology to support professional record keeping and documentation. Students are exposed to a language that is understood across many disciplines and that allows professionals to communicate accurately.

Unit II: Foundations for Massage Benefit

5 Research Literacy and Evidence-Informed Practice
6 Indications and Contraindications for Therapeutic Massage
7 Hygiene, Sanitation, and Safety

Massage therapy has become an evidence-informed practice. Chapter 5 further explores what this means and explains the scientific basis for evidence that supports the benefits of therapeutic massage. This chapter also focuses on research literacy, empowering students to look deeper into their practice and its value. Chapter 6 begins the process of decision making in terms of indications and contraindications to massage. Chapter 7 presents information on sanitation, hygiene, and safety, ensuring the reader understands the importance of protecting the client from harm.

Unit III: The Massage Process

8 Body Mechanics
9 Preparation for Massage: Equipment, Professional Environment, Positioning, and Draping
10 Massage Manipulations and Techniques
11 Assessment Procedures for Developing a Care/Treatment Plan

Chapter 8 covers the very important content of body mechanics and ergonomics. It is necessary for massage therapists to be able to use their bodies effectively, efficiently, and wisely to have a successful massage career. Chapter 9 describes massage equipment and supplies, positioning and draping procedures, various massage environments, and other information ancillary to a successful massage practice. Chapters 10 and 11 focus on technical skills. Each section builds on the previous one, beginning with the basics and expanding assessment methods to support therapeutic applications. As the methods and techniques of therapeutic massage are presented, the reader learns how and why they work and when to use them to obtain a particular physiologic response. Upon completion of this unit, the learner should be able to provide an outcome-based massage.

Unit IV: Beyond the Basics

12 Complementary Bodywork Systems
13 Massage Career Tracks and Practice Settings
14 Adaptive Massage
15 Wellness Education
16 Case Studies

Chapter 12 introduces the concept of adjunct methods, such as hydrotherapy and essential oils. Massage application systems that have become specialized, such as lymphatic drainage, connective tissue, and myofascial release, and approaches to treating trigger points are presented in the next section of the chapter. An overview of Eastern and cultural approaches based on traditional Chinese medicine, Ayurveda, and others is covered in the next section. Reflexology is also included in this content. Finally, a discussion on the adjunct methods based on biofields (often called *energy work*) is provided, as well as technical skill from the polarity system, which provides a model for this type of bodywork.

Chapter 13 focuses on three main career tracks—wellness/spa, medical care, and athletics. Chapter 14 describes how to adapt massage to address the needs relevant to particular populations, from pregnant mothers and infants to hospice patients and people with physical impairments. Chapter 15 explores the issues of wellness and nutrition. Massage therapy is a physically taxing field of work. An MT must stay strong and healthy to do a good job and to continue feeling rewarded by the work.

Finally, Chapter 16 sets the stage for putting the material and your study to work through the use of comprehensive case studies based on the clinical-reasoning model, outcome-based massage, and treatment plan development. This chapter presents 20 case studies that integrate the information from both this textbook and the student's science studies, such as those covered in *Mosby's Essential Sciences for Therapeutic Massage*. The case studies cover the majority of common conditions seen by massage professionals in day and destination spas, as well as in wellness, health, fitness, sport, and medical settings. If students study the process of clinical reasoning carefully, these case examples will enable them to address almost all other conditions encountered in professional practice. The entire book focuses on developing clinical-reasoning skills for this profession.

Appendices

Helpful appendices are located at the end of the book. These include an updated appendix on indications and contraindications and common pathology. A new quick muscle reference guide appendix has been added. An appendix on human trafficking is provided. A basic pharmacology for massage reference written especially for this textbook by a clinical pharmacist is found on the Evolve site.

AN ADAPTABLE DESIGN

It is not necessary to have multiple textbooks for each course. Chapters in *Mosby's Fundamentals of Therapeutic Massage* can be used in multiple ways to provide content for courses within the curriculum. The textbook can be taught in a sequential manner from Chapter 1 to Chapter 16, or it can be adapted to fit the order of topics within the chosen curriculum. Another approach is to cluster the chapters into units as previously described or modules such as the following:

- Chapters 1–4 as the professionalism and ethics unit
- Chapters 5–6 as the research literacy unit
- Chapters 7–12 as the guide on how to build massage application skills
- Chapters 13–16 can then act as an integration unit.

Another organizational approach is as follows:

- Chapters 1–6 cover the practical and critical-thinking skills, which can simultaneously be taught with
- Chapters 7–12, so that the student learns hands-on skills with thinking skills, all in a coordinated manner.
- Chapters 13–14 can be presented as practice specialization content.
- Chapters 15–16 focus on integration of skills, such as clinical experience. Chapter 15 (as well as many of the exercises provided throughout the text) promotes introspection, understanding, and topics that are supportive to the general well-being of the therapist, and Chapter 16 offers a wide variety of case studies.

When combined with *Mosby's Essential Sciences for Therapeutic Massage*, *Mosby's Fundamentals of Therapeutic Massage* provides a complete textbook resource for a relevant, accurate, and outstanding massage therapy curriculum. Designed for teachers and students by someone who is a teacher and massage therapist, it is our hope that the textbook, all the ancillaries, and instructor support materials serve both teachers and students in the journey of becoming extraordinary massage therapy professionals.

Acknowledgments

My thanks to all of the professionals who have influenced the content and clarity over multiple editions of this text to ensure accurate presentation of information.

A specific acknowledgment to Ann Blair Kennedy and her fellow researchers for use of the massage therapy practice framework found in the papers:

- **A qualitative study of the massage therapy foundation's best practices symposium: Clarifying definitions and creating a framework for practice** Kennedy, Ann Blair. PhD diss., University of South Carolina, 2015.
- **Process for massage therapy practice and essential assessment** Kennedy, Ann Blair, Jerrilyn A. Cambron, Patricia A. Sharpe, Ravensara S. Travillian, and Ruth P. Saunders. Journal of bodywork and movement therapies 20, no. 3 (2016): 484–496.

The content and clarity provided by Dr. Kennedy and fellow researchers informed this edition of the textbook.

There are several people who deserve special recognition for their efforts in the publication of this edition.

A special thank you to:

All of the individuals on my support team at Elsevier.

The clients I have had for more than four decades, the athletes I work with for a day or throughout their careers—for constantly challenging me to figure out what to do with all their assorted bumps, bruises, sprains, strains, breaks, performance stresses, and personalities.

And to all the students I have worked with, for keeping me honest and humble.

It truly has been a team effort.

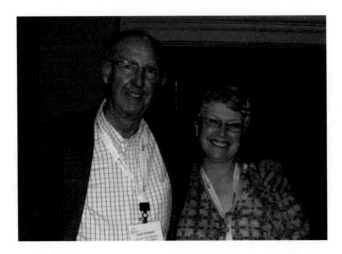

Leon Chaitow, ND, DO (1937–2018), wrote the forewords for each edition of this textbook. When he passed in 2018, he left both an extensive and rich legacy and sorrow and longing for my teacher, mentor, and friend. I fully expected he would also write the foreword for this new eighth edition. Instead this edition is dedicated to Dr. Chaitow.

From the foreword in the sixth edition.
"Since the first edition in 1995, author Sandy Fritz has emphasized critical thinking and clinical reasoning as the foundation of the text. These skills are the cornerstone of evidence-informed practice. The range of topics, and their depth of exploration—combined with the unique, practical, easy-to-follow delivery of information—makes it a universally useful resource for anyone in the manual therapy professions in general, and massage therapists in particular, and not just in their early training stages. There is much to learn for experienced therapists since the author has focused on bringing the very latest in clinical and practical research and understanding into the text. For more than 20 years, this textbook has evolved with and guided the professional advancement of massage therapy."
Leon Chaitow, ND, DO

Fritz Gives You the Fundamentals and More!

Welcome to the Eighth Edition

For content you can trust, this text delivers:

ALL CHAPTERS HAVE BEEN REVISED AND UPDATED to reflect changes in curriculum standards and to include new research.

CHAPTERS ARE DIVIDED INTO 15- TO 30-MINUTE TEACHING AND STUDY SECTIONS

- ELAP and MTBOK knowledge, skills, attitudes, and terminology content.
- Content is aligned with the MBLEX and the NCBTMB Board Certification Exam.
- Detailed and competency-based chapter and section objectives.

PROFESSIONAL TOUCH

SECTION OBJECTIVES

Chapter objective covered in this section:

1. Identify personal interpretations of touch and their influence on professional interactions.

Using the information presented in this section, the student will be able to:

- Distinguish between professional and nonprofessional forms of touch
- List factors that influence the communication of touch
- Define bias and implicit bias

CHAPTER OBJECTIVES

After completing this chapter, the student will be able to:

1. Identify personal interpretations of touch and their influence on professional interactions.
2. Describe professional touch.
3. Define professionalism.
4. Define therapeutic massage.
5. Explain the rich heritage and history of therapeutic massage.
6. Explain the influence of historical events and global culture on the current development of therapeutic massage.
7. Self-assess for leadership qualities.
8. Analyze a professional practice framework.

CHAPTER OUTLINE

- Spiral and scaffolded approach to learning is embedded where first the basic facts of a subject are presented. As the learner progresses through the textbook, the basic content is reinforced, expanded, and framed in increasingly more complex ways, which supports critical thinking and content retention.
- ONGOING AND EXPANDED emphasis on critical-thinking and clinical-reasoning skills development.

Therapeutic Massage as a Profession **CHAPTER 1** 3

of following a straight line. It may be confusing because one question leads back to another.

One of the many ways your brain learns is by circling around and around through information, collecting an increased understanding with each revolution. Eventually, the understanding begins to turn the circle into a spiral as comprehension leads to creative application (Fig. 1.1). In straight-line learning, a piece of information is presented once, then the next piece is presented, and then the next, and so on, much like driving down a road from point A to point B. Except for elementary sequential information, straight-line learning is not very effective. We do not learn efficiently by experiencing something only once. Even if we go back and repeat the linear A-to-B sequence repeatedly, the brain begins to ignore the information because it is too familiar (Fig. 1.2).

Repetition is necessary to learn anything. However, to keep the brain interested, the repetition somehow must be different each time. Think of a piece of music. You can hear the repetition of a melody in a few lines of music, but you can also hear where the composer has changed a note or two. You enjoy hearing the repetition of a good melody, but you also enjoy it when it is changed slightly because this prevents you from becoming bored with it. This is called *novel repetition* (Fig. 1.3); that is, the same information is given over and over, but always a little differently and in a circular format. As you learn about massage therapy, this type of repetition eventually spirals into the ability to become a creative and skilled massage therapist. As you read and study this textbook, notice how learning spirals, novel repetition, and asking questions are teaching you to use critical thinking and eventually teaching you to become your own teacher to support lifelong learning.

In massage, which is a professional, structured, therapeutic touch, education begins with questions.

- What is the significance of touch?
- What is professional touch?
- What motivates me to study therapeutic massage?
- What is therapeutic?
- How am I served by touching others?
- When did touch become professional?
- Why did touch become professional?
- Do therapeutic forms of touch have to be provided by a professional?
- In what way is professional therapeutic touch different from casual touch, friendship touch, family touch, intimate touch, or erotic (sexual) touch?
- How do different individuals, social groups, or cultures view touch?
- In what way does the past affect the present and guide the future development of the massage therapy profession?

Questions continue to arise, and the answers are not necessarily simple. As we seek to serve our clients, eventually we are faced with these questions and many others. Some of the questions mentioned previously are explored in this text, especially as they relate to the professional practice of therapeutic massage. Some are not explored directly; rather, both questions and answers evolve as a learner's knowledge and experience increases. Although this text does not always provide definitive answers, it does provide information to help you find your own.

What will your questions be? How will your answers influence those you touch? How will your answers touch you? These are huge issues to consider at the beginning of any course of study. As you begin to think about them, you might feel interested, excited, overwhelmed, or maybe even frightened as you come to realize how necessary, beneficial, complex, and powerful touch can be. These important questions are posed at the beginning of this study likely before you have sufficient information to develop effective answers. Remember that understanding

FIG. 1.1 Spiral learning.

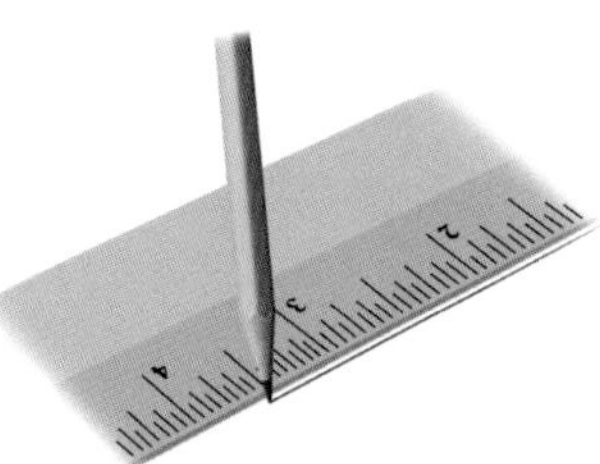

FIG. 1.2 Straight-line learning.

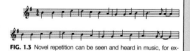

FIG. 1.3 Novel repetition can be seen and heard in music, for example.

- UPDATED Chapter 5 : *Research Literacy and Evidence-Informed Practice*, which focuses on the expanding role students can play in learning more about the growing body of science within the massage field.

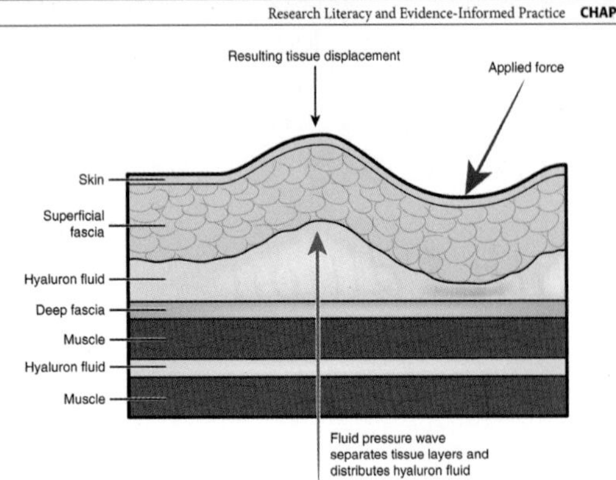

FIG. 5.3 Example of how applied force from massage can displace tissue and fluid between tissue layers to create a fluid pressure wave; this both separates tissue layers and distributes hyaluron-based fluid to restore sliding among tissue layers.

work has provided a biomechanical model that helps decipher the role of fascia in musculoskeletal disorders (Arumugam and Harikesavan, 2021).

Researchers think that the richly innervated fascia may be maintained in a taut resting state, called *fascial tone*, as a result of the different muscular fibers that pull on it (somewhat like a trampoline). This resting state enables the free nerve endings and receptors in the fascial tissue to sense any variation in the shape of the fascia (and therefore any movement of the body) (Schleip et al., 2005; Stecco et al., 2007a; Ganjaei et al., 2020). Deep fascia is designed to sense and assist in organizing movements. When body parts move in any direction, a myofascial tensional rearrangement occurs in the corresponding fascia (Schoenrock et al., 2018).

The mechanical forces generated by massage and other forms of manual therapy may stimulate fascial mechanoreceptors, which in turn may trigger tonus changes in connected skeletal muscle fibers (Chaudhry et al., 2008; Frey et al., 2009).

It is likely that the stiffness felt after periods of inactivity is related to the fascial system. If the amount of hyaluronan is reduced or if hyaluronan is not equally distributed, the tissue sticks or slides less efficiently (Bordoni and Zanier, 2014). Mechanical force applied by massage may separate tissue layers and allow for even hyaluronan distribution (Fig. 5.3).

Interestingly, reduced sliding of the various layers limits the functionality of the endocannabinoid system (McPartland et al., 2014; Buscemi et al., 2021). There is a close relationship between the endocannabinoid and endorphin system and fibroblasts. This relationship is believed to manage inflammation and pain information originating in the fascial tissue. This is a complex interaction because fascia continuously remodels daily.

If defective sliding results from a scar, the fascial continuum enables pain symptoms (Zugel et al., 2018). *Densification*, or a thickening of the ground substance, can develop into fibrosis (Pavan, 2014). Fibrosis or fibromatosis results from a disorder of connective tissue that is affected by hyperplasia and hypertrophy of the fibroblasts; this can occur as a result of a chronic inflammatory environment or nonphysiological mechanical stress and immobility; calcification phenomena can also be observed (Cao et al., 2013). The systemic effects associated with mechanical-load responses of the soft tissue remain difficult to isolate but suggest that anatomical areas with low pain can be selected for manual treatment, potentially causing body-wide benefit.

Another research focus related to functional mobility is postexercise stiffness, known as *delayed-onset muscle soreness* (DOMS). After unaccustomed exercise, which results in DOMS, the levels of the enzyme creatine kinase increase, indicating that muscle damage has occurred. Olszewski et al. (2009) and Zainuddin et al. (2005) found that massage was effective at alleviating DOMS by approximately 30% through the effect of reduced swelling. They also found that massage treatment had important effects on plasma creatine kinase activity, citing a significantly lower peak value at 4 days after exercise. Despite these changes, massage application had no effect on muscle function.

In a different study, Bakowski et al. (2008) found that massage administered 30 minutes after exercise could have a beneficial influence on DOMS by reducing soreness, but that it did not affect muscle swelling or range of motion.

- REVISED CHAPTER ON BUSINESS AND PROFESSIONAL SKILL clearly describing career focus both as self-employed or employee.

e and injury are usually caused by ineffective of the body while giving massage. Chapter 8 anics and contains possibly the most important eventing burnout. It is reasonable to expect that t can work 40 hours a week and perform 25–30 ssage during that time. This is a full-time mas-

n is common in our society. The economy people have to adapt to limited resources. It xpect that entry-level massage therapists can y if employed and net profit if self-employed before income taxes of $35,000–$45,000 if they can work full time and provide the 25–30 actual hours of massage sessions each week. A self-employed massage therapist would need a business gross of $70,000–$90,000 a year to have a net profit of $35,000–$45,000. Again, it is important to begin your massage career with realistic expectations. However, it is also important to realize that with experience and increased client retention, the income can increase as the overhead decreases or if the employer increases wages for a productive and valued employee. Massage therapy is a service business, and income stability depends on client satisfaction, retention, and a full appointment schedule. If a client cancels an appointment, it creates a reduction in income. If you are employed, the business owner must absorb the loss of income. If you are self-employed, you have to deal with the deficit. The burnout issue occurs when income barely covers personal expenses, and there is no financial safety net. It is stressful to live from paycheck to paycheck.

Emotional stress is a major cause of burnout. For massage therapists, this is characterized by taking better care of others than we do of ourselves. Burnout can be a problem in most service professions. Taking care of others is a big job. If we do not take care of ourselves also, we soon have nothing to give others or ourselves. Each of us must take care of our physical needs, such as resting, eating well, getting regular massages, and paying attention to our emotional needs. Surround yourself with people who believe in you. Take care of your spiritual needs, which connect the value of what you want to accomplish with a much higher purpose. Follow the wellness guidelines presented in Chapter 15.

The actual application of massage is basic, repetitious touch, which sometimes can get boring. It is important to keep yourself excited about the benefits of such repetitious applications of touch. One of the best ways to do this is to continue your education. Classes make you think and bring you together with other massage professionals. These are good opportunities to share and learn together. State-licensed massage schools and professional organizations are the best sources for massage education. It also is important to get away from massage for a bit. Having a hobby or creating downtime creates balance. Take care of yourself, and let others take care of you. Take a vacation, a walk, or a long warm bath, and burnout will be less of a problem.

After a person begins to live life—including their career life—with purpose, the energy to develop the career focus becomes available. Living with purpose is the key to motivation. It means drawing strength from knowing that what we have to offer is valuable (Proficiency Exercise 3.3).

PROFICIENCY EXERCISE 3.3

Separate into small groups and take turns describing a time when you were burned out. Explain what steps you took to get out of the burnout phase.

Self-Employment, Employee, or Combined Practice

This chapter does what generic business texts and websites cannot do: it shares the experience gained from walking the career path in therapeutic massage, both as an employee and as a self-employed professional. Throughout the text, you are encouraged to ask questions about your massage education, to use clinical reasoning as a problem-solving method, and to challenge information. You are urged to seek authoritative sources carefully and to compare information from many experts. The same principles apply in your massage career. You can work full time or part time, be either self-employed or an employee, and you can either have a career or hold a job in massage. Do not think that you must be self-employed and working full time to have a career.

Employee or self-employed? Each of these two options has its advantages and disadvantages. One person may feel that the independent decision making involved in self-employment is an advantage, whereas a person who has difficulty producing independent ideas would consider this a disadvantage. Only you can decide which, or a combination of both, is best for you.

In the past, most massage therapists were small-business owners. Few employment opportunities existed. But times have changed. The profession has seen a steady increase in jobs and career opportunities in the more traditional employee market, in which the massage practitioner goes to work for an individual or a company at a wage-based income (Box 3.8).

The employee market exists within personal service, fitness, wellness centers, recreational industries, and medical establishments. The most rapid expansion of employment opportunities is occurring in the spa and franchise setting. Franchises and business chains are spreading quickly and offer employment options. A wellness center is an establishment that offers health services for the body and mind, with massage therapy being a major offering. The fitness industry is another source of employment. Many health clubs offer the services of a massage professional. The recreation industry (e.g., hotels, cruise ships, retreats, and resort centers) also is an active employer of massage practitioners. The independent massage therapy clinic offers opportunities for employment when the owner or manager of the clinic handles all business responsibilities and hires massage practitioners to do the work. Massage professionals are working for physicians, physical therapists, mental health professionals, and other health care professionals. It is possible to have two part-time positions working for two different employers. For ethical purposes, the employers should be providing massage service to two different client populations; for example, one job may be at a franchise and the other for a home health service. Always disclose dual employment arrangements to both employers.

Successful self-employment requires an entrepreneurial spirit. An *entrepreneur* is a person who organizes, operates, and assumes the risk of a business venture. Not everyone is cut out for self-employment. The hours are long, and 100%

Box 8.2 Massage Equipment General Ergonomic Recommendations

Working With a Massage Table

- As a general rule, the table height should be at the hip joint or pubic bone. Depending on the therapist's torso, arm, and leg length ratios, the correct height for the table will be 2 to 3 inches higher or lower. An individual with long arms may need a shorter table than a person with short arms. A person with a short torso, short arms, and long legs often needs a taller table. There will be some variations to this when it comes to various massage techniques. The lighter the technique application, the higher the table height or it should be as close to the hip joint height as recommended earlier.
- Typically, a female needs a taller table than a male of the same height.
- A table that is 28 to 30 inches wide provides adequate space for the client to lie down comfortably, but it is not so wide that the therapist must reach for the client in the middle of the table. When moving around the table while performing massage, minimize the potential for overreaching by positioning your body as close to the client body area you are working without breaching any physical touch boundaries. An ergonomics rule of thumb is to move your body as close to the work task as possible to keep the body in its most ideal operational position. Referring to the OSHA recommendations as pictured in Box 8.4, it emphasizes this concept. When ergonomists evaluate job tasks, they are looking for the safest and best practices in movement (Pheasant, 1991).
- The knees and hips are used to lift portable tables. The therapist should not bend forward at the waist when lifting the massage table. Some tables have shoulder straps, wheel bases, and other devices to aid in transport by redistributing the weight load.
- Consistently carrying the table on only one side of the body may be harmful. Alternate carrying arms; for example, carry in with the left arm, carry out with the right. The best ergonomic solution is to use a table cart whenever possible to transport a portable table.
- For the most adaptability for massage pressure and technique application, height variability, and best body positioning for each client on your table, use an electric lift/hydraulic table whenever possible.

Sitting on a Chair or Stool at a Massage Table

- Sitting and providing massage is an option especially when lighter pressure is the focus, if there are extended periods of standing or static positioning, or if you are working on a specific finite area on a client's body.
- Sitting for part of the massage session provides posture variation and allows for a bit of a break or rest for larger muscle groups that are sustaining your upright standing position.
- The massage table is generally lower when providing massage while seated. Be sure that you are able to fit your flexed knees completely under the table while minimizing your reach when working seated.
- If using a rolling chair or stool, make sure the wheels can lock so the chair/stool does not roll back when force is applied into the client's body. Alternatively, the massage therapist's feet and legs may need to hold the chair/stool in place, which is still acceptable provided the foot and leg positioning used is similar to standing positions (e.g., transverse and longitudinal stances). Be sure that the stool or chair is an appropriate size for your use, such as making sure that you fit comfortably in the seat pan and the height is adjustable to where your knees can be in a comfortable, flexed, 90-degree position. Also, use a stool that has back support whenever possible for the best neutral seated positioning (Pheasant, 1991).

Working on a Floor Mat

- Table body mechanics also apply for working on a mat on the floor. The main notable difference is that the center of gravity is lower, necessitating greater core strength.
- When working on a floor mat, there is greater potential for torso bending and twist due to the lower center of gravity as mentioned earlier. To assume the most ideal position, be sure to position your body as close to the client body area you are working on to reduce overreach or bending when possible.
- Movement around the client is different when the person is on a floor mat rather than a massage table. The weight-bearing balance points on the floor are from the knees instead of the feet.
- Padding on the knees may be required. Kneepads are a good, available option for protective equipment for the therapist.
- The mat must be large enough so that the massage therapist can keep their knees on the mat while doing the massage.

Working With a Massage Chair

Specially designed massage chairs help with positioning the client so that compression can be applied correctly. However, due to the variations of client size in relation to the size and shape of the massage therapist, prolonged use of a massage chair to deliver massage can increase the risk of strain in the massage therapist's body. Whenever possible, utilize a stool or chair to take a seated position when performing chair massage, such as when working on the forearms or hands of a seated client.

The center of gravity is moved by "leaning" on the client, just as someone would comfortably lean against a wall or on a table. During massage application, you lean forward from the ankle as body weight is transferred to the client in the direction in which you will apply pressure, and your back leg is used for translating weight forward and the front leg for balance (Fig. 8.2 and Proficiency Exercise 8.1).

Even though a force is either a push or a pull, the practitioner seldom "pushes" against the client. Pushing requires a tense body and the use of muscle contraction to exert pressure. It is important that the practitioner use body weight. Although muscle strength is not a big factor, leverage is essential (Magee and Zachazewski, 2007). By leaning to transfer weight, the practitioner can substantially reduce muscle tension in the shoulders, neck, wrists, hand, elbows, and lower back and efficiently apply mechanical forces during the massage. When pushing, create a hinge moment with the upper body in front of the base of support (leaning in against the

- Chapter 8 : *Body Mechanics*, which takes a closer look at adapting massage application based on body shape and gender. Therapeutic massage is a physically labor-intensive therapy that requires time to perform, with an emphasis on ergonomics and correct body mechanics.

- Features and activities that motivate and make you think.

PROFICIENCY EXERCISE 6.3

1. Using the reference section in Appendix A, list five regional/local contraindications to massage that you have encountered (or that you think you may encounter) with clients.
   a.
   b.
   c.
   d.
   e.
2. List the five general or relative contraindications. you think you will encounter most often.
   a.
   b.
   c.
   d.
   e.

- Reality-based examples embedded throughout the textbook, helping readers understand content.

FIG. 10.28 Examples of percussion. A, Hacking. **B,** Cupping. **C,** Fist beating. **D,** Beating over the palm. **E,** Slapping. **F,** Finger tapping.

Heavy percussion should not be done in the kidney area, directly over joints, or anywhere pain or discomfort is present. The following are methods of percussion (Fig. 10.28):

1. *Hacking.* Hacking is applied with both wrists relaxed and the fingers spread, with only the little finger or the ulnar side of the hand striking the skin surface. The other fingers hit each other with a springy touch. Point hacking can be done by using the fingertips in the same way. Hacking is done with the whole hand on the larger soft tissue areas, such as the upper back and shoulders. Point hacking is used on smaller areas, such as the individual tendons of the toes, or over motor points.
2. *Cupping.* To perform cupping, the fingers and thumbs are positioned as if making a cup. The hands are turned over, and the same action used in hacking is performed. When done on the anterior and posterior thorax, cupping is good for stimulating the respiratory system and for loosening mucus. If the client exhales and makes a monotone noise during cupping, enough intensity is used so that the tone begins to break up, changing from "AAAAAAAAAAAAH-HHHHH" to "AH AH AH AH AH AH."
3. *Beating* and *pounding.* These moves can be performed with a soft fist with the knuckles down or with the fist held vertically and the action performed with the ulnar side of the palm. This technique is used over large muscles, such as the buttocks and upper leg muscles.
4. *Slapping (splatting).* For this technique, the whole palm of a flattened hand contacts the body. This is a good method for causing the release of histamine, thereby increasing vasodilation and its effects on the skin. It also is a good method to use on the bottoms of the feet. The broad contact of the whole hand disperses the force laterally instead of downward, and the effects remain in the superficial tissue. Kellogg (2010) called this movement *splatting.*
5. *Tapping.* For this technique, the palmar surface of the fingers alternately taps the body area with light to medium pressure. This is a good method to use around the joints, on the tendons, on the face and head, and along the spine (Proficiency Exercise 10.8).

PROFICIENCY EXERCISE 10.8

1. Play a drum or watch a drummer. Pay attention to the action of the arms and wrists and the grasp of the drumsticks. Notice that the drummer holds the drumsticks loosely.
2. Get a paddleball or yo-yo and see what actions it takes to make these toys work. Play with a rattle or tambourine.
3. Use the foam from the compression exercises and practice the different methods and intensity of percussion (light to heavy, slow to fast).
4. While shaking your hands quickly, use hacking to strike the foam or a practice client. Without stopping, change hand positions so that all the methods are used.
5. Design a stimulating massage with various applications of percussion. Notice which qualities of touch are most reflected with these methods.

- END-OF-CHAPTER MULTIPLE-CHOICE QUESTIONS FOR DISCUSSION AND REVIEW with answer and rationales on the EVOLVE site. This feature supports the critical-thinking process and preparation for licensing exams.

dicated if the ______.
ma in the lower legs after a plane flight
bout care at the local outpatient clinic
ly
g a new medication
history of car accidents. During
hey were seriously burned. What
would benefit the massage therapist?
care

b. Whole person care
c. Biopsychosocial care
d. PEACE and LOVE care

15. A massage therapist is developing a care plan for a client scheduled to have knee replacement surgery in the next month. What would be the best approach to care sequence?
a. Current: relaxation. Immediately after surgery: functional mobility. Six weeks post-surgery: acute pain management. Twenty-four months post-surgery: stress management.
b. Current: well-being/palliative. Immediately after surgery: restorative. Six weeks post-surgery: stress management. Twenty-four months post-surgery: therapeutic change.
c. Current: condition management. Immediately after surgery: well-being/palliative. Six weeks post-surgery: therapeutic change. Twenty-four months post-surgery: restorative.
d. Current: pain management. Immediately after surgery: functional mobility. Six weeks post-surgery: therapeutic change. Twenty-four months post-surgery: well-being/palliative.

16. A massage client is requesting pain management for shoulder arthrosis, stress management to support restorative sleep, and reduced migraine headache frequency. Which type of contraindication is most likely to require the massage therapist to adapt to provide the best care for this client?
a. Relative
b. Absolute
c. Total
d. Local

17. What would be the most common suggestion for a massage dosage when the approach to care is condition management related to nonspecific low back stiffness?
a. As needed, 15- to 60-minute sessions
b. Weekly, 60-minute sessions, ongoing
c. Twice a week or weekly, 60-minute sessions, ongoing
d. Daily, twice a week or weekly, 15- to 60-minute sessions, 12 weeks

18. A massage therapist is justifying a massage therapy care plan recommending ongoing weekly massage sessions for an individual with an autoimmune condition. What would be the best indication for massage?
a. Support productive allodynia
b. Manage chronic inflammation
c. Reverse joint pain
d. Reduce tendency to hyperalgesia

19. A client recently completed a successful course of chemotherapy and radiation therapy, and cancer is in remission. They are experiencing ongoing discomfort related to the treatment. What is most likely occurring?
a. Brachial plexus impingement
b. Phantom pain
c. Viscerally referred pain
d. Neuropathic pain

20. Which of the following people would primarily seek a massage therapy outcome of relaxation, a well-being approach to care, and have a regional contraindication?
a. A client with resilience and with contact dermatitis on their arm
b. A client taking antianxiety medication and is hypermobile
c. A client who has had multiple right shoulder dislocations and is a competitive athlete
d. A client taking an anticoagulant medication and is otherwise healthy

Write Your Own Questions

Write at least three multiple choice questions. Make sure to develop plausible wrong answers and be sure that the correct answer is clearly correct. Then write a rationale for each question. The more questions you write, the better you will understand the material. Exchange questions with classmates or discuss in class. The questions from all the learners can be combined to create a review quiz.

Case Studies **CHAPTER 16** 691

A general full-body massage session will be used, with a depth of pressure sufficient to elicit the relaxation response. All massage manipulations will be used except friction and percussion because friction causes pain and percussion is generally a stimulating method. The rhythm will be slow and even, meeting the client's body rhythms and then slowing over the course of the session. The direction of massage will be primarily toward the heart but with changes as necessary to address connective tissue bind. Lymphatic drainage methods will be used on the right shoulder. Muscle energy methods will be used, especially to address the eye and neck reflexes and to lengthen all short muscles identified during the assessment.

Because the major tension is in the neck and shoulders, having the client roll eyes in large circles or roll head in small circles while broad-based compression is applied to the tender areas, especially the occipital base muscles, will help. Kneading and skin rolling with myofascial techniques, coupled with lymphatic drainage, will increase pliability in the areas of thick and short connective tissues. Active trigger points in muscles will be addressed with the least invasive measures possible to reduce the guarding response and pain behaviors because pain increases sympathetic arousal. Positional release will be the primary choice and will be applied to the indicated areas in the serratus anterior and intercostal muscles.

Muscles that are inhibited will be encouraged to function through the use of limited tapotement (i.e., not so much as to arouse the nervous system) at the attachments of these muscles.

Joint movement methods will focus on reducing the internal rotation of the right arm and the external rotation of the right leg. Integrated muscle energy methods will be the primary method used and will combine these patterns so that the muscle imbalances can be treated in sequence. The abdominal massage sequence will ease constipation, but caution is required because of heartburn. Prone and supine positioning will also need to be monitored to identify if it creates a heartburn sensation. Side-lying may be a better option.

Teaching the client simple breathing and relaxation exercises, as described in Chapter 15, is appropriate.

CASE 2. MUSCLE TENSION HEADACHE

A 26-year-old female is in good health except for frequent headaches that radiate pain from the back of her skull around her ears and over her eyes. Migraine and cluster headaches have been ruled out. The diagnosis is muscle tension headaches. Because no medical reason has been found for the headaches, they are assumed to be stress related. They do not follow any cyclic pattern. A relationship to the menstrual cycle has not been indicated.

The client has a temporary job as a server while she finishes college. She spends a lot of time sitting, reading, and working at the computer. She notices increased tension in her neck, shoulders, and lower back when she has to spend a lot of time with her studies. She swims three times a week for exercise and is careful with her diet. She has a moderate intake of caffeine and alcohol, and she smokes. She is not under any medical care.

Because common over-the-counter analgesics such as aspirin and acetaminophen bother her stomach, she is seeking an alternative to manage the pain. She has tried chiropractic care, with limited success, and often experiences a headache right after an adjustment. She has heard that massage can help these types of headaches. A friend referred her, indicating that she would be comfortable with a middle-aged female therapist with a home-based practice. The client has completed an informed consent process and has agreed to treatment.

Assessment

Observation

The client is nearsighted and wears glasses. She repositions her glasses often, and she squints in the bright light. She is polite and soft-spoken. She appears frustrated and tired of the inconvenience of the headaches. She is neatly groomed and organized; she provides a list of all the treatments that have been tried, including a food diary and schedules, in an attempt to identify the cause of the headaches. Her weight is normal for her height. She has long, thick hair that she wears in a ponytail.

Interview and Goals

The client's history reveals that she has had headaches for as long as she can remember. She has a headache severe enough to interfere with daily activities about 10 days out of a month. The headaches last about 12 hours, and the pain is a 7 on a scale of 1 to 10 (1 being slight, 10 being extreme). She does not remember any injury or surgery or any childhood diseases other than the normal ones. She had the headaches during adolescence. She generally ignores the headaches, but they are becoming draining. The family history provides no insight. There is a family history of cancer. She wore braces for 3 years and recently had them removed. She has worn glasses and has had long hair since her early teens. She admits to being a perfectionist.

Her goals for the massage are to reduce the frequency and intensity of the headaches.

Physical Assessment

Posture
No obvious postural asymmetry.

Gait
No obvious gait distortions.

Range of Motion
Slightly limited in all directions in the neck with moderate reduction of capital flexion. Temporomandibular joint (TMJ) opens only to two fingers' width (three is normal).

Palpation
Near Touch
Neck near the occipital base and the lower back are warm.
Skin
All areas are normal except for goose bumps and dampness at the occipital base and lower back. Tissue texture is symmetrical and normal. The examiner is unable to lift a skinfold over the entire length of the spinal column.

- UNIQUE TO THIS TEXT: **The final chapter in this book contains 20 case studies that help the student appreciate the complexities of a therapeutic relationship, all in a competency-based format.**

- *FOCUS ON PROFESSIONALISM* **feature throughout the text that reinforces the importance of professional and ethical behavior.**

FOCUS ON PROFESSIONALISM

Massage therapy must never interfere with or contradict the physician's care plan, nor should the massage therapist assume the role of counselor. If the health care professional must be contacted directly, the massage professional should always work through the receptionist. Leave whatever information is needed with the front desk; if the doctor believes that speaking with the massage therapist directly is important, they will call. Ongoing interaction with the physician follows guidelines for consultations described in Chapter 2.

The reason for referral and the date of referral must be noted on the client's record, along with the signs and symptoms. If the client responds in any unusual way, such as by panicking or refusing to go to the doctor, this must be indicated in the client's record.

As mentioned, most disease processes present with a few basic symptoms (see Appendix A). A client should always be referred for diagnosis if the symptoms listed in Box 6.8 do not have a logical explanation (e.g., if the client has been up late or working long hours, they will show symptoms of fatigue). Massage practitioners should use common sense tempered with accurate information and caution (Proficiency Exercise 6.3).

MENTORING TIP

Massage practitioners should not rely on lists of specific contraindications, but rather should use a set of medical and therapeutic guidelines pertinent to clinical applications and research developments. Unfortunately, such guidelines are not consistent in current literature. You will have to learn to make appropriate, informed decisions for each client. As mentioned earlier, this text is targeted to the entry-level massage therapist; therefore the recommendations are conservative. With increased experience and education, the massage therapist develops the ability to work with more complex client situations.

Contraindications are unique to each client and to each region of the body. The ability to reason clinically is essential to making appropriate decisions about the advisability of, modifications to, or avoidance of massage interventions. It is important to understand when to refer a client for diagnosis and when to obtain assistance in modifying the approach to the massage session so that it will best serve the client. Remember—when in doubt, refer!

- *MENTORING TIP* feature from the experiences of the author to promote introspection and classroom discussion.

- *LEARN MORE* feature that provides information in the text and links on the website to expand on selected content. The information and links guide the reader in exploration of the many helpful resources from a variety of US government and affiliated agencies, nonprofit organizations, and sources for valid research.

LEARN MORE ON THE WEB

It is impossible to learn everything in school and from just one textbook. You need to become your own teacher. This list of informational websites will get your started, but you will have to keep the process going. The US government's official web portal, USA.gov, makes it easy for the public to get US government information and services on the Web. The main sites are CareerInfoNet, CareerOneStop, the Small Business Association, Business USA, the Centers for Disease Control and Prevention, the Social Security Administration, the US Department of Commerce, the US Department of Labor, and the US Equal Employment Opportunity Commission. Links to specific topics that are especially relevant are on the Evolve site.

- EXPANDED CONTENT AND ENHANCED ONLINE EVOLVE SITE THAT PROVIDES A COMPREHENSIVE REVIEW PROCESS FOR LICENSING EXAMS, PARTICULARY THE MBLEX
  - EXPANDED Web-based content on the EVOLVE site, including 3 hours of case studies, demonstrations, animated footage, and more!
  - *QUICK CONTENT REVIEW IN QUESTION FORM*, which is a student Evolve resource that reinforces key concepts in the chapter and allows learners to quiz themselves as a review and for learning strategies.
  - MBLEX PRACTICE EXAMS
  - HOURS OF SCIENTIFIC ANIMATIONS
  - ANATOMY LABELING EXERCISES

AND BEYOND THE BASICS—The content in the textbook also covers the information in the content outline and job task analysis for the National Certification Board for Therapeutic Massage and Bodywork's BOARD CERTIFICATION EXAM.

- TEACH lesson plan manual for instructors, which is available on Evolve at http://evolve.elsevier.com/fritz/fundamentals/.

Contents

Appendices

Contents in Brief

UNIT I

Professional Practice

To be a successful massage therapist, you will need two types of skills. These can be classified as soft skills and hard skills. Both will be essential to your career.

Soft skills include abilities developed in communication, etiquette, friendliness, teamwork, problem solving, interpersonal skills, and leadership.

Hard skills are specific teachable abilities that can be measured. The massage skills, as well as some business and documentation skills, are considered hard skills.

Soft skills are related to social and emotional intelligence. Daniel Goleman, a psychologist, wrote a book in 1995 titled *Emotional Intelligence,* and he and others have continued to investigate and describe the importance of human interaction. Soft skills relate to social neuroscience; that is, the study of what happens while people interact. We now know that social and emotional intelligence is multifaceted, and the soft skills in this unit are just as important for career success as the massage (hard) skills you will learn in Units 3 and 4.

The information in the first four chapters of this textbook combine to address the spectrum of soft skills, including the mindset, behavior, and interpersonal skills needed to function as a massage therapist in a professional setting. In addition, hard skills needed for business procedures and documentation are presented. Unit 2, Foundations for Massage Benefit, supports Unit 1 and bridges to Unit 3, The Massage Process, and Unit 4, Beyond the Basics. So, let's begin Unit 1, Professional Practice, starting with Chapter 1, Therapeutic Massage as a Profession.

LEARN MORE ON THE WEB

This feature appears at the end of each chapter and leads you to valuable information provided by various departments of the US government (and sometimes those of other countries). Unless specifically noted, the content in the LEARN MORE features is in the public domain and free for you to use. For example, soft skills such as communication, attitude, and teamwork are extremely important in a service profession such as massage. The US Department of Labor has many resources to expand your knowledge on these topics. Use the search term soft skills.

CHAPTER

1 Therapeutic Massage as a Profession

http://evolve.com/Fritz/fundamentals/

CHAPTER OBJECTIVES

After completing this chapter, the student will be able to:

1. Identify personal interpretations of touch and their influence on professional interactions.
2. Describe professional touch.
3. Define professionalism.
4. Define therapeutic massage.
5. Explain the rich heritage and history of therapeutic massage.
6. Explain the influence of historical events and global culture on the current development of therapeutic massage.
7. Self-assess for leadership qualities.
8. Analyze a professional practice framework.

CHAPTER OUTLINE

KEY TERMS

Autonomy	Occupation
Code of ethics	Patterns
Culture	Profession
Diversity	Professional
Equity	Professional autonomy
Expressive touch	Professional touch
Healing	Professionalism
Implicit bias	Service
Inclusion	System
Leadership	Therapeutic applications
Massage	Touch technique
Mechanical touch	Vocation

You are embarking on a journey that will lead you to your goal of becoming a massage professional. You are beginning an active learning process. Three important words were just used to describe how you will proceed with your education:

- *Active* means that you are participating in your education by doing something.
- *Learning* means that you are using experiences to gather and evaluate information, determining its meaning and value. In addition, you are encoding memory (what you have learned) into a web of nerve connections that makes the information retrievable and usable.
- *Process* means that you are using an ongoing series of actions that produces a measurable and desirable outcome. In this case, the outcome is that you become a highly skilled and knowledgeable massage therapist.

Education is just as much about asking questions as it is about seeking answers. Information accumulated during an educational process, coupled with the ability to formulate insightful and productive questions, allows learners to make thoughtful decisions. Are decisions answers? Do answers come from thoughtful situational decisions? Are answers valid?

Some questions seem to have easy answers. For example, "What is the color of grass?" Quickly we jump to the answer "green"; however, is that always the correct answer? Depending on the region and the season, grass turns brown. Because many questions can have several answers, validity sometimes can be difficult to determine. In what way is the professional application of touch influenced by the practitioner's ability to make thoughtful decisions and find answers that best serve the situation at a particular moment? As you read this discussion, you might get the feeling that it is written in circles instead of following a straight line. It may be confusing because one question leads back to another.

One of the many ways your brain learns is by circling around and around through information, collecting an increased understanding with each revolution. Eventually, the understanding begins to turn the circle into a spiral as comprehension leads to creative application (Fig. 1.1). In straight-line learning, a piece of information is presented once, then the next piece is presented, and then the next, and so on, much like driving down a road from point A to point B. Except for elementary sequential information, straight-line learning is not very effective. We do not learn efficiently by experiencing something only once. Even if we go back and repeat the linear A-to-B sequence repeatedly, the brain begins to ignore the information because it is too familiar (Fig. 1.2).

Repetition is necessary to learn anything. However, to keep the brain interested, the repetition somehow must be different each time. Think of a piece of music. You can hear the repetition of a melody in a few lines of music, but you can also hear where the composer has changed a note or two. You enjoy hearing the repetition of a good melody, but you also enjoy it when it is changed slightly because this prevents you from becoming bored with it. This is called *novel repetition* (Fig. 1.3); that is, the same information is given over and over, but always a little differently and in a circular format. As you learn about massage therapy, this type of repetition eventually spirals into the ability to become a creative and skilled massage therapist. As you read and study this textbook, notice how learning spirals, novel repetition, and asking questions are teaching you to use critical thinking and eventually teaching you to become your own teacher to support lifelong learning.

In massage, which is a professional, structured, therapeutic touch, education begins with questions.

- What is the significance of touch?
- What is professional touch?
- What motivates me to study therapeutic massage?
- What is therapeutic?
- How am I served by touching others?
- When did touch become professional?
- Why did touch become professional?
- Do therapeutic forms of touch have to be provided by a professional?
- In what way is professional therapeutic touch different from casual touch, friendship touch, family touch, intimate touch, or erotic (sexual) touch?
- How do different individuals, social groups, or cultures view touch?
- In what way does the past affect the present and guide the future development of the massage therapy profession?

Questions continue to arise, and the answers are not necessarily simple. As we seek to serve our clients, eventually we are faced with these questions and many others. Some of the questions mentioned previously are explored in this text, especially as they relate to the professional practice of therapeutic massage. Some are not explored directly; rather, both questions and answers evolve as a learner's knowledge and experience increases. Although this text does not always provide definitive answers, it does provide information to help you find your own.

FIG. 1.1 Spiral learning.

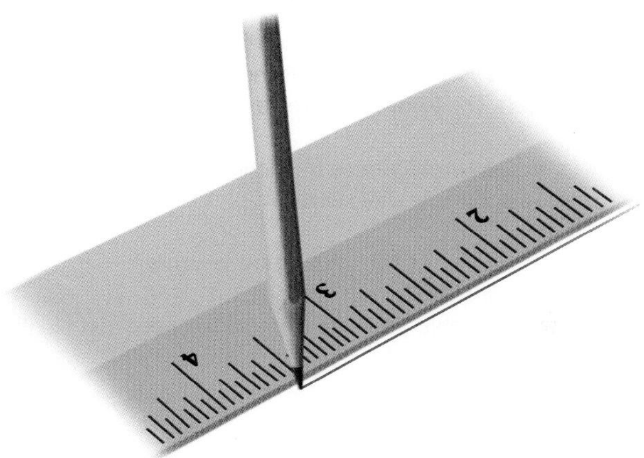

FIG. 1.2 Straight-line learning.

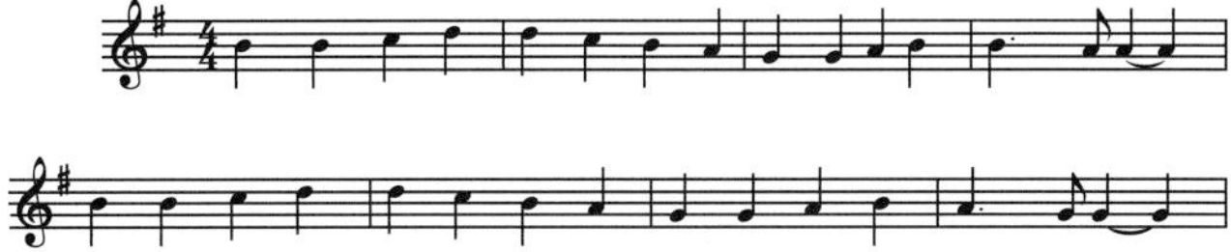

FIG. 1.3 Novel repetition can be seen and heard in music, for example.

What will your questions be? How will your answers influence those you touch? How will your answers touch you? These are huge issues to consider at the beginning of any course of study. As you begin to think about them, you might feel interested, excited, overwhelmed, or maybe even frightened as you come to realize how necessary, beneficial, complex, and powerful touch can be. These important questions are posed at the beginning of this study likely before you have sufficient information to develop effective answers. Remember that understanding evolves. Your awareness of these questions will help guide you in your study of therapeutic massage.

Essential to understanding the development of answers is embracing the importance of respect, not only for yourself but also for all those with whom you interact, both personally and professionally (Proficiency Exercise 1.1).

PROFESSIONAL TOUCH

SECTION OBJECTIVES

Chapter objective covered in this section:

1. Identify personal interpretations of touch and their influence on professional interactions.

Using the information presented in this section, the student will be able to:

- Distinguish between professional and nonprofessional forms of touch
- List factors that influence the communication of touch
- Define bias and implicit bias

A **profession** is defined as an occupation or vocation that requires training and specialized study of a complex set of knowledge and skills through formal education and/or practical experience. An **occupation** can be defined as a productive or creative activity that serves as one's regular source of livelihood. A **vocation** is a strong altruistic motivation to follow a specific occupational career pathway to be of service to others. Vocational education trains for an occupation. In the professional sense, our vocation should be based on a sense of life purpose. A **professional** is a person who engages in a profession and is committed to adhering to the standards expected of a qualified and experienced person in a specific work environment. **Professionalism** is the adherence to professional status, methods, standards, and character (see the discussion on ethics in Chapter 2). **Autonomy** means the ability to practice massage therapy independently (focus on professionalism).

PROFICIENCY EXERCISE 1.1

My Touch History

On a piece of paper, write a brief touch history of yourself. Then explain the ways your history may influence your delivery of professional touch. The following example is provided as a model.

Culture

I grew up in the United States in Michigan. I lived in a small town that was primarily Caucasian.

Subculture

My family was a blue-collar, working-class family.

Genetic Predisposition

I am most comfortable with a large personal space and plenty of time alone.

Gender

Female

Age

60+

Biases

People's lifestyles should be moderate instead of exorbitant.

People should be able to self-teach and figure things out.

Caucasian older males are controlling.

Life Events

I experienced touch trauma from a grandfather and uncles, who would tickle me until I could not stand it.

I gave birth to three children and am a single parent.

I had a special friend who was blind.

I had unexpected open-heart surgery.

My eldest son was killed in a tragic accident at age 33.

Spiritual Path

I initially had an unstructured Protestant focus. I developed a specific fundamentalist path in early adulthood. I embraced many paths as truth in later years as I evolved from the practice of religion to the development of personal spirituality.

Ways My Touch History May Influence My Delivery of Professional Touch

I had to learn a lot about unfamiliar cultures because my exposure to a diverse population was limited while I was growing up. I have to be careful to understand a person's culture before I approach to touch them. I am most comfortable with blue-collar, working-class people. I am more relaxed and find myself willing to spend more time when I touch someone from this population. I feel overwhelmed if I am touched too much and tend to limit initiated touch from the client. I am a woman, and I learned during my gender role development to fulfill others' needs before my own. I often overextend myself for a client instead of setting time limits. I am hypersensitive to light touch and tend to avoid giving light touch when I give a massage. I am understanding of the numerous demands on a single parent and tend to touch one in similar circumstances with sympathy instead of empathy. I have to be careful of boundaries when I touch stressed, overwhelmed single parents. I am casual when touching someone with a disability. I have experienced life-threatening illness, tragedy, and loss. This has changed my life perspective, and if I am not careful, I can discount what may seem to me to be the more minor struggles of others. I seek to understand various spiritual paths and deeply wish to respect issues of touch within each discipline. I tend to assume that one must actually make physical contact during healing and must remind myself that this is not everyone's truth.

Your Turn

Culture

Subculture

Genetic Predisposition

Gender

Age

Bias

Life Events

Spiritual Path

Ways My Touch History May Influence My Delivery of Professional Touch

FOCUS ON PROFESSIONALISM

The actions of every massage therapist affect the massage profession as a whole. There is an expectation of behavior when one claims to be a massage therapist. Behaviors include appearance, speech, actions, and advancement of knowledge and skills through lifelong learning. As professionals, we need to walk the talk. Each of us has a responsibility to the entire massage community. As professionals, we must always act like professionals even during personal time if we are in public view. Social media is an example of a situation in which professional commitment can be confused. If a posting to social media does not comply with accepted and expected professional behavior, especially when directly related to massage therapy, the conduct could be considered unethical. For example, it is very unprofessional if a picture of a massage therapist in revealing clothing or discussing involvement in questionable behavior (e.g., driving under the influence) is included with posts about massage appointment availability. Think about it.

To understand the concept of professional touch, we look at specialized training that allows a person to provide a service to another. Professionals may sell a product, but a profession usually is built around a skilled ability to provide a service, such as the professional touch of therapeutic massage. A **service** is something done for another that results in a specific outcome; for example, the car is fixed, the garden is tended, communication skills are taught, emotional problems are sorted out, bodily functions are restored, and spiritual or life paths are discovered. In return, income (livelihood) is received for that service.

When a professional relationship exists, certain agreed-on criteria apply. The person providing the service is skilled (educated) and operates within certain standards of practice, including technical application and ethical conduct. **Professional touch** is skilled touch delivered to achieve a specific outcome, and the recipient reimburses the professional for services rendered. A professional relationship is focused on providing a client with a set of skills that focuses on a specific outcome. If professional and/or personal roles overlap, such as with dual and multiple roles, the professional relationship becomes confusing.

The aspect of skilled or schooled touch leads to the idea of structured touch. Professional touch is not random but purposeful. It is organized according to systems and patterns. A **system** is a group of interacting elements that function as a complex whole. Professional touch, such as that provided by a massage practitioner, requires education in the many systems of the body; the application of massage and other forms and styles of soft tissue methodology; and an understanding of the influence of massage on body systems. Communication and interpersonal skills, including systems of social and cultural interaction, are also part of the education of the therapeutic massage professional.

Patterns are created by the replication of structures and functions that entwine and influence each other. Patterns can be identified if we can see a big enough picture. The pattern may be missed if the focus is too small. For example, muscle tension can be identified in an individual muscle of the arm, or it can be seen as part of an interacting pattern of movement during walking. The ability to see both the individual segments or pieces and the ways the pieces interact in patterns is a necessary skill for the individual application of professional touch.

Inherent in the understanding of skilled and structured touch is the idea of the therapeutic application of touch. The term **therapeutic application** describes the act of applying a method for a particular purpose or use. Something therapeutic provides the structure for wellness, well-being, quality of life, beneficial change, or support for current healing practices. A walk in the woods or a conversation with a compassionate friend can be therapeutic. Various bodywork modalities, medical and mental health practices, and empowering spiritual rituals can be therapeutic. **Healing** is the restoration of well-being, and therapeutic applications promote a healing environment.

Touch

We need to consider the nature of touch to understand the role of professional touch and the evolution of therapeutic massage throughout history. It is important to look at the idea of professionalism in the physical, emotional, social, cultural, and, in some instances, spiritual dimensions of touch. The roots of the word *massage* (Box 1.1) concern touch and the various applications of touch. It is important to explore the ideas behind the structure of touch. We must differentiate the therapeutic value of touch in the professional sense from forms of touch shared between people in life circumstances outside the professional environment. These themes are expanded on throughout this chapter, and in some instances, the information is further developed in future chapters.

Science of Touch

Anatomically and physiologically, touch is the collection of tactile sensations that arise from sensory stimulation, primarily of the skin but also of deeper structures of the body, such as the muscles and associated connective tissue. Cutaneous mechanoreceptors are localized in the various layers of the skin, where they detect a wide range of mechanical stimuli, including light brush, stretch, vibration, movement of hair, and pressure. Touch responses involve a very precise coding of mechanical information with interpretation of the stimuli in the central nervous system (Roudaut et al., 2012; Forstenpointner et al., 2022).

The skin is an amazing organ. It has many functions, but the most notable for this discussion is its function in touch. The skin is the largest sensory organ of the body. From the outside,

Box 1.1 How Massage Got Its Name

The term *massage* is thought to be derived from several sources. The Latin root *massa* and the Greek roots *massein* and *masso* mean "to touch, handle, squeeze, or knead." The French verb *masser* also means "to knead." The Arabic root *mass* or *mass'h* and the Sanskrit root *makeh* translate as "to press softly."

we are always touched first on our skin, and in many ways, through the skin, we touch ourselves from the inside. Many internal somatic soft tissue structures (e.g., muscles, connective tissue) and visceral structures (e.g., the lungs, heart, and digestive organs) project sensation to the skin (see Chapter 6 for a discussion of viscerally referred pain patterns). The autonomic nervous system (see Chapter 4), which regulates the visceral and chemical homeostasis of the body, is highly responsive to skin stimulation in support of well-being. Mood (the way a person feels) is often reflected in the skin as we touch ourselves from the inside. We blush with embarrassment, flush with excitement, or grow pale with fear.

The anatomy of the skin is described in most comprehensive anatomy texts. The anatomical parts that make up the skin—the epidermis (top layer), the dermis (inner layer), and the interlacing connective tissues of these layers—and the massive network of nerves both receive and relay information from the central nervous system. This vast network combines with the rich complex of circulatory vessels that supply the skin. Yet even in their complexity, the anatomy and physiology of the skin cannot explain the experience of touch. In some way, the pressure, vibration, temperature, and muscle motion that move the skin enliven us with sensations and experiences of pleasure, connectedness, joy, pain, fear, sadness, longing, and satisfaction.

We must be touched to survive. Touch is a hunger that must be fed; it is the essence of our survival, not simply a matter of well-being. The importance of touch has been well described in the books of Ashley Montagu, particularly *Touching: The Human Significance of the Skin*, which is recommended reading for all learners of therapeutic massage. Dr. Tiffany Field has conducted scientific research on touch at the Touch Research Institute at the University of Miami's Miller School of Medicine, and additional research has been done at various locations (see Chapter 5). Initially, much of this research was devoted to infant development, primarily in premature babies. Dr. Field has greatly expanded our understanding of the importance of touch by studying many different groups of people, including infants, elderly people, people currently well but under stress, and very ill people. Research supports the belief that touching in a structured way is incredibly important for all living beings (Kopf, 2021).

Scientific study and technology have enabled us to describe some of the physiological responses to touch, such as changes in the concentration of hormones, alterations in the activity of the central and peripheral nervous systems, and regulation of body rhythms (these mechanisms are discussed more extensively in later chapters) (Yu et al., 2022). Scientists at the Washington University School of Medicine in St. Louis, Missouri, have identified a neural circuit and neuropeptide in mice that transmits the sensation of pleasant touch from the skin to the brain (Liu et al., 2022). However, information falls short of helping us understand the experience of touch. For all its scientific interpretations, the experience of touch is much more than the sum of its parts. Touch understanding remains elusive to researchers. A part of the brain called the *insula* processes actual physical contact and attaches affective interpretation of the meaning of the touch—or, more simply, being touched and what the contact implies: compassion, rebuke, connection, danger, anger, appreciation, admiration, or love. One such touch complexity involves mirror-touch synesthesia, in which individuals can feel the same sensation another person feels. This phenomenon may be related to the mirror neurons present in the motor areas of the brain. These specialized cells may support emotion recognition by activating somatosensory representations to simulate and eventually help us understand how others feel (Banissy & Ward, 2013; Schaefer et al., 2021).

Confounding the touch experience are various virtual touch interface systems now found in virtual learning simulations, as well as video games. Haptics is the science of applying touch (tactile) sensation and control to interaction with computer applications. Haptic technology is a tactile feedback technology that recreates the sense of touch by applying forces, vibrations, or motions to the user. The reality of the virtual experience makes one wonder if we actually have to be physically touched to feel touched.

The Experience of Touch

Touch often is the concrete experience of more abstract sensations. For example, something that can be seen may not necessarily be real (e.g., watching a movie), but when something can be touched, it is tangible. The concept of tangible is changing. The first edition of this textbook (1995) was available only in the traditional paper book format. This edition is available in both paper and electronic formats. You may have one or the other or both. Is one more real than the other? Interesting question.

You will learn to listen to a client give their history and to observe during a physical assessment. However, not until you touch the client and feel the person will you begin to understand that individual's body. The client can sense through your touch if you understand the information the body provides. Touch is a fundamental, multilayered, and powerful form of communication, the most personalized form of communication we know.

Touch as Communication

In many ways, touch is a more emotionally powerful form of communication than speech. Verbal communication uses specific words with specific meanings to relay a message. Touch communication is more ambiguous, relying on the interpretation of its meaning through experience and current circumstances. Delivering a clear, concise verbal message is difficult enough when both parties—the one delivering the message and the one receiving it—agree on the meaning of the words. It is much more challenging to deliver a touch message in which many factors are involved in the interpretation of the message. The potential for misunderstanding increases. Often, with both verbal and touch communication, the message intended is not necessarily the one received.

The communication of touch is influenced by personal, family, and cultural contexts. Each person defines an area around themselves as personal space, and the distance encompassed by this personal space differs from person to person and culture to culture. Therapies using touch enter this personal space; therefore the professional must be sensitive to the numerous factors that influence people's responses when their personal space is entered. **Diversity** refers gender, age, ethnicity, physical ability, neurodiversity, and more. **Equity** is fair treatment for all people and **inclusion** values and respects all individuals and encourages them to contribute their unique perspectives and ideas.

Cultural Influences

A **culture** is defined by the arts, beliefs, customs, institutions, and all other products of human work and thought created by a specific group of people at a particular time. To say that people of a certain culture act a certain way is stereotyping; individuals always vary. However, tendencies can be defined by culture, and this may provide a way to begin initial touch interaction until the person's uniqueness is better understood.

Cultures are no longer isolated by distance. Modern-day travel supports the intermingling of people from many parts of our world. We are a global society with multiple languages, beliefs, and practices. It is necessary to be culturally aware and respectful. It is not necessary to endorse or adopt cultural beliefs and practices into our own individual behavior and belief systems to be culturally respectful. Culture is important, yet it may be considered stereotypical to define a person by their culture. Because we live in a global community, we are likely to interact with people from other parts of the world. Exploring the vast diversity of cultural norms and traditions is beyond the scope of this text. However, as a professional, you are responsible for developing an understanding of the social, cultural, and spiritual ways of the client population you serve while avoiding stereotypes. You can do this in several ways. Begin with online research about a particular culture. In your practice, ask relevant and courteous questions, and let your clients teach you about themselves and their culture. Most of all, be open and receptive to what your clients say and make sure you respect your clients' cultures.

Gender Identity and Diversity

Gender can be considered a spectrum. Gender diversity has existed throughout history and all over the world. Gender identity is a social construct and is the way people perceive themselves. A person's gender identity can be consistent with, or different from, the sex assigned at birth. Sexual orientation relates to emotional, romantic, or sexual attraction to other people and is different from gender identity. The language a person uses to communicate their gender identity requires a broader gender vocabulary. The vocabulary of gender continues to evolve, and there is no universal agreement about the definitions of many terms. Respectful professional behavior involves becoming and remaining current with language that reflects individual identity.

Gender neutrality emphasizes the equal treatment of all people with an emphasis on people as individuals. In gender neutralism, the emphasis is on transcending the perspective of gender in our professional interactions with clients. As massage professionals, our personal gender identity and sexual orientation are private and not expressed in our professional roles. Professionals strive to be nonjudgmental, which is an ongoing process of self-examination and education. The clients served are people to be respected. As with cultural diversity, the client is the best source of information. In your practice, ask relevant and courteous questions, and let your clients teach you about themselves.

Influence of Age on Touch

Age differences can be a factor in the interpretation of touch. Some may consider touching young people appropriate but may be more cautious about touching older people. A younger person touching an elder may be acceptable, but the dynamics are different when two people of the same age touch. The touch of a young practitioner may be interpreted differently from the touch of an older practitioner, even if the skill and experience levels are equivalent.

Influence of Life Events and the Interpretation of Touch

Life events can influence the response to touch experiences. People who have undergone painful and extensive medical interventions, especially at an early age, may process touch differently from those who have not had these experiences. People who have experienced touch trauma are influenced by those events, and individuals who have experienced isolation respond uniquely to touch. People who grew up with excessive touch stimulation outside the context of trauma (e.g., being part of a large family in small living quarters or being an only child with many adoring family members) may develop certain touch responses. Having a healthy, appropriate touch history also influences a person's interpretation of touch. Any of these experiences and many more affect the way a person understands another's experience of touch.

Spiritual Touch

Touch also can have a spiritual context. Many spiritual rituals incorporate touch, especially those that involve concepts of healing of the body (that which is organic), the mind (that which is of thought), or the spirit (that which is transcendent and sacred). Each person deserves respect for their personal truth and individual spiritual path.

Diversity and Touch

Generalities are useless in discussing cultural orientations to touch because we cannot stereotype all people from a specific culture as holding to similar customs. The same difficulties with stereotyping occur concerning gender, age, and one's life or spiritual path. On any given day or even at any given moment, the need, desire, interpretation, and appropriateness of touch given and received can change. These changes occur because a person is in a constant state of flux in responding and adapting to encountered events. The type of relationship between people and its duration influence touch. For example, a first-time client may not be receptive to the deeper pressure used in some applications of massage, especially if the goal of the session is relaxation. However, several sessions later that same client may be responsive to deeper pressure in some areas if related to reducing pain or increasing mobility. A client may be ticklish to light touch initially in the session, but after relaxing may find that same touch pleasurable.

PROFICIENCY EXERCISE 1.2

In the space provided, answer these questions:

1. What do I do when I am touch hungry?
2. Who and what touches me in a safe, respectful, and healing way?

A person's response to and need for the delivery of touch cannot be predetermined. However, each individual, including you, has been influenced by many factors regarding the appropriate procedure for touch and ultimately the interpretation of the meaning of a touch.

We need to explore and challenge our biases which consist of attitudes, behaviors, and actions that are prejudiced in favor of or against one person or group compared to another. **Implicit bias** is a form of bias that occurs automatically and unintentionally; it affects judgments, decisions, and behaviors. Removing these biases is a challenge, especially because we often don't even know they exist. Understanding what implicit biases are and how to recognize them in ourselves and others are all incredibly important in working towards overcoming such biases. There are educational courses available to help people overcome implicit bias. As professionals, we must be aware, sensitive, and open to an appreciation of the wide variety of influences that affect professional touch while also diligently seeking an understanding of our own desires, motivations, and responses to touch. After all, it is impossible to touch clients without them in turn touching us. A touch given is at the same time a touch received (Proficiency Exercise 1.2).

PROFESSIONAL CLASSIFICATIONS OF TOUCH

SECTION OBJECTIVES

Chapter objective covered in this section:

2. Describe professional touch.

Using the information presented in this section, the student will be able to:

- Identify factors that constitute appropriate and inappropriate touch in the professional setting.

Touch involves many nuances and forms. As a student of massage therapy, it is necessary to appreciate the complexity of the simple act of touching.

Physical and Psychological Perspectives on Professional Touch

When a person is touched, sensation is received and internalized. Professional touch is not overtly an act of exerting power and dominance. Although the ability to receive touch is powerful, the difference in the power base between those who give touch and those who receive it must be considered. This interplays with the appropriateness or inappropriateness of touch. Careful attention must be paid during professional touch to manage the issue of power and dominance ethically.

Forms of Inappropriate Touch

Inappropriate touch in some way devalues the individual receiving the touch. This type of touch intention is often based on some sort of internal conflict in the individual doing the touching. Inappropriate touch of any kind is not to be allowed in a professional setting. The three forms of inappropriate touch in massage therapy are hostile or aggressive touch, erotic (sexual) touch, and invasive touch.

Hostile or Aggressive Touch

Hostile or aggressive touch occurs when a potential for conflict or a power struggle exists. Professionals who use touch need to be aware of the underlying energy directed toward the client to prevent this intention in the touch. The obvious is easy; if you are angry with a client, it is best not to touch at that moment. Likewise, if a client is angry with you, it is best not to touch them until the emotions change. A more subtle aspect of professional interactions is the undercurrent of conflict. For example, the client may arrive late for the appointment, or the massage therapist may be hurried or angry about something at home. In these cases, the practitioner inadvertently may be more aggressive than necessary during the massage.

The perception that one holds power over another underlies hostile or aggressive touch. Careful attention must be paid to this idea of power in the therapeutic relationship between the professional and the client. In the professional relationship, a power difference between the professional and the client exists simply because of the knowledge base that defines the profession. Knowledge is power, and most of the time, the professional knows more about the service rendered than the client does.

In body therapies such as therapeutic massage, the client's physical position often creates an environment that fosters a power differential. Clients usually lie down or are seated, and the professional is standing and physically above the client, generating the impression of authority and dominance.

During massage, we need to sustain a focus on how and where the client's body is being touched and the client's perceptions of the touch. There is a difference for clients between submitting to and enduring a massage and receiving and integrating a massage. The massage environment also can influence the perception of the massage. An environment (including the staff) that may be harsh appears hostile. A location in an area considered unsafe or an office in which the background noise includes sirens from emergency vehicles, arguments, or gossiping will diminish the ability of the client and the therapist to relax.

Erotic (Sexual) Touch

The intention of erotic, or sexual, touch is sexual arousal and expression. The issue of erotic touch cannot be sidestepped in the study of massage therapy or any other body-oriented treatment in which touch is a primary aspect of the therapy. Complex physiological and mental aspects of both the client and the practitioner influence the ideas of erotic touch.

The pleasure of being touched is inherent in many forms of massage and bodywork. Pleasure is an important therapeutic tool. In later chapters, you will learn that chemicals in the body create pleasure moods and that feelings of connectedness increase during massage. These chemical responses are one of the main reasons for the therapeutic benefit of massage methods. Constant attention must be paid to the understanding and interpretation of the feelings generated during professional touch so that pleasurable touch does not evolve into or become misinterpreted as erotic touch.

Psychotherapists and other health care professionals also must be aware of the potential for sexual feelings in the context of the professional environment. Professionals are people with complex, intertwined needs, desires, and means of expressing themselves. However, it is inappropriate for professionals to foster or express any type of erotic feelings with a client, either within the therapeutic environment or outside that environment.

Invasive Touch

Invasive touch can be both intentional and unintentional. As a massage professional, you are responsible for understanding personal and cultural rules about where and when to touch.

Different areas of the body reflect different tactile issues. Some areas of the body called erogenous zones have many nerve endings and are more sensitive when touched. The largest distribution of erogenous zones is in the genital area. Other common erogenous zones include breasts and nipples, lips, mouth, tongue, buttocks, and inner thighs. These areas are considered no-touch zones, in terms of professional therapeutic massage touch. Orifices, including the anus, genitals, mouth, ears, and nose, are taboo in most societies. The ventral (front) surfaces of the body, including the breasts, are more sensitive than the dorsal (back) surfaces. We see this pattern in massage; much of the massage session is devoted to the back of the torso and the legs while the client is lying face down, with the front of the body "protected" by the massage table. Therapeutically, this creates difficulties, because soft tissue dysfunction also occurs on the front of the body, where sensations of touch are more apt to elicit emotional responses and feelings of vulnerability.

Often the least intrusive form of touch is laying a hand on a person's upper back near the shoulder, whereas having the hands massaged can feel very intimate and connected. The head also is an area sensitive to touch. Although children often are touched on the head and face, adults are seldom touched casually in these areas. Adults often respond emotionally to touching of the face and head.

Areas of a person's body that have experienced trauma (e.g., accidents or surgery) carry more emotional charge and therefore are more sensitive to the interpretation of touch.

The appropriateness or inappropriateness of touch, then, is about when, how, and with what intent we touch (Lederman, 1997; Zur & Nordmarken, 2011; McGuirk, 2012; Warwick, 2022).

Forms of Appropriate Touch

Nontherapeutic forms of touch that people often encounter include inadvertent touch, such as when people are jostled together in an elevator, and socially stereotyped touch, which involves highly ritualized touch that carries a consensual meaning within a culture, such as a handshake.

Therapeutic forms of touch involve touch that communicates information or expresses feeling as part of the therapeutic relationship (McParlin et al., 2022). This form of touch is not so much about creating a specific outcome as it is about delivering information, expressing comfort, or understanding (Smith et al., 1998; Swade, 2020; Hargie, 2021). Some examples of this type of touch are touching a client's shoulder to direct them to the massage room or holding a client's hand as they thank you for the session.

Touch Technique

Touch technique is the basis of therapeutic massage methods. Touch is the tool for massage. **Massage** is the use of various forms of touch to achieve a specific outcome. This type of touch can be considered technical touch. In terms of touch technique, a therapeutic intent exists. The intention of touch therapy can be classified in two ways:

1. **Mechanical touch**, which is used to achieve a specific anatomical or physiological outcome (e.g., using massage to increase the range of motion of the shoulder).
2. **Expressive touch**, which is used to support and convey awareness and empathy for the client as a whole person (e.g., using massage for general relaxation and pleasure to comfort a client after a particularly hard day at work) (Lederman, 1997; Dekeyser & Leijssen, 2005; Stonehouse, 2017).

The professional's intention influences the interpretation of touch. A client with a mechanical restriction in the shoulder might find a more expressive form of touch uncomfortable because it might feel too intimate for the circumstances. Stressed, overworked clients may find a mechanical approach distant and impersonal because they are seeking empathy and understanding along with physical changes.

As we develop as professionals, both forms of touch technique must be perfected. Mechanical touch skills increase as we learn anatomy, physiology, and effective delivery of specific forms of massage (these topics are covered throughout the textbook). Development of the expressive form of touch technique is more complex and involves the professional's personal growth, interpersonal and communication skills, and understanding of their own life experiences.

Humans are much more alike than different, especially as we consider the effects of therapeutic massage on anatomy and physiology. We can also find nuggets of wisdom in cultural practices even if, as an individual, we do not embrace the totality of the beliefs. It is not feasible to discuss all cultural variations in this textbook, but a thread of cultural awareness runs throughout the book, especially when massage-related practices have influenced the current practice of therapeutic massage.

The desire for physical contact is an instinctive and physiological need for well-being. Well-being is the foundational outcome of massage therapy. Professional therapeutic touch often feeds touch hunger for people in a safe, professional environment. Massage professionals serve others by providing touch. Professional touch provided through therapeutic massage, coupled with an understanding of the various needs and diversity of the population we serve, is complex. It is common to feel as if there is too much to know. It is important in professional development to honor personal and professional limits and to set appropriate personal and professional boundaries. When touch is the primary treatment method, it is even more important to understand the interpersonal dynamics of the therapeutic relationship (McParlin et al., 2022). (Professional boundaries are discussed further in Chapter 2.)

Massage professionals must embrace the expansive and abstract experience of touch. The concrete experience of caring most often is conveyed through touch. That knowing, or "felt sense," experienced both by the client and the practitioner often is internalized through professional touch. We must show our willingness as practitioners to be open personally to sharing the experience with the client, at the same time being professional enough to respect the client and maintain the focus of the experience for the individual. If we are going to be able to provide this type of touch experience for others, how do we take care of our personal touch needs? What happens to you if your hunger for safe, nurturing (nutritious) touch is not met? To do this, each of us who uses touch professionally must be aware of self-care, and we must develop resources and support people (and pets and plants) who touch us in a safe, respectful, and healing way.

> *"No one cares how much you know, until they know how much you care."*
>
> —— **Theodore Roosevelt**

PROFESSIONALISM AND THERAPEUTIC MASSAGE

SECTION OBJECTIVES

Chapter objectives covered in this section:

3. Define professionalism.
4. Define therapeutic massage.

Using the information presented in this section, the student will be able to:

- Compare therapeutic massage with professional development criteria.
- Describe the two professional development trends in therapeutic massage wellness and medical care.
- Compare various definitions of massage and massage therapy.
- Justify the use of the term *massage therapist*.

A profession is a paid occupation, especially one that involves prolonged training, a formal education, and specific qualifications to practice. A profession has these characteristics:

- A specialized body of knowledge
- Extensive training
- An orientation toward service
- A commonly accepted code of ethics
- Legal recognition through licensure
- Verification of advanced training with board certification
- Membership in a professional association

Each of these areas related to a profession will be compared to the current status of massage therapy.

Specialized Body of Knowledge

Massage therapy methods are grounded in a specialized body of knowledge, which is presented in this textbook. Historical foundations and current research validate this body of knowledge. One important source is the *Massage Therapy Body of Knowledge* (MTBOK), created by the MTBOK Stewards, who include representatives from the American Massage Therapy Association, the Associated Bodywork & Massage Professionals, the Alliance for Massage Therapy Education, the Federation of State Massage Therapy Boards, the Massage Therapy Foundation, and the National Certification Board for Therapeutic Massage and Bodywork. Another important source is the Entry Level Analysis Project (ELAP), a research project supported by several professional massage therapy associations. A lifetime of study could easily be devoted to therapeutic massage methods.

Extensive Training

Before considering massage therapy in relation to the criteria of extensive training, it is necessary to discuss massage practice and the required education. It is this area that may or may not support massage therapy as a profession.

Inconsistencies continue regarding the duration of massage training and the information and technical skills that should be included in that training. The *Massage Therapy Body of Knowledge* and the *Entry-Level Analysis Project* provide recommendations for knowledge, skills, and abilities applicable to entry-level education. The entry-level recommendation is 625 contact hours based on the ELAP curriculum content. This is not considered extensive training based on criteria for a profession.

In massage therapy, two main categories of practice have emerged, with six distinct practice settings:

- Wellness and health promotion
  - Spa setting
  - Massage franchise/wellness center
  - Sports and fitness setting
  - Independent massage practice
- Medical care
  - Clinical/medical/rehabilitation settings
  - Independent massage practice with clients who have medical conditions

These categories and practice settings overlap extensively. However, categorizing information is useful when we are attempting to understand the big picture. Because massage therapy has a history of multiple practice settings and one person can practice in multiple settings, the situation can become complex. Therefore we start with a simple approach.

The entry-level education required in the wellness/health promotion categories of therapeutic massage can be considered the basic educational requirement and foundation for practice, with licensure as the credential. Continuing professional development can be validated through board certification provided by the National Certification

Board for Therapeutic Massage and Bodywork (NCBTMB). Specific information can be found on the NCBTMB website.

The National Center for Education Statistics (NCES) collects, analyzes, and reports statistics about American and international education. This organization categorizes education as occupational or academic.

- *Occupational/vocational education* is specifically designed to educate for a career/job. Certificate programs typically are 1 year or less of formal study. A certificate—also called a *diploma*—refers to an award granted for the successful completion of a subbaccalaureate postsecondary program of study. These certificates are usually awarded in a career education field and may cover the same coursework as an associate's degree, but without the general education requirements. Health sciences, into which massage therapy education is typically categorized, is the predominant field in which subbaccalaureate occupational credentials, either certificates or an associate's degree, are achieved.
    - Associate's degree: A degree granted for the successful completion of a subbaccalaureate program of study, usually requiring the equivalent of at least two but less than four full-time academic years of college-level study. An associate's degree covers the content of occupational/vocational education but also requires additional general education, math, and writing courses to round out the program.
- *Academic study* involves the achievement of a baccalaureate degree or higher. A bachelor's degree is granted for the successful completion of a baccalaureate program of studies, usually requiring the equivalent of at least 4 but not more than 5 full-time academic years of college-level study (Hudson 2018).

Because most massage therapy education results in a diploma or certificate, massage therapy education is typically occupational and vocational. There are a few exceptions for which an associate's degree is available. In educational settings, occupational education is used to describe shorter, nonacademic programs that lead to paraprofessional careers, whereas professional education usually describes postgraduate programs leading to degrees. Occupational education is an excellent way to develop a career and in no way indicates less professionalism than an academic degree. However, the criteria for a profession often involve academic degree education. This may be changing. Current trends in education for career development are focusing more on vocational training because it is the source of most employment and career opportunities.

An important move toward the availability of an academic degree has occurred because college credits toward a bachelor's degree are now awarded based on the advanced credential of board certification. A bachelor's degree in applied science in massage therapy is available from Siena Heights University in Adrian, Michigan, which awards 45+ college credits toward the 120 total credits required to achieve this degree. In the future, other community colleges and universities may develop similar partnerships based on board certification. Individuals who already have professional academic degrees are obtaining massage therapy training and combining the two skills to function effectively in the health and athletic worlds; some examples of these combinations are nurse/massage therapist, athletic trainer/massage therapist, respiratory therapist/massage therapist, physical therapy assistant/massage therapist, occupational therapist/massage therapist, and social worker or psychologist/massage therapist. Because entry-level massage therapy education is occupational, the career pathway can begin at a lower educational cost and investment of time. Then ongoing education is pursued as part of professional development.

Let's return to the basic classifications of massage therapy practice:

- Wellness and health promotion
    - Spa setting
    - Massage franchise/wellness center
    - Sports and fitness setting
    - Independent massage practice
- Medical care
    - Clinical/medical/rehabilitation settings
    - Independent massage practice with clients who have medical conditions

All of these areas provide opportunities both for entry-level practice and advanced education and career specialization.

Entry-Level Practice

Spa and Wellness Setting

Growing interest in health and wellness is driving annual growth in the spa and wellness sector. The evolving spa environment encompasses a range of massage services for wellness-based massage; these services can overlap with sports and fitness massage and massage related to health care in the so-called medical spa. This text (coupled with your science studies) provides the skills necessary to develop a successful career in the spa environment, especially with supervision in the fitness-focused spa or medical spa. The spa setting also can be considered a massage specialty requiring additional education and experience. Career development in this setting usually follows the employee pathway. Chapter 13 provides specific information about the spa as a career track. Check out Chapter 3 for more information about career success as an employee.

Massage Franchise/Wellness Centers

Many massage therapy franchises have entered the massage market. This business concept is fast becoming the largest employer of massage therapists. Franchises typically offer a subscription-based membership model for clients. A *wellness center* is an establishment that offers health services for the body and mind. Wellness centers usually offer massage therapy, hydrotherapy and thermotherapy, yoga, meditation, fitness, personal training, nutrition consulting, and skin care services. Some wellness centers offer services such as chiropractic, acupuncture, or holistic medicine.

Career development follows the employee pathway. Because franchises and wellness centers manage all the marketing and business responsibilities, they provide an excellent entry-level opportunity; they also support employees who pursue the experience and professional development necessary for career advancement. The content of this textbook (coupled with your science studies) effectively prepares you to work in this setting.

Sports and Fitness Setting

The sports and fitness career path covers a spectrum of massage outcomes, ranging from wellness to medical intervention typically (but not exclusively) based on issues related to environments that support exercise and sports performance. The importance of exercise in the management of most lifestyle-related diseases, such as diabetes, obesity, cardiovascular disease, mental illness, and many more, is well documented. Massage can support physical changes related to exercise and can help manage the discomfort related to physical activity and injury for those beginning an exercise program. Massage can also be beneficial for the extensive performance demands required of entertainers, competing athletes, military personnel, and first responders. Information in this text, presented in the appropriate scientific context, provides the foundation for working in this setting. However, professional development and experience are necessary for a practitioner to become confident and proficient in this area.

Clinical/Medical/Rehabilitation Setting

Massage provided in a medical care setting is becoming more common for massage practice. The name of this type of practice remains a little ambiguous; it currently is labeled the clinical/medical/rehabilitation career path. The ELAP documents use the term *health care-oriented massage*. The term *clinical massage* is defined as massage therapy practice that involves more extensive use of assessment, focused techniques, and applications with the intention of achieving clinical treatment outcomes. Stress-related issues and pain management are major reasons hospitals and other health care facilities offer massage. Other primary reasons for providing massage include:

- Palliative care
- Aid to physical therapy
- Mobility/movement training

The common thread in clinical/medical care-oriented massage careers is integration with medical care systems. This type of massage treatment may focus on stress management and prevention, management of chronic disease and pain, acute care palliation, presurgical and postsurgical care, prenatal care, elder care, and hospice care. People who receive medical care are usually called *patients*. All massage recipients are considered *clients,* but not all clients are classified as medical patients.

Independent Massage Practice

The independent practice setting is the most complex because an independent practice can be structured in many ways. Typically, the massage therapist is self-employed.

These career paths can serve as entry-level jobs; however, the demands of the clients and complex outcomes for the massage typically require a commitment to advanced education and experience. This textbook, coupled with science studies, can prepare you to practice massage therapy successfully in these settings if you commit to focused study and competency in the entire content presented. This means that reading the information once is not enough. You must study, review, practice, and then review some more until you have integrated the information into your massage therapy skills.

This text provides the necessary foundation for general massage in the clinical/medical/rehabilitation setting and the medical care-oriented massage career pathway. Continuing education provides the information that enables the practitioner to become confident and proficient in providing this type of massage therapy (Chapter 13 describes this content in depth).

It does not seem reasonable to expect entry-level educational programs of 500–1000 contact hours to provide sufficient time for the complex integration of clinical reasoning methods; extensive physical assessment procedures; and the study of pathology, pharmacology, and psychology, as well as other information the massage professional needs to work effectively with other medical care professionals and with complicated, multifaceted medical concerns. The same can be said for sports massage or working with athletes. To work effectively with athletes, the professional must have an in-depth education in the dynamics of sports activity, the injury process, and rehabilitation.

After this lengthy description, the question related to a profession requiring extensive training and how that relates to massage therapy remains unclear.

Orientation to Service

The definition of service that best applies to this discussion is "to meet a need." Massage can be described as a vocation and reflects the concept of orientation to service. An additional concept in a service orientation is that although reimbursement is expected for services rendered, the desire to meet a need takes precedence over financial return. Observation of those who practice massage professionally and of the attitudes of current learners indicates that providers of therapeutic massage tend to be oriented toward service, sometimes to the detriment of sound business practices. Although caring for the people we serve is important, it is just as important to generate the necessary and appropriate income to support the professional practice and a modest lifestyle for the professional. Finding a balance between professional fees charged to clients and reasonable income for the massage therapist is an ethical, professional, and personal issue. (Massage costs and realistic expectations for income at the entry level are discussed in depth in Chapter 3). However, it is necessary to discuss the gray areas related to professional ethics, setting fees, and earning an income.

The cost of a massage session and whether the client pays for the massage directly determines how frequently someone will receive a massage. Is it ethical for massage fees to be high enough that most of the population cannot afford massage regularly? Should massage fees be set low enough for most of the population to regularly receive massage? How much financial sacrifice should clients make to get the massage help they need? Should a less expensive massage session have a lower quality than a more expensive massage session? What should that fee range be? What should the wage be for entry-level employment? Is a sliding fee scale based on a client's income fair? Should a massage therapist earn the same income as a medical care professional with much more formal education? Is it ethical for an employer to expect a massage therapist to work for minimum wage as base pay, with additional income per client and gratuities? Is it ethical for a massage therapist to expect to earn more income yearly than the employer? Should an employer's annual income be double, triple, or even more than the employee's? Is it fair for a self-employed massage therapist to earn more than a massage employee? Is it ethical for one massage therapist to charge more or less than others in their geographical region? Should an entry-level massage therapist just completing school earn as much as an experienced massage therapist? What obligation does the massage community have to those living in poverty situations, in which finding money to pay for massage is unrealistic? What is a living-wage income necessary for an individual to meet basic living costs in a particular region of the country?

There are no easy answers to these questions, and to a certain extent, individuals will need to find their own balance between income and an orientation toward service. Massage therapists cannot serve others if they cannot take care of themselves and their families. We must earn a reasonable income that at least meets the standard for what is considered a "living wage." The living wage is defined as the wage needed to cover basic family expenses (basic needs budget) plus all relevant taxes. A living wage is more than minimum wage. It is a market-based approach that draws upon geographically specific data related to a family's likely minimum costs for food, childcare, health insurance, housing, transportation, and other necessities (e.g., clothing, personal care items). The living wage is the amount of income needed to provide a decent standard of living. A useful tool for calculating a living wage has been developed by Dr. Amy K. Glasmeier and the Massachusetts Institute of Technology. It can be found at the Living Wage Calculator website (https://livingwage.mit.edu/).

Commonly Accepted Code of Ethics

A code of ethics is an agreed-on set of behaviors developed to promote high standards of practice. As you study the rest of this textbook, you will see that although there is general agreement about what a code of ethics for massage therapy entails, no agreement has been reached on a specific code of ethics to serve the entire massage community. (This information is discussed in Chapter 2).

Legal Recognition by Licensure

Currently, all US states (except three at this writing), the District of Columbia, at least half of Canadian provinces, and many other countries have formal licensing or legislated registration for massage professionals. In states that regulate massage therapy, massage therapists must meet the legal requirements to practice, which may include fulfilling a minimum number of hours of initial training and passing an examination. In states that do not regulate massage therapy, this task may fall to local municipalities. Most states that license massage therapists require a passing score on the Massage & Bodywork Licensing Examination (MBLEx), which is administered by the Federation of State Massage Therapy Boards (FSMTB). Entry-level education should prepare you for meeting licensing requirements.

Verification of Advance Training With Board Certification

It is common practice for professionals to become board certified, which verifies that the professional has completed the requirements for certification under the standards of an independent regulatory body. Board certification is much more than licensure. Board certification is an additional, voluntary process that one goes through to demonstrate competency in a specialty area.

Membership in a Professional Association

Several organizations represent the therapeutic massage profession. In addition, each of the various bodywork methods (e.g., reflexology, shiatsu, polarity) has its own professional organization. Although diversity is good for a profession and supports professional development, the lack of coherence in the field of therapeutic massage often confuses us as well as the public and other professionals. Developments in this area will be interesting to watch.

Massage Therapy as a Profession

The question remains: does massage therapy meet the criteria of a profession? Good question. The most logical answer is "almost." The need for academic degrees for career success is being questioned, and occupational education is being promoted. If massage therapy is to be considered a profession, then some level of educational standards must be endorsed. Professional organizations remain competitive instead of collaborative, but that is changing. The biggest obstacle is a lack of clarity about what massage therapy actually entails. There is no agreed-upon definition of massage and massage therapy.

Defining Massage

A valid definition of massage must encompass the foundational methods used by various approaches and must be written concisely. Massage is a form of manual therapy using applied mechanical forces to peripheral tissues as part of the therapeutic delivery. The effects of mechanical forces on the human body are of great interest to two groups of professionals: scientists who study neural systems involved in mechanosensation and clinicians who use force-based manipulations such as massage therapy, spinal manipulation, or acupuncture (Langevin, 2021). Massage cannot be considered a single skill; a more appropriate concept is a collection of skills (Fig. 1.4). In addition, the definition of therapeutic massage depends on individual governmental laws and the definition of massage

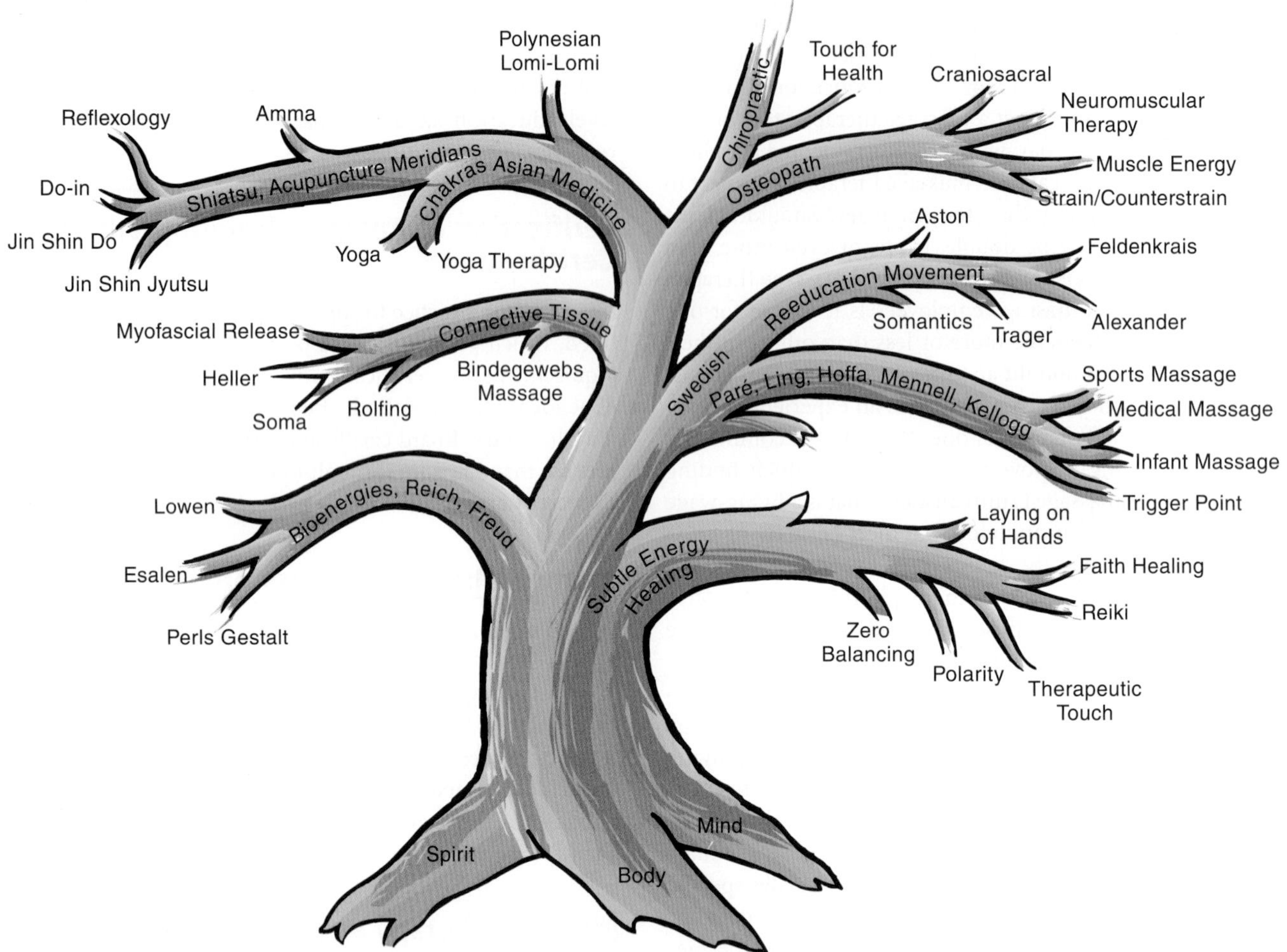

FIG. 1.4 The therapeutic massage tree. Although massage encompasses a wide diversity in its uses and applications, all forms of therapeutic massage methods stem from the same roots.

included in those laws. Defining massage accurately and completely is difficult because of the many forms and styles of massage and bodywork currently practiced. Four important developments in the massage profession have occurred since 2010 that have influenced the definition of massage:

- The Coalition of National Massage Therapy Organizations was formed and includes:
  - Alliance for Massage Therapy Education (AFMTE)
  - American Massage Therapy Association (AMTA)
  - Associated Bodywork & Massage Professionals (ABMP)
  - Commission on Massage Therapy Accreditation (COMTA)
  - Federation of State Massage Therapy Boards (FSMTB)
  - Massage Therapy Foundation (MTF)
  - National Certification Board for Therapeutic Massage and Bodywork (NCBTMB)
- The coalition members worked together to fund and support the *Massage Therapy Body of Knowledge* (MTBOK, https://www.afmte.org/education/mtbok/) and the *Entry-Level Analysis Project* (ELAP, https://elapmassage.org/).
- The FSMTB developed a Model Practice Act (https://www.fsmtb.org/media/1126/model_massage_therapy_practice_act.pdf) and reached an agreement with the National Certification Board that the MBLEx would be the only licensing examination.
- The NCBTMB validated credentialing of massage practice beyond licensure through the board certification credential.

These four events have moved the massage community toward unification and have created a clear pathway for the standardization of massage education, licensing at the entry level, and career development through board certification. Much work remains to be done, but progress is evident. The two projects, MTBOK and ELAP, identify what massage therapy is and what the educational requirements need to be to standardize and advance the massage profession. Until the publication of the MTBOK document and the two extensive ELAP reports, there was no consensus on the knowledge, skills, and attitudes that provide the foundation for massage therapy as a profession. Box 1.2 presents several definitions of massage, including the definition established by the MTBOK, ELAP, the FSMTB Model Practice Act, and the definition of massage therapy used by the National Center for Complementary and Integrative Health (NCCIH).

The unofficial consensus is that massage therapy is a health and wellness profession. The practice of massage therapy involves a client/patient-centered session, intended to fulfill therapeutic goals. Massage therapy also meets the

Box 1.2 What's in a Name? Definitions of Therapeutic Massage

Massage Therapy Body of Knowledge (MTBOK)[a]
Massage therapy is a health care and wellness profession. The practice of massage therapy involves a client-centered session that is intended to fulfill therapeutic goals and in which the therapist has no personal agenda. Massage therapy also meets the well-researched need for touch and human connection. Massage therapy is about one human being touching another with clear intention, focused attention, and an attitude that is compassionate and nonjudgmental. During a session, the massage therapist incorporates a wide variety of techniques and approaches to address the client's varied focuses, which may include any or all of the following: treating an injury or condition; relaxation; reducing stress; wellness; enhancing personal growth; encouraging awareness of the body; or facilitating balance and interconnection of the body, mind, and spirit.

Entry Level Analysis Projects (ELAP) Definitions[b]
Bodywork: A broad term that refers to many forms, methods, and styles, including massage, that positively influence the body through various methods, which may or may not include soft tissue deformation, energy manipulation, movement reeducation, and postural reeducation.
Massage: The ethical and professional application of structured, therapeutic touch to benefit soft tissue health, movement, posture, and neurologic patterns.
Wellness-oriented massage: Massage performed in wellness- or relaxation-oriented environments to facilitate stress reduction, relaxation, or wellness.
Health care-oriented massage: Massage performed in medical or health care-oriented environments to facilitate therapeutic change, condition management, or symptom management.

Federation of State Massage Therapy Boards (FSMTB)[c]
Section 104. Practice of Massage Therapy
The practice of massage therapy means the manual application of a system of structured touch to the soft tissues of the human body, including but not limited to: (1) assessment, evaluation, or treatment; (2) pressure, friction, stroking, rocking, gliding, kneading, percussion, or vibration; (3) active or passive stretching of the body within the normal anatomic range of movement; (4) use of manual methods or mechanical or electrical devices or tools that mimic or enhance the action of human hands; (5) use of topical applications such as lubricants, scrubs, or herbal preparations; (6) use of hot or cold applications; (7) use of hydrotherapy; and (8) client education.

National Center for Complementary and Integrative Health (NCCIH, formerly the National Center for Complementary and Alternative Medicine [NCCAM])[d]
Massage therapy encompasses many techniques. In general, therapists press, rub, and otherwise manipulate the muscles and other soft tissues of the body. They most often use their hands and fingers but may also incorporate their forearms, elbows, or feet.

[a]Alliance for Massage Therapy Education https://www.afmte.org/education/mtbok/.
[b]Coalition of National Massage Therapy Organizations http://www.elapmassage.org/.
[c]Federation of State Massage Therapy Boards https://www.fsmtb.org/media/1126/model_massage_therapy_practice_act.pdf.
[d]From the National Center for Complementary and Integrative Health https://nccih.nih.gov/health/integrative-health.

well-researched need for touch and human connection. Massage therapy is about one human touching another with clear intention, focused attention, and the attitudes of compassion and nonjudgment.

If we are to consider ourselves *therapists*, we must understand the implications of that title and determine how we should conduct ourselves in behaving as therapists. Other options for an occupational title exist, such as *technician* and *practitioner*. Because the massage therapy community has determined that we are professionals, we are obligated to conduct ourselves as professionals. For help in this matter, massage therapy professionals can consider their scope of practice (see Chapter 2). According to the Federation of State Massage Therapy Board's Model Practice Act,

> The practice of Massage Therapy means the manual application of a system of structured touch to the soft tissues of the human body, including but not limited to: (1) Assessment, evaluation, or treatment; (2) Pressure, friction, stroking, rocking, gliding, kneading, percussion or vibration; (3) Active or passive stretching of the body within the normal anatomic range of movement; (4) Use of manual methods or mechanical or electrical devices or tools that mimic or enhance the action of human hands; (5) Use of topical applications such as lubricants, scrubs, or herbal preparations; (6) Use of hot or cold applications; (7) Use of hydrotherapy; (8) Client education.

Confusion continues over the similarities between massage and bodywork. Massage therapy is a bodywork system, but not all bodywork systems are massage. Other bodywork and somatic practices, such as shiatsu and structural integration, have separately developed systems and philosophies, scopes of practice, and educational requirements. With most of these massage and bodywork systems, the outcomes for the client are similar. The most common outcomes people seek from bodywork are relaxation/well-being, stress management, pain management, and support for mobility and physical performance (function). As a specific professional practice, massage therapy can achieve all these client goals through the use of methods considered massage by the Model Practice Act (MPA). Other bodywork systems, in achieving these outcomes, use different methods or have a different philosophy and specific language. Later in the text, you will learn that the methods of application for most bodywork systems, including massage therapy, interact with the same physiology of the body and therefore are more alike than different. Again, based on the explanation provided in the MPA, bodywork methods in which the body is not physically touched are not massage therapy. Practitioners who manipulate soft tissue in any way, regardless of the name of the method described in the MPA, are considered massage therapists for licensing purposes.

The full scope of practice of the massage therapy profession goes beyond the minimum entry-level competency. Everyone who learns a skill needs to start at the beginning. Because you are reading this text, which is written as an entry-level textbook, you are just starting the process of achieving entry-level competency. Just as there is an entry level, there also are advanced levels of professional development that you can strive to achieve, which would allow you to practice massage therapy within the full scope of practice.

The final element addressed by the MTBOK project and the ELAP was an agreed-on terminology (taxonomy). Until the release of these documents, massage terminology was inconsistent and sometimes confusing and frustrating. Now we have the foundation for a language that we all can learn and understand. That terminology is used in this text.

This textbook and a companion textbook, *Mosby's Essential Sciences for Therapeutic Massage,* include the ELAP content recommendations and MTBOK content. In addition, these textbooks present information you will need to prepare for advanced levels of learning, including preparation for the credential Board Certified in Therapeutic Massage and Bodywork (BCTMB), the highest attainable credential in the massage therapy and bodywork profession. Board certification is a separate credential above and beyond entry-level massage therapy state licensure.

Clarifying Definitions for the Massage Therapy Profession

An ongoing issue in the massage therapy community is the lack of agreed-upon definitions of massage, massage therapy, and massage therapy practice. According to the study "Clarifying Definitions for the Massage Therapy Profession: The Results of the Best Practices Symposium 2016," a large part of the lack of clarity in definition may be due to the common practice of using the terms *massage* and *massage therapy* interchangeably when, in fact, they appear to be two separate concepts (Kennedy et al., 2016a). The study's authors offered the following definitions, which guide this textbook.

- *Massage:* Massage is a patterned and purposeful soft-tissue manipulation accomplished by the use of digits, hands, forearms, elbows, knees, and/or feet, with or without the use of emollients, liniments, heat and cold, hand-held tools, or other external apparatus, for the intent of the therapeutic change.
- *Massage therapy:* Massage therapy consists of the application of massage and non–hands-on components, including health promotion and education messages, for self-care and health maintenance; therapy, as well as outcomes, can be influenced by: therapeutic relationships and communication; the therapist's education, skill level, and experience; and the therapeutic setting.
- *Massage therapy practice:* Massage therapy practice is a client-centered framework for providing massage therapy through a process of assessment and evaluation, plan of care, treatment, reassessment and reevaluation, health messages, documentation, and closure in an effort to improve health and/or well-being. Massage therapy practice is influenced by the scope of practice and professional standards.

Once massage has been defined, then what do we call the people who provide massage? The confusion continues. Are we massage professionals, myomassologists, neuromuscular therapists, or soft tissue practitioners? Are we bodyworkers, and is massage a form of bodywork? Are we massage professionals, with other forms of bodywork becoming subcategories of massage? There are hundreds of massage-type methods. The term *bodywork* has been used to cover the scope of the development of various types of hands-on modalities. The ongoing confusion caused by the ambiguity of the difference between massage and bodywork is a major obstacle to the advancement of massage as a profession. Massage is more accurately described as a form of manual therapy (Degenhardt et al., 2023).

The terms *masseuse* (female) and *masseur* (male), although appropriate and respected in other countries, are related to the sex trade in the United States. "Massage parlor" still indicates a front for prostitution. The therapeutic massage community continues to grapple with this unfortunate and incorrect association. Only with ongoing diligence in professional development—both individually and throughout the profession—will massage therapists be able to move beyond this awful association.

Technician? Practitioner? Therapist?

A *technician* is perceived differently from a therapist, particularly in terms of education level. A technician can be defined as one who has expertise in a technical skill or process. A technician has the least training and the most limited scope of practice in a professional group.

The next educational level is the *practitioner.* A practitioner can be defined as one who practices an occupation or a profession. A practitioner operates from a greater knowledge base and within a larger scope of practice than a technician. Another term that could be used is *paraprofessional.*

A *therapist* can be defined as one who treats illness or disability. A therapist requires the highest educational background and has the broadest scope of practice.

The massage community currently does not use these designations as they are defined in this text, but the public and the health care professions often do. What is the public's perception, then, if massage therapist is our title? The terms *massage therapist* and *massage practitioner* are used interchangeably in this text because both are used as identifiers for a massage professional. According to some legislation, those using the term *massage therapy* or equivalent terms need only be licensed. This provides a loophole for unlicensed people to provide massage and charge fees for the service. In these instances, the term *technician* or some other bodywork-based name is used. The term *massage therapist* seems to be emerging as the common descriptor of an educated and licensed professional who accepts the accountability it implies.

HISTORICAL PERSPECTIVES AND THE FUTURE OF MASSAGE

SECTION OBJECTIVES

Chapter objectives covered in this section:

5. Explain the rich heritage and history of therapeutic massage.
6. Explain the influence of historical events and global culture on the current development of therapeutic massage.
7. Self-assess for leadership qualities.

Using the information presented in this section, the student will be able to:

- Trace the general progression of massage from ancient times to today.
- Discuss the trends and potential future of massage theory and relate them to personal career development.

To understand professional, structured, therapeutic touch, the learner must explore historical influences and the evolution of massage from its ancient foundations through projections for the future (Fig. 1.5).

A knowledge of history helps massage therapists develop a sense of professional identity and pride in their profession. Historical perspectives help members of a profession identify the profession's strengths and weaknesses. As learners of massage read historical books about massage, they discover that the fundamental body of knowledge has changed little over the centuries; in fact, the most currently prevalent concepts in massage were written many years ago. Massage has stood the test of time, proving itself a vital, health-enhancing technique and a rehabilitative discipline. Currently, the massage therapy community is at a defining moment; it is growing in acceptance and support based on valid scientific evidence. In the future, beginning massage professionals will learn from our history.

Many people have played important roles in tracing the historic journey of therapeutic massage and bodywork methods. Specific acknowledgment must be given to Richard Van Why, who compiled the Bodywork Knowledgebase, a collection of more than 100 historical books and more than 4000 research and journal articles on therapeutic massage and related methods. Much of the information in this chapter comes from this work. If it were not for van Why's diligence, much of the history of massage would be scattered in research libraries and would be unknown to us today. Fran Tappan, a true expert in massage who wrote respected textbooks, and Patricia J. Benjamin also deserve credit for historical perspectives about massage. Special appreciation is also extended to Judi Calvert for her diligent work in maintaining massage therapy historical records and teaching about the history of massage.

This chapter consolidates historical information about massage. Because the references used overlap extensively, text citation has been kept to a minimum. With gratitude and respect for those who have devoted their lives to compiling this history, both those mentioned and the many more who are not, let us begin the journey by looking to the past.

History of Massage

Certain animal behaviors, such as applying pressure, rubbing, and licking, indicate that massage is used instinctively to relieve pain, to respond to injury, and to comfort. Massage has always been one of the most natural and instinctive means of relieving pain and discomfort. When a person has sore, aching muscles, abdominal pain, a bruise, or a wound, the impulse is to touch and rub that part of the body to obtain relief.

Touch as a method of healing appears to have numerous cultural origins (see Box 1.3). Therapeutic massage has strong roots in Chinese folk medicine, but it also has many aspects in common with other healing traditions, such as Indian herbal medicine and Persian medicine. The art of massage is believed to have been first mentioned in writing around 2000 BC (Tappan and Benjamin, 2004), and it has been discussed extensively in books since about 500 BC. The historical medical literatures of Egypt, Persia, and Japan are full of references to massage. The Greek physician Hippocrates advocated massage and gymnastic exercise. Asclepiades, another eminent Greek physician, relied exclusively on massage in his practice.

Throughout history, many systems and supporting theories for the management of musculoskeletal pain and dysfunction have come and gone. In each case, the scientific thinking of the day provided the validation for massage. Over the years, scientific research has changed the philosophy of massage theory, and current research continues to further define the physical effects of therapeutic massage. Trends today show an increase in the popularity of massage and body-related therapies for stress reduction and chronic musculoskeletal pain.

Ancient Times

According to research reports, most ancient cultures practiced some form of healing touch. Often a ceremonial leader, such as a healer, priest, or shaman, was selected to perform the healing rituals. The healing methods frequently used were herbs, oils, and forms of hydrotherapy. Archaeologists have found many prehistoric artifacts depicting the use of massage for healing and cosmetic purposes. Some speculate that massage used for pain relief incorporated concepts of counterirritation, such as scraping, cutting, and burning of the skin, as part of the process. These methods produce a sensation that masks a distressful sensation, such as pain. Massage may have been used as a cleansing procedure, along with fasting and bathing, in preparation for many tribal rituals.

In China, massage has been known by three names: *anmo* and *amma*, the ancient names, meaning "press-rub," and *tuina*, of more recent origin, meaning "push-pull." These Chinese methods were administered by kneading or rubbing down the entire body with the hands and using gentle pressure and traction on all the joints.

The practice of acupuncture involved the stimulation of specific points along the body, usually done by the insertion of tiny, solid needles, but massage and other forms of pressure also were used. Such practices were also found in indigenous healing practices in which sharp stones were used to scratch the skin's surface. Today, scientists are investigating physiological reasons for the value of these ancient practices.

Knowledge of massage and its applications already was well established in Chinese medicine at the time of the Sui dynasty (AD 589–617). The Japanese came to know massage through the writings of the Chinese. Massage has been a part of life

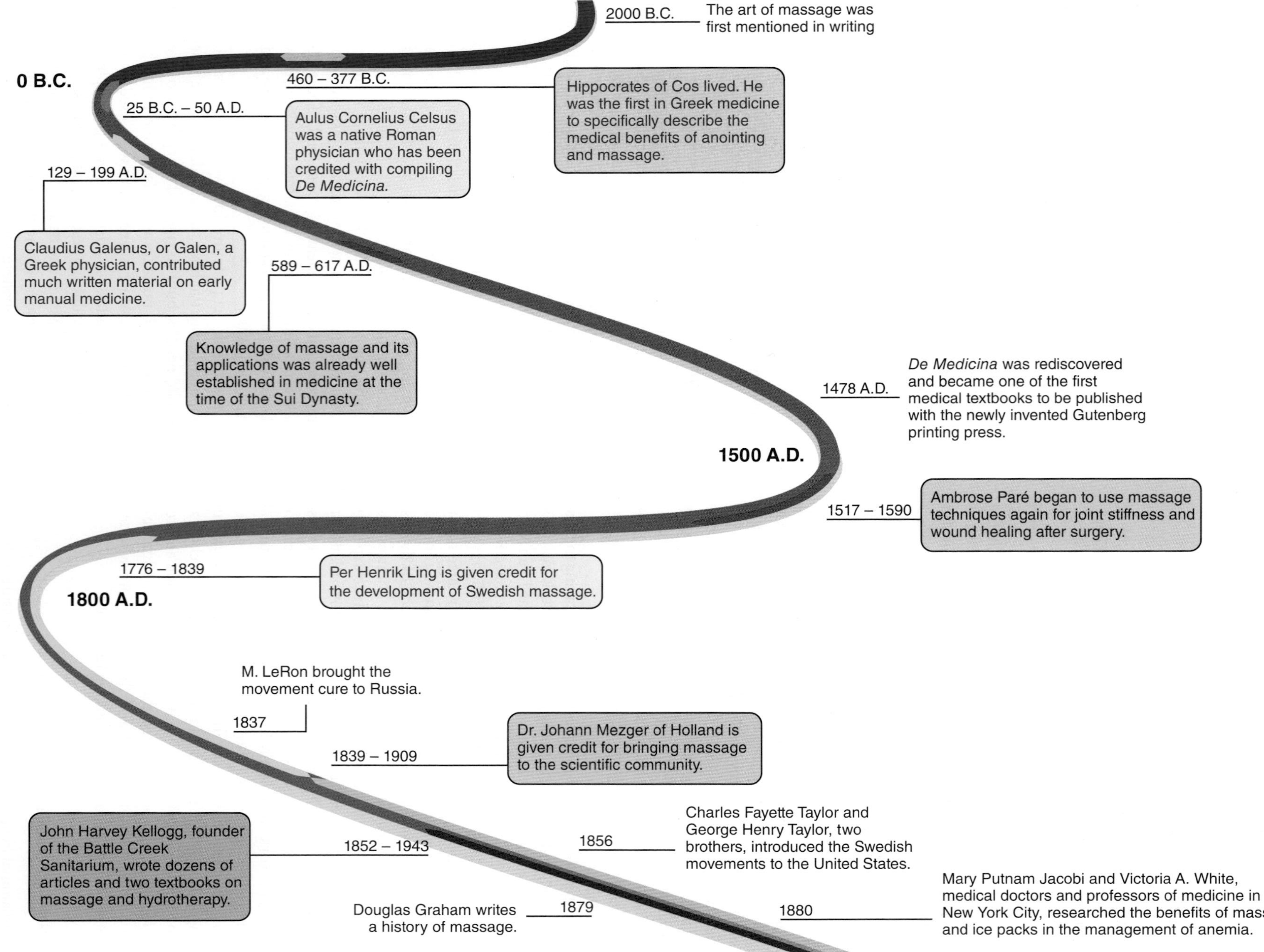
2000 B.C. The art of massage was first mentioned in writing
0 B.C.
460 – 377 B.C.
Hippocrates of Cos lived. He was the first in Greek medicine to specifically describe the medical benefits of anointing and massage.
25 B.C. – 50 A.D.
Aulus Cornelius Celsus was a native Roman physician who has been credited with compiling *De Medicina*.
129 – 199 A.D.
Claudius Galenus, or Galen, a Greek physician, contributed much written material on early manual medicine.
589 – 617 A.D.
Knowledge of massage and its applications was already well established in medicine at the time of the Sui Dynasty.
1478 A.D. *De Medicina* was rediscovered and became one of the first medical textbooks to be published with the newly invented Gutenberg printing press.
1500 A.D.
1517 – 1590
Ambrose Paré began to use massage techniques again for joint stiffness and wound healing after surgery.
1776 – 1839
Per Henrik Ling is given credit for the development of Swedish massage.
1800 A.D.
M. LeRon brought the movement cure to Russia.
1837
1839 – 1909
Dr. Johann Mezger of Holland is given credit for bringing massage to the scientific community.
1852 – 1943
John Harvey Kellogg, founder of the Battle Creek Sanitarium, wrote dozens of articles and two textbooks on massage and hydrotherapy.
1856
Charles Fayette Taylor and George Henry Taylor, two brothers, introduced the Swedish movements to the United States.
Douglas Graham writes a history of massage.
1879
1880
Mary Putnam Jacobi and Victoria A. White, medical doctors and professors of medicine in New York City, researched the benefits of massage and ice packs in the management of anemia.

FIG. 1.5 Historical timeline of massage.

1886 — Charles K. Mills, a prominent neurologist and massage advocate in Philadelphia, levied sharp criticism concerning the uneven quality of lay practitioners of massage.

1894 — The massage scandals are revealed by a commission of inquiry of the British Medical Association in the *British Medical Journal.*

1894 — The Society of Trained Masseuses is formed.

1900 A.D.

early 1900s — Polarity therapy was created by an American physician, Randolph Stone.

1916 — Dr. James B. Mennell divides the effect of massage into two categories: mechanical and reflex actions.

1918 — The polio epidemic renews interest in massage.

1920 — Chartered Society of Massage and Medical Gymnastics is formed.

1920s — Connective tissue massage is developed by Elizabeth Dicke, and *lymph drainage* or *manual lymphatic drainage* is developed by Emil and Estrid Vodder.

1932 — Mary McMillan, a lay practitioner, writes an influential textbook, *Massage and Therapeutic Exercise.*

1934 — Reich settled in the United States and is considered by many to be the founder of psychotherapeutic body techniques.

early 1940s — Licensing for physical therapy begins.

1943 — The American Association of Masseurs and Masseuses was formed.

late 1940s and early 1950s — Cyriax published the first edition of *Textbook of Orthopedic Medicine.*

1950 A.D.

1950s — Francis Tappan and Gertrude Beard write important articles and books on massage techniques.

1956 — Margaret Knott and Dorothy Voss write the book *Proprioceptive Neuromuscular Facilitation.*

1960 — The humanistic movement begins.

1960 — An emphasis on physical fitness by President John F. Kennedy begins interest in sports massage.

1970s — Acupressure receives attention.

late 1980s — The professional organization Associated Bodywork and Massage is formed.

late 1980s — Melzack proposes a theory to explain this endorphin release in the prestigious journal, *Clinics in Anesthesiology*. His theory of hyperstimulation analgesia was the first in recent decades inspired by findings concerning massage.

1991 — The Touch Research Institute is created.

1991 — The National Institute of Health establishes the Office of Alternative Medicine.

1992 — National Certification Examination for Therapeutic Massage and Bodywork is first administered.

1993 — The *New England Journal of Medicine* reports the use of alternative and complementary forms of health care/

1994 — *Alternative Medicine: Expanding Medical Horizons: A report to the National Institutes of Health on Alternative Medical Systems and Practices in the United States* is published.

1990s — David Palmer formalizes the concept of "on-site or chair massage."

1995 to present — The available research information about therapeutic massage continues to increase.

FIG. 1.5, cont'd

Box 1.3 Popular Methods of Massage and Bodywork

This list of massage styles, systems, founders, and developers is not meant to be all inclusive, because the information changes almost daily. Rather, it is meant to show the wide variety of therapeutic massage approaches and how confusing this seemingly endless list can become.

Asian

- Amma, acupressure, shiatsu, jin shin do, do-in, hoshino, tuina, watsu, Tibetan point holding, Thai massage

These methods derive from traditional Chinese medicine concepts, from offshoots of this Chinese base, and from other Asian modalities (e.g., Ayurveda). The efficient use of the therapist's body and the performance of these techniques on a clothed client have many benefits. The effects of compressive manipulations and stretches that focus on specific areas of the body elicit responses in the nervous, circulatory, and muscular systems and affect the energetic flows in the client's body. The philosophy of these systems is grounded in ancient concepts that have stood the test of time.

Structural and Postural Integration

- Bindegewebs massage, Rolfing, Hellerwork, Looyen work, Pfrimmer deep muscle therapy, Soma bodywork, Bowen therapy

These techniques focus more specifically on the connective tissue structure to influence posture and biomechanics. These systematic approaches are effective because they are grounded in the fundamentals of physiology and biomechanics.

Neuromuscular Methods

- Neuromuscular techniques, muscle energy techniques, strain/counterstrain, orthobionomy, Trager, myotherapy, proprioceptive neuromuscular facilitation, reflexology, trigger points

These are the European approaches based on the work of Dr. Stanley Leif and Dr. Boris Chaitow, and the Western methods based on the work of Dr. Janet Travell, Dr. John Mennell, Dr. Raymond Nimmo, Dr. Lawrence Jones, Dr. Milton Trager, Eunice Ingham, William Fitzgerald, Arthur Lincoln Pauls, Bonnie Prudden, and others. Dr. Leon Chaitow wrote extensively on these concepts and taught in the United States and Europe. Many of the techniques are similar to those found in Rolfing, Asian methods, and Swedish/classical massage and exercises. As the name implies, the approach is a nervous or reflexive method. Connective tissue also is affected. Common threads running through all the styles are the basic concepts of activating the tonus receptor mechanism, reflex arc stimulation, positional receptors, and applications of stretching.

Manual Lymphatic Drainage

- Vodder lymphatic drainage

Emil Vodder developed an excellent system that uses the anatomy and physiology of lymphatic movement with both mechanical and reflexive techniques to stimulate the flow of lymphatic fluid. Others have contributed to the understanding of lymphatic drain procedures, including Bruno Chickly and Lyle Lederman. The variations of this system sometimes are called *systemic massage.*

Energetic (Biofield) Methods

- Polarity, therapeutic touch, Reiki, zero balancing

These systems, which are based on ancient concepts of body energy patterns, were recently formalized by Dr. Randolph Stone, Dr. Dolores Krieger, Dr. Fritz Smith, and others. Subtle energy medicine is under study by Dr. Elmer Green at the Menninger Foundation in Topeka, Kansas, and elsewhere by other researchers. Polarity and similar energetic approaches use near touch or light touch to initiate reflexive responses, often with highly effective results. There is controversy about how these methods are integrated into or separate from massage. Some are based in more of a spiritual context.

Craniosacral and Myofascial Methods

- Craniosacral therapy, myofascial release, soft tissue mobilization, deep tissue massage, connective tissue massage

These systems focus more specifically on the various aspects of both mechanical and reflexive connective tissue functions. Dr. William Garner Sutherland was the first to formalize the concept of tiny movement of the cranium and dura. Dr. John Upledger and physical therapist John Barnes have expanded on and formalized his work. Both light and deep touch are used, depending on the method. The cross-fiber friction methods of Dr. James Cyriax fall into this category. In particular, methods that target connective tissue have ongoing research, and currently methods are explored at international fascia congress and meeting symposiums.

Applied Kinesiology

- Touch for health, applied physiology, educational kinesiology, three-in-one concepts

Dr. George Goodheart formalized the system of applied kinesiology within the chiropractic profession. The approach blends many techniques but works primarily with the reflexive mechanisms. A specific muscle testing procedure is used for evaluation; this process acts as somewhat of a biofeedback mechanism. Some of the corrective measures use Asian meridians and acupressure; others rely on the osteopathic reflex mechanisms defined by Chapman, Bennett, and McKenzie that seem to correspond to traditional Chinese acupuncture points. Dr. John Thie and others modified these techniques for use by massage professionals and the public.

Integrated Approaches

- Sports massage, infant massage, equine/animal massage, on-site or seated massage, prenatal massage, geriatric massage, massage for abuse survivors, Russian massage

Many styles of massage that focus on a specific group of people use combinations of methods based on physiological interventions. Founders and teachers of integrated methods include every massage professional who designs a massage specifically for an individual client and every devoted massage instructor who attempts to combine and explain methods to learners.

in India for almost 3000 years. The Chinese introduced the methods in India during trading forays. As has Chinese acupuncture, hatha yoga, which was developed in India, has reappeared in modern forms of body therapy, with its life force energy concepts of prana, chakras, and energy balance.

The ancient Egyptians left artwork showing foot massage. Before Greek athletes took part in the Olympic games, they underwent friction treatment, anointing, and rubbing with sand. The use of touch as a mode of healing is recorded in the writings of the Hebrew and Christian traditions. The "laying on of hands" was particularly prominent in 1st-century Christianity. Massage with oils (anointing) goes back even further in Jewish practices. The ancient Jews practiced anointing for its ritual, hygienic, and therapeutic benefits. The Jewish culture honored rubbing with oils to such an extent that the root word for rubbing with oils and for the Messiah is the same *(ma-shı-ah).*

The ancient Mayan people of Central America, the Incas of South America, and other Indigenous people of the American continents also used methods of joint manipulation and massage.

Hippocrates of Cos (460–377 BC) was the first physician in Greek medicine specifically to describe the medical benefits of anointing and massage, along with the chemical properties of oils used for this purpose. He called his art *anatripsis,* which means "to rub up." Of this art, he said, "The physician must be acquainted with many things and assuredly with anatripsis, for things that have the same name have not always the same effects, for rubbing can bind a joint that is too loose or loosen a joint that is too hard." Hippocrates' methods survived virtually unchanged well into the Middle Ages. Many techniques similar to those methods, especially traction and stretching principles, are still in use today. Claudius Galenus, or Galen, another Greek physician (AD 129–199), contributed a substantial amount of written material on early manual medicine, including many commentaries on Hippocrates' methods (Cantu and Grodin, 2001).

Massage came to the Romans from the Greeks. Julius Caesar (100–44 BC) had himself "pinched all over" daily to relieve his neuralgia and prevent epileptic attacks (Tappan and Benjamin 2004). Aulus Cornelius Celsus (25 BC–AD 50), a Roman physician, has been credited with compiling *De Medicina,* a series of eight books covering the body of medical knowledge of the day. Seven of the books deal extensively with prevention and therapeutics using rubbing, exercise, bathing, and anointing. This work was rediscovered during the late Middle Ages by Pope Nicholas V (1397–1455). In 1478, *De Medicina* was one of the first medical textbooks to be published with the newly invented Gutenberg printing press. It was one of the most popular medical textbooks during the Renaissance.

The Middle Ages

In the Middle Ages, while Europe was mired in superstition and feudal chaos, the Islamic countries became the intellectual center of the world. The *Canon of Medicine* is a 14-volume medical encyclopedia written by Persian scientist and physician Avicenna (Ibn Sina, 981–1037), as he was known in the West. Avicenna's real name was Abu-Ali Husayn Ibn-Abdullah Ibn-Sina. Ibn Sina completed the canon of medicine in 1025. The book was based on a combination of Islamic medicine, the writings of the Roman physician Galen, Chinese materia medica, and many other sources from the time. The canon is considered one of the most famous books in the history of medicine and remained a medical authority up until the 18th and early 19th centuries. Ibn Sina described evidence-based medicine and the importance of research, both of which are important topics in the massage profession today. He is regarded as a pioneer of aromatherapy for his invention of steam distillation and extraction of essential oils (Isham Ismail, 2006; Masic et al., 2008; Afnan, Soheil Muhsin 2009).

Massage developed differently in the East and the West. In the East, as part of the Islamic empire, it represented a continuation of Greco-Roman traditions. In the West, the Greco-Roman traditions disappeared, but massage was kept alive by the common people and became part of folk culture. In this form, massage was an important part of the healing tradition of the Slavs, Finns, and Swedes. Because massage was integrated into the health practices of the common people, it was often associated with supernatural experiences and observances. This association alienated massage from what little scientific approach there was during this time. Practitioners of folk medicine often were persecuted, and the Church claimed that the practitioners' healing powers came from the devil.

Not until the 16th century did massage regain its respectability in Europe. One of the founders of modern surgery, the French physician Ambrose Paré (1517–1590), began to use massage techniques again for joint stiffness and wound healing after surgery. In his work, Paré described three types of massage strokes: gentle, medium, and vigorous. His ideas were passed down to other French physicians who believed in the value of manual therapeutics.

Nineteenth Century

Per Henrik Ling

Per Henrik Ling (1776–1839) often is credited with developing Swedish massage, but he did not invent it. The term *Swedish massage* is inaccurate; the more appropriate name is *classical massage.* Ling proposed an integrated program for the treatment of disease using active and passive movements; he called this program Swedish gymnastic movements. The curriculum of the Royal Central Gymnastic Institute founded by Ling in 1813 did not teach massage as we know it. Legend has it that Ling's interest in these methods was sparked by the gout in his elbow. He developed a system that used many of the positions and movements of Swedish gymnastics, and in so doing, he healed his diseased elbow. Ling's program was based on the newly discovered knowledge of the circulation of the blood and lymph. (Interestingly, the Chinese had been using these methods for centuries.)

In his system, Ling divided movements into active, duplicated, and passive forms. Active movements were performed by the person's own effort; these movements correspond to what commonly is called exercise. Duplicated movements were performed by the person with the cooperation of a gymnast (therapist); they involved active efforts by both parties in which the action of the one was opposed by the action of the other. Duplicated movements correspond to what today is commonly called resistive exercise. Passive movements were performed for the person by the active effort of the gymnast alone. They consisted of passive movements of the extremities, which today we call range-of-motion work and stretching.

Ling taught many physicians from Germany, Austria, Russia, and England, who spread his teachings to their own countries. He was recognized by his contemporaries and later followers not so much as a great innovator but rather as a keen observer who adopted methods only after testing their effectiveness. He combined many techniques into one coherent system. By the time of Ling's death in 1839, his system had achieved worldwide recognition.

Modern Revival of Massage

Per Henrik Ling and others who practiced the Swedish movement cure deserve credit for reviving massage after the Middle Ages. Initially, nonprofessionals spoke to physicians in a language they did not share, which made communication difficult. Dr. Johann Mezger of Holland (1839–1909) is credited with bringing massage to the scientific community. He presented massage to fellow physicians as a form of medical treatment. The French terms *effleurage*, *pétrissage*, and *tapotement* were not used by Ling. Mezger's followers in Holland began to use these names, although historical references do not explain why French terms were chosen. So often history is confusing, and the issue of who deserves credit for what becomes clouded.

As physicians talked to one another about massage, its popularity began to grow. The physicians sought common ground between their methods and massage, both to justify their current view of massage and to expand it. Lay magazines and medical journals published manuscripts on massage. The successful experience and testimony of distinguished people, especially monarchs and diplomats, further bolstered the image of massage and increased public and medical acceptance. Many physicians were drawn to study massage because they had a strong scientific interest in its effects. They conducted animal studies and well-designed clinical trials, which further persuaded physicians of the value of the method and increased the interest of the medical community. The same has held true for massage in this century through studies conducted under grants from the National Institutes of Health (NIH) and other respected entities.

The Swedish movement quickly spread to other European countries. The first institute outside Sweden was established in Denmark. In 1837, two years before Ling's death, his disciple, M. LeRon, brought the movement cure to Russia and established a clinic in St. Petersburg.

Massage in the United States

In the United States, the first waves of European immigration came from northern Europe, which had accepted massage earlier because of its therapeutic benefits. The immigrants produced many great writers and teachers of massage, along with eager, trusting clients.

Two brothers, Charles F. Taylor and George H. Taylor, introduced the Swedish movement system to the United States in 1856. They had learned the skills from Dr. Mathias Roth, an English physician who studied directly with Ling. Roth, also a leader in the homeopathic movement, felt that massage worked on the same principles as homeopathy: the law of similars and the concept of "like cures like."

Dr. John Harvey Kellogg (1852–1943), founder of the Battle Creek Sanitarium in Michigan, wrote dozens of articles and two textbooks on massage and hydrotherapy and edited and published a popular magazine, *Good Health*.

In his 1879 history of massage, Douglas Graham described Lomilomi, a form of massage practiced in Hawaiian culture. He stated that it was used as a hygienic measure to relieve fatigue or was performed simply for the pure pleasure of it. Graham continued to write on massage and its use in almost every area of medicine until his death in the late 1920s.

In 1889, a letter from a physician in Kansas appeared in a New York medical journal. The physician said that he had thought massage was just "a novel method of therapeutics" until he had read a passage from Captain James Cook's diary of his third voyage around the world near the end of the 18th century. Cook had described how his pseudosciatic pain was relieved in an elegant and generous ritual by a Tahitian chief and his family, who used a type of massage method called *romee*. General massage, as the forerunner of wellness-based massage, emerged in the late 1800s as part of a treatment for nervous disorders, which consisted of complete rest, usually combined with a systematic diet, massage, and other health practices, especially at a spa or sanatorium (Benjamin 2015).

Massage as Medical Care

Massage endured even during the challenging time of the late 1800s. Institutes of massage appeared in France, Germany, and Austria by the middle of the 19th century. Between 1854 and 1918, the practice of massage developed from an obscure, unskilled trade to a field of medical health care from which the profession of physical therapy began. Treatments consisted of massage, mineral baths, and exercise.

Dr. David Gurevich, a Russian physician and instructor of Russian medical massage, believed that the long-standing interest in massage and its continuing development are strong proof of its usefulness and necessity. According to Dr. Gurevich, ancient Slavic tribes practiced massage, especially in combination with therapeutic bathing, or hydrotherapy. Beginning in the 18th century, many great Russian scientists and physicians (Mudroff, Manasein, Botkin, Zakharin, and others) contributed to the development of the theory and practice of massage. I.Z. Zabludovski wrote more than 100 books, textbooks, and scientific articles devoted to the methods of massage and its physiological basis in therapy, postsurgical care, and sports.

An institute of massage and exercise was founded in Russia at the end of the 19th century, and many courses in massage also were started. Massage gradually progressed from an auxiliary method of therapy to an independent therapeutic method that was used effectively with other types of treatments (Gurevich, 1992).

Licensing for physical therapy began in the early 1940s. Louise L. Despard's *Text-Book of Massage and Remedial Gymnastics* was one of a handful of textbooks on massage recommended in 1940 as essential reading for all learners of massage by the Massage Round Table of the American Physical Therapy Association.

Mary McMillan, an English lay practitioner of massage, wrote an influential textbook, *Massage and Therapeutic Exercise,* in 1932. She had extensive experience in the field. From 1911 to 1915, she was in charge of massage and therapeutic exercise at the Greenbank Cripples Home in Liverpool, England, and from 1916 to 1918, she served as director of massage and remedial gymnastics at the Children's Hospital in Portland, Maine. During World War I, she served in the military as a rehabilitation aide (Tappan and Benjamin, 2004).

Frances Tappan's outstanding contributions to massage and physical therapy are formalized in her textbook, *Healing Massage Techniques*. Sister Kenny used massage in the treatment of polio. Ida Rolf's massage system grew to become the technique of Rolfing. Dr. Dolores Krieger has made major contributions to energetic approaches through her system of therapeutic touch.

Twentieth Century

1900 to 1960

In the early 1900s, Dr. Randolph Stone, an American physician, devised polarity therapy. Stone studied many body systems, both ancient and modern, including acupuncture, hatha yoga, osteopathy, chiropractic techniques, and reflexology. From his investigations, he concluded that magnetic fields regulated and directed the physiological systems of the body. Influenced by Eastern philosophy and medicine, Stone believed that all aspects of the universe were expressed in opposite poles (e.g., male and female, positive and negative electrical charges); therefore he called his therapeutic method polarity.

In 1907, Edgar F. Cyriax began a distinguished publishing career that spanned almost 40 years. He was the last great proponent of Ling's Swedish movement cure, which Cyriax called mechanotherapeutics.

A textbook published in 1900 by Albert Hoffa and revised in 1913 by Max Bohm describes the more classic massage techniques, such as effleurage, pétrissage, tapotement, and vibration. Most therapists still learn these methods as standard massage techniques in entry-level programs.

The polio epidemic of 1918 sparked a more widespread interest in massage because victims and their families were desperate for any helpful remedy. Research on the benefits of massage in preventing the complications of paralysis began at this time.

Connective tissue massage (CTM) as a specific system was developed in the 1920s by German physiotherapist Elizabeth Dicke, whose work was later expanded on by Maria Ebner. CTM was first used because Dicke herself suffered from a prolonged illness caused by an impairment of the circulation in her right leg. As with Ling, her search for self-healing added much to the development of massage.

During this time, Emil Vodder, a Danish physiologist, and his wife, Estrid, developed a technique of light massage along the course of the surface lymphatics; they called the technique lymph drainage or manual lymphatic drainage. This technique was and still is used to treat chronic lymphedema and other diseases of the lymphatic and peripheral vascular systems.

The American Association of Masseurs and Masseuses was formed in Chicago in 1943 and subsequently was renamed the American Massage Therapy Association (AMTA). Another professional organization, the International Myomassetics Federation, was formed later through the efforts of Irene Gauthier, a notable massage instructor, and others.

James H. Cyriax, the son of Edgar Cyriax, became an orthopedic surgeon at St. Thomas Hospital, a prestigious teaching institution in London. The younger Cyriax gained fame through his development of transverse friction massage. In the late 1940s and early 1950s, he published the first edition of his now classic *Textbook of Orthopedic Medicine*. His work is especially significant in the area of massage because it recognized, categorized, and provided differential diagnoses for pathological conditions of the body's soft tissues. The concept that dysfunction of soft tissues, including periarticular connective tissue, can be a source of nociceptive signaling in the nervous system is a working theory of soft tissue manipulation today. Cyriax also was the first to introduce the concept of end feel in the diagnosis of soft tissue lesions.

Dr. Herman Kabat researched neuromuscular concepts based on the work of neurophysiologists and Pavlov's conditioning of reflexes. The Sherrington law of successive induction provided the foundation for the development of rhythmic stabilization and slow reversal techniques. By 1951, research had begun on a new method, which was formalized in 1956 in the book *Proprioceptive Neuromuscular Facilitation*, written by Margaret Knott and Dorothy Voss.

Frances Tappan and Gertrude Beard also authored important articles and books on massage techniques during the 1950s. Their texts are still available, and serious learners of massage can benefit from reading these classic works. Frances Tappan influenced the profession of massage through interviews, conferences on the future of massage, and consultation with many leaders in the field.

1960 to the Present: The Most Recent Revival of Massage

The most recent revival of massage began around 1960 and has continued to this day. Recognition of chronic diseases that are resistant to surgical or drug treatment has increased. Neither the acute care concept nor a single-solution approach seems to work with these cases. A more complex way of envisioning and treating these diseases has had to be developed, and massage is one approach that has proven effective over time.

The humanistic movement that began during the 1960s spilled over into medicine and allied health. Concerns about "bedside manner," "genuineness," and the benefits of touch again raised the issue of the legitimacy and value of massage for its nurturing effect alone. Later, the Esalen movement and Gestalt psychology inspired psychologists and psychotherapists to explore massage and other movement therapies. Many controlled clinical studies in medicine, nursing, physical therapy, and psychology inspired more academic and clinical interest in massage.

In 1960, increased medical awareness that lack of exercise contributed to cardiovascular disease and other disorders prompted President John F. Kennedy to emphasize physical fitness, especially for children. This new interest grew into the physical fitness movement of the late 1960s and led the health sciences into a movement toward preventive medicine. The benefits of sports were rediscovered, as a result, historic literature in the field of massage was brought to light, such as Albert Baumgartner's book, *Massage in Athletics*, which discussed the relationship between massage and exercise and the value of massage in conditioning and stress control.

Acupressure received more attention than any other bodywork method during the 1970s and 1980s. Contemporary medical, physical therapy, and nursing literature examined it closely on the basis of controlled clinical trials. Through writings on nursing and rehabilitative medicine, a body of knowledge emerged on the benefits of massage in preventing and treating decubitus ulcers and in the overall management of heart rate and blood pressure in people suffering from acute and chronic manifestations of cardiovascular disease.

The fields of pain research and pain management supported more research. Ronald Melzack, a professor of psychology in the anesthesiology department of McGill University Medical School and one of the initial proponents of the gate control theory of pain, published the results of several controlled clinical trials on the value of ice massage and manual massage for the relief of dental pain and low back pain. Melzack found these techniques effective in preventing or reducing pain, and he proposed a theory for the neural mechanisms by which they operated. In the late 1980s, in the prestigious journal *Clinics in Anesthesiology*, Melzack proposed a theory of hyperstimulation analgesia, which was the first in recent decades inspired by findings concerning massage. The theory argues that certain intense sensory stimuli, such as puncture with a needle or exposure to extreme cold or pressure when applied near the site of an injury, sends a signal to the brain through a faster channel than that used by the pain signal it was attempting to treat, thereby disrupting the pain (van Why, 1992). Over the years, Melzack has expanded this pain theory. In 2004, in a lecture presented at the World Congress of the World Institute of Pain, Melzack (2005) presented the topic, "Evolution of the Neuromatrix Theory of Pain":

The neuromatrix theory of pain proposes that pain is a multidimensional experience produced by characteristic "neurosignature" patterns of nerve impulses generated by a widely distributed neural network—the "body-self neuromatrix"—in the brain. These neurosignature patterns may be triggered by sensory inputs, but they may also be generated independently of them. Acute pains evoked by brief noxious inputs have been meticulously investigated by neuroscientists, and their sensory transmission mechanisms are generally well understood. In contrast, chronic pain syndromes, which are often characterized by severe pain associated with little or no discernible injury or pathology, remain a mystery. Furthermore, chronic psychological or physical stress is often associated with chronic pain, but the relationship is poorly understood. The neuromatrix theory of pain provides a new conceptual framework to examine these problems. It proposes that the output patterns of the body-self neuromatrix activate perceptual, homeostatic, and behavioral programs after injury, pathology, or chronic stress. Pain, then, is produced by the output of a widely distributed neural network in the brain rather than directly by sensory input evoked by injury, inflammation, or other pathology. The neuromatrix—genetically determined and modified by sensory experience—is the primary mechanism that generates the neural pattern that produces pain. Its output pattern is determined by multiple influences, of which the somatic sensory input is only a part, which converges on the neuromatrix.

Lorimer Moseley, a clinical and research physiotherapist from Australia, has developed theories relating to chronic pain based on the neuromatrix approach. According to Moseley, pain is a multisystem output that is produced when an individual-specific cortical pain neuromatrix is activated. Pain is an output of the brain that is produced whenever the brain concludes that body tissue is in danger and action is required. When pain becomes chronic, less input (both nociceptive and non-nociceptive) is required to produce pain (Moseley, 2003). Pain research is ongoing, and massage therapy is an effective intervention for many types of chronic/persistent pain.

In 1988, the AMTA spearheaded a proposal for the development of a national certification process. The proposal stirred up much controversy and was hotly debated. With the participation of other professional massage and bodywork sources, the National Certification Examination for Therapeutic Massage and Bodywork was devised in 1992. In 2014, the National Certification Board for Therapeutic Massage and Bodywork discontinued the National Certification Examination and credential and upgraded to the Board Certified credential, which reflects commitment to excellence beyond licensure.

In the late 1980s, the professional organization Associated Bodywork and Massage Professionals was formed to serve the needs of a growing and diverse group of bodywork therapists.

The 1990s saw a significant shift in the massage profession, and the groundwork was laid for the major events that influence massage practice today.

RECENT EVENTS AND CURRENT PROFESSIONAL TRENDS: 1990 TO NOW

Before 1985, massage professionals worked primarily in independent settings with little or no supervision. The best of this situation was the freedom to serve clients' needs without the constraints of regulation. The worst was the lack of consistent training and the confusion among other professionals and the public about what constituted therapeutic massage.

Frustration with massage parlor and sex trade regulations enacted to control prostitution and the desire of many massage professionals to enter the mainstream of public awareness pushed the massage therapy profession to begin seeking an alliance with the existing medical care structure to justify the validity of massage. In some instances, this movement into the existing health care world created turf battles over which profession would provide massage therapy. Both legitimate and reactionary questions and concerns were expressed by the physical therapy and nursing professions.

The public's desire for physical fitness had reached its peak during this time, and the concept of "sports massage" provided an avenue for mainstreaming massage therapy. During the 1990s, the mainstream approach shifted from sports to corporate America. David Palmer can be given credit for formalizing the concepts of on-site and chair massage. These two trends allowed the public to see massage in a way much different from the preconceived notions of a "feel good" luxury of the wealthy or a front for prostitution.

As research continues to validate massage therapy and as massage evolves into a distinct professional course requiring a credible, standardized education, the turf battles in the health care system seem to be quieting down. Health care is moving in the direction of multidisciplinary teams in which many different professionals work together. As this process continues, nurses and physical therapists probably will find themselves supervising massage paraprofessionals and working as partners with more comprehensively trained massage therapists who have earned a degree.

In 1990, the AMTA established the Massage Therapy Foundation and its mission, which is to bring the benefits of massage therapy to the broadest spectrum of society through the generation, dissemination, and application of knowledge in this field. The foundation is now a dynamic independent organization. Current trends indicate that research will be the most important process for the future of the massage profession, and the Massage Therapy Foundation is positioned to be an ongoing leader in the massage profession.

In 1991, the Touch Research Institute at the University of Miami opened under the direction of Dr. Tiffany Field. More than any other single development in the 1990s, the research produced by the institute has moved massage into the mainstream as an accepted health care practice.

Also in 1991, the NIH established the Office of Alternative Medicine. Two years later, the *New England Journal of Medicine* reported on a national survey on the use of alternative and complementary forms of health care. Massage was the third-most-used treatment. In line with this trend, in 1994 the NIH published the report *Alternative Medicine: Expanding Medical Horizons. A Report to the National Institutes of Health on Alternative Medical Systems and Practices in the United States.*

The credibility and acceptance of natural approaches to health and illness are developing, and knowledge bases are beginning to overlap. Three areas in osteopathic medicine that currently apply to massage are muscle energy techniques, positional release and strain/counterstrain techniques, and neuromuscular techniques. Dr. Leon Chaitow, who died in 2018, was the most noteworthy educator and author of these methods. Like Ling, Chaitow was an expert synthesizer of the best of many concepts. He developed a strong foundation in manual medicine working as an assistant to his uncle, Dr. Boris Chaitow, the co-developer of neuromuscular technique, along with his cousin, the legendary Dr. Stanley Lief (Chaitow, 1988). Dr. Leon Chaitow has authored many books that have enriched the body of knowledge of soft tissue methods, including therapeutic massage.

Other authors and professionals worthy of mention include Ida Rolf, developer of the Rolfing system; Dr. Milton Trager, developer of Trager; and Dr. Janet Travell, coauthor with David Simons of the most comprehensive texts written on the subject of trigger points. (Travell and Simons are the authors of the two-volume text *Myofascial Pain and Dysfunction: The Trigger Point Manual.*)

Research continued to validate the benefits of massage through the 1990s. After years of struggle for acceptance and validation, massage moved into the mainstream in the mid-1990s. Since 1995, the amount of information available on therapeutic massage has increased dramatically. Many new books are on the market, and websites for therapeutic massage have been created on the Internet. As a result of advances in technology, massage education now can be provided through a variety of formats. In the late 1990s, concern related to quality massage therapy education resulted in the formation of the Commission on Massage Therapy Accreditation (COMTA) to accredit both educational institutions and programs offering instruction in massage therapy and bodywork. In 2002, COMTA was recognized by the US Department of Education as a specialized accrediting agency.

In 2007, a historical research event occurred that changed our understanding of how massage supports beneficial change. The International Fascia Research Congress was held at Harvard University. The congress was conceived and organized by a multidisciplinary committee of science researchers and practicing health care professionals who share a common focus on and interest in the human body's soft connective tissue matrix. The congress meets every 2 years.

Also in 2007, the massage therapy professional community began to explore the possibility that the profession's leadership organizations might work together to develop a consensus on a defined terminology and scope of practice issues. The leadership group included representatives of six organizations: the AMTA, the ABMP, the FSMTB, the MTF, the NCBTMB, COMTA, and, a bit later, the AFMTE. The AFMTE is a nonprofit organization established to serve as an independent voice, advocate, and resource for the entire education sector from entry-level massage training programs through post-graduate studies. These six organizations work together as the Coalition of National Massage Therapy Organizations, which established the ELAP study and published its findings. The goals of ELAP were to define the knowledge and skill components of entry-level education and recommend the minimum number of hours schools should teach to prepare graduates for safe and competent practice in the massage profession. Completed in December 2013, the project published two documents that describe ELAP workgroup findings and recommendations: "The Core: Entry-Level Analysis Project Report (Final Report)" and "The Core: Entry-Level Massage Education Blueprint (the Blueprint)." These documents are available to download at elapmassage.org.

The ELAP information is important to massage therapy learners. The education for entry-level massage therapy learners should follow ELAP guidelines. The FSMTB incorporated the ELAP-recommended 625 contact hours as the minimum requirement for program length as part of the Model Practice Act for licensing massage therapists. The Model Practice Act has gained little traction in the United States but still functions as a guide for regulations development.

Other countries are involved in advancing the massage therapy profession. Canada has expanded education requirements for Registered Massage Therapists. Each province has different requirements for practicing massage therapy in its jurisdiction. The provincial associations affiliated with the Massage Therapy Alliance of Canada (MTAC), in addition to European countries, are working toward expanded training and support the development of massage therapy competencies and national accreditation of massage therapy education programs (http://www.massagetherapycanada.com/).

Massage therapy organizations in the United Kingdom, Australia, and New Zealand also embrace a consistent and uniform level of ethical, professional, and quality standards, and work continues to support professionalism in education and practice. The Complementary and Natural Healthcare Council (CNHC) is the regulatory body for massage therapies and other complementary therapies in the United Kingdom. Registration is a voluntary system, supported by the Department of Health. In Australia, national competency standards were introduced for massage therapy in 2002 as part of the Health Training Package. These qualifications sit within the Australian Qualifications Framework (AQF), the national system of qualifications encompassing higher education, vocational education and training, and schools.

Licensure and Board Certification

Most US states now license massage therapists. The FSMTB supports its member boards in their work to ensure that the practice of massage therapy is provided to the public safely and effectively by guaranteeing the provision of a valid, reliable licensing examination to determine entry-level competence. Educational requirements set through state licensure average 500–1000 clock hours. ELAP determined that 625 hours of education is the minimum time necessary to train competent entry-level massage professionals. How the FSMTB will encourage individual states to change from current licensing practices to adopt the Model Practice Act remains to be seen. Legislative initiatives and changes move slowly.

Now that there is a level of agreement about entry-level education for massage practice in the United States, the massage community is turning its attention to the validation of advanced massage therapy practice. Schools of massage therapy have begun to work with colleges and universities to develop articulation agreements that allow graduates of their programs to complete degrees in massage. The first of these articulation agreements was reached in 1995 between the Health Enrichment Center in Lapeer, Michigan, and Siena Heights University in Adrian, Michigan, to grant both associate and bachelor's degrees in applied science in massage therapy. Some private massage schools have increased their educational requirements to enable them to grant associate's degrees. More community colleges are developing certificate programs in therapeutic massage, and some of these programs can lead to an associate's degree in applied or general science. Board certification, offered by the NCBTMB, was launched on January 1, 2013. Therapists achieving this credential will have the proper foundation to better serve clients and demonstrate a commitment to raising the standards of the profession, which have remained stagnant for the past 20 years. As in other professions, board certification will be an additional differentiator to advance a massage career.

An important development is the availability of a bachelor's degree in massage therapy from Siena Heights University, the same university that has supported massage therapy since 1995 through articulation agreements with individual massage therapy schools. Announced in 2014 in a progressive initiative, the university will accept board certification from the NCBTMB for college credit.

As the future unfolds, committed researchers and those who apply the research to the practicalities faced by massage therapy practitioners will probably become the driving force for the advancement of massage therapy.

As mentioned, the Alliance for Massage Therapy Education (AFMTE) was established in 2010. This organization brings together directors and administrators from massage therapy schools, along with massage school teachers and those who provide continuing education seminars and advanced training in the field. All are committed to the advancement of quality education. The major contribution of the Alliance is the development of teaching standards for massage therapy educators and teacher certification. With the AFMTE supporting quality in education and the MTF supporting research, the two working together will ensure that massage therapy follows the path of excellence into the future.

In 2016, these research articles were published by Crawford and colleagues (see the References list for the full citations):

- The Impact of Massage Therapy on Function in Pain Populations: A Systematic Review and Meta-Analysis of Randomized Controlled Trials. Part I, Patients Experiencing Pain in the General Population. https://doi.org/10.1093/pm/pnw099.
- The Impact of Massage Therapy on Function in Pain Populations: A Systematic Review and Meta-Analysis of Randomized Controlled Trials. Part II, Cancer Pain Populations. https://doi.org/10.1093/pm/pnw100.
- The Impact of Massage Therapy on Function in Pain Populations: A Systematic Review and Meta-Analysis of Randomized Controlled Trials. Part III, Surgical Pain Populations. https://doi.org/10.1093/pm/pnw101.

This research supports the use of massage therapy and a nonpharmaceutical intervention for pain management. The release of these papers coincided with the recognition of problems in prescribing opiate-based medications and the resultant US opioid epidemic.

The search for alternate treatments for pain has brought awareness of massage therapy forward. For more information on the opioid crisis, explore the US Department of Health and Human Services website (https://www.hhs.gov/) using the search term *opioid epidemic*.

Advances in Licensing Portability

The Council of State Governments partnered with the Department of Defense and the Federation of State Massage Therapy Boards to support the mobility of licensed massage therapists through the development of an interstate compact. IMpact is the interstate occupational licensure compact for massage therapy. If states enact legislation, IMpact will enable licensed massage therapists to practice in all states that join the compact, rather than get an individual license in every state in which they want to practice. Each compact member state agrees to mutually recognize the practitioner licenses issued by every other state in the Massage Therapy Compact. In 2023, the Interstate Massage Compact was finalized and made available for enactment by individual states.

The COVID-19 Pandemic

The COVID-19 pandemic significantly affected the massage therapy community. The World Health Organization (WHO) declared the outbreak a pandemic on March 11, 2020. The effects of the pandemic affected nearly all aspects of society. Governments responded to the pandemic with a range of strategies, including forced quarantines and nationwide lockdowns. The professional identity of massage therapists was challenged when predominately classified as nonessential health care providers during the COVID-19 pandemic (Fogarty et al., 2022). Many jurisdictions completely closed massage therapy unless under the order of a medical doctor, osteopath, or chiropractor (Tague et al., 2021). Public notices on practice closures were classified using the offensive term “massage parlor” based on the North American Industry Classification System (NAICS). NAICS is the standard used by federal statistical agencies to classify business establishments and to collect, analyze, and publish statistical data related to the US business economy. Activism from the massage therapy community resulted in significant changes. NAICS updates, which took effect on January 1, 2022, eliminated the references to massage parlors, replaced the terminology with massage wellness spas/centers, and stated that massage therapy provided as an integrative health therapy should remain included under the large umbrella of “other” health practitioners.

Pandemic lockdowns affected massage therapy education. Entry-level massage therapy schools scrambled to shift education to remote delivery using technology platforms. An upside of this is the understanding that portions of the massage therapy curriculum can be provided electronically which will influence future educational delivery. Educational mandates included in legislation will need to be revised to support this development.

Diversity, Equity, and Inclusion

Emerging as a prominent issue is the need to examine diversity, equity, and inclusion within the massage therapy profession. Diversity includes all the ways in which individuals or groups of people differ from one another. Equity is the fair treatment of all. Inclusion is the act of creating environments in which any individual or group can be and feel welcomed, respected, supported, and valued to fully participate. The diversity of the massage therapy profession and those who seek massage therapy treatment are not topics that are often discussed. The massage therapy community must work together to address these inequities, striving to identify and eliminate barriers that have prevented the full participation of marginalized groups (Balogun & Kennedy, 2020).

Career Options

The career pathway in massage therapy is shifting from self-employment at the entry level to finding employment as a massage therapist. Shifting from employment to self-employed may occur after practicing for a few years. Massage therapy as a career is unique because massage therapists have autonomy in professional practice and can provide massage therapy services in a variety of settings. **Professional autonomy** means having the authority to make decisions and the freedom to act in accordance with one’s professional knowledge base. Autonomy means the ability to practice massage therapy independently, without physician oversight, especially in the wellness and health promotion sector. It is important that massage therapists be recognized as contributors to care in the medical setting without losing their ability to practice independently. Some health care insurance plans and managed care systems are beginning to look at ways to include massage therapy in their covered services. Sports massage for amateur and professional athletes is becoming the norm, with massage therapists working side by side with athletic trainers and coaches.

In the wellness and health promotions sector, spas, franchises, and wellness centers are bringing awareness of massage therapy to the general public. The various franchised entities and spa industries are among the fastest-growing employers of massage professionals.

As the world becomes a global community, the ever-increasing exchange of information will enrich the knowledge base of therapeutic massage. Research has shown that various massage and bodywork methods are more alike than different. A shift has occurred from the confusing proliferation of massage and bodywork styles to an understanding of massage application provided to achieve outcomes such as stress and pain management, increased mobility, and enhanced performance.

The abundant massage and bodywork methods will likely continue to combine into a consolidated system of therapeutic massage without losing the rich diversity of professional expression. Terminology and education are becoming increasingly standardized, yet we have maintained the integrity of the individual applications of massage and bodywork. For those now entering the field of massage therapy, success depends not on how many distinctive styles of massage you know but on your commitment to critical thinking, understanding the nature of human connection, and practicing until perfected the skilled application of the fundamental aspects of massage. The pressure to learn many ways to perform massage will evolve into skilled massage application based on evidence-informed professional practice. The move from opinion and experience-based practice to the more objective evidence-informed practice of massage is an ongoing theme in this text.

Two tracks of massage service likely will continue to standardize: wellness and health massage practices outside the medical care system, and medical/clinical massage practice within the medical care system. Although similar, these trends allow a vast diversity in the types of services available. Critical-thinking skills, research literacy, experience, and empathy are the markers of career success.

Massage therapy is a female-dominated occupation. This trend remains steady. As gender becomes less of an issue in our society and people primarily seek quality services, this may begin to shift. People begin their massage careers at a variety of life stages. As a first career, many recent high school graduates are seeking vocational skills and are attracted to massage therapy. The entry point at a certificate/diploma level and education in a year or less allows the education to be affordable and attainable. Some in this demographic use massage therapy as a jumping point to other health occupations and professions. As more full-time practice becomes common, these individuals may find that massage therapy can be a lifetime career. In early and middle adulthood, part-time practice and supplemental income are attractive to those who are managing multiple life demands and want to be involved in the health services field. There exists a growing trend of people in their 50s and 60s becoming massage therapists as a career change instead of retirement, or as a way to be involved in a helping occupation to fulfill work satisfaction needs and augment income. These individuals often work well into their later years, taking advantage of the flexible schedules and ability to work part time.

Some questions must be answered if we are to continue moving forward. For example:

- Will we be willing to accept research findings and let go of myths and misinformation about massage?
- Will we learn to use critical-thinking skills to develop outcome-based massage sessions to achieve client goals?
- Will we learn to collaborate with other professionals in multidisciplinary teams?
- Will we agree on terminology about massage so that we can communicate with each other?
- Will we let go of the differences that divide us and reach for the similarities that bring us together?
- Will we commit to expertise through educational excellence, professional practice, and ethical behavior?
- Will we demand that educators and professional organizations be current, proficient, and committed to training future generations of massage therapists?
- Will we respect our history, understand our traditions, and strive to bring those values into the future?

The Future

The future is bright and promising, especially if we pay attention to our past and remember the words and wisdom of an old Russian physician: "Massage is massage." We ourselves constitute one of the biggest threats to the future of massage. The profession currently remains fragmented and educational standards are inconsistent; however, the pieces are finally in place for unification. All bodywork professions must come together to work for the common good. As the massage profession moves forward and reclaims its heritage as an important health service, it is important to look back so that we can see the strengths and weaknesses of the professional journey.

Honoring those who have dedicated so much of their lives to developing the body of knowledge of therapeutic massage is also important. Many today are dedicating a significant part of their lives to the professional advancement of therapeutic massage. Patricia Benjamin, PhD, captured the history of massage in her 2015 book, *The Emergence of the Massage Therapy Profession in North America.* When the history of massage is written in the future, these names will appear with the information they have organized and contributed. We are all contributors to the future of massage, and we all will become part of its history (Proficiency Exercise 1.3).

PROFICIENCY EXERCISE **1.3**

In the space provided, answer these questions:

1. What do you want the future of massage to bring?
2. How are you going to assist in the development of that future?

MENTORING TIP

Massage therapy can be an autonomous health service. Benefits of massage support health and wellness and can manage many conditions that diminish well-being, such as stress, pain, and limits in physical function. Massage therapy supports a healthy lifestyle that includes moderate exercise and restorative sleep. Therapeutic massage achieves the best results through maintenance and prevention support for regular clients. This type of practice is based on a range of outcomes and categories of care, primarily palliative care, and condition management. Therapeutic change (i.e., "fix it") is rare. The education required for autonomous practice needs to be rigorous, especially in safety and the need for referral. Study related to pathology is not intended to enable the massage therapist to fix or cure a condition but rather to recognize, adapt, and refer. This is a huge accountability issue. In a medical environment, other medical professionals are involved and are primarily responsible for diagnosis, oversight, and recommendation for massage care. There is a built-in support structure. *Not so* in an autonomous practice. We are accountable. Our assessment, including history taking and documentation, must be impeccable. Critical-thinking skills are necessary.

Massage therapy also has a support role managing the same type of conditions within a medical environment. Medical intervention can expand into prevention, especially with physiological monitoring and early detection. However, most medical intervention is pathology based. When pathology is detected, medical intervention is important and will have a better outcome if health and well-being are supported during medical treatment. In this role, massage therapy is integrated as supportive care and supervised either in the medical environment or by communication with the medical care team. This is not autonomous practice. There is an increased knowledge component in the medical environment but not necessarily related to specific massage application. It is important to be able to provide massage adapted to a more complex and fragile client.

In addition, massage therapists will need to understand the implications of massage based on a variety of medical interventions such as medication, surgery, rehabilitation, and mental health counseling. Health maintenance and promotion to support well-being can play just as important a part in the long-term plan for a client who has a complex health status but no longer requires active medical intervention.

Massage therapists also will have much to learn when adapting to a medical environment. For example, they will have to understand infection control, the strict privacy requirements of the Health Insurance Portability and Accountability Act (HIPAA), how to use different types of equipment, and so on.

LEADERSHIP

Leaders guide progress toward the future. Think about the people who have influenced or motivated you to make major decisions. They were leaders because they caused you to act. How did they influence you? Was it by example? Did they share their experiences of failure and success? Did others talk about them? Did you read their biographies or autobiographies?

Leaders in the therapeutic massage profession must be able to motivate themselves and others to pursue excellence. They must also be forward thinkers, not only by paying attention to the historical past and the current moment but also by projecting into the future and preparing for it now. As massage therapy continues to expand into multiple environments such as sports and fitness facilities, chiropractic offices, multidisciplinary health care practices, wellness centers, massage franchises, and the spa industry, it will be increasingly important for massage therapists to develop leadership skills to support the changes in the profession that inevitably will occur.

Leadership involves influencing others for good, rousing others to action, and inspiring them to become the best they can be, as a group works together toward a common goal. Numerous elements build effective leadership. For example:

- Trust promotes good relationships and confidence.
- A willingness to understand change and recognize that disruptions are inevitable is crucial.
- The ability to shift gears paves the way for change.
- Humility is a focus on being open, teachable, and flexible.
- Commitment seeks to develop vision and values in a leader and moves leaders to stand for something greater.
- Focus gives leaders the ability to achieve and direct their time and energy to important goals and objectives.
- Compassion is the desire to understand and care for others, such as staff, family, clients, or community.
- Integrity demands that leaders be responsible for seeking to create quality assurance in their service for clients, as well as in all their relationships.
- Peacemaking leaders bring calmness by listening, learning from others, and seeking good solutions rather than making quick decisions.
- Endurance refers to courage, perseverance, and strength when situations, people, or an environment become chaotic or difficult.

Do you have the desire and motivation to become a leader? This is an important question. Real leadership is a gift given to the present and the future. To be a leader, you must first know how to follow. You also need to be willing to work behind the scenes without expecting credit or status for your efforts. How might you develop the leadership qualities of trust, willingness, humility, commitment, focus, compassion, integrity, peacemaking, and endurance? The individuals discussed in the history of massage were and still are leaders. Who are the leaders in the massage community now? What are they doing to support your future as a massage therapist? Will you become a leader in the future?

MENTORING TIP

Status Recognition, Professional Position

Because therapeutic massage education is vocational and career focus is occupational, some in the massage field are concerned about our status as health professionals. Status does not relate to where or to whom you provide massage. There is no more status designation for a massage therapist working in a medical setting than for a massage therapist working in a spa, massage franchise, or wellness center. There is no more status in working with sick clients than with well clients. There is no more status in working with celebrities than in working with blue-collar workers.

Achieved status is acquired and earned based on merit and the value of your contribution. Those who have achieved status can be valuable teachers and mentors. Respect is important for those who have contributed to the understanding and advancement of massage therapy practice. Unfortunately, status often is measured externally based on education, income, and occupation rather than commitment, contribution, and compassion. Respect and status will come to you as a massage therapist when you earn it through professional and ethical behavior, study, commitment, compassion, work, and experience.

MASSAGE THERAPY PRACTICE FRAMEWORK

SECTION OBJECTIVES

Chapter objective covered in this section:

8. Analyze a professional practice framework.

Using the information presented in this section, the student will be able to:

- Define massage, massage therapy, and massage therapy practice.
- List the seven components of a client-centered massage therapy practice framework.
- Explain the steps involved in implementing the massage therapy practice framework in professional practice.

In 2010, the Massage Therapy Foundation's Best Practices Committee held a 2-day symposium during which the participants' discussion focused more on the processes of massage therapy than on specific conditions. Three overarching themes were identified during the symposium discussions:

1. How massage should be defined
2. The multidimensional nature of massage therapy
3. The factors that influence massage therapy practice

Recall these definitions, which were presented earlier:

- *Massage:* Massage is a patterned and purposeful soft tissue manipulation accomplished by the use of digits, hands, forearms, elbows, knees, and/or feet, with or without the use of emollients, liniments, heat and cold, hand-held tools, or other external apparatus, for the intent of therapeutic change.
- *Massage therapy:* Massage therapy consists of the application of massage and non–hands-on components, including health promotion and education messages, for self-care and health maintenance; therapy, as well as outcomes, can be influenced by: therapeutic relationships and communication; the therapist's education, skill level, and experience; and the therapeutic setting.
- *Massage therapy practice:* Massage therapy practice is a client-centered framework for providing massage therapy

through a process of assessment and evaluation, plan of care, treatment, reassessment and reevaluation, health messages, documentation, and closure in an effort to improve health and/or well-being. Massage therapy practice is influenced by the scope of practice and professional standards and ethics.

The influence of the researchers who worked to produce these definitions will extend beyond this text, and this author is especially grateful for their diligence, ongoing work, and support of therapeutic massage. A special thanks is due to Ann Blair Kennedy for her leadership and guidance as we move toward the future of massage therapy practice (Kennedy et al., 2016a and b).

The Framework

A conceptual model can help you visualize the concepts and processes, especially at the beginning of your studies. This practice framework can be applied (Fig. 1.6); however, keep in mind that an individual massage therapy session or a series of sessions is intended to be flexible and adaptive. This textbook (plus science studies) covers the content needed to implement this practice framework. The content is integrated throughout the entire book. The framework is client centered and moves through the steps of assessment and evaluation, plan of care, treatment, reassessment and reevaluation, health messages, document/charting, and closure. The process is influenced by the massage therapy scope of practice and professional standards and ethics (see Chapter 2).

Client-Centered Practice

Massage therapy practice should be client centered. The partnership between the massage therapist and the client is based on the client's goals, values, wants, and needs. The massage therapist provides accurate information about massage to help the client give informed consent and participate in the decision-making process for goal setting and session implementation.

Massage Therapy Assessment and Evaluation

The process begins with the assessment (Fig. 1.7). A thorough health history begins the assessment process; this includes repeat clients (e.g., the massage therapist inquires how the health history has changed since the last session). (The assessment process is covered in Chapters 4 and 11).

The next step is to investigate the client's goal or goals for the session (or sessions). Possible goals include relaxation/well-being, stress or pain relief, or improvement in function. Each goal has a series of assessment questions, or the therapist may decide to use a validated instrument; (examples are provided in full on the Evolve website content for this chapter.) (This step is covered in Chapters 5, 6, and 14.)

Well-Being Assessment

The foundational goal is well-being. This category is for clients who have no particular goal for the session, who simply enjoy massage, and/or who feel it enhances their life and helps maintain good health. It is important to have clients rate their current health to monitor changes over time. Tracking changes over time may help massage therapy practice become more evidence based and scientific over time; additionally, tracking clients consistently may help improve outcomes over time.

Stress Assessment

Questions related to stress begin with asking the client to rate their stress, either on a simple 0-to-10 scale or using a valid and reliable stress scale. Ask how the client feels stress in the body. Does the client have headaches, tight neck and

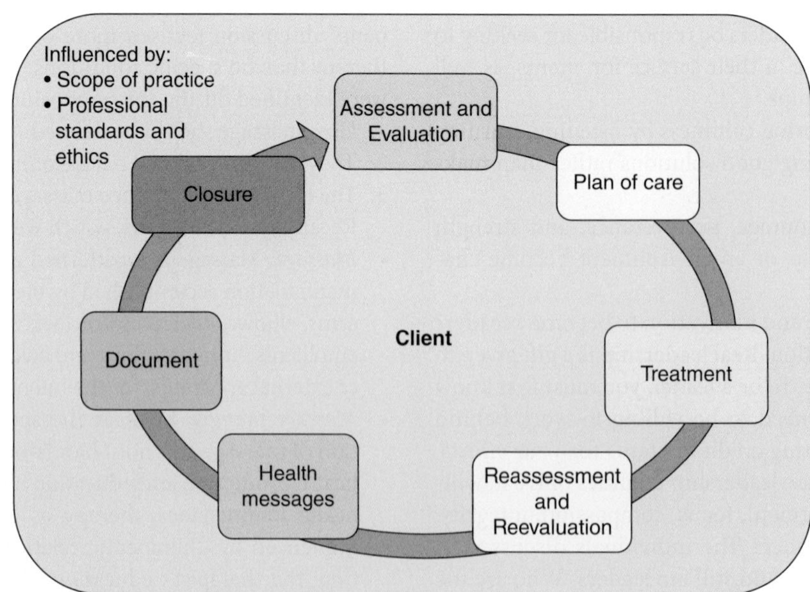

FIG. 1.6 Process for massage therapy practice. Kennedy AB, Cambron JA, Sharpe PA, Travillian RS, Saunders RP. Clarifying definitions for the massage therapy profession: the results of the Best Practices Symposium. *Int J Ther Mass Bodywork.* 2016;9(3):15.

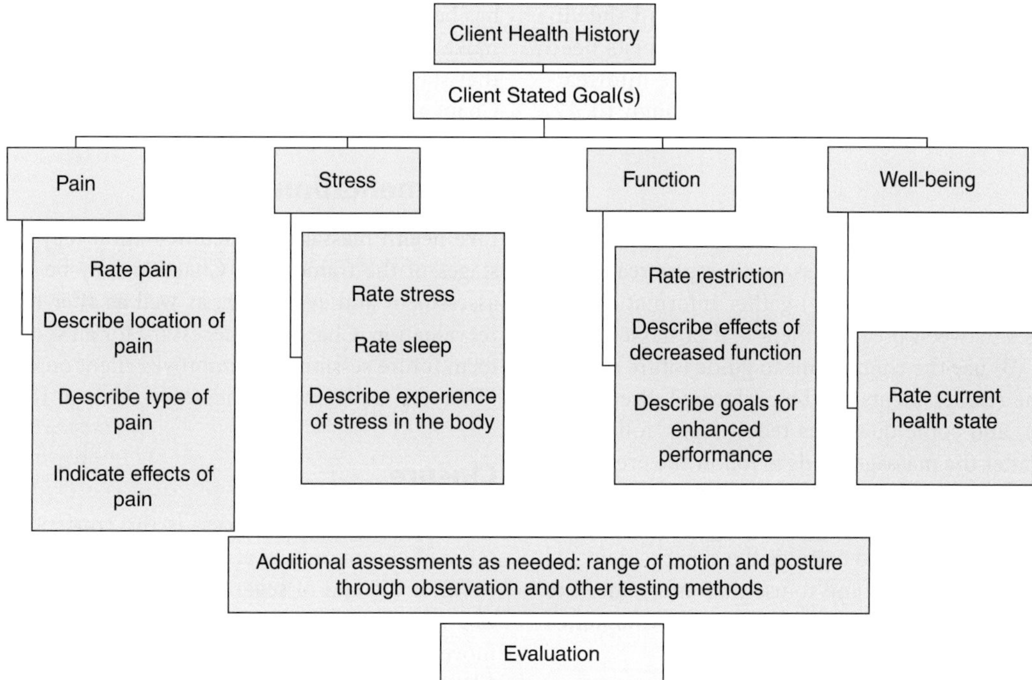

FIG. 1.7 Process of assessment. Kennedy AB, Cambron JA, Sharpe PA, Travillian RS, Saunders RP. Process for massage therapy practice and essential assessment. *J Bodyw Mov Ther*. 2016;20(3):484–496.

shoulders, or lower back pain? Ask the client to rate their sleep quality. These questions can help guide the treatment options and may help facilitate change.

Pain Assessment

Questions related to reducing pain include having the client rate their pain or using other assessment instruments to measure subjective pain levels. Next, inquire about the location of the pain in the body, and then about the type of pain. Finally, ask about the effects of the pain and what work, activities, and/or movements are hindered by the pain.

Function Assessment

To help get a better idea of how function is impaired, the therapist should ask the client to rate their level of restriction and specify what activities are affected by the impairment. Valid and reliable function scales also may be used, and some scales can be used specifically for certain impairments.

Additional Assessments

Massage therapists do not want limitations placed on possible ways to assess their clients. Examples of other methods of assessment include range of motion, orthopedic assessment, posture assessments, and similar methods; all of these are recommended to guide the planning for the massage session. These assessments are based on the therapist's education and experience within their scope of practice.

The follow-up to all these categories is to ask questions about what may be contributing to the client's problems. These contributing factors may give the massage therapist insight into the session planning and the expected outcomes. This follow-up also allows the therapist to provide health messages and assign clients "homework" to help improve their outcomes.

Evaluation

The evaluation process reviews the assessment data and helps in clinical decision making and treatment/session planning. After the assessments, the therapist makes judgments; these judgments guide care planning and the type of interventions to be used during the session. (This step is covered in Chapters 9, 11, 14, and 16.)

Plan of Care

After completing the evaluation process, the therapist determines the best way to address the client's needs and goals. These decisions must consider the client's input and goals, the best available evidence, and the therapist's own professional experience. When creating the plan of care, the therapist must bear in mind all cautions, contraindications, and any need for referral; these are important aspects of the care plan. (This step is covered in Chapters 5 through 7, 11, 14, and 16.)

Treatment/Massage Application

For our purposes, "treatment" is simply a term for the hands-on portion of massage therapy; the planned and patterned soft tissue manipulation. During the massage session, the massage therapist continues to assess and evaluate the client's responses, making changes to the treatment based on those findings. The session implementation is adapted according to this ongoing assessment and the client's feedback during the session. Massage therapists need to be mindful that the client's goals may change midtreatment. (This step is covered in Chapters 4, 7 through 10, 12, and 16.)

REASSESSMENT AND REEVALUATION

After the massage session, the massage therapist reassesses and reevaluates. This is done to (1) gather information; (2) identify changes between preassessment and postassessment measures; and (3) use the conclusions to guide future session planning. Some reassessments can be performed directly after the session, and some questions require later follow-up. Reassessment after the massage needs to follow the preassessment process, but it is important for the therapist to document whether the client's original goal changed during treatment. Reevaluation is intended to judge the changes detected based on the massage session and to use that information to guide ongoing treatment. (This step is covered in Chapters 4 through 6, 11, 14, and 16.)

Health Messages

Providing clients with health messages is an important part of massage therapy. Some therapists refer to this as giving "homework" to their clients to help maintain or improve the outcomes of the treatment session. These messages may be incorporated into the practice at various stages; they may be provided during the assessment when the therapist asks about contributing factors, during treatment, and/or after treatment has been completed. It is important for massage therapists to make sure they give clear and correct information and that they stay within their scope of practice. (This step is covered in Chapters 4 through 7 and 15.)

Documentation

Like health messaging, documentation may occur at various stages of the framework. Charting may be done during the assessment and evaluation, as well as after reassessment and reevaluation. Charting is necessary for all sessions; it helps inform future sessions and improves client outcomes over time. (This step is covered in Chapters 4, 11, and 16.)

Closure

The final step in the process is the concept of closure. This sense of closure occurs at the end of a session, but it may also occur at the end of several sessions. This formalized ending, to a session or therapy as a whole, helps clients detach and move along in their day and their life. (This step is covered in Chapters 1, 2, and 9.)

SUCCESS AS A MASSAGE THERAPIST

The path to success as a massage therapist also has been studied by researchers Ann Blair Kenny and Nicki Munk (2017). As you journey through this textbook, be aware of the massage therapy practice model (see Fig. 1.6) and the success model (Fig. 1.8). The possibilities are exciting, and the future is bright (Fig. 1.9).

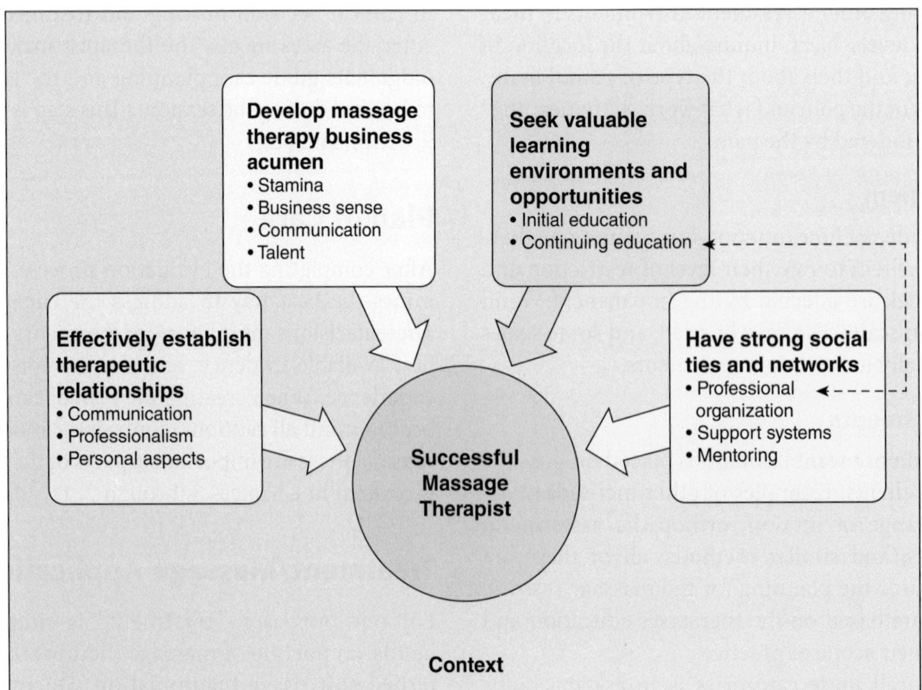

FIG. 1.8 Becoming a successful massage therapist. Kennedy AB, Munk N. Experienced practitioners' beliefs utilized to create a successful massage therapist conceptual model: a qualitative investigation. *Int J Ther Mass Bodywork.* 2017;10(2):9–19.

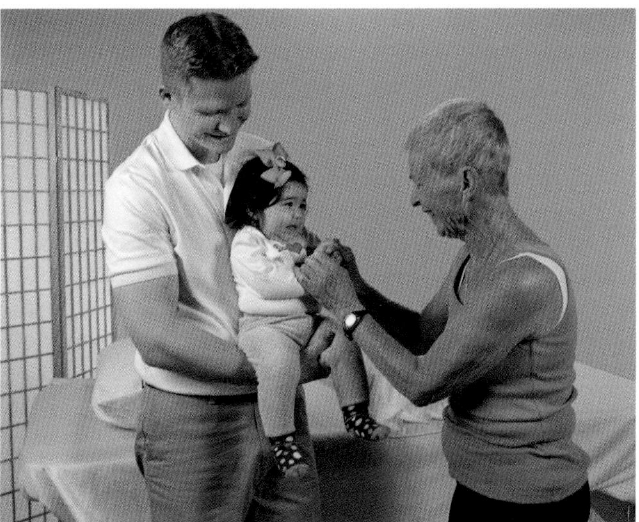

FIG. 1.9 A bright future: teaching the next generation.

Foot in the Door

Laying a foundation is important as you begin the process of developing your career as a massage therapist. Your entry-level education serves as this foundation. How committed are you to learning these basic skills? Sometimes learners become impatient with the early material, such as fundamental draping skills, sanitation, equipment maintenance, and so forth. However, the foundation you create for yourself must be solid and sound. If you intend to be an excellent massage therapist, the process begins right now, with your commitment to your education. Then, when you graduate, you will be able to present yourself to future clients, co-workers, and employers with self-confidence, professionalism, and even leadership skills that will help you get your foot in the door.

SUMMARY

This chapter begins with questions and discusses the nature of touch in the professional setting and its importance. The reader should now be aware of how culture, gender, age, life events, spirituality, and diversity all may influence the experience of touching and being touched. Inappropriate forms of touch were identified, appropriate forms of professional touch were presented, massage therapy as a profession was analyzed using standard criteria, and the importance of massage as a vocation and an occupation was highlighted.

The history of massage from ancient times to the present was explored, as were projections for the future. A timeline highlighted many key dates. The foundation has been laid for the study of therapeutic massage, and a platform for leadership has been created. You have a conceptual model to help you visualize the concepts and processes related to study and how the knowledge fits into professional practice. Chapter 2 expands on the area of professionalism, including the broader political and legal issues you will encounter. It also focuses on soft skills, such as communication, conflict management, professional boundaries, and—most importantly—professional ethics.

Evolve

Visit the Evolve website: http://evolve.elsevier.com/Fritz/fundamentals/

Evolve content designed for massage therapy licensing exam review and comprehension of content beyond the textbook.

Evolve content includes:

- Content updates
- Science and pathology animations
- Body spectrum coloring book
- MBLEx exam review multiple-choice questions

In each chapter, you will find:

- Answers and rationales for the end-of-chapter multiple-choice questions
- Electronic workbook and answer key
- Chapter multiple-choice question quiz
- Quick content review in question and answer format
- Technique videos when applicable
- Learn more on the web

REFERENCES

Afnan, Soheil Muhsin. Avicenna. *His Life and Works*. The Other Press; 2009.

Balogun O, Kennedy AB. Equity, diversity, and inclusion in the massage therapy profession. *Int J Ther Massage Bodywork*. 2020;13(3):1.

Banissy MJ, Ward J. Mechanisms of self-other representations and vicarious experiences of touch in mirror-touch synesthesia. *Front Human Neurosci.* 2013;7. Article 112. Retrieved from: http://www.ncbi.nlm.nih.gov/pmc/articles/PMC3615185/pdf/fnhum-07-00112.pdf.

Benjamin PJ. *The Emergency of the Massage Therapy Profession in North America*. Curties-Overzet Publications; 2015.

Cantu RI, Grodin AJ. *Myofascial Manipulation: Theory and Clinical Application*. 2nd ed. Aspen Publishers; 2001.

Chaitow L. *Soft Tissue Manipulation*. Healing Arts Press; 1988.

Crawford C, Boyd C, Paat CF, et al. The impact of massage therapy on function in pain populations: a systematic review and meta-analysis of randomized controlled trials. Part I, Patients experiencing pain in the general population. *Pain Med*. 2016;17(7):1353–1375. Available at: https://doi.org/10.1093/pm/pnw099.

Crawford C, Boyd C, Paat CF, et al. The impact of massage therapy on function in pain populations: a systematic review and meta-analysis of randomized controlled trials. Part II, Cancer pain populations. *Pain Med*. 2016;17(8):1553–1568. Available at: https://doi.org/10.1093/pm/pnw100.

Crawford C, Boyd C, Paat CF, et al. The impact of massage therapy on function in pain populations: a systematic review and meta-analysis of randomized controlled trials. Part III, Surgical pain populations. *Pain Med*. 2016;17(9):1757–1772. Available at: https://doi.org/10.1093/pm/pnw101.

Degenhardt B, van Dun PLS, Jacobson E, Fritz S, Mettler P, Kettner N, Franklin G, et al. Profession-based manual therapy nomenclature: exploring history, limitations, and opportunities. *J Man Manip Ther*. 2023:1–15.

Dekeyser M, Leijssen M. Studying Body-Oriented Responses: From the Therapist to the Client and Back Again. Book of Abstracts. *Presented at the International Meeting of the Society for Psychotherapy Research*, Montreal, Canada; 2005. Retrieved from. http://www.academia.edu/492962/Studying_Body-Oriented_Responses_From_the_Therapist_to_the_Client_and_Back_Again.

Fogarty S, Hay P, Calleri F, Fiddes L, Barnett R, Baskwill A. Impact of the COVID-19 Pandemic on the Professional Identity of Massage Therapists: The Reporting of a Quantitative Strand of a Mixed-Methods Study. *J Integr Complement Med*. 2022;28(2):124–135.

Forstenpointner J, Elman I, Freeman R, Borsook D. The omnipresence of autonomic modulation in health and disease. *Prog Neurobiol*. 2022:102218.

Gurevich D. *Historical Perspective*; 1992 (unpublished article).

Hargie O. *Skilled interpersonal communication: Research, theory and practice*. Routledge; 2021.

Hudson L. *Trends in Subbaccalaureate Occupational Awards: 2003–2015 Stats in Brief. NCES 2018-010*. National Center for Education Statistics; 2018.

Isham Ismail Z. *Glory years of Muslim medicine*. New Straits Times; 2006. http://www.highbeam.com/doc/1P1-132973038.html.

Kennedy AB, Cambron JA, Sharpe PA, Travillian RS, Saunders RP. Clarifying definitions for the massage therapy profession: the results of the Best Practices Symposium. *Int J Ther Massage Bodyw.* 2016a;9(3):15.
Kennedy AB, Cambron JA, Sharpe PA, Travillian RS, Saunders RP. Process for massage therapy practice and essential assessmentb. *J Bodyw Mov Ther.* 2016b;20(3):484–496.
Kennedy AB, Munk N. Experienced practitioners' beliefs utilized to create a successful massage therapist conceptual model: a qualitative investigation. *Int J Ther Massage Bodyw.* 2017;10(2):9–19.
Kopf D. Massage and touch-based therapy: Clinical evidence, neurobiology and applications in older patients with psychiatric symptoms. *Z Gerontol Geriatr.* 2021 Dec;54(8):753–758. doi:10.1007/s00391-021-01995-4. Epub 2021 Nov 23. PMID: 34812896; PMCID: PMC8609249.
Langevin HM. Fascia mobility, proprioception, and myofascial pain. *Life.* 2021;11(7):668.
Lederman E. *Fundamentals of Manual Therapy Physiology, Neurology, and Psychology.* Churchill Livingstone; 1997.
Liu B, Qiao L, Liu K, Liu J, Piccinni-Ash TJ, Chen ZF. Molecular and neural basis of pleasant touch sensation. *Science.* 2022;376(6592):483–491.
Masic I, Dilic M, Solakovic E, et al. Why historians of medicine called Ibn al-Nafis second Avicenna. *Med Arh.* 2008;62:244–249.
McGuirk J. The place of touch in counseling and psychotherapy and the potential for healing within the therapeutic relationship. *Inside Out.* 2012;68(Autumn). Irish Association of Humanistic and Integrative Psychotherapy. Retrieved from: http://iahip.org/inside-out/issue-68-autumn-2012/the-place-of-touch-in-counselling-and-psychotherapy-and-the-potential-for-healing-within-the-therapeutic-relationship.
McParlin Z, Cerritelli F, Rossettini G, Friston KJ, Esteves JE. Therapeutic Alliance as Active Inference: The Role of Therapeutic Touch and Biobehavioural Synchrony in Musculoskeletal Care. *Front Behav Neurosci.* 2022;16:897247. doi:10.3389/fnbeh.2022.897247. Published 2022 Jun 30.
Melzack R. Evolution of the neuromatrix theory of pain. The Prithvi Raj Lecture. Presented at the Third World Congress of World Institute of Pain, Barcelona 2004. *Pain Pract.* 2005;5:85–94.
Moseley GL. A pain neuromatrix approach to patients with chronic pain. *Man Ther.* 2003;8(3):130–140.
Schaefer M, Joch M, Rother N. Feeling touched: empathy is associated with performance in a tactile acuity task. *Front Hum Neurosci.* 2021;15:593425.
Smith EWL, Clance PR, Imes S. *Touch in Psychotherapy.* Guilford Press; 1998.
Stonehouse D. The use of touch in developing a therapeutic relationship. *Br J Health Assist.* 2017;11(1):15–17.
Swade T. *The Touch Taboo in Psychotherapy and Everyday Life.* Routledge; 2020.
Tague C, Seppelfrick D, MacKenzie A. Massage Therapy in the Time of COVID-19. *J Altern Complement Med.* 2021;27(6):467–472.
Tappan FM, Benjamin PJ. *Tappan's Handbook of Healing Massage Techniques: Classic, Holistic, and Emerging Methods.* 4th ed. Prentice Hall; 2004.
van Why RP. *History of Massage and its Relevance to Today's Practitioner.* The Bodywork Knowledgebase; 1992. Self-published.
Warwick L. "Depends who it is": Towards a relational understanding of the use of adult-child touch in residential child care. *Qual Soc Work.* 2022;21(1):18–36.
Roudaut Y, Lonigro A, Coste B, Hao J, Delmas P, Crest M. Touch sense: functional organization and molecular determinants of mechanosensitive receptors. *Channels (Austin).* 2012;6:234–245. Retrieved from: http://www.ncbi.nlm.nih.gov/pmc/articles/PMC3508902/pdf/chan-6-234.pdf.
Yu H, Miao W, Ji E, et al. Social touch-like tactile stimulation activates a tachykinin 1-oxytocin pathway to promote social interactions. *Neuron.* 2022;110(6):1051–1067.
Zur O, Nordmarken N. *To Touch or Not to Touch: Exploring the Myth of Prohibition on Touch in Psychotherapy and Counseling.* Zur Institute; 2011. Retrieved from. http://www.zurinstitute.com/touchintherapy.html.

MULTIPLE-CHOICE QUESTIONS FOR DISCUSSION AND REVIEW

The answers, with rationales, can be found on the Evolve site.

Use these questions to stimulate discussion and dialog. You have to understand the meaning of the words in the question and possible answers. Each question provides you with the opportunity to review terminology, practice critical-thinking skills, and improve your multiple-choice test-taking skills. Answers and rationales are provided on the Evolve website. Remember that it is just as important to know why the wrong answers are wrong as it is to know why the correct answer is correct.

1. Professionalism is defined as _____.
   a. An occupation that helps people
   b. A service provided for others
   c. An intricate system that is structured and systematic
   d. Adherence to professional status, methods, standards, and character
2. A productive or creative activity that serves as one's regular source of livelihood is a(n) _____.
   a. Service
   b. Therapeutic application
   c. Healing
   d. Occupation
3. If a massage therapist is describing how much their career choice satisfied their need to help people who are seeking a healthy lifestyle, they are speaking of massage as a _____.
   a. Vocation
   b. Professional job
   c. Cultural communication
   d. Technique
4. A middle-aged client is reluctant to work with a 22-year-old massage therapist. This is an example of _____.
   a. Gender issues
   b. Genetic predisposition
   c. Age issues
   d. Body sensitivity
5. Culture is defined by _____.
   a. Race, as determined by skin color, nationality, educational standard, economic status, and gender roles
   b. Arts, beliefs, customs, institutions, and all products of human work and thought created by a specific group of people at a particular time
   c. What you study, the profession you choose, the family you grew up in, and whom you marry
   d. The workplace, including the people, environment, physical location, and fiscal management
6. Which is a form of touch technique?
   a. Socially stereotyped touch
   b. Mechanical touch
   c. Inadvertent touch
   d. Ritualized touch
7. When a professional operates from many bases of knowledge while interacting with clients therapeutically, the concern is _____.
   a. Expressive touch
   b. Gender diversity
   c. Dual roles
   d. Wellness promotion
8. The term _____ has been used to cover the scope of the development of various types of hands-on modalities.
   a. Massage
   b. Bodywork
   c. Technician
   d. Practitioner

9. Who wrote a definitive text on trigger points?
   a. Dr. James B. Mennell
   b. Randolph Stone
   c. Wilhelm Reich
   d. Dr. Janet Travell
10. The ability to make decisions and the freedom to act in accordance with one's professional knowledge base allowing independent practice of massage therapy describes:
   a. Autonomy
   b. Leadership
   c. Legislation
   d. Research
11. Which massage trend developed in the 1990s supported acceptance of the benefits of massage?
   a. An increase in valid research
   b. Deregulation of massage education
   c. An increase in the variety of massage and bodywork methods
   d. Resistance to integrating massage into traditional health care settings
12. _____ involves influencing others for good, inspiring them to become the best they can be, and working together toward a common goal.
   a. Practice framework
   b. Leadership
   c. Licensure
   d. Intuition
13. A massage therapist is frustrated with the dress code at the place of employment. All massage employees are required to wear the uniform provided by the employer. Which of these statements supports the employer's rule?
   a. A vocation is a strong altruistic motivation to follow a specific occupational career pathway to be of service to others.
   b. A professional is a person who engages in a profession and is committed to adhering to the standards expected of a qualified and experienced person in a specific work environment.
   c. Professional autonomy means having the authority to make decisions and the freedom to act in accordance with one's professional knowledge base.
   d. A service is something done for another that results in a specific outcome.
14. An individual response to professional therapeutic touch _____.
   a. Is consistent with cultural influences
   b. Cannot be predetermined
   c. Is gender specific
   d. Depends on the outcomes
15. Scientific study and technology have identified the physiological responses to touch but have not fully explained _____.
   a. The experience of touch
   b. Touch communication
   c. How sensation is received
   d. How touch is related to sexual arousal
16. A massage practitioner has just finished a massage session with a difficult client who insists on deep pressure even when increased pressure is not indicated. Which of these could be a factor in the next massage session?
   a. Hostile or aggressive touch
   b. Erotic touch
   c. Invasive touch
   d. Expressive touch
17. A client has children in the same school as the massage therapist. The therapist and the client have attended the same meetings on school safety and emergency response. Which of these needs to be monitored during the massage session?
   a. Orientation to service
   b. Health promotion
   c. Scope of practice
   d. Dual role
18. A massage graduate is preparing for licensure in their state. Which of these applies?
   a. MBLEx
   b. Board certification
   c. College degree
   d. ELAP
19. A massage practitioner chooses to be involved with the promotion of massage therapy benefits in their city. Part of this process is recruiting and organizing other massage therapists to participate in scheduled events. Which of these describes the massage therapist's role?
   a. Leadership
   b. Motivation
   c. Inclusion
   d. Status
20. Which part of the massage therapy practice framework most involves clinical decision making?
   a. Assessment
   b. Treatment/massage application
   c. Documentation
   d. Plan of care

Note: The multiple-choice questions for discussion and the review sections found at the end of each chapter support preparation for the massage therapy licensing exam that you will take upon completion of your education. An excellent review strategy is to create multiple-choice questions. You will get better at this activity as you progress through the textbook. For this first chapter, the following short segment provides guidelines on how to develop a multiple-choice question. Use this information to create multiple-choice questions for all the remaining chapters.

Designing Multiple-Choice Questions

A multiple-choice question has two parts: a stem that identifies the question or problem, and a set of alternatives or possible answers. One of the answers is the best answer to the question. The other possibilities are called *distracters*, which are plausible but incorrect answers to the question. In the stem:

- Use your own words and avoid using sentences directly from the textbook.

- Think about the stem as a focused problem that one of the possible answers will solve.
- Include only the information necessary to identify the best answer. Keep the stem concise.

In the answer choices:

- Create a, b, c, and d options.
- Make sure the answer options are similar in length.
- Make sure the best answer is clearly correct.

Creating distracters can be difficult. However, you will learn the most by creating plausible wrong answers.

Hints for creating wrong answers:

- Use true statements that do not answer the questions.
- Use false information that appears to be related to the problem in the stem.
- Use similar language but make sure the terms are clearly incorrect.
- Trivial details should not make a statement false.
- Avoid using "all of the above" or "none of the above" as answer options.

Write Your Own Questions

Write at least three multiple-choice questions, one of each type: factual recall and comprehension, application and concept identification, and clinical reasoning and synthesis. Make sure to develop plausible wrong answers and be sure that the correct answer is clearly correct and then write a rationale for each question. The more questions you write, the better you will understand the material. Exchange questions with classmates or discuss in class. The questions written by all your peers can be combined to create a review quiz.

CHAPTER 2

Ethics, Professionalism, and Legal Issues

http://evolve.com/Fritz/fundamentals/

CHAPTER OBJECTIVES

After completing this chapter, the student will be able to:

1. Define ethics; also, develop and explain a code of ethics and the standards of practice for therapeutic massage.
2. Define a scope of practice for therapeutic massage.
3. Define evidence-based practice and evidence-informed practice.
4. Complete an informed consent process.
5. Practice procedures to maintain client confidentiality.
6. Describe basic functions of the Health Insurance Portability and Accountability Act (HIPAA), the training in its rules, and its requirements.
7. Integrate ethics into maintaining professional boundaries and the therapeutic relationship.
8. Explain and demonstrate qualities of the therapeutic relationship.
9. Use a problem-solving approach to ethical decision making.
10. Use basic communication skills to listen effectively and deliver an I-message.
11. Identify and resolve conflict in the professional setting.
12. Identify legal and credentialing concerns of the massage professional.
13. Identify and report unethical conduct by colleagues.

CHAPTER OUTLINE

KEY TERMS

Active listening
Aspirational ethics
Clinical reasoning
Code of ethics
Confidentiality
Conflict
Consultation
Countertransference
Credentials
Decision
Defensive climate
Dilemma

Dual role
Ethical behavior
Ethical decision making
Ethics
Evidence-based practice
Evidence-informed practice
Implicit bias
Informed consent
Initial treatment plan
Jurisprudence
Mandatory ethics
Mentoring
Model Practice Act
Open-ended questions
Peer support
Power differential
Practices
Principles
Reciprocity
Reflective listening
Right of refusal
Scope of practice
Standard of care
Standards of practice
Supervision
Supportive climate
Therapeutic alliance
Therapeutic relationship
Transference

As a student of therapeutic massage, you must develop the ability to make professional decisions that are well thought out and can be justified. *Justified* means having an acceptable reason for the action taken based on sound reasoning and information that can be defended. *Defended* means to support the decision by proving its validity. Chapter 1 presented a foundation for professionalism and future trends. This chapter will help you begin asking necessary questions about professional behavior and to find effective ways to answer those questions for yourself.

FOCUS ON PROFESSIONALISM

Implicit Bias Awareness

Implicit bias is an automatic reaction we have towards other people. These attitudes and stereotypes can negatively impact our understanding, actions, and decision making resulting in unintentional discrimination. Professional ethical behavior involves self-reflection. People have unconscious or conscious biases about perceived gender, race, age, income, and education level. These biases contribute to negative associations about others and may lead to less-than-optimal ethical behavior. Project Implicit is a 501(c)(3) nonprofit organization and international collaborative of researchers who are interested in implicit social cognition. The mission of Project Implicit is to educate the public about bias and to provide a "virtual laboratory" for collecting data on the internet. Project Implicit scientists produce high-impact research that forms the basis of our scientific knowledge about bias and disparities. understanding attitudes, stereotypes, and other hidden biases that influence perception, judgment, and action. Learn more at (https://www.projectimplicit.net).

The following weblink will take you to The Implicit Association Test (IAT), which measures implicit attitudes and stereotypes about groups (race, age, disability, sexuality, religion, and weight to name a few (https://www.implicit.harvard.edu).

Innovation, productivity, and decision making are enhanced when we embrace differences from gender identity and sexual orientation to race and ethnicity, age, physical ability, and neurodiversity. Knowledge and innovation are born of diversity of people, ideas, thought, culture, and perspective. In science and health—where knowledge can change a life or the destiny of our planet—diversity is essential.

These professional development topics and skills are addressed in this chapter:

- The scope of practice for massage professionals
- Ethical conduct and standards of practice for massage professionals
- The therapeutic relationship
- Communication and conflict management skills to support professional interaction
- Professional record keeping supporting professional achievement
- Provisions of the Health Insurance Portability and Accountability Act of 1996 (HIPAA)
- Licensing and other legal concerns of the massage professional
- Credentialing beyond licensure
- Peer support, supervision, and mentoring

This information provides the structure for professional and ethical decision making. It can help you develop the level of professionalism essential to the successful practice of therapeutic massage (Focus on Professionalism).

Ethics and professionalism have a unique language. These definitions clarify some of the terminology used in this chapter.

Countertransference is an inability on the part of the professional to separate the therapeutic relationship from personal feelings and expectations for the client; it is personalization of the professional relationship by the professional.

Dual role results when scopes of practice overlap (e.g., one professional provides support in more than one area of expertise) or the personal and professional relationships overlap.

Ethics is the science or study of morals, values, and principles, including the ideals of autonomy, beneficence, and justice. Ethics comprises principles of right and good conduct.

Ethical behavior is right and correct conduct based on moral and cultural standards as defined by the society in which we live.

Ethical decision making is the application of ethical principles and professional skills to determine appropriate behavior and resolve ethical dilemmas.

Fidelity is concerned with building trusting relationships; the keeping of promises.

Fiduciary duty is an obligation to maintain trust and the legal responsibility to act solely in the best interest of another party.

Informed consent is a consumer protection process; it requires that clients be informed of the steps of treatment, that their participation be voluntary, and that they be competent to give consent. Informed consent is also an educational process that allows clients to make knowledgeable decisions about whether to receive a massage.

Jurisprudence relates to the theory and practice of the law. A jurisprudence examination is a test taken to demonstrate knowledge of a specific piece of legislation such as a massage therapy law.

Mentoring is a professional relationship in which an individual with experience and skill beyond those of the person being mentored provides support, encouragement, and career expertise.

Peer support is the interaction among those of similar skill and experience to encourage and maintain appropriate professional practice.

Principles are basic truths or rules of conduct; they are generalizations that are accepted as true and that can be used as a basis for ethical conduct.

Scope of practice is the knowledge base and practice parameters of a profession.

Standards of practice are principles that serve as specific guidelines for directing professional ethical practice and quality care, including a structure for evaluating the quality of care. They are an attempt to define the parameters of quality care.

Standard of care is an assessment and treatment process that a clinician (massage therapist) should follow for a certain type of clinical circumstance performed at the level at which similarly qualified practitioners manage the client's care under the same or similar circumstances.

Supervision is the situation in which a person oversees others and their professional behavior. The supervisor may be from a different discipline (e.g., a nurse) or may be a massage therapist with more skill and experience than those supervised. Supervisors usually are in a position of authority. They are actively involved in such areas as the development and approval of treatment plans, review of clarity, scheduling, discipline, and teaching.

Therapeutic alliance is an interpersonal provider–client model that addresses the continuum of compliance, adherence, and collaboration in therapeutic relationships.

Therapeutic relationship is created by the interpersonal structure and professional boundaries between professionals and their clients.

Transference is the personalization of the professional relationship by the client.

ETHICS AND STANDARDS OF PRACTICE

SECTION OBJECTIVES

Chapter objective covered in this section:

1. Define ethics; also, develop and explain a code of ethics and the standards of practice for therapeutic massage.

Using the information presented in this section, the student will be able to:

- Develop a personal and professional code of ethics using the eight ethical principles.
- Explain the standards of practice for therapeutic massage.

ETHICS

Culture, time, location, events, politics, religion, scientific knowledge, and many other factors affect the way we interpret behavior. Ethics defines the behavior we expect of ourselves and others and society's expectations of a profession. Simply defined, *ethics* is "what is right." Our society determines that a person has acted ethically when the right thing has been done. However, what is the right thing? No one individual or group has the answer. Often the best that can be offered in discussions of ethics are questions and guidelines based on principles of conduct established by a group.

Ethics has social, professional, and personal dimensions. Separating these elements is not easy in theory or in practice. We behave according to a complex and continually changing set of rules, customs, and expectations. For this reason, ethical behavior must be a dynamic process of reflection and revision.

Ethics is not just a varied collection of do's and don'ts; rather, it is a system of principles, interrelated in a reasonable, coherent way, which makes our society and our lives as civilized and happy as possible. Conflicts and uncertainties are inevitable. For this reason, in applying ethics, we must learn more than a list of guidelines, more than just what to do in this or that particular case; we must also develop a set of priorities and a way of thinking about them. To use ethics in decision making, we must be able to think critically about what we have learned to capture the spirit of being ethical. Although morals and values are ultimately a personal concern, ethics reflects one's professional and social character.

The purpose of practicing our profession ethically is to promote and maintain the welfare of the client. Laws often reflect the minimal standards necessary to protect the safety and welfare of the public, whereas codes of ethics represent the ideal standards set by a profession. Through their behavior, professionals can comply both with the law and with professional codes. If compliance with the law is the only motivation in ethical behavior, the person is said to be practicing **mandatory ethics**. However, a professional who strives for the highest possible benefit and welfare for the client behaves with **aspirational ethics** (Corey et al., 2011).

As professionals we must constantly be alert not only to gross violations of ethical principles but also to the subtler ethical violations that occur when the client's welfare is not the primary determining factor of professional behavior. An example of the latter is hesitating to refer a client to a more qualified massage professional because referral means the loss of a paying client. Often this type of unethical conduct goes unnoticed, yet the client's welfare is compromised. This situation is further complicated because the practitioner may not recognize the breach in ethical behavior. *Mentoring* (career support by someone more experienced), *supervision* (monitoring by one with more expertise), *peer support* (interaction and exchange of information among fellow professionals), and *meticulous objective personal reflection* on professional behavior can bring to light these subtler types of ethical violations. Professionals can monitor their own behavior by repeatedly asking themselves whether they are doing what is best for the client and whether their behavior is ethical.

Professional growth involves change in our knowledge, skills, attitudes, and beliefs. A professional **code of ethics** is a set of norms (acceptable behavior) adopted by a professional group to direct choices and behavior in a manner consistent with professional responsibility. Many elements in the profession of massage enhance the lives of its practitioners, such as respect, authority, and prestige. In return, professionals must be willing to adjust their personal behavior for the professional good. We have to gauge our personal and professional behavior not only by what is right and good for us as individuals but also by what is appropriate for the client and the profession as a whole (Focus on Professionalism).

FOCUS ON PROFESSIONALISM

As a learner you have professional responsibilities. There are skills you need in order to most benefit from your education and advance as a massage therapist. Use the following list to do a self-assessment. If you identify areas that need improvement and development assistance, be self-responsible and find the help you need. There are many ways to improve your learning abilities.

1. Basic academic skills
   - Read and write English at a basic 10th-grade level and perform basic math. Use technology at a basic level, including internet access, email, and general navigation. Find tutoring assistance when needed.
2. Goal-setting skills
   - Determine your personal goals related to school, career, or health. Write long-term, intermediate-term, and short-term goals and evaluate those goals to see whether they realistically can be achieved. Identify tasks, actions, and obstacles involved in achieving the goals. Develop a step-by-step plan to achieve a goal using a timeline.
3. Time management skills
   - Write monthly, weekly, and daily schedules and weekly and daily to-do lists. Plan ahead and prioritize tasks to meet deadlines. Plan sufficient time to complete each task. Evaluate tasks and commitments for importance. Eliminate and reduce nonessential activity. Simplify daily life activities. Recognize procrastination and avoid it.
4. Study skills
   - Take effective notes from reading assignments and classroom lectures and discussions. Complete homework on or before homework deadlines. Identify and use a variety of study and test-taking strategies. Form and participate in study groups. Ask questions that are well thought out and relevant to the topic. Make accurate decisions about what to study for specific recall and what to study for background and general purposes.
5. Critical- and creative-thinking skills
   - Identify and define problems and gather relevant information from a variety of sources to generate possible solutions. Analyze possible solutions using collected information, prior knowledge, and intuitive feelings to select the best solution and implement it. Evaluate new solutions to make adaptations or refinements. During the process, ask questions that are well thought out. Look for patterns among objects, ideas, processes, and concepts. Compare and contrast ideas or processes to identify the interrelationship of the parts in a whole. Break down the problems and possible solutions into small parts. Put parts together in multiple ways to form a variety of options.
6. Interpersonal skills
   - Establish healthy, mutually beneficial relationships with others. Treat others with respect and listen to their points of view. Offer to help others. Ask for help when needed. Seek and consider feedback from others while functioning effectively without ongoing reassurance from others. Seek critical appraisal from those with more knowledge and experience. Work cooperatively with others, including people with different points of view. Reflect to gain insight and learn from past experiences and be accountable for choices, actions, and outcomes. Manage conflicts effectively using appropriately assertive behaviors. Balance the needs of self with the needs of others.

From the Coalition of National Massage Therapy Organizations. (2013). The Core: Entry-Level Massage Education Blueprint. Available at: ELAP-elapmassage.org.

Ethical Principles

These ten principles guide professional ethical behavior.

1. *Respect* (esteem and regard for clients, other professionals, and oneself)
2. *Client autonomy and self-determination* (the freedom to decide and the right to sufficient information to make the decision)
3. *Veracity* (the right to the objective truth)
4. *Proportionality* (the principle that benefit must outweigh the burden of treatment)
5. *Nonmaleficence* (the principle that the professional shall do no harm and prevent harm from happening)
6. *Beneficence* (the principle that treatment should contribute to the client's well-being)
7. *Confidentiality* (respect for privacy of information)
8. *Justice* (the principle that ensures equality among clients)
9. *Fidelity* (building of trusting relationships keeping of promises).
10. *Fiduciary duty* (an obligation to maintain trust and the legal responsibility to act solely in the best interest of another party)

These broad concepts direct the development of standards of practice.

Standards of Practice

Standards of practice provide specific guidelines and rules that form a concrete professional structure. For example, in standards of practice, the ethical principle of respect translates into professional behavior, such as maintaining the client's privacy and modesty, providing a safe environment, and being on time for appointments. The principle of client autonomy and self-determination requires informed consent and ready access for clients to their files.

Standards of practice direct quality care and provide a means of measuring the quality of care.

Code of Ethics and Standards of Practice for Therapeutic Massage

Because the massage therapy profession is not yet united in terms of professional affiliation and techniques, presenting a code of ethics or providing agreed-on standards of practice for the massage professional is difficult. Because each of the professional groups that constitute the massage profession have developed individual codes of ethics and standards of practice, this text offers a comprehensive compilation of many ethical codes and standards of practice, developed through professional organizations, licensing requirements, and the standards of practice of other health professions (Boxes 2.1 and 2.2). An attempt has been made to include all points presented in the various ethical conduct codes and standards of practice statements.

Box 2.1 Code of Ethics and Standards of Practice for Massage

Ethical Principles

The four basic principles that constitute the code of ethics for massage professionals are:

- *Respect for the dignity of people:* Massage professionals must maintain respect for the interests, dignity, rights, and needs of all clients, staff, and colleagues.
- *Responsible caring:* Competent, quality client care must be provided at the highest standard possible.
- *Integrity in relationships:* At all times, the professional must behave with integrity, honesty, and diligence in practice and duties.
- *Responsibility to society:* Massage professionals are responsible for and accountable to society and must conduct themselves in a manner that maintains high ethical standards.

Standards of Practice

The principles of the code of ethics form the basis of these standards of practice for massage professionals.

1. Respect all clients, colleagues, and health care professionals through nondiscrimination, regardless of age, gender, race, national origin, sexual orientation, religion, socioeconomic status, body type, political affiliation, state of health, personal habits, and life-coping skills.
2. Perform only those services for which the massage professional is qualified. Massage professionals must represent honestly their education, licensing, certification, professional affiliations, and other qualifications. They may apply a treatment only when a reasonable expectation exists that it will be advantageous to the client's condition. The massage professional, in consultation with the client, must continually evaluate the effectiveness of treatment.
3. Respect the scope of practice of other health care and service professionals, including physicians, chiropractors, physical therapists, podiatrists, orthopedists, psychotherapists, counselors, acupuncturists, nurses, exercise physiologists, athletic trainers, nutritionists, spiritual advisors, and cosmetologists.
4. Respect all ethical health care practitioners and work with them to promote health and healing.
5. Acknowledge the limitations of personal skills and, when necessary, refer clients to an appropriately qualified professional. The massage professional must consult with other knowledgeable professionals when:
   - A client requires diagnosis and opinion beyond a therapist's capabilities of assessment.
   - A client's condition is beyond the massage professional's scope of practice.
   - A combined health/medical care team is required.

   If referral and communication to another health/medical care provider are necessary, they must be done with the client's informed consent.
6. Use appropriate caution when working with any individual who has a specific disease process and seek supervision by a licensed medical professional when needed.
7. Be adequately educated and understand the physiologic effects of the specific massage techniques used to determine whether any application is contraindicated and to ensure that the most beneficial techniques are applied to a given individual.
8. Avoid false claims about the potential benefits of the techniques rendered and educate the public about the actual benefits of massage. Strive to maintain an evidence-based/-informed practice.
9. Acknowledge the importance and individuality of each person, including colleagues, peers, and clients.
10. Work only with the informed consent of a client, and professionally disclose to the client any situation that may interfere with the massage professional's ability to provide the best care to serve the client's best interest.
11. Show respect by honoring a client's process and following all recommendations and by being present, listening, asking only pertinent questions, keeping agreements, being on time, draping properly, avoiding "no touch" zones, and customizing the massage to address the client's needs. The client's consent is required for work on any part of the body, regardless of whether the client is fully clothed, fully draped, or partly draped. (Draping is covered in Chapter 9).
    - It is the responsibility of the massage professional to ensure the privacy and dignity of the client and to determine whether the client feels comfortable, safe, and secure with the draping provided.
    - The client may choose to be fully draped or clothed throughout the treatment.
    - A female client's breasts are not undraped unless specified by referral from a qualified medical care professional and the massage professional is working under the supervision of such a medical professional.
    - The genitals, perineum, and anus are never undraped.
12. Provide a safe, comfortable, and clean environment.
13. Maintain clear and honest communication with clients and keep client communications confidential. Confidentiality is of the utmost importance. The massage professional must inform the client that the referring physician may be eligible to review the client's records and that records may be subpoenaed by the courts.
14. Conduct business in a professional and ethical manner in relation to the clientele, business associates, acquaintances, government bodies, and the public.
15. Follow city, county, state, national, and international requirements.
16. Charge a fair price for the session. Gratuities are appropriate if within reasonable limits (i.e., similar to percentages for other service providers, such as 15%–20%). A gift, gratuity, or benefit that is intended to influence a referral,

Continued

Box 2.1 Code of Ethics and Standards of Practice for Massage—cont'd

decision, or treatment may not be accepted and must be returned to the giver immediately.

17. Keep accurate records and review the records with the client.
18. Never engage in any sexual conduct, sexual conversation, or any other sexual activities involving clients.
19. Avoid affiliation with any business that uses any form of sexual suggestiveness or explicit sexuality in advertising or promoting services or in the actual practice of service.
20. Practice honesty in advertising, promoting services ethically and in good taste, and advertising only techniques for which the professional is certified or adequately trained.
21. Strive for professional excellence through regular assessment of personal strengths, limitations, and effectiveness and through continuing education and training.
22. Accept the responsibility to oneself, one's clients, and the profession to maintain physical, mental, and emotional well-being and to inform clients when one is not functioning at full capacity.
23. Refrain from using any mind-altering drugs, alcohol, or intoxicants before or during professional massage sessions.
24. Maintain a professional appearance and demeanor by practicing good hygiene and dressing in a professional, modest, and nonsexual manner.
25. Undergo periodic peer review.
26. Respect all pertinent reporting requirements outlined by legislation regarding abuse.
27. Report to the proper authorities any accurate knowledge and its supportive documentation regarding violations by massage professionals and other health, medical or service professionals.
28. Avoid interests, activities, or influences that might conflict with the obligation to act in the best interest of clients and the massage therapy profession and safeguard professional integrity by recognizing potential conflicts of interest and avoiding them.

Box 2.2 Occupational Definitions and Scopes of Practice

The scope of practice described for the following professions is derived from regulations typically established to govern these occupations. The regulations predominantly used for these descriptions are the administrative rules of the Michigan Occupational Regulations' Department of Licensing and Regulation and the Occupational Regulations section of the Michigan Public Health Code.

Acupuncture

Acupuncture is a form of primary health care based on traditional Chinese medical concepts. It uses acupuncture diagnosis and treatment, in addition to adjunctive therapies and diagnostic techniques, to promote, maintain, and restore health and prevent disease. Acupuncture includes but is not limited to insertion of acupuncture needles and application of moxibustion (medicinal herbs burned on or near the skin) to specific areas of the human body.

Athletic Training

Athletic training is the study of athletic performance, injury prevention, and rehabilitation. It includes training regimens; evaluation and assessment of injury; treatment, rehabilitation, and reconditioning of athletic injury; therapeutic exercise; and use of therapeutic modalities.

Chiropractic

Chiropractic is the discipline within the healing arts that deals with the nervous system, its relationship to the spinal column, and its interrelationship with the other body systems. Chiropractic uses radiography to detect spinal subluxation and misalignment and adjusts related bones and tissues to establish neural integrity through techniques that use the inherent recuperative powers of the body to restore and maintain health. Examples of these techniques include the use of analytic instruments, the provision of nutritional advice, and the prescribing of rehabilitative exercise. Chiropractic does not include the performance of incisive surgical procedures or any invasive procedure that requires instrumentation or the dispensing or prescription of drugs or medicine.

Cosmetology

Cosmetology is a service provided to enhance the health, condition, and appearance of the skin, hair, and nails through the use of external preparations designed to cleanse and beautify. It includes the application of beautification processes, such as makeup and skin grooming.

Dentistry

Dentistry is the discipline of diagnosis, treatment, prescription, and surgery for disease, pain, deformity, deficiency, or injury of human teeth, alveolar processes, gums, jaws, and dependent tissues. Dentistry also is concerned with preventive care and the maintenance of good oral health.

Esthetics

An esthetician is a person who works to clean and beautify the skin. Estheticians, also called skin care therapists, specialize in cosmetic treatments of the skin, and perform treatments such as facials, superficial chemical peels, body treatments, and waxing.

Medicine

Medicine is the diagnosis, treatment, prevention, cure, or relief of human disease, ailment, defect, complaint, or other physical or mental condition by attendance, advice, device, diagnostic test, or other means.

Naturopathy

Naturopathy is the combination of clinical nutrition, herbology, homeopathy, acupuncture, manipulation, hydrotherapy, massage, exercise, and psychological methods, including hypnotherapy and biofeedback, to maintain health. Naturopathic physicians use radiography, ultrasound, and other forms of

Box 2.2 Occupational Definitions and Scopes of Practice—cont'd

diagnostic testing but do not perform major surgery or prescribe synthetic drugs.

Nursing

Nursing is the systematic application of substantial specialized knowledge and skill, derived from the biological, physical, and behavioral sciences to the care, treatment, counsel, and health education of individuals who are experiencing changes in the normal health process or who require assistance in the maintenance of health and the prevention or management of illness, injury, and disability.

Osteopathic Medicine

Osteopathic medicine is an independent school of medicine and surgery that uses full methods of diagnosis and treatment in physical and mental health and disease, including the prescription and administration of drugs and vitamins; operative surgery; obstetrics; and radiologic and electromagnetic diagnostics. Osteopathy emphasizes the interrelationship of the musculoskeletal system with other body systems.

Physical Therapy

Physical therapy is the evaluation or treatment of an individual by the use of effective physical measures, therapeutic exercise, and rehabilitative procedures, with or without devices, to prevent, correct, or alleviate a physical or mental disability. It includes treatment planning, the performance of tests and measurements, interpretation of referrals, instruction, consultative services, and supervision of personnel. Physical measures include massage, mobilization, and the application of heat, cold, air, light, water, electricity, and sound.

Podiatric Medicine

Podiatric medicine is the examination, diagnosis, and treatment of abnormal nails and superficial excrescences (abnormal outgrowths or enlargements) on the human feet, including corns, warts, callosities, bunions, and arch troubles. It also includes the medical, surgical, or mechanical treatment and physiotherapy of ailments that affect the condition of the feet. It does not include amputation of the feet or the use or administration of general anesthetics.

Psychology

Psychology is the rendering to individuals, groups, organizations, or the public service involving the application of principles, methods, and procedures of understanding, predicting, and influencing behavior for the purpose of diagnosis, assessment, prevention, amelioration, or treatment of mental or emotional disorders, disabilities, and behavioral adjustment problems. Treatment is provided by means of psychotherapy, counseling, behavior modification, hypnosis, biofeedback techniques, psychological tests, and other verbal or behavioral methods. Psychology does not include the prescription of drugs, performance of surgery, or administration of electroconvulsive therapy.

SCOPE OF PRACTICE

SECTION OBJECTIVES

Chapter objective covered in this section:

2. Define a scope of practice for therapeutic massage.

Using the information presented in this section, the student will be able to:

- Understand the scope of practice of various health and service professionals.
- Explain what constitutes the practice of medicine.
- Explain the difference between medical or rehabilitative massage and wellness massage.
- Develop a scope of practice for massage that respects the scope of practice of other professionals.

As mentioned earlier, the scope of practice of a profession defines the knowledge base and practice parameters of that profession. The scope of practice is defined and regulated by the government agency that has jurisdiction over the location of the practice. The individual practitioner is responsible for becoming fully informed about and compliant with these regulations. Each health and service profession has a unique knowledge base, yet members of many professions share a common knowledge and methodology. Because of this shared information, the lines defining a profession's scope of practice are not always clear, and overlap can occur.

The Massage Therapy Body of Knowledge presented a recommendation for scope of practice for massage therapy (Massage Therapy Body of Knowledge [MTBOK] Stewards, 2010). The Entry Level Analysis Project (ELAP) findings only imply a scope of practice based on the knowledge and skills that should be included in entry-level education. The Federation of State Massage Board's Model Practice Act recommends a scope of practice (Coalition of National Massage Therapy Organizations, 2013; Federation of State Massage, 2014). State, provincial, and municipal laws specify scopes of practice. The descriptions of the massage scope of practice are similar, but there is no single universally endorsed version. Each massage therapist must be in compliance with the regulatory mandates where they intend to practice.

The scope of practice evolves with the professional, from entry-level beginner to experienced practitioner, following a commitment to careerlong learning and professional practice. A professional must be able to evaluate an acquired body of knowledge and determine the parameters of ethical practice within the scope of practice. True professionals understand the limits of their knowledge and technical skills. Even if a massage therapy scope of practice includes a variety of methods and approaches, unless you have the specific knowledge and technical skill obtained through education and experience, those specific approaches are outside your personal scope of practice (Fig. 2.1). Massage therapists must also consider other professionals for whom massage is part of their scope of practice. Cosmetologists and estheticians can provide massage as part of their licensed services. Massage also is within the scope of practice for physical therapists, athletic trainers, nurses, acupuncturists, chiropractors, naturopaths, and physicians (both osteopathic and MD). The difference is that for massage therapists, massage is the primary practice method; other professionals use massage as a supplement to other methods.

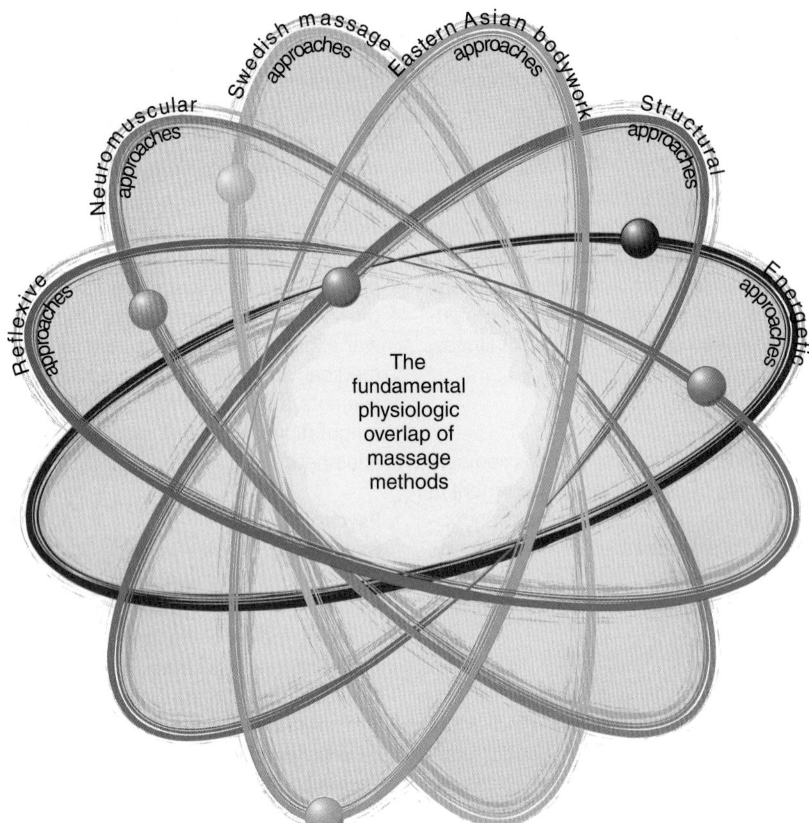

FIG. 2.1 The fundamental physiologic overlap of massage methods.

Professionals with more education are allowed to do more within their specialized fields. Those with less education work under supervision or within a limited scope of practice. The scope of practice for therapeutic massage should complement but not infringe upon the boundaries of the work of these professionals. We hope that the future of integrated health care will allow more flexibility and overlap of professional practice for the benefit of clients (Fig. 2.2).

Unique Scope of Practice Parameters for Therapeutic Massage

Therapeutic massage is unique in that it can be used in two distinct professional areas: wellness and health promotion, and medical care. There is extensive overlap between the two categories, which complicates the knowledge, skills, and abilities needed to support a professional scope of practice. Massage professionals participate in various levels of care and support, each requiring more education and expanded levels of competence. Recall the definitions of these terms from Chapter 1:

- Massage: Massage is a patterned and purposeful soft tissue manipulation accomplished by the use of digits, hands, forearms, elbows, knees, and/or feet, with or without the use of emollients, liniments, heat and cold, handheld tools, or other external apparatus, for the intent of therapeutic change.
- Massage therapy: Massage therapy consists of the application of massage and non–hands-on components, including health promotion and education messages, for self-care and health maintenance; therapy, as well as outcomes, can be influenced by: therapeutic relationships and communication; the therapist's education, skill level, and experience; and the therapeutic setting.
- Massage therapy practice: Massage therapy practice is a client-centered framework for providing massage therapy through a process of assessment and evaluation, plan of care, treatment, reassessment and reevaluation, health messages, documentation, and closure in an effort to improve health and/or well-being. Massage therapy practice is influenced by scope of practice and professional standards and ethics.

Also recall from Chapter 1 that massage therapy has two main categories of practice and six distinct practice settings. All the practice categories are equally important, and each requires a commitment of ongoing professional development.

- Wellness and health promotion
- Spa setting
- Massage franchise/wellness center
- Sports and fitness setting
- Independent massage practice
- Medical care
- Clinical/medical/rehabilitation settings
- Independent massage practice with clients who have more complex problems and/or medical conditions

The wellness and health promotions sector is the largest and most diverse practice category with the most autonomy. The medical sector is more contained, primarily limited to medical settings, focuses on support care, and is much less autonomous, with medical oversight involved. Typically massage care provided in the medical category is short term, and

Normal Adaptation
Client displays resourceful functioning with good ability to respond to and recover from stress.
Massage Training
500+ hours of education.
Health Care Supervision Required?
No.
Support Professionals
Fitness trainers, cosmetologists, wellness educators, prevention and healthy lifestyle–focused health care and mental health professionals.
Ineffective and Strained Adaptation
(Scope of practice encompasses normal adaptation)
Client displays ability to function with effort and reduced ability to respond to and recover from stress. Recovery time is increased. Client demands extraordinary function of body.
Massage Training
1000+ hours of education.
Poor Ability to Adapt
(Scope of practice encompasses technician and practitioner levels)
Client displays function breakdown — substantially reduced ability to respond and recover or extensive healing period required such as with surgery and trauma.
Massage Training
2000+ hours of education.
Health Care or Athletic Trainer Supervision Required?
Possibly. No for wellness service and mild dysfunctional patterns. Moderate to identifiable dysfunctional pattern — Yes, but indirect; attention to referral needs is important.
Support Professionals
Athletic trainers — exercise physiologist, health care and mental health professionals — spiritually based support.
Health Care Supervision Required?
Yes. Direct supervision for all clients in this category; Possibly for dysfunctional category; No for wellness clients.
Support Professionals
Entire multidisciplinary team — health care/mental health professionals — spiritually based support.
Comprehensive scope of practice for therapeutic massage
Wellness personal service scope of practice for therapeutic massage
Dysfunctional and athletic patterns scope of practice for therapeutic massage
Illness/trauma scope of practice for therapeutic massage

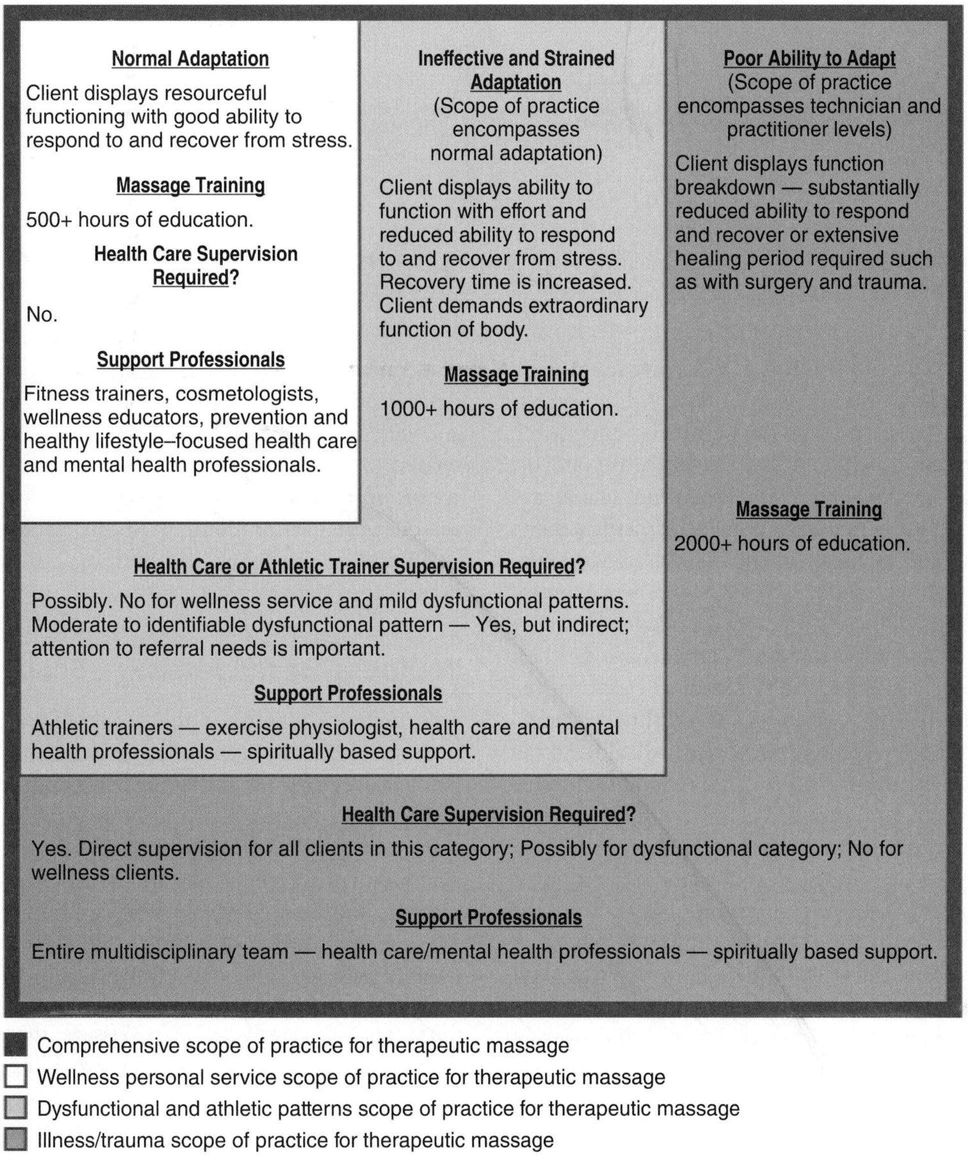

FIG. 2.2 The most expansive scope of practice for therapeutic massage is represented by the entire box *(outlined in dark blue).* Within this scope of practice are levels of professional function based on training and experience. The scope of practice for an entry-level position in therapeutic massage is represented by the Normal Adaptation box *(white box).* The next higher level of professional practice, the massage practitioner, is depicted in the Ineffective and Strained Adaptation Ability box *(light violet box).* The third and highest level of professional practice requires the most education and experience; it is depicted in the Poor or Inability to Adapt box *(light purple box).* Note that each level encompasses the one next to it. As the model shows, the scope of practice expands with experience and education effectively with all groups.

the intention is for clients to improve enough to be served in a more health maintenance and condition management care plan within the wellness and health promotions sector.

Within each practice category and practice setting, these outcomes are addressed: well-being/relaxation, stress management, pain management, and physical function. The main differences between the two categories of wellness and health promotion and medical care are the complexity of the clients' conditions, the increased risk of adverse effects, the need for adaptation to medical settings, the level of interdisciplinary interaction, and medical professional oversight. Additional education to function in the medical sector is not about advanced methods. Increased knowledge is necessary to identify cautions and contraindications that pose a risk for a complex client, understanding the implications for massage based on medical intervention and adaptation to the medical setting.

The two categories can overlap, and this is where most of the confusion about massage practice occurs. To help you sort out the practice overlap confusion, let's consider a model of health and disease.

Salutogenesis and the Wellness Continuum

Salutogenesis is a term coined by Aaron Antonovsky, a professor of medical sociology. The salutogenic mode involves a continuum, with movement toward health. The pathogenic

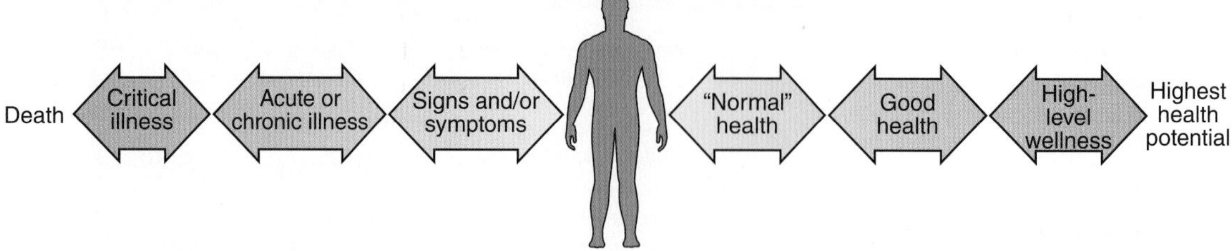

FIG. 2.3 The Illness to Health Continuum. From Chitty K., Black B.P. (2007). *Professional Nursing.* 5th ed. St. Louis: Saunders.

model, which is based on disease, is also a continuum, with movement away from disease. Massage therapy slides on the continuum, with a primary focus on well-being and health promotion rather than on factors that cause disease and the treatment of pathology. However, the full spectrum of massage therapy outcomes (well-being/relaxation, stress management, pain management, and physical function) have value in supporting medical treatment, sliding the scope of practice toward the more medical end of the continuum. The scope of practice is clear at either end, but as the middle is approached, the complexity of the client's condition and the medical care involved determine whether the massage therapist can function independently, with recommendations from the medical team but outside the medical environment, or with oversight within the medical structure as part of the medical treatment plan.

This concept of practice was described by John W. Travis, MD, in 1972 (Fig. 2.3). Dr. Travis describes medicine as typically treating injuries, disabilities, and symptoms to bring the individual to a "neutral point" where there is no longer any visible illness. However, the wellness paradigm requires moving the state of well-being further along the continuum toward optimal physical, emotional, and mental states. The concept assumes that well-being is a dynamic rather than a static process. Dr. Travis wrote and self-published the *Wellness Workbook* in 1977, which is now in a third edition.

A salutogenic approach, complemented by the illness–wellness continuum, focuses on factors of health and well-being rather than disease, and this is relevant to our understanding of the scope of practice for massage therapists. Well-being moves beyond problems and symptoms toward joy, happiness, enthusiasm, and hope. Within that framework, massage therapy may find clarity in the public health model, more so than in the medical model. The difference between public health and medicine is that medicine emphasizes disease treatment and care, whereas public health emphasizes disease prevention and health promotion. The primary goal of medicine is to provide treatment and medical care for individuals who have already developed a disease. Public health deals with preventing disease and promoting health at the community or population level.

Specialization and Scope of Practice

Regardless of the practice category and practice setting, specialization is an option. Specialization requires additional education and skills in a particular area, such as spa services, palliative care in hospice, elder care, athletics, pain management, prenatal and postnatal/postpartum clients, fitness, orthopedics, oncology, well-being, working with animals, addiction rehabilitation, scar tissue management, and active military and veterans. These specializations can be population focused, related to a practice environment, or method/approach and condition/outcome specific. Chapters 12 through 14 provide career specialization content. Specialization is always a step beyond entry level, and the additional knowledge and skills expand the scope of practice.

Wellness-Based Massage Scope of Practice

This textbook describes the scope of practice of wellness massage to be a nonspecific approach that focuses on assessment procedures for detecting contraindications to massage and determining if referral to other health care professionals is needed. A plan of care is focused on the development of a health-enhancing physical state for the client. The plan for the massage session is developed by combining the skills of the massage practitioner with intake and assessment information, desired massage outcomes, and direction from the client to provide an individualized massage session aimed at normalizing body systems. This normalization is accomplished through:

- External manual stimulation of the nervous, circulatory, and respiratory systems, connective tissue, and muscles to achieve:
  - Generalized stress reduction
  - A decrease in muscle tension
  - Symptomatic relief of pain related to soft tissue dysfunction
  - Other benefits similar to those of exercise
  - Other relaxation responses produced by therapeutic massage to increase the client's well-being and quality of life.

The wellness scope of practice is considered entry-level practice credentialed by licensure to protect the public safety and well-being. The ELAP education recommendations target this level of scope of practice.

The Medical Care-Based Massage Scope of Practice

This textbook describes the scope of practice for clinical massage delivered within the medical care setting and for massage provided in conjunction with specific athletic training protocols and rehabilitation care as: massage therapy developed to maintain, rehabilitate, or augment physical function; relieve or prevent physical dysfunction and pain; and enhance the well-being and quality of life of the client. The care program is developed in conjunction with various health care and medical professionals working together to support the client during medical treatment, rehabilitation, and a return to functional capacity, moving toward improved health status and well-being. The medical care scope of practice incorporates all of the knowledge and skills described in the wellness-based massage scope of practice with added education and experience in adaptation to reduce the client's risk in the medical setting. Specialization is likely indicated based on target population.

The information in this text can carry the student from the world of wellness massage into the world of medical health services primarily working to manage dysfunctional conditions, such as pain and chronic disorders, and to support those who may benefit from a generalized approach to massage, such as an athlete. Chapter 16 presents a series of case studies and treatment plans that provide a model of massage applications in both professional worlds.

Limits of Practice

A massage professional's ability to practice has legal limits. A scope of practice established by legislation both defines and limits the ability to practice massage. Respectful practice of therapeutic massage limits the scope of practice so that the practitioner does not encroach on the scope of practice of other professionals.

Each professional also has personal limits that affect the scope of practice. These limits involve the type and extent of the person's education, personal biases, life experiences, specific interests in terms of the type of client served, and any physical limitations, such as size and endurance levels.

Both personal and professional practice limits are valid and valuable. They allow us to set and maintain boundaries that support a variety of professionals especially in an integrated and multidisciplinary wellness or medical setting. Limits of practice free us from falling into the trap of believing we must be all things to all people; we cannot be, and it is ethical to acknowledge the limits of practice and to collaborate with other professionals.

Massage professionals who provide health services at the level of supportive wellness care require fundamental information about general wellness processes. Massage professionals should be able to provide health messaging related to stress management, including effective breathing, progressive relaxation, and quieting responses (meditation-type activities); they should be able to give general dietary recommendations; and they should emphasize the importance of appropriate exercise programs.

Massage professionals are able to function autonomously in a wellness scope of practice. A properly trained massage professional can recognize a client who is not functioning effectively, not recovering from the stress of daily activities, and beginning to fall into dysfunctional patterns. As the client's problems become more complicated, requiring increased expertise, referral and collaboration with supervision is indicated. Clients in this category benefit from a specifically designed care/treatment plan that includes a means of measuring the outcomes of care objectively. Realistic and attainable short- and long-term goals are developed, and time frames are set for the achievement of these goals. The general goals of the massage professional are to help the client move toward normal functioning, regain personal control of the body/mind/spirit systems, and achieve and maintain optimal health.

Body/Mind/Spirit Connection

The body, mind, and spirit share a definite link. The physical body functions involve anatomy and physiology, including the body's chemical responses. Feelings are body functions.

The cognitive process of the mind interprets physical sensations and sets physical responses in motion. Emotions seem to be the result of the interplay between body and mind. Behavior is the action that results from the physical-emotional-cognitive combination.

The spirit provides the strength, hope, faith, and love that create a reason for being. Each of these areas of functioning influences and interacts with the others.

In reality, the body, mind, and spirit cannot be separated; however, together they involve too much information to allow a professional to become an expert in all areas of human function. Professional skill levels, the parameters of the scope of practice, and avoidance of dual and multiple roles in the professional relationship artificially divide the body, mind, and spirit functioning of the person seeking assistance. This is undesirable, but it is often unavoidable. An excellent solution is for professionals to work together. A multidisciplinary, integrative approach to care is best, with professionals working together to support a comprehensive care plan that addresses all the client's needs. Most hospice programs are excellent models of multidisciplinary teams.

Honoring Scope of Practice

As a massage professional, you can determine whether you are within your scope of practice by making sure your responses to the client are from a body and massage perspective. When a client expresses distress, shares personal information, or requests specific information, first determine whether the issue is most specifically a body, mind, or spirit issue. If it is a mental or spiritual issue, use listening skills and acknowledge the situation, but do not attempt to problem-solve or provide professional intervention. If the situation presented is a physical concern (i.e., affects the body), decide whether the information falls within the scope of therapeutic massage and respond accordingly.

The severity or complexity of a situation determines whether simple empathetic listening, without advice being given, is sufficient or whether a professional referral is indicated. Often the physical stress of the circumstances can be managed by massage approaches while the client seeks additional help from supportive resources and professionals who can deal more specifically with the source of the problem. Massage therapists recognize when to refer individuals to these professionals.

Medical, athletic training, coaching, and cosmetology professionals have committed a significant part of their lives to formal schooling, licensing procedures, and continual experiential and formal education. The information they have acquired is specific to their professional discipline yet also quite broad. Although massage techniques may not be common knowledge among many professionals, the importance and power of touch are. Many of these professionals understand that massage practitioners use touch skills these other professionals may be unable to provide. To develop and support a cooperative, multidisciplinary philosophy of care, massage professionals must respect the dedication of the professionals with whom they work by maintaining the appropriate scope of practice for therapeutic massage.

Massage professionals benefit from being able to adapt massage therapy to various health and medical care, sports and fitness training, and personal service needs; in doing so, they are best able to serve both the professionals with whom they work and the clients they serve. In a multidisciplinary team setting (e.g., the spa environment, which may employ wellness professionals, fitness and sports professionals, and medical professionals), it is important to be able to communicate effectively with any professional with whom you work; this requires you to be familiar with the language and terminology used in that profession. It is important to be able to explain massage therapy interventions in terms familiar to the professionals on the team as well as explain the ways you, as a massage therapist, intend to support them in providing appropriate care.

Consultation

As the scope of practice blends between the wellness and medical practice spectrum, multiple health and wellness professionals are working together in multidisciplinary centers or through networking. Consultation is how we professionally communicate in these settings.

Consultation is exchanging information and experience about something in order to reach a better understanding or to make an informed decision (Noble et al., 2022). A productive consultation is all about the right questions being asked and answered. Consultation is an organized process

- Gather all relevant information
- Identify the issues
- Develop pertinent questions
- Organized meeting agenda
- Schedule meeting (recommend 15 minutes maximum)
- Use time efficiently
- Stay on topic
- Listen and take notes
- Ask clarifying questions
- Schedule follow-up meeting if needed.

EVIDENCE-BASED/EVIDENCE-INFORMED PRACTICE

SECTION OBJECTIVES

Chapter objective covered in this section:

3. Define evidence-based practice and evidence-informed practice.

Using the information presented in this section, the student will be able to:

- Explain the importance of an evidence-based/evidence-informed practice as an aspect of professional behavior.
- List the skills necessary to perform massage from an evidence-based and evidence-informed professional foundation.

As massage therapy becomes a common part of an integrated health and medical care system, the massage therapy profession will be expected to maintain high levels of professional practice. **Practices** are defined as skills, techniques, and strategies that can be used by a practitioner. One area in which massage therapists must become educated is evidence-based practice and evidence-informed practice. **Evidence-based practice (EBP)** is defined as "the conscientious, explicit, and judicious use of current best evidence in making decisions about the care of individual patients" (Sackett et al., 2000). Evidence-based practices are validated by some form of documented scientific evidence. This includes findings established through controlled clinical studies, meta-analyses, and systematic reviews (Chapter 5); however, other methods of establishing evidence may be valid as well. For many years, the term *evidence-based* has been used freely by health care professionals. More recently the term *evidence-informed* is used.

Although the evidence-based process was defined for physicians, it has been adopted by many professions and used to develop clinical practice guidelines.

Clinical practice guidelines are systematically developed statements that assist practitioners and clients in making decisions about appropriate health care by providing evidence-informed recommendations. Expert opinion and consensus statements guide clinical decision making where/when evidence is insufficient to inform practice. The massage therapy community has not developed clinical practice guidelines. However, a massage practitioner may encounter these types of procedures if part of integrated health care.

Standard of Care

A *standard of care* is the assessment and treatment process that a clinician (e.g., massage therapist) should follow based on similarly qualified practitioners in the same or similar circumstances. The massage therapy community, with the support of the Massage Therapy Foundation, has committed to developing best practices guidelines. Best practices guidelines are standards of care determined and practiced by our profession.

A role of the Massage Therapy Foundation is to develop an inclusive process to identify evidence-based/evidence-informed practice guidelines, backed by systematic academic and peer review and clinical research when available. This process is in its infancy and will evolve over time.

Evidence-informed practice (EIP) allows for innovation while incorporating the lessons learned from the existing research literature. Ideally, evidence-based and evidence-informed programs and practices coexist, but professionals need to be clear about each category when describing method validity. If a method is evidence based, the assumption is that benefit has been confirmed. If a method is evidence informed, the validity of the claimed result is less reliable. The EIP model provides a framework to provide and justify effective care (Woodbury and Kuhnke, 2014; Guy and Majumder, 2022; Sarkies et al., 2022; Kumah et al., 2022).

Evidence-informed practice uses:

- The best available research
- Logical, plausible suppositions (a *supposition* is an educated guess or hypothesis)

- Expert opinion consensus, meaning that a majority of experts agree
- Practice knowledge based on clinical experience

Currently, not enough high-quality research is available for therapeutic massage practice to be considered completely evidence based; however, the research is improving. In Chapter 5, we discuss the research current as of this text's publication. Massage therapy is moving closer to being evidence based, but it is more accurate to describe massage methods and outcomes as evidence informed.

Evidence-based/evidence-informed practice requires that decisions about health care be based on the best available, current, valid, and relevant evidence. These decisions should be made by those receiving care, informed by the knowledge of those providing care, within the context of available resources. To function in the evidence-based/evidence-informed health care structure, you must be able to:

- Find, read, and analyze research (this is called *research literacy*)
- Analyze the accuracy of clinically based evidence of massage benefit when research is not able to validate fully the massage result
- Use clinical reasoning to apply the information to massage practice
- Apply information derived from the clinical reasoning process to develop outcome-based massage sessions
- Justify decisions related to indications and contraindications to massage applications for individual clients
- Address each client in a client-centered manner, individualizing the massage for that particular client based on valid evidence

Developing an evidence-based/evidence-informed massage practice is a process. It is important to begin now, at the start of your education, to use the best available research evidence, clinical reasoning, experience, and professional knowledge to provide the best massage care for each individual client. Evidence-based/evidence-informed practice is a mark of professionalism. Research literacy, clinical reasoning, and outcome-based massage applications are discussed throughout this textbook, especially in Chapter 5. Evidence changes as more sophisticated research emerges. Massage therapists need remain current and be willing to evolve with the information.

Evidence in Evidence-Based/Evidence-Informed Practice

Evidence can be generated from a range of sources, including but not limited to:

- Academic journals (e.g., the Journal of Bodywork and Movement Therapies and the International Journal of Therapeutic Massage & Bodywork: Research, Education, & Practice)
- The Massage Therapy Foundation
- Research and systematic reviews of research
- The Internet (e.g., PubMed, Google Scholar, Medline)
- Data gathered from other massage therapists, especially in the form of case reports
- Knowledge gained from experienced massage therapists and other health care professionals

Evidence-informed practice includes:

- Practice knowledge and experience
- The expert opinions of colleagues and other professionals
- Intuitive or gut feelings
- The wishes and experiences of clients
- Evidence from research in massage or other, similar disciplines

You may want to use evidence to:

- Explain and justify your reasons for a decision
- Help you choose among different approaches
- Explain what the research says about the massage services a client is receiving
- Raise your awareness about a condition or illness

Once evidence has been gathered, these questions are to be answered:

- How relevant is the evidence to what we are seeking to understand or decide?
- How does the evidence represent the population that concerns us?
- How reliable and valid is the source of the evidence?

The original concept was evidence-based practice, meaning that quality evidence was available to support actions. However, in many disciplines, such as massage, research cannot always be related to practice. When we provide therapeutic massage for a client, we want to be as evidence based as possible and evidence informed when definitive evidence does not exist.

Professional and ethical behavior dictates that massage professionals must disclose to clients and others the current status of research and must not make definitive claims for methods that have not yet undergone the scrutiny of qualified researchers. Also, it is okay that we may never truly understand the multilayered benefits of compassionate touch.

INFORMED CONSENT

SECTION OBJECTIVES

Chapter objective covered in this section:

4. Complete an informed consent process.

Using the information presented in this section, the student will be able to:

- List and explain the nine components of informed consent.
- Determine whether a client can provide informed consent for a massage.
- Prepare written client information materials to support the informed consent process.
- Complete two types of informed consent forms.

Informed consent is a protection process for the consumer. It requires that clients understand what will occur, that they participate voluntarily, and that they be competent to give consent. Informed consent is also an educational procedure that allows clients to decide knowledgeably whether they want to receive a massage, whether they want a particular therapist to work with them, and whether the professional structure, including client rules and regulations, is acceptable to them. Informed consent supports professional ethical behavior. It reflects the ethical principle of client participation and self-determination in a client-centered approach.

Clients must be able to provide informed consent and demonstrate that they understand the information presented to them (Proficiency Exercise 2.1). Parents or guardians must provide informed consent for minors. Guardians must provide informed consent for those unable to do so (e.g., clients with dementia). Ethical decision making becomes important in gray areas, such as when a language barrier exists, and the massage professional is not sure the client understands or when any form of intoxication or prescription drug use alters the client's judgment.

True informed consent presents the opportunity to evaluate the options available and the risks involved in each method; it also requires the massage professional to include information about the inherent and potential benefits and hazards of the proposed treatment, the alternatives available, and the probable results if treatment is not provided. Clients have the legal right to choose from a range of suggested options and to receive enough information to allow them to pick the most appropriate approach for them. Credentials and personal and professional limitations that may affect the client–therapist relationship are disclosed. Clients also need information about recourse options if the outcomes of the massage are undesirable. As professionals, we are ethically bound to ensure that the client makes choices based on a solid understanding of the information presented. The professional is responsible for providing the client with this information (Box 2.3).

PROFICIENCY EXERCISE 2.1

Gather in groups of three and write about a specific situation in which informed consent would be difficult to obtain from a client. For example, the client has diminished hearing, or you do not speak the client's language. The groups should then exchange responses and role-play potential situations wherein one learner acts as the massage practitioner, another as the client, and the third evaluates the way the situation is managed. Try different situations until each learner has had a chance to play each role.

Box 2.3 Informed Consent

The following questions should be answered at the outset of the professional relationship:

- What are the goals of the therapeutic program?
- What services will be provided?
- What behavior is expected of the client?
- What are the risks and benefits of the process?
- What are the practitioner's qualifications?
- What are the financial considerations?
- How long is the therapy expected to last?
- What are the limitations of confidentiality?
- In what areas does the professional have mandatory reporting requirements?

Intake Procedures

Single or random massage sessions targeting relaxation and well-being goals do not necessarily require a comprehensive intake procedure. Instead, possible contraindications to massage are identified. The informed consent process informs the client of the limitations of a single massage session and describes the approaches used in the single-session massage experience (Proficiency Exercise 2.1).

A comprehensive intake procedure, including an informed consent process, is necessary when addressing how defined outcomes will span a series of sessions. The **initial treatment plan** states the therapeutic goals, duration of the sessions, number of appointments needed to meet the agreed-on goals, cost, general classification of intervention to be used, and an objective method for measuring progress and identifying when goals have been reached (the forms used for these procedures are presented in Chapters 4 and 11).

A form with all the pertinent information is signed by the client and kept in the massage practitioner's files. Maintaining a record of signed informed consent forms is an important legal issue; in many jurisdictions, touching a person without the person's consent is an action that can be prosecuted as battery.

The following is a possible sequence for obtaining informed consent.

1. The massage professional provides a general explanation of massage, supported by written information (often in the form of a brochure) about indications, benefits, contraindications, potential risk for adverse effects and alternative approaches that provide benefits similar to those of massage.
2. The massage professional informs the client about the scope of practice for massage; reporting measures for professional misconduct and recourse policies; the professional's training, experience, and credentials; and any limiting factors that may affect the professional relationship, including lack of training in a particular area and any special circumstances related to the massage professional (e.g., hearing or vision difficulty) that may need to be considered. The client is given written information covering these topics, often in the form of a brochure, to enhance the understanding of this discussion.
3. The massage professional then discusses business and professional policies and procedures, including the logical consequences of noncompliance by the client. These policies include handling of payment, returned checks, additional charges, gratuities, late arrival, scheduling, sexual impropriety, draping, hygiene, sanitation, confidentiality, and rights of refusal. The client also is given pertinent written information about these topics, such as a professional policy statement (Box 2.4).
4. After these procedures, the client signs an informed consent form. The client should not be overwhelmed with extensive, detailed information; however, it is important to provide enough information for the individual to make an informed choice. Informed consent is a continual process, and client education and involvement always supported and encouraged.

Initial Care/Treatment Plan

As mentioned previously, if the client is working toward specific outcome goals that will require several appointments, an

Box 2.4 Developing a Client Brochure and Policy Statement (Electronic or Paper-Based)

A massage professional should cover these important points when developing a client brochure and policy statement. If you will be working as an employee (spa franchise or health and sport center), the business will have policy statements and brochures. This information is posted to the business website. Use this list to ensure that the employer-provided information is sufficient.

Type of Service

- Explain the type of massage you provide.
- Explain the benefits and limitations of this particular style of massage.
- Specify whether you specialize in working with a particular group, such as older adults, athletes, or people with specific problems, such as headaches or back pain.
- Indicate any situations or conditions with which you do not care to work, such as pregnancy or certain medical conditions. Provide a brief explanation to avoid implying discrimination; for example, "Because I do not have specific training in geriatric care, I refer clients over the age of 80."

Training and Experience

- If your state requires licensing or if you are board certified, provide documentation.
- State how long you have been in practice.
- Provide information about continuing education you have pursued.
- Provide information about any additional education (e.g., you are also an athletic trainer).
- Provide the names of any professional organizations of which you are an active member.

Appointment Policies

- Request personal information such as last name, address, phone number, etc.
- Have new clients fill out the intake form in advance.
- Clients pay in advance with a credit card.
- Client etiquette which is the customary code of polite behavior
- Inappropriate behavior and consequences
- Specify the length of an average session. Include time spent on intake and exit interviews and actual hands-on massage.
- Inform the client of the days you work and your hours and whether you provide mobile/on-site residential or business work.
- Inform the client that the first appointment for intake will be longer than subsequent appointments.
- State whether you take walk-in appointments or only work by appointment.
- Describe an optimum appointment schedule, such as weekly or every other week.
- Be clear about the cancellation policy and your policy for late appointments.
- Explain to the client any change in or restriction on physical activity before or after the session.

Client and Practitioner Expectations

- Explain in detail what happens at the first massage session (i.e., paperwork, health history, and other preliminaries).
- Make sure clients know they can partly undress or undress down to their underclothes and that they are always covered and draped during the session.
- Explain policies related to massage for the chest, abdomen, inner thigh near the groin, and gluteal regions.
- Explain the order in which you massage (face up or face down to begin), the parts of the body on which you work and in what order, whether you use oils or creams, if a shower is available before or after the massage, and if bathing at home before the massage appointment is expected.
- If specific products are used for massage, including lubricants and essential oils, explain how you will inform the client before exposure to prevent an allergic reaction.
- Make sure clients understand that they should tell you immediately if anything feels uncomfortable.
- If you have low lighting and music during the session, be sure the client is comfortable with that atmosphere.
- Make sure the client understands when a reaction might be expected, such as tenderness when direct-pressure methods are used.
- Tell clients that before the session, you will discuss with them the goals for the massage and the proposed styles and methods of massage, and that consent must be given for all massage procedures.
- Inform the client that your profession has a code of ethics and explain your policy on confidentiality.
- Let clients know that if they are uncomfortable in any way, a friend or relative may accompany them.
- Inform clients that they can stop the massage at any time and do not need to give a reason for doing so. Inform clients that the massage therapist can stop the massage at any time if they feel uncomfortable or unsafe with the behavior of the client or if other circumstances indicate that the session should end.

Fees

Make sure your fee structure is clearly defined regarding:

- What the fees are
- Different fees for variations in the length of a session
- Additional fees for add-on services
- Whether a series of sessions can be bought at a discount
- If there is a cost savings membership plan and the details of billing
- How often you raise your fees
- Whether you have a sliding fee scale
- Whether you take only cash or will accept money orders, checks, or credit cards
- Whether you bill
- Whether you accept insurance
- How often insurance covers your services

Sexually Inappropriate Behavior

- Sexual behavior by the therapist toward the client or by the client toward the therapist is always unethical, inappropriate, and may be a crime. It is always the responsibility of the therapist or health professional to ensure that sexual misconduct does not occur.
- A client who feels that the massage therapist has acted inappropriately should feel free to address this issue immediately. When necessary, the client has the right to inform

Continued

Box 2.4 Developing a Client Brochure and Policy Statement (Electronic or Paper-Based)—cont'd

the police, in addition to the massage therapist's licensing board, certification body, and professional organization. Contact information for these organizations should be provided.

- A person who asks someone to commit an illegal act has committed the criminal act of solicitation. If a person is looking to pay for sex and makes this request by words or gestures, the person can be arrested for solicitation of prostitution. If either the client or the massage therapist is solicited for sex for pay, this is an illegal act, and the police should be called.
- Clearly state that flirting, inappropriate touching, and sexual innuendos will not be tolerated. The police will be called for any indication of solicitation (seeking to engage another to commit a crime) and assault (unlawful contact with another person or the threat to do so).

Recourse Policy

Describe the policy to be followed when a client is unhappy or dissatisfied. Explain how you issue a refund (full or partial). Let the client know that if the matter is not managed satisfactorily, a professional organization or licensing board is available where complaints can be registered. Contact information for this organization should be provided.

NOTE: Some employers and massage professionals make client policy and procedure booklets available on the business website. It is helpful for the client to review this information before the scheduled appointment.

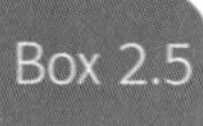

Box 2.5 Development of the Initial Care or Treatment Plan

First, the client's goals and desired outcomes for the massage sessions are determined. The client agrees to proceed with the next part of the session, which consists of history taking using a client information form and a physical assessment using an assessment form (see Chapters 4 and 11). The information is evaluated to develop a care plan for the client. Care plans usually consist of a series of sessions.

A care or treatment plan is developed that spells out:

- Specific outcomes (i.e., the therapeutic goals)
- The frequency of visits (number of appointments per week or month) and the duration of visits (e.g., 30, 50, or 90 minutes)
- The estimated number of appointments needed to achieve the therapeutic goals (e.g., 10 sessions, 15 sessions, ongoing)
- General methods to be used (e.g., therapeutic massage, muscle energy methods, neuromuscular methods, connective tissue methods)
- Objective progress measurements (e.g., pain reduced [based on a scale of 1–10], 50% increase in range of motion, sleep improved by increasing 1 hour per night, episodes of tension headache reduced from four per week to one per week, feelings of relaxation maintained for 24 hours)

The client provides (informed) consent for the care or treatment plan by signing the appropriate form.

initial treatment plan is completed (Box 2.5). Specific details on completing this process are provided in Chapter 4.

The process of assessing needs, identifying goals, and developing a treatment plan takes 30 minutes to 1 hour and constitutes the initial intake procedure. In complex circumstances, this process can extend over the first two or three sessions. It is appropriate to charge for the intake session, which is an important part of the professional interaction. The treatment plan may evolve or change during subsequent sessions as the client's needs change during the therapeutic process. The initial treatment plan is the massage practitioner's best educated guess as to how the therapeutic relationship will proceed.

When massage is used in a very nonspecific way, especially if the client will be seen only once or if a series of massage sessions is not appropriate, the massage professional need not perform an extensive assessment or develop a comprehensive treatment plan. Instead, the practitioner should predetermine the outcome of the session by informing the client that, under these circumstances, no specific work can be done, and that massage can provide relaxation and general normalizing of the body. A short history and physical assessment are done to detect any contraindications to massage. A condensed version of the client policy statement is prepared and provided in written form. The client always provides formal written consent for the massage. An example of an informed consent process is presented in Box 2.6.

CONFIDENTIALITY

SECTION OBJECTIVES

Chapter objective covered in this section:

5. Practice procedures to maintain client confidentiality.

Using the information presented in this section, the student will be able to:

- Establish and maintain client confidentiality.
- Complete a release of information form.

Confidentiality is the principle that the client's information is private and belongs to the client. It is built on respect and trust. In professional terms, confidentiality concerns client information and files. Client information is never discussed with anyone other than the client without the client's written permission. During peer counseling or supervision, client confidentiality extends to the professionals we consult. Even when the client's name is withheld, a unique situation often is enough to breach confidentiality requirements.

Client files must represent information accurately and only as it relates to the service offered. Personal information about a situation that involves a muscle or skeletal complaint need not be recorded. For example, a client describes having a headache and says that a coworker is disruptive and the manager does nothing about it, which they feel contributes to the tension aggravating the headache. The only part recorded in the client's

Box 2.6 Informed Consent Process

A new client arrives for a massage. The massage therapist asks if the client read the polices statements on the therapist's website and also shows the client an informational brochure briefly explaining massage, the current evidence that supports benefit and the general contraindications, and the procedures and process of massage. The client reads the information. The massage professional then discusses the information with the client. In general terms, the massage professional explains alternatives to massage, such as exercise and meditation, which provide benefits similar to massage.

The massage professional then tells the client about their professional background; for example, they graduated from a state-licensed massage therapy school 2 years earlier after a training program of 625 hours; is licensed and recently achieved Board Certification by the National Certification Board for Therapeutic Massage; has been in professional practice part time for 2 years and averages eight massages a week; has taken additional training in myofascial approaches, pain management, and massage for older adults (approximately 50 contact hours for each). The client is given information on methods of reporting misconduct by the massage therapist to state agencies, national professional organizations, and the police.

The massage therapist gives the client the policy and procedures booklet or statement and is asked to read it. The massage professional goes over the booklet with the client, point by point, assuring the client understands the massage therapist's rules and requirements. The massage professional makes sure to discuss the requirements to report abuse and any threat of deadly harm, in addition to the release of files by court order.

The massage professional then hands the client a consent form (such as this example).

I, (client's name) ______________________, have received a copy of the policies for Massage Works operated______. I have read Massage Works' policies, and I understand them. The massage procedures, information about massage in general, general benefits of massage, contraindications to massage, and possible alternatives have been explained to me. The qualifications of the massage professional and reporting measures for misconduct have been disclosed to me.

I understand that the massage I receive is for the purpose of relaxation and well-being, stress reduction, and relief from muscular tension, spasm, or pain and to support functional movement. If I experience any pain or discomfort, I will immediately inform the massage practitioner so that the pressure or methods can be adjusted to my comfort level. I understand that massage professionals do not diagnose illness or disease or perform any spinal manipulations, nor do they prescribe any medical treatments, and nothing said or done during the session should be construed as such. I acknowledge that massage is not a substitute for medical examination or diagnosis and that I should see a health care provider for those services. Because massage should not be performed under certain circumstances, I agree to keep the massage practitioner updated as to any changes in my health profile, and I release the massage professional from any liability if I fail to do so.

Client's signature ______________________

Date ____________

Therapist's signature ______________________

Date ____________

Consent to Treat a Minor

By my signature I authorize (therapist's name) ____________ ____________ to provide therapeutic massage to my child or dependent.

Signature of Parent or Guardian ______________________

Date ____________

For clients who will have several sessions, the next step is completion of the initial care or treatment plan (presented in detail in Chapter 4).

Modified Informed Consent Form for Single Session

For clients who will be seen only once or are receiving a promotional introductory massage (e.g., the professional is working on a cruise ship, doing sports massage at an event, or doing promotional chair massage at a health fair), the following modification to informed consent can be made.

I, (client's name) ______________________, have received a copy of the policies for (name of business) ___ ______________________, operated by (owner) ______________________. I have read the rules and policies, and I understand them. The general benefits of massage and contraindications to massage have been explained to me. I have disclosed to the therapist any condition I have that would contraindicate massage. Other than to determine contraindications, I understand that no specific needs assessment has been performed. The qualifications of the massage professional and reporting measures for misconduct have been disclosed to me.

I understand that the massage I receive is for the purpose of relaxation and well-being. If I experience any pain or discomfort, I will immediately inform the massage practitioner so that the pressure or methods can be adjusted to my comfort level. I understand that massage professionals do not diagnose illness or disease or perform any spinal manipulations, nor do they prescribe any medical treatments. I acknowledge that massage is not a substitute for medical examination or diagnosis and that I should see a health care provider for those services.

I understand that a single massage session or massage used on a random basis is limited to providing a general, nonspecific massage approach using standard massage methods and does not include any methods to specifically address soft tissue structure or function.

Client's signature ______________________

Date ____________

Therapist's signature ______________________

Date ____________

Consent to Treat a Minor

By my signature I authorize (therapist's name)____________ ____________ to provide massage work to my child or dependent.

Signature of Parent or Guardian ______________________

Date ____________

NOTE: It is becoming more common for this informed consent information to be provided and signed electronically.

file is their belief that emotional tension is contributing to the headache. Including more of the story would be considered a breach of confidentiality because it makes a permanent record of an event that may be made public if the client's files are ordered released to the court.

Confidentiality also pertains to public recognition. Massage practitioners should not acknowledge a client in public unless the client recognizes and greets the professional first; to do so may place clients in the position of having it revealed that they were seeking professional massage therapy services, a fact they may want kept private.

Potential Limits of Confidentiality

Clients must be told during initial informed consent procedures that files may be ordered and released to the court. Massage therapists have no professional exemptions. Clients must be made to understand these limits to confidentiality during the informed consent procedures.

Clients also must be informed that confidentiality will be breached under laws *Duty-to-Warn or Duty-to-Protect Laws* that require professionals to report abuse and threat of deadly harm. Mandatory reporters may include social workers, teachers and other school personnel, childcare providers, physicians and other health care workers, mental health professionals, and law enforcement officers. Depending on juristical regulation massage therapists may be classified as mandatory reporters. The California Supreme Court stated, "The protective privilege ends where the public peril begins."

If information is disclosed to you that a child, an elderly person, or a person who may be physically or mentally unable to report abuse or protect themselves is being harmed, as a professional, you must report this alleged abuse to the appropriate government agencies. If a client threatens deadly harm to another person or themselves, professionalism requires reporting this information to the police or an appropriate agency. If the massage therapist is working in a supervised setting such as a medical care facility, reporting occurs through supervisory channels. Because the massage professional is not specifically trained to identify or diagnose those who may harm themselves or others, all threats must be taken seriously. In these most difficult situations, the massage professional should seek legal counsel on ways to proceed.

To allow professionals to exchange information, the client must sign a release-of-information form (Box 2.7).

Box 2.7 Release of Information Form

This is an example of a release of information form.

I, (client's name) ______________________, grant permission for (therapist's name) ______________________, a massage therapist, to provide or exchange information with (other professional's name) ______________________ about the following conditions ______________________ for the time frame beginning (dates) ______________ and ending ______________. This permission may be revoked at any time either verbally or in writing.

Client's signature ______________________

Date ______________

A copy of the release-of-information form is kept in the client's file, and the original is sent to the consulting professional. The use of the term *exchange information* in the form allows each professional involved to share pertinent information; otherwise, each professional must obtain a release-of-information form from the client to share information about that client.

HEALTH INSURANCE PORTABILITY AND ACCOUNTABILITY ACT OF 1996 (HIPAA)

SECTION OBJECTIVES

Chapter objective covered in this section:

6. Describe basic functions of the Health Insurance Portability and Accountability Act (HIPAA) and the training in its rules and requirements.

Using the information presented in this section, the student will be able to:

- Explain the purpose of HIPAA and list the three primary areas it covers.
- Define the chain of trust.
- Store records in a HIPAA-compliant manner.
- Locate additional information about HIPAA.
- Describe the training for meeting HIPAA requirements.

The Health Insurance Portability and Accountability Act was signed into law by President Bill Clinton on August 21, 1996. Conclusive regulations were issued on August 17, 2000, to be instituted by October 16, 2002. HIPAA requires that the transactions of all patient health care information be formatted in a standardized electronic style. In addition to protecting the privacy and security of patient information, HIPAA includes legislation on the formation of medical savings accounts, the authorization of a fraud and abuse control program, the easy transport of health insurance coverage, and the simplification of administrative terms and conditions. HIPAA encompasses three primary areas, and its privacy requirements can be broken down into three types:

- Privacy standards
- Patients' rights
- Administrative requirements

Not all massage practices need to be compliant with HIPAA regulations. A practice that must comply is called a *covered entity.* A covered entity is one of the following:

- Health care provider
- Doctors
- Clinics
- Psychologists
- Dentists
- Chiropractors
- Nursing homes
- Pharmacies
- Health plan or health care clearinghouse
- Health insurance companies
- Health maintenance organizations (HMOs)
- Company health plans
- Government programs that pay for health care, such as Medicare, Medicaid, and the military and veterans' health care programs

Massage therapists are more likely to have to comply with HIPAA regulations if they practice in a medical care environment. The confidentiality requirements to protect client privacy have the greatest effect on massage practice. Because massage therapists obtain a client health history, maintain client records, and may communicate with other health and medical care professionals, including transmitting records (electronically or not), it is prudent to function in compliance with HIPAA's requirements regardless of whether one is a covered entity.

Chain of Trust

If patient/client data are shared with a third party, a certain level of trust must be established to ensure that the external parties to whom data are passed can guarantee that they will maintain data integrity and confidentiality; this is called the *chain of trust.* A chain-of-trust agreement must take the form of an approved and formal contract in which the responsibilities of the individual parties are clearly outlined.

Security measures include the following:

- Obtain written consent from the client for email communication that specifically relates to health records. Put a confidentiality notice on all faxes and emails. Avoid using this type of communication for confidential information.
- Do not leave files where they are accessible to unauthorized individuals.
- Keep appointment books private, and practice password-protected software management.
- Do not discuss any medical information with a third party without written authorization from the client.

Data Storage

Massage therapists also need to inform clients of how electronic record keeping is used. This is important because more massage therapists are using electronic practice management software that includes HIPAA-related content. A HIPAA declaration that clearly describes the process for management of a client's records must be available for the client to read and sign. This document should include:

- Use of the client's information
- The type of storage method used to secure the client's files
- Situations in which disclosure of information may be required
- Information on how clients can obtain copies of their records

The HIPAA notice must be posted where it is clearly visible to clients, and each client should be given a copy of this notice. All personnel involved with the client should be trained in HIPAA procedures.

Protected Health Information

HIPAA defines protected health information (PHI) as confidential, personal, identifiable health information about individuals that is created or received and is transmitted or maintained in any form. "Identifiable" means that a person reading this information could reasonably use it to identify an individual. A piece of health-related information becomes PHI if it has these elements (among others):

- Name
- Address
- Email address
- Birth date (except year)
- Social Security number

Massage therapists must keep up to date on the HIPAA requirements.

Training in HIPAA Requirements

Massage professionals must obtain the appropriate training for HIPAA compliance. Different work environments have different compliance procedures; therefore employment-related compliance training is important.

HIPAA's Privacy Rule stipulates that all members of the enterprise workforce receive training that is appropriate to their organizational roles. The "workforce" includes employees, volunteers, trainees, and other individuals who work for a covered entity, regardless of whether it pays them. Some staff members must be trained in applying specific policies and procedures, such as providing the notice of information practices or obtaining authorizations. Others may require only an overview of HIPAA's background, objectives, principles, and general regulatory requirements.

New employees who join the organization must receive training within a reasonable period. Often, the practical course is to include HIPAA privacy training in new employee orientation programs, particularly because privacy principles easily fit into discussions of the organization's mission and infrastructure. Workforce members who change jobs or receive new responsibilities must receive additional training if their new job duties include new patient privacy-related responsibilities. Further, the Privacy Rule requires retraining for each member of the covered entity's workforce whose functions are affected by a material change in policies or procedures.

Covered entities must also document that privacy training has been provided. Although members of the workforce are not required to sign a certificate after training, documenting the completion of training by each worker is useful for future verification purposes.

The privacy provisions do not prescribe the nature of the required training; the Department of Health and Human Services has left the design, approach, and specific content to the discretion of the covered entity. However, it is recommended that, at the very least, the following topics be covered with all members of the workforce:

- Principles and objectives of HIPAA's Privacy Rule
- Background (e.g., what constitutes PHI)
- Need for privacy of PHI
- Overview of HIPAA privacy regulations, including penalties
- Individual's rights regarding privacy
- Individual's rights regarding control of uses and disclosure of PHI
- Individual's right to request access, accounting, and amendment
- New organizational privacy policies and procedures
- Sanction policy
- Notice of privacy practices

- Authorizations for use and disclosure
- Privacy officer's role and contact information
- Complaint policies and procedures
- Cooperating with investigations or audits
- Reporting of violations and the whistleblower policy
- The organization's commitment to patient privacy

More specialized training in detailed HIPAA requirements and internal procedural changes must be tailored for workforce groups directly affected by these requirements or changes in the course of their work. Up-to-date information about HIPAA is found on the US Department of Health and Human Services website. Use the search term *HIPAA*.

PROFESSIONAL BOUNDARIES

SECTION OBJECTIVES

Chapter objective covered in this section:

7. Integrate ethics into maintaining professional boundaries and the therapeutic relationship.

Using the information presented in this section, the student will be able to:

- Develop strategies for maintaining professional boundaries with clients.
- Explore personal prejudices, biases, fears, and limitations that may interfere with the ability to provide the best care for a client.
- Help a client recognize personal boundaries in the massage process.

Professional boundaries are those rules and limits that prevent the lines between massage practitioner and client from becoming blurred. Boundaries provide a framework for relationships both personal and professional, minimize misunderstanding and conflict, and help prevent burnout. Boundaries are all about respect for ourselves and others.

Professional boundaries are determined by legal, ethical, and organizational frameworks to maintain a safe working environment for the client and massage therapy professional. Many ethical dilemmas are related to boundary issues.

We need to identify our personal boundaries to be able to develop professional boundaries. We bring to our adulthood varying experiences that shape what we feel is correct and define our personal boundaries. As professionals, we are responsible for finding the client's comfort zone. This responsibility begins with learning our personal and professional comfort zones. Anything that prevents us from being able to touch a person in a respectful, nonjudgmental way must be considered so that we can decide whom we may best serve as massage professionals. Hindrances include personal bias and prejudices regarding body size, color, gender, and attitude. For example, some people do not relate well to children. It is ethical for such professionals to refer children to someone else for professional care. Others may be uncomfortable with those of a specific gender, and again, it is best to refer such clients elsewhere. We may be uncomfortable with the prospect of working with people who have certain types of diseases. If this is the case, our touch may be uncomfortable for these people. A potential client may have a personal behavior that drives us crazy (e.g., sniffing, speaking loudly, snapping chewing gum). The behavior interferes with our ability to be the best massage professional for that particular client.

PROFICIENCY EXERCISE 2.2

On a piece of paper, write at least one page about your personal biases, prejudices, and fears about people. Be honest in listing the physical and behavioral aspects of others that you find difficult.

It is important that you be honest with yourself. Only by accepting that we have these areas of challenge will we be able to best serve potential clients.

It is important, therefore to explore professional boundaries by looking honestly at our fears, frustrations, prejudices, biases, and personal and moral value systems. These emotions and beliefs are very personal and often deeply held. The anchors for many of these beliefs may not be easily understood at a conscious level. Acknowledging factors that define and limit our personal and professional boundaries does not necessarily involve changing or even understanding why we feel a certain way. Changing belief systems is a complex process that often requires professional help. Although personal growth is encouraged, the expectation that we can overcome all our limitations is unrealistic. Instead, it is important to recognize when our personal boundaries will affect the professional relationship. We work closely with our clients, using touch as the primary medium of treatment. (The essential quality of touch communication was explored in Chapter 1). We must be honest with ourselves and about ourselves to be able to respect the individual needs and space of our clients (Proficiency Exercise 2.2).

Ethnicity, Culture, and Religion

Ethnicity refers to cultural factors, including nationality, regional culture, ancestry, and language. Race is primarily associated with the physical features of a person. Physical characteristics are a nonissue for the massage therapist; therefore race should be a nonissue.

Ethnicity is reflective of much more, and the massage therapist should seek to understand and respect ethnicity, nationality, heritage, culture, and identity. If the massage therapist is unable to accept a client's ethnicity, then boundaries become a concern.

Religion relates to groups of people's relationship to that which they regard as holy, sacred, divine, or worthy of reverence. Religion can be explained as a set of beliefs concerning the cause, nature, and purpose of the universe, usually involving devotional and ritual observances, and often containing a moral code governing the conduct of human affairs. A client's religion must be respected, and the massage therapist's religion, although personally important, should not be an aspect of the therapeutic relationship. If it is an essential aspect of the practitioner's presentation, then boundary issues can occur.

Gender Identity and Sexual Orientation

Gender identity and one's biological sex are not the same. Biological sex is determined by chromosomal, hormonal, and anatomical characteristics used to classify an individual as female, male, or intersex, which is atypical combinations of features that usually distinguish male from female. Gender identity is an individual's innermost concept of self as male, female, a blend of both, or neither; in other words, how individuals perceive themselves and what they call themselves. It can mirror an individual's biological sex or be entirely different.

Gender identity and sexual orientation are different as well. Sexual orientation is someone's emotional, romantic, or sexual attraction to other people. Common categories of sexual orientation include heterosexual, bisexual, gay person, and asexual.

People who are transgender are diverse in their gender identities, gender expressions, and sexual orientations. You cannot tell someone's preferred gender from how they look. The responsibility of the massage therapist is to be respectful. A person's sexual orientation—whether client or massage therapist—is not part of the massage therapy interaction; therefore it is not a factor in the therapeutic relationship.

A person's sense of self is important and needs to be honored. In the massage therapy setting, the massage therapist should not emphasize gender identity. A more gender-neutral appearance and behavior is appropriate.

Social Stratification

Social standing and social class are formal or informal classifications of status. Often the differentiation of these two is based on power, prestige, and wealth. It is unethical to be influenced by perceived status. Status-based classification is a subtle but insidious form of discrimination; it is the unjust or prejudicial treatment of different categories of people. Celebrity status is an example of what may be considered high status. A factory worker may be considered to have a lower status. Preferential treatment of some clients is the concern. Professional boundaries should not be influenced by an individual's status. Massage therapists need to be mindful of providing preferential treatment to clients based on social standing. We must also monitor our own sense of status, which should not be based on whom we have as clients.

Ageism

The concept of age identity refers to the inner experience of a person's age and the aging process. The following are common categories of aging:

Infancy/childhood: birth to 10 years
Adolescence: 10–20 years
Early adulthood: 20–40 years
Middle adulthood: 40–60 years
Mature adulthood: 60–80 years
Late adulthood: 80+ years

Ageism is stereotyping of and discrimination against individuals or groups on the basis of their age. Ageism can take many forms, including stereotyping, discriminatory practices, and practices that perpetuate stereotypical beliefs (Beard et al., 2016). Those in early adulthood can be minimalized by older people, who think the younger ones are not mature enough for certain levels of responsibility. Those in early or middle adulthood can be condescending to mature adults, thinking that they are too old to learn or comprehend.

Types of Professional Boundaries

Healthy boundaries are the foundation of healthy relationships. Types of professional boundaries important in the massage therapy practice are:

Physical Boundaries

Physical boundaries clearly define that your body and personal space belong to you and are protected, that you have the right to not be touched, privacy, and your physical needs are met.

A physical boundary can be defined as the personal space within an arm's length perimeter. It also can be thought of as the personal emotional space designated by morals, values, and experience. Some people are not good at defining personal boundaries or respecting others' boundaries. Certainly, boundaries are defined by more than physical space, but for our purposes, a respect for personal boundaries simply begins with staying an arm's length away from another until invited to come closer. Personal space can be defined by extending the arm directly in front of the body and turning in a circle; the area within that space is that individual's personal space. Cultural differences may change this boundary, but for therapeutic massage, we will consider this a person's personal space range (see Touch in Chapter 1). No one should ever enter this space uninvited (i.e., without informed consent).

Emotional Boundaries

Emotional boundaries protect the right to have your own feelings and differentiate those feelings from others. Emotional boundaries support emotional safety by respecting other's feelings and avoid oversharing personal information that is inappropriate for the nature of the relationship. What is shared between close friends is different than what is shared with coworkers or clients.

Political and Religious Boundaries

People have many different opinions, political beliefs, and religious views. You can believe whatever you wish in your personal life. However, in the professional setting it is important to not impose those views on others and to avoid discussions about religion or politics.

Time Boundaries

Time boundaries are how you schedule your time, how you prioritize your time, what your time is worth. Set clear rules that regulate the length of time that you spend with a client and manage timekeeping for both you and your client. Also explain how and when to contact you during designated business hours.

Social Media Boundaries

Social media use can blur professional boundaries. While the point for many in using social media is connecting with current and new potential contacts, you do not have to accept all friend/connection requests. Posts should center on professional topics. Be mindful if content sharing is appropriate and respectful, offensive, or harmful. Just because something isn't illegal does not mean it's okay to share. Examples include name-calling, cyberbullying, and spreading rumors. Oversharing on social media can lead to problems with coworkers and clients.

Personal Relationship Boundaries

Avoid forming social relationships with current or ex-clients. Clearly explain that the professional relationship is different than a friendship. If they need to see you, it should be done during work hours within a work setting.

Assertive Communication

Assertive communication is direct, respectful, and requires clear listening and expression. Assertiveness can be understood as a relational style that treads a middle path between being passive and being aggressive.

Be clear: communicate in a straightforward way that explicitly states your thoughts and feelings.

Be consistent: what you say today reflects what you said yesterday, rather than changing daily without explanation.

Be courteous: respect your listener and communicate in a manner that does not pass judgment on them or presume ill-intent.

- Be honest about what you are trying to say, and in particular what you feel.
- Use a firm but not aggressive tone of voice, keep the volume steady and no louder than necessary.
- Make relaxed but steady eye contact without staring them out.
- Make sure your body language is confident but relaxed. Stand tall but relaxed; relax your shoulders.
- Acknowledge what the other person has said and let them know that you have heard it.

It is difficult to speak assertively when emotionally reactive. If you can slow yourself down and remember the goal is a successful exchange, rather than a win/lose exchange, your communication in all relationships will be more satisfying, less stressful, and more successful.

Once we are aware of our boundaries, then we need to help our clients establish their boundaries. We should be respectful in our approach and explain therapeutic boundaries carefully. What is acceptable for us may be offensive for someone else. We may offend someone unintentionally because of differences in our personal and moral value systems. It is important for the massage therapist to help the client define a personal boundary (Box 2.8). Sometimes people who have been emotionally, physically, or sexually abused have not had the chance to define or recognize physical and personal boundaries.

Once a client's boundaries have been defined, we must respect them. If a professional cannot respect a client's boundary needs, the professional should refer the client to a massage therapist better able to deal with those needs.

It is equally important that the client understand the therapist's personal and professional boundaries; therefore the therapist must be honest in creating a personal code of ethics and must clearly communicate the professional boundaries to the client. Boundaries are discussed with the client during the initial informed consent procedures and are included in writing in the client policy statement. (Communication skills for the professional are presented later in this chapter.)

Even when a massage professional is conscientious about establishing boundaries with the client during the initial intake procedure, those boundaries can become blurred as the professional interaction progresses, or something may occur that the professional had not considered. When this happens, the situation must be dealt with immediately; waiting only allows the problem to escalate, leading to the development of conflict. Blurred boundaries create an environment conducive to the development of ethical dilemmas. Professional boundaries are situational and must be identified and established with each client. Clear professional boundaries support an effective therapeutic process for both the client and the professional.

Box 2.8 Determining a Client's Boundaries

An effective way to determine a client's boundaries is to ask questions. For example, the massage professional might ask the client:

- Is there any part of your body that you would rather not have massaged?
- Do you prefer any particular kind of music? Here are some selections to choose from.
- I am a smoker, and I know the smell lingers. Will that bother you? (What will you do if the client says yes?)
- I have three massage lubricants. Which would you prefer?

Right of Refusal

Clients have the right to refuse the massage practitioner's services; this is called the **right of refusal**. The client has the right to refuse or to stop treatment at any time. When this request is made during treatment, the therapist must comply even though prior consent was obtained.

Professionals also have a right of refusal. Massage professionals may refuse to massage or otherwise treat any person if a just and reasonable cause exists. Obviously, lack of appropriate knowledge or skills is a reason for refusal and referral. It is more ambiguous situations that cause concern. Massage professionals also are bound by a nondiscrimination code of conduct. You may refuse to work with anyone as long as you explain the reasons, specifically that these reasons ultimately would affect the quality of care for the client; this is called *disclosure.*

Touching someone with whom you are uneasy is difficult, whatever the reasons. If you honestly explain the situation, the client can make the decision.

A massage professional has the right to refuse to treat any area of a client's body and to terminate the professional relationship if they feel that the client is sexualizing the relationship or if the professional feels adversely influenced in any way by the client.

Refusal becomes more difficult when clearly defined discrimination issues are involved. This might occur if a professional limits their practice to a particular ethnic group or refuses to provide services to someone with a legally classified disability. In these cases, the massage practitioner is wise to seek legal counsel to determine the extent of professional liability.

Professional Application

People who get into trouble regarding boundaries have often confused their personal life with their professional life. Setting boundaries does not mean you act entitled. It's about self-care for mental wellness, mutual respect, and clear-cut communications. Healthy boundaries support individual well-being. However, individual boundaries should not be burdensome to others. It is important to self-evaluate the effects of individual boundaries on professional relationships.

For example: An employed massage therapist sets a work-related time boundary for massage scheduling, they can only be scheduled from 10:00 am to 2:30 pm on Mondays and Tuesdays. The employer and the reception staff have difficulty filling this schedule since these are typically slow business days and slow times of the day. This work schedule is desirable for the massage therapist but burdensome for the employer. It may be that this boundary for the massage therapist is not compatible with the needs of the work setting. The massage therapist does not need to change their boundary but may need to find a better fit for employment.

Reinforcing and maintaining boundaries isn't always easy. It can feel uncomfortable to say no to people but saying "no" is about protecting your boundaries. When reinforcing boundaries and saying no, be firm, courteous, and straightforward. You can learn to set boundaries without being confrontational, and you can reinforce those boundaries kindly and mindfully.

THE THERAPEUTIC RELATIONSHIP

SECTION OBJECTIVES

Chapter objective covered in this section:

8. Explain and demonstrate the qualities of the therapeutic relationship.

Using the information presented in this section, the student will be able to:

- Define and recognize potential transference and countertransference issues.
- Explain the professional power differential.
- List factors that create dual or multiple roles.
- Explain to clients the feelings of intimacy that can arise between them and the massage professional.
- Diffuse sexual feelings during the massage session.
- Recognize and avoid sexual misconduct activities.

In the therapeutic setting, specific parameters define the professional relationship between the client and the massage professional. The therapeutic relationship has an inherent **power differential**, which stems from the difference in knowledge and skills between the client and the professional. Even when services are exchanged between peer professionals, the power differential exists because one is placed in the position of controlling the situation. This power imbalance must be minimized as much as possible without denying its existence.

Client expectations about massage benefits and the relationship with the massage therapist influence client satisfaction. Outcome expectations refer to the expected benefits of massage. Role expectations refer to the expected behaviors of the massage therapist—what clients expect massage therapists will do before, during, and after the massage session (Boulanger et al., 2012).

The Development and Validation of the Client Expectations of Massage Scale, a study done by Karen T. Boulanger and associates (2012), found that massage therapy clients have four categories of expectations about massage. Three of these expectations involve massage therapist behavior, and one relates to the specific effects of the massage application. Clients expect massage therapists to be professional and confident as a massage therapist, skilled as a teacher of self-help methods, and personable and friendly—but not a friend. Clients also expect that massage methods address their outcomes such as pain or stress management.

It is important for massage therapists to assess for realistic and unrealistic client expectations and to inform the client about the importance of expectations related to the therapeutic relationship and the benefits of massage. If unrealistic expectations are allowed to develop, therapeutic relationship issues can perpetuate. Another important finding from this same study is the importance of appropriate conversation between the client and the massage therapist. Conversation at the beginning of the massage session that relates to assessment and determining outcomes for the massage is important. During the massage, conversation needs to be limited to client comfort such as pressure and warmth or related specifically to instructions and feedback about a massage intervention. Conversation at the end of sessions needs to identify results related to the massage, self-help, and scheduling for the next appointment. Avoid chatting about general or personal topics with the client. This type of conversation is inappropriate and results in a reduced level of client satisfaction and benefit from the massage. A final takeaway from this study is that clients will be more satisfied with the massage session when reasonable expectations are met rather than when high expectations are not met, and the therapeutic relationship is not maintained.

Transference

Issues of transference and countertransference diminish the effectiveness of the therapeutic relationship. *Transference* is the personalization of the professional relationship by the client. When a person seeks out a professional, the important issues of power, trust, and control in the therapeutic relationship become the professional's responsibility. Clients often seek a sense of control outside themselves to help reestablish or replace their loss of an internal sense of control. The client is in a vulnerable state when doing this. This situation is more common with people who are ill or under considerable stress, but even a healthy client is vulnerable in the therapeutic setting. The reality of today's society is that although most people cannot be diagnosed as sick, most have not achieved true wellness either. Although we ideally speak of wellness massage to help a client maintain or achieve optimal wellness, the truth is somewhat different.

Unfortunately, few people seek massage as a quality-of-life activity and to enhance their health. Most of the clients we serve, even outside the health care setting, are not optimally well. They just are not sick yet. Most seek massage services because they do not feel good and want to feel better. Massage is most beneficial when received regularly, and a retention client structure, regardless of work setting, provides the most stable income for the massage therapist. The cost and time burden to a client may not be justifiable for well-being goals even though these outcomes are possibly the most important provided by massage. Clients with pain management, functional movement, and performance goals will be more likely to schedule regularly and make up the majority of clients in a retention-based massage practice. A therapeutic relationship with these clients is more prone to boundary issues. The more disorganized, disempowered, and lacking in internal resources clients are, the more susceptible they are to transference.

Transference occurs when the client sees the therapist in a personal light instead of a professional manner. If the client becomes dependent on the professional unrealistic expectations may develop. Manifestations of transference include demands for more of the therapist's time, bringing the therapist personal gifts, attempting to engage the professional in personal conversation, proposals of friendship or sexual activity, and expressions of anger and blame. If the client's expectations are not met, the person may blame the professional. If the client's expectations are met or exceeded, the person may project the credit to the therapist instead of acknowledging their own efforts. In both cases, the professional takes on a superhuman image that sooner or later crumbles, often leaving the client disillusioned and disempowered.

Managing transference is a common ethical dilemma. The massage professional must understand and separate the client's appropriate, genuine feelings from the transference issues. For example, a client may be angry if the therapist continually arrives late for the appointment; this is a justified feeling, not transference. Also, the client may genuinely appreciate the massage therapists skill and may express that appreciation, but this does not constitute transference unless it interferes with the boundaries of the therapeutic relationship.

The massage professional has the ultimate responsibility for the therapeutic relationship and the direction of the therapeutic process.

Countertransference

Countertransference is the inability of the professional to separate the therapeutic relationship from personal feelings and expectations for the client; it is the professional's personalization of the therapeutic relationship. Countertransference presents itself in feelings of attachment to the client, such as excessive thinking about a client between visits, a feeling of professional inadequacy if the client does not make anticipated progress, a sense of the client as being special or sexual feelings; it also can manifest as favoritism, anger, or revulsion toward a client. Countertransference often is fed by the personal needs of the therapist, such as:

- The need to fix people
- The need to remove pain and discomfort
- The need to be perfect
- The need to have the answer
- The need to be loved

The client's problems may serve as a reflection of the professional's personal life experiences. The massage professional is wise to consider their own personal needs and develop a reliable sense of self-awareness. Without a high level of self-awareness on the part of the professional, the focus of the massage session may shift from meeting the goals of the client to meeting the needs of the therapist. The massage therapist may lose objectivity and empathy in the therapeutic relationship.

During appropriate therapeutic interactions, a bond forms between the therapist and the client. Many terms, such as *unity*, *connection*, or even *in the zone*, can be used to describe this intangible experience. *Attunement* means to bring into a harmonious or responsive relationship. In massage therapy, *rapport* is another term that can be used to describe the concept of attunement.

Scientists have discovered cells in the brain, called *mirror neurons,* which support human connection (Heyes and Catmur, 2022). Mirror neurons play a role in the imitation necessary for learning and the ability to empathize with others. An important aspect of the professional relationship is understanding the condition of another person while remaining nonjudgmental. Vittorio Gallese, who identified mirror neurons, describes intentional attunement as a state that generates a peculiar quality of familiarity with other individuals (Gallese, 2005; Gallese et al., 2007; Bonini et al., 2022).

The amygdala is the part of the brain that underlies empathy and allows for emotional attunement. Facial expressions, voices, gestures, and body movements transmit emotions. Humans especially tend to subconsciously mimic and model the facial expressions, vocalizations, postures, and movements of others, especially when an interdependent or survival relationship exists. Understanding the communication of body language processed by mirror neurons is a fundamental aspect of attunement. With this mechanism we do not just see an action, an emotion, or a sensation in another; we feel what one would feel during a similar action and are able to determine the intentions and emotions behind that action (Keysers et al., 2018; Decety and Holvoet, 2021). The therapeutic relationship is grounded in all these concepts.

If the client's personal situation is similar to that of the massage practitioner, especially with regard to life challenges, the practitioner may subconsciously offer advice which more pertains to themselves rather than the client. For example, both the professional and the client may be facing difficult marital issues or dealing with the recent loss of a parent or relocation to a new city. This dynamic can be detrimental to the client because it breaches the professional relationship and fosters psychologically unhealthy behaviors between the massage practitioner and the client. An environment of sympathetic dependence often results, and this dynamic is a basis for countertransference. As professionals, we do have empathy for our clients; however, sympathy is different. Bluntly said, empathy is about the client, and sympathy is really about you.

Practitioners personalize the professional relationship when they assume too much responsibility for the outcome of the session for the client or when they project a personal situation onto the client process. Countertransference issues often reflect unresolved issues on the part of the professional. Identifying countertransference in the therapeutic relationship can point out areas the practitioner may wish to explore and resolve with a qualified professional. It is important to remain as objective as possible. The goal is not for the massage professional to be flawless before beginning practice; rather, the goal is to maintain professional boundaries and be aware of how personal challenges may interfere with the therapeutic relationship.

Managing Transference and Countertransference

Transference can be expected in some form in the therapeutic relationship. As it arises, it is the massage professional's responsibility to reinforce the boundaries of the professional relationship. The practitioner should explain to clients why these feelings may occur and help them redirect the transference activity to the appropriate people or situations in the client's life. This becomes difficult when the client does not move through the transference stage toward more self-directed resources and coping strategies or when the client has extremely limited resources and coping mechanisms. Such clients may need to be referred to another professional, with appropriate disclosure for the reason for referral, to help them understand that the boundaries of the professional relationship are being breached and that the existing situation is inappropriate.

The professional is always responsible for self-monitoring for the development of countertransference issues and for seeking supervision or professional support, such as problem solving with peers and/or a mentor or counselor, if necessary, to resolve personal issues. When the professional faces the realization that countertransference has occurred, the first step in resolving these issues has been taken. It is a breach of professional boundaries to allow countertransference issues to develop and linger or to be acted on. In extreme cases, the client may need to be referred to a different therapeutic massage professional, with appropriate disclosure on the part of the therapist, so that the client does not take the need for referral personally. For example, massage professionals can tell a client that they are beginning to exceed their professional ability to best serve the client's outcomes. They recommend that a massage therapist with different skills will best serve the client's continued progress. They then offer a list of suitable massage professionals.

Peer support, supervision, and mentoring are important for the massage professional dealing with transference and countertransference. Supervision and mentoring support professional development. Those mentoring the massage professional do not necessarily need to be massage therapists. Various health care professionals grapple with similar issues. Mental health professionals in particular must frequently consider transference and countertransference issues. If supervision and mentoring are not part of your professional practice, it may be helpful to seek out a qualified mental health professional and establish a professional relationship with that person to sort out these particular issues.

Peer support also is important. Interacting regularly with other massage practitioners creates an environment that promotes healthy work practices through both technical information and guidance on solving interpersonal dilemmas. When sharing with peers, be attentive to the confidentiality of your clients.

The Therapeutic Alliance

A way to manage transference and countertransference and maintain appropriate professional boundaries is to establish a therapeutic alliance. A therapeutic alliance can be described by three elements: developing a trusting relationship through building rapport, establishing a need in clients' minds to be actively engaged in self-help activities, and identifying a massage approach and appointment schedule the client will find beneficial. The process of developing a therapeutic alliance with clients supports massage practice using a client-centered approach to care and respects client boundaries. Questions should be limited to information that relates to the massage session. If the client wants to tell you a personal story, listen respectfully but avoid giving advice or asking for any additional information.

MENTORING TIP

Maintain an appropriate level of self-disclosure. Clients really do not want to know that much about your personal life. If they ask personal questions, it is usually because they are nice people and are attempting to get comfortable with the situation, especially early in a therapeutic relationship. When a client pays for a massage, the agreement is that that time is all about the client, not about you. Do not talk about yourself unless you are providing information about something going on with you that may affect the massage. Example: You take a medication that has dry mouth as a side effect. You can inform the client that dry mouth from a medication means that you may need to sip water during the session. That's it. The client does not need to know anything else. If they ask what medication or why you take it, you can offer a bit more information, but be very brief. You can say, "It is a medication for hypertension, and now let's focus on you."

Dual or Multiple Roles

A dual role exists when scopes of practice overlap, and one professional provides support in more than one area of expertise; it may also occur when personal relationships overlap with professional services. Dual or multiple roles develop when professionals assume more than one role in their relationship with their clients. These roles develop in many ways. Providing massage in the professional environment for family members is a classic example of a dual role, as is providing professional services for a personal friend.

Dual and multiple roles are difficult to manage in the professional relationship and can be a breeding ground for ethical dilemmas. The human experience encompasses body, mind, and spirit. The body is our anatomy and physiology. The mind is our beliefs, learning, behavior, and thinking. The spirit is our hope and faith. As soon as one professional assumes professional authority with the body and the mind, the body and the spirit, or the spirit and the mind, the therapist can be said to be assuming a dual role (or multiple roles if the authority is assumed in all three areas). In this situation, the professional holds more power in the relationship than is appropriate, and the client begins to become disempowered. The power differential is increased. This allows a dangerous power shift that supports the development of transference and countertransference. It often leads to enmeshment and dependence on the part of the client and burnout on the part of the therapist. Managing the inherent power differential of the therapeutic relationship is difficult enough without increasing the likelihood of transference and countertransference or the breach of professional boundaries by assuming dual and multiple roles.

In the professional therapeutic massage relationship, mental and spiritual issues need not be dealt with directly. The focus of massage is the body. When interacting with your client, maintain the focus of the work on the body while using attentive listening, empathetically acknowledging the client's circumstances, and always being alert to the possible need for referral. Interacting professionally in the area of the mind or spirit may breach the professional contract for massage therapy services, which focuses on the body. Always recognize and appreciate the wholeness of the person. Remain within the scope of massage therapy and collaborate with a variety of professionals to deal with other areas. With this approach the client remains empowered in the process of achieving wellness.

A dual role also can arise in more subtle situations. The sale of products to a client, bartering of services, excessive personal disclosure by the therapist to the client, shared social interaction, or shared professional services all create situations in which the power balance of the therapeutic relationship can become problematic. As in all ethical dilemmas, decisions about conduct are gauged against the client's welfare. The clinical reasoning process is an effective way to analyze an ethical dilemma and develop a plan to address the issue.

Massage Therapy and Intimacy

To dispel in advance any sexual innuendo associated with many of the terms used in the following paragraphs, definitions from *Merriam-Webster's Dictionary* are provided at this point for clarification (Merriam-Webster, 2014):

Intimacy: The state or fact of being intimate.

Intimate: Inmost, essential, internal, most private, or personal; closely acquainted or associated; familiar.

Essential: Intrinsic, fundamental, basic, and inherently primary.

Sensory: Connected with the reception and transmission of sense impressions (through the nervous system).

Stimulation: The act of exciting or increasing activity.

The work of a massage practitioner is sensory stimulation; therefore by its very definition, body stimulation is sensual and may become intimate. When a person encounters the essential touch that a sensitive and confident massage practitioner provides, that person's whole system responds. For many, the closest things to essential touch ever experienced are parenting activities and sexual interaction. Because our bodies constantly react to new situations through comparison to past experience, a client's response system understandably might interpret these feelings as sexual arousal or as maternal or paternal. Furthermore, for many adults, the only familiar routine they have for expressing these feelings is a sexual one. It is easy to see why the client might misinterpret the sensations and feelings associated with massage, confusing them with sexual responses or a parenting role.

The massage professional must understand the physiological aspects of therapeutic massage and recognize that the same massage techniques that alleviate stress and promote relaxation also stimulate the entire sensory mechanism, which may include a sexual arousal response. Within the parameters of professional ethics, it is always considered unethical for the client or the practitioner to interact on a sexual level, whether verbally or physically. However, it is essential that both client and practitioner understand why the urges and sensations of sexuality may present themselves. A more thorough knowledge of the physiological and psychological network leads to a better understanding of the responses by both client and practitioner. The practitioner is then better able to alter the session to maintain a proper professional relationship.

The lumbar nerve plexus (nerve bundles) and the sacral nerve plexus conduct sensory information to and from the abdominal area, the lower extremities, and the buttocks and also to and from the genital area. Stimulation of a nerve plexus area is not confined to local perception but rather is diffused throughout the area. For example, when the lower abdominal area is stroked, the nerve signals of the genital area also are influenced. The entire sexual arousal response is part of the relaxation response through the output from the parasympathetic autonomic nervous system. Therefore each time a client relaxes out of the fight-or-flight responses of the sympathetic autonomic nervous system into the more relaxed response, the predisposing physiological factors are present for sexual arousal. This reaction also occurs for practitioners as they begin to relax while performing the massage.

On a physiological level, parasympathetic stimulation activates most of the benefits of massage for stress reduction. This neurological state is also favorable to sexual arousal. These physical responses are all connected, but the sexual response is usually short-lived and quickly replaced by feelings of deep relaxation as the massage continues. Responses vary with each client, and the sexual response may be totally bypassed. However, physical sexual arousal may occur in females and males (e.g., engorgement of erectile tissue with blood and shifts in breathing), and the massage practitioner needs to understand both the physiology of this situation and ways to deal with it ethically (Box 2.9).

Box 2.9 Diffusing Feelings of Sexual Arousal

1. Recognize the physiology and interrupt it; change what you are doing.
2. Be aware of your own psychological state and change it; become more alert.
3. Adjust the intent of the session to stimulate a more sympathetic output response by using compression, joint movement, and active participation by the client.
4. Change the music, lighting, and conversation and the client's position.
5. Stop working with your hands and use your forearms.
6. Explain the feelings in a professional manner using clinical terminology.

The practitioner is responsible for putting the whole issue of sexuality into perspective, understanding it clearly, and explaining the "feelings" to the client on a physiological level. The practitioner also is responsible for monitoring the client's responses and acting appropriately to adjust the physiology and change the pattern of the massage to diffuse the sexual energy. This is easily accomplished by altering the approach of the session. It is common knowledge that sexual arousal is not purely physical and depends on both psychological and tactile responses; in these ways, the practitioner can modulate the client–practitioner responses.

The *Merriam-Webster Dictionary* defines *intercourse* as "connection or reciprocal action between persons or nations; the interchange of thought, feelings, products, services, communication, commerce, and association" (Merriam-Webster, 2014). Massage becomes an intercourse in the purest sense. Essential intimacy is the circle that begins to develop between practitioner and client. People want this type of intimacy; it is the type of interaction that promotes survival and health. Essential touch is vital, fundamental, and crucial to well-being. It is the touch of a litter of puppies sleeping in one big pile. It is combined with the sexual interchange between lovers. However, it does not require sexual expression to be considered essential intimacy.

Touch Intimacy

Remember that, as was explained in Chapter 1, the intention of a touch is a determining factor in the interpretation of the touch. The touch of the massage professional is not focused on sexual arousal and release or parenting. The interpersonal communication skills of the practitioner determine the professional interaction and monitor responses. Keep discussions light. Change the topic. Change the environment.

The moments of intimacy must be dealt with carefully. Misunderstanding the psychological or physiological responses, the client may interpret them as an indication of feelings of romantic love or that the therapist is a new best friend. Clients manifest this response in different ways. Usually clients want to bring the professional into their lives, perhaps through invitations to lunch, a desire for more frequent sessions, or a proposal for a relationship. Do not allow this to happen. The practitioner must maintain professional space and monitor personal feelings. Keep the balance by confining the intimacy of massage to the therapeutic environment.

Having little or no understanding of all these subtle interactions, the client cannot be blamed for wanting more attention from the massage practitioner. The moments of togetherness that are shared are special and can range from a great deal of laughter to sharing work-related experiences. The session can accomplish something as simple as relieving the day's tension or as complex as overcoming years of pain. Make no more and no less of the interaction.

Clients may look to the professional for emotional support beyond the ethical scope of practice for massage. Encourage them to find the support they require from another source. If a client needs assistance with coping skills, refer the person to someone who is qualified to help. Credit counselors, ministers, rape crisis counselors, marriage counselors, counselors for sexual dysfunction, physicians, and many other caregivers can provide the help clients may need. The massage practitioner's intention is to support and accept the client in a nonjudgmental manner, listen, and blend touch skills to benefit the client.

Sexual Misconduct and Sexual Harassment

Sexual misconduct is any type of sexual activity that occurs between the professional and the client. Although sexual misconduct has been relatively well defined (Box 2.10), conduct that is invasive but not blatantly sexual remains a gray area.

Box 2.10 Guidelines on Sexual Misconduct

- The therapist will respect the integrity of each person and therefore not engage in any sexual conduct or sexual activities involving clients.
- The therapist will not date a client.
- The therapist will not commit any form of sexual impropriety or sexual abuse with a client.
- Whatever the behavior of the client, it is always the responsibility of the massage therapist not to engage in sexual behavior.

Sexual Impropriety

Sexual impropriety includes:

- Any behavior, gestures, or expressions that are seductive or sexually demeaning to a client
- Inappropriate procedures, including but not limited to:
  - Disrobing or draping practices that reflect a lack of respect for the client's privacy
  - Deliberately watching a client dress or undress
- Inappropriate comments about or to the client, including but not limited to:
  - Sexual comments about a client's body or underclothing
  - Sexualized or sexually demeaning comments to a client
  - Criticism of the client's sexual orientation
  - Discussion of potential sexual performance
  - Conversations about the sexual preferences or fantasies of the client or the massage therapist
  - Requests to date

Sexual Abuse

Sexual abuse includes:

- Therapist–client sex, whether initiated by the client or not
- Engaging in any conduct with a client that is sexual or reasonably may be interpreted as sexual, including but not limited to:
- Genital-to-genital contact
- Oral-to-genital contact
- Oral-to-anal contact
- Oral-to-oral contact (except cardiopulmonary resuscitation [CPR])
- Oral-to-breast contact
- Touching or undraping the genitals, perineum, or anus
- Touching or undraping the breasts
- Encouraging the client to masturbate in the presence of the massage therapist
- Masturbation by the massage therapist while the client is present
- Masturbation of the client by the massage therapist

A joke told between friends may be inappropriate in the professional setting. A statement about appearance may be taken as a compliment or could be interpreted as a sexual remark. Something that is appropriate with one client may not be acceptable with another. Practitioners can find it overwhelming to try to second-guess what is appropriate for clients. The best defense against confusion is communication. Ask questions and provide clients with information about acceptable behavior in the professional setting.

Sexual harassment occurs in the work setting between peers or with supervisors. Unwelcome sexual interaction (physical or verbal) in conjunction with employment status or work environment constitutes sexual harassment. Sexual harassment is clearly defined by law, whereas sexual misconduct often is more subtle and more difficult to prosecute unless clearly coerced sexual acts have been committed (Focus on Professionalism).

FOCUS ON PROFESSIONALISM

A brief mention about human trafficking. More comprehensive information can be found in the appendices at the end of the textbook. Unfortunately, massage remains a cover for prostitution and in many cases human trafficking. Human trafficking is modern-day slavery and involves the use of force, fraud, or coercion to obtain some type of labor or commercial sex act. General information and specific antitrafficking resources can be found at the Blue Campaign (https://www.dhs.gov/blue-campaign). This is the unified voice for the efforts of the US Department of Homeland Security (DHS) to combat human trafficking. Working in collaboration with law enforcement, government, nongovernmental, and private organizations, the Blue Campaign strives to protect the basic right of freedom and to bring those who exploit human lives to justice. Department of Homeland Security (https://www.dhs.gov/blue-campaign/what-human-trafficking).

Human trafficking is a hidden crime; victims rarely come forward to seek help because of language barriers, fear of the traffickers, and/or fear of law enforcement. Those who solicit illicit sexual services are committing a crime and should be immediately reported to the police. Illicit sexual services fronting as massage often involve human trafficking.

Maintaining the Professional Environment

The therapeutic relationship is a unidirectional focus in which the knowledge and skills of the professional are used to assist the client in achieving therapeutic outcomes. To preserve the unidirectional focus, certain crucial professional boundaries must be maintained. For example, it is important to maintain professional space. Box 2.11 presents some simple ways to accomplish this.

As the therapist closes the session and leaves the client's space, it is important to change both physiology and body language. When greeting a client and providing the massage, the therapist's body language is open, inviting, connecting, and moving toward the client (Fig. 2.4). When it is time to close the session, the therapist's body language moves away from the client, pulls in toward the therapist, separates, and indicates that the session is finished (Fig. 2.5). Separating well from the client is a skill that gives both the client and the massage therapist a sense of closure. It often helps to establish a "time to go" ritual by always saying good-bye the same way. Clients who linger after the session may not know how to leave or may not recognize that it is time to leave. A "time to go" ritual helps considerably.

One example of a leaving ritual is to keep a box labeled "A thought to take with me" that contains fun, empowering quotes on note cards. Have the client pick a card from the box. Put the information for the next appointment on the back of the card, hand it to the client, and say good-bye. When the session is finished, the therapist needs to refocus as the room is prepared for the next person.

Managing Intimacy Issues

Effectively managing intimacy issues can seem like an overwhelming task. However, do not be afraid of the special professional intimacy of therapeutic massage. Instead, educate clients by answering their questions intelligently, basing your answers on the facts of physiology, and encouraging them to use this information to interact more resourcefully with others. If you begin to feel physically and emotionally receptive to a client, take steps to diffuse the situation. Later, review the session to evaluate your personal feelings. Was it a fleeting warm feeling? Is there just something about this particular person? Could it have been a hormonal response? Oxytocin, the bonding chemical, may be a big influence in couples bonding and parental feelings. This hormone is stimulated during skin contact such as massage. Were you feeling alone and needing to be connected? If the problem arises from something lacking in life, empower yourself to search out the cause and change circumstances so that personal reactions are kept out of the therapeutic setting.

Remember, as massage professionals when we touch, we also are being touched. The exchange is unavoidable, and we also need to monitor our own feelings and expressions of intimacy. If we do not deal effectively with these responses, the feelings associated with them could become uncomfortable. The client may react by discontinuing the massage sessions, or the therapist may effectively detach from the client and possibly stop seeing the client altogether. In the latter case, the client may feel abandoned.

If a professional relationship cannot be maintained with a client, stop providing therapeutic massage and refer the client to someone else. Give an honest, simple explanation so that the client understands it was not something they said or did that prompted the referral. Professional ethics cannot safeguard us from being human; however, behavior becomes unethical when the problem is not acknowledged, and resourceful action is not taken to solve it.

If a client refuses or is unable to change an inappropriate response to the massage, the client is refused further treatment. Explain to the client that the situation is uncomfortable and massage therapy can no longer be provided. The dismissal is done gently but assertively, and the client is told the decision is final.

Care must be taken in situations that could become difficult, and any situation in which behavior could be questioned must be avoided. One such situation concerns male massage

Box 2.11 Maintaining Professional Space

1. At the start of a professional relationship, a formal informed consent process must be completed.
2. In most instances, the time frame for working with a client should not exceed 90 minutes; 45–60 minutes is the norm. If more time is spent with the client, it becomes difficult for both the professional and the client to maintain the original intent and focus of the session, and the result is an environment that fosters transference and countertransference.
3. Professionals should wear clothing that sets them apart from clients; this is one of the benefits of a uniform. A name tag that identifies one as a massage therapist also is helpful. Wearing a uniform or maintaining a professional style of dress that is different from casual clothing provides a visual message that reflects professionalism. The clothes must be unrevealing and present an understated and neutral appearance. Therapists must be conscious of their appearance and make sure it is kept as nonsexual as possible.
4. The therapist should avoid assuming a dual role and multiple scopes of practice. The professional contract is for a specific type of intervention. General information about lifestyle or health issues can be provided, but the contract is for massage. This is a consideration even if the professional is credentialed in more than one area or discipline. Often the therapist needs to decide which professional hat to wear.
5. The professional environment should be neutral and must not indirectly imply any content other than therapeutic massage. Choices made in decorating the space or in reading material can be seen as creating an environment that fosters a dual role by promoting a specific mental, spiritual, nutritional, or exercise approach.
6. Selling products to clients can become an issue because of the perceived authority influence and power differential of the professional. Closely related products, such as self-massage tools that are made available for the client's convenience, as opposed to products sold for profit making, often present less of a problem than something like nutritional products. The client may like the services of the massage therapist but does not want to feel pressured into buying products. These situations must be managed with careful reflection because ethical dilemmas often result from the sale of products.
7. Privacy can be preserved by using a dedicated smartphone or similar device with a specific business number and returning calls or texts within set hours. If financially possible, have a receptionist or secretary monitor phone calls.
8. Maintain regular appointment hours. Begin and end sessions on time.
9. If you go to clients' homes, be extra cautious about entering a home alone. It is important to screen your clients carefully. The initial intake interview is a good opportunity to do this. Have the client come to your location, where you have more professional control over the screening process. Individual circumstances dictate when the following recommendations are necessary; however, remember it is better to be safe than sorry.
   - An on-site massage session for a bedridden elderly person will have a different level of concern than a female massage therapist providing on-site massage to a single male client, or vice versa. At the very least, make sure someone always knows where you are and check in with someone periodically throughout the day. If you are anxious about doing an on-site massage session, consider referring the client to someone else or team up with a fellow massage practitioner and both perform the massage.
   - Hire someone to go with you to the client's home. This person does not need to be a massage professional. This person remains within hearing distance of the place where the massage is given and can function as a witness should the client claim inappropriate behavior by the massage professional. This person also provides protection from any type of entrapment or illicit advances against the massage practitioner. It is appropriate to charge for this protection, and it is reflected in the fee structure.
   - It is also important to use your cell phone when entering a home or other location where less control is available to the massage practitioner. Call a prearranged number and then provide the name, address, and phone number of the client, the time of arrival, and the expected time of departure. You can call in and then tell them you will text them the location information if it is different from that provided on the appointment sheet. Tell this person that you will call (not text) just before you leave. Leave instructions to call the authorities should you not call at the agreed time. Make sure that your client hears this conversation.
10. Think carefully before setting rules about client conduct, rescheduling, and payment methods. Make sure you are willing to enforce your policies. If you are not, do not make them. Record this information clearly and concisely and make sure the client reads it. Posting it on the wall provides additional reinforcement.
11. Do not spend personal time, such as lunch, with clients. In rare situations, the professional may choose to forgo the professional relationship to develop a personal relationship. This decision can be considered a breach of professional ethics and is almost always a professional and personal mistake. The initial relationship structure was built on the basis of one who serves and one who is served. Rarely is an effective transition made to a relationship of mutual support. Both people usually end up disappointed.

therapists who want to do home-based appointments for females who are alone in the house. A good solution is to pair up with a female practitioner and provide these massage sessions as a team. It is important that a parent or legal guardian be in the room when massage services are given to a minor under 18 years of age. The touch of a massage professional should be safe touch.

Safe is defined as "not apt to cause danger, harm, or hurt; to be free of risk" (Merriam-Webster, 2014). Physiologically, safe means a state of homeostasis rather than the fight-or-flight

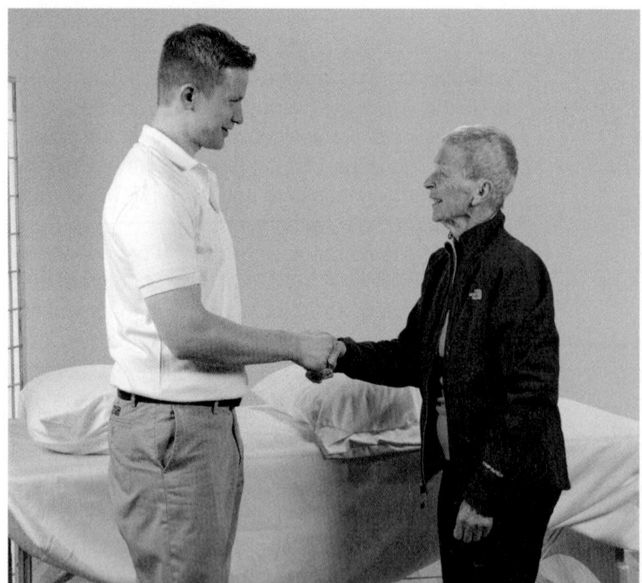

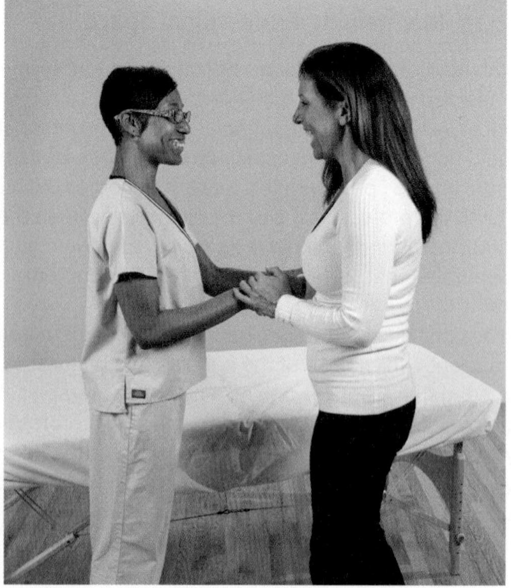

FIG. 2.4 The Body Language of Greeting. When greeting a client, the massage professional leans toward the person and gently draws the individual into the space of the massage session.

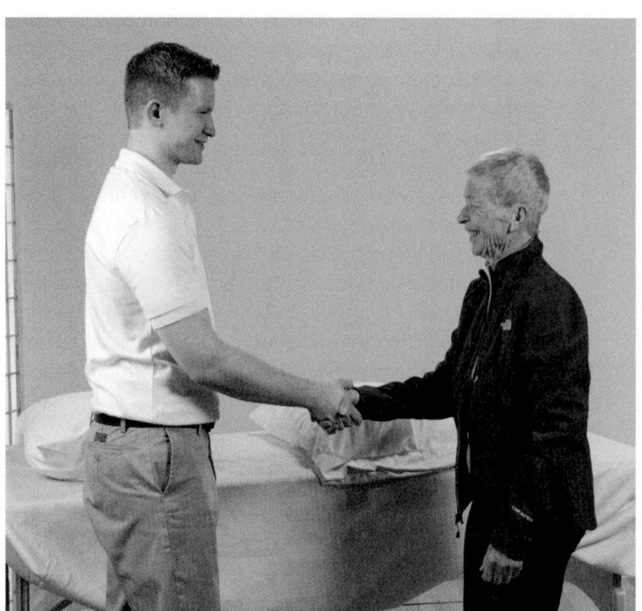

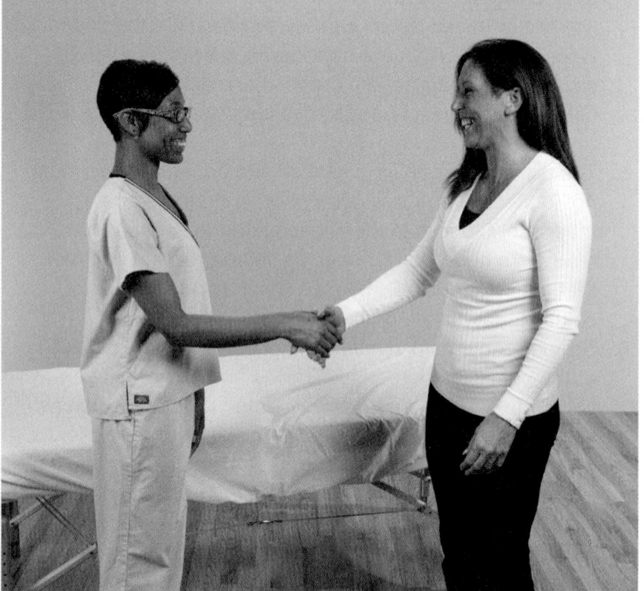

FIG. 2.5 The Body Language of Closure. When the massage is complete, the massage professional gently withdraws from the client by using body language that moves away from the person.

responses of the sympathetic autonomic nervous system or intense retreat/withdrawal responses of the parasympathetic autonomic nervous system (see Chapter 5). Being safe means having the ability to maintain well-being in a situation and to alter responses easily and to cope with the demands of everyday life. The therapeutic massage professional must consider everything, including personal beliefs and fears that may make touch unsafe for clients.

Sexual Solicitation

A client who is seeking sexual interaction is a different case. If this occurs, the massage professional explains succinctly that neither sexual release nor any other kind of sexual interaction is provided; the therapist then dismisses the person immediately and leaves the area to go to a safe place. Asking for sexual activity is solicitation, and it is illegal. You can call the police. A person who asks someone to commit an illegal act has committed the criminal act of solicitation. When a person is looking to pay for sex and makes this request by words or gestures, the person can be arrested for solicitation of prostitution. It also is important to note that a person who offers to perform a sex act for money can be arrested for prostitution.

Uniqueness of Long-Term Clients

Maintaining the delicate professional balance between client and practitioner is especially difficult with long-term clients. The nurturing approach of the massage practitioner fosters an environment in which friendships can form. Regular clients do become important, both as people and in their roles as clients. Massage practitioners must always be honest with themselves about the development of personal feelings for a client. Remember, this is a relationship, and professional relationships can last a long time. These people become important to us. When clients move away, we miss them. When a client dies, we grieve. When clients rejoice, so do we. And when clients do not need us anymore, we celebrate. Clients touch our lives. They are our best teachers. How can we not care about them?

By using this educational material to explore these issues, you can move forward in your development as a massage therapist while maintaining a safe and professional environment. The essence of this work is human touch. By dealing with personal intimacy issues, not only can the massage professional provide essential touch for the client, but the client also learns to establish proper boundaries. It must always be kept in mind that each individual massage practitioner represents the entire massage therapy profession. Demonstrating respect for the self demonstrates respect for the profession as a whole.

Consider all the dynamics of the therapeutic relationship, but do not be afraid of empathy, compassion, connection, and caring. Do not become so professionally detached that the client does not connect with you, the person, and you with them.

If problems develop, and answers become ambiguous or inconsistent, the following questions can help structure a problem-solving approach to make ethical decisions (Proficiency Exercise 2.3).

- Can I manage the professional power differential from a position of respect and empowerment for the client?
- Do I have the knowledge and skills to respond effectively to the situation?
- Am I avoiding dual or multiple roles with the client?
- Am I maintaining the boundaries of the therapeutic relationship?
- Am I within the established scope of practice for therapeutic massage?
- Am I respecting the scope of practice of other professionals?
- Do I have the highest good of the client in mind?
- Is what I am doing supporting the highest good of the massage therapy community?
- And perhaps the most telling: Would I want anyone else to know what I am doing?

PROFICIENCY EXERCISE 2.3

Working in groups of three, write down specific situations in which sexual misconduct or feelings of intimacy may develop. Exchange responses with other groups and role-play a situation, with one learner acting as the massage practitioner, one playing the client, and the third evaluating the way the situation was managed. Try different situations until each learner has had a chance to play each role.

ETHICAL DECISION MAKING

SECTION OBJECTIVES

Chapter objective covered in this section:

9. Use a problem-solving approach to ethical decision making.

Using the information presented in this section, the student will be able to:

- Implement an eight-step decision-making process.

When ethical dilemmas occur, massage professionals are expected to engage in a conscientious decision-making process that is clear and detailed enough to bear public scrutiny. A **dilemma** occurs when there may be multiple ways to address a situation and it is difficult to decide what to do.

Decisions should be thought-out responses based on principles, information, and the complexities of the situation. Effective decision making requires a person to:

- Define the situation or problem
- Consider the facts of what occurred or would influence the situation
- Generate possible solutions or courses of action
- Evaluate the logical consequences of cause and effect (pros and cons) and the effect on people of each potential solution or course of action
- Make a decision about what to do

Each decision is unique. The best decision for one person will not work for another. Most of the time, there is no specific right way or wrong way to do something. A few rules in the professional setting are absolutes: a professional does not breach sexual boundaries with a client; clients are to be referred when the skills required are out of the scope of practice or training of the professional; all care must focus on giving help and avoiding harm; and clients are to be given complete information about the treatment. However, most ethical dilemmas are about more ambiguous situations and require a thoughtful approach to decision making.

Ethics is not only about answers; it is also about the willingness to ask the questions and to seek help when needed. It is said that professionals do not let personal judgments interfere with professional care, but what do we do when, for example, we cannot keep our mind on our work because of a client's body odor? What do we do when a client schedules appointments more frequently than necessary because the client likes being with us? How do we manage a client who refuses to seek medical intervention when indicated? These are just a few of the many questions you may find yourself asking throughout your professional massage therapy career. Where does a massage therapist go for help to work through these dilemmas?

As stated previously, mentoring, supervision, and peer support are helpful to a professional grappling with ethical dilemmas that fall into the more common situational gray areas.

- A *mentor* is concerned with the successful career growth of those they mentor. A mentor is usually one in the profession of therapeutic massage with more career experience. Because a mentor does not have the hire, fire, and discipline role, the relationship is more individually focused, with freedom to discuss issues without fear of inadequacy or retribution.

- *Supervision* involves periodic review of a professional's actions by one in authority in the work setting. This can be direct supervision, in which the supervising professional actually observes the professional at work, or reflective supervision, in which the supervisor discusses the professional practice with the massage therapist. Supervision can help identify potential ethical concerns and assist in ethical decision making.
- *Peer support* provides a format for discussion, brainstorming, and reflection for the professional practice. Two or three heads are better than one in the process of ethical decision making.

Problem-Solving Approach to Ethical Decision Making

Problem solving to reach an effective decision is not an easy task. A generic model created from many different problem-solving methods is presented here for the purpose of ethical decision making. The model is developed from a critical-thinking perspective. Critical thinking uses the scientific method as a framework for making informed and evidence-based decisions. This model is used throughout the text in regard to what may be called clinical reasoning, which involves taking the client's health history, performing a physical assessment, developing a care or treatment plan, choosing methods to implement the treatment plan, and charting. Most of this information is presented in Chapter 4, with additional refinement throughout this text.

Massage therapists with well-developed clinical reasoning are able to generate, implement, and evaluate approaches to care. **Clinical reasoning** involves why and how to provide massage. The difference between critical thinking and clinical reasoning is this: *critical thinking* is a process that can be applied to many situations, both in the massage therapy profession and in everyday life; *clinical reasoning* is a form of critical thinking that targets a specific therapeutic practice, such as massage therapy. The decision-making process described can be used for both critical thinking and clinical reasoning.

We are most comfortable believing that our decision-making abilities are comprehensive, objective, intuitive, and workable. For some, this actually may be the case; however, years of teaching and self-exploration have shown that most people have never learned comprehensive decision-making skills. To complicate matters, different people, when gathering information, are naturally attracted to certain types of information and are influenced by certain types of criteria when evaluating possible solutions. Some experts believe that this attention focus is a genetic predisposition, and others believe that it is learned behavior. Regardless, most people, unless specifically trained, effectively consider only about half of the relevant and available information when making a decision. This can lead us to making decisions that do not serve us well.

A problem-solving model not only leads us through the steps we more naturally would take but also reminds us to take note of important information we might tend to overlook when making a decision (Box 2.12). When this process is followed diligently, it eventually becomes a habit. In the beginning, the process may feel cumbersome and uncomfortable. The parts of the process that we do not understand or find frustrating often are the areas on which we do not naturally focus. These are the areas, then, that need the most practice (Proficiency Exercise 2.4).

The decision-making process presented in Box 2.12 acknowledges the importance of factual data, intuitive insight, concrete and objective cause and effect, and the feelings, experiences, and influences of the people involved.

COMMUNICATION SKILLS

SECTION OBJECTIVES

Chapter objectives covered in this section:

10. Use basic communication skills to listen effectively and deliver an I-message.
11. Identify and resolve conflict in the professional setting.

Using the information presented in this section, the student will be able to:

- Identify a person's preferred communication pattern.
- Develop and use an I-message to deliver information and listen reflectively.
- Follow a suggested communication pattern for resolving ethical dilemmas and conflict.
- Identify three barriers to effective communication.

Communication is the act of exchanging thoughts, feelings, and behavior. Many ethical and professional dilemmas result from communication difficulties. To make ethical decisions and resolve ethical dilemmas, we must communicate effectively. Effective communication is often a difficult process for both the professional and the client. Without a direct communication approach, ethical dilemmas tend to escalate into conflict, and all individuals involved suffer in the process. Professionals seek to establish genuine positive regard for all clients and to relate to each with sensitivity to that person's uniqueness.

As described in Chapter 1, touch is a powerful mode of communication. The intent of professional touch may be influenced by many factors, including countertransference and the thought process of the therapist at the moment of the touch. The way touch is interpreted by the client is often influenced by the unspoken intent of the therapist; therefore it is important to monitor thoughts and feelings while professionally communicating through touch. Professional ethics demands that if feelings of criticism or negativity arise related to a client, we be aware of it and work to prevent it from interfering with our commitment to compassionate, quality care. Direct, honest communication that focuses on the concrete facts of the situation rather than the person's emotional behavior, accompanied by a gentle, respectful approach, opens the door for resolution.

Putting ethical principles into action requires some basic communication skills. Communication skills are required to retrieve information, maintain charting and client records, and provide information effectively so that the client can give informed consent. Using the following communication skills can help the professional maintain ethical practices in the therapeutic relationship.

The strongest message is delivered through the kinesthetic mode, or body language. As we express ourselves through our bodies, others visually receive the messages and/or feel our touch. Congruence in what is heard, what is seen, and what is

PROFICIENCY EXERCISE 2.4

Be a Critical Thinker

NOTE: Learning this process can be difficult, but it is important. It is okay to be confused and frustrated, but practice eventually will result in understanding. Proficiency exercises are important to do. In the beginning, it is okay if you just attempt to do them. In time, they get easier. On a separate piece of paper, go through the six steps.

Decision Making Using the Problem-Solving Model with Peer Support

Identify an ethical dilemma with which you are dealing or make up a dilemma that you believe you will deal with in the future. Describe the dilemma by answering the following questions on a piece of paper.

Step 1

Identify and define the situation.

Key Questions

What is the problem?

What happened in factual terms?

What caused the situation?

What was done or is being done?

What has worked or not worked?

Who is involved and what responsibilities do they have?

Step 2

Divide into groups of four. Choose who will present the facts of their dilemma to the group. This presentation should not take longer than 5 minutes. Each of the other three group members will play a role in the decision-making process.

One of the three remaining group members now provides input from step 2 of the problem-solving model by suggesting possible solutions, using the following questions as a guide. For the purpose of this exercise, limit the possibilities to three or four. Spend 3–5 minutes on this part of the exercise and remember to stay in your role; it confuses the process when you bounce between steps 3 and 4.

Key Questions

What are the possibilities?

What does my intuition suggest?

What are the possible contributing factors?

What are possible approaches for corrective action?

What might work?

What are other ways to look at the situation?

What do the data suggest?

Provide three possible solutions to the dilemma.

Step 3

The next person uses logic to evaluate each of the possible solutions presented in step 2, using the following questions as a guide. Spend 3–5 minutes on this part of the exercise. Again, stay in your role; do not work with steps 2 or 4.

Key Questions

What are the costs, resources needed, and time involved?

What is the logical progression of the pattern, contributing factors, and current behaviors?

What are the logical causes and effects of each solution identified?

What are the pros and cons of each solution suggested?

What are the consequences of not acting?

What are the consequences of acting?

Step 4

The last person evaluates each of the possible solutions generated in step 2 in terms of the people involved, using the following questions as a guide. Spend 3–5 minutes on this part of the exercise. Stay with the process; do not become chatty or conversational.

In terms of each possible solution considered in step 2, what is the effect on the people involved: client, practitioner, and other professionals working with the client?

Key Questions

How does each person involved feel about the possible solutions?

Does the practitioner feel qualified to work with such situations?

Does a feeling of cooperation and agreement exist among all parties involved?

Step 5

Now, the person who originally presented the ethical problem chooses a solution and develops an implementation plan. Again, spend 3–5 minutes on this part of the exercise. Write the solution with the implementation plan on a piece of paper.

Step 6

Rotate the roles so that each member of the group plays all four roles. It will take 1 hour to complete the entire exercise with all participants taking turns playing the four roles. After the entire process has been completed, answer these questions:

What was the easiest part of the process for me?

What was the hardest part of the process for me and what made it difficult?

What was the most difficult part of the process for the group?

What might help the group problem-solve more effectively?

How would I implement the process by myself without a peer support group?

felt is important. When congruence is lacking, the kinesthetic message seems to have the strongest effect.

The tone of voice is more important than the words spoken. Tone is kinesthetic and auditory because of the pressure waves emitted. We hear and feel the sound waves from tone of voice.

The words are the least effective part of the communication pattern. Words can have mixed meanings, depending on each person's interpretation. It is important to make sure that each of the people communicating is working from the same definition of a word. For example, the massage practitioner's definition of the word *disrobe* may be different from the client's definition. To a massage professional, disrobe may mean to remove external clothing but keep underwear on; the client interprets the same word as meaning to take off all clothing. During the informed consent process, the massage professional may say, "It is out of my scope of practice to diagnose or

Box 2.12 Problem-Solving Model for Decision Making

Learning how to make good professional decisions is important; the key to this is practice, practice, practice.

Step 1: Gather the facts to identify and define the situation.
Key questions: What is the problem? What happened in factual terms?
- What has happened?
- What caused the situation?
- What was done or is being done?
- What has worked or not worked?
- Who is involved and what responsibilities do they have?

Step 2: Brainstorm possible solutions.
Key question: What might I do? or What if?
- What are the possibilities?
- What does my intuition suggest?
- What are the possible contributing factors?
- What are possible approaches for corrective action?
- What might work?
- What are other ways to look at the situation?
- What do the data suggest?

Step 3: Logically and objectively evaluate each possible solution identified in step 2; look at both sides and the pros and cons.
Note: This objective analysis of the possible solutions generated in step 2 is important. The ability to analyze objectively is an essential skill for effective professional practice. In addition, this area of processing becomes important in dealing with conflict situations that may arise from ethical dilemmas, because the focus of this information is a process. Processes can be evaluated and altered; people's feelings usually cannot. A professional who has not developed the ability to evaluate a situation logically and objectively will have difficulty identifying where processes have broken down. Remember, change an action and people's feelings change.

Key question: What would happen if I...? (Insert each brainstormed idea from step 2.)
- What are the costs, resources needed, and time involved?
- What is the logical progression of the pattern, contributing factors, and current behaviors?
- What are the logical causes and effects of each solution identified?
- What are the pros and cons of each solution suggested?
- What are the consequences of not acting?
- What are the consequences of acting?

Step 4: Evaluate the effect of each possible solution on the people involved.
Key question: How would each person involved feel if I...? (Insert each brainstormed idea from step 2.)
- In terms of each solution being considered, what is the effect on the people involved: client, practitioner, and other professionals working with the client?
- How does each person involved feel about the possible interventions?
- Does the practitioner feel qualified to work with such situations?
- Does a feeling of cooperation and agreement exist among all parties involved?

Step 5: Choose a solution and develop an implementation plan after carefully processing steps 1 through 4.
Implementation plans are step-by-step procedures that detail what must be done to carry out the decision.

Example

A solution arrived at using the previous steps might be: I will learn more about asthma so that I can work more effectively with my client. The implementation plan would be as follows:
- Use the Internet/Medline Plus to learn about asthma.
- Search for research about massage and asthma on PubMed.
- Contact the local asthma support group for information.
- With the release of information form on file, contact the client's physician for specific recommendations.
- Talk with my friend who is a respiratory therapist.
- Compile the information into a massage benefit report to develop the massage approach.
- Discuss the report with my client.

Step 6: Implement the plan and set a date for reevaluation.
Just doing it is sometimes the hardest part.

Step 7: Determine the logical consequences if the plan is not followed.
It is important to determine what will happen if one of the parties in a decision that affects more than one person does not meet their commitment. Make sure to document this (write it down). For example, a decision is made between a massage therapist and a chronic no-show client that the client will be charged for the full session unless they call 24 hours in advance to cancel the appointment. Both parties agree, but the very next session, the client does not show and does not call. Because the consequence has been agreed on in advance (i.e., the client will be charged for the full session), the possibility of escalation of the conflict is diminished.

Step 8: Reevaluate and make necessary adjustments; then implement the refined plan.
Remember, decisions are not static; reevaluation may show you ways to alter, refine, or change them.

treat any specific condition." The massage practitioner defines the word *treat* as meaning to provide remedial or rehabilitation procedures. The client interprets the word *treat* as any type of method used.

To encourage effective communication, begin by identifying a person's communication pattern; that is, the words used, tone of voice, and body language. Use neutral topics such as the weather or a community event to generate general discussion. During this time, adjust your communication pattern to meet the person's communication style. Shift your body language, word choice, and tone to match the client's before attempting to deliver a message.

When communicating feelings, be specific. Words such as *upset* are too ambiguous; instead, use words such as *afraid, angry, annoyed, discouraged, embarrassed, irritated, rejected, accepted, appreciated, capable, determined, compassionate, glad, grateful*, *proud*, *loved*, and *trusted*. Define the words you use. Do not assume that what you mean by a word is what your listener understands it to mean. For example, a massage therapist tells a new client, "It is important for you to tell me if the method being used *bothers* you, such as it tickles, is too deep or light, feels ineffective, is painful, or any other uncomfortable sensation." The word *bothers* was defined in this example.

Listening

Effective listening involves the development of focusing skills. *You cannot listen effectively if you are distracted, planning what you will say next, or preparing your response.* **Reflective listening** involves restating the information to indicate that you have received and understood the message. **Active listening** may clarify a feeling attached to the message but does not add to or change the message.

Listening does not involve any form of response, such as giving advice, resolving the problem presented, or in any other way interjecting information about what was said. Effective listening occurs when we listen to understand instead of to respond. Understanding the message and agreeing with the content of the message are not the same thing; the basis for this confusion most likely evolved from our feeling of being most understood when someone agrees with us. Understanding can occur regardless of whether agreement exists. Much time is wasted, and conflict is encouraged when people equate understanding with agreement.

EXAMPLE

As a student you may not agree with the author's (my) position on the importance of wearing a uniform in the professional setting. Because you have a different opinion does not mean that the textbook is wrong or that you are wrong; the two positions are simply different. You can understand that I am basing my information on the existing standards of professionalism and my previous experience; however, you can choose not to follow the recommendation. I, as the author of the text, can understand that a valid case can be made for not visually creating distinction (a uniform) between the professional and the client; however, I would not agree with your decision if you decided not to wear a uniform. Sometimes this is called "agreeing to disagree," but this approach still seems to have the context of right or wrong, whereas simply being understood feels nonjudgmental and essential (Mentoring Tip).

MENTORING TIP

We must have an ongoing self-evaluation process. This often takes the form of honestly seeking answers to some hard questions. We need to seek answers from ourselves and others who care enough about us to give us accurate information. Check out these questions related to communication:

- What are my conversational downfalls? Do I interrupt? Do I speak too loudly or too softly? Am I hard to understand?
- Am I bossy or overbearing? Do I come across as a know-it-all? When I am honest with myself, what do I do that annoys others? What do others do to annoy me? Do I nitpick, tease, gossip, criticize, complain, and whine?

MENTORING TIP—Cont'd

- What are my conversational strengths? Am I really a good listener? Do I listen more than I talk? Do I really listen or just pretend to? How do I let others know that I really do understand? How do I support a team effort? Do I laugh good-heartedly? How do I recognize when someone else needs my support? Do I provide effective feedback and suggestions that are logical and valid? How do I do that? How do I express my opinions and feelings?
- What are the defense mechanisms I use when stressed? Defense mechanisms include sarcasm, denial, making excuses, blaming, crying, stomping off, refusing to talk, bringing up the past, being a victim ("poor me"), lying, exaggerating, and pouting.
- Which of these behaviors bothers me when others act out? How do I respond to others' defensive behavior? How do others respond to my defensive behavior? How may these behaviors interfere with my massage career?

When someone gives you information in response to questions such as these, be thankful the person cares enough to respond. Evaluate the validity of the information. Don't let your feelings get hurt. Take action to improve.

Delivering Information With I-Messages

I-messages share feelings and concerns. You-messages put a person down, blame, criticize, and provoke anger, hurt, embarrassment, and feelings of worthlessness. I-message patterns require the four elements of information used in effective decision making (Box 2.13):

- Describe the behavior or problem you find bothersome (facts)
- State your feelings about the situation (effect on people)
- State the consequence (logical cause and effect)
- Request the preferred behavior or action (possibilities)

It takes practice to use the simple I-message communication pattern well.

After an I-message has been delivered, request a response using open-ended questions. **Open-ended questions** encourage the sharing of information and cannot be easily answered in one word. Open-ended questions begin with where, when, what, how, and which. Avoid why questions because they en-

Box 2.13 I-Message Pattern

The steps for creating an I-message are as follows:

1. Describe the behavior or problem you find bothersome (facts).
2. State your feelings about the situation (effect on people).
3. State the consequence (logical cause and effect).
4. Request the preferred behavior or action (possibilities).

The pattern is:

When ______________ happens, I feel ______________.
The result is ______________, and what I would prefer is ______________.

When delivering I-messages, remain pleasant, respectful, and honest. Be aware of your body language, tone of voice, and quality of touch.

courage defensive reactions. When listening to the response, use active and reflective listening.

The I-message format also can be an effective listening tool. While listening, organize the information using these questions:

- What happened, or what are the facts?
- What feelings are being expressed?
- What was the logical outcome?
- What are the possibilities for solution or resolution?

When listening reflectively, repeat the information back to the client: "What I heard you say was: When ____ happened, you felt ___. The result was ___, and what you prefer is ___. Did I understand correctly?" If a person leaves out information (as commonly occurs), you will not be able to fill in that blank. In that case, a clarifying question can be formed, such as, "What would you prefer?" or "What was the logical outcome of the situation?"

A common ethical dilemma for massage therapists is clients who tend to arrive late for their massage appointment. The conversation in the Example box demonstrates how I-messages and active and reflective listening skills can be used.

EXAMPLE

The client walks through the door, exclaiming: "Wow! Traffic was heavy, and I know I'm late again. Sorry. I sure am ready for my hour massage session!"

The massage therapist responds with reflective and then active listening: "So, what I'm hearing is that you were stuck in traffic and that's why you were late. Is this the same traffic issue that resulted in your being late last week as well?"

Client: "Yes, the road construction is really slowing people down."

Massage therapist: "I can appreciate the reason for the delay and that you are apologetic. I also understand that you are expecting the full massage session. However, when clients are late for the massage, I feel frustrated because my schedule will not allow me to provide a full 50 minutes of massage. Today I will do my best to address your goals in the time we have left. I hope you can find a way to avoid the construction or allow more time to get here so we can have all the time allowed for your massage."

Client: "Well, I'm doing the best I can to be on time, and my neck really is stiff. Can't you push the schedule back so I have the full time? I really need it."

Massage therapist: "I'm aware that your neck is your problem area, but my next client has already called to confirm. I will modify my approach so the neck is targeted. Now let's get started so we use the remaining time efficiently. Next week I am sure you'll be here at 4:00 p.m. Or we could consider a different day or time."

Conflict and Conflict Resolution

Conflict is a struggle between at least two interdependent parties who perceive incompatible goals, scarce resources, and/or interference from the other party in achieving their goals. Conflict arises when one or more people view the current system as not working. At least one person is sufficiently dissatisfied with the status quo to be willing to own the conflict and speak up in the hope of being able to improve the situation. Through conflict, we have opportunities to do things differently in the future. Conflict arises from a number of factors, such as:

- Varied perspectives on a situation
- Differing belief systems and values, which have arisen from the involved parties' accumulated life experience
- Differing objectives and interests
- Concern about the effect of the dispute on the relationship
- Time concerns
- Expense
- Effect on others
- Lost opportunities
- Stress
- Lack of closure
- Uncertain compliance

Conflict and conflict resolution play important roles in individual and social evolution and development. Many cultures value harmony, compatibility, satisfaction, and independence. Because of these values, the tendency in the past has been to avoid conflict. Conflict should also be recognized as existing at two levels. In addition to the typically obvious interpersonal dispute among individuals, some conflict almost always exists within us. This inner conflict may be evidenced by confusion, inconsistency, or lack of congruity.

People in conflict have both common ground and differences. Common ground comprises ideas, results, and expressions of shared benefit. Areas of common ground include:

- Overlapping interests
- Interdependence
- Points of agreement

The common ground can serve as the starting point for conflict resolution.

Conflict resolution does not necessarily resolve tensions between people. Conflict resolution may simply align matters sufficiently to allow each person to make progress toward their goals rather than stall in an uncertain and stressful state of disagreement.

Many people have long operated by the myth that the best way to resolve conflict is to "do battle," and the one who "wins" ends the conflict. This approach is more about power and control than conflict resolution. Doing battle and winning or losing supports a corresponding belief that every situation involves a right and a wrong. If we respond to conflict this way, we have limited our awareness and understanding of the nature of conflict and of alternative means of responding to conflict, such as mediation and negotiation. The decision-making process in this text presents a format for mediated and negotiated types of conflict resolution.

Types of Conflicts

Various types of conflicts exist. If we can pinpoint the type of conflict, we are more likely to be able to resolve it.

Relationship Conflicts

Relationship conflicts, often called *personality conflicts*, occur as a result of strong negative emotions, misperceptions or stereotypes, poor communication or miscommunication, or repetitive negative behaviors. Relationship problems often lead to an unnecessary escalation in destructive conflict. Conflict resolution supports the safe and balanced expression of the perspectives and emotions of each person involved, leading to acknowledgment and understanding of that individual's point of view and personality traits.

Personality traits are generally classified as behaviors, attitudes, and actions individuals use in combination to function in society. Personality traits have been categorized into personality styles. Evaluations exist for identifying different personality styles and using these evaluation tools can be helpful to better understand ourselves and others. A word of caution: use personality evaluations only as a guide. People are much too complex to be defined by personality styles. Two personality evaluations worth exploring are the Big Five Personality Domains and the 16 Personalities and Myers-Briggs Type Indicator. You can learn more about these systems and other personality inventories on the Internet. These types of evaluations may help individuals with differing perspectives interact more productively.

EXAMPLE

Two massage therapists have worked together for 2 years. Just recently a new massage therapist has been hired. This individual prefers to eat lunch alone and remain in the massage room during breaks. Conflict develops when the original massage therapists begin to describe their new coworker as stuck up and a snob.

Data Conflicts

Data conflicts occur when people lack information necessary to make wise decisions, are misinformed, disagree on which data are relevant, interpret information differently, or have collected data differently. Some data conflicts may be unnecessary because they are caused by poor communication among the people in conflict. Other data conflicts may be incompatibilities associated with data collection, interpretation, or communication. Most data conflicts have "data solutions," and once the information has been corrected, the conflict will resolve unless it has developed into a relationship conflict.

EXAMPLE

Conflict can occur because of a scheduling problem. Two clients arrive for their appointments at the same time. When the clients check their appointment cards, one realizes that they entered the appointment in their calendar on the wrong day.

Interest Conflicts

Interest conflicts are caused by competition over perceived incompatible needs. Conflicts of interest result when one or more people believe that to satisfy their needs, the needs and interests of an opponent must be sacrificed. This often occurs during times of scarcity or when it is perceived that there is not enough of something to go around. Interest-based conflicts may occur over such things as money, physical resources, or time; over procedural issues, such as the way a dispute is resolved; or over psychological issues, such as perceptions of trust and fairness and the desire for participation and respect. For an interest-based dispute to be resolved, those involved need to define and express their individual interests so that all these interests may be addressed jointly. Interest-based conflict is best resolved through maximum integration of the parties' respective interests, positive intentions, and desired experiential outcomes. A third person, such as a mediator, is often necessary to successfully resolve this type of conflict.

EXAMPLE

Four massage therapists have been working at the same massage franchise for a year and have had full schedules. Business has been slow for the past 3 months, and they are now competing with each other for clients.

Values Conflicts

Values give meaning to our lives. Values explain what is "just" or "unjust." Differing values need not cause conflict. People can live together in harmony with different value systems. Values disputes arise only when people attempt to force one set of values on others or lay claim to exclusive value systems that do not allow for divergent paths. It is no use to try to change values and systems during relatively short mediation. However, supporting each participant's expression of their values and beliefs for acknowledgment by the other party can be helpful. Belief systems are more likely to change. Values are like the ethical principles described earlier, whereas belief systems are like standards of practice. Belief systems are often superimposed on us during our developmental childhood years. We are taught what is right or wrong, good or bad. Because we learn our belief systems, we can change them through education and a willingness to be open to new possibilities.

EXAMPLE

A massage therapist strongly believes most health conditions can be controlled without medication. This practitioner has a new client who uses a variety of medications to manage anxiety. The massage therapist is finding it difficult to refrain from telling the client that anxiety can be managed with lifestyle changes and that medication is not necessary. The conflict is based on differing belief systems.

Ways of Dealing With Conflict

Five common methods can be used to deal with conflict. Learning about the alternative means of handling conflict gives us a wider choice of actions to use in any given situation and makes us better able to respond to the situation. Although the methods described in the following sections are the common ways of increasing the chance of success, the reality is that we use each of these ways of dealing with conflict at least some of the time. We approach conflict in the way we believe will be most helpful to us. Our style for dealing with conflict changes with the circumstances. Conflict-handling behavior is not a static procedure; rather, it is a process that requires flexibility and constant evaluation to be truly effective. In all conflict situations, remain focused on the issue not the individual.

Denial or Withdrawal

With denial or withdrawal, a person attempts to eliminate conflict by denying that it exists and refusing to acknowledge it. Usually, the conflict does not go away but rather grows to the point that it becomes unmanageable. When the issue and the timing are not critical and the issue is short-lived and will resolve itself, denial may be a productive way to deal with conflict. The effectiveness of this approach depends on knowing when to use denial.

EXAMPLE

The receptionist in the spa where you work tends to schedule massage sessions for one massage therapist with whom they are personal friends more than they schedule the other massage therapists. However, the receptionist is moving to another city in a month and will be leaving this job. This situation is going to resolve on its own without intervention.

Suppression or Smoothing Over

A person using suppression plays down differences and does not recognize the positive aspects of managing the conflict openly. Instead, the situation is acknowledged (unlike with denial), but it is glossed over. The source of the conflict rarely goes away. However, suppression may be used when preserving a relationship is more important than dealing with a relatively insignificant issue.

EXAMPLE

A client chews gum during the massage, and the massage therapist finds this behavior annoying. The massage therapist has mentioned that chewing gum can interfere with the client's ability to relax, but the client chews gum anyway. The massage therapist learns to ignore the behavior.

Power or Dominance

Power is often used to settle differences. It may be inherent in a person's authority or position. It may take the form of a majority (as in voting) or a persuasive minority. Power strategies result in winners and losers. The losers do not support a final decision in the same way the winners do. Future meetings of a group may be marred by the conscious or unconscious renewal of the struggle previously "settled" by the use of power. In some instances, especially when other forms of handling conflict are not effective, power strategies may be necessary. Parents often say to children, "Because I said so." This use of power works in the short term but over time results in deeper relationship conflict.

EXAMPLE

A massage therapist has just begun to work for a chiropractor who employs three other therapists. The chiropractor mandates a dress code of blue scrubs with the company logo and white athletic shoes. The new therapist does not want to wear the required uniform and complains to the massage supervisor, who simply says, "Wear the uniform with a good attitude, or you will be let go."

Compromise or Negotiation

Compromise (i.e., "You give a little, I'll give a little, and we'll meet each other halfway") has some serious drawbacks. Such bargaining often causes both sides to assume initial inflated positions, because they are aware that they are going to have to "give a little" and want to reduce the loss. The compromise solution may be watered down or weakened to the point that it will not be effective. There may be little real commitment by any of the people involved. Still, in some cases, compromise makes sense, such as when resources are limited or a speedy decision needs to be made.

EXAMPLE

The fitness center where two massage therapists work is remodeling, and for 1 month the massage rooms will be unavailable. There are two rooms that can be used instead, but one is small. One massage therapist has rented space with the fitness center for 3 years and the other for 2 years. After a staff meeting, it is agreed that the massage therapists will rotate, with each taking a shift in the small room, even though the massage therapist with 3 years thinks they should have the large room.

Integration or Collaboration

The integration or collaboration approach suggests that all involved in the conflict recognize the interests and abilities of the others. Each individual's interests, positive intentions, and desired outcomes are thoroughly explored in an effort to solve the problems in a maximizing way. Participants are expected to modify and develop their original views as work progresses. This sounds like the ideal way to manage and resolve conflict; however, for collaboration to be successful, those involved need a nonthreatening and collectively supportive system. This process takes time, openness, and energy. It is often necessary to use an independent, unbiased mediator to negotiate collaboration.

EXAMPLE

The owner of an independent holistic health clinic that rents space to massage therapists who function as self-employed sells the facility and business to an individual who wants to change the business model to an employee system. The new owner would like to hire the massage therapists who are currently renting rooms within the business, but there is resistance. The new owner schedules a day-long meeting to discuss the issues and identify workable solutions.

Conflict Climate: Defensive or Supportive

A **defensive climate** reflects the type of atmosphere characteristic of competition; it is an atmosphere that inhibits the mutual trust required for effective conflict management. A **supportive climate** reflects collaboration; it is an environment that leads to mutual trust and to an atmosphere conducive to managing differences. In the best case, the participants in conflict resolution come to appreciate that the issue causing conflict does not need to limit their discussions. Participants are encouraged to express the full breadth and depth of their interests, with each participant seeking to identify a "value" that each can bring to the discussion and the maximized satisfaction of underlying interests and intentions.

Conflict is important. If managed well, it identifies and supports effective change. Conflict can foster avoidance, or it can expand our experiences. Making good decisions about managing and resolving conflict can pave the way for greater understanding and well-being.

During the process of resolving a conflict, written documentation should be maintained about the nature of the conflict, the type of resolution attempted, the success of the conflict resolution, and the outcome. Because conflict already exists, interpretation of the requirement for resolution can become confused. Objective documentation that is agreed on by those involved helps maintain clarity. If the conflict cannot be resolved independently, documentation of the nature of the conflict is extremely important in case the situation escalates to legal action.

Communicating When Dilemmas Arise

The following pattern can be used to resolve ethical dilemmas.

1. Carefully examine the facts, possibilities, logical causes and effects, and your feelings about the situation.
2. Speak with a mentor, a peer, or a supervisor about the situation in a peer review or support context.
3. Plan a time to talk about the situation with the other person or people involved.
4. Begin the conversation by identifying the problem as you see it.
5. Use the standard I-message format to provide information and professional disclosure about your inability to work with or be comfortable with the situation.

In the following example, a massage professional uses an I-message to talk with a client about the client's body odor:

> *"When a client seems to have a distinctive body odor that I am aware of [facts], I feel distracted from my work [effect on people]. As a result, because of my inability to focus, the client does not receive the best massage [logical cause and effect]. I would like to see if we can resolve this situation. If I can't deal with the situation better, I may find it to your benefit to refer you to someone who is not as sensitive to odors as I am [possibilities]."*

The client's body language and tone of voice may indicate embarrassment. The therapist then uses another I-message:

> *"When I find it necessary to speak with someone about issues as personal as this [facts], I feel uncomfortable and embarrassed because I am afraid I will embarrass or hurt the person [effect on people]. It is difficult for me, but I want you to have the best possible care [logical cause and effect]. What information do you have that can help me [possibilities and open-ended question]?" Ending with an open-ended question encourages a problem-solving discussion.*

It is essential to determine who has the problem. This can be done easily by deciding who will have to implement the solution to resolve the problem. Sometimes both parties own a part of the problem, with each needing to implement a portion of the solution for total resolution. Continuing with the example of body odor, the therapist identifies and owns the problem by saying, *"The difficulty is in my sensitivity to odors."*

Next, information is gathered, and possible solutions are devised. The client continues to express embarrassment through body language and states that they are aware of the problem and tells you that body odor has been a problem related to taking medication for a health problem. The client showered before coming to the session and thought the odor was gone.

> *The massage practitioner responds using reflective listening: "If I understand correctly, you are taking a medication that causes the body odor [facts], and others are aware of the odor [impact on people], but you felt the odor was gone since you showered before coming to the session [logical cause and effect]."*
>
> *The therapist asks, "Do you have any suggestions?" The client replies, "Could you use a scented oil or a room scent?" The client also says that he can speak to their physician and continue to shower just before coming for the session (generating possible solutions).*
>
> *The therapist explains that using scented oil may be a problem because of sensitive skin and that using a room scent bothers other clients. The therapist asks, "Would it bother you if I wore a mask treated with a scented oil?" The client indicates that would be fine (evaluating possible solutions in terms of logical outcomes and pros and cons, as well as people's feelings).*
>
> *The therapist says, "How about if I try the mask next time you are here, and we will talk about it after the massage? If this doesn't work, we will see if we can come up with another solution. If nothing works, I will help you find a good therapist who can better serve your needs and is not so sensitive to odors." The client agrees (deciding on and implementing a plan, setting a date for reevaluation, and agreeing on logical consequences).*

After a decision has been made and agreed to, it should be well defined, and all parties should agree as to what will happen if the solution to the problem is not implemented effectively. The plan and the agreed-on consequences should be written down.

The therapist closes with an I-message: *"I feel relieved [effect on people] that we were able to discuss my sensitivity to odors [facts]. This conversation has encouraged me to be more honest with myself and my clients [logical cause and effect]. I hope that I will be able to continue to communicate effectively with you [possibilities]. Thank you for being open with me."*

A week later, the plan is carried out, and the therapist finds that using the mask is distracting but effective. A sense of humor and understanding on the part of both the therapist and the client continue to support an effective solution (reevaluate and make the necessary adjustments).

Barriers to Effective Communication

Effective communication is a skill. It can be learned. Effective communication is essential in the therapeutic relationship. Professionals diligently seek to improve their communication skills. Some factors function as barriers or blocks that interfere with productive communication.

Time

It takes time to communicate effectively. This is why writing is sometimes a more effective form of communication. When writing, we should make time to consider the words and reflect on what is being said. The person responding to the written message also has time to reread and reflect on the message. We also need to make time to speak with someone by scheduling the time and place where open communication can occur.

Old Patterns

Falling into old patterns and old conditioning limits effective communication. It is important to "know thyself," and we must recognize personal triggers to old reactionary patterns in communication. Sometimes we need to leave a situation and come back to it so that we can respond instead of reacting. Issues with self-esteem and confidence can result in falling into past behavior patterns.

Avoidance

People generally procrastinate about addressing conflict until it is unavoidable. They avoid people who display strong emotion because it makes them feel uncomfortable. Personal and emotional triggers often lead to avoidance.

Language, Culture, and Communication

We live in a global society with many languages and beliefs. To communicate, people need to understand the language used and respect the cultural traditions. Sometimes an interpreter is needed.

CREDENTIALS AND LICENSING

SECTION OBJECTIVES

Chapter objective covered in this section:

12. Identify legal and credentialing concerns of the massage professional.

Using the information presented in this section, the student will be able to:

- Describe the difference between government and private credentials.
- Determine whether a credentialing program is valid.
- Explain the basic roles of local and state laws and legislation and their influence on therapeutic massage.
- Contact local, state, or provincial government agencies to obtain information about laws pertinent to the practice of therapeutic massage.

Credentials

Credentials are a form of official verification, earned by completing an educational or examination process that confirms a certain level of expertise in a given skill. Standardization of the massage profession has resulted in different methods of proving one's skills to practice therapeutic massage. The only credentials required for the practice of therapeutic massage are those specified by government agencies (Box 2.14). All others are voluntary.

Many massage organizations and training programs have developed their own types of credentials. These credentials are valid because they indicate a level of professional achievement. A school diploma, which is granted on completion of a course of study, is an example. This is an important document for a massage professional, but it is not a legally required credential unless stipulated by the law. For instance, a massage professional may need a diploma from a state-regulated school to take licensing examinations in states that license massage therapists.

Anyone can offer private certificates. Many individuals or organizations will give a certificate of completion for attending a class. These types of certificates are common in continuing education. These certificates do not have any legal value but do verify ongoing education.

The educational requirement for taking a licensing examination is described in the law. As previously described, the formal education range is 500 contact hours to more

Box 2.14 Credentials and Regulations

Licensing: Common

- Requires a state or provincial board of massage or similar agency
- Requires all who practice the profession to be licensed
- Legally defines and limits the scope of practice for a profession
- Requires specific educational courses and/or an examination
- Protects the use of a title (e.g., only those licensed can use the title of massage therapist)

Government Certification: Rare

- Administered by an independent board
- Voluntary but required for anyone using the protected title (e.g., massage therapist); others can provide the service but cannot call themselves massage therapists
- Requires specific educational courses and an examination

Government Registration: Uncommon

- Administered by the state Department of Registry or other appropriate state agency (not to be confused with private registration processes)

Voluntary Verification: Rare

- Does not necessarily require specific education such as a school diploma; other forms of verification of professional standards, such as years in practice, are often acceptable
- Does not provide title protection

Exemptions: Uncommon

- Means that a practitioner is not required to comply with an existing local or state regulation
- Excuses practitioners who meet specified educational requirements from meeting current regulatory requirements
- Does not provide title protection

than 1000 contact hours. The Federation of State Massage Boards offers the MBLEx licensing examination, which covers the information and competencies required by the law and as indicated by the most recent job survey. Experts develop the question bank. Each examination is computer generated from the test bank, and the examinations are administered regularly in convenient locations. The licensing examination does not include a practical demonstration of skills. The questions are multiple choice. Most of the questions are not answered with a regurgitation of factual data but rather require effective decision-making skills to identify the best answer. Some states in the United States have also required additional test components, such as a jurisprudence examination. *Jurisprudence* is a term used to indicate the theory and practice of a law. A jurisprudence examination is a test taken to demonstrate knowledge of a specific piece of legislation, such as a massage therapy law.

Valid credentialing beyond licensing is voluntary and important. The National Certification Board for Therapeutic Massage and Bodywork offers board certification. Board certification is designed to measure professional experience and ongoing education necessary to work confidently in complex practice situations. It is based on critical thinking and clinical reasoning. Board certification confirms that a massage therapist is no longer a new graduate and has gained additional education and experience as a massage therapist. Board certification in therapeutic massage and bodywork should be a professional goal.

The Difference Between Certificates and Certification

A *certificate* provides recognition of the completion of classes in a specialty area of practice or set of skills. Certificates can be issued by anyone without any form of oversight. Certificates of attendance or participation are provided to individuals who have attended or participated in classes, courses, or other education/training programs or events.

Certification recognizes professionals who meet established knowledge, skills, or competencies. Certification is provided by a designated standard-setting organization that participates in oversight by other external credentialing bodies. The content assessed during a certification process is identified through a defensible, industry-wide process. Certification requires an ongoing maintenance process to meet standards for ongoing use of the credential.

The easy way to remember the differences is that schools and continuing education classes do not offer certification—they offer certificates. Certification requires applicants to take qualification exams provided by designated credentialing organizations.

It is unethical to say that you are certified after taking a course and have received a certificate. You can only be certified when you complete the appropriate prerequisites to participate in a certification examination process, maintain the credential with continuing education, and recertify on a regular basis.

Laws and Legislation

The main purpose of a law or an ordinance is to protect the safety and welfare of the public. Laws and ordinances are not passed to protect the interests of a small group (i.e., a special interest group). Sometimes massage therapists become frustrated by the procedures they have to follow to be in compliance with laws that govern massage therapy. Remember, the law is specifically designed to protect the public, and everything required is intended to serve that purpose.

Many but not all health professionals are regulated at the state level through licensing. If the government feels that a particular activity could cause harm to the public, it seeks to control and limit the individuals who can participate in the activity. (For example, physicians, nurses, chiropractors, physical therapists, dentists, builders, electricians, cosmetologists, and plumbers all are licensed.) Requirements for a knowledge base and the amount and type of education are determined and verified by testing. The scope of practice is described in the law that governs the licensed professional. Currently almost all states of the United States have some type of state licensing for the professional practice of therapeutic massage. Licensing requirements in the European and Asian countries, Canada, New Zealand, Australia, and other countries vary to such an extent that it is impossible to cover all that information in this chapter. However, there is a global trend to legally regulate the practice of therapeutic massage. A word of caution: therapeutic massage is not consistently regulated by law. Because of this inconsistency, massage professionals must carefully research the governmental controls and laws that apply in the areas where they plan to practice massage therapy.

State and Local Regulation

The types of legislative controls that massage therapists most often encounter are state or provincial controls and local controls. A province is a political unit of some countries, such as Canada. It typically is a large area made up of many small local units of government. In the US, states are the equivalent of provinces. States are further subdivided into counties, local townships, and cities.

In the United States, all states that have enacted massage licensing laws are eligible to belong to the Federation of State Massage Therapy Boards (FSMTB). A massage therapy board oversees the practice of individuals who use the title of massage therapists, or otherwise represent themselves to be massage therapist. A board of massage therapy evaluates the qualifications of applicants for licensure and grants licenses to those who qualify. The board establishes rules and regulations to ensure the integrity and competence of licensed massage therapists and investigates complaints for unprofessional conduct. Professional licensing protects the health and safety of the public from fraudulent and unethical practitioners. The board is the link between the consumer and the licensed massage therapist and promotes the public health, welfare, and safety.

The FSMTB developed an examination specifically for state licensing of massage professions, the Massage & Bodywork

Licensing Examination (commonly known as the MBLEx, as noted earlier). Launched in 2007, this examination supports states in developing legislative guidelines for massage therapists.

If a state does not choose to license a particular profession (occupational licensing), local governments (usually townships and cities) can choose to regulate activities within their jurisdiction. Again, local laws, usually called *ordinances,* are in place to protect the public's safety and welfare.

The local government does regulate where the professional may work. This is done through zoning ordinances and establishment licenses. Professionals such as physicians, lawyers, and accountants are often required to locate their place of business in a particular zone or area of land use. Land use is usually determined on a master plan that directs the way the local government wants to see the area grow and develop. It is important to designate areas as residential (living), industrial (manufacturing), retail business districts (commercial), professional offices (office), parks (recreational), and farming (agriculture). Without such zoning, a loud industrial operation could disturb the quiet living in a residential area. Local governments are also concerned with the safety of the buildings in their areas. Monitoring the safety of buildings is the responsibility of the building inspector.

Many old laws and local massage ordinances were written to control prostitution by preventing the practice of massage. This type of ordinance is easy to recognize because it specifies medical examinations for sexually transmitted disease and other degrading requirements. Although the situation is improving, local ordinances of this type are still found in states where the profession of massage has not yet been licensed.

If the state licenses massage, the local government usually treats the massage professional like any other licensed health or service professional. Business operations are allowed in the proper zoning location, usually an area of office or commercial zoning.

Local governments often discourage any type of business operation in residential areas but, with special restrictions, will designate which types of businesses can be operated from a home. These home occupations usually are service oriented rather than retail oriented (the sale of goods) and limit traffic to and from the home. To establish a home office, the massage therapist may need to have a special and separate area in the home, including a separate entrance. Another requirement might be that no employees other than the family in the home may be hired. Sometimes only those with a special need, such as a disability that prevents working outside the home, are eligible for a home office permit. Usually a special permit is required for a home office; each local government is different. Many massage practitioners choose to work from a home office. A massage practice is a business that fits well within these special requirements.

The bottom line is the massage professional must comply with the existing standards of practice, both required and voluntary (Box 2.15) If a difficult state law or local ordinance is encountered, massage therapists can work together to change the regulation.

Box 2.15 Steps for Complying with Licensing Requirements

1. Find out whether your state or province requires licensing. Contact the Occupational Licensing Division of the Department of Licensing and Regulation for this information. If state licensing is required, find out what educational requirements must be met to take the examination.
2. If your state does not have licensing, contact the local government for the area where you intend to work to inquire about local ordinances. Obtain a copy of the ordinances and read them carefully. Especially look for the educational, zoning, and facility requirements. Whether you live in a city, township, or similar government unit, the clerk's office is the department that usually has this information.
3. Investigate carefully for your school of massage training. Contact the state Department of Education and confirm that the school is licensed and in compliance with state regulations.
4. Before renting, buying, or setting up your massage practice, contact the local government about zoning requirements and building codes. If you are considering a home office, check the zoning ordinances to make sure you will be in compliance. Again, your city or township officials (usually the clerk) are your best sources of information.
5. Special zoning permits require a public hearing. Your neighbors are notified by mail, and the hearing is advertised in the newspaper. Contact the zoning department to find out what action is required. Whether you are establishing your business in a home office or a business zone, contact the neighbors to explain your business and find out their response. Without their approval, or at least lack of opposition, you are unlikely to obtain a permit. Attend the hearing at all costs. Remember: No permit = no business. Zoning permits may require 6–8 weeks to complete. If you start your business without proper permits, you could be shut down at any time by government authorities.
6. Before you rent space or begin your business, contact the local government and apply for any necessary permits or business licenses including establishment licenses related to the location a massage therapist practices massage. Make sure you meet all regulations. Fees can run anywhere from $25 to $500.
7. Make sure the employer you are considering working for is in compliance with the previous requirements.

Reciprocity

Reciprocity is the right of exchange of privileges between governing bodies. Some states have similar licensing requirements for professionals. When this is the case, a state may accept a different state's license. This is not common for many professionals, and it is even less common for massage therapists.

Individual state licensing or any type of certification does not secure the right to practice massage in any location outside that of the government issuing the license.

Regulations, standards of practice, codes of conduct, scopes of practice, and so forth are methods of setting the rules for cooperative professional relationships. All organized groups have rules that permit effective interaction among members. Respect is important and working together as a team is essential in professional practice. Let us hope that the massage therapy profession is an example of cooperation, respect for other professions, and ethical standards of practice that provide for internal professional regulation and compliance with external governmental control.

DEALING WITH SUSPECTED UNETHICAL OR ILLEGAL BEHAVIOR

SECTION OBJECTIVES

Chapter objective covered in this section:

13. Identify and report unethical conduct by colleagues.

Using the information presented in this section, the student will be able to:

- List and explain the four steps involved in reporting unethical behavior.

Addressing unethical behavior and violations of standards of practice by colleagues can present a difficult dilemma. Everything covered in this chapter is an important consideration when dealing with inappropriate behavior by others (Proficiency Exercise 2.5). When concern develops about the conduct of a colleague, an approach that combines self-reflection, peer support, mentoring, supervision, and effective communication skills is the best way to deal with these situations.

Self-Reflection

Carefully reflect on the personal motivation causing the concern. It is important that motives for confronting a fellow professional be based on a genuine concern for the therapist and the therapist's clients, in addition to the higher good of the profession as a whole. Make sure the situation is purely one of professional ethical concern and not a reaction based on personal values or moral beliefs.

PROFICIENCY EXERCISE 2.5

Working in groups of three, imagine and then develop a specific situation in which a colleague has acted unethically. Exchange responses with a different group and role-play to resolve the situation. One learner acts as the massage practitioner, one plays the colleague, and the other evaluates the way the situation is managed. Role-play different situations until each learner has had a chance to play each role. Use the problem-solving model and communication/conflict management skills while role playing.

Mentoring and Peer Support

Discuss the situation with your mentor or a colleague in a peer support situation while maintaining the confidentiality of the suspected party. Explore the motives supporting your concern.

Talking With Those Involved

If others share your concern, speak directly to the colleague. Often the person is not aware of the breach of standards of practice or that the behavior appears to be unethical. Peer support and bringing the concern to the person's attention may help resolve the problem.

Formal Reporting

Depending on the seriousness of the infraction and the colleague's response, you may have to file a formal complaint through the professional organization or the legal system in your area. Ask yourself the following questions:

- How do I feel about the various laws that influence my professional practice?
- Which type of law could I find myself breaking? Fraud? Negligence? Malpractice? Defamation of character? Invasion of privacy? Software theft or piracy?
- What makes me vulnerable to breaking this type of law?
- What would I do and how would I feel if I were accused of malpractice or breaking some other law? What if I was at fault?
- What would I do and how would I feel if I were falsely accused of breaking a law?
- Have I ever reported someone for breaking a law? How did I feel? Proud, scared, nervous, or regretful? Have I ever falsely accused someone of anything? Was it an accident or mistake? Did I pass on wrong information? Was I being spiteful? How do I feel when I think about this (Box 2.16)?

Your responses to these questions can be an indication of where you may encounter dilemmas when confronted with illegal and unethical situations. Ignoring unethical behavior in colleagues is unprofessional. A willingness to be involved with profession-wide ethical concerns supports professional integrity as a whole (Corey et al., 2011). Carefully document the concerns and the process of intervention. Follow all ethical principles in these types of situations.

Foot in the Door

When you graduate from massage therapy education, you will be competing with others for clients, a job, and status. What will set you apart from the rest and make the future clients, employers, and others who could influence your career skills notice you? Naturally, your massage skills need to be excellent. However, your people skills are just as important. It is necessary to behave in an ethical and responsible manner as a massage professional. Communicate effectively (including being quiet). Make responsible decisions about client care and peer/professional relationships. Use critical thinking skills. Always conduct yourself professionally. These actions will give you an advantage over those who do not prioritize professionalism. Not only will you get your foot in the door, but you will also move to the head of the line.

Box 2.16 Lawsuits

Litigation

Litigation is the process of a lawsuit. A *lawsuit* is a legal action in a court. The person or party that institutes the suit in court is the *plaintiff.* The person accused of the wrongdoing is the *defendant.*

During malpractice litigation in a massage therapy practice, the client may be the plaintiff. The massage therapist or person who is being sued is the defendant. Other individuals in the massage office likely will be named as a defendant, a fact witness, or an expert witness in the legal proceedings.

Negligence

Negligence is the performance of an act that a reasonably careful person under similar circumstances would not do or the failure to perform an act that a reasonably careful person would do under similar circumstances. Negligence is an act of omission (i.e., neglecting to do something that a reasonably prudent person would do) or commission (i.e., doing something that a reasonably prudent person would not do). To prove negligence, it is necessary to prove that there has been a breach of duty owed, including deviation from the standard of care. In a massage negligence case, it is often necessary to provide expert testimony. To prove negligence, the plaintiff must show that there is an obligation to provide care according to a specified standard, that there was failure to meet that standard, that the failure to meet the standard led to injury, and that there was actual injury to the client.

Good Samaritan Law

During the past three decades in the United States, every state has passed some form of legislation that grants immunity for acts performed by a person who renders care in an emergency situation. This concept, called the Good Samaritan law, was considered necessary to create an incentive for medical care providers to provide medical assistance to the injured in cases of automobile accidents or other disasters without the fear of possible litigation. This law is intended for individuals who do not seek compensation but rather are solely interested in providing care to the injured in a caring and safe manner with no intent to do bodily harm. This law does not provide protection for a negligent health care provider who is being compensated for services.

Malpractice

Professionals usually consider *malpractice* a form of negligence, but in a broader sense, it can mean any wrongdoing by a professional. Malpractice can refer to any professional misconduct, evil practice, or illegal or immoral conduct (not just negligence). Malpractice can be unintentional or intentional.

Defamation of Character

Defamation of character is the communication of false information to a third party about a person that results in injury to that person's reputation. The communication can be verbal (slander) or written (libel). The false statement may be about a person's product, business, profession, or title to property. A massage professional should make statements about a client or other professional only as it relates to the rendering of massage care and only to other massage care providers involved in that care.

Invasion of Privacy

Invasion of privacy is a tort that refers to several wrongs involving the use of otherwise confidential information. In the case of a massage therapy practice, a tort may involve publishing or otherwise using information related to the private life or affairs of a person without that person's approval or permission, prying into private affairs, or appropriating the plaintiff's identity for commercial use.

To avoid this situation, you must remember that any information a client gives to you or office staff remains confidential within the office. No information about a client should be shared outside the office. When a client requests a transfer of massage treatment records, a signed authorization to transfer should be completed by the client. In the health/medical care setting, the massage therapist must follow the regulations of the Health Insurance Portability and Accountability Act (HIPAA).

Computer Security

The massage therapist may be exposed to activities that may cause illegal or unethical activity while using a computer. Computer security refers to safeguards that are implemented to prevent and detect unauthorized access or deliberate damage to a computer system and data. A computer crime is the use of a computer to commit an illegal act.

In a massage office, the most common activity that can violate computer integrity is software theft, or piracy. Some people make an illegal copy of a disk or tape instead of paying for an authorized copy. Software theft is a violation of copyright law, and it is a crime. For large users, such as massage schools or other health care institutions, most software companies provide a site license and multiple-copy discounts. Although most massage offices use personal computers rather than a mainframe, the potential for gaining unauthorized access to data still exists, especially in a hospital-type setting. If you inadvertently gain access on the computer to unauthorized or confidential data, you should exit the file, including the data, and report to the appropriate supervisor that you accidentally entered a confidential file. To make changes in a confidential file without authorized permission constitutes an unethical and possibly illegal act.

Fraud

Fraud is a deception that is deliberately practiced to secure unfair or unlawful gain. Fraud is related to money. One of the most common practices of fraud in health/medical care is obtaining fees through third-party payments by misrepresentation. Third-party insurance reimbursement for massage services is not common, but the trend is increasing. It therefore is important to understand some of the problems that occur with health insurance reimbursement. Another issue of importance is identity theft. Identity theft occurs when someone wrongfully obtains another's personal information without their knowledge to commit theft or fraud.

SUMMARY

A tremendous amount of information has been covered in this chapter. Years of experience confirm that when a massage therapist encounters difficulty in the professional setting, the problem is seldom about a technical skill and almost always about an ethical dilemma. Wise learners will review this chapter repeatedly during their study and will seek support in reviewing the information periodically as they mature in their professional practice after graduation. The fundamentals of ethics and professionalism remain fairly constant even if the details of behavior and legalities change. Ethical and professional behavior form the cornerstone of leadership development and the important ability to think critically.

Decision-making skills, achieved by using the problem-solving model and by developing effective communication and conflict management skills, will prove to be some of the most valuable information in this text. Both decision making and communication are learned skills, and massage professionals must practice them to gain proficiency. And, as with any skill, when you first begin to use them, you will feel awkward and uncomfortable. That's okay. You probably will have the same feeling as you practice all the new skills in this text, such as body mechanics, draping procedures, and all the massage manipulations and techniques. Practice is essential to perfect the skills required of a massage professional.

Evolve

Visit the Evolve website: http://evolve.elsevier.com/Fritz/fundamentals/.

Evolve content designed for massage therapy licensing exam review and comprehension of content beyond the textbook. Evolve content includes:

- Content Updates
- Science and Pathology Animations
- Body Spectrum Coloring Book
- MBLEx exam review multiple choice questions

FOR EACH CHAPTER FIND:

- Answers and rationales for the end-of-chapter multiple-choice questions
- Electronic Workbook and Answer Key
- Chapter multiple choice question Quiz
- Quick Content Review in Question Form and Answers
- Technique Videos when applicable
- Learn More on the Web

REFERENCES

Beard JR, Officer A, de Carvalho IA, et al. The World report on ageing and health: a policy framework for healthy ageing. *Lancet.* 2016;387(10033):2145–2154.

Bonini Luca, Rotunno Cristina, Arcuri Edoardo, Gallese Vittorio. Mirror neurons 30 years later: implications and applications. *Trends Cognitive Sci.* 2022;26(9):767–781.

Boulanger KT, Campo S, Glanville JL, et al. The development and validation of the client expectations of massage scale. *Int J Ther Massage Bodywork.* 2012;5(3):3.

Coalition of National Massage Therapy Organizations: Alliance for Massage Therapy Education, American Massage Therapy Association, Associated Bodywork & Massage Professionals, Inc., Commission on Massage Therapy Accreditation, Federation of State Massage Therapy Boards, Massage Therapy Foundation, and National Certification Board for Therapeutic Massage & Bodywork, Inc. *The Core: Entry-Level Massage Education Blueprint*; 2013. Retrieved July 1, 2014, from ELAP-elapmassage.org.

Corey G, Corey MS, Callanan P. *Issues and Ethics in the Helping Professions.* 83rd ed. Brooks/Cole; 2011.

Decety J, Holvoet C. The emergence of empathy: A developmental neuroscience perspective. *Dev Rev.* 2021;62:100999.

Federation of State Massage. *Therapy Boards. Model Practice Act. All rights reserved. Copyright* 2014. Retrieved from https://fsmtb.org/Model_Practice_Act.pdf.

Gallese V. "Being like me": Self-other identity, mirror neurons and empathy. In: Hurley S, Chater N, eds. MIT Press; 2005. *Perspectives on imitation: from cognitive neuroscience to social science.* 1:101–118.

Gallese V, Eagle MN, Migone P. Intentional attunement: Mirror neurons and the neural underpinnings of interpersonal relations. *J Am Psychoanal Assoc.* 2007;55(1):131–175.

Guy SD, Majumder S. Fulfilling the potential of evidence-based research: The collaborative nature of implementation. *Public Policy Aging Rep.* 2022;32(1):36–38.

Heyes C, Catmur C. What happened to mirror neurons? *Perspect Psychol Sci.* 2022;17(1):153–168.

Keysers C, Paracampo R, Gazzola V. What Neuromodulation and Lesion studies tell us about the function of the mirror neuron system and embodied cognition. *Curr Opin Psychol.* 2018;24:35–40.

Kumah EA, McSherry R, Bettany-Saltikov J, van Schaik P. Evidence-informed practice: simplifying and applying the concept for nursing students and academics. *Br J Nurs.* 2022;31(6):322–330. doi:10.12968/bjon.2022.31.6.322.

Massage Therapy Body of Knowledge (MTBOK) Stewards. Massage therapy body of knowledge (MTBOK), version 1, May 15, 2010. Retrieved March 21, 2011, from http://www.mtbok.org.

Merriam-Webster, Webster Online. Retrieved July 1, 2014, from http://www.merriam-webster.com.

Noble LM, Manalastas G, Viney R, Griffin AE. Does the structure of the medical consultation align with an educational model of clinical communication? A study of physicians' consultations from a postgraduate examination. *Patient Educ Couns.* 2022;105(6):1449–1456. doi:10.1016/j.pec.2021.10.001.

Sackett DL, Straus SE, Richardson WS, et al. *Evidence-Based Medicine: How to Practice and Teach EBM.* 2nd ed. Churchill Livingstone; 2000.

Sarkies MN, Jones LK, Gidding SS, Watts GF. Improving clinical practice guidelines with implementation science. *Nat Rev Cardiol.* 2022;19(1):3–4. doi:10.1038/s41569-021-00645-x.

Woodbury MG, Kuhnke JL. Evidence-based Practice vs. Evidence-informed Practice: What's the Difference? *Wound Care Canada.* 2014;12:18–21.

MULTIPLE-CHOICE QUESTIONS FOR DISCUSSION AND REVIEW

The answers, with rationales, can be found on the Evolve site. Use these questions to stimulate discussion and dialog. Each question provides you the opportunity to review terminology, practice critical-thinking skills, and improve multiple-choice test-taking skills. Answers and rationales are on the Evolve website. Remember: it is just as important to know why the wrong answers are wrong as it is to know why the correct answer is correct.

1. The knowledge base and practice parameters of a profession are called _____.
   a. Scope of practice
   b. Informed consent
   c. Dual role
   d. Therapeutic relationship

2. A client, a professional dancer, is basically healthy but is seeking massage to manage minor injury and support recovery. Which scope of practice description best describes these outcomes?
   a. Wellness/normal function
   b. Health care services
   c. Dysfunction and athletic performance
   d. Illness/trauma
3. A massage professional is careful to provide an informed consent process for each client and updates informed consent regularly. Which of these ethical principles is being followed?
   a. Confidentiality
   b. Justice
   c. Proportionality
   d. Client autonomy and self-determination
4. Taking a client's history and providing a physical assessment to develop a massage care plan is called _____.
   a. Intake assessment
   b. Brochure and policy statement
   c. Release of information
   d. Chart
5. A massage professional has worked hard to develop a policy statement and has included types of service offered, information on training and experience, appointment policies, client and practitioner expectations, sexual appropriateness and zero tolerance policy, and recourse policy. What did the professional forget to include?
   a. Number of appointments to meet therapeutic goals
   b. Fee structure
   c. Objective progress measurements
   d. Methods of clinical reasoning
6. A client informs a massage professional that another massage practitioner in the practice is soliciting clients to move to a new private practice the therapist is starting. The massage professional knows that everyone in the massage practice signed a contract agreeing not to behave in this manner. After the massage therapist carefully considers the situation and discusses the issue with a peer in another state who is in a similar situation, what is the next step in dealing with this type of unethical behavior?
   a. Formal reporting
   b. Contacting a lawyer
   c. Talking with those involved
   d. Speaking to fellow workers
7. A massage therapist is frustrated with their supervisor over being told to chart each massage using new forms. When the massage therapist voiced concerns, the supervisor stated there was no point in arguing–they could either follow the policy or leave. Which of these terms describes the conflict resolution method the supervisor used?
   a. Power/dominance
   b. Denial
   c. Collaboration
   d. Negotiation
8. A massage professional becomes angry with a client who complains about personal problems during the massage. The massage practitioner is displaying _____.
   a. Transference
   b. A therapeutic relationship
   c. Ethical behavior
   d. Countertransference
9. A massage professional does not regularly drape all clients in a modest and professional manner. Which of these statements best describes this conduct?
   a. The massage professional practices a dual role.
   b. The massage professional has breached a standard of practice.
   c. The massage professional is involved in misuse of the scope of practice.
   d. The massage professional needs additional training in draping.
10. A massage professional works with three main populations: athletes, those with chronic pain, and clients supporting personal well-being. The therapist uses a variety of methods. Which of these terms best describes the massage application style being used?
    a. Structural and postural approaches
    b. Applied kinesiology
    c. Integrated approaches
    d. Myofascial methods
11. A massage professional has been working with a particular client for 12 months. Recently the client has been experiencing increasing difficulties with the family communications. The biggest problem is stress and tension between child and parent. Discussions during massage are centered around solving this problem. Which of these statements best describes this situation?
    a. The massage professional is having difficulty maintaining informed consent.
    b. Scope of practice violations, particularly with psychology, are occurring.
    c. The client should be referred for acupuncture or chiropractic.
    d. The client is engaged in countertransference.
12. A massage professional with entry-level training has been seeing a client recently diagnosed with diabetes. The massage professional is becoming more uncomfortable providing massage as the client displays more symptoms. What is occurring?
    a. The massage professional is in a dual role now that the client is ill.
    b. The client is more demanding of the professional.
    c. The massage professional has failed to abide by the definition of massage.
    d. The massage professional is functioning outside the personal scope of practice.
13. Which of these actions is a violation of confidentiality?
    a. Maintaining client records in a secure location
    b. Asking the client questions about work environment
    c. Approaching and speaking to a client in a restaurant
    d. Speaking to a client's chiropractor with appropriate releases

14. Which of these would be an appropriate disclosure to a client?
    a. The massage professional has a cold
    b. Business financial concerns
    c. Discussion about a mutual acquaintance
    d. Domestic partner difficulties
15. A massage professional has been asked to work with a support group for people with cerebral palsy. The therapist is well trained and has 7 years of experience but is uncomfortable around people with disabilities, especially if communication is a problem. Which of these is grounds for the massage professional to refuse the request?
    a. Lack of skills
    b. Lack of peer support
    c. Inability to serve without bias
    d. Only wishes to work with females
16. A massage professional with 15 years of experience but minimal continuing education is in charge of a massage clinic. A recent massage graduate has obtained a position at the clinic. The new graduate notices that their current skills, particularly in charting and critical thinking, are more sophisticated than those of the supervisor but is hesitant to discuss the issue. What is the best description for this situation?
    a. Power differential
    b. Dual role
    c. Maintenance of a professional environment
    d. Reciprocity
17. Which of these is the best example of transference?
    a. A massage professional is biased toward a client because of political beliefs.
    b. A massage professional is receiving small gifts from a client expressing affection.
    c. A massage professional asks a client to attend a meeting about a nutritional product.
    d. A client is angry with the massage professional for being late for the last three appointments.
18. Which of these would be the best explanation for a client who is confused over an incident of becoming mildly sexually aware during the last massage?
    a. The massage practitioner was sexualizing the massage.
    b. The client was sexualizing the massage.
    c. The client was experiencing parasympathetic sensations.
    d. The massage practitioner was massaging erotic zones.
19. A massage therapist is angry with a coworker about the scheduling of the massage room. The therapist is busier than their coworker and wants to schedule more time on Saturdays. What type of conflict is this?
    a. Relationship conflict
    b. Data conflict
    c. Interest conflict
    d. Value conflict
20. A massage professional is troubled over a client's responses during the last four massage sessions. There is nothing specific about the client's behavior, but something has changed in the client's response to the massage. What could be helpful to the massage professional?
    a. Credentialing review with certification
    b. Managing intimacy issues
    c. Changing body language
    d. Decision making with peer support

Write Your Own Questions

Write at least three multiple choice questions, one of each type: factual recall and comprehension, application and concept identification, and clinical reasoning and synthesis. Make sure to develop plausible wrong answers and be sure the correct answer is clearly correct. Then write a rationale for each question. The more questions you write, the better you will understand the material. Exchange questions with classmates or discuss them in class. The questions from all the students can be combined to create a review quiz.

CHAPTER 3

Business Considerations for a Career in Therapeutic Massage

http://evolve.elsevier.com/Fritz/fundamentals/

Note: Most calculations used in this chapter are based on the 2022 Massage Profession Research Report, published by the American Massage Therapy Association (AMTA), the US Department of Labor's Employment and Training Administration, and the Bureau of Labor Statistics. Fees, income, and expenses vary depending on demographics and cost of living. Depending on demand, fees, income, and expenses may increase or decrease. The figures used in this chapter are examples. The same calulation formulas can be use for a variety of fees and business factors. Additional information is available at CareerOneStop (www.careeronestop.org), a site sponsored by the Department of Labor. The AMTA research report can be accessed on the association's website (www.amtamassage.org).

CHAPTER OBJECTIVES

After completing this chapter, the student will be able to perform the following:

1. Describe the influence of inspiration, intention, and intuition as they relate to developing a career in therapeutic massage.
2. Determine one's personal motivation for pursuing a career in therapeutic massage.
3. Create a career mission statement and attainable career goals.
4. Identify business risks and develop a risk management plan.
5. Describe client retention.
6. Self-evaluate the attributes necessary for client retention.
7. Develop and maintain a client scheduling system for massage practice.
8. List the types of client and business records.
9. Define time management.
10. Create a personal and business budget.
11. Obtain professional and business insurance.
12. Self-analyze the potential for burnout.
13. List the pros and cons of employee and self-employed status.
14. Create a résumé and cover letter.
15. Prepare for an employment interview.
16. List elements included in an employment agreement.
17. Explain how employment wages are calculated.
18. Estimate the employer wage expense ratio to gross business profits.
19. Self-evaluate the potential for an increase in wages.
20. Explain unemployment benefits, resignation, termination, and layoff.
21. List the skills needed to achieve employee success.
22. List the elements of business development when self-employed.
23. Develop a business plan.
24. Design a marketing strategy and advertising materials for a massage business.
25. Develop a business management, accounting, and record-keeping system.
26. Describe the process for setting fees and determining income.

CHAPTER OUTLINE

KEY TERMS

Burnout	Payroll taxes
Career	Risk management
Employee	Self-employed
Job	Self-employment taxes
Marketing	Start-up costs
Motivation	

Chapter 3 builds on Chapters 1 and 2 and describes the soft and hard skills needed for career success from the business perspective. The information presented in this chapter is unique to therapeutic massage and will guide the learner toward additional learning opportunities and will generate classroom discussion. Because massage therapists have autonomy in professional practice and can develop a career in multiple ways, this chapter is presented in three distinct segments:

- First discussed is information that all massage therapists need, regardless of career pathway, to help decide which career pathway is best for you upon graduation: to work as an employee or to become self-employed.
- Next the content will focus on the employment career pathway.
- Then the focus will be on self-employment including business development.

Regardless of whether you choose to be an employee as a part of the team or to be self-employed with your own business obligations, everyone benefits from understanding the requirements of business development and operations. As an employee, you are better able to understand the commitment, risks, and responsibilities of business ownership. The chapter takes the position that the nuts and bolts of business are no different for the massage profession than for any other professional service business. Detailed information on topics such as marketing methods, financial record keeping, and tax requirements can be found easily on the internet, especially on the Internal Revenue Service (IRS) website (https://www.irs.gov/). Resources on the business aspects of massage therapy also are available, and professional organizations often provide business information. Fortunately, there are many resources where you can learn more on this topic. The Small Business Association (SBA) (https://www.sba.gov/) is the best place to begin. Almost all the information needed to start and manage a successful massage business is there for you for free. You can even access business mentors through the SCORE program. SCORE is a network of volunteer, expert business mentors. While serving as a resource partner of the SBA, SCORE has helped more than 10 million entrepreneurs by offering mentoring, workshops, and educational resources since 1964. Check out the content now, then explore in depth when you really need the information after graduation.

BUSINESS OF THE MASSAGE THERAPY CAREER

SECTION OBJECTIVES

Chapter objectives covered in this section:

1. Describe the influence of inspiration, intention, and intuition as they relate to developing a career in therapeutic massage.
2. Determine one's personal motivation for pursuing a career in therapeutic massage.
3. Create a career mission statement and attainable career goals.
4. Identify business risks and develop a risk management plan.
5. Describe client retention.
6. Self-evaluate the attributes necessary for client retention.
7. Develop and maintain a client scheduling system for massage practice.
8. List the types of client and business records.
9. Define time management.
10. Create a personal and business budget.
11. Obtain professional and business insurance.
12. Self-analyze the protentional for burnout.
13. List the pros and cons of employee and self-employed status.

Using the information presented in this section, the student will be able to perform the following:

- Define inspiration, intention, and intuition.
- Perform simple exercises to increase intuitive awareness.
- Understand the importance of motivation in successfully developing a career.
- Explore personal strengths and weaknesses that would aid or impede the development of a successful career.
- Write a career mission statement.
- Analyze your career plan for business risks and develop a risk management plan.
- Set career goals.
- Define client retention.
- Explain the relationship between client retention and career success.
- Explain the importance of regular massage to clients.
- List major reasons for clients to schedule regular massage sessions.
- Develop and use an appointment scheduling system.
- Identify problems that may arise with client retention.
- Develop a personal application of methods to prevent burnout.
- Develop your personal list of pros and cons for self-employment and employee status.
- Identify ethical concerns with a combined practice.
- Define independent contractor status and misclassified employees.

There are skills that all massage therapists need for career success. There is knowledge that influences career decision making and practice. Some concepts are general overarching themes. Some of the information is specific. All the information is important for career development in the massage therapy profession.

One of the unique aspects of a massage therapy career is the variety of options for career development. Most occupations have one or two paths from education to work. Massage therapy has many paths, including self-employment, traditional employment, full time, part time, mobile or in office, home office, or a combination of these. We can work in a spa, one of the many massage therapy-based franchises, wellness centers, medical care and sport environments (see Chapter 13), and with many clients with different goals. We can provide massage in multiple environments, using a variety of methods uniquely combined to meet the needs of individual clients. The career focus can evolve as we gain experience. All these choices make the career aspect of a therapeutic massage practice much more complex than most other occupations. If, for example, someone trains to become a medical assistant, the path to employment is fairly clear. On completion of education and training, the individual will seek employment in a health/medical facility. There is no option for self-employment or a variety of practice settings. Because of the extensive variety of career development options available to massage therapists, this chapter explores multiple possibilities for entry-level positions in the massage practice that you can look into upon completion of your education.

Inspiration, Intention, Intuition

As you progress through your educational journey, the goal is to be prepared to have a successful massage therapy career—

whatever that means to you. Figuring out how your career plan begins and how it will progress involves the following elements:

- Inspiration: Ideas that manifest the dream
  - Inspiration occurs when a certain combination of ideas suddenly reveals a simple underlying pattern. When this happens, you typically have an intellectual, emotional, and physical response that often results in clarity and in motivation to bring ideas into tangible form. People seem to be wired to see a pattern and make sense of it. Inspiration is difficult to explain but easy to recognize because it enlivens us and creates passion and energy. Inspiration is the big picture, and in its simplicity, the complicated becomes uncomplicated. It is like a cookie. The cookie is the whole, and the flour, sugar, eggs, butter, and vanilla are the pieces. They do not form a cookie until combined and baked. Being inspired can be likened to the moment of clear understanding that results in a deep sense of peace. More than the "a-ha" moment or gut feeling of intuition, being inspired is the beginning of purpose.
- Intention: Goals
  - Intention determines what you want. For example, if you are looking for a red ribbon, you will eventually find it because you are focused on it. We have all experienced a moment when we find what we are looking for, but we have to know what it is we seek. If you have been inspired to be a massage therapist, you will seek skills and knowledge and will find a teacher and a school. The same process occurs when building a massage clientele. If you are inspired to work for a specific group, such as the military, first responders, or performers, you will seek what you need to build the practice.
- Intuition: Following inner guidance
  - Intuition is the conscious awareness of the collected and integrated subconscious information that is processed through the environment, experience, and circumstances. Intuition, sometimes called gut instinct, is an important guide, and the intuitive process is more concrete than it appears. Although science does not totally understand the phenomenon, there is little doubt that intuition is an aspect of survival mechanisms based on physiological function. With development, intuition can become a valuable source of information for important personal and professional decision making. You may experience intuition as a feeling, a gut reaction, images that reoccur, a dream, or an internal voice with a message. You need to figure out how your inner self communicates with your conscious self. You can get in touch with your intuition in several ways.
  - Ask the question: What is the next step I need to take to progress in my career? At some level of consciousness, you already know what you need to do. Trust yourself. Gather factual information about the area you are exploring, and then let the process happen. Intuition cannot be forced; you need to be patient. You can do several things to build a factual database, including reading, asking people questions, and talking to experts.
  - Be quiet, and perform repetitive mundane tasks, such as weeding the garden, folding laundry, meditating, knitting, doing dishes, soaking in a tub, or going for a walk. Let the thoughts flow.
  - Be aware of the thoughts and dreams that come to you. For example, how did you decide on which massage training program to attend? Did you research the various schools? What criteria influenced your choice—cost, location, schedule, reputation? How did the final decision moment feel? Was it solid or iffy? As you develop your massage career, the same process may occur in deciding what location to rent or which position to take.

As you learn to recognize, develop, and trust inspiration, intention, and intuition, you will achieve a level of confidence with professional decision making. Although these concepts appear abstract, they are not. We all have these abilities that evolved from basic survival mechanisms. To survive, we need to have an instinct about what is safe, what path to take, and with whom to build relationships for mutual benefit. The gut instinct, new idea, and a-ha moment are manifestations of the gestalt whole of knowing. All it takes is a little practice, increased awareness, and observation of the results. These internal mechanisms of self-awareness become powerful tools for professional development.

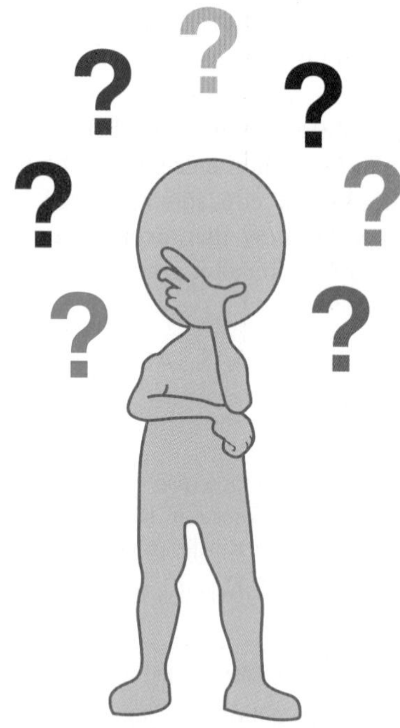

Career and Employment

Consider the difference between a career and a job. A **career** is commonly defined as a chosen pursuit, a life's work. A **job** is a regular activity performed for payment. Therapeutic massage can be either a job or a career. Which do you want? The answer to that question determines in large part how you proceed with your professional development. This text in general, and this chapter in particular, views therapeutic massage as a career. A career can evolve whether you are self-employed or you work for someone else as an employee. If you choose to work for someone else, your employer will take care of most details of developing and managing a business. The employer also takes risks involving uncertainty and potential loss, especially financial risks for business success. You, as an employee, can concentrate on being an excellent massage therapist and supporting the business by being an excellent employee. If you choose to be self-employed, you must be an excellent massage therapist, be willing to take financial and professional risks, and also be able to manage all business-related responsibilities, but you have ultimate control over how your business is managed. Someday you may want to be an employer or rent space to self-employed massage therapists, each of which provides space for others to manifest their career dreams.

Motivation

To succeed at anything, a person must be motivated. Motivation is an internal drive that provides the energy to do what is needed to accomplish a goal. Without the motivation to stick to the commitment, people give up during difficult times. This is especially true of small businesses with single owners, a category that includes most solely owned massage businesses.

Motivation begins with knowing what you want. Plans must be developed, but the massage professional must be willing to change them if a strategy is not working. If success is the goal, quitting cannot be an option. The following are some important points:

- *Know thyself.* No one should persist with something that goes against their core values, no matter how successful the process may be for someone else.
- *Follow your dream.* Success flows from desire and motivation. Desire and motivation are the driving forces for the dreams that come from deep within us to bring us joy and healing. Hard times and hard work are part of the process of building a new career. If we follow our dreams and live our purpose, the hard work provides a rewarding, intrinsic sense of satisfaction.
- *Accept that experience is the best teacher.* We learn from our mistakes as well as from our successes. Implementing plans is the only way to find out whether they work. It may become obvious over time that another approach is more advantageous, but being afraid to make mistakes will limit you as a professional.
- *Ask "What's in it for me?"* To succeed in any endeavor, we need to recognize the benefits to be gained from the process. This is an important consideration in any decision. It is not a selfish attitude; rather, it is a smart approach. People will not put energy into something that does not give them satisfaction. This concept also applies to money. Business is business, and earning money is part of any successful business operation. However, money itself is a poor source of motivation. Motivation is a more deeply felt sense that comes from the heart and soul.
- *Recognize that self-concept matters.* People have ideas about who they should be, and these often conflict with what we have been told and believe that we are. Self-esteem is very important for career success. A successful career is built on who we are, not on what others want us to be. Develop your ability to use all aspects of yourself to the best advantage.
- *Believe in your product.* Understand and be able to explain the benefits of therapeutic massage. It is most acceptable to explain the benefits of massage in terms of physiological responses that all people share. Explanations of this type are easy for most people to understand.
- *Provide a quality product.* The massage practitioner must be skilled. Clients pay for the benefits they experience from massage. Client retention is based on your ability to continue to produce those benefits. To be truly successful, the practitioner must put the person, not their condition, first. People seek caring, nurturing, and nonjudgmental touch as much as technical skill.

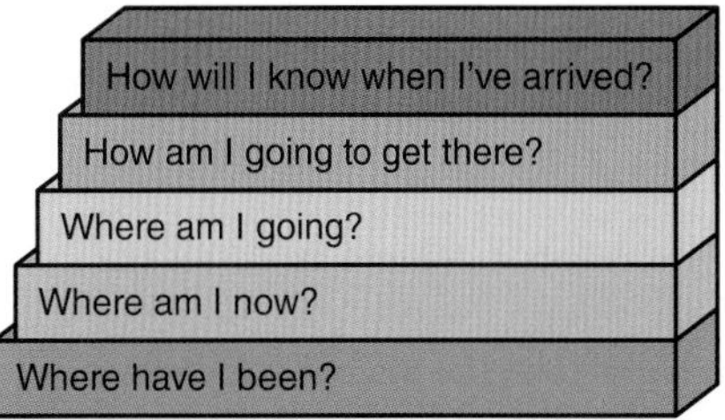

FIG. 3.1 Job preparation. Questions to ask yourself when preparing for a job search. From Finkbeiner BL, Finkbeiner CA: *Practice management for the dental team,* ed 6, 2006, Mosby.

Career Mission Statement

Whether you intend to be self-employed, approach a massage career as an employee, or blend the two, it is important to have a plan. To make the plan workable, you need to know where you are in the present, what your path has been, and what you have learned from accumulated experiences (Fig. 3.1). This information is the foundation for future plans. Consider these possibilities:

- The career pathway as an employee, regardless of environment (spa, franchise, wellness center, or health/medical facility), is a viable entry-level option for massage professionals. Many new massage therapy graduates begin by working part time and then build their clientele over the first year.
- A career plan option is to move gradually into a new massage career by working at it part time while letting the business grow slowly (and keeping your non-massage full-time job).
- Another option is to commit to the new massage career full time, either as an employee or through self-employment. If you choose full time, it is necessary to build your client base. In the first months you may have a lower income until enough clients seek your massage service. You should have enough money saved up to meet basic needs for about 1 year.

You need to decide what fits you. This is the type of information that becomes formalized when you develop a career plan. In all career planning, the important thing is to find and fill a need. What is the need using therapeutic massage that you, as a therapeutic massage practitioner, are willing to fill? The answer to this question becomes the basis of your mission

PROFICIENCY EXERCISE 3.1

Write a career mission statement.

statement. A mission statement expresses the intent of the career plan. To develop a mission statement, you will answer this question: What will be the main focus of my career?

Here are some examples of mission statements:

- My career mission is to serve the blue-collar labor population in my area by providing therapeutic massage and self-help education at a reasonable cost, with flexible appointment hours, and at an easily accessible location in a small office setting.
- My career mission is to serve military veterans through both volunteer services with various community outreach programs and employment by an organization that serves disabled veterans.
- My career mission is to work with amateur and professional athletes, supporting recovery and performance by creating a flexible work schedule and being able to travel with the clients.
- My career mission is to develop a small retention client base while working from a home office.
- My career mission is to obtain employment as a massage therapist with one of the massage franchise businesses and learn how to become a manager as well as progress to the position of supervisory massage therapist for the company (Proficiency Exercise 3.1).

Development of your formal career plan begins while you are still in school. The first step of the career plan is to become educated in the skills needed to carry out the mission statement. Another part of the career plan is the development of a financial plan to support the educational process and the first year of professional practice, which is a time when income may be low. While in school, learners should use the expertise of teachers and fellow students to explore career options. Career plans can change as you career progresses. A career plan evolves.

Goal Setting

Once the "big picture" concepts of the career plan are identified by the mission statement, smaller steps to implement the plans are identified. These are goals. Goals are important because they provide direction and landmarks for achievement. An effective model for goal setting is called SMART. This approach has its roots in the management theories of Peter Drucker, who presented them in the 1950s. The acronym SMART stands for *specific, measurable, attainable, relevant,* and *time-bound* (Box 3.1). There are many goal-setting methods, and an internet search will provide information on additional approaches. Your goals and the decisions made to achieve your goals will change over time. Plan for change.

Risk Management

A business risk is a future possibility that may prevent you from achieving a business goal. Risk is part of business and career development. **Risk management** in business refers to the practice of identifying potential risks in advance, analyzing them, and taking precautionary steps to reduce or avoid the risk. Risk management helps you identify and prepare for the risks facing your career path. A process for planning for potential risks involves the following:

- Identifying the risks
- Putting plans in place to deal with risk, such as the following:
  - Unexpected illness or injury prevents you from working: have a savings account in place for emergencies or having disability insurance.
  - Employer goes out of business: maintain an up-to-date résumé and letters of recommendation, and know what businesses typically hire massage therapists in your area.
  - Competing business opens: maintain ongoing support for client retention and have a prepared marketing strategy in place, such as a short-term coupon package for loyal clients.

As you make career decisions and evaluated risk, a question to ask is: "What is the worst possible thing that could happen as a result of this decision?" List what comes to mind. Think ahead to possible solutions should the worst happen and try to determine whether you could survive that experience. What will you gain if you take the risk? It is important to take calculated risks. If these risks are small and entered into slowly, you can change strategies if needed. The clinical reasoning model used throughout this text is an invaluable tool for setting attainable goals.

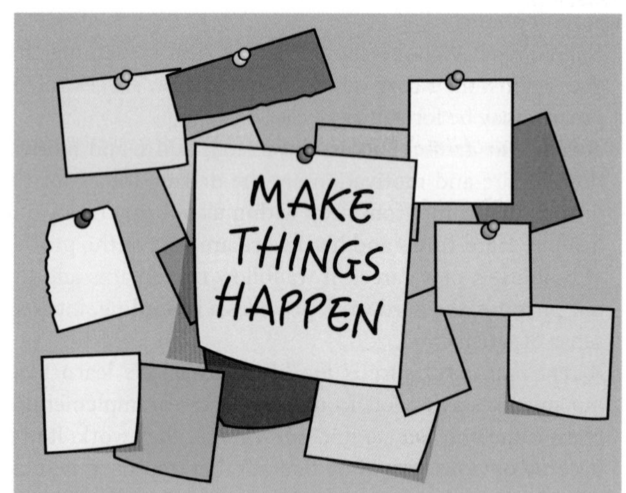

Seeking Help

The massage therapist brings more than massage skills to a career in therapeutic massage. Each professional also brings personal strengths and weaknesses, successes and failures, and experiences and learning. Using all our strengths is important. Recognizing the areas in which we are not as strong is even more important, because these limitations can influence career success. It is important to identify where we will need help.

Although experts, authorities, and mentors are beneficial, no single individual has all the answers or knows the whole truth. Each of us must find our own answers. Truth is personal, empowering, and freeing. Many motivational audio

Box 3.1 Using the Clinical Reasoning Model to Set Goals

- State your goals in the present tense. Make sure you are the main character. Use the pronouns *I* and *me*.
- Make sure your goals are realistic and attainable. Can you achieve these goals using your own resources with little help from others? If the activity of a specific person is necessary to achieve your goal, rethink it. What other people may be able to be part of the goal? Avoid depending on only one other person.
- Speak positively. Avoid words such as *should, would, could, try*, and *never*.
- Set target deadlines for yourself; they will give you something to work toward.
- Make sure your goals are small steps toward your ultimate plan. For example, graduating from school is too big to be a goal; it is more like a mission statement. Completing all the exercises in this chapter within 4 weeks is an attainable goal.

Gather facts to identify and define the situation.
Key questions:
What is the desired outcome?
What are the facts?
My business mission is to serve the blue-collar labor population in my area by providing therapeutic massage and self-help education at a reasonable cost, with flexible appointment hours, and at an easily accessible location.
I will need a group of 20 people for a client base.
Brainstorm possible goals.
Key questions:
What might I do?
What if … ?
What are the possibilities?
What does my intuition suggest?
What if I contact the XYZ Manufacturing Plant as a potential population?
What if I contact the ABC Packing Company as a potential population?
Evaluate each possible goal identified in step 2 logically and objectively; look at both the pros and the cons.
Key questions:
What would happen if … ? (Insert each idea brainstormed in step 2.)
What are the costs, resources needed, and time involved?
What are the logical causes and effects of each possibility identified?
What are the pros and cons of each goal suggested?
What are the consequences of not acting?
What are the consequences of acting?
What would happen if I contacted the XYZ Manufacturing Plant?

- I would need a massage room on site.
- Travel time to work would be 45 minutes.
- Pro: This plant has 300 employees, a large potential client base.
- Con: This plant has a history of worker turnover.

What would happen if I contacted the ABC Packing Company?

- I could work at my existing office site.
- I am 15 minutes from work on foot.
- Pro: This company is in a growth phase.
- Con: This company has only 50 employees.

Evaluate the effect of each possible goal on the people involved.
Key questions:
How would each person involved feel if … ? (Insert each idea brainstormed in step 2.)
For each goal, what would be the effect on the people involved: client, practitioner, and other professionals working with the client?
How does each person involved feel about the possible goals?
Does a feeling of cooperation and agreement exist among all parties involved?
How might people feel if I contact the XYZ Manufacturing Plant?

- *This company is quite traditional. The president is sometimes resistant to change. I am socially acquainted with the plant manager, and they might like the idea.*

How might people feel if I contact the ABC Packing Company?

- *This company is very progressive in terms of human resources. I have a personality conflict with one of the vice presidents but have a good rapport with the other members of the human resources department.*

Choose a goal and develop an implementation plan after carefully processing steps 1 through 4. On the basis of this process, I believe the most attainable goal is to contact the ABC Packing Company.

Implement the plan and set a date for reevaluation.
Implementation plans are step-by-step procedures that detail what must be done to achieve the goals; these procedures can be considered subgoals.
Steps for implementing the goal of contacting the ABC Packing Company:

- Develop a presentation packet (1 week).
- Send a letter of inquiry (tomorrow).
- Make an appointment for an interview (2 weeks).

Now let's evaluate the goal-setting example using SMART goals: specific, measurable, attainable, relevant, and time-bound.

Specific: My business mission is to serve the blue-collar labor population in my area by providing therapeutic massage and self-help education at a reasonable cost, with flexible appointment hours, and at an easily accessible location.
Measurable: I will need a group of 20 people for a client base.
Attainable: I have a personality conflict with one of the vice presidents but have a good rapport with the other members of the human resources board. I could work at my existing office site. I am 15 minutes from work on foot. This company is in a growth phase but has only 50 employees.
Relevant: This company is very progressive in terms of human resources. The goal matches my career mission statement. I can continue to work with my existing clients.
Time-Bound:
Develop a presentation packet (1 week).
Send a letter of inquiry (tomorrow).
Make an appointment for an interview with human resources (2 weeks).
Distribute an information packet to employees (3 weeks).
For 1 week offer 15-minute massage samples on site immediately before the shift schedule, at breaks and lunch, and at end of the shift schedule, and begin scheduling massage sessions (4 weeks).

The analysis using SMART goals indicates that the goal development is sound but a little weak in measurability. How will the massage therapist know whether progress is being made on achieving the goal? Is it possible to quantify or put numbers to the outcome? What do you think could be done to improve the goal plan?

programs, books, and speakers are available that can be used for inspiration. The overlapping themes, which can be found in most of these sources, are the kernels of truth:

- Whatever we believe—with emotion and feeling—becomes our reality.
- What we do with confidence can become our self-fulfilling prophecy.
- We attract into our lives that which harmonizes with our dominant thoughts.

Career success requires a team. Some will be paid for their help, such as a lawyer. Others will volunteer to help, like family and friends. Regardless, we all need help, and it is important to choose help wisely.

Value

Many massage professionals underestimate the value of their service, whereas others overestimate it. People usually live according to an equal exchange for services rendered or for goods received. Equity (fairness and justice) is an important factor when you are thinking about money and how much to charge for a service or what your wage or salary should be. It is important to charge what a massage is worth in benefit and time value. If the fee is too high, the professional does not support those stable weekly and biweekly clients who are the mainstays of a massage practitioner's clientele. However, if fees or wages are too low, the business will not generate enough income for the business operations and make a realistic profit.

You can have a reality check on income potential and fees for services by calculating how much you could afford to pay for massage at least two times a month or 24 massage sessions per year based on your personal budget. Currently the average cost range for massage is $60–$120 per session. This is approximately $1500–$2500 per year. Can your personal budget support this level of massage expenditure?

Your value as a massage therapist is measured in more than income. Recall from Chapter 2 that a professional has an orientation toward service. Satisfaction received from helping someone is also a measure of our value. At the same time, we need to make enough money to satisfy our personal needs and quality of life so we can serve others.

Comparing Self-Employment and Employee Incomes

It is difficult to compare self-employed business profits to employee wages. The career models are very different. Those self-employed pay **self-employment taxes**, whereas the employer pays a portion of these taxes for an employee. This alters income calculations. Generally, for every $1 of net profit, the self-employed person loses 15 cents. Every $1 of employee wages results in a gain of about 7 cents. This adds up to more than $4000 which self-employed must pay in self-employment taxes, compared with the employee gain of more than $2000 that the employer has paid in payroll taxes. Employee wages reflect massage session time during work hours, whereas the self-employed must account for both the massage time and all of the business responsibilities.

A realistic way to compare employee and self-employed income, based on the same volume of clients, is to look at the income subject to income taxes. When this comparison is made and if the same number of massage session hours are performed, the income is about the same regardless of whether the practitioner is an employee or is self-employed.

Self-Employed Income

If you intend to be self-employed, plan on spending 30–50% of the gross income of your business (all income generated by business activities) on overhead expenses and setting aside one-third of the net income (gross income minus business expenses) to pay income and self-employment taxes. Always remember that each hour spent doing massage requires at least 30–60 minutes of business and facility management time. Giving twenty 1-hour massage sessions is at least 40 hours of work if a person is self-employed.

EXAMPLE

The average fee for a 60-minute massage session is $70. If the massage therapist completes five sessions, the gross business income is $350. Of that amount, 50% goes to overhead and self-employment taxes. The profit for the day is $175, and the massage therapist earns $35 per massage session. However, the workday is longer for self-employed practitioners, with a conservative estimate at 8 hours. Therefore the hourly rate is about $20 per hour.

Employee Income

Employee income is based on hourly wages or a fixed yearly salary. It is rare for massage therapists to be paid a salary, so the focus here will be on hourly wages. An employer must pay at least the federal minimum hourly wage, or state minimum wage if higher. There are two common ways wages are calculated for massage therapists. Both are confusing because massage therapists seldom work a common 9 a.m. to 5 p.m., 5 days a week, Monday through Friday schedule at a set hourly rate of pay.

A common method to calculate wages is to use a flat fee or percentage of fee for each massage performed, often called a massage hour. This type of arrangement is considered *piece rate pay*. The massage therapist is paid an amount for each massage. The typical rate per massage hour for an entry-level practitioner is $25–$35. If massage therapists have a full schedule of massage sessions, they will make a good wage. Also, the business is protected from paying a high hourly wage to an underperforming massage therapist. The problem with this type of wage calculation is that the employer is only responsible for paying minimum wage for all hours scheduled during the pay period. Pay-per-massage income depends on the number of client's seen during the pay period. Typically, more than 10 massage sessions need to be completed in a 40-hour pay period, over 7 days, for the massage therapist to make more than the minimum wage per hour.

EXAMPLE

*These figures DO NOT include gratuities.

Suppose that a massage therapist completes 25 massage sessions at $27.50 each for a total of $687.50 for the 40-hour pay period. Dividing $687.50 by 40 hours provides the hourly rate of $17.18. This amount is more than minimum wage, so the employer is following federal and state labor laws.

The second method to calculate employee wages is for the employer to pay a base hourly rate for every hour scheduled and an additional piece rate for each massage hour performed. The base rate is often the minimum wage. A fair piece rate is the same as the minimum wage. So if the minimum wage is $12.75 per hour, then the additional piece rate is another $12.75.

A typical 8-hour workday with 5 massage hours can be calculated as follows: 8 hours × $12.75 base pay = $102 plus an additional $12.75 × 5 massage hours = $63.75 for a total of $165.75 for the workday. This calculates out as $20.72 per hour or $33 per massage. If during the same workday the massage therapist provided 4 massage hours (rather than 5), the pay will be $153 per day or $19.12 per hour or $38 per massage.

As you can see, the pay structure of base pay + piece rate favors the employee. An employer cannot afford to pay a full-time base rate to an underperforming massage therapist. This is why the "paid by piece" per massage hour wage calculation is common. A paid per massage hour rate also appears as if the massage therapist is being paid more but this is misleading. It is typical for the wages earned for "per massage hour" calculated out for all hours on the clock to be less than base pay + piece rate.

Massage therapists rarely work a 40-hour work period. Consensus on full time practice is 20–25 massage hours in a 30-hour work period. Most massage therapists work ¾ time or 20–25 clock hours providing 15–20 massage hours. If a massage schedule is 5 hours massage in a 6-hour schedule, the hourly rate increases. When the income earned in this schedule is recalculated, a typical 6-hour workday with 5 massage hours can be calculated as follows: 6 hours × $12.75 base pay = $76.50 plus an additional $12.75 × 5 massage hours = $63.75 for a total of $140.25 for the workday. This calculates out as between $23 and $24 per hour or $28–$30 per massage. If during the same workday the massage therapist provided 4 massage hours (rather than 5), the pay will be $127.50 per day or $21.25 per hour or $33–$32 per massage hour.

Employee wages compared to self-employed net profit are about the same. The sample calculations may not reflect all therapeutic massage practices but provide a reliable comparison.

Regardless of whether you are an employee or have your own business, based on all the time and resources it takes to manage a business, you can realistically expect to make no less than $15–$20 per hour (not including gratuities) at *entry level* for all of your time on the clock or time spent satisfying business responsibilities. This income is on par with other occupations with similar education and credential requirements. Massage therapy requires a vocational, certificate/diploma-based education. Logically, earning comparisons should be for similarly educated occupations (Box 3.2).

Box 3.2 Health Care Occupations

Employment in healthcare occupations is projected to grow 16% from 2020–2030, much faster than the average for all occupations, adding about 2.6 million new jobs. Healthcare occupations are projected to add more jobs than any of the other occupational groups. This projected growth is mainly due to an aging population, leading to greater demand for healthcare services.

The median annual wage for healthcare practitioners and technical occupations (such as registered nurses, physicians and surgeons, and dental hygienists) was $75,040 in May 2021, which was higher than the median annual wage for all occupations in the economy of $45,760.

Healthcare support occupations (such as home health aides, occupational therapy assistants, and medical transcriptionists) had a median annual wage of $29,880 in May 2021, lower than the median annual wage for all occupations in the economy.

BLS provides summary data, including employment projections, for healthcare occupations not shown in the table on this page. That information is available on the Data for Occupations Not Covered in Detail page.

From https://www.bls.gov/ooh/healthcare/home.htm.

Gratuities

Gratuity is a more formal word than *tip*. Gratuity is a way of expressing gratitude. The appropriateness of tipping in the massage therapy community is debated and controversial. The decision about whether or not to leave a tip is entirely at the customer's discretion. In many work settings, a tip of between 15% and 20% is considered the norm. If you work in service sectors such as a spa, on a cruise ship, or at a massage franchise, tipping is common and appropriate. If you are working in a medical environment or are self-employed, it is less likely you will receive gratuities. It is likely that the massage fees in these environments would be higher. All gratuities belong to the massage therapist and would be reported as income on one's personal tax return. Gratuities are not considered regular pay if you are an employee and are added additional income. The employer will include them in your paycheck (Box 3.3).

Full-Time and Part-Time Practice

Typically, full-time practice for a massage therapist employee is a 30- to 40-hour workweek with an average of 25 actual massage hours. The remaining non-massage work hours are for turnover time between clients, charting, facility tasks such as laundry and cleaning, and a 30-minute food break and 15-minute rest break.

A full-time solo self-employed massage therapist would have the same number of massage session hours as an employee, 25 actual massage hours, but the non-massage hours increase. The typical full-time workweek for self-employment is at minimum 40 hours and more likely 50 hours.

Many massages therapists work part time. Part-time work varies from a few hours per week to half time and three-quarters time. This type of schedule is actually more common than a full-time massage practice. The massage session hours range from 10–15, and the actual work hours range from 15–20.

Box 3.3 Make It Simple

If you are self-employed in a private solo practice, you can expect to make for personal use 50% of whatever fee is charged; the other 50% covers all overhead and self-employment business tax expenses. Gratuities are included as additional income. You will have to pay income taxes on the net income.

Example: The massage fee is $80. Of this amount, $40 must be allotted to pay for overhead expenses and self-employment taxes and $40 for personal use and to pay income taxes. It would take 2 hours to earn the $40, resulting in $20 per hour.

If you are an employee, it is likely that the best the employer can do is pay a wage based on 30%–35% of whatever fee is charged for the massage, and the employer will have to deduct appropriate payroll and income taxes.

Example: The massage fee is $80. You would make $24–$28 for the 1-hour massage session. Based on five massage sessions in a 6-hour day, you would earn $20–$22 per hour. Your employer also pays a portion of payroll taxes, deducts the employee's portion of payroll taxes, and withholds income tax. After deductions of about 15% of wages, you take home $20–$24 of the massage fee. Gratuities are additional income and claimed separately when filing year-end income taxes.

Working part time does not change income per clock hour or income per massage hour. Working part time makes more financial sense for an employee because there are no business overhead costs to cover. Many employers are happy to have part-time massage therapists and will accommodate individual scheduling requests when possible. The employer is more likely to adapt to individual part-time scheduling if the massage therapist will work peak, high-demand hours, which are weekends and some evenings.

Part-time, sole practitioner, self-employed massage therapists may work from a home office or go to a client's location to keep overhead costs low. It is also possible to rent workspace and/or share space with other massage therapists. This arrangement helps manage overhead costs (Box 3.4).

Client Base

The number of clients you see each week and how you schedule them is the client base. You typically do not have the same clients each week. It is more likely that your schedule, based on full-time practice and a 1-hour massage session, will look like this:

- Five weekly clients (take really good care of regular clients!); 20 clients who get a massage every other week (i.e., 10 during the first week and 10 the second); and 20 clients who come once each month (5 each week).

This schedule includes a total of 20 clients per week who are regulars, the sustaining base of a successful full-time professional practice. This leaves five sessions per week open for referrals, the occasional client, and the first-time client. These people are your future, and it is important to impress them the first time you see them with your professional behavior and massage expertise. These individuals may become regulars or tell people about the excellent massages they had. If you are exceptional and provide a safe and neutral environment, you will eventually fill the remaining five appointments. The base of clients required to support a massage practice (self-employed or employee) is between 75 and 100 solid contacts.

Box 3.4 Compare Full- and Part-Time Practice

Similar for employees or those who are self-employed.

Work Schedule

Full-time: 25 hours massage; 30–40 hours per week; 20–25 clients per week

Three-quarters time: 18 hours massage; 20–25 hours per week; 16–18 clients per week

Half-time: 12 hours massage; 15–20 hours per week; 10–12 clients per week

Income

Full-time income $40,0000–$45,000 subject to income tax per year

Three-quarters time income $30,000–$33,750 subject to income tax per year

Half-time income $20,000–$22,500 subject to income tax per year

NOTE: Most massage therapists work half to three-quarter time by choice.

Client Retention

A successful massage practice, regardless of whether the therapists are employed or self-employed, is built on clients who receive therapeutic massage regularly. This is client retention. Clients who get a massage on a weekly, biweekly, or monthly basis are the mainstay of a massage business. To maintain a retention client structure, the massage professional must provide a quality massage; offer clients consistent, personal attention; deliver exceptional service; and charge affordable fees. Clients who are happy with the massage services are the best source of word-of-mouth advertising. Retention rates are higher for educated clients; therefore it is necessary to provide accurate and up-to-date information about massage.

The development of a regular client base is possible with therapeutic massage because massage benefits wear off if massage is not continued. Also, the benefits of massage are cumulative and better sustained with regular appointments. In Chapter 5, research is presented that supports the importance of regular massage sessions.

Clients are more apt to commit to a regular schedule of massage in the following circumstances:

- They notice measurable benefits related to their goals.
- They understand the physiological reasons for the results of massage.
- They experience a safe, professional, and ethical massage environment.

Clients who maintain a regular appointment schedule typically want to achieve quantifiable (measurable) and qualifiable (experiential) goals. Common goals, which are also called outcomes, are relaxation, stress management, pain management, and support for functional mobility and physical performance. Long-term care/treatment plans are important for these clients. If the massage therapist does not have the knowledge and

FOCUS ON PROFESSIONALISM 3.1

If retention is a problem and at least half of first-time clients do not reschedule massage sessions at least on a monthly basis, the massage practitioner needs to evaluate their skills and professional interaction with clients. Consider asking the following questions:

- Were my communication skills effective?
- Did I establish rapport with the client?
- Did I look and act professionally?
- Did I offend the client?
- Did something about my appearance make the client uncomfortable?
- Was my hygiene impeccable?
- Could an offensive environmental or body odor have been a problem?
- Was the massage environment safe, clean, and comfortable?
- Did I talk too much during the massage?
- Did I use the appropriate massage methods and pressure levels?
- Did the massage I provided meet the client's goals?
- Did something about my behavior make the client uncomfortable?
- Are my fees reasonable for the demographics?
- Do my fees support retention?

skills to help the client achieve these goals, the client will not be satisfied and will not return for massage.

Clients should be encouraged to schedule a standing appointment, such as every Thursday at 1 p.m. If the client is not able to commit to a regular appointment schedule, then they should be asked to reschedule after each appointment. A client should be reminded of the appointment schedule by telephone, text, or email. Literature should be available that explains the benefits of regular massages (Focus on Professionalism 3.1).

Massage therapy is typically paid for by the client out of pocket. The amount of financial resources that can be allocated to massage on a monthly basis must be considered when setting a standing appointment schedule. Standing appointments should account for three-fourths of the practice's schedule. Based on an average of 20 clients each week, this means that 15 sessions would be standing appointments. The most common pattern is an appointment every other week (twice a month). This schedule is affordable for most out-of-pocket payers. Some clients will get a massage regularly on a monthly basis. This is one of the reasons for a membership model in the massage practice. A monthly fee is paid, which pays for the first session of the month, and additional services in the month are often discounted for members. For the sake of profitability and productivity, the massage therapist should foster the standing appointment system. Also you will only need 100 loyal clients to maintain a profitable and successful massage business regardless of whether you are an employee or are self-employed.

Problems With Client Retention

The business owner (you if self-employed) has the responsibility to bring people into the business. This is done using advertising and marketing. It is the massage therapist's responsibility to ensure clients want to return. If there is a problem with client retention, it is usually because of some issue related to the massage therapist. Although it might be due to the facility or location, this is rare. The massage therapy occupation is female dominated, with almost 90% of massage therapists identifying as women. This makes it harder for massage therapists identifying as male to develop a retention client base. Although male massage therapists may need more time to build a retention clientele, it should still occur. Yes, it is impossible to please everyone, and not every client is going to be satisfied with a massage therapist's approach. However, most problems with client retention are directly related to an issue specific to the massage practitioner. This means that if you are not steadily retaining clients to build your client base, the problem is *you*.

Most problems with client retention are related to the massage therapist's skill, personality, hygiene and appearance, professionalism, attentiveness to client goals, ability to listen, and other factors. Clients really do not like massage therapists to talk much during the massage, especially if they talk about themselves. Clients will avoid massage therapists who smell, so be sure to take exceptional care of your personal hygiene,

EXAMPLE

- Client A finds massage beneficial but will only commit to a massage every other week. The best time for them is Wednesday evening at 7:30 p.m. Client A has a standing appointment.
- Client B has been receiving massage randomly for 6 months. The client calls and schedules a massage when they have time and then hopes for an opening in the schedule. The last couple of times, the client was not able to get in for a massage because openings were not available. The client has been receiving massage on average once every 3 weeks. The massage therapist suggests a regular appointment schedule of once a month. Then the client can call for additional sessions but will be assured of the monthly massage appointment. Because of a random work schedule, the only time available for a standing appointment is Fridays at 5 p.m. This time works for the massage therapist as well. Client B now has a standing schedule and could possibly move into a twice-a-month standing schedule.
- Client C will not commit to a standing appointment but wants to receive massage regularly. After each massage session, the client should be asked to schedule the next massage. If a pattern of appointments occurs, such as on Tuesday or Thursday, and a time or frequency repeats, such as 9 a.m. or 10 a.m., this should be pointed out to the client by saying, "I noticed that for the past 3 months, your massage sessions have occurred primarily on Tuesdays and Thursdays and before noon. You have also averaged a massage every 2 weeks. Have you considered scheduling a standing appointment so that you could be assured I am available, and you could plan the massage in your schedule? I have space available Tuesdays at 10:30 a.m. on the second and fourth Tuesdays." Client C is being encouraged to schedule standing appointments based on their pattern of massage usage.

including mouth hygiene. Bad breath will keep clients from returning. Avoid scented products including essential oils, unless requested by or used for specific clients. Just because you like the smell does not mean anyone else will. Also, smoking leaves a problematic odor on your clothing and hands. Non-smoking clients will often avoid massage therapists who smoke. Other behaviors that will influence client retention are issues with voice modulation (either too soft or too loud) and facility decorations and music that express religious or political views. Clients do not like pushy product sales and may be annoyed by upselling additional service (add-ons). Scrutinizing ourselves and being honest about our massage skills, appearance, hygiene, communication skills, environment, and so forth can be difficult. However, we must perform this evaluation to support client retention. Without client retention, we decrease our opportunity for career success (Box 3.5).

Scheduling for Productivity

Most massage businesses develop a schedule that includes extended business hours beyond the traditional workday. They may include early morning, evening time, or weekend days. Prime time is the period most often requested by clients. Prime time in most massage therapy businesses is after 3 p.m. weekdays and on weekends.

Massage therapy is a business, and one of the most effective ways to be profitable is to increase productivity. This is a real concern because massage is time intensive. Overlapping booking is not possible as it is with spa treatments or medical service. There is a limit to the number of clients one massage therapist can work with in a day. If your body mechanics are effective, you should be able to schedule five massage sessions per day and maintain basic business procedures if self-employed. It is more efficient to do this as an employee because someone else is managing much of the business; you can schedule clients with minimal time between because the front desk staff is handling the check-in and check-out procedures.

A full-time practice for a single self-employed massage therapist requires a minimum of 40–50 scheduled business hours per week, including massage sessions, buffer periods, facility management (e.g., cleaning), various marketing activities, and business activities (e.g., paying bills, billing clients, ordering supplies, returning calls). Buffer periods are scheduled time slots within the work period for breaks and catch-up. If you practice in a setting where you do not have to manage the office (i.e., you are an employee in a business with a receptionist), you will need less buffer time. Instead, you will likely be scheduled with two break periods and a lunch or dinner period.

You are expected to stay on schedule so that clients do not have to wait. Sessions are usually scheduled at 30 minutes, 60 minutes, 90 minutes, or 120 minutes. These are session times for scheduling purposes and not the amount of time spent actually giving the massage. A massage session includes the initial interview with the client (along with preassessment procedures and goal setting for the session), the post-massage assessment, time for the client to disrobe and settle onto the massage table, and then time for the client to redress and exit the massage area. These activities take between 10 and 15 minutes, meaning that a 60-minute therapeutic massage session is about 50 minutes on table, and a 90-minute session is 75 minutes on table. The 30-minute session is typically performed over clothing, so 20 minutes of actual hands-on-the-client time occurs. Between sessions you must be able to effectively prepare the massage area, wash your hands and arms, and greet the next client.

Box 3.5 Client Rights

Massage therapy clients are entitled to the following:

- To be treated with adequate, appropriate, compassionate care at all times and under all circumstances
- To be treated without discrimination based on race, religion, color, national origin, sex, age, handicap, marital status, sexual preference, or any condition covered by Americans with Disability Act (ADA)
- To be informed of all aspects of treatment
- To be informed of appointment and fee schedules
- To review their financial and clinical records
- To obtain a thorough evaluation of their needs
- To be treated as a partner in care and decision making related to treatment planning
- To receive current information and be assured of quality treatment
- To be able to refuse treatment and to be informed of the medical/massage consequences of that refusal
- To expect confidentiality of all records pertinent to their massage care
- To be informed if the massage therapist participates in different third-party payment plans
- To be able to request and expect appropriate referrals for consultation
- To expect continuity of treatment
- To be charged a fair and equitable fee
- To have appointment schedules and times maintained
- To be treated by a staff of professionals who maintain good health and hygiene
- To be respected for requesting a second opinion
- To be respected as human beings who have feelings and needs

Important Factors in Scheduling Appointments

You will deal with a variety of situations in scheduling appointments. Management of the appointment schedule requires a well-defined plan, an established appointment sequence. The massage therapist's biological clock will influence scheduling. Some people are early birds, and others are night owls. It is important to understand your body rhythms to best use your time. Not all people are at their best at all times of the day. Some people do not reach their peak period until 1 or 2 p.m., when the early birds who were dynamic at 8 a.m. have begun to lose energy. Others work best in the evening. This becomes an important factor in determining when to schedule clients. Because massage is a service business, you also need to consider when clients are available for massage sessions. The massage schedule can begin as early as 6 a.m. and continue well into the evening, depending on when clients are available and how their needs fit your schedule.

Habitually Late Clients

A small number of clients persist in being late for their appointments. You should stress the importance of being on time for the appointment by explaining to the client, "Your massage sessions require all the time allotted, and being on time for your appointment is therefore important to you." Your business policy should address the ramifications for clients who are late. Often the policy is that the late client pays for the full session but only receives what time is left in the appointment.

Clients Who Arrive on the Wrong Day

Clients may arrive on the wrong day or at the wrong time. The error may be the client's, or you might have written the wrong date on the appointment card. You should ask to see the appointment card, and if the client has made the mistake, indicate the actual date and time of the appointment. If you or another staff member made the error, an apology is necessary, and the massage therapist should still see the client if at all possible. The built-in buffer system in the daily schedule should make this possible. You may be able to contact the scheduled clients, explain that an "unexpected change has occurred in the schedule," and delay their arrival. Regardless of who is responsible for the error, you should remain tactful and helpful in correcting the mistake.

Drop-in and Walk-in Clients

It can be disruptive when a client drops by the business and say, "I was just in the area and thought I'd drop in and see if I could get a massage." If one of the open appointments is available, the individual can be seen. Otherwise, tactfully inform the client that you see clients by appointment only and tell the person when the next appointment is available.

This practice does not apply to the many walk-in (convenience) massage clinics established in the past few years. One of the prime objectives of these clinics is to accommodate clients without appointments.

Canceled Appointments and No-Shows

Sometimes, a client absolutely must cancel an appointment or is prevented from keeping the appointment by some unforeseen circumstance. Most clients respect the massage therapist's time, and the massage therapist should be understanding when a cancellation occurs. Other clients, unfortunately, seem always to find an excuse for canceling an appointment. Although the initial reaction of most massage therapists is to charge for canceled appointments, this becomes difficult to accomplish and can result in poor public relations. However, it is becoming the norm for a credit card to be on file to book an appointment, and the business has the option to charge if the cancelation policy is not followed. The typical cancelations policy is 24 hours' notice without a fee. Sometimes the fee for the entire massage session is charged; in other cases, the client will be charged a percentage of the fee. It is prudent to issue a reminder notice—such as a text, email, or call—24 hours before the day of the appointment. It is acceptable to charge the massage rate for those people who do not call and do not show up for a scheduled appointment.

Dovetailing

Dovetailing means working a second client into the schedule during another scheduled client's treatment. Many health care professionals and some service professionals (e.g., cosmetologists) can accomplish this. Massage therapists should not attempt this type of scheduling.

Entering Appointments

Commonly an electronic scheduling system is used. Appointments should include the following information:

- Client's full name and home and business phone numbers to confirm the appointment or to reach the client in case of an emergency
- Time of appointment
- Type or goal of the massage if appropriate
- Length of the appointment
- Payment information
- Special notations (e.g., new client)

If a paper appointment book is used, the entry is made in pencil to allow changes. It must be accurate, complete, and legible.

Reminder Calls, Emails, or Texts

It is common practice to remind clients of appointments. Even clients with regular appointments should be reminded. Commonly a reminder call is made, but many prefer electronic reminders such as email or text message.

Canceling Appointments

On occasion the massage therapist may need to cancel an appointment with a client. It is important to inform clients as soon as possible when canceling appointments. Have client contact information easily accessible so that contact can be made efficiently. If the massage professional knows in advance when they will be unavailable, such as for a planned vacation or family event, the clients should be told well ahead of time and reminded frequently. If the cancellation is due to an unexpected event, contact clients immediately or plan for someone to contact all clients to cancel. This would be the task of a receptionist if you are employed. It is appropriate to provide a brief reason for the cancellation, such as unexpected family responsibility or illness. Canceling appointments should be a rare event (Box 3.6).

Records

All massage professionals, whether employees or self-employed, must keep accurate, comprehensive client files. The success of your professional life depends on it. This topic will be covered in Chapter 4. Business records must also be maintained. Many commercial software record-keeping systems are available for both types of records. A wise course is to choose one and use it consistently. The current trend toward electronic data storage and various types of user-friendly software supports this option. There are a variety of software programs that specifically target massage therapy business needs. These programs include schedulers; calendars; subjective, objective, assessment, and plan (SOAP) or other types of note forms; inventory tracking; financial records; and anything else you

Box 3.6 Appreciate the Front Desk/Reception Staff

The term *front desk* is used to identify office reception area where guests/clients are greeted, information is provided, phones are answered, appointments are made, fees are paid, records are maintained, and more. A *receptionist* is the person who is employed to manage the front desk. As the initial point of contact, receptionists help form a visitor's first impression of a business. The receptionist also handles conflict if clients are not satisfied. An excellent receptionist contributes to business success. A poor receptionist can create confusion, conflict, and lead to business failure. The receptionist in a service-based business is very important but underappreciated. Massage therapists who are fortunate enough to have the support of a quality front desk staff need to be respectful and helpful.

could ever need to manage a sole proprietor-based massage business. You can actually manage a small massage business using smart phone/tablet technology and the huge selection of apps available. Device internet allows access to cloud-based storage systems, solving the problem of lack of storage space and backup limitations on the device. Monetary transactions can be handled with systems such as Square, Google Pay, Zelle, Venmo, or PayPal (Box 3.7).

Box 3.7 Categories of Records

The massage therapist must decide which records to keep, how to organize and store them, how long they legally must be retained, and when to dispose of them. In general, records can be categorized as vital, important, useful, or unimportant and as active or inactive.

Vital Records

Vital records are essential documents that cannot be replaced. They include client clinical and financial records and the practice records, such as rental agreement, insurance policies, and tax records. These records should be kept in a fireproof, theft-proof vault or safe, and copies often are kept in a protected, offsite location, such as a safe deposit box at a bank.

Important Records

Important records are extremely valuable to the operation of the office, but they are not vital. They include accounts payable and receivable, invoices, canceled checks, inventory and payroll records, and other federal regulatory records. Such records may be needed for a tax audit or if a question arises about a financial transaction. Important records should be retained for 5–7 years. Most offices keep them for about 7 years or in accordance with federal or state regulations.

Useful Records

Useful records include employment applications, expired insurance policies, petty cash vouchers, bank reconciliations, and general correspondence. This category is difficult to define because one office may consider a document useful, whereas another may find it indispensable. These records usually are retained for 1–3 years.

Unimportant Records

Unimportant records are the documents that lie around, have little importance, and take up space. They include items such as notes to yourself, reminders of meetings, outdated announcements, and pamphlets. Common sense dictates when these materials may be discarded.

Time Management

A vital aspect of a successful massage therapy practice is time management. There is more to working efficiently than just knowing how to perform a specific task. Understanding the relationship of time to production is also important. All these concepts together make up time management. Time management involves planning and scheduling your work and avoiding wasted time. Behaviors that waste time are failing to plan and budget time, giving in to interruptions, failing to follow through and complete a task, hesitancy making decisions, performing unnecessary work, and failure to delegate. Other time wasters are social media, lack of privacy, and desk clutter.

To determine the effectiveness of your own time management, you must assess the way you are working. Determine ways to use your time more effectively or confirm that you are already using your time efficiently. Evaluation of time management is an ongoing process and can be done routinely by recording the way you spend your time, analyzing how you spend your time, and determining which activities can be adjusted to make you more effective. You need discipline to schedule your activities daily, weekly, monthly, and for the long range, and you must adhere to the schedule. Efficient time management requires that you organize individual tasks, maintain daily schedules, analyze daily tasks, schedule major projects, establish deadlines, and organize workflow.

It is essential that you are at work on time. Regardless of whether you are an employee or are self-employed. There is nothing that frustrates clients more than a late massage therapist. Being habitually late for work is going to interfere with your career success. A no-show for work is also inexcusable. Yes, a serious and unexpected emergency might occur, but this is rare. If you have family that requires ongoing care, such as children or elder parents, it is necessary to secure reliable support care while you are at work. You must also have reliable transportation.

Maintaining Daily Schedules

To efficiently maintain a daily schedule, it is necessary to use a calendar of activities and tasks and a to-do list, determine priorities, show flexibility, use free time wisely, and review the schedule. It is important to review scheduling with the receptionist or supervisor if you are an employee.

The use of a calendar, personal appointment book, and the office appointment book is necessary in maintaining a daily schedule. You can use electronic or paper systems. A desk or electronic calendar provides a method for keeping track of your daily schedule, and it is used for short- and long-range scheduling. Make entries neatly if done manually, be consistent in making entries, and avoid making confidential entries if you use an electronic calendar that is accessible to others.

- A to-do list should provide a summary of all pending tasks, not just those to be done on a specific day. This list need not include routine daily tasks, such as opening and closing the office or opening mail. Delete each task upon completion, and transfer tasks not completed to a list for the following day.

- Determine priorities by ranking each task on the list by its priority or its level of urgency and importance. Items on the list can be ranked by giving a "1" to tasks that must be completed immediately, "2" to tasks that must be completed that day, and "3" to tasks that may be done whenever you have time.
- Be flexible in your plans for the day because emergencies arise, and new priority tasks will be identified. In addition to the routine to-do list, another list could be kept that details various tasks that should be completed when time permits. This list provides tasks to do during a slow period or when no clients are scheduled.
- Do not overschedule or underestimate how long some tasks will take. It is better to under schedule than overschedule. Life, both personal and professional, will be much more enjoyable and less stressful when your time is efficiently managed.

Managing Money

Whether you are an employee or are self-employed, success depends on money management. If you are an employee, money management involves earned income for personal expenses. If you are self-employed, there is business money management as well as personal money management.

Budget

A budget is a money management plan. It is an estimation of income and expenses over a period of time. Budgets can be made for a person, a family, or a business. The personal budget becomes the platform for determining income to support one's lifestyle. Make two budgets: one for the minimal income needed for personal expenses and one realistic optimal budget. Another way to think of this is to ask yourself these questions: What is the least amount of money I need for baseline necessary expenses? What is the most money I need to establish and maintain the economic lifestyle I desire?

Abundance, Enough, Not Enough: Balance

There are many definitions of *abundance, enough,* and *scarcity* (not enough). A few definitions are needed to develop an understanding of a money relationship.

Balance is as much as is needed (enough). If enough is just right, scarcity is not enough, and abundance is more than enough. Scarcity (or not enough) is easiest to understand. Most have experienced the sensation of not enough time. Some have experienced not enough food. When really hungry, we feel empty. However, not enough does not mean without. The thing we want is available, but not enough of it to feel satisfied.

If there is enough, we are satisfied, but is there enough to share? If there is more than enough, we may save for a time when there may not be enough, or we may feel generous and distribute the excess. For example, if we have just enough to eat, we will be satisfied, but if we share, we will not be full. Will we share when resources are scarce and there is not quite enough but there could be enough if everyone contributed a small amount?

How do we know when enough is enough? What happens when the pursuit of one thing in abundance—money or athletic performance, for example—results in not enough time for friends, children, relaxing, or sleeping? Most disease can be described in terms of too much in one area that results in not enough in another. In massage, if you spend too much time working on the back, there is not enough time to adequately massage the rest of the body. It all becomes a management issue (i.e., practice of managing, handling, supervision, or control).

There is a difference between a need and a want. A need indicates that something is necessary for life, such as nutritious food, clean water, a specific medication, or shelter. A want is something we do not need, but it brings a sense of satisfaction. When truly hungry, we need and want food. We can meet the need with beans, rice, and spinach mixed together in a quantity that can fit in an individual's hands cupped together, or we can meet the need with something we want, such as a pint of ice cream, or a whole bag of candy. Many of the current diseases plaguing affluent societies come from meeting a need with a want. Too much of a good thing becomes a bad thing. Obesity and the resulting diabetes stem from overeating the wrong types of foods. To counteract obesity caused by too much of the food we want and not enough exercise, we need to shift the balance. Reducing food and creating scarcity on purpose as well as increasing exercise so there is enough movement will result in a reduction of what we do not need: excess body fat. Easily said but sometimes very hard to do.

We do need some fat reserves, and in a similar manner, we do need money reserves. It is important to save appropriately so there is enough during times of scarcity. For example, there are natural slow times in the massage business. When the weather becomes nice in the spring or around holidays, people may get a massage less often. For a couple of weeks, business is slow, and income diminishes. Financial management anticipates the seasonal fluctuation in income, and money from periods of abundance is saved for times of relative scarcity. It is a balance.

Abundance is more than enough. Abundance can be wonderful or not. Abundance means that we have more than we need, but when we have more than we need, what do we do with it? Use it anyway? Save it? Hide it? Share it? A combination of all four options? Only you can answer this, and how you answer the question can provide insight into your relationship with money. Abundance is a worthwhile goal. Financial abundance is one aspect to consider. Financial abundance means that we can achieve some of our wants; for example, ice cream for dessert along with the beans, rice, and spinach; clean water pumped to the house instead of having to carry it from a distant well; and owning a house with a garden instead of living in a car or shelter. Abundance means that we can set aside resources to sustain ourselves when there are times of scarcity. Saving money is like preserving food during the abundance of the fall harvest to feed ourselves during the winter.

We all need to consider our future needs and wants, as well as the needs of those who depend on us, such as our children.

It is important to regularly save from the current abundance in some sort of investment retirement plan. Investments grow and produce income. Investments can include savings accounts that earn a small amount of interest and purchasing property that will increase in value. All massage professionals, whether self-employed or employed by others, should set up an individual retirement plan. After taxes have been paid, 10% of income could be invested in a long-term growth asset. A local bank or insurance company may have access to stable mutual funds. Individual retirement accounts (IRAs) also are available. Some employers offer investment plans. Money can be invested in compound interest-bearing accounts in many ways. This takes discipline, but aging is inevitable, and planning for that time now is important. Investment means that we are doing something productive with our abundance when the resources are more than enough.

Another investment to consider is providing one massage per week for someone who really needs it but truly cannot afford the massage fees. Consider this recommendation as a "pay it forward" investment. The person receiving the massage always has something to return to the massage professional. The client will feel better when giving back. It could be garden produce or knitted slippers. Maybe it is a smile of appreciation and gentle wishes, which can be worth more than gold.

We can hide abundance, but hiding is a secret. People may hide income so that they do not have to pay taxes. In businesses that have cash payments or if receiving cash gratuities it is tempting to "pocket" the cash. That money cannot grow because it cannot be seen. If you are paying taxes, it means that you have earned abundance in income. Those who make an income below a certain level (i.e., barely enough) do not have to pay much in income taxes, whereas those who have more than enough income pay on the abundance. Taxes can be seen as a form of sharing abundance. The tax laws are convoluted and not always fair, but the concept is sound. If you are paying taxes, you are making at least enough money to meet survival needs.

EXAMPLE

Budget examples are given for a single person who is 30 years old living in an area of moderate cost-of-living expenses. All amounts are averages and estimates and represent income subject to income taxes. Figures are adapted from the Internal Revenue Service (IRS). This would be an example of "enough" income.

Monthly expenses:

- Food, clothing, and other items: $700
- Transportation (monthly loan or lease payments, monthly operating costs): $800
- Housing and utilities: $1200
- Health care (insurance and out of pocket): $400
- Total monthly expenses: $3100
- Total yearly expenses after taxes: $37,200
- Yearly income needed: $45,000 ($22 per hour)

Now let's look at four income levels: Not Enough, Barely Enough (breakeven), Enough, and Abundance:

- Not enough/scarcity: poverty-level annual income: $13,500 (approximately 30% of barely enough) and minimum wage–based annual income $25,000 (approximately 80% of barely enough)

EXAMPLE—Cont'd

- Barely enough (breakeven), no monetary abundance; this is considered a living wage and meets needs only: $32,000 yearly income at $15.38 per hour employee based on 40-hour workweek
- Enough $45,000 (approximately 25% more than barely enough)
- Abundance: $60,000 (almost double barely enough)

There is satisfaction in identifying each end of your personal economic curve and continuum. Determine your budget for a breakeven point as well as what an abundance budget would look like. Once you have a base income amount, you will know what you need to earn. This is going to be different for everyone related to personal circumstances. Where someone lives makes a difference. Cost of living varies depending on the area. The high-end living wage factored for New York City and San Francisco is $50,000–$65,000 a year subject to income tax. The low end is factored based on multiple rural areas and is $30,000 a year subject to income tax. The *living wage* is the minimum income standard for financial independence and determines a minimum subsistence wage for persons living in the United States. You can use the Massachusetts Institute of Technology (MIT) living wage calculator to find your living wage. The Living Wage Calculator was first created in 2004 by Dr. Amy K. Glasmeier at MIT (http://livingwage.mit.edu/).

(Proficiency Exercise 3.2).

Medical Insurance or Third-Party Reimbursement Income

Insurance reimbursement for massage is uncommon and occurs for massage therapy about 10% of the time. Usually a physician must indicate massage as a medical necessity. Some massage professionals do well with insurance reimbursement. Workers' compensation and smaller insurance companies are more apt to pay. For the United States, changes to the health care delivery system present a variety of challenges as new provisions are implemented. The effect on the massage therapy profession will continue to be determined separately in each state. As with almost all aspects of professional practice, insurance coverage has its pros and cons. The documentation requirements for collecting insurance are extensive, and it is necessary to submit claims electronically. Most massage professionals are unable to bill the insurance company directly for reimbursement. If the massage therapist is an employee of a licensed medical professional or of a managed care corporation with access to insurance billing codes and is working under direct supervision, the massage services may be available for billing. In this situation, the massage therapist receives an hourly wage or salary. The burden of collecting from the insurance company falls on the physician, chiropractor, physical therapist, dentist, psychiatrist, or corporate entity, not on

PROFICIENCY EXERCISE 3.2

Make a budget based on your current living situation. Use the MIT Living Wage Calculator and identify the living wage in your area (http://livingwage.mit.edu/).

the massage practitioner. However, the massage practitioner needs to be able to perform effective assessments, write appropriate treatment plans, and maintain charts.

Occasionally a client can collect from the insurance company by providing a prescription for massage from the physician and a receipt showing payment, the diagnostic code from the physician, and a description of the procedure. It is important to have the insurance company preapprove payment for therapeutic massage. This is done by having the client contact the insurance company before any massage begins. Documentation on the benefits of massage, the physician's prescription, and any other information required by the insurance company are presented for review. This usually is the client's responsibility. On the basis of this information, the insurance company determines whether the client will be reimbursed for the massage services and notifies the client in writing of the decision. The client pays the massage professional directly, and the massage professional provides the receipt with the physician's diagnostic code, the procedure used, and the duration of the session. Responsibility for collecting insurance reimbursement falls to the client.

A client may also be able to use funds in a health savings account, a type of savings account that allows individuals to set aside money on a pretax basis to pay for qualified medical expenses. It would be the responsibility of the client to determine if therapeutic massage is a qualified expense.

In some areas, licensed massage therapists may be able to bill insurance companies directly. Although this situation is not common, if you live in a jurisdiction that does allow direct billing by massage therapists, be realistic about the responsibilities required to maintain a positive working relationship with insurance companies. To bill you will need a National Provider Identifier (NPI) number. This is a unique 10-digit identification number issued to health care providers in the United States by the Centers for Medicare and Medicaid Services (CMS). The NPI is a Health Insurance Portability and Accountability Act (HIPAA) administrative standard. The NPI was created to improve the efficiency and effectiveness of the electronic transmission of health information. All health care providers who are HIPAA-covered entities, whether individuals or organizations, must obtain an NPI. HIPAA-covered entities include the following:

- Health care providers that conduct certain transactions in electronic form
- Health care clearinghouses
- Health plans (including commercial plans, Medicare, and Medicaid)

For more information and to access a tool to help you determine whether you are a covered entity, refer to https://www.cms.gov/Regulations-and-Guidance/Administrative-Simplification/HIPAA-ACA/AreYouaCoveredEntity.html. To apply for an NPI number through a web-based application process, visit the National Plan and Provider Enumeration System (NPPES) at https://nppes.cms.hhs.gov/?NPPES/Welcome.do#/ on the CMS website. Individual providers must create a username and password through the Identity & Access (I&A) Management System, log in to the NPPES using that username and password, and follow the instructions.

Typically, insurance claim form 1500 is used to submit the billing. This form can be found on the web using search term: insurance claim form 1500. If you are able to bill insurance companies, contact each company individually, speak with a representative, and ask for information on the best way to work with the company (See Chapter 13 for more information about massage therapy in the medical care environment.)

Professional and Business Insurance

All massage practitioners need professional liability insurance, often called malpractice insurance. The term *malpractice* refers to professional negligence or maleficence. Negligence is an unintentional wrong. A negligent person fails to act in a reasonable and careful manner and consequently causes harm. Maleficence is causing deliberate harm. Clients expect a certain level of professional education, standards of practice, and responsibility for conduct. Unfortunately, in the highly litigious climate of today's world, the best protection against a lawsuit is insurance. Insurance reduces the risk of having a liability claim filed against you personally. Accurate, comprehensive records are the next best protection; anything that seems even slightly important must be documented (see Chapter 4).

The best place to obtain professional liability insurance is through the professional organizations. Those that have been in existence for many years are the American Massage Therapy Association and the Associated Bodywork and Massage Professionals. Insurance costs are usually part of the dues structure of these organizations, an arrangement that makes insurance available at a reasonable cost. Insurance may also be obtained from other professional sources at a reasonable yearly fee. Private companies also provide professional liability policies, but they may be quite expensive. Employees may be asked to have the employer added to the policy as an *additional insured.* Those that rent space to massage therapists may also request to be added as an additional insured. This is a common practice because if a client is going to claim injury or misconduct, the lawsuit is often filed against anyone associated.

For business owners, premise liability insurance also is needed; this is often called "trip and fall" insurance. It can be obtained through professional organizations or from a local insurance agent. Because home business offices are not covered under a homeowner's policy, additional coverage in the form of a business rider is needed. The insurance agent also can discuss fire and damage insurance on equipment. The sale of products requires product liability insurance. The more complicated a business, the more comprehensive the insurance coverage must be. The insurance agent and the insurance representative of the professional organization can provide additional information.

Burnout

When a person is burned out, motivation is lost. **Burnout** occurs when you use up your energy faster than you can replenish it.

There are three main reasons for burnout in the massage profession:

- Physical fatigue and injury
- Financial strain
- Emotional stress

Physical fatigue and injury are usually caused by ineffective and excessive use of the body while giving massage. Chapter 8 targets body mechanics and contains possibly the most important information for preventing burnout. It is reasonable to expect that a massage therapist can work 40 hours a week and perform 25–30 actual hours of massage during that time. This is a full-time massage practice.

Financial strain is common in our society. The economy has changed, and people have to adapt to limited resources. It is reasonable to expect that entry-level massage therapists can earn a wage/salary if employed and net profit if self-employed before income taxes of $35,000–$45,000 if they can work full time and provide the 25–30 actual hours of massage sessions each week. A self-employed massage therapist would need a business gross of $70,000–$90,000 a year to have a net profit of $35,000–$45,000. Again, it is important to begin your massage career with realistic expectations. However, it is also important to realize that with experience and increased client retention, the income can increase as the overhead decreases or if the employer increases wages for a productive and valued employee. Massage therapy is a service business, and income stability depends on client satisfaction, retention, and a full appointment schedule. If a client cancels an appointment, it creates a reduction in income. If you are employed, the business owner must absorb the loss of income. If you are self-employed, you have to deal with the deficit. The burnout issue occurs when income barely covers personal expenses, and there is no financial safety net. It is stressful to live from paycheck to paycheck.

Emotional stress is a major cause of burnout. For massage therapists, this is characterized by taking better care of others than we do of ourselves. Burnout can be a problem in most service professions. Taking care of others is a big job. If we do not take care of ourselves also, we soon have nothing to give others or ourselves. Each of us must take care of our physical needs, such as resting, eating well, getting regular massages, and paying attention to our emotional needs. Surround yourself with people who believe in you. Take care of your spiritual needs, which connect the value of what you want to accomplish with a much higher purpose. Follow the wellness guidelines presented in Chapter 15.

The actual application of massage is basic, repetitious touch, which sometimes can get boring. It is important to keep yourself excited about the benefits of such repetitious applications of touch. One of the best ways to do this is to continue your education. Classes make you think and bring you together with other massage professionals. These are good opportunities to share and learn together. State-licensed massage schools and professional organizations are the best sources for massage education. It also is important to get away from massage for a bit. Having a hobby or creating downtime creates balance. Take care of yourself, and let others take care of you. Take a vacation, a walk, or a long warm bath, and burnout will be less of a problem.

After a person begins to live life—including their career life—with purpose, the energy to develop the career focus becomes available. Living with purpose is the key to motivation. It means drawing strength from knowing that what we have to offer is valuable (Proficiency Exercise 3.3).

PROFICIENCY EXERCISE 3.3

Separate into small groups and take turns describing a time when you were burned out. Explain what steps you took to get out of the burnout phase.

Self-Employment, Employee, or Combined Practice

This chapter does what generic business texts and websites cannot do: it shares the experience gained from walking the career path in therapeutic massage, both as an employee and as a self-employed professional. Throughout the text, you are encouraged to ask questions about your massage education, to use clinical reasoning as a problem-solving method, and to challenge information. You are urged to seek authoritative sources carefully and to compare information from many experts. The same principles apply in your massage career. You can work full time or part time, be either self-employed or an employee, and you can either have a career or hold a job in massage. Do not think that you must be self-employed and working full time to have a career.

Employee or self-employed? Each of these two options has its advantages and disadvantages. One person may feel that the independent decision making involved in self-employment is an advantage, whereas a person who has difficulty producing independent ideas would consider this a disadvantage. Only you can decide which, or a combination of both, is best for you.

In the past, most massage therapists were small-business owners. Few employment opportunities existed. But times have changed. The profession has seen a steady increase in jobs and career opportunities in the more traditional employee market, in which the massage practitioner goes to work for an individual or a company at a wage-based income (Box 3.8).

The employee market exists within personal service, fitness, wellness centers, recreational industries, and medical establishments. The most rapid expansion of employment opportunities is occurring in the spa and franchise setting. Franchises and business chains are spreading quickly and offer employment options. A wellness center is an establishment that offers health services for the body and mind, with massage therapy being a major offering. The fitness industry is another source of employment. Many health clubs offer the services of a massage professional. The recreation industry (e.g., hotels, cruise ships, retreats, and resort centers) also is an active employer of massage practitioners. The independent massage therapy clinic offers opportunities for employment when the owner or manager of the clinic handles all business responsibilities and hires massage practitioners to do the work. Massage professionals are working for physicians, physical therapists, mental health professionals, and other health care professionals. It is possible to have two part-time positions working for two different employers. For ethical purposes, the employers should be providing massage service to two different client populations; for example, one job may be at a franchise and the other for a home health service. Always disclose dual employment arrangements to both employers.

Successful self-employment requires an entrepreneurial spirit. An *entrepreneur* is a person who organizes, operates, and assumes the risk of a business venture. Not everyone is cut out for self-employment. The hours are long, and 100%

Box 3.8 Methods to Calculate Wages: Analyze the Two Examples

Base hourly pay + Per piece rate

Example

First, calculate regular pay: $10 (i.e., minimum wage) 40 hours = $400

Add the per piece rate for massage sessions: 20 sessions × $10 = $200

Total gross wages for the weekly pay period: $600

Average hourly: $600 divided by 40 hours = $15 per hour

Average per massage: $30

Gratuities not included in pay but reported on W-2: $100

Business gross: 20 massage sessions × $60 session fee = $1200

Employer wage burden: 50%

Piece rate: Rate paid per unit of production × Number of units completed in the pay period

Example

Regular pay $25 per massage × 20 massage session in a 40-hour pay period = gross pay $500

Average hourly: $500 divided by 40 hours = $12.50

Average per massage: $25

Gratuities not included in pay but reported on W-2: $100

Business gross: 20 massage sessions × $60 session fee = $1200

Employer wage burden: 40%

By comparing these two examples you can see that the per piece rate favors the employer and the hourly + piece rate favors the employee.

What adjustments would need to be made to the hourly + piece rate to bring the wage burden to 40%? How might these figures appear if rates were 10%, 25%, or 50% higher? How would the calculation change if the fee for massage was $80, $100, or $120?

commitment is required. Self-employed people must be self-starters with a broad range of professional and business skills. Some people think that self-employed individuals get to be their own boss; however, this is not so; instead of one or two bosses, every client becomes the boss.

Besides an entrepreneurial spirit, self-employment requires a deep internal commitment. If you have the commitment, drive, skill, and discipline necessary for self-employment and are willing to make the 100% commitment (and more) it takes to build and maintain a massage therapy practice, self-employment may be the best option for you.

To determine whether self-employment is the best career choice, answer the following questions:

- How disciplined am I?
- Do I wait until the last minute to do a job?
- Am I on time, or do I usually run late?
- Do I keep myself organized?

After you have answered the questions, ask trusted friends and family members to answer the same questions about you. Tell them you need honest responses. The insight of others is valuable as you make important decisions about your career.

The very skills that make a wonderful massage therapist—intuition, sensitivity, an ability to respond to the moment—can be a source of difficulty in meeting the business requirements of planning ahead, keeping bills paid on time, carefully planning business strategy, and staying in one place long enough to carry out the business plan. If you do not have either the self-discipline or the skills necessary for self-employment, employee status may be the better choice.

This information should not discourage an individual from self-employment as a career vision. It should, however, provide a dose of reality and prepare an individual for the committed and complex journey of being self-employed. It is frustrating for those with the entrepreneurial spirit to be constrained in the structure of someone else's business dream.

Advantages and Disadvantages of Self-Employment

There are advantages to self-employment. Some feel that self-employment offers more freedom to self-direct the business structure, in addition to flexibility in scheduling work hours and long-term financial security. The business income could be increased by subletting the office space (make sure any rental agreement allows for this). Retail and non-massage services such a sauna can add income. Likewise, after the first few years, advertising and marketing expenses decline because you have established a repeat business with clients who return regularly for massage, and net income increases.

Disadvantages include numerous responsibilities both for business concerns and for client services, isolation, lack of peer support and supervision if working alone, and the inability to leave the business for any length of time. Income can vary, and no group benefits are available, such as insurance packages or paid vacations. Membership in professional associations can offset the benefits issue because group insurance programs are available through them.

Advantages and Disadvantages of Employment

There are many advantages to being an employee. When choosing a career option, consider that, as a therapeutic massage employee, you are not responsible for any of the business concerns and can focus most of your professional energy on client services. In addition as an employee you also have many government protections such as Equal Employment Opportunity laws, the Department of Labor's Unemployment Insurance (UI) programs, and the Department of Labor–enforced Fair Labor Standards Act (FLSA), which sets basic minimum wage and overtime pay standards. Employers must also pay payroll taxes for each employee to cover potential unemployment benefits and future Social Security and Medicare costs. Employers also have to withhold income taxes. Employee status usually involves working with other professionals in some way, creating an environment of support and mentoring. Some businesses may offer benefits and paid vacations. Income usually is stable. Employees who have established long-term relationships with their employers often get pay increases.

The disadvantages of being an employee might include adherence to business rules and regulations, less flexibility in work scheduling, being in an environment where other employees behave unprofessionally, and having to share a workspace. It is also possible that the employer does not run an ethical and efficient business. The owner or manager may have a difficult personality. If you are an excellent employee, you deserve to work for an excellent employer. If you realize that the employer is not creating an excellent business environment, discuss the situation with the employer and if the situation does not improve, provide notice and leave. Also, if you are not an excellent employee and the business does not benefit from having you in the workplace, the employer has the right to terminate your employment.

The Combined Career Pathway

Because massage therapists are able to work in a variety of settings, a combined practice is an option—part employee and part self-employed. Just remember to be ethical and loyal to your employer. Always tell the employer that you also work as a self-employed practitioner on the side. Do not attempt to move clients from the employer's business to a self-employed private practice. When developing a combined career path, make sure that the private practice is distinctly different from the employer's business.

EXAMPLE

- Employee in a medical pain clinic and self-employed providing on-site massage athletes.
- Employee in a local spa and self-employed providing massage to a few homebound clients.
- Employee in a massage franchise and self-employed at home if living at least 30 minutes from the franchise location.
- Employee at a chiropractic office and self-employed providing mobile massage to a couple of families who are not patients of the chiropractor.

There is no one preferred career path. You decide. The next section in the chapter provides specific information related to employment (Proficiency Exercise 3.4).

Clarification Related to Independent Contractor Status

Confusion exists related to the work status of independent contractor (I/C). Independent contractors are self-employed and are contracted by a business to provide a specific service or complete a specific task. Employers may attempt to use the classification to simplify or avoid federal and state labor and tax laws. Almost all massage therapists classified as independent contractors are misclassified employees.

Whether a worker is an independent contractor or employee depends on the facts in each situation. California has a good description. To qualify a worker as an independent contractor in California, the hiring party must demonstrate the following:

A. The worker is free (contractually and in fact) from the control and direction of the hirer in connection with the work; *and*

B. The worker performs work that is not the hiring entity's usual business; *and*

C. The worker is customarily engaged in an independently established trade, occupation, or business of the same nature as the work performed for the hiring entity.

There is no such thing as a "1099 employee." The "1099" part of the name refers to the fact that independent contractors receive a form 1099 at the end of the year, which reports to the IRS how much money was paid to the contractor. In contrast, employees receive a W-2. Often a company may choose to designate certain service providers to be independent contractors instead of employees, but this is not always up to the parties to decide. In many situations, workers who are deemed to be independent contractors by agreement between the company and the worker are still considered to be employees by law. When that happens, the IRS, the department of labor, and state agencies will reclassify the worker to be an employee and treat the employer as if it simply violated its legal obligations in how it handled that employee. As a result, the consequences for misclassifying a worker can be quite severe. Workers who believe they have been improperly classified as independent contractors by an employer can use Form 8919, Uncollected Social Security and Medicare Tax on Wages, to figure and report the employee's share of uncollected Social Security and Medicare taxes due on their compensation.

BOTTOM LINE: It is unlikely that a massage therapist can be considered an independent contractor. Just because pay is per massage does not make you an independent contractor. Career pathways are employee, self-employed, or a combination of both and *not* independent contractor.

PROFICIENCY EXERCISE 3.4

Develop your personal lists of pros and cons for self-employment and employee status.

Self-Employment

- Pros, cons

Employee Status

- Pros, cons

MENTORING TIP

Employee? Self-employed? Combining both? It can be overwhelming. There is no right way. As a longtime massage therapist and educator, I do have a recommendation, however. There are good employment opportunities available. Right out of school the most important things to concentrate on are your massage skills and client interactions. Employment offers the opportunity to focus on becoming an excellent massage therapist. Employment can be a stepping-stone to becoming self-employed. Be responsible and ethical to the employer who gave you your space to begin your career if this is your plan. You may also find career satisfaction as part of an employment team. Be open to the possibilities.

A happy medium is the combined career pathway. You can maximize the advantages and minimize the disadvantages. The concern of the combined career concept is that the employer, who supported you at the beginning of your career, often ends up with an unequal deal as the self-employed aspect of your massage practice grows. The combined practice only works when it is a win-win situation. Should the time come when it is time to leave the employer and focus on being on your own, communicate, be responsible, be respectful, and be thankful.

EMPLOYEE-SPECIFIC FOCUS

SECTION OBJECTIVES

Chapter objectives covered in this section:

14. Create a résumé and cover letter.
15. Prepare for an employment interview.
16. List elements included in an employment agreement.
17. Explain how employment wages are calculated.
18. Estimate the employer wage expense ratio to gross business profits.
19. Self-evaluate the potential for an increase in wages.
20. Explain unemployment benefits, resignation, termination, and layoff.
21. List the skills needed to achieve employee success.

Using the information presented in this section, the student will be able to perform the following:

- List and describe the qualities of an excellent employee.
- Write a résumé and cover letter.
- Describe an interview.
- Dress appropriately for an interview.
- Respond confidently to an interviewer's questions.
- Follow up appropriately after an interview.
- Negotiate and justify an employment agreement.
- Calculate wages and determine fair wages.
- Justify a wage increase.
- Define unemployment benefits, resignation, termination, and layoff.
- Self-evaluate employee performance.
- Evaluate employer performance and provide feedback to an employer.

If you decide that you are better suited to achieving success as an employee, commit to being an excellent employee. Many employers complain about the quality and commitment of their employees. The massage/bodywork industry is no different. If you choose to be an employee, the information in this text should help you understand the commitment and responsibility required of an employer to create an environment that allows you to pursue your career as a massage professional free of business responsibilities. Investigate each position in which you are interested. It is important to understand the job description, the hours that will be spent on the job, and obligations to the employer. Once you have obtained a massage therapy position, commit to career growth. You need to meet the expectations of the clients, improve your skills, and build relationships with people at work. In other words, you have to be an excellent employee with a good work ethic. When you do this, you invest in yourself. You develop excellent work habits one day at a time, one behavior at a time. Attitude is more than a state of mind. It is the way you look at life. Employers want friendly people with positive attitudes, and you learn to think positively about yourself by doing positive things. Make yourself valuable, and you will be valued.

The Résumé and Cover Letter

The résumé and cover letter are your first introduction to an employer. Remember that first impressions are important. Make sure these two documents are formatted correctly and that the spelling and grammar are correct. If the documents are presented on paper, use quality paper stock; if they are delivered electronically, follow all the correct procedures. Above all else, make sure everything written is true and honestly presented.

Developing a Résumé and Cover Letter

A résumé is a compilation of professional and personal data about a person. Your résumé is your professional story. A cover letter for your résumé is like an introduction to the hiring company. It tells them who you are, the position for which you are applying, how you found out about the position, and a brief explanation of why you should be called for an interview. Cover letters are always targeted to a specific employer. Before writing a cover letter, investigate the company and learn as much as you can about the vision and mission of the business. Find out about the business organization and who the people in positions of authority are. In writing the cover letter, use action verbs that are descriptive and concrete, that really sell your experience, skills, and abilities. The cover letter should be one-half to three-fourths of a page long and should be printed on plain, white or ivory, professional-grade paper or delivered in appropriate electronic form.

The format and delivery of a résumé and cover letter have changed in recent years mostly because of electronic communication. Make sure when you develop a résumé and cover letter that you are using the most current recommendation. Reliable places to find help are the public library and your local chamber of commerce. Also search the internet for recommendations. College and university sites are helpful. This section of the chapter provides general guidelines, but the actual résumé and cover letter development needs to be current and targeted. Sample résumés would be dated and therefore have not been included here. You will need to be proactive to make sure that your résumé and cover letters are updated regularly, follow current format recommendations, and are delivered correctly to potential employers.

Log on to CareerOneStop, sponsored by the US Department of Labor, Employment and Training Administration (www.careeronestop.org), and search for the term *résumé* for up-to-date guidance on résumé and cover letter creation. Following is a method to create a résumé and cover letter:

1. Gather all data, including the following:
   - Personal contact information, such as full name, email, cell phone and other contact numbers, website if applicable, and social media contacts, such as LinkedIn.
   - Employment information past and present: The résumé should list not only massage experience but also other work experience. You will need names, addresses, and other contact information, names of supervisors, dates of employment, and details of job duties. Described what you learned from the job that can contribute to your massage career. For example, if you worked in food service as a server, you have experience in customer service.
   - Education and training: You will need details about schools, training programs, military experience, diplomas, degrees, continuing education, and self-education. Data include names of schools or providers, contact

information, dates of attendance and completion, and relevance to your massage career, especially if education is not specific to massage therapy. For example, courses in communication or psychology contribute to professional skills.
2. Find and download a couple of résumé and cover letter templates. Many free templates are available. The software on your computer may have templates for résumés and cover letters. Internet sites offer free templates. Be cautious, however; many of these sites want you to buy services, but the templates are still usable.
3. Plug the information gathered in step 1 into the templates and play around with the content and organization until you develop a couple of samples that you like.
4. Take all the data from steps 1 and 2 and the samples you made in step 3 to someone who can help you improve what you created in step 3. Start with staff at your public library and chamber of commerce. There may be staff at your school. Remember, seeking help is a good thing (Proficiency Exercise 3.5).

The Interview

The interview allows the employer to get to know the person applying for the position. When you apply for a job, you are the applicant. The interview also allows the applicant to ask questions about the company and the available position, building on the information accumulated to prepare for the interview. Through the interview process, the employer develops a good sense of the applicant's communication skills, which are demonstrated when the applicant answers questions, provides feedback on possible situations, and asks questions about the position and company.

PROFICIENCY EXERCISE 3.5

Using an employment website like Indeed, Glassdoor, or ZipRecruiter, pick a massage position that interests you. Draft a résumé and cover letter that you would use if you were to apply for the position.

Communication

Some think that effective communication is one of the most important skills an employee can have. To communicate effectively during the job interview, you can research the company, the setting, and the position for which you are applying. Write down questions to ask during the interview process. This is a good way to prepare for the interview.

During the interview, speak clearly, professionally, simply, and loud enough to be heard. Maintain relaxed eye contact and avoid fidgeting. Ask relevant, concise questions. Practice asking these questions before the interview. Also, write down the interviewer's answers to questions about the position and the company for future reference; this is another way of showing the employer that the applicant truly wants the position.

Dressing for Success

The applicant's attire and shoes should be neat and clean at the interview. Conservative business dress is appropriate for the job interview, even if a uniform is usually worn. The applicant should bring a uniform and massage supplies to the interview in case the interviewer wants a demonstration massage. Attention to the details of one's appearance is crucial to the success of an interview. The following tips can help you present a professional appearance (Fig. 3.2):

- Wear plain tailored business attire. A suit is a good choice for both genders.
- The clothing should fit well but not be tight or revealing.
- Skirt length should be modest and about knee length.
- Wear clean, polished, conservative dress shoes.

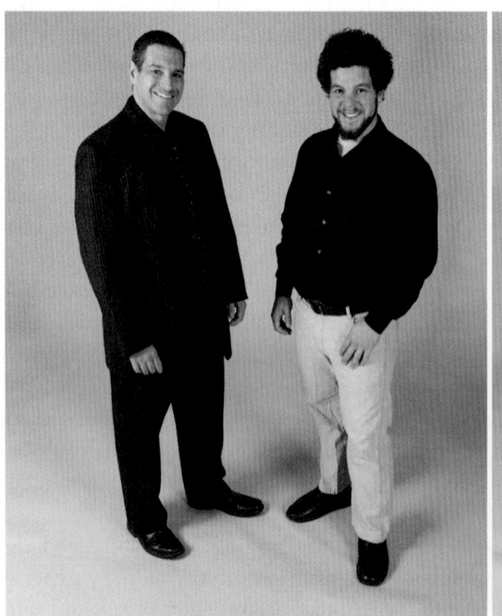
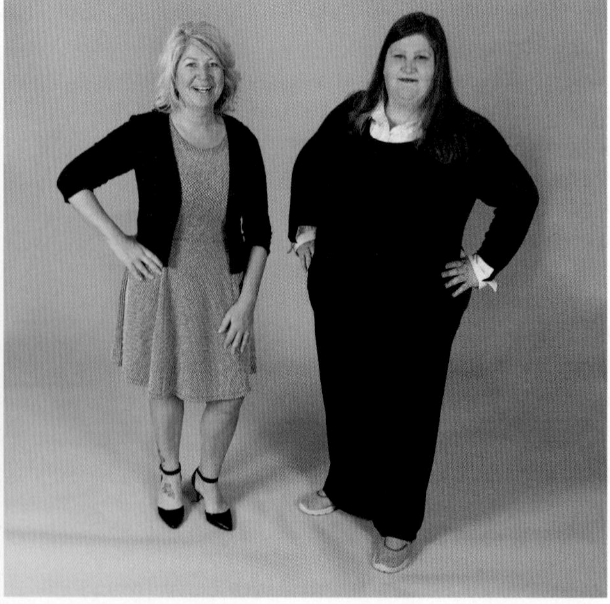

FIG. 3.2 Examples of business dress.

PROFICIENCY EXERCISE 3.6

Develop a set of questions you might use to interview a massage therapist if you were going to hire them to work in your business. Pair up with a classmate and take turns practicing being the interviewer and the interviewee. Repeat the activity but role-play an interview with a potential employer. Repeat again, but this time pretend that a potential client is asking questions to a massage therapist to decide whether or not to book a massage session.

- Use little makeup and apply conservatively.
- Facial hair needs to be neat and trimmed.
- Wear a well-groomed conservative hairstyle.
- Make sure your fingernails are clean, trimmed, with no nail polish.
- Wear no cologne, perfume, or essential oils.
- Make sure you have well-brushed teeth and fresh breath.
- Do not have gum, candy, or other objects in your mouth.
- Wear minimal jewelry.
- Make sure you do not have any body odor.
- If you will be performing a massage as part of the interview, bring an appropriate uniform to the interview and change before giving the massage.

Interview Questions

When the interviewer asks questions, make eye contact when you answer and be confident (Proficiency Exercise 3.6). The following are just a few questions that could be asked during the interview. You need to prepare and rehearse responses to these types of questions in advance:

- What do you consider your greatest strengths and weaknesses?
- Describe a time when you were faced with problems or stresses at work that tested your coping skills. What did you do?
- How do you deal with competition?
- What would you consider an ideal work environment?
- What are your long-range career objectives, and what steps have you taken toward realizing them?
- How well do you work with people? Do you prefer working alone or as part of a team?
- What do you think are the qualities of an effective leader?
- What do you do when people disagree with you? How do you manage conflict?
- In which of your massage skills are you most confident?
- Do you have or anticipate obtaining additional training in massage, and what are you interested in?
- Is there a specific type of client you want to work with?
- What type of massage do you enjoy?
- Do you want to work full time or part time, and what do these designations mean to you?
- What can you offer to the company to improve services?

Questions to Ask the Employer

You need to prepare questions to ask your potential employer about the position and the company in order to be sure this is the right job for you. Your opportunity to ask questions usually comes at the end of the interview. The initial interview is not the best time to discuss and negotiate wages. Wait until the next step of the interview process.

Possible questions include the following:

1. Can you tell me more about the day-to-day responsibilities other than massage therapy?
2. What do you think are the most important qualities in successful massage therapists you have employed?
3. What are the strengths and weakness of the current massage therapy and support staff?
4. What are the goals for this business over the next 5 years?
5. What do you think the current massage therapists like best about working for this company?
6. What is the typical career path for someone in this role?
7. What are the next steps in the interview process?

Remember: Don't ask about salary or benefits just yet. Wait until you are in the final steps of the interview process to negotiate the actual employment contract.

Closing the Interview

You should have an idea of what you will say when leaving the interview. Make sure you state the skills you have that would make this job a definite fit for you and the reasons your strengths make you right for the position. You may want to ask the interviewer if you could send some references or set up an appointment to give the person a massage. Respectfully asking when the decision will be made reinforces your desire for the position. Verifying how you should contact the employer to follow up (phone or email) shows that you are considerate and polite. Finally, make a parting comment, such as "Thank you for taking the time to speak with me about the massage therapy position. I look forward to speaking with you again soon." After the interview, send a thank-you note for the interview opportunity and again express your interest in the position. A handwritten note is the most professional way to thank the employer, but if time is an issue (e.g., the decision will be made quickly), an email may be more appropriate.

It is common to get nervous during an interview. Rehearsals help. Have classmates, instructors, and friends conduct practice interviews. Reverse roles and play the role of interviewer. Go to as many interviews as possible. Even if you do not get the position, the experience is valuable.

Negotiating the Terms of Employment

A contract of employment is an agreement between an employer and employee and is the basis of the employment relationship. Most employment contracts do not need to be in writing to be legally valid, but it is better if they are. Starting work proves that you accept the terms and conditions offered by the employer. Employee handbooks are often included in employment agreements. Unless the text of an employee handbook clearly indicates otherwise, an employee handbook can be considered a legally binding document between an employer and its employees. There are many laws requiring employers to notify employees of certain workplace rights, but there are actually no federal or state laws specifically requiring an employer to have an employee handbook, and plenty of employers choose not to have one.

Many states are considered "at will." At-will employment means that both the employee and the employer can end the employment relationship at any time, for almost any reason.

You should be provided with the following information:

- Title and job description
- Compensation
- Terms of employment
- Employee responsibilities
- Employee benefits
- Employment absence
- Dispute resolution
- Nondisclosure agreements
- Noncompete agreements
- Grounds for termination

You can negotiate with the employer to discuss the terms of employment. Before completing the final employment agreement, make sure to investigate common terms in your area for employment, including wages and other forms of compensation paid to massage therapists. When the employee and employer have agreed on the pay rate, the pay rate should be put in writing and signed by both parties.

Understanding Wages and Payroll

There is a difference between entry-level compensation and pay rates for those with experience. It is also important to understand how much an employer can really afford to pay.

Employee Income and Wage Calculations

According to the US Bureau of Labor Statistics, annual wage for massage therapists was $49,860 per year (September 2023). The median wage is the wage at which half the workers in an occupation earned more than that amount and half earned less. The lowest 10% earned less than $29,040, and the highest 10% earned more than $90,530.

This is about $22–$25 per hour (not per massage hour) based on a 40-hour workweek. Remember that the employee portion of payroll taxes and income taxes must be paid on this amount.

When practitioners work for an hourly wage, they are usually paid for the time spent at the job location, regardless of whether massage is given. A workweek is a period of 168 hours during seven consecutive 24-hour periods. It may begin on any day of the week and at any hour of the day established by the employer. Generally, for purposes of minimum wage and overtime payment, each workweek stands alone; there can be no averaging of 2 or more workweeks. Employee coverage, compliance with wage payment requirements, and the application of most exemptions are determined on a workweek basis.

In general, "hours worked" includes all time an employee must be on duty, or on the employer's premises, or at any other prescribed place of work, from the beginning of the first principal activity of the workday to the end of the last principal work activity of the workday. Also, employees may be "on call," meaning available to work with limited notice. The Fair Labor Standards Act (FLSA), enacted in 1938, has defined the federal guidelines that govern whether or not you will be paid for on-call hours. The underlying question that determines if you will be compensated is "Does the time you spend on call qualify as "hours worked" when calculating overtime and minimum wage?" When employees make themselves available in the worksite for on-call assignments, employers must pay them for the time they spend there because these on-call hours are spent in restricted conditions where an employee cannot use time for personal purposes. However, when an employee is on call at home, time is spent in "non-restricted conditions," where the employee is free to use the time however they wish. The employer can require certain things of at-home on-call employees; for instance, that they are accessible by phone or pager and that they refrain from drinking alcohol while working. Nevertheless this time does not qualify as "hours worked" and will not be compensated. Once you arrive at your job site and begin working, you are entitled to be paid for your time.

Gross Pay and Net Pay

Gross pay for an employee is the amount used to calculate the employee's wages. It is the total amount the employer owes the employee for work during one pay period. Gross pay includes regular hourly and per piece compensation and any overtime paid to the employee during the pay period. A pay period is 7 consecutive days, and it can be paid weekly, biweekly, or monthly.

Hourly gross pay is calculated by multiplying the number of hours worked in the pay period by the hourly pay rate. Overtime pay is also included in the gross pay calculation. An employee signs in and out of work using some sort of electronic or paper record. Regular pay is calculated by multiplying the total hours worked in the pay period by the employee's hourly pay rate. Employee overtime hours (any hours over 40 in the pay period) are calculated at 1.5 times the pay rate. If a piece rate is used in addition to an hourly rate, it is calculated and added to the gross pay. Gratuities are entered in different places on the employee's annual W-2 form, and they are not included in gross pay. The W-2 form is the form that an employer must send to an employee and the IRS at the end of the year. The W-2 form reports an employee's annual wages and the amount of taxes withheld from their paycheck. Each pay period, the employer provides a paycheck or, more commonly, an electronic direct deposit to the employee's bank account. A pay stub is the part of a paycheck that lists details about the employee's pay including taxes and other deductions taken out of an employee's earnings. The pay stub can be electronic or paper. Information provided includes the following elements:

- Total gross: The money you made.
- Total net: The amount, after all taxes and deductions, that you will actually take home.
- Hours worked: If you are an hourly employee, this will be the exact number of hours you have worked.
- Total deductions: All of the money taken out for insurance, taxes, and more.

The amount on an employee's W-2 form (annual wage and tax report) is different from gross pay. The amount on line 1 of the W-2 is "wages, tips, other compensation" and includes all compensation including tips and taxable employee benefits. Again, the "gross" amount refers to the pay an employee would receive before withholdings are made for such things as taxes, contributions, and savings plans. An hourly employee's hours per week vary based on the weekly schedule. Employees must be paid, at the least, the minimum wage. This wage varies from state to state. Employers must pay their hourly employees either the state or federal minimum wage, whichever is higher. Hourly employees are paid for the number of hours they work per week up to 40 hours at a determined rate. Per federal law, hourly workers are entitled to overtime pay for hours worked over 40 hours per workweek.

Employer Payroll Burden Relative to Percentage of Gross Business Income

In a health service business like massage therapy, wages are the biggest expense. In a dedicated massage therapy business, where all income is produced by massage fees, not only are the massage therapists paid wages but so are members of the support staff such as receptionists, maintenance staff, and office staff. Also, payroll expenses for an employer are more than simply the wages. Employers must follow labor laws related to wages. The minimal legal burdens for an employer related to payroll are Social Security tax, Medicare tax, federal unemployment tax, and state unemployment tax. The absolute most a business can have in wage expenses and maintain business stability is 40% of gross business income. Remember, the employer has to pay other business expenses as well, such as rent, utilities, supplies, advertising, and more. These costs can easily be 50% of gross business income, leaving a 10% profit margin. In this situation, the business is in financial stress. A more financially secure situation is for wage expenses to be 35% of gross business income with 25% going to massage therapy wages and 10% to support staff wages. Overhead costs should be maintained at 40%. This leaves a 25% profit, of which half should be saved as a buffer fund for unexpected expenses and the other half going to the business owner income.

If you work for a business, you want it to be strong and profitable. If the fee for a massage session is $70, the most the employer can allocate for wages is $28 for that service, and a portion of that would need to cover support staff and payroll taxes. With this in mind, if you are offered $22–$25 per massage hour, you can better understand the economics from the employer's perspective.

Many massage therapy business owners push wage expenses to 50% of gross business income to offer higher wages. The owner ends up with a lower profit and may not be maintaining a sufficient buffer account in case of unexpected expenses. It is likely that a potential employer is a small business owner working very hard and makes no more than the massage therapist. Realize that massage franchises are also individually owned and operated.

Hiring Process

Once you are hired there is information the employer must have, and you will need to fill out forms and provide information. Mandated information for an employee includes the following:

- The employee must prove that they are eligible to work in the United States, as verified by completing Form I-9, Employment Eligibility Verification.
- The employer is required to get each employee's name and Social Security number (SSN) and to enter them on Form W-2.
- The employer needs to know how much income tax to withhold from employees' wages. Form W-4, Employee's Withholding Allowance Certificate indicates the amount of income tax withholding.

Raises

Pay increments may be discussed when you begin work, and you may find that raises are given after 6 months or 1 year of successful employment. To avoid any misunderstanding, determine how and when these raises can be obtained before accepting the job. Few employers would consider performing extensive treatment with clients before informing them of the anticipated fees. Similarly, you should not be working unless you are aware of your potential earning capacity and anticipated promotions. It is wise to obtain written verification of employment conditions and responsibilities and a wage scale before beginning work. However, if pay increments have not been discussed and you have completed a year of employment, you might wonder when and how the subject can be raised (Box 3.9).

Before approaching the employer about a raise, you should do a self-evaluation to determine that you are justified in making such a request. A wage increase conference should be a two-way discussion that allows you to identify your assets for the job and explain your performance success and that allows the employer to relate the performance to a monetary amount that will reward your performance and inspire increased productivity.

If you have given serious thought to the factors mentioned in Box 3.9, and you feel you deserve a raise, how do you approach the employer? Select an opportunity when the work schedule allows enough time for a discussion of the subject. Do not wait until the end of the day, when the employer is tired and ready to leave the office. It also is not wise to start the day by asking for a raise, especially if the schedule is rather heavy.

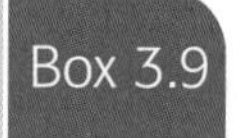

Questions to Consider Before Asking for a Raise

- Have I performed my duties well enough to deserve a raise?
- Have I improved or advanced my skills since beginning the job?
- Have I been cooperative with other members of the team?
- Have I continued to maintain good client management skills?
- Can I verify that my attendance and punctuality have been above average?
- Have I continually maintained professional ethics, safe practice, and quality standards?
- Can I verify that the practice's productivity has increased because of my performance?
- Do economic factors in the practice and in the economy support a raise?

Now apply these same criteria to the rationale for raising fees for massage services if self-employed.

Let the employer know why you believe you deserve a raise. If the employer asks why you should have one, be prepared to answer. For example, cite the rising cost of living, transportation costs, insurance, increased business production because of your efforts, or compensation for good performance.

Employees often do not assert themselves enough to make the employer aware that a raise should be given. If you become passive and content with a pay rate, naturally you will continue to be paid at this rate; however, if your professional skills are an asset and because of these skills the employer realizes a profit, you should be given a raise. If the employer cannot raise your pay rate, consider the benefits as alternatives to a pay increase.

If you are unsuccessful in getting a raise, it is appropriate to ask for the reasons. Express your appreciation for the employer's understanding and consideration and think about your alternatives. If you receive a raise, be sure to thank the responsible person.

Income matters should be treated confidentially and are not discussed with other staff members. Wage and compensation problems destroy positive attitudes and productivity and should be resolved as quickly as possible.

Employee Benefit Packages

Employee benefits are employee compensation packages that include extras such as medical insurance, retirement savings plans, paid vacation days, and more. Employers offer employee benefits to attract and retain top talent, as well as improve employee productivity and engagement. Benefits are added value to the employee in addition to wages. Remember benefits are a cost to the employer.

The costliest benefit is medical insurance. The cost can be prohibitive for a small business owner. Small business owners are not required to offer health insurance if they have fewer than 50 full-time employees.

There are disadvantages of employer-provided medical insurance. One is that the coverage ends when an employee leaves the job. Another is that the coverage does not necessarily meet individual needs. There are advantages for obtaining and paying for your own medical insurance. Medical insurance using the Health Insurance Marketplace (https://www.healthcare.gov/) is affordable. When you apply for coverage in the Health Insurance Marketplace, you will find out if you qualify for a "premium tax credit" that lowers your premium (the amount you pay each month for your insurance plan). By completing an application through the Marketplace, you can review plans and rates available to you. Assistance signing up for a Marketplace plan is available from navigators, certified application assisters, and licensed health insurance agents who have completed training and registration with the Marketplace. Health insurance agents must also be licensed with DIFS. These individuals cannot charge you for their assistance. Visit https://localhelp.healthcare.gov/ to find assistance in your area.

Unemployment Benefits

As an employee, you may be eligible for state and federal government unemployment benefits. Three situations can occur that may lead to you leaving an employment position. You can leave by your choice, you can be terminated (fired), or you can be laid off. If you leave by choice, it is on your terms, and you should plan in advance. If you are fired, you should have known that your job performance was problematic because employers are required to inform the employee with a series of warnings and interventions. If you are laid off, this is typically the result of some sort of downsizing of the organization, usually due to lack of business. This is a difficult situation for the employee and employer. There are times when no matter how hard someone works and even when they are doing all the correct things to support a productive business, larger issues such as an economic downturn may occur. Be supportive of the employer. If business improves, it is likely that you will be called back to work. There may even be some sort of contribution you can make to increase business, especially if you enjoy the people you work with and believe in the business. When employers have to lay off employees, they usually provide positive letters of recommendation and offer references for employees who get other jobs. If you are an employee who has been laid off through no fault on your part, you are eligible for unemployment.

According to the US Department of Labor, the basic eligibility requirements to qualify for unemployment are as follows:

- Be unemployed through no fault of your own (the law imposes disqualifications for certain types of separations from employment).
- Be physically and mentally able to work full time.
- Be actively seeking work by making reasonable efforts to find employment each week.

According to the US Department of Labor, the general rule is that a person who voluntarily leaves suitable work without good cause attributable to the employer is not eligible for unemployment benefits. For good cause to be attributable to the employer, it must relate to the wages, hours, or working conditions of the job. A change in conditions created by your employer or a breach of your employment agreement that is substantial and adversely affects you may be good cause to quit. If the job itself adversely affects your health or aggravates or worsens a medical condition, it may be good cause to quit.

Regardless of the cause, in most cases, a good cause attributable to the employer may be found only if you took reasonable steps to inform your employer of your dissatisfaction and sought to remedy the problem before you left. If you quit, it is your burden to prove that there was good cause for leaving. When applying for benefits after quitting a job, you will be scheduled to attend a predetermination hearing to establish whether you had good cause for leaving. Your employer will be notified of this hearing and will be invited to attend or to send a written statement.

Resignation

Leaving a job can be an obstacle for some individuals, especially when the job change is from one massage practice to another in the same general locale. When you change jobs, make sure the change is to your advantage. Circumstances over which you have no control may be the reason for a change in jobs. However, a massage therapist who frequently changes jobs with inadequate notification or reason soon gains a poor professional reputation. Whatever the reason for terminating the job, do it ethically:

- Give the reason for leaving the job.
- Give sufficient notice, at least 2 weeks or longer if your job requires an extensive training period for a new massage therapist.
- Write a letter of resignation as a follow-up to your verbal resignation.
- Do not discuss leaving the job with other members of the team until you are ready to inform the employer that you will be leaving. The grapevine is a poor method of transmitting such information.
- If you leave a job where serious conflicts exist, it is best to leave these conflicts where they originated and not carry the feelings to another job. When beginning a new position, you should not make negative comments about a former employer. This is simply good ethics.
- Determine what is ethical for clients who wish to follow you to a different location. Discuss this topic openly with the employer. This may be problematic if you signed a non-compete agreement, meaning you have agreed to avoid providing massage services within a certain distance for a specified time. It is to your advantage to avoid signing a non-compete agreement; however, the employer may require one, as it protects the interest of the business.

Being Terminated/Fired or Laid-Off

There must be a reason for being fired. It is important to evaluate what happened that caused the employee-employer relationship to fail. Be honest with yourself. What did you do or not do that created the problem? Learn from the experience and be determined to not make the same mistakes again. According to the US Department of Labor, if you are fired or suspended, you may be disqualified for benefits if the employer can prove one of the following:

- Willful misconduct in the course of your employment. The term *willful misconduct* means deliberate misconduct in willful disregard of the employer's interest or a single knowing violation of a reasonable and uniformly enforced rule or policy of the employer, when reasonably applied, provided such violation is not a result of the employee's incompetence. In the case of absence from work, an employee must be absent without notice or good cause on three separate instances within a 12-month period.
- Illegal activity during the course of your employment including conduct that is a felony under the law or larceny (stealing) of property or service that is valued at more than $25 in the course of your employment.

If you are fired, it is the employer's burden to prove that there was willful misconduct. When applying for unemployment benefits after being discharged or suspended from a job, you will be scheduled to attend a predetermination hearing to determine eligibility. Your employer will be notified of this hearing and will be invited to attend or to send in a written statement.

At-Will Employment

In many employment situations, the law generally considers the employment relationship to be terminated at the will of either party. Recall that in at-will employment, either the company or the employee can terminate the employment relationship at any time, with or without cause, with or without notice. This does not mean that employers can arbitrarily fire employees without good faith communication, fairness, and nondiscriminatory practices. Generally, states allow at-will employees terminated through no fault of their own to qualify for unemployment benefits. Individual circumstances are unique and would need to be addressed by appropriate agencies.

The Work Environment

Each staff member and all business owners and managers make up a team that is working together for success. An unpleasant work environment is often why employees are dissatisfied and why businesses fail. It takes committed employees and employers working together to create a productive and nurturing work environment (Box 3.10).

Typically, in the massage therapy world, business owners function just as they do in any small business. The owner is also the day-to-day manager. If the owner is not also the manager of the business, a business manager may be hired to run the day-to-day operations. Often managers are also required to actually do some of the activities related to business operations. Managers are busy and involved in multitasking. Business managers in a small company report directly to the owner. The manager is in the middle with the owner on one side and employees on the other. The owner delegates authority to the manager to make decisions and act related to the business, but the manager typically has limits on independent action without approval from the business owner. Business managers often hire and manage employees, putting them in the position of employer. When this is the case, the characteristics of a great employer apply to the manager. It is common for managers to feel as if they are pulled in multiple directions and multitasking, especially if the manager has front desk responsibilities as well. Although not desirable or productive, it is common for managers to be frazzled. An employee should respect the managers and work out conflicts with them. However, if the manager is unresponsive or performing poorly, the employee can communicate directly with the owner of the business.

Following are characteristic traits of great employees and employers. When there is a commitment to teamwork and cultivating these behaviors, the work environment will be a positive and productive place to have a massage therapy career.

Characteristics of a Great Employee

The assumption is that you are committed to evolving as an excellent massage therapist. As a new graduate, you need to practice and practice more. You also need to be a committed lifelong learner. The following characteristics and behaviors are related to your professional behavior as an employee. Valued employees do the following:

- Have a strong work ethic
- Set and achieve workplace goals

Box 3.10 Chain Versus Franchise

On the surface, chains and franchises can seem the same, but they are different forms of business ownership/operation. These two business models are often confused in the massage therapy community.

Chain

A chain store is one of several locations that share a brand, central management, and standardized business practices and sell the same merchandise. A chain business model is often used in a local area for restaurants and in a regional area for retail and grocery stores. There are a variety of chain stores from big-box retailers to specialty shops to supermarkets to restaurant chains. Examples of well-known chain stores include Walmart, Target, Home Depot, and Kroger. Chains do not function as local small businesses. Each location in the chain does not have a different owner. Instead, each is owned by the corporate office and has a manager. It is the chain model that can undermine local businesses. Although there may be some spas and wellness centers that function as a small regional chain, the chain business model is rare in massage therapy.

Franchise

Independent owners operate individual stores in a franchised business concept. A franchisee functions as a local small business. Investors may purchase more than one franchise, but many owner/operators typically run just one location. A franchisee buys the right to market and sell certain products and services from a franchisor (the person who sells the franchise) through a legal agreement. Fees and royalties (a share of the income) are then paid to the franchisor over a specific period of time. The franchisee is in charge of operations, finances, and human resources for that specific location. The franchise business model was introduced into the massage community in the early 2000s. The business model was misunderstood then and continues to be misunderstood today. Many speak of massage franchises as if they are all one unified entity. Not true. Franchising is a business model for a small independent business owner. The franchise business model's popularity has to do with its proven track record of success and the relative ease in which people can become franchise business owners. A franchise business provides a detailed, step-by-step business blueprint. There are rules the owner of the franchise must follow to honor the brand, provide similar services for consumer reliability, and support brand marketing. Some rules include the use of approved signage and marketing materials, design of the facility, types of services offered, and products used. Franchisors also provide ongoing business support to their franchisees. Franchising is more like a community of individual business owners working together with a franchisor serving as support and quality oversight. Massage franchises provide career opportunities for practitioners to work as employees.

- Are dependable and on time
- Consistently follow through with workplace tasks
- Have a positive attitude and sense of humor
- Avoid workplace drama and gossip
- Are appropriately assertive without being demanding, overbearing, and abrasive
- Are self-motivated and work effectively with little direction
- Are team oriented and support collaboration
- Are effective communicators who understand the benefits of conciseness and clarity
- Maintain perspective and avoid catastrophizing
- Manage conflict directly and effectively by focusing on issues and not the people.
- Are able to keep from getting upset or offended by the things other people say and do
- Are flexible/able to adapt in a meaningful way
- Are open to feedback without defensiveness
- Support and help implement positive change
- Are problem solvers
- Help others
- Are kind
- Do what is needed without having to be told; function beyond the job description
- Understand that they succeed when the business and everyone involved is successful (Box 3.11)

Characteristics of a Great Employer

If you are committed to being an excellent employee, then you deserve to work for an excellent employer. Remember that employers are human beings just like you. They can have great days, good days, and bad days. The employer is taking the majority of the business risks and has multiple responsibilities that you may not realize. The employer may or may not be a massage therapist. They may need to learn more about massage therapy or may have never given a massage and don't understand what it is like to be a massage therapist. The employer is managing multiple aspects of the business and has a broader understanding of the entire business process. You will want your employers to be excellent business professionals because creating an excellent and successful business is their primary role. Your goal as a massage therapist is to become an excellent massage practitioner and an excellent employee. This is different and more contained than the employer. Avoid a narrow perspective. Imagine yourself in the owner's position as you consider how effective they are. There are qualities to consider when evaluating the employment position. These same qualities can be used to evaluate and provide feedback to your employer as your career progresses. Feedback is necessary for you to grow as a massage therapist and for the business to be successful. Broaden your perspective when providing feedback to the employer, owner, or manager. If you have a concern, spend time clarifying the issue and offer viable suggestions to solve the problem. Do not just complain. Do not complain behind the employer's back. Do not complain to co-workers. If you have an issue, go to the employer. You can expect your employer to do the following:

- Be open to feedback that is professionally provided
- Listen attentively to you
- Investigate your concerns
- Consider your suggestions and be open to ideas
- Provide ongoing updates about the business status

Box 3.11 Employee Dos and Don'ts

Dos
- Do get to work on time.
- Do look and act like a professional.
- Do be consistent and accurate with the recording and documentation requirements of the business.
- Do be courteous and supportive.
- Do be professionally assertive and communicate openly with your employer.
- Do develop a sense of commitment and loyalty to your employer.
- Do take your responsibilities seriously.
- Do improve your skills.
- Do own your mistakes and correct them.
- Do be willing to extend yourself in the short term for everyone's long-term gain.
- Do be a team player.
- Do be flexible and creative.
- Do use problem-solving skills to resolve potential conflict.
- Do commit to the job.
- Do use correct grammar, pronounce words correctly, and expand your vocabulary.
- Do explain technical terms in understandable language without being demeaning.
- Do make clients feel important; discuss issues of interest to them.
- Do perform proper introductions of the clients and staff members.
- Do introduce yourself to a new client and extend a warm welcome.
- Do say "Thank you" when a client is helpful, has cooperated during treatment, or has complimented you.
- Do send thank-you notes for referrals or other thoughtful acts.
- Do respect the client's privacy.

Don'ts
- Don't gossip.
- Don't complain without providing a viable solution.
- Don't be dishonest.
- Don't behave unethically.
- Don't behave irresponsibly.
- Don't show up to work late.
- Don't call in at the last minute to say that you are unable to work.
- Don't leave cleaning and other responsibilities undone.
- Don't eat or drink in front of clients.
- Don't talk with your mouth full.
- Don't use slang or vulgar language.
- Don't speak too loudly.
- Don't answer the phone too casually in a business setting.

- Clearly communicate expectations and rules, and enforce fairly
- Maintain flexibility and adapt when possible
- Have a sense of humor
- Respect your work-life balance needs
- Create a team-based environment, and willingly help with business tasks if needed
- Create and maintain a great employee experience, including the provision of up-to-date and ergonomically supportive treatment rooms, equipment and needed supplies, and a healthy work environment
- Effectively manage workplace conflict and deal efficiently with non-productive staff behavior.
- Continually support business success and plan for the future

If your employer is performing well in these areas, tell them. Employers need feedback, support, and confirmation just as much as you do. If improvement is needed, communicate directly with the employer. Describe the issue in writing and explain concisely what is occurring and why it is a problem. Consider all aspects of the issue and seek a beneficial solution. Sometimes there isn't one. Doing your best under the circumstances is required.

EXAMPLE

- The workplace is noisy because of new construction in an adjacent office. This falls under the category "Creates and maintains a great employee experience, including the provision of up-to-date and ergonomically supportive treatment rooms, equipment and needed supplies, and a healthy work environment." However, in this situation there is nothing the employer can do.
- An employee is thought to be stealing from other employees. You want the person to be let go immediately. This falls under the category "Effectively manages workplace conflict and deals efficiently with nonproductive staff behavior." The employer cannot just fire someone without cause, even in an at-will employment state. The information described is hearsay and there is no evidence. If stealing is occurring, the employer could call the police to investigate, but this is not the solution you offered.

Do not hesitate to communicate with your employer. Be respectful, relevant, focused, accurate, and willing to listen to all sides of the situation. If the employer is performing poorly in multiple areas and not working toward improvement, then it may be time to leave and seek a more fitting work environment. You do not need to be angry, create a scene, convince others to leave with you, or post anything on social media. Just leave and move on (Box 3.12) (Proficiency Exercise 3.7).

SELF-EMPLOYED-SPECIFIC FOCUS

SECTION OBJECTIVES

Chapter objectives covered in this section:

22. List the elements of business development when self-employed.
23. Develop a business plan.
24. Design a marketing strategy and advertising materials for a massage business.
25. Develop a business management, accounting, and record-keeping system.
26. Describe the process for setting fees, determining income, and doing insurance billing.

Using the information presented in this section, the student will be able to perform the following:

- Develop an effective business name.

- Determine average start-up costs, overhead expenses, and yearly income.
- Develop a word-of-mouth and a multimedia marketing plan.
- Develop an informational brochure, business card, and media story.
- Negotiate lease agreements.
- Define business finances.
- List accounting steps.
- Create a plan for a business start-up.
- Use a step-by-step procedure to set up business management practices.
- Design a fee structure for therapeutic massage services.
- Determine criteria for massage fees in a particular geographical area.
- Explain the process of insurance reimbursement.

Regardless of the career path you follow (self-employed or employee), to be successful you must understand the fundamentals of the business structure. The foundation of a successful business is planning and implementation. Just as massage therapy is based on a few key underlying principles, so is business. This all begins with a business plan. Writing a business plan teaches you about the detail required to finance, own, operate, and succeed in business. Even if you plan to work for a business owner, developing a business plan for a "pretend" business prepares you to be a better employee, because you will understand the commitment and responsibilities required of your employer.

An excellent resource for business topics is the Small Business Association (SBA), an independent agency of the US government with the mission of helping Americans start, build, and grow their own businesses. Make sure to use the extensive resources this organization offers.

Box 3.12

What Employers Dislike About Employees

- Being late to work or taking extended breaks
- Being unprepared
- Being a know-it-all or being overly aggressive
- Whining and complaining
- Causing drama
- Calling in sick when you are not really sick/contagious
- Coming to work when you are really sick and contagious
- Saying, "Not my job"
- Using your electronic devices when other tasks need to be done
- Not following the rules and acting entitled (believing oneself to be inherently deserving of privileges or special treatment)

What Employees Dislike About Employers

- Practicing favoritism
- Micromanaging
- Not understanding massage therapy
- Treating staff disrespectfully
- Behaving in ways that are unreasonable, selfish, manipulative, and bullying
- Engaging in public correction and blaming
- Refusing to talk to people on the phone/in person
- Not being present in the business
- Not helping or pitching in when busy
- Breaking the rules employees are expected to follow
- Acting entitled

PROFICIENCY EXERCISE 3.7

Using the Characteristics of a Great Employee list, evaluate yourself as an employee based on past employment experiences. Then evaluate an employer you recently had against the Characteristics of Great Employer list.

The Business Plan

A business plan generally consists of the following elements:

- Executive summary: This is the most important part of the business plan and should be devised last, once the other parts are well into development or are complete. The material from those parts helps create an executive summary that includes a mission statement, possible locations, services, market summary, number of employees, and so on. (In your case, the point of the executive summary is to demonstrate concisely the focus of your proposed massage business, your expertise, and your competitive edge in the market.)
- Market analysis: This section includes a description of the industry (in your case, therapeutic massage), a survey of the competition, and a description of the target market.
- Company overview: This section covers the way the different parts of the proposed business will work together and gives the reasons this is a recipe for success.
- Description of management and organization of staff: Whom the owner plans to hire and who will be in charge of certain duties.
- Ownership information: This part of the business plan reviews subjects such as the owners' names, percentage of ownership, and owner influence.
- Business structure: Sole proprietorship (DBA), LLC (limited liability company/corporation).
- Funding requests: This section explains how much money will be needed for start-up or expansion costs and the proposed uses of borrowed funds.
- Financials: This section covers the financial history of the enterprise (if applicable), in addition to short- and long-term goals and forecasts.

A resource partner with the SBA, Service Corps of Retired Executives (SCORE), is also a valuable business resource. Working and retired executives and business owners donate time and expertise as business counselors providing free advice. These mentors enjoy sharing their knowledge and want to see other entrepreneurs succeed. Both in-person and online counseling are available. Owners of start-up businesses can talk to a SCORE mentor as much as they need or want; no limit has been placed on any of SCORE's services. In fact, many may find long-term mentoring to be a great help.

The format for developing a business plan is evolving just like with résumés and cover letters. Business plan samples are easily found on the internet. Just as recommended for résumé development, gather the data, download a sample business plan template from the Web, develop a draft, and then polish the document with the assistance of experts such as SCORE volunteers who want to help.

Business Structure/Entity

Choosing the right type of legal entity for your business is important, as it will determine the rules and regulations you're bound to as well as how your company is taxed. This chapter is structured around the sole proprietorship with guidance for a limited liability corporation.

A sole proprietorship (one owner) is the simplest way to set up a massage therapy business. The other common business entity for massage therapy practice is a limited liability corporation (LLC).

Partnerships, cooperatives, and corporations are complicated business structures, and the need for them should be discussed with an attorney.

Partnership

A partnership is when two or more people operate a business as co-owners to share risk, debt, and income. All co-owners (partners) act on behalf of each other in the business. In a general partnership, all partners share equal rights and responsibilities. Problems in a business partnership are the natural result of differing individual preferences which can lead to disagreements. General partners are 100% liable for the actions of other partners. If one general partner makes a mistake, all general partners are liable for that mistake and any accompanying debt or other obligations that go along with that mistake. For these reasons, the partnership business model is not recommended.

Cooperative

A cooperative is a business or organization owned by and operated for the benefit of those using its services. Profits and earnings generated by the cooperative are distributed among the members. Typically, an elected board of directors run the cooperative while regular members have voting power to control the direction of the cooperative. Members can become part of the cooperative by purchasing shares. This business entity may become more common as wellness centers and interdisciplinary practices emerge.

Corporation

Corporations offer the strongest protection to its owners from personal liability, but the cost to form a corporation is higher than other structures. Corporations have a completely independent life separate from its shareholders. Corporations also require more extensive record-keeping, operational processes, and reporting. Corporation types include:

- C corporations involve one or more people. Owners are not personally liable.
- S corporations involve one or more people, but no more than 100, and all must be US citizens.
- B corporations involve one or more people. Owners are not personally liable.
- Nonprofit corporations involve one or more people. Owners are not personally liable. This entity is tax-exempt, but corporate profits can't be distributed. Nonprofits are often called 501(c)(3) corporations.

Sole Proprietorship

A sole proprietorship is the most basic type of business to establish. Sole proprietorships are easy to form, and they provide complete control of your business with no distinction between the business and the owner. You are entitled to all profits and are responsible for all the business's debts, losses, and liabilities. There are several benefits to choosing a sole proprietorship business structure. It is inexpensive to start, and there are minimal fees associated with registering a sole proprietorship. If you're a sole proprietorship you'll need to file a DBA if you want your company to operate under a name that's not your full, legal name. DBA stands for "doing business as," also referred to as your business's assumed trade or fictitious name. DBA requirements vary by state, county, city, and business structure. In general, registering a DBA comes with paperwork and filing fees anywhere from \$10–\$100. You'll either go to your county clerk's office to file your paperwork or you'll do so with your state government. The DBA sole practitioner is an efficient option when there are no employees.

Limited Liability Company

A limited liability company, or LLC, is a legal entity used to own, operate, and protect a business. LLCs provide the same legal and financial protections of corporations but can be simpler to operate. When you form an LLC, you gain the exclusive right to use your name as a business entity name in your state, and you also create a public record of your use of the name. Setting up an LLC may cost a few hundred dollars. Many states require LLCs to file annual reports and pay annual fees and taxes that can vary between \$10 and \$800 or more.

A corporate veil is when a business is incorporated so that its owners, shareholders, and employees will not be held personally responsible if the business can't pay its debts. The main reason for an LLC is to avoid personal liability. However, personal liability is still a possibility such as when a member acts fraudulently, illegally, or recklessly and such action(s) harms the business or someone else.

Business Name

Careful consideration is needed to create a business name that clearly and concisely reflects the intention of the business.

When deciding on a name for your business, you should do the following:

- Create a name that appeals to you but also to the client target you are trying to attract.
- Create a comforting or familiar name with pleasant memories so that clients respond to the business on an emotional level.
- Create a short, descriptive, concise name that is easy to pronounce and easy to remember.
- Imagine how the name would look on business cards, on a website, and in advertisements.
- Determine whether a logo can be designed that reflects the intention of the name.

On the other hand, when creating a business name you should avoid:

- Embarrassing misspellings, abbreviations, and potentially offensive undertones.
- Implied associations with organizations or people with whom the business is not connected.

Start-Up Costs

Start-up costs are the initial expenses required to begin a business. In addition to the start-up costs amount, you should have a minimum cash reserve equal to the amount of money needed to cover basic business and personal living expenses for 6 months to 1 year. Many people begin a business without these cash reserves and do fine. Others give up the business venture because they do not have enough money to pay bills. This situation forces them to find other jobs. Keeping a cash reserve allows you to focus on developing your business with less financial worry (Proficiency Exercise 3.8).

Starting small, with the bare essentials, keeps start-up costs under $5000.

- A basic portable table should not cost more than $500. Plan on investing in an electric lift massage table as soon as possible.
- Business cards and a simple brochure are needed, as are client-practitioner statements, policy and procedure booklets, receipt books, and client information forms. You will want practice management software that will run on a mobile devise or tablet and sync to your business computer. The total cost for these is about $500.
- A computer, smart phone and data plan, and internet cost about $1000.
- Membership in one of the professional organizations also provides liability insurance; the membership and insurance usually cost less than $300.
- Linens and supplies should cost about $300.
- Opening a bank account, plus miscellaneous expenses, takes about $500.
- An expenditure of $1000 for website and initial advertising is reasonable.
- Renting a small office can push up the start-up costs to about $7000–$10,000. This includes the expenses detailed previously plus office costs, such as rent (about $1000, because renting office space often requires payment of the first and last months' rent up front), office furniture, and utility hook-ups (another $1000). Developing a home office will also have similar initial start-up costs.

Massage Business Location

There are many places where you can provide massage services. You can go to client's location, work from home, rent a small office, or rent space in an existing business. All have advantages and disadvantages, and it is important to carefully consider what works best for the business you want to create. Your business location needs to reflect the personality of your business intention. For example, if your business intention is to offer a quiet, serene space, then a location in a gym or near a fire station may not be the best idea. Carefully locate your business where people in your target market can find you. If you want to target people who are retired, then locate the business near where this population lives. Take advantage of the visibility offered by having your massage office near a restaurant or shopping area. If you want to develop a pain management massage practice, locate near medical facilities. Consider street visibility and signage. People need to be able to see your business location. Make sure there is convenient parking available. If you locate your business where there is limited foot traffic and visibility, you need additional marketing plans to let your target market know where you are located. This is especially true of a mobile on-site practice and a home office practice.

PROFICIENCY EXERCISE 3.8

1. Talk with a couple of self-employed massage practitioners and ask them what it cost to start their massage businesses.
2. Use professional massage publications and other resources to complete a sample start-up costs worksheet.

Renting Space

Many massage therapists rent space for the business. The main options are a private office, space in an existing business, or shared space. Rental fees vary, depending on the business location and the area of the country. The person/business you rent from is the property owner (landlord). The person renting the property is called a tenant. The agreement between a property owner and a tenant is called a lease or rental agreement.

You can also sublease space. A sublease is a lease or rental agreement between a tenant who already holds a lease to a commercial space or property and another party—called the sublessee or subtenant—who wants to use part of that space. A sublessee pays rent to the original tenant, who is commonly called the sublessor. The property owner must approve of the sublease (Focus on Professionalism 3.2).

A property can have regulations related to the workspace, such as access times, type of signage, use of common and exclusive areas, and suitability of the facility for specific types of professional practice. Property owners must follow all zoning and health and safety regulations. A property owner must give notice to the tenant and receive permission from the tenant before entering exclusive areas of a rented premises. This rule does not apply if there is a bona fide emergency, such as a fire or some other danger to the premises.

If you rent traditional office space, it is likely that you are working directly with the property owner or their manage-

FOCUS ON PROFESSIONALISM 3.2

Subleasing space to a massage therapist is how some businesses are responding to the misclassification issue of employees versus independent contractors. Be perfectly clear when subletting a space that you are a sole practitioner, self-employed, and the person/business you are renting from has absolutely no control over how you conduct business so long there are no legal or zoning violations. You pay a predetermined rental fee for the space by the hour, day, week, or month. You collect your own fees. The only control the sublessor has is related to the facility, such as music volume, use of scents that permeate outside of the space, fire safety, and so on. You do not pay a percentage of each service as rent. This type of arrangement is considered a fee-splitting, percentage-based, revenue-sharing arrangement between a clinic and its health care practitioners and may violate Stark, antikickback, and fee-splitting laws.

ment company. A traditional office has only exclusive space, not shared space. A main building, with multiple offices, may have common areas such as a parking lot and a central lobby.

If you rent a space that is part of another office/business facility, it is likely you are subleasing. For your protection make sure the property owner allows subleasing prior to signing any sort of agreement.

It is becoming common for massage therapists to sublease a massage room in a larger facility. The facility and business types that sublet to massage therapists are wellness centers, chiropractors, spas and salons, and individually owned massage centers (not franchises). You can sublet a room for exclusive use or shared space by the hour, day, or week. If renting exclusive space, it is likely you will bring all supplies and equipment and permanently set up in the rental room. If renting shared space by the hour or day, the main equipment (e.g., massage tables) may be included as part of what is called furnished space, but you will bring all linens and supplies.

The information must be presented as a written legal agreement, or contract. Massage professionals should never rely on oral or handshake contracts. They should always have all business agreements in writing (Box 3.13).

Marketing and Advertising

Marketing encompasses the advertising and other promotional activities required to sell a product or service. Advertising is a must when starting a new business, and many forms of advertising are very costly. For massage, some types of advertising work better than others. When you develop any written material or advertising, make sure you provide potential clients with the answers to these basic questions:

- Who? (You)
- What? (Therapeutic massage)
- Where? (Address and phone number)
- When? (Appointment times)
- How? (They can reach you by phone, text, email, or web page)

Fig. 3.3 describes internal and external marketing procedures.

The Target Market

In developing a business, it is important to know the market. Many opportunities are open for the massage business, ranging from the service approaches of stress reduction massage to

Box 3.13 Rental Samples

Office Space Rental (Not Sublease)

In this type of rental space is exclusive. For a sole proprietor with no employees or with only a receptionist, 300–400 square feet will be adequate. An office space should not be less than 200 square feet with designated restrooms. There are two basic types of leases: a full-service lease and a net lease.

A full-service lease requires the property owner to be responsible for paying the expenses associated with the property, including property taxes and insurance, repairs and maintenance, and utilities. This is the most common commercial lease and the best type of lease for the tenant.

A net lease is a lease agreement in which the property owner charges a lower annual rent as compared to a full-service lease but can include monthly "usual costs" such as property taxes, property insurance, and common area maintenance (CAM) fees.

Commercial office leases typically range from 1–5 years. Monthly rent can range from $500 to more than $2000 per month.

Exclusive Use Sublease

In this type of rental, the actual massage space is not shared even though it is located in a shared facility. You are able to personalize the area and leave equipment and supplies in the rental space. You can lock the door. You will set up space with your own equipment such as a massage table, office furniture such as a desk and chairs, and a storage cabinet. Ideally the space with have an exclusive restroom. More commonly, restroom access is part of the common area. Make sure the space is large enough, at minimum 120 square feet; 140–160 square feet is recommended. Avoid dimensions where width or length is less than 10 feet; 12-foot room dimensions are better.

A suggested formula for figuring a fair monthly rent involves calculating the percentage of the total square footage of the sublet space related to the total space of the facility.

Example

The room you want to rent is 12 × 12 feet, or 144 square feet. You are renting exclusive space with shared common areas to include a restroom and waiting area. The business occupies 2000 square feet. The 12 × 12 room is about 7% of the total available space. The owner pays $2800 per month for rent ($14 per square foot); 7% of $2800 is $196. It is common to double the business owner's square footage costs. In this example $196 × 2 = $392 a month with a likely rent of $400 a month. A 1-year lease is common.

NOTE: If the lessor's rent is higher, then it is reasonable to expect that the sublessee's rent will also be proportionally higher.

Shared Space Rental

Example

The room you want to rent is 10 × 12 feet with a hydraulic table, hot towel cabinet and stand, sink, small desk, and two chairs.

Full days currently available: Tuesday, Thursday, Saturday

Half days currently available: Monday (morning), Wednesday (afternoon/evening), Friday (morning/evening)

Facility hours: 8 a.m. to 8 p.m. Monday through Saturday and 9 a.m. to 6 p.m. on Sunday

Rates:

1 day/week = $200/month with 6-month lease

2 days/week = $350/month with 6-month lease

3 days/week = $600/month with 12-month lease

Included in lease agreement: Exclusive locker for on-site storage of linens and supplies, all utilities including wireless, use of the washer/dryer, reception area/waiting room, restrooms, and break room and weekly general cleaning

Day rate (not available on Sunday):

$45 for half day: 9 a.m. to 2 p.m. or 3 p.m. to 8 p.m.

$75 for full day: 9 a.m. to 7 p.m.

Day usage includes furnished massage room, access to wireless, reception/waiting room, restroom, and breakroom. The room is completely vacated each day.

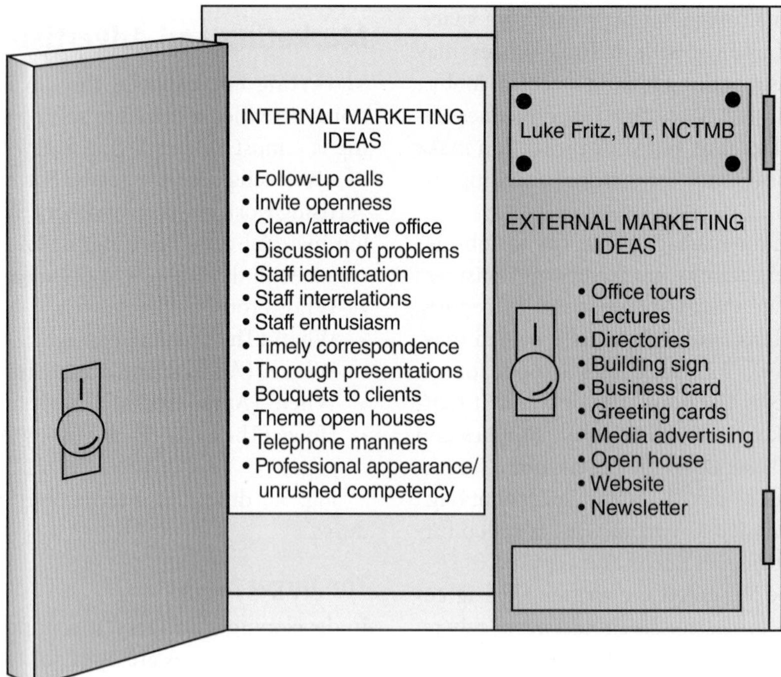

FIG. 3.3 Internal and external marketing procedures. From *Fritz S: Business and professional skills for massage therapists, 2009, Mosby.*

the allied health opportunities of working in clinical settings. There is no typical massage business. Successful massage professionals can be found practicing in many formats. A business could be developed entirely at one location or in three or four locations. A massage therapist may work one day at a local manufacturing business for the employees and the next day may do home (on-site) visits for local business people. The third day could be spent teaching a self-help massage class for the local community education program. On the fourth day, the therapist may see clients at a full-service cosmetology establishment in the morning and that evening provide on-site massage for a local support group dealing with stress.

With all the available possibilities, the massage practitioner is wise to narrow the focus on one, two, or three specific markets to keep advertising and promotional activities manageable. Answering the following questions begins the process of narrowing and developing a target market for a therapeutic massage business:

- Where do you plan to work?
- What potential client groups or populations are available within a half-hour drive of the location?
- What type of massage or bodywork do you enjoy giving?
- What group or type of people do you want to help most?
- How are you going to reach those potential clients?
- When do you want to be available to do massage?

By the fifth year of business, the practitioner usually has established a solid focus, a narrow target market, and a consistent clientele.

Word of mouth is the best advertising. Meeting people and talking with them are far more effective than other forms of advertising. Having satisfied clients who tell other potential clients about you is even better. In the beginning, the massage therapist must talk with many people to develop a client base. Building a clientele takes time. It is important not to become discouraged because, if you want to succeed, quitting is not an option.

The massage therapist should persist in handing out business cards and brochures and giving demonstrations until the clients are found. Placing an ad in a local publication or on social media and then sitting in an office waiting for clients to call does not work. Success comes by arranging to speak at service clubs and churches in the area or by volunteering to work at local events. Businesses may want to offer a stress management class. Local school districts often have adult education classes, and short classes that teach simple massage routines are popular. Charitable organizations often have auctions, which are wonderful opportunities to give away gift certificates for massage.

Being visible in the community helps generate business. A regular base clientele of about 100 is sufficient to support a thriving therapeutic massage business. Some clients will have weekly standing appointments, others will have appointments biweekly, and the rest will visit monthly or occasionally. It may be necessary to talk to 2000 people to find 100 clients.

There are two main marketing obstacles for wellness massage:

- Convincing the public that regular massage is beneficial to a lifestyle program that focuses on managing stress and striving for wellness
- Helping would-be clients justify the fees for massage

To overcome these obstacles, it is important to provide education and an experience, such as a complimentary massage, so that potential clients understand the value of massage.

MENTORING TIP

Recommendations for identifying and connecting with target markets

1. Range: How far/long will people (or you, if mobile) travel for massage sessions? The typical range is 30 miles/30 minutes. Map out the 30-minute circle from your home base.
2. Demographics: High/low-income range, age, culture, urban/suburban/rural. For example, using the United States Census Bureau (https://www.census.gov/), an area has a median household income of $65,000. Population growth is minor. Age: 35 years and older. Growing population of 65+, large military veteran population. Expanding hospital and medical complex, and so forth.
3. Target market: A particular group of consumers at which a product or service is aimed. The target market must be relevant to range and demographics. Example for my demographic based target markets include retired population including military veterans, Hospital employees, farmers. Biggest determinate is disposable income which influences fees.
4. "Ideal" client base: a particular group of consumers at which a product or service is aimed: An ideal client is a person who is the best client for you to work with. You will not really find "ideal" clients, but you will find clients who have degrees of your "ideal" client. The client base needs to be compatible with your range, demographics, and target market. The clients need to be willing to follow your business policies. Example: Retention clients that schedule weekly/biweekly/monthly. Self-pay with sufficient income to pay $75–$85 per 60-minute session. Primary outcome goals: well-being and improved quality of life, stress, and pain management. Flexible schedule for weekday and daytime appointments.
5. Marketing: Marketing as a discipline involves all the actions a business undertakes to draw in customers and maintain relationships with them. Marketing occurs within the range, demographics, target market, and determined ideal client base. Example: social media in local groups, participation in local service organizations and chamber of commerce. Networking with local medical centers, chiropractors and physical therapists, membership program, referral program.
6. Providing: The massage therapy service must meet client's expectations put forth in the marketing. The environment must be inviting and comfortable and clean. The perceived value of the session must meet the value exchanged in fees paid. The client's goals are addressed.
7. Sustaining: The business must make sufficient money to pay expenses, taxes and generate personal income. The business needs to meet your personal and professional goals. The business commitment must be resilient to endure the risks, ups and downs, and unexpected events. The business needs to be stable—which usually means retention clients seen over and over and over. Burnout needs to be managed.

There are no short cuts, magic methods, or fancy concepts.

Brochure and Business Card

Even as technology dominates, these paper marketing pieces are important. The content of the brochure and business card are the foundation for a business website.

PROFICIENCY EXERCISE 3.9

1. Locate three professional websites, brochures, and business cards. Evaluate them against the criteria listed in this section.
2. Develop a sample professional brochure and business card for your future business. Share these samples with your classmates and critique each other's work.

Develop a Client-Practitioner Agreement and Policy Statement

In developing a client-practitioner agreement and policy statement, you need to be specific about certain types of information. On a separate piece of paper or on the computer, use the following list to assemble the information a client needs to know. When you are done, you will have a comprehensive outline to use in creating a booklet or website piece. Compare your results with those of your classmates.

1. The types of services offered
2. Descriptions of the services offered
3. The practitioner's qualifications (training and experience)
4. The financial and time investment required of the client
5. The client's role in health care
6. Appointment and cancellation/no-show policies
7. Client and practitioner expectations and informed consent
8. Fees
9. Policy for sexually inappropriate behavior
10. Recourse policy

The brochure is the primary tool for educating the public and potential clients about the services offered. The brochure should provide the following specific information (Proficiency Exercise 3.9):

1. *The nature of the services offered.* The brochure should explain clearly that therapeutic massage is a general health service. It should state that no specific treatment of any kind is given for preexisting physical or mental problems. It also should make clear that all specific problems of a medical, structural, psychological, or dietary nature will be referred to the appropriate licensed professional. The brochure should clearly and prominently state that any sexual overtures, behavior, or requests are considered criminal solicitation, and the police will be called.
2. *A description of the services offered.* The brochure should give a simple explanation of the process of a massage. It should include a full description of the types of services offered and the procedures followed in rendering those services. It should explain that the client will always be properly draped or can choose to remain dressed. It should clearly state that the client may stop the session at any time and may choose not to have any area of the body touched or to have any particular technique used.
3. *The qualifications of the practitioner.* The massage professional's credentials, education, training, and experience should be outlined in a manner that allows potential clients to verify the practitioner's competence. The massage licensing number is included.
4. *The client's financial and time investment.* The brochure must provide a realistic statement of costs and fees. It

should emphasize that the effects of massage are temporary, and that massage is best used as a maintenance system. The brochure should state that the massage practitioner will teach the client self-help practices if requested. It also should make clear that the best results from massage are maintained when treatment is given on a weekly or biweekly basis, and that therapeutic massage, when used only occasionally, provides only temporary effects.
5. *The client's role in health care.* The brochure should address the importance of the client's responsibility for their personal health care. It is important for the client to realize that the massage practitioner is a facilitator in the wellness process.

The business card should be similar to the brochure in design. The card should be simple and direct and include your massage licensing identification number, but it should not list all your credentials. It is convenient to put the information about the next appointment date on the back of the card. Information on the business care should include the following:

- The name of the business and massage therapist's name and license number
- Services offered: only list the basic categories such as therapeutic massage and whether you have obtained additional education in a population specialization (e.g., specializing in pain management)
- Appointment times and locations
- How they can reach you (by phone, text, email, or website)

Developing a Client-Practitioner Agreement and Policy Statement

It is essential to have the client read a client-practitioner agreement and policy statement (see Chapter 2). This is the document in which you set forth the professional rules for the client. People usually do quite well with information presented to them in a clear, concise, upfront way. The potential for conflict increases if the rules are not understood and agreed on or if they are changed too often midstream. The client-practitioner agreement and policy statement will prevent conflicts by clearly stating all policies. This agreement is more comprehensive than the marketing brochure and becomes part of the informed consent process; however, it is not protection against a lawsuit. Its value is that it can do the following:

- Clarify for the client the nature of the service rendered
- Help protect against unwarranted and unrealistic client expectations
- Serve as a constant reinforcement of the scope and limits of the practitioner's practice within acceptable legal parameters
- Serve as a valuable factual tool if required in court action

The agreement or policy statement should be presented in simple, easily understood language. It gives the practitioner an opportunity to define the professional practice. The client-practitioner agreement has little value if it does not accurately describe the type of service offered to the public.

Website

The Web offers significant advantages over traditional advertising media in that it is dynamic, interactive, and relatively inexpensive. It can be used to showcase your specific skills, book appointments, and educate potential and current clients about the benefits of massage. A good website not only entices visitors but also ensures that they keep coming back for repeat visits. Establishing a website is an easy process. You can create your own using services offered by the professional massage organizations or hire a professional website designer. Your website should have some basic features:

- Loads pages quickly
- Clearly identifies you and your business
- Has the best template for your personality and business profile
- Is easy to navigate and read
- Has relevant content that is kept current

Make sure the website provides the name of your business and your professional name, the business's phone number and address, a link for directions and a map to your location, brief descriptions of the types of massage skills you have, and an electronic version of the brochure and client–practitioner agreement and policy statement. Make sure the website's directory is clear and that clients can easily find important information. Some designs support online scheduling, which is recommended.

Website set-up costs and ongoing fees to maintain the website are part of business expenses. Hosting (site location) and domain (name) registration are the main costs. Domain registration costs about \$10, and hosting fees can range from \$10–\$25 per month. Developing a simple site is not difficult, but unless the massage professional is already skilled in website design, they probably would be better off hiring a professional. As noted earlier, it is possible to include appointment scheduling features on the website. Various massage therapy organizations provide support for website development.

Media

Media advertising is a changing environment. With a variety of online sources, the internet is now the main mode of advertising. Local newspapers still exist as well, and they often run stories about new businesses. Many larger papers are now delivering their product over the internet. Media advertising (internet, newspaper, radio, and television) is expensive and not the best idea initially. Remember that massage is a local business. Clients typically will drive only 30 minutes to have a massage. If you are providing an on-site massage service, you may not want to drive long distances. Therefore any media marketing needs to target your local area.

When providing a story to the media, the massage professional should write their own draft article to prevent embarrassing mistakes. Including photographs of the professional giving a massage is a great idea. Providing the journalist who will write the final article with copies of other good news stories about therapeutic massage also is beneficial.

Social Media

Social media are the online platforms and sites that provide a way for people to connect and share content with friends and like-minded people. Using social media to market massage therapy is useful and cost effective. Social networking sites have changed over the years and will continue to change based on technological developments and usage trends such as mobile-based social media. There are a variety of sites such as Facebook, Instagram, and Twitter where massage therapists can market themselves. Facebook is the top social network on the Web. LinkedIn is the social network for career development. Individuals can promote themselves and their businesses, outline their education and work experience, make connections with other professionals, interact in group discussions, post job ads, or apply for jobs on the site.

It is important to maintain professional behavior when using social media to market massage therapy. The lines between personal and business worlds are easily blurred through social media. It is detrimental to your professional development to allow this to occur. Remember that each of us represents the entire massage profession. How you appear and what you post on social media affects perceptions of massage therapy. Mixed messages are confusing. We all need to be careful where we post and what we post on social media and make sure we use clear, professional messages.

EXAMPLE

A massage therapist has a Facebook page dedicated to the massage practice and also has a personal Instagram site. The massage therapist thinks the personal and professional worlds are separate and posts on Instagram pictures taken at family gatherings where the therapist was involved in risky behavior and at parties in where they were wearing revealing clothing. The posts on the personal site are casual, sometimes with sexual innuendo, and use crude language. Even though the therapist's professional page on Facebook is well done and maintained, people will still connect the personal and professional sites. Social media allows us to search for people as well, and both sites will pop up. People will know you are a massage therapist, but when comparing the content they will be confused about your professional behavior, and this will reflect on the massage profession as a whole.

Coupon Websites

Coupon websites are essentially online advertising sites that use direct marketing. There are many coupon websites, but for massage businesses, the most familiar is Groupon. Coupon websites develop large customer databases by collecting the name, contact details, and location of each person who purchases from them. Coupon websites have customer databases that can be sorted according to customer location. The discount offer will go out to subscribers in the business area, advertising your business to a large local audience. Local customers are more likely than others to visit your business, and more likely to become repeat customers.

Unlike many forms of advertising, coupon websites do not require you to pay anything to run your offer. The coupon discounts vary, but it is likely that you will trade profit for advertising. It is common to lose money on coupons. The sites do work to get your name in front of thousands of people. But remember, you need to be able to cover the cost of honoring all the coupons sold. It is one thing to make a manageable loss on a coupon offer in order to attract new customers. It is another to lose so much money that it takes months to recover your losses. The main point of many coupon offers is to draw new customers into a business, with the goal of converting them into repeat customers. Before beginning a coupon offer, develop a strategy to encourage new customers to return.

The coupon websites make money by keeping from 20–60% of the value of each coupon purchased. They then forward the business its share of the coupon's purchase cost. Some websites pay the business a share of every coupon purchased, whereas others pay only a share of each voucher that is redeemed. Be informed about all of the ramifications of using coupon websites.

Management

Management consists of all the activities required to maintain a business, particularly record keeping and financial disbursement. The KISS principle (keep it simple and specific) is an excellent concept to help organize the details of business practices. Of course, a business operation can be set up in many ways. A business consultant and an attorney are usually the best advisers. The simplest business arrangement, the sole proprietorship DBA, is detailed in this textbook. The steps in setting up this arrangement are as follows:

1. Obtain all necessary licenses.
2. Comply with business location regulations.
3. Determine the legal structure of the business.
4. Register the name of the business.
5. Register for tax purposes.
6. Arrange for insurances.
7. Open business banking accounts.
8. Maintain business finances.
9. Set up investments.
10. Maintain business records.

See Proficiency Exercise 3.10 at the end of this section.

Obtaining Licenses

Massage professionals usually deal with two distinct types of licenses: professional licenses and business licenses. A professional license shows that you have achieved the skills required to practice your profession. It may be issued by the state or by a local government body (see Chapter 2) and may be required for all who practice massage. Most states now license massage therapists or are in the process of developing licensure. However, difficulties occasionally arise with local licensing if state licensing is not in place. If you encounter this problem, it is important to organize a group of massage professionals and other supporters in the local community to work to change any local control that does not support massage as a profession.

If a state licenses massage practitioners, the professional usually must show proof of a certain level of education and pass some sort of licensing test. The best way to find out about licensing in any state is to contact the Department of Licensing and Regulation at the state capital. Usually the licensing department for massage is in the Occupational License Department. This agency can provide the necessary information.

A business license, which is obtained from the local government, allows that government body to regulate the types and

PROFICIENCY EXERCISE 3.10

Using the information in this section and the following outline, develop a checklist for your personal business management plan. The first item is done as an example to get you started.

1. Obtain licenses.
   - Check with the state about license requirements.
   - Obtain a copy of the licensing forms.
   - Complete and return the forms.
   - Check with local government about requirements for a business license.
     a. Obtain a copy of the licensing forms.
     b. Complete and return the forms.
   - Check with local government about requirements for a professional practice license or ordinance.
     a. Obtain copy of the licensing forms.
     b. Complete and return the forms.

Your Turn

2. Choose a business location and confirm appropriate zoning.
3. Establish the legal structure of the business.
4. Register the name of the business.
5. Register for tax purposes.
6. Arrange for insurance.
7. Open business banking accounts.
8. Set up investments.
9. Keep records.
10. Develop a client-practitioner agreement and policy statement.

locations of business operations. If a profession is licensed, the professional may need to show a copy of the license to obtain a business license. Any required forms should be filled out carefully. If you need help with the forms, ask the personnel at the agency. When asking for help be polite and considerate of their time, but do not hesitate to ask for the assistance.

Business Location Regulations

When deciding where to locate your business, remember that each community has specific zoning regulations. These regulations protect the investment of those who own property. For example, without zoning, someone could put a junkyard next to a home. Usually the zoning that a massage business requires is general office or commercial zoning. Because of difficulties with local ordinance control of massage establishments, some restrictions may apply to locations for a massage business. Some jurisdictions require a specific massage establishment license. An establishment is site, premises, or business where massage therapy is practiced by a licensed massage therapist. To obtain this information, the practitioner should visit local government offices and ask to see the zoning ordinances.

A permit or business license may be needed. It is important that the business owner develop a good working relationship with government officials. These officials usually have a sincere concern for their communities, and the massage professional must respect this. Occasionally these officials need to be educated about therapeutic massage. Be patient, cheerful, and cooperative. Difficulty with massage parlor ordinances has diminished substantially, but the problem still exists. We hope that growing public awareness about therapeutic massage eventually will resolve this problem.

Home-Based Business

Massage therapy can be a successful home-based business. Investigate local government, neighborhood associations, and rental agreements to identify any restrictions on home offices. Because clients will be in a home office, building codes related to barrier-free access, restrooms, and the like will be applicable. Sometimes it is more cost effective to lease space than convert a section in the home. Because laws vary by city or county, knowing what is legal for your locale will help to prevent problems and allow you to adapt your business accordingly. You should contact your local government or zoning office or consult with lawyers, insurance agents, and accountants, who will be able to advise you. After the legal concerns are addressed, other factors may be considered:

- How can you develop a management plan for using household space which best accommodates your family and your business?
- How is having your business in your home affecting your family?
- Do you have a plan for integrating family and business space needs?

Mobile/On-site Massage Practice

For a mobile/on-site massage session, the practitioner travels to the client's home or business, and travel and setup time are added to the fee. Because the therapist is already organized to do massage, other sessions at the same location can be provided at the regular rate. If a person is housebound for health reasons, the massage therapist commonly takes this into consideration when setting the fee. The massage professional who has only a mobile/on-site business saves on facility rental and utility costs, which may influence the on-site fee structure. Remember that time is money, and an on-site massage takes longer than one in the office. The added fees for travel and setup cost can be calculated many ways. If round-trip travel time is about an hour, then a simple method is to double the standard massage fee. If $75 is the fee in your office setting, then the mobile session fee would be $150.

The mobile massage practice based on retention clients has the least overhead and is the most lucrative way to practice massage therapy. Those massage consumers with a household income of between $75,000 and $100,000 are most likely to have a massage in their home or office. In addition those receiving massage in their location will often request an hour and half (90-minute) session, increasing the fee.

Registering for Tax Purposes

Federal, state, and local taxes must be paid. A business is assigned a unique identification number in order to differentiate it from all others, much the same way a Social Security number is a unique identifier for each person. A tax identification number or TIN is the business version of a Social Security number, and small business owners often get TINs so they can conduct business and keep their personal finances separate from business finances. A TIN is made up of nine digits that

FOCUS ON PROFESSIONALISM 3.3

You must claim all income including cash payments and gratuities (tips). There are individuals who will hide cash income by not claiming it as income, and this practice is more than unprofessional—it is illegal. You do not want to get into tax trouble. It is expensive, time consuming, degrading, and not worth it. Pay your taxes on time, including any property taxes, employment taxes, and income taxes. Also, do not attempt to practice massage without the proper zoning and business permits. You can go to someone's home to do a massage and be just fine, but if that same client comes to your home, you must be compliant with all regulations.

the government uses to identify a person or business. Individuals use Social Security numbers as their TINs. For a business entity, the name for a TIN is the employer identification number. It can be called an EIN or TIN.

The tax ID number or TIN must be included on all tax forms that the owner submits for the business. Banks also require tax ID numbers when opening business accounts.

For a sole proprietorship, a separate tax identification number isn't required for tax purposes. This is because the sole proprietor's Social Security number is the same thing as the business's ID for tax purposes. No separate paperwork needs to be filed for this. The coverage is automatic since the owner and the business are technically the same entity.

Other types of businesses, such as partnerships or corporations, must apply for a separate tax ID number if they want to conduct business. Because two or more people are involved in a partnership, a partnership can't use just one person's Social Security number. A corporation, because it's a unique entity, is already separate from the individual owner or owners and needs its own TIN number.

A separate tax ID number isn't required for a sole proprietor to do business unless that sole proprietor wants to hire employees. Then an EIN is required. The EIN is necessary for tax forms when paying employees' taxes on behalf of a sole proprietorship's workers. When the W-2 is prepared for each employee, the EIN is shown on that form. As a business owner, you'll need an EIN to open a business bank account, apply for business licenses, and file your tax returns.

Your business will need an EIN to apply for Small Business Administration (SBA) loans, An EIN looks like the following format: XX-XXXXXXX. The first two numbers of an EIN are separated from the last seven numbers. A social security number is XXX-XX-XXXX.

A sales tax identification number may also be needed. Information about federal taxes can be obtained from the Internal Revenue Service (IRS). State tax information can be obtained from the Department of the Treasury in any state. Information about local taxes can be obtained from both the county and local government offices. The IRS has many publications and counseling services that help explain the payment of business taxes. You are strongly urged to seek the advice of a business attorney or certified public accountant regarding tax requirements.

Budgeting for Taxes

One-third of the gross income of a business is usually needed to cover various taxes. Recall that gross income is the money brought into the business before any expenses have been deducted. Tax money must be set aside every month and left untouched. One of the biggest problems new business owners have is non-payment of taxes because the tax money was spent on overhead expenses. The best protection is to pay the government first, because the penalties are high and tax laws are difficult. A professional tax preparer can help a great deal with management of your taxes. Depending on projected income, it may be necessary to pay installments on taxes. These installments are called quarterly estimates (Focus on Professionalism 3.3).

Opening Business Banking Accounts

A business account can be opened at a local bank. A DBA (doing business as) or EIN is usually required to use a business name. If the massage professional is disciplined enough to maintain a low balance on a credit card, a business credit card is a good idea. The monthly statement is a valuable record of business expenses.

Online banking has become increasingly common. It is also possible to set up automatic payments for regular expenses such as rent and utilities. Automatic payments simplify the bookkeeping process. Regularly monitor your account balance to make sure you have enough money in the account to cover all automatic payments. When setting up business accounts, you would be wise to work with a bank representative to learn about all the available options.

Business Transactions

All income from the business is deposited into the business account, which serves as a record of gross business income. Bartering is the exchange of massage services for other goods or services without using money, and the value is included in gross income. All expenses are paid from this account, which provides a record of business deductions. What is left over is called the net business income. Income taxes are paid quarterly on the net income. A wise professional will contact an experienced bookkeeper or accountant to help set up the payment schedule for taxes.

After all business expenses and taxes have been covered, the massage professional may write themselves a paycheck (called a draw check) or electronically transfer money from the business bank account to the personal bank account. Personal expenses can be paid from this account. Personal and business money must not be mixed.

Avoid using cash to pay for business expenses, and if cash is used, receipts must be saved and filed. Use automatic withdrawal from the bank account to pay regularly occurring expenses such as facility rent, internet services, and cell phone data plans. Use a designated business credit card to pay all other expenses, such as travel expenses, and then set up automatic withdrawal from the bank account to pay off the credit card each month. Estimate how much will be charged to the credit card each month and place a limit on how much can be charged to the card. A limit of $1000 should be sufficient to cover monthly expenses and any emergency expenses. Pay off the credit card each month. Monthly statements from the bank and credit card company provide information about business expenses for tax purposes.

Information should be organized monthly on a spreadsheet so that when it is time for the tax preparer to calculate the business and personal taxes, everything can be verified. Financial management software will do this. This paper trail is important for a properly run business, and it must be established. It is likely your paper trail will be an electronic trail. Make sure that a backup is maintained and that hard copies of important documents are kept in a safe place. Copies of all important documents should be stored in a location other than that of the originals.

Comprehensive client files, either paper or electronic, must be kept in order (see Chapter 4). Payment records also are kept in the client files. Note whether payment was made by cash, credit card, or check. If a check is used, note the check number. If cash is paid, note the receipt number. If a monthly billing system is used, post the date the bill was sent and the date the payment was received, along with the payment form (i.e., debit or credit card or check). All credit card information should be recorded, and records must be kept current. Computer practice management software will handle these tasks. Back up regularly. There are cloud-based backup systems that will complete this task for a reasonable charge as well.

Business Finances

Money coming into the business is income, and money going out indicates the expenses. Money may flow into a business as cash sales, credit card sales, or other methods. Money may go out of a business when supplies are purchased, bills are paid, and so on. Expenses are the costs that occur as part of a business's operating activities.

- Income (revenue): How much money are you generating from sales of your products or services?
- Expenses (costs): How much money are you spending on business costs such as rent, utilities, supplies, advertising, office materials, business taxes, and the cost of employing yourself (including insurance and self-employment taxes)?

If you have more revenue coming in than costs going out, you are making a profit. If it is the other way around, you have a loss.

Accounting skills are essential when starting and operating a new business, so it is important that you understand basic accounting concepts and terminology.

Accounting

Accounting provides you with various pieces of information regarding your business operations. There are two accounting methods for keeping track of your business's income and expenses: cash and accrual. Almost all small businesses use the cash accounting method. In cash accounting, income is not counted until the cash is actually received, and expenses are not counted until they are actually paid (Box 3.14).

Box 3.14 Business Finances

There are three main financial statements used for accounting.

Balance Sheet

The balance sheet outlines the financial condition of your business at a specific point in time. The balance sheet provides a financial perspective by highlighting what you own (assets) and what you owe to other parties (liabilities).

Assets: are what your business owns. They are bought to increase the business's value and can generate cash flow. They include accounts receivable, inventory, and prepaid expenses.

Fixed assets are property and equipment owned by your business that are not normally intended for sale and are used repeatedly, such as buildings and machines.

Liabilities: When you owe someone else, you could say that you are liable to that person or company. Therefore we call these amounts liabilities. Liabilities are the company's debts or obligations that arise during the course of business operations. Bank debt, loans, and accounts payable are examples of liabilities.

Income Statement

The income statement is used to track sales and expenses during a particular period. It is sometimes called a profit and loss statement and tells you whether your business is profitable or not. It shows your income earned and expenses incurred. The resulting difference between your income and your expenses is called your net profit. Income minus expenses equals net profit. Net profit is subject to self-employment taxes and income taxes. Net profit is similar to an employee's wages.

Cash Flow Statement

A cash flow statement shows the beginning cash balance, plus cash inflows, minus cash outflows, which equals the ending cash balance. A cash flow statement should never have a negative ending cash balance. If you have a negative ending cash balance it means you are bankrupt or out of cash.

There are only a few sources of cash inflow, such as cash collected for massage services or selling products, cash collected that was owed on account, loans made to the business, or personal money put into the business. These cash inflows are added together to produce the total sources of cash for the time period the statement covers.

The cash flow statement also lists cash leaving the business to pay bills or to take money out to pay yourself. These cash outflows are added together to produce the total uses of cash for the time period the statement covers.

The ending cash balance is the difference between your cash inflows and your cash outflows for the period.

Bookkeeping

Bookkeeping refers to the recording of financial records. Maintaining accurate financial records should be a business priority. Bookkeeping systems are used to record your financial transactions and can range from simple to complex as needed depending on your business requirements. The two basic bookkeeping systems are single-entry and double-entry. A double-entry accounting system is more complex than a single-entry system. It tracks the debit and credit for each transaction the business makes. A single-entry accounting system is the simpler of the two and sufficient for a single owner sole massage practice. Similar to a personal checking account, it keeps track of what goes in and what goes out of the account.

Bookkeeping is one of the least popular administrative tasks for small business owners. There are several options for small business owners to handle their accounting responsibilities:

Before deciding that you are going to handle the accounting responsibility, carefully consider if you really will attend to the details and time it takes to maintain business financial records. If you are going to be the one to do the bookkeeping, use electronic accounting software.

If you are focused on growing your business and do not have the time or expertise to handle the bookkeeping duties yourself, pay someone else to do it so you can focus on other important aspects of your business. Outsourcing involves hiring a professional services firm to handle the bookkeeping and accounting for you. Most outsourcing is handled electronically via the internet. Regardless of which option you choose, always remember that it is your business and staying intimately familiar with your finances is critical to your long-term success.

Tax Accounting

Self-employed individuals generally are required to file an annual return and pay estimated taxes quarterly. They usually must pay self-employment tax (SE tax) as well as income tax. SE tax is a Social Security and Medicare tax primarily for individuals who work for themselves. It is similar to the Social Security and Medicare taxes withheld from the pay of most wage earners. In general, anytime the wording "self-employment tax" is used, it only refers to Social Security and Medicare taxes and not any other tax (like income tax). (Proficiency Exercise 3.11). Most self-employed massage therapists function well with the sole proprietorship model. If you are a sole proprietor, you will use the follow types of tax forms:

- Income Tax 1040, US Individual Income Tax Return and Schedule C (Form 1040), Profit or Loss From Business or Schedule C-EZ (Form 1040), Net Profit From Business
- Self-Employment Tax Schedule SE (Form 1040)
- Estimated Income Tax 1040-ES, Estimated Tax for Individuals

PROFICIENCY EXERCISE 3.11

1. Respond to the following questions either on paper or in a small group discussion.
   What are your income expectations for your first year of practice after graduation? Three years after graduation? Five years after graduation? How are you going to achieve these income goals? How many hours a week do you plan on devoting to your career? A standard 40-hour workweek consists of 25 massage hours and 15 non-massage hours: cleaning, laundry, paying bills, and maintaining computer records. Do you want charge more for massage sessions and provide fewer sessions to reach your income goals? Do you want to charge less for massage sessions and work with more people? Review the responses to these questions with fellow students as well as a variety of employers and self-employed massage therapists.
2. Investigate the fee structure for massage therapy in your area.

GENERATING INCOME

A business must make a profit. To do this, clients pay you for massage therapy services. What you charge for massage services is the fee structure. A concern for the client is how much the massage will cost. When deciding how much to charge for massage services, it is helpful to investigate what other massage practitioners within a 1-hour radius of your business location are charging. Consider setting your fees in the midrange of current fees in the area. Incentives and coupons can be offered to generate interest in the business. However, attempting to undercut the competition by charging very low fees usually is unwise because you will not be able to maintain the low fee structure for an extended period. Also, this is not considered an ethical business practice.

Setting and Reviewing Service Fees

The current (as of publication) range for a massage session fee is \$30–\$40 for a 30-minute massage session and \$60–\$90 for a full hour session. These fees represent the current national average and can vary up or down depending on the location. Massage fees are often set by length of appointments. Adding adjunct methods such as hot stones, aromatherapy or other services adds 10%–20%. Fees are lower in the Midwest, and highest in coastal regions and urban centers. While there is typically little difference in fees among spas, gyms or specialty clinics, rates at hotel and resort spas are typically 30%–50% higher. A typical session includes about 10 minutes for pre- and post-massage procedures. For example, a 60-minute massage session has about 50 minutes of massage time reflecting the typical therapeutic hour used in health care and allows scheduling on the hour.

A way to determine the fees appropriate for your area or target market is to calculate the average hourly wage of the people in your target market and multiply that by four (up to a maximum hourly fee, which usually is about \$150). The justification for this structure is that people may understand the value of working 4 hours to provide self-care.

EXAMPLE

If the employees of ABC Packing Company make \$15 per hour, the fee for a 1-hour massage session would be \$60. This group of individuals would generally only be able schedule a massage once a month, which is not enough to support cumulative benefits. Client benefits from massage are achieved by regular sessions at minimum every 2 weeks, and once a week is better based on research to determine massage frequency (dosing) for achieving and maintaining results (see Chapter 5).

The challenge in fee setting for this potential client group is to find a fee range that will support regular massage and generate a moderate income for the massage therapist. When an individual's income is in the low to moderate range, there is less money available to pay for massage. These

EXAMPLE—Cont'd

individuals will have to budget carefully to pay for massage because living expenses use a larger percentage of income. The massage fee of $60 per 1-hour massage two times a month can be justified both for the client with this level of income and the massage therapist. It will require creativity and commitment to serve individuals in this income range. The client will need to budget about $5 a day to save $120 a month for massage. Most of us mindlessly spend $5 a day on coffee, fast food, and other nonessentials. Clients will need to value massage enough to mindfully save $5 each day instead of mindlessly letting the money slip away. The questions are then: Is the massage you are selling worth the fee based on solid benefits that make the client's life easier? Can you educate the client about massage benefits enough so they will diligently budget the funds?

If you are self-employed and consistently fill 25 appointments per week with loyal clients paying $75 per massage, yearly gross income is about $90,000. However, overhead costs drop because there is little need to pay for advertising and there is little wasted time. The massage business is efficient. Instead of overhead being 50% of gross, it is realistic for business operating costs to drop to 30% of gross for a net yearly income of about $63,000 subject to self-employment and income tax.

Alternate fee setting method: In this method the massage practitioner begins with their desired net income + estimated self-employment and income taxes (20%). Then that amount is doubled to determine gross business income needed. Next the massage therapist determines number of massage session they want to schedule. That number is divided into gross business income to determine massage fees.

Example: Desired net income $45,000 per year + $9000 taxes = $54,000 needed for business profit. Business profit is doubled to estimate gross business income of $108,000 per year. The massage therapist determines they want to perform 20 massage sessions per week (50 weeks) which factors out to 1000 massage sessions per year. $108,000 is divided by 1000 to determine massage fee or $108 per massage. The next question is if the demographic and targeted clients will pay this amount. Maybe and maybe not. If this type of calculation method does not result in a reasonable fee for the demographic and target market, then adaptation is needed.

Fee Discounts

Fee discounts offer ways that the base massage fee can be adjusted to entice new clients, encourage referrals from current clients, reward client loyalty, and modulate fees based on income or need. This can be done in a variety of ways. A client can pay for 10 massage sessions in advance with a $5 discount for each massage. The package deal saves the client $50 over the standard fees. Another option is to give a $5 discount to anyone who books a weekly appointment (Focus on Professionalism 3.4).

Fee Increase

It is important to review fees yearly. A good time is at the end of the year when taxes are filed (this usually happens in April, so May is a good time to raise rates). Clients should be notified at least 30 days in advance of any price changes. Just like asking for a raise when employed, raising fees needs to be justified, or the clients may seek massage elsewhere. What are the reasons for the fee increase?

FOCUS ON PROFESSIONALISM 3.4

How to Make More Money

If you have a professional dream that includes making more money than that described in Box 3.15, what are you going to do about it?

You could charge more per massage. This is possible if your services are worth it. If you are going to increase fees, then you need to provide excellent massage and client services. You also have to be cautious of losing clients once fees are increased. What fee would you and could you pay for a massage on a regular basis? Would you pay what you want to charge for a massage? Answering this question is often a reality check.

You can reduce overhead. For example, instead of a commercial office you might consider a home office. Even more cost effective is the mobile on-site massage practice. When your schedule is full, your advertising fees decrease.

You can increase the number of clients you see. To do this, your body mechanics and attention to ergonomics need to be excellent. Increasing client appointment availability from 20–25 clients will result in a substantial increase in income. What will it take to get retention commitment from clients so that your appointment schedule is consistently full?

You can expand income by creating an environment in which you can earn income by being an employer. Or you could sublet your massage space to another massage therapist during the hours you are not there.

Supplementing income with more passive services such as hydrotherapy (e.g., hot tub, sauna) or through product sales is a possibility.

Most important, you have to want to provide massage to be successful. It is like anything else; you can do something for a while even if you do not like it, but eventually your clients will be able to tell that you do not want to be there, and you will not have the motivation to persevere.

Cancellation/No-Show Fees

Clients who cancel their appointments or just do not show up for the massage session are a problem for the massage therapist, whether self-employed or working as an employee. Many types of professionals who work by appointment will charge a fee if the person does not cancel the appointment at least a day in advance and will charge a "no-show" fee. The policy for cancellation and no-show fees must be disclosed to clients before providing massage services.

Membership Models

This method of setting fees is to have two price schedules: one for members and one for non-members. This is a common model in the franchise-based business structure. A monthly fee is charged and typically automatically withdrawn on a credit card. The monthly fee includes one massage session. Members then receive discounts on massage services received that month. For example, if the monthly membership fee is $75, this also reflects the cost of the first massage received that

Box 3.15 Generating Income

Determine what you need to have as a desirable but realistic income. Because you are self-employed, you have the freedom to set your fees however you want. Begin with the outcome: for example, $50,000 (net business profit with self-employment taxes already paid) subject to income tax. Now estimate your needed business gross by doubling your desired income: $50,000 × 2 = $100,000 a year is what you need to generate as business gross income. Now determine how many massage sessions you want to do a week. Using 20 sessions a week based on the hour-long session × 50 weeks (2 weeks for vacations and holidays) equals 1000 sessions a year. Divide $100,000 by 1000 and you have the fee you will need to charge. The session fee is $100. Now you need to develop the type of marketing strategy, client base, and retention plan to find the clients who will consistently fill your schedule so that you have 20 clients each week paying $100. What will it take for you to implement this type of fee structure?

If your income expectations are $40,000 a year with 25 clients a week, the fee is very different: $40,000 × 2 = $80,000 business gross; 25 clients × 50 weeks = 1250 client sessions a year; $80,000 divided by 1250 session = $64 for the massage session fee.

There is no one way to figure fees. The bigger question is, what will people pay for massage in the target market? Demographics and part of the country influence fee structures. Cost of living in various areas is also a determining factor. For example, a massage therapist currently earning $35,000 in Detroit, Michigan, would need to earn $34,000 to maintain the same standard of living in Salt Lake City, Utah. Cost of living in San Diego, California, is 49% higher than it is in Detroit. A salary of $50,000 in Los Angeles, California, could decrease to $21,604 in Memphis, Tennessee, while allowing the practitioner to maintain a similar standard of living. If you live in Fairbanks, Alaska, and charge $70 for an hour-long session, you may have to reduce fees to about $50 if you move to Mobile, Alabama, and wish to maintain the same standard of living. You can charge whatever you want for your massage service, but if people will not or cannot pay the fee, you will not make money. Do an internet search using the term "cost of living comparison calculator," and explore the variations in cost of living.

month. Then any additional massage sessions that month are $65, yielding a savings of $10. This model supports more frequent massage use by the client (Box 3.15).

Foot in the Door

This chapter has explored a career in massage therapy from multiple directions, weaving together many examples and describing two main career pathways that can overlap as you move toward success. The ability to manage the details of the business of massage adds to your potential for success. If your career path leads you to work as an employee, not only will you need to attend to your own responsibilities, but you also must support those in the office or clinic who manage the business details. Stop for a moment and consider the responsibilities of the office manager, receptionist, bookkeeper, accountant, marketing manager, and those who maintain the facility. Wow! How do all the bills get paid and the floors stay clean? Think about your massage school and all the tasks that need to be done just so you can learn about massage therapy in a clean, pleasant environment.

Clients expect a well-run business. As an employee, you will want to work for a well-run business; if you decide on self-employment, you will need to maintain a well-run business. When considering what door you want your foot in, evaluate the attention the organization pays to the effectiveness of the business.

SUMMARY

This chapter is full of details, regulations, requirements, obligations, paperwork, and responsibilities. The concept of paperwork is primarily based on electronic methods, but the thinking process remains the same. Take advantage of all the resources on government websites. Success takes time; it does not usually happen overnight. Persistence, flexibility, and determination are your keys to a successful business practice. Make your goals realistic while nurturing professional dreams. Remember, motivation is how we strive for success. Define success not only by the amount of money you make but also by the value obtained from providing professional therapeutic massage services. Take care of yourself to prevent professional burnout so that you can continue to serve your clients in this wonderful and needed profession.

Both self-employment and working for someone else are viable avenues for success. Each has its pros and cons. It is important to make good decisions about what is best for you. Initially, commitment to being an excellent employee can provide you with valuable experience without all the additional responsibilities of maintaining a business structure. Whatever path you choose, commit to excellence.

LEARN MORE ON THE WEB

It is impossible to learn everything in school and from just one textbook. You need to become your own teacher. This list of informational websites will get your started, but you will have to keep the process going. The US government's official web portal, USA.gov, makes it easy for the public to get US government information and services on the Web. The main sites are CareerInfoNet, CareerOneStop, the Small Business Association, Business USA, the Centers for Disease Control and Prevention, the Social Security Administration, the US Department of Commerce, the US Department of Labor, and the US Equal Employment Opportunity Commission. Links to specific topics that are especially relevant are on the Evolve site.

Evolve

Visit the Evolve website: http://evolve.elsevier.com/Fritz/fundamentals/.

Evolve content designed for massage therapy licensing exam review and comprehension of content beyond the textbook. Evolve content includes:

- Content Updates
- Science and Pathology Animations

- Body Spectrum Coloring Book
- MBLEx exam review multiple choice questions

FOR EACH CHAPTER FIND:

- Answers and rationales for the end-of-chapter multiple-choice questions
- Electronic Workbook and Answer Key
- Chapter multiple choice question Quiz
- Quick Content Review in Question Form and Answers
- Technique Videos when applicable
- Learn More on the Web

MULTIPLE-CHOICE QUESTIONS FOR DISCUSSION AND REVIEW

The answers, with rationales, can be found on the Evolve site. Use these questions to stimulate discussion and dialogue. Each question provides you the ability to review terminology, practice critical thinking skills, and improve multiple choice test taking skills. Answers and rationales are on the Evolve site. It is just as important to know why the wrong answers are wrong as it is to know why the correct answer is correct.

1. A massage professional is considering a position at a local day spa. The owner of the business offered an employee position at an hourly wage or paid per massage. What is the advantage of the hourly wage?
   a. Variable income
   b. Stable income
   c. Subject to the employer's regulations
   d. Independent ability to set work hours
2. Expenses used to begin new business operations are called ______.
   a. A business plan
   b. Reimbursement
   c. Investments
   d. Start-up costs
3. A massage therapist is developing a promotional campaign to increase massage business since taking on a part-time massage employee. What is this called?
   a. Marketing
   b. Business plan
   c. A résumé
   d. Management
4. A massage practitioner has just redesigned the business website and has included the types of massage provided, the massage process, information about the practitioner's qualifications, and client responsibilities. What was forgotten?
   a. Tax structures
   b. Type of premise liability insurance
   c. Fees
   d. Client-practitioner agreement
5. A client notices that the massage office is clean, neat, and efficient and that licenses and certifications are posted on the wall. The client is impressed with the massage practitioner's abilities in ______.
   a. Applications of massage
   b. Communication skills
   c. Marketing
   d. Management
6. A massage professional wants to see whether the location for an office being considered for rental is in an appropriate business distinct. Where does one find this information?
   a. Local zoning office
   b. Facility rental agreement
   c. State licensing bureau
   d. County clerk's office
7. Gross employee wages minus taxes equals ______.
   a. Deductions
   b. Deposits
   c. Net income
   d. A draw
8. The type of insurance needed to protect the business in case a client falls while at the location is ______.
   a. Malpractice
   b. Premise liability
   c. Product liability
   d. Disability
9. A massage practitioner has obtained required licenses and permits for the business location. The type of business set up was a sole proprietorship with a DBA. The business checking account was opened, and a tax plan was developed with an attorney. A local insurance agent has set up appropriate premises insurances. Membership in a professional organization supplies the professional liability insurance. A marketing plan is in place, and client-practitioner agreements are printed and ready. What was forgotten?
   a. Retirement investment plan
   b. Zoning approval
   c. Salary structure
   d. Business plan
10. Which of the following is a major difference between being self-employed and being an employee?
    a. Responsibility for overhead costs
    b. Time management
    c. Type of massage provided to clients
    d. Motivation for career success
11. Which of the following is a legal requirement for setting up a massage business?
    a. Retirement investments
    b. Licenses
    c. Business cards
    d. Competitive fees
12. A massage therapist needs protection in case a client is injured during the massage. What is this called?
    a. Sole proprietorship insurance
    b. Policy statement insurance
    c. Professional liability insurance
    d. Disability insurance
13. A massage therapist is an employee. Which of the following does the employer have to provide at year end?
    a. Form 1099
    b. Form W-2
    c. Form I-9
    d. Form W-4

14. What is the name of the taxes a sole proprietor pays to contribute to Social Security and Medicare?
   a. Income tax
   b. Property tax
   c. Self-employment tax
   d. Corporate tax

15. A massage practitioner is applying for a position at a massage franchise. Which of the following is provided along with the job application?
   a. Social Security number
   b. HIPAA documents
   c. Résumé
   d. NPI number

16. A self-employed massage professional has been working 8- to 9-hour days for 2 years, seeing 25 clients per week and managing business operations. Lately, the professional has been tired and out of sorts and does not attempt to rebook clients who cancel. What is the most logical explanation for this behavior?
   a. Motivation
   b. Coping mechanisms
   c. Burnout
   d. Infection

17. A massage practitioner has been let go from four massage therapy clinics. The practitioner is having difficulty understanding the nature of the problem. The last employer took the time to discuss the issue with them. Which of the following would be the most likely reason for the employment difficulties?
   a. Refusing to gossip
   b. Lack of credentials
   c. Time management difficulties
   d. Start-up costs

18. A massage practitioner who is having difficulty maintaining a full-time practice has consulted a marketing expert and implemented various marketing and advertising strategies. There is a good response to the coupons and promotional programs, so what is the problem?
   a. Client retention
   b. The résumé
   c. The DBA business structure
   d. Licenses

19. A massage therapist has moved from the West Coast to the Midwest. Which of the following may need to be reevaluated in terms of the clients' demand for massage?
   a. Record keeping
   b. Self-concept
   c. Experience
   d. Fee structure

20. Which of the following career paths would most likely be appropriate for insurance reimbursement?
   a. Day spa
   b. Sports maintenance
   c. Pain clinic
   d. General fitness

Exercise

Write your own questions. Make sure to develop plausible wrong answers and be sure that the correct answer is clearly correct. Then write a rationale for each question. The more questions you write, the better you will understand the material.

CHAPTER 4

Massage and Medical Terminology for Professional Record Keeping

http://evolve.com/Fritz/fundamentals/

CHAPTER OBJECTIVES

After completing this chapter, the student will be able to:

1. Explain massage terminology as presented by the Massage Therapy Body of Knowledge (MTBOK) and Entry-Level Analysis Project (ELAP) documents.
2. Apply quality-of-life terminology to client massage outcomes.
3. Explore cultural terminology and use it respectfully.
4. Recognize gender- and age-biased language and use gender- and age-neutral terminology.
5. Describe the importance of people-first terminology.
6. Use medical terminology to identify the three-word elements used in medical terms and to comprehend unfamiliar medical terms.
7. Define anatomical and physiological terminology for bones, joints, and muscles.
8. Define anatomical and physiological terminology for the nervous, cardiovascular, lymphatic, and immune systems.
9. Define anatomical and physiological terminology for the respiratory, digestive, endocrine, and integumentary systems.
10. Use the information in this chapter for effective professional communication and documentation.

CHAPTER OUTLINE

KEY TERMS

Abbreviations	Language
Anatomic tools	Muscle tone
Approach	Nomenclature
Bending	Patient
Care or treatment plan	People-first language
Charting	Prefix
Client records	Pressure
Compression	Progress or session notes
Contraindication	Qualifiable
Cultural competency	Quality of life (QOL)
Cultural humility	Quantifiable
Database	Root word
Deformation	Shear stress
Disability	SOAP notes
Documentation	Suffix
Force	Taxonomy
Forms/styles	Tension stress
Friction	Terminology
Gender	Tissue load
Goals	Torsion
Indication	Well-being

Communication is information exchange through a common language system of symbols, signs, or behavior. Communication is essential for cooperation and collaboration. There is a communication problem in the massage therapy community and in the overarching manual therapy disciplines, health and medical care providers, and the researchers in the scientific community. The problem is that there is no commonly agreed-on language. Fortunately, the language of science is more universal, but even with agreed-on medical terminology and terms used in anatomy and physiology, confusion exists. In September 2019, the National Center for Complementary and Integrative Health (NCCIH), the Eunice Kennedy Shriver National Institute of Child Health and Human Development/National Center for Medical Rehabilitation Research, the National Institute of Neurological Disorders and Stroke, the National Institute on Aging, and the National Institute of Biomedical Imaging and Bioengineering sponsored a workshop to highlight current knowledge of biological mechanisms of force sensing and biomechanical force-based manipulations, with the following goals: (1) to identify research gaps and barriers in the field of force-based manipulations; (2) to discuss new research opportunities in this field; (3) to promote collaborations among neuroscientists, manual therapists (e.g., chiropractors, physiotherapists/physical therapists, osteopathic physicians, massage therapists), physiologists, mathematicians, and engineers to advance cutting-edge research related to force-based manipulations; and (4) to discuss the need for common terminology. The meeting report is available at https://files.nccih.nih.gov/force-workshop-summary-110920-508-updated.pdf.

One of the high-priority research areas is:

1. Terminology and measurement of force-based manipulations: Develop common terminology and metrics to characterize, uniformly define, and quantify the types of mechanical forces applied in various manual therapies.

Force-based manipulations are the passive application of mechanical force to the outside of the body with therapeutic intent, rather than active movement or exercise, as part of pain management care (e.g., low back pain), rehabilitation care, or general wellness and disease prevention.

Using agreed-on terms to describe massage therapy has become ever more important as massage therapists increasingly interact with all types of health care professionals. In addition a common language helps the general public better understand the purposes and benefits of massage therapy. Until the development of the Massage Therapy Body of Knowledge (MTBOK) in 2010, numerous terms and definitions were used to describe the same or similar massage methods or skills. However, this confused legislators, clients, educators, learners, and people in general. Fortunately, the MTBOK document began the process of consensus massage therapy language that we all can learn to speak. The terminology usage in the Entry-Level Analysis Project (ELAP) documents has further advanced the cross-disciplinary language of massage and bodywork therapy. The ELAP documents have been incorporated into the Model Practice Act developed by the Federation of State Massage Boards and used in the licensing examination (MBLEx). Therefore it is important to explore this terminology in depth.

The health care community uses language from the World Health Organization's Quality of Life documents and assessment instruments. This language will help refine and clarify documentation procedures. Communication with people from many cultures is a reality for massage therapists. Professionals must be culturally literate. Massage therapists must communicate respectfully with all individuals, regardless of culture, race, gender, or age. The concept of "people-first" language will help provide guidelines for communication with others, regardless of life circumstances.

The massage professional must be able to accurately maintain client records. The ability to record information accurately and concisely depends on correct use of terminology and an organized approach to charting procedures. This chapter provides an outline of the medical terminology most often encountered by the massage professional, particularly as it relates to charting and record-keeping procedures.

The chapter also consolidates the vast array of medical terminology, focusing on the elements specifically useful to the massage professional. You can master the information in this chapter more easily if you also use a medical terminology textbook, a medical dictionary, and the internet. The website MedlinePlus (https://medlineplus.gov/) is especially useful.

The expanding and changing knowledge base of therapeutic massage makes it almost impossible for anyone to remember all the details required for professional practice. This chapter includes a list of the terms most often encountered by the massage professional. Definitions for these words are available in a medical terminology text or medical dictionary (paper or electronic), and you can reinforce your learning by looking them up. Exploring medical terminology automatically provides an overview of anatomy and physiology. Although this section is not meant to replace an anatomy and physiology text, it provides a quick reference for documentation procedures, including record-keeping and charting skills.

Used with a standard anatomy and physiology textbook and class instruction, this section can help the learner or professional focus on information specific to the field of massage. The recommended anatomy and physiology text is *Mosby's Essential Sciences for Therapeutic Massage: Anatomy, Physiology, Biomechanics, and Pathology, Seventh Edition*, by Sandy Fritz and Luke Fritz (Mosby, 2025), which was developed specifically for therapeutic massage learners. However, the information in this chapter can be used with any comprehensive anatomy and physiology book.

The information presented here is especially pertinent to an understanding of massage as it relates to anatomy, physiology, pathology, and client records. Because the basis for medical terminology is scientific language, understanding this information will help massage learners understand massage therapy research, in addition to articles and books on subjects related to massage. Learning the names of muscles, bones, joints, and other anatomical structures lays a firm foundation for understanding and correctly using medical terminology.

MASSAGE THERAPY TERMINOLOGY

SECTION OBJECTIVES

Chapter objective covered in this section:

1. Explain massage terminology as presented by the Massage Therapy Body of Knowledge (MTBOK) and the Entry-Level Analysis Project (ELAP) documents.

Using the information presented in this section, the student will be able to:

- Define terms used in the creation of the MTBOK document.
- Define and use ELAP massage and bodywork terminology.

Box 4.1 How We Communicate

Language is made up of socially shared rules that include:
- Sounds and symbols that convey meaning
- Word definitions (i.e., vocabulary)
- The ability to make new words
- Agreed-on sequences of words used to communicate (i.e., grammar)
- Terminology: language specific to a specialized knowledge (i.e., medical terminology)
- Taxonomy: the science of classification according to a predetermined system
- Nomenclature: a system of names; a *vocabulary* is a system of names with explanations of their meanings; a *classification* is a systematic organization of things

The terminology used in massage therapy is still inconsistent. Although similar words are used, the meanings of those words do not always coincide. The definitions for the massage therapy vocabulary in this textbook are based on traditional definitions, common knowledge, and the MTBOK and ELAP documents (Box 4.1).

Massage Therapy Body of Knowledge

The terms and definitions provided by the MTBOK document provide a common ground for a language for massage.

Entry-Level Analysis Project Terminology

The following section presents the terminology used in the ELAP documents, modified by additional definitions and explanations of the words used and the relationship to massage therapy. The shift from vague and outdated historical or developer-named massage and bodywork methods is a major advancement. The ELAP-recommended descriptors are grounded in general sciences related to physics, engineering, biotechnology, and the physical behavior of materials both organic and inorganic. The tissues of the body can be considered organic and inorganic materials and respond in similar fashion. Shifting to this language structure is a major step in supporting cross-discipline communication and creating clarity. For you to understand and then use the language and concepts described, it is necessary to elaborate on the definitions. In the future, this type of terminology will be commonplace, but at the time of this edition of the textbook, the ELAP terminology is just beginning to be used to describe massage therapy. An attempt has been made to be as concise and simple as possible and to relate the content to therapeutic massage. Because some of the language structure is based in sciences, background must be provided, or the language will have little meaning.

Language Used in the ELAP Documents

Anatomic tools: Palms, forearms, fingertips, knuckles, and other body parts used to apply force to soft tissue.

Force: Power that internally or externally causes the movement of the body to change or soft tissue structures to deform. In physics, a force is any external effort that causes an object to undergo a certain change concerning its movement, direction, or shape. For example, when a muscle contracts, it creates a force that is transferred to the tendon to pull on the bony attachment, resulting in movement. When a massage therapist moves joints passively, they create the force, and the body part moved has changed direction. During massage, the massage therapist generates the force when the tissue is pressed, pushed, or pulled and has changed shape. There are different types of force, but for massage application, we need to understand mechanical/physical applied force. A mechanical/physical applied force (a push or a pull) has both magnitude (how much) and direction (which way). Its magnitude is measured in pounds (or in Newtons). For example, a push against tissue might be 1 pound per square inch.
Key concept: A force is a push or a pull.

Friction: A force that acts in an opposite direction to movement. Friction is a force that holds back the movement of a sliding object. During massage, lubricants reduce friction so the anatomic tool used to provide massage can slide. Too much lubricant = too much slide. Not enough lubricant = too much friction, and instead of slide, the tissue is pushed or pulled. Most massage methods should move and change the shape of the tissue, which occurs with pushing or pulling. If just the right amount of lubricant is used, then the tissues can be moved, but the friction is not uncomfortable.

Pressure: In massage, we often use the word *pressure* to indicate magnitude. Light pressure = small magnitude and deep pressure = increased magnitude. Pressure is the amount of force applied into the tissue. Pressure during massage is usually applied down into the client's body at an angle of 45–90 degrees. Pressure applied within the 45-degree range orients more horizontally, and pressure applied closer to the 90-degree range is more perpendicular.

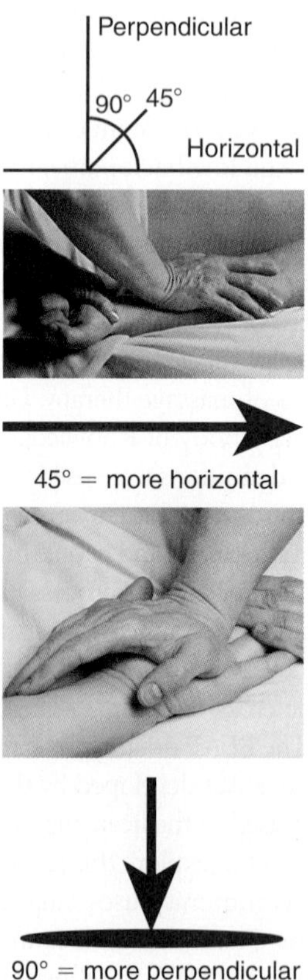

Pressure is also determined by the contact area. Using a large or broad contact during massage, such as the forearm, distributes the force, and the pressure will be more comfortable than pressure applied with a narrow contact, such as the tip of the finger or the elbow. Pressure applied in a small contact area concentrates the force application, which therefore is more specific and more apt to cause injury and pain sensations.

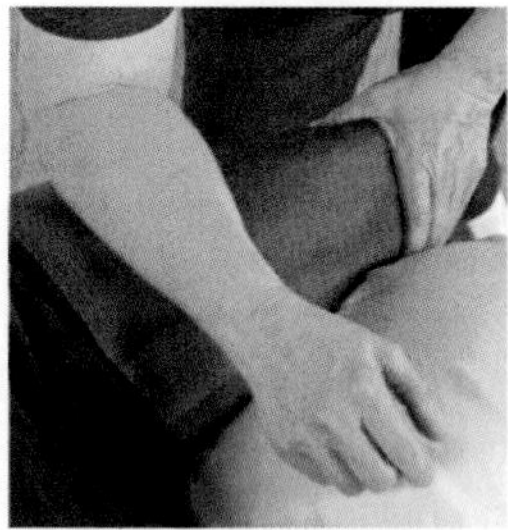

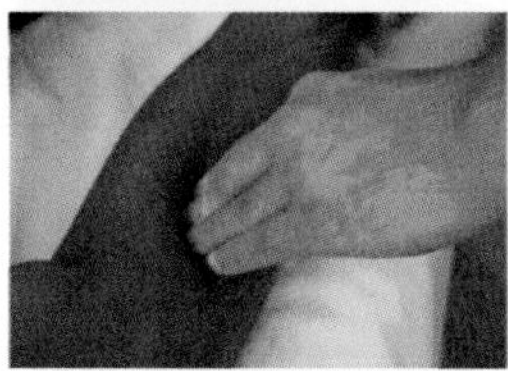

Key concept: During massage, therapists apply mechanical/physical force when we push or pull on the body tissues. For example, we use methods to push or pull, such as gliding, kneading, twisting, and elongation. When methods slide on the tissue, there is friction. The intensity (magnitude) depends on how strong the push or pull is and how much friction is resisting the motion. These two factors determine the amount of pressure.

An important consideration with force is that it is a vector quantity. A vector quantity always has three variables:

- Point of application
- Magnitude
- Direction

During massage application, the massage method is modified by where it is applied (point of application), how intense it is (magnitude), and the direction in relation to the tissues. Remember, an applied mechanical/physical force causes motion or a change in shape.

Key concept: If the force is applied to an object, the object will move if it can. If movement is not possible, the object will change shape. During massage, we usually want the tissue to change shape, so that means it cannot move while the massage method is applied. When tissue changes shape, it typically gets flatter, longer, twisted, or bunched up. Sometimes we want movement as well, such as when a joint is moved.

If we are going to understand how a force application causes movement, then we must briefly explore Newton's Three Laws of Motion (Box 4.2).

External forces: Forces that create loads on soft tissue by pushing or pulling on the body in a variety of ways. A belt around your waist is creating an external compressive load. Gravity is an external force. Massage is an external force.

Internal forces: Forces that create loads on soft tissue, such as misaligned joints or poor body mechanics, cause soft tissue to shorten, tighten, lengthen, and/or weaken, which may load surrounding tissue; for example, a tight muscle or tendon could compress a nerve running close by and cause pain or dysfunction. Increased pressure in the stomach from overeating is also an example of an internal force.

Tissue load: Forces load soft tissues during massage application. **Tissue load** creates *stress* in tissues, and tissues exposed to force are considered to be *loaded*. During massage application (applied force), if there is too much load, the tissue might fail and be injured; too little load and tissues may not respond as desired. The change in shape of tissue in response to the load is called the *strain*. Too much strain, and the tissues can be damaged. Not enough strain, and the tissues may not respond and adapt.

Box 4.2 Newton's Three Laws of Motion

The first law states an object at rest tends to stay at rest, and an object in motion tends to stay in motion, with the same direction and speed. Motion (or lack of motion) cannot change without unbalanced force acting. This means a force must act on the object that is stronger (of greater magnitude) than what is moving it or keeping it still. For example, a child attempts to pick up a box on the floor, but it is too heavy for them to move; this means the child's force application is too small. However, if an adult can lift the box, then the adult's applied force is stronger than the forces created by gravity and the weight of the box.

The second law shows that if you exert the same force on two objects of different mass, you will get different accelerations (changes in motion). The effect (acceleration) on the smaller mass will be greater (more noticeable). Mass is the amount of something there is. In the body, the leg has a greater mass than a finger.

The third law says that for every action (force), there is an equal and opposite reaction (force). Forces are found in pairs. When you push against a wall, it pushes back. Acting forces encounter other forces in the opposite direction. If the opposite forces are equal, no movement or shape change will occur. If one force is stronger (magnitude), it will overpower the weaker force, and something will move or change shape as in the previous example of moving the box. This law will become important when learning about how to apply massage methods without hurting yourself in Chapter 8, Body Mechanics.

EXAMPLE

The goal of the massage is to increase the pliability of the soft tissue in the calf. The massage therapist will choose an anatomic tool (forearm), to apply a force (push and pull) at the back of the leg just below the knee (point of application) using moderate pressure (magnitude) and push the tissue toward the ankle (direction). The applied force loads the tissue, causing stress, and the tissue changes shape due to the strain.

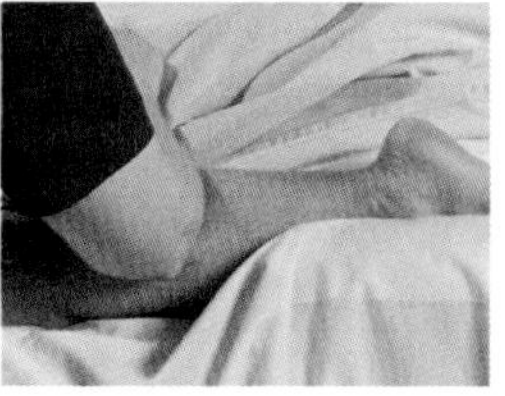

Categories of force load: The five types of loads that can act on soft tissue are tension, compression, shear, bending, and torsion. These five loads fall into two categories: simple loads and combined loads.

Simple loads: One specific type of load that results in one specific type of stress

- Simple (or primary) force load outcomes: compression stress, tension stress, and shear stress

Combined loads. Different types of loads acting at the same time

- Combined force load outcomes: torsion stress and bending stress

Simple loads:

- Compression

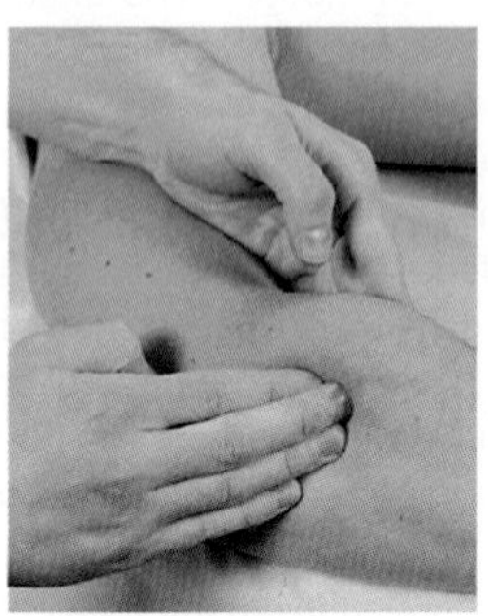

Compression pushes or presses soft tissue, making it shorter and thicker. Another way to understand compression is two pushing forces, directly opposing each other, that squeeze or press an object and try to squash it—for example, placing a ball of clay on the table and squashing it to make it flat. In this example the clay is subjected to a compressive load. The result is compressive stress. The flatting of the clay is the strain. Gravity is a force that is "pushing down" on the body while the reaction force of the chair, massage table, or floor, for example, is "pushing up." Gravity creates compressive stress.

- Tension

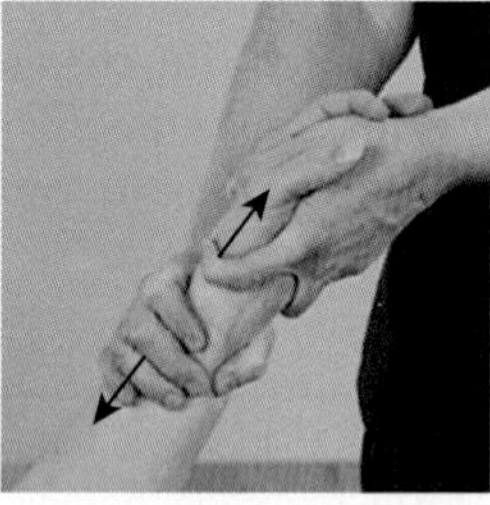

Tension stress (or tensile stress) occurs when two forces pull on an object in opposite directions so as to stretch it and make it longer and thinner and try to pull it apart. For example, stretching out a rubber band puts it in tension or subjects it to a tensile load. The primary load a muscle tissue experience is a tension load. When the muscle structure contracts, it pulls on the tendons at both ends, which stretch a little. Thus the tendons are under tensile stress.

- Shear

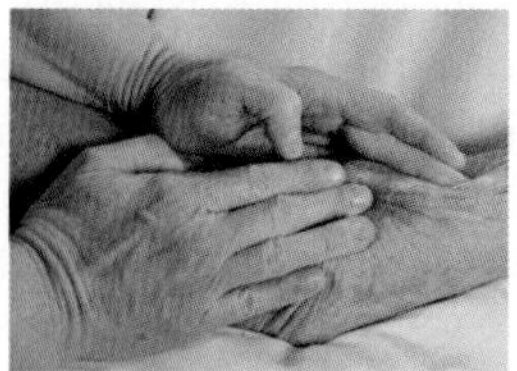

Shear stress is two forces acting parallel to each other but in opposite directions so that one part of the tissue is moved or displaced relative to another part. Shear causes two objects to slide over one another. When a massage therapist's palm or forearm moves across the client's body during massage, shear stress is created. Sliding creates friction.

Combined loads:

- Torsion

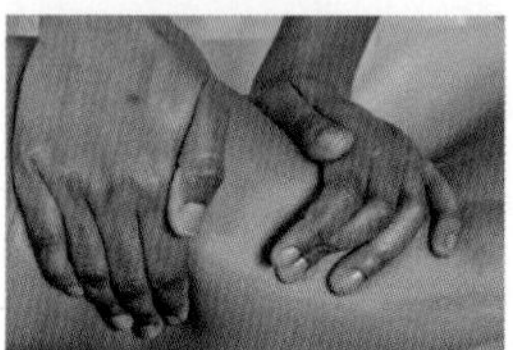

Torsional loading, which we usually just call torsion, occurs when forces cause a twist around a longitudinal axis (think of wringing water out of a sponge). The stresses that occur during torsion including shear, compressive, and tensile stresses. Torsion actually produces shear stresses inside the material.

- Bending

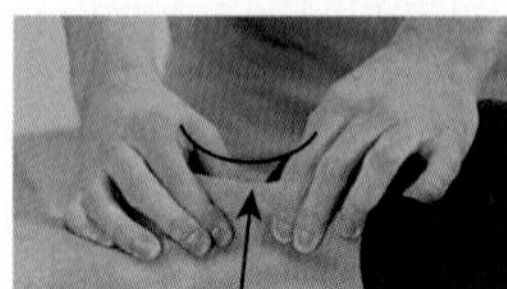

Bending loads produce tensile and compressive stresses. Think about bending a wire with both hands: you are actually creating a compressive stress on one side and a tensile stress on the other.

Soft tissue deformation: Deformation means the tissue changes shape. As deformation occurs, internal forces in the material oppose the applied force. If the applied force is not too large, these internal forces may be sufficient to resist the applied force completely, allowing the substance to assume a different shape and return to its original shape when the load is removed. A larger applied force may lead to a permanent deformation of the substance or even its structural failure. This is what happens when a bone breaks or a tendon is strained. How much tissue deformation can occur is a function of the tissue properties, such as how stiff or pliable it is, how long the force is applied (time), if the tissue is cold or warm (temperature), and the type of load, such as pulling to stretch. For example, bone is resistant to stretching but can break if bent. Depending on the magnitude of the applied stress and its duration, the deformation may become so large that the tissue is injured. During massage, we need to monitor the tissue to make sure that the force applied does not injure the tissue. One theoretical proposed mechanism for massage benefit is based on various studies that have looked at the plastic, viscoelastic, and piezoelectric properties of connective tissue. Sensory receptors of the nervous system are embedded in the soft tissue. These receptors are stimulated when tissues change shape, sending information to the spinal cord and brain about movement, position, and potential tissue damage. Vessels that carry blood and lymph are also embedded in the soft tissue, and movement and tissue shape changes either supports or interferes with fluid movement. Even though the concept of push–pull force application may seem simple when thinking about the benefits of massage, it is amazing how much is affected by an intelligent and skilled mechanical force application. These concepts are discussed throughout the textbook (Box 4.3).

Soft Tissue Deformation Methods

This section discusses the terminology for the way forces are applied during massage. Each of these methods has the potential to load tissue and create a variety of mechanical stresses, such as compression, tension, shear, torsion, and bending stress.

- Compression Methods

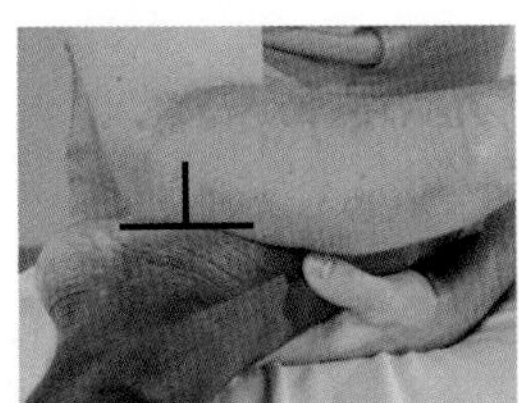

Examples: Approximation (pushing ends of tissues together), pushing tissue against another tissue, applying pressure into tissue; direct pressure techniques: often used interchangeably with static compression and ischemic compression

- Gliding Methods

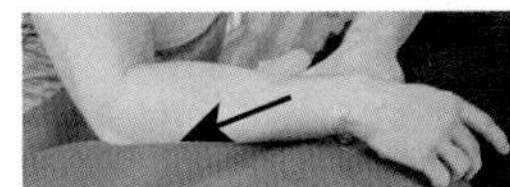

Examples: Stroking, Swedish/classical effleurage, a stroke applied in a smooth, continuous motion that does not lose contact with the client's skin

- Torsion/Twisting Methods

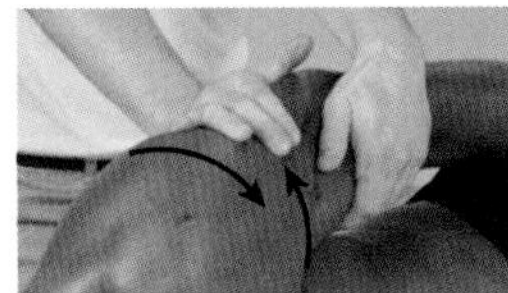

Examples: Kneading, skin rolling, pulling, wringing, fascial torquing, Swedish/classical pétrissage

- Shearing Methods

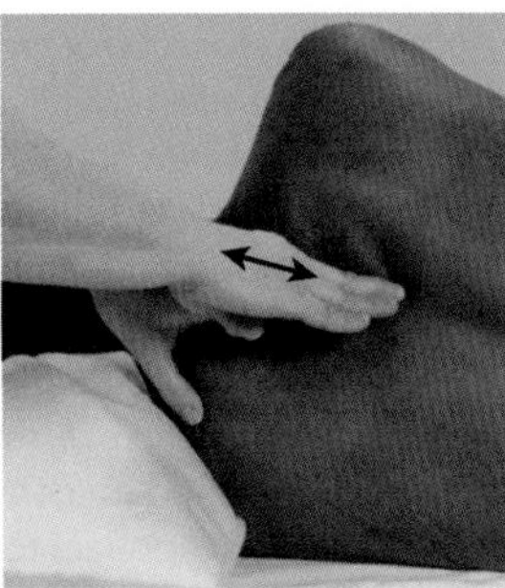

Examples: Superficial friction, linear friction, circular friction, cross-fiber friction, muscle layer separation

- Elongation Methods

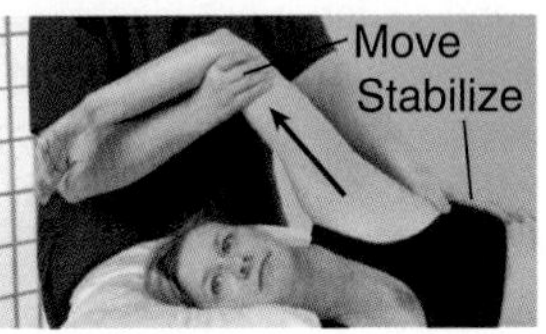

Examples: Crossed hands stretch, fascial spreading, pin and stretch, arm pulling, leg pulling, traction

- Oscillating Methods

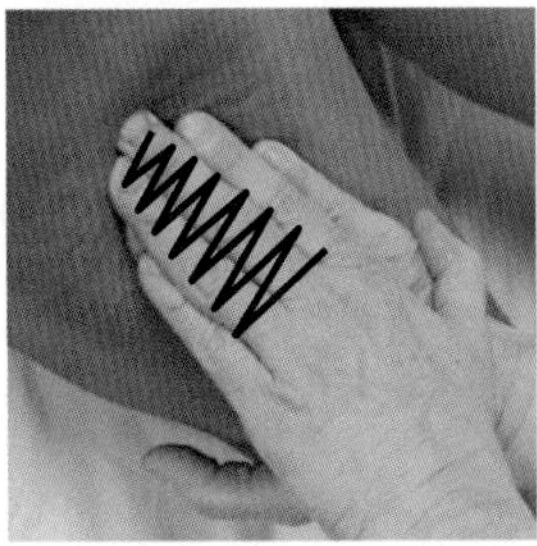

Examples: Vibration, rocking, jostling, shaking

- Percussive Methods

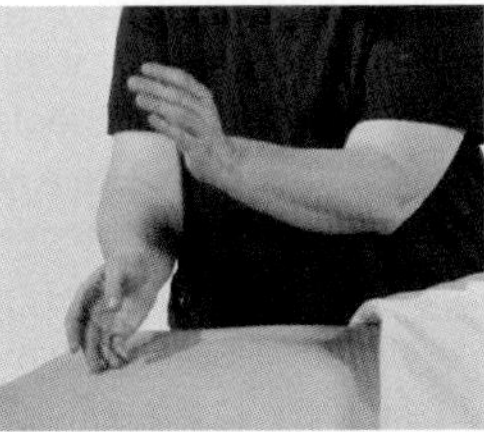

Examples: Tapping, hacking, cupping, slapping, beating, pounding, clapping

- Static Methods

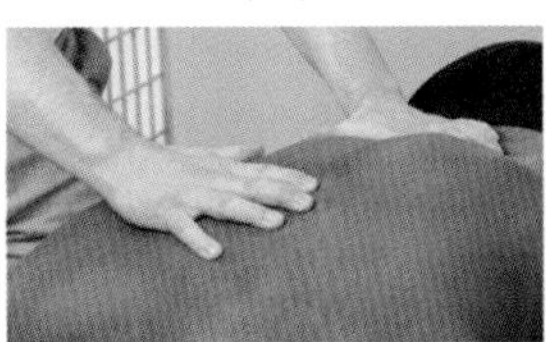

Examples: Holding, direct pressure

Box 4.3 Why Soft Tissue Can Deform

Soft tissues in the body are usually colloids. A *colloid* is a solution that has small particles able to remain evenly distributed throughout a fluid. A *fluid* is a substance that can flow. A fluid is either a liquid or a gas. There are different types of colloids, but most relevant for massage application are sols, gels, and emulsions, which act like soft tissue. Examples of sols are paints, cell fluids, and blood; examples of gels are jellies and connective tissue ground substance; examples of emulsions are milk and mayonnaise.

Thixotropy is a property exhibited by certain gels (semisolid, jellylike colloids). A thixotropic gel appears to be solid and maintains a shape and a stiffness unless influenced by a mechanical force. It then acts as a sol (a semifluid colloid) and becomes more pliable. Thixotropic behavior is reversible, and when allowed to stand undisturbed, the sol slowly reverts to a gel.

Viscosity is how thick or thin a fluid substance is. For example, honey is viscous, and water is not viscous. A substance that is more viscous is also more pliable, meaning it is easily bent, folded, twisted, or manipulated. For example, connective tissues in our body are thixotropic; they become more fluid (pliable) when stirred up (massaged) and more solid (stiff) when they remain undisturbed. Colloids stiffen if a strong and abrupt force is applied but soften if the force is applied slowly and evenly. During massage, when a force is applied quickly, tissue behaves more stiffly, and when the load is applied slowly, tissue becomes more pliable.

Elastic means that a substance changes shape in response to an applied force but will return to the original shape when the force is removed. *Hysteresis* means if the force magnitude (strength) remains within elastic limits, tissues return to their initial state when the force is removed.

Plastic applies to substances soft enough to be molded yet capable of hardening into the desired fixed form. Soft tissues have elastic and plastic qualities. When soft tissues are deformed beyond the elastic stage, they act more plastic, and the shape will be permanent. For example, a gymnast may stretch (deform) ligaments around joints so much that the length change is permanent, and the positions required to perform are achievable.

Viscoelasticity is the property of a substance that exhibits both viscous and elastic characteristics when undergoing deformation. By definition, a viscoelastic material exhibits the characteristics of both a liquid and a solid. A great example is Silly Putty. If you roll Silly Putty into a ball, it will hold its shape like a solid, but left to sit, it will eventually begin to flow and spread onto a surface, forming a flat plane, like a liquid.

Creep occurs as a result of constant stress over an extended period applied to a viscoelastic material. In materials science, creep is the tendency of a solid material to move slowly or deform permanently under the influence of mechanical stresses. Creep is a slow response to maintained stretch with gradual elongation. It can occur as a result of long-term exposure to high levels of force loading the tissue, as long as the tissue does not fail, meaning it breaks. Creep deformation does not occur suddenly; instead, strain accumulates as a result of long-term stress. Think about the gymnast example in which consistent stretching (tension stress) causes creep in the ligaments. Creep is responsible for many soft tissue changes and can be the cause of soft tissue dysfunction.

Piezoelectricity is the electrical charge that accumulates in certain solid materials such as crystals, certain ceramics, and biological matter, such as bone, and various proteins in response to applied force creating mechanical stress. The word *piezoelectricity* means electricity resulting from pressure. When a bone or cartilage is compressed, a tendon or ligament is stretched, or skin is stretched, small electric pulsations are created. The colloidal gel component of soft tissue, which makes up the ground substance that embeds all of the connective tissue/collagen in the body, is influenced by electrical fields. There is a hypothesis yet to be proven that these small electric fields may be one of the factors that might influence the gel-to-sol (melting) transition of connective tissue when massage loads the tissue, deforming collagen.

Adhesiveness is the property of sticking together. An adhesive is any substance applied to the surfaces of materials that binds them together and resists separation. The term *adhesive* may be used interchangeably with glue. All surfaces, except those that are highly polished, have pores. If the adhesive flows into these pores, a mechanical bond is formed.

Layers of tissue slide against themselves, and tissues secrete slippery substances to reduce the friction between sliding structures, preventing bonding or sticking together. A lubricant reduces friction. This means that the surfaces no longer rub directly on each other but slide past on a layer of something slippery.

Friction is what happens when any two things rub against each other. When tissues slide over other tissues, friction occurs. Repeated fiction causes heat and can make the slippery substance sticky. Tissues that are stuck together when they should be sliding over each other will alter the function of the tissue.

Adhesions are bands of scarlike tissue that form between two surfaces inside the body and cause them to stick together. As the body moves, tissues or organs inside are normally able to shift around each other. This is because these tissues have slippery surfaces. Inflammation (swelling), surgery, or injury can cause adhesions to form and prevent this movement. The extracellular matrix provides a framework for cell adhesion, supports cell movement, and serves to compartmentalize tissues into functional units. Basic components of connective tissues and extracellular matrix relative to the understanding of adhesiveness are:

- Collagens are the most abundant components of the extracellular matrix and many types of soft tissues.
- Elastin is another major component of certain soft tissues, such as arterial walls and ligaments. Elastin is the main component of elastic fibers in matrix tissue, where it provides elastic recoil and resilience to a variety of connective tissues.
- Fibronectin is a core component of many extracellular matrices. Fibronectin is an adhesive (sticky) molecule that plays a crucial role in wound healing, particularly in extracellular matrix (ECM); it also works with another cell type, called a *myofibroblast*, to pull the edges of a wound together and stabilize the tissue. Myofibroblasts are secretion of extracellular matrix, development of adhesion structures with the substrate, and formation of contractile bundles composed of actin and myosin. Myofibroblasts are reparative connective tissue cells that contribute to the reconstruction of injured tissue by secreting new ECM and by exerting high contractile force.

In a more pathological role, fibronectin contributes to the development of fibrotic disease. Fibrosis is characterized by an excessive deposition of connective tissue that leads to the impairment of tissue structure or function and is considered a chronic inflammatory tissue-repair response. Rapid repair comes at the cost of tissue contracture, the result of the myofibroblasts' inability to regenerate tissue.

- Movement Methods

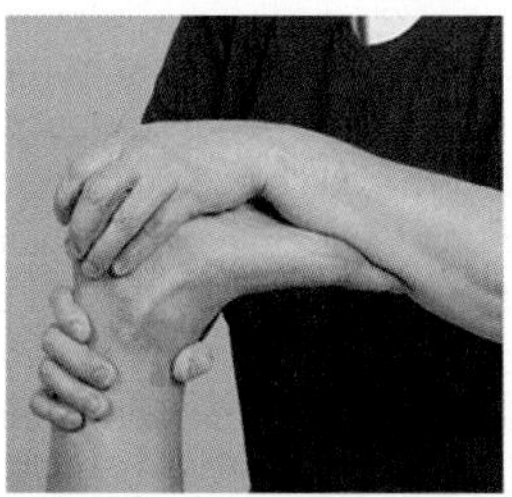

Examples: Active/passive joint movement, stretching

- Hot and Cold Methods

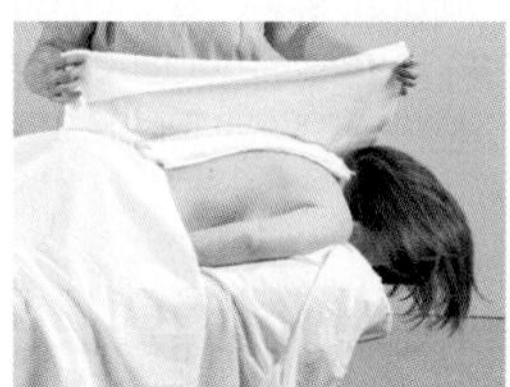

Note: Hot/cold methods do not specifically deform soft tissue but are listed as an adjunct method common to massage therapy. Examples: thermotherapy/cryotherapy, hydrotherapy, hot stones, hydrocollator, hot pack, warm pack, cold pack, ice massage, footbath, ice immersion, paraffin dip

Approaches—A way of thinking and problem solving during massage.

Examples: Wellness/relaxation approaches, clinical/treatment-oriented approaches, structural integration approaches, neuromuscular approaches, myofascial approaches, movement approaches, psychological mind/body approaches, energetic approaches, Eastern approaches

Forms/styles—A particular procedure or cultural approach used to do massage and bodywork.

Examples: Swedish/classical massage, craniosacral therapy, reflexology, manual lymphatic drainage, Esalen massage, seated massage, Lomi, Russian massage, Ayurvedic massage, Thai massage, Tuina.

Core Concepts in Massage and Bodywork Application

- **Quality of touch:** Examples include warm, soft, dry, open, and confident hands/forearms that sink into the tissue at just the right depth; continuity of massage sequence.
- **Therapeutic intention:** Focus on client- and goal-centered interactions. Centeredness (examples: attentiveness, palpation skills, confidence, continuity in contact).
- **Pacing and leading:** The idea that the massage therapist adapts to and matches the client's personal pace (speed) in movement and breathing rate when entering the session to establish connection and then leads the client toward client outcomes by altering the speed and rhythm of massage application and breathing.
- **Rhythm:** In the application of massage/bodywork methods, the idea that strokes should be applied in regular patterns at a regular pace or tempo to elicit the parasympathetic nervous system response. Strokes delivered in uneven patterns or at an irregular pace are jarring for the nervous system, and the client has more difficulty relaxing.
- **Engaging the tissue:** During massage/bodywork application, clear communication regarding the agreed-on session goals, the approaches that work best, and the agreed-on depth of pressure leads to a massage/bodywork session that is therapeutic and satisfying for the client.
- **Therapeutic edge:** The particular pace, depth, and intensity of work for the specific client that allows for achieving outcomes. The place where the client feels the "good hurt/therapeutic discomfort"; a technique feels "close to the limit," but the client also feels that the tissue is changing in a positive way; the stroke feels appropriate and satisfying.
- **Flow and continuity:** In massage/bodywork application, the idea that methods flow from one technique to another and from one body area to another through smooth transitions.
- **Stroke length in massage and bodywork sessions:** Strokes are used that connect body areas and completely cover appropriate areas without compromising body mechanics; strokes should travel the length of muscles or muscle groups when possible.
- **General versus specific work:** The idea that broad and general application methods lead to more specific or focused methods and then back to broad, general methods as the session closes and that there is a difference between what a client experiences with general work versus specific, focused work in just one area; for example, to work in layers (e.g., therapists often work superficial to deep and back to superficial, avoiding changing the depth of application sporadically).
- **Resistant tissue is not forced:** Slow down and wait for the tissue to deform, make sure tissue is warmed up sufficiently, find the therapeutic edge, work in layers.
- **Working at oblique angles:** Most often therapists work (apply forces) at oblique angles no greater than 45 degrees; this ensures that blood vessels, lymph vessels, and nerves will not be pinched. Sometimes (using caution) therapists push straight down.
- **Palpatory sensations:** Sensations that signal soft tissue is changing; knowledge that informs touch, such as the ability to name body landmarks in a particular region; kinesthetic discrimination skills, or the ability to sense, feel, and interpret normal and altered qualities of the body's tissues, such as temperature, texture, fiber direction, density, depth, hydration, and tone; communication skills (e.g., the ability to use correct terminology and name sensations so that perceptions of tissue can be categorized and analyzed more easily).
- **Felt sense:** An internal somatic knowing, difficult to express using words.
- **Sequencing:** Refers both to the sequence of strokes (the order in which strokes are applied to a particular body area) and to the overall sequence of the massage (the order in which body areas are massaged).
- **Transitioning:** Smooth and enjoyable movement from one type of technique to another type of technique, or the efficient progression of skills, such as the change from undraping a body area to the introduction of the therapist's hands onto the client's body.

- **Variety in massage/bodywork application:** Therapists use a variety of methods to work in layers and to engage the interest of the client, and also because muscles in particular areas respond better to certain methods and techniques; in addition, using a variety of methods reduces stress on the therapist's body that might be produced through overly repetitive motions.
- **Use of breath during sessions to benefit the client:** Used to help the client relax; breath can support the release of tension, reduce sensations of pain, and positively influence lymphatic movement.
- **Clients communicate perceptions about massage with therapists:** The massage therapist assists the client in describing what is expected during massage. For example, a client might request "deep tissue massage" but simply mean that they want the tissue engaged to the therapeutic edge.
- **Trauma-informed approach:** The understanding of and responsiveness to the impact of trauma. It promotes positive outcomes by emphasizing physical, psychological, and emotional safety and enhances wellbeing by empowering individuals to define their needs and goals and make choices about their care and services. A trauma-informed approach requires constant attention, caring awareness, sensitivity, and possibly a cultural change **according to at least four basic principles:**
  1. Realize the prevalence of traumatic events and the widespread impact of trauma.
  2. Recognize the signs and symptoms of trauma.
  3. Respond by integrating knowledge about trauma into policies, procedures, and practices.
  4. Seek to actively resist re-traumatization.

  https://www.ahrq.gov/

The ELAP terminology is not perfect, but combined with the MTBOK terminology, it provides a language based on descriptions instead of obscure and confusing terms that have multiple meanings depending on who is using them. Massage terminology will continue to be revised and refined for clarity in communication. It is necessary for the massage professional to remain current with these changes (Focus on Professionalism).

FOCUS ON PROFESSIONALISM

Changes in language use is occurring in multiple areas. There is increasing attention to respectful language related to culture, diversity, and gender. There is ongoing terminology refinement in the scientific community. Effective communication relies on clear language with consistent meaning. Jargon consists of special words or expressions that are used by a particular profession or group and are difficult for others to understand. Slang is a specialized vocabulary used by a certain group. The similarities end there. Unlike jargon, slang is not used by professionals and is, in fact, avoided by them. Because slang is based on popularity and the present, it is constantly changing and evolving with social trends and groups. Jargon, slang, and unique naming needs to be avoided. Attention to respectful language use and updated terminology is an ongoing process for the massage professional.

QUALITY-OF-LIFE TERMINOLOGY

SECTION OBJECTIVES

Chapter objective covered in this section:

2. Apply quality-of-life terminology to client massage outcomes.

After completing this section, the student will be able to:

- Define quality of life.
- Use quality-of-life terminology in massage practice.

Quality of life (QOL) is a broad, multidimensional concept that usually includes subjective evaluations of both positive and negative aspects of life. Although health is one of the important domains of overall quality of life, there are other domains as well—for instance, jobs, housing, schools, the neighborhood. Culture, values, and spirituality are also key aspects of overall quality of life that add to the complexity of its measurement.

In December 2010, the US Department of Health and Human Services launched Healthy People 2020 (Fig. 4.1), which has four overarching goals (US Dept of Health and Human Services, 2010):

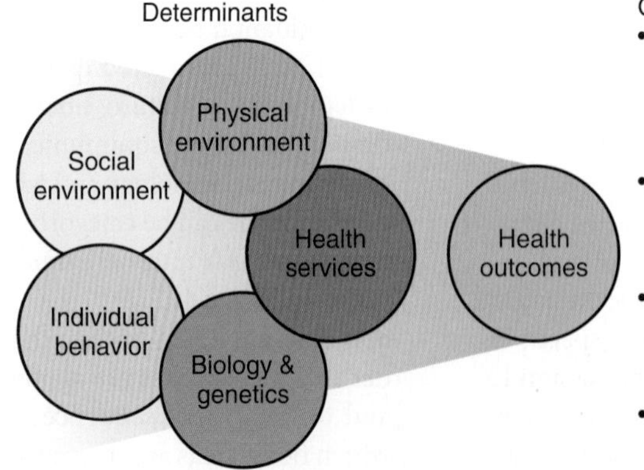
Healthy People 2020
A society in which all people live long, healthy lives
Determinants
Physical environment
Social environment
Health services
Health outcomes
Individual behavior
Biology & genetics
Overarching Goals:
• Attain high-quality, longer lives free of preventable disease, disability, injury, and premature death.
• Achieve health equity, eliminate disparities, and improve the health of all groups.
• Create social and physical environments that promote good health for all.
• Promote quality of life, healthy development and healthy behaviors across all life stages.

FIG. 4.1 Healthy People 2020. The vision, mission, and overarching goals provide structure and guidance for achieving the Healthy People 2020 objectives. Social determinants of health have a major impact on people's health and well-being — and they're a key focus of Healthy People 2030. (From the US Department of Health and Human Services [HHS]:Healthy People 2020: the Vision, Mission, and Goals of Healthy People 2020. https://healthypeople.gov/2020/Consortium/HP2020Framework.pdf.)

- Attain high-quality, longer lives free of preventable disease, disability, injury, and premature death
- Achieve health equity, eliminate disparities, and improve the health of all groups
- Create social and physical environments that promote good health for all
- Promote quality of life, healthy development, and healthy behaviors across all life stages

Every decade, the Healthy People initiative develops a new set of science-based, 10-year national objectives, with the goal of improving the health of all Americans. The development of Healthy People 2030 includes establishing a framework for the initiative—the vision, mission, foundational principles, plan of action, and overarching goals—and identifying new objectives.

Well-Being

There is no consensus on a single definition of well-being, but there is general agreement that at a minimum, **well-being** includes the presence of positive emotions and moods (e.g., contentment, happiness), the absence of negative emotions (e.g., depression, anxiety), satisfaction with life, fulfillment, and positive functioning. Massage therapy is said to support wellness as a factor in well-being. According to the Centers for Disease Control and Prevention (CDC), factors in the physical and social environment that influence well-being include (CDC, 2019):

- Physical well-being
- Economic well-being
- Social well-being
- Emotional well-being
- Psychological well-being
- Life satisfaction
- Engaging activities and work
- Longevity
- Healthy behaviors
- Mental and physical illness
- Social connectedness
- Productivity

When clients tell a massage therapist that they want to feel better, these factors related to well-being are involved. The massage professional also must have a sense of well-being to be of service to clients.

Standard of Living

Standard of living generally refers to the level of wealth, comfort, material goods, and necessities available to a certain socioeconomic class in a certain geographic area. An evaluation of standard of living commonly includes these factors:

- Income
- Quality and availability of employment
- Class disparity
- Poverty rate
- Hours of work required to purchase necessities
- Gross domestic product (GDP)
- Inflation rate

Standard of living has a huge impact on whether a client can justify the expense of massage therapy even when it contributes to well-being. The massage therapist's income determines their standard of living. This was discussed extensively in Chapter 3.

The World Health Organization (WHO) is the directing and coordinating authority for health within the United Nations system. WHO undertook the task of identifying, defining, and assessing the spectrum of life quality. The WHO Quality of Life (WHOQOL) project was initiated in 1991. The definition of quality of life presented by WHO is "individuals' perceptions of their position in life in the context of the culture and value systems in which they live and in relation to their goals, expectations, standards and concerns."

The categories of QOL have been described and presented in a language that can be used to communicate clearly with clients, peers, and others. Interestingly, the common outcome goals for massage therapy intervention are related to QOL categories. WHO has called these categories *domains* (Box 4.4).

The language established by WHO, the CDC, and other documents concerning QOL provides a structure for critical thinking, clinical reasoning, communication, and documentation (which is described later in the chapter).

Box 4.4 World Health Organization Quality of Life Domains[a]

This information is summarized from the World Health Organization (WHO) Quality of Life (QOL) User Manual.

Domain I: Physical

Pain and Discomfort

Pain is judged to be present if a person reports it to be so, even if there is no medical reason to account for it. The assumption is made that the easier the relief from pain, the less the fear of pain and its resulting effect on quality of life.

Examples:

- Unpleasant physical sensations such as stiffness, aches, long-term or short-term pain, and itches
- Constant threat of pain
- Extent to which these sensations are distressing and interfere with life

Energy and Fatigue

Energy is the enthusiasm and endurance that a person has to perform the necessary tasks of daily living, as well as other chosen activities, such as recreation. Lack of energy becomes fatigue.

Examples:

- Feeling really alive
- Adequate levels of energy
- Fatigued but functioning with effort
- Disabling tiredness due to illness, problems such as depression, and overexertion

Sleep and Rest

Restorative sleep is necessary for quality of life. Problems with sleep and rest affect the person's quality of life. If sleep is disturbed, reasons can be due either to the person's life and circumstances or to factors in the environment, such as noise or interruption.

Continued

Box 4.4 World Health Organization Quality of Life Domains[a]—cont'd

Examples:
- Difficulty going to sleep
- Waking up during the night
- Waking up early in the morning
- Being unable to go back to sleep
- Lack of refreshment from sleep

Domain II: Psychological

Positive Feelings

A person's view of and feelings about the future are seen as an important part of life. Does the individual experience enjoyment of the good things in life?

Examples:
- Contentment
- Balance
- Peace
- Happiness
- Hopefulness
- Joy

Thinking, Learning, Memory, and Concentration

A person's view of their ability to think with clarity of thought and ability to gather and absorb new information and make informed decisions that affect quality of life.

Examples:
- Thinking
- Learning
- Memory
- Concentration
- Confidence
- Confusion
- Forgetfulness

Self-Esteem

Self-esteem is how people feel about themselves and their perception of self-worth. This might range from feeling positive about themselves to feeling extremely negative about themselves.

Examples:
- Feeling of self-efficacy
- Satisfaction with oneself
- Self-control
- Ability to get along with other people
- Educational experience and success
- Ability to respond to change
- Sense of dignity
- Self-acceptance

Body Image and Appearance

The focus is on the person's satisfaction with the way they look and the effect it has on their self-concept, including the extent to which "perceived" or actual physical impairments, if present, can be corrected (e.g., by makeup, clothing, artificial limbs). How others respond to a person's appearance is likely to affect the person's body image considerably.

Examples:
- The person's view of their body
- Is the appearance of the body seen in a positive or negative way?

Negative Feelings

Although negative feelings are normal, how often, how much, and to what extent a person experiences negative feelings reflect quality of life and affect the person's day-to-day functioning.

Examples:
- Despondency
- Guilt
- Sadness
- Tearfulness
- Despair
- Nervousness
- Anxiety
- Lack of pleasure in life

Domain III: Level of Independence

Mobility

The focus is on the person's general ability to go wherever they want to go without the help of others, regardless of the means used to do so.

Examples:
- Ability to perform mobility tasks (e.g., walking, running, reaching, pushing)
- Ability to get from one place to another
- Ability to move around the home
- Ability to move around the workplace
- Access to transportation services

Activities of Daily Living

The focus is on a person's ability to conduct activities needed to perform on a day-to-day basis.

Examples:
- Ability to perform usual daily living activities
- Self-care
- Wellness level exercise
- Family care
- Work activities
- Caring appropriately for property
- Participation in hobbies and other recreational activities

Dependence on Medication or Treatments

When an individual feels dependent on medication or some sort of treatment, quality of life is affected. A person's real or perceived dependence on medication or integrative and complementary medicines and treatments such as acupuncture, massage, and herbal remedies for supporting their physical and psychological well-being can either enhance or hinder quality of life.

Examples:
- Medications or treatment side effects
- Medication or treatment benefits
- Time expended in obtaining treatments
- Convenience of obtaining medication or treatments
- Medication or treatment costs and ability to pay
- Perception of medication or treatment cost/benefit ratio

Working Capacity

Work is defined as any major activity in which the person is engaged. Quality of life can depend on a person's use of their available energy for work, satisfaction with the work, and ability to work.

Examples:
- Work for pay
- Desire to work but not employed
- Unpaid work
- Voluntary community work
- Full-time study
- Care of children
- Household duties

Box 4.4 World Health Organization Quality of Life Domains[a]—cont'd

Domain IV: Social Relationships

Personal Relationships

The extent to which people feel they can share moments of both happiness and distress with loved ones and a sense of loving and being loved affect quality of life.

- Experience companionship, love, and support
- Ability to hug and touch and display other forms of physical affection
- Ability to be hugged and touched and to receive physical affection
- Desire for intimate relationship, both emotionally and physically
- Commitment to caring for and providing for other people
- Ability and opportunity to love, to be loved, and to be intimate

Social Support

Social support occurs when family and friends share in responsibility and work together to solve personal and family problems.

Examples:

- Support of family and friends
- Ability to depend on support in a crisis
- Availability of practical assistance from family and friends
- Approval and encouragement from family and friends

Sexual Activity

For many people, sexual activity and intimacy are intertwined. How a person is able to express and enjoy sexuality appropriately and without guilt or value judgment is an aspect of quality of life.

Examples:

- Healthy sexual expression is practiced
- The individual is physically able to participate in sexual behavior
- Supportive sexual partners are available
- Sexual activity is expressed in intimate relationships
- The individual is able to choose to participate in sexual relationships
- The individual is free to express the creative forces of sexuality in a nonphysical way

Domain V: Environment

Physical Safety and Security

A threat to safety or security might arise from multiple sources, such as other people, political oppression, and natural disasters, and affects quality of life.

Examples:

- Sense of freedom
- Feeling of safety and security
- Lack of safety and security
- Protection from physical harm

Home Environment

Home is the principal place where a person lives; keeps most of their possessions; and, at a minimum, sleeps. The quality of the home is assessed on the basis of being comfortable, as well as affording the person a safe place to reside.

Examples:

- Crowdedness
- Amount of space available
- Cleanliness
- Opportunities for privacy
- Availability of facilities such as electricity, toilet, running water
- The quality of the construction of the building
- The quality of the immediate neighborhood

Financial Resources

A person's perspective on financial resources is an influence on quality of life.

Examples:

- Resources that meet the need for a healthy and comfortable lifestyle
- What the person can afford or cannot afford
- A sense of satisfaction/dissatisfaction with income
- Income that allows independence
- Financial resources that are inadequate to support independence
- The feeling of having enough

Health and Social Care: Availability and Quality

A person's view of the health and social care in the near vicinity, access to that care, and the quality of the care are aspects of quality-of-life experience.

Examples:

- Time it takes to get help
- The availability of health and social services
- The quality and completeness of care
- Access to volunteer and community support organizations
- Access to governmental support organizations
- Access to police, fire, and rescue services

Opportunities for Acquiring New Information and Skills

The ability of a person to fulfill a need for information and knowledge, whether this refers to knowledge in an educational sense or to local, national, or international news, is relevant to a person's quality of life.

Examples:

- Opportunity to learn new skills, acquire new knowledge
- Access to libraries, schools, and organizations involved in learning
- Access to media (television, radio, Internet) to be in touch with what is going on

Participation in and Opportunities for Recreation and Leisure

Quality of life is found in a person's ability, opportunities, and inclination to participate in leisure, pastimes, and relaxation.

Examples:

- Access to parks and recreational facilities
- Ability to see friends and spend time with family
- Time to read, watch television, be entertained, or do nothing

Physical Environment (Pollution/Noise/Traffic/Climate)

A person's view of their environment can improve or adversely affect quality of life.

Examples:

- Noise
- Pollution
- Climate
- General aesthetic of the environment

Transport

The availability of transport allows the person to perform the necessary tasks of daily life as well as the freedom to perform chosen activities.

Examples:

- Available and easy to find
- Reliable
- Affordable

Continued

Box 4.4 World Health Organization Quality of Life Domains[a]—cont'd

- Easy to use
- Multiple modes of transport available (e.g., bicycle, car, bus)

Domain VI: Spirituality/Religion/Personal Beliefs

Spirituality/Religion/Personal Beliefs

A person's personal beliefs affect quality of life. Beliefs can enhance or degrade quality of life.

Examples:

- Ability to cope with difficulties in life
- Give structure to experience
- Ascribe meaning to spiritual and personal questions
- Provide a sense of well-being
- Ability to be hopeful
- Lack of spiritual, religious, and personal beliefs, sometimes leading to despondency
- Rigid, imposed spiritual, religious, and personal beliefs, sometimes disempowering

[a]WHO reports are available at Publications (who.int) (https://www.who.int/publications/). From the World Health Organization (WHO). https://www.healthypeople.gov/2020/about/qolwbabout.aspx; data from WHO. [1998]. *WHOQOL User Manual.* pp 61–71. Geneva, Switzerland: WHO.

EXAMPLE

Quality-of-life terminology can become a useful tool for performing and documenting client history and assessment as the initial database for the client is developed. The terminology is also helpful for framing questions used during the history-taking process and developing outcome-based goals for massage (see Box 4.4). For example, the energy and fatigue content from Domain I can be used as part of the subjective aspect of gathering data from the client.

Domain I – Energy and Fatigue

Energy is the enthusiasm and endurance that a person needs to perform the necessary tasks of daily living, as well as other chosen activities, such as recreation. Lack of energy becomes fatigue.

Levels

- Feeling really alive
- Adequate levels of energy
- Fatigued but functioning with effort
- Disabling tiredness caused by illness, problems such as depression, or overexertion

Questions to Ask

- How would you explain your endurance for performing daily tasks?
- Please describe your energy level today.

Possible Answers

- Really alive and full of energy
- Adequate
- Fatigued but functioning
- Unable to function because of fatigue

Follow-Up Questions

- What would you be able to do differently if your fatigue decreased and your energy increased?
- What do you believe is causing you to be fatigued?
- How might massage help you have more energy?
- Would an appropriate outcome goal for massage be to reduce stiffness and improve sleep?

The language in each of the domains in Box 4.4 can be used to form useful questions as you communicate with your clients.

The language can also be used to educate clients.

Domain IV—Social Relationships

Social support: When family and friends share in responsibilities and work together to solve personal and family problems, this provides social support. For example:

- Support of family and friends
- Ability to depend on support in a crisis
- Availability of practical assistance from family and friends
- Approval and encouragement from family and friends

If a client has been diagnosed with a chronic pain condition, coping mechanisms can be described in this way:

Massage therapy can be helpful in managing chronic pain. In addition the support of family members and friends and their ability to help, especially in a crisis, can be an important aspect of coping. I would be happy to teach some basic massage methods to some of your family members or friends so that they can help you between massage sessions.

CULTURAL COMPETENCY, GENDER-NEUTRAL LANGUAGE, AND AGE-APPROPRIATE TERMS

SECTION OBJECTIVES

Chapter objectives covered in this section:

3. Explore cultural terminology and use it respectfully.
4. Recognize gender- and age-biased language and use gender- and age-neutral terminology.

Using the information presented in this section, the student will be able to:

- Define cultural competency.
- Define cultural humility.
- Use resources to develop cultural competency and humility.
- Define gender neutral.
- Identify language based on the life span.

Cultural Competency

Massage therapy is provided within a global community. As described in Chapter 1, we need to interact with others in a professional and respectful manner, and an appreciation of culture is one factor in this level of communication. *Culture* is often described as the combination of a body of knowledge, a body of beliefs, and a body of behavior. It involves a number of elements, including personal identification, language, thoughts, communications, actions, customs, beliefs, values, and institutions that are often specific to ethnic, racial, religious, geographic, or social groups. Learning to be culturally competent supports respectful responses to the health beliefs, practices, culture, and language of diverse populations. The Bureau of Educational and Cultural Affairs (ECA) of the US Department of State fosters mutual understanding between the people of the United States and the people of other countries to promote friendly and peaceful relations. The ECA accomplishes this mission through academic, cultural, sports, and professional exchanges that engage youth, learners, educators, artists, athletes, and rising leaders in the United States and more than 160 countries.

Again as described in Chapter 1, **cultural competency** requires exploration into one's own culture and a sincere curiosity about other cultures to develop the ability to interact genuinely and respectfully with others. Each individual has a unique culture, yet in this global society we all need to strive to be multicultural. Our global society requires that we be intellectually and emotionally committed to the basic unity of all human beings. Human beings and our cultures are much more similar than different. Professionals do not stereotype or define others by ethnicity, size, language, religion, economic status, and so forth. Cultural diversity is a beautiful aspect of the human experience, and massage professionals appreciate the differences that exist among people of different cultures. **Cultural humility** is a lifelong commitment to self-evaluation and self-critique of the power imbalances in the client and massage therapist therapeutic relationship related to diversity. Two specific areas are important for professional interaction:

- Value clients' cultural beliefs
- Recognize complexity in language interpretation

To develop cultural competency and humility, we all need to be more aware of our own cultural beliefs and be more responsive to culturally diverse clients. We can participate in cultural events in our local areas. We can foster professional relationships with health professionals from other cultures. The openness and willingness to learn can lead to self-awareness and, over time, change beliefs and attitudes that limit the resourceful and productive relationships of us all.

Gender-Neutral and Age-Appropriate Terms

Gender-neutral language or gender-inclusive language is language that avoids bias toward a particular sex or social **gender**. Words such as humankind, people, partner, spouse, significant other, parent, sibling, child are examples. Gender-neutral pronouns, most commonly they/them/theirs, are acceptable whether speaking of an individual or group of people.

Another concern is respectful language for those over age 65. Since the early 20th century, at least 30 years has been added to the average life expectancy. The term "older adults" currently is considered politically correct; "seniors" and "elders" are tolerable. "Elderly" is not recommended because it implies frail and in poor health. All people have a life span that ends at death. There are stages within the life span. The experiences of each life stage prepare us for the next phase of the life span. There are realistic developmental expectations of behavior and accomplishment as we mature. Unfortunately, there are also stereotypes based on age that may become discriminatory. The aging process is ongoing, and the passage from one period to the next seems subtle and gradual. The common life span stages are:

Neonatal (birth–1 month)	Young adulthood (18–29)
Infancy (2–23 months)	Adulthood (18+)
Childhood (birth–12 years)	Thirties (30–39)
Preschool age (2–5)	Middle age (40–64)
School age (6–12)	Senior/older adults (65+)
Adolescence (13–17)	Elder (85+)

There are many other ways to name the stages of the life span. As with all communication and interaction with others, it is important to consider the individual first and avoid preconceived ideas about a group of people, which is called *stereotyping*. We are all unique in important ways, even when we are similar in culture, gender, and age.

Stay up-to-date with trends in respectful language by using the following websites.

- MedlinePlus: https://medlineplus.gov/populationgroups.html.
- US Department of Health & Human Services: https://www.hhs.gov/aging/index.htmlCultural Competency Resources https://www.hhs.gov/programs/topic-sites/lgbtqi/enhanced-resources/competency-resources/index.html.

PEOPLE-FIRST TERMINOLOGY

SECTION OBJECTIVES

Chapter objective covered in this section:

5. Describe the importance of people-first terminology.

Using the information presented in this section, the student will be able to:

- Define disability.
- Define people-first language.
- Use appropriate language related to the diverse population of individuals with disabilities.

The Americans with Disabilities Act (ADA) defines **disability** as a physical or mental impairment that substantially limits one or more major life activities. Although the term *disability* itself implies a negative, it is the most objective term in English. Disability is a general term used for an attribute or a functional limitation that interferes with a person's ability to, for example, walk, lift, or learn. It may refer to a physical, sensory, or mental condition, such as depression, irritable bowel syndrome, Lyme disease, posttraumatic stress syndrome, diabetes, multiple sclerosis, and other conditions that restrict the activities of daily living. **People-first language** literally puts the person first instead of the disability. By referring to an individual as a person with a disability instead of a disabled person, you are providing an objective description instead of a label.

Nondisabled is the preferred term when the context calls for a comparison between people with and without disabilities. Use *nondisabled* or *people without disabilities.*

- Do not use the terms *able-bodied*, *normal*, or *whole.*
- Do not use the term *handicapped*, because many people with disabilities consider it offensive.

Some people prefer *identity language* to people-first language as a way to signal their disability pride. A person might proudly say, "I am autistic." Still, the guiding principle remains:

- Give people with disabilities the dignity and respect that all people want by using people-first language.
  Follow these guidelines for respectful communication:
- Put the person first, not the disability. This person-first language puts the focus on individuals, not their functional limitations.
- Emphasize abilities, not limitations. For example, saying "uses a wheelchair" rather than "confined to a wheelchair." Emphasize capabilities and avoid negative words that portray the person as passive or suggest a lack of something, such as *victim, invalid*, or *defective*.
- Do not focus on a disability unless it is essential to services provided.
- Avoid condescending terms such as *special, handicapable, differently abled*, and *challenged*. Although *special* is used in the names of some educational programs and organizations, the use of *special needs* is offensive to many adults with disabilities.
- Avoid sensationalizing and negative labeling. Saying *afflicted with, crippled with, victim of*, or *suffers from* portrays individuals with disabilities as helpless objects of pity and charity. Do not portray successful people with disabilities as heroic overachievers or long-suffering saints.
- A disability is not an illness. People with disabilities can be healthy.
- Do not refer to people with disabilities as patients unless their relationship with their doctor is under discussion or they are being referenced in the context of a clinical setting.
- Respect the person. Do not use offensive words such as *retard, freak, lame, subnormal, vegetable*, and *imbecile*.

Disability Terms

According to the World Health Organization, disability has three dimensions:

- Impairment in a person's body structure or function, or mental functioning; examples of impairments include loss of a limb, loss of vision or memory loss.
- Activity limitation, such as difficulty seeing, hearing, walking, or problem solving.
- Participation restrictions in normal daily activities, such as working, engaging in social and recreational activities, and obtaining health care and preventive services.

Additional information is available at Disability and Health Overview | CDC https://www.cdc.gov/ncbddd/disabilityandhealth/disability.html.

Although opinions differ on some words, this list offers preferred terms for many visible and invisible disabilities, illustrated with person-first language. The list was modified from the World Report on Disability (2011).

- *Autism spectrum disorders (ASD)* refers to a group of complex disorders of brain development that may cause difficulty with social interactions, problems with verbal and nonverbal communication, and repetitive behaviors. In terms of symptoms, people with an ASD can have severe limitations in one area with no limitations in others. Use "child with autism" or "person on the spectrum." Do not say autistic.
- *Blind* describes a condition in which a person has loss of sight for ordinary life purposes. A person is legally blind when vision with best correction is no better than 20/200. Low vision and vision loss are generic terms for vision loss caused by macular degeneration and other conditions. *Low vision* usually denotes someone who is legally blind but can still see large print, bright colors, light and shadow, and large shapes, whereas vision loss refers to those who have lost vision after birth. Say *person who is blind, person who has low vision*, or *person who is legally blind*. Ask which term best suits the person. *Visually impaired* and *visually challenged* are considered negative terms.
- *Brain injury or traumatic brain injury (TBI)* describes a condition in which there is long-term or temporary disruption in brain function resulting from injury to the brain. Difficulties with cognitive (thinking remembering, learning), physical, emotional, and/or social functioning may occur. Use *person with a brain injury* or *employee with a traumatic brain injury*. Do not say *brain damaged*.
- *Cleft palate or lip* describes a specific congenital disability involving the lip and gum. Say *person who has a cleft palate*. The term *harelip* is anatomically incorrect and stigmatizing.
- *Congenital disability* describes a disability that has existed since birth but is not necessarily hereditary. Use *person with a congenital disability* or *disability since birth*. Do not say *birth defect* or *deformity*.
- *Deaf* refers to a profound degree of hearing loss that prevents understanding speech through the ear. *Hearing impaired* or *hearing loss* are generic terms used by some individuals to indicate any degree of hearing loss, from mild to profound, although some dislike the negative term *impaired*. *Hard of hearing* refers to a mild to moderate hearing loss that may or may not be corrected with amplification. A person who has hearing difficulties may have speech difficulties too, but deafness does not affect mental abilities. Say *person who is deaf* or *person who is hard of hearing*. People who have some degree of both hearing and vision loss prefer the term *deaf-blind*. Also acceptable is *person with combined vision and hearing loss* or *dual sensory loss*. As a group, this population typically refers to itself as the *Deaf* or *Deaf community* (with a capital D) rather than *people who are deaf*. They identify with a specific community made up of those who share a common language, American Sign Language, and culture. Never use *deaf and dumb*.
- *Developmental disability* is a broad term that describes any physical and/or mental disability that starts before age 22. Examples include cerebral palsy, autism spectrum disorders, and sensory impairments. People with developmental disabilities have a wide range of functioning levels and disabilities. Although the term *intellectual disability* is often used in conjunction with developmental disability, people with a developmental disability do not have an intellectual disability. Say *she has cerebral palsy, he has autism*, or *they have a developmental disability*. Do not say *she is mentally retarded*.
- *Disfigurement* refers to physical changes caused by burns, trauma, disease, or congenital conditions. Do not say *burn victim*. Say *burn survivor* or *child who has burns*.

- *Down syndrome* describes a chromosomal disorder that causes a delay in physical, intellectual, and language development. Say *person with Down syndrome.*
- *HIV/AIDS* is a disease of the immune system. Over time, HIV (human immunodeficiency virus) can weaken the immune system to a point where the body becomes susceptible to certain illnesses that healthy immune systems resist. People with HIV are diagnosed with AIDS (acquired immunodeficiency syndrome) when one or more specific conditions are met. Use *person living with HIV* or *people who have AIDS.* Do not use *AIDS victim.*
- *Intellectual disability* refers to limitations in intellectual functioning and adaptive behaviors that require environmental or personal supports for the individual to live independently. Although *mental retardation* was previously an accepted clinical term, many consider it an insult, so people who have this condition, their families, and related organizations have campaigned to end its use. Say *people with intellectual disabilities.* Do not use *retarded, mentally retarded,* or *subnormal.*
- *Learning disability* describes a neurologically based condition that may manifest as difficulty learning and using skills in reading (called *dyslexia*), writing (dysgraphia), mathematics (dyscalculia), and other cognitive processes due to differences in how the brain processes information. Individuals with learning disabilities have average or above-average intelligence, and the term does not include a learning problem that is primarily the result of another cause, such as intellectual disabilities or lack of educational opportunity. Say *person with a learning disability.* Do not use *slow learner* or *retarded.*
- *Postpolio syndrome* is a condition that affects some people who have had poliomyelitis (polio) long after recovery from the disease. It is characterized by new muscle weakness, joint and muscle pain, and fatigue. Say *person with postpolio syndrome.* Do not use *polio victim.*
- *Psychiatric disability* refers to a variety of psychological conditions. Say *person with a psychiatric disability or mental illness.* In a clinical context or for medical or legal accuracy, use *schizophrenic, psychotic,* and other diagnostic terms. Note, too, that *bipolar disorder* has replaced *manic depression.* Words such as *crazy, maniac, lunatic, schizo,* and *psycho* are offensive and should never be applied to people with mental health conditions.
- *Seizure* describes an involuntary muscle contraction, a brief impairment, or loss of consciousness resulting from a neurologic condition such as epilepsy or from an acquired brain injury. Say *person with epilepsy* or *teen with a seizure disorder.* The word *convulsion* should be used only for seizures involving contraction of the entire body. Do not use *epileptic, fit, spastic,* or *attacks.*
- *Service animal or service dog* describes a dog that has been individually trained to do work or perform tasks for people with disabilities. In addition to guiding people who are blind, they may alert people who are deaf, pull wheelchairs, alert and protect a person who is having a seizure, remind a person with mental illness to take prescribed medications, or calm a person with posttraumatic stress disorder during an anxiety attack. Miniature horses are also considered service animals under the Americans with Disabilities Act (ADA), although monkeys no longer are. Do not use *seeing eye dog.*
- *Short stature* describes a variety of genetic conditions causing people to grow to less than 4'10" tall. Say *person of short stature,* although some prefer *little people. Dwarfism* is an accepted medical term but should not be used as general terminology. Do not refer to these individuals as *midgets* because of the term's circus sideshow connotations.
- *Speech disability* is a condition in which a person has limited or impaired speech patterns. Use *child who has a speech disability.* For a person without verbal speech capability, say *person without speech.* Do not use *mute* or *dumb.*
- *Spinal cord injury* describes a condition in which there has been permanent damage to the spinal cord, resulting in some degree of paralysis. *Quadriplegia* denotes loss of function in all four extremities, whereas *paraplegia* refers to loss of function in the lower part of the body only; in both cases, the individual might have some function in the affected limbs. Although people with spinal cord injuries often refer to themselves as a para or a quad, communicators should use *person with paraplegia, person who is paralyzed,* or *person with a spinal cord injury.* Don't say *cripple* or *handicapped.*
- *Substance dependence* refers to patterns of substance use that result in significant impairment in at least three life areas (e.g., family, employment, health) over any 12-month period. Although such terms as *alcoholic* and *addict* are medically acceptable, they may be derogatory to some individuals. Acceptable terms are *people who are substance dependent* or *person who is alcohol dependent.* Individuals who have a history of dependence on alcohol and/or drugs and are no longer using a substance may identify themselves as *recovering* or as a *person in recovery.*
- *Survivor* is used by people to affirm their recovery from or conquest of an adverse health condition such as *cancer survivor, burn survivor, brain injury survivor,* or *stroke survivor.* Don't call them victims.

Additional terms related to the Americans with Disabilities Act (ADA):

- *Accessibility:* Describes the degree to which an environment, service, or product allows access by as many people as possible, in particular people with disabilities.
- *Accessibility standards:* A standard is a level of quality accepted as the norm. The principle of accessibility may be mandated in law or treaty and then specified in detail according to international or national regulations, standards, or codes, which may be compulsory or voluntary.
- *Affirmative action:* The proactive recruitment of people with disabilities.
- *Appropriate technology:* Assistive technology that meets people's needs, uses local skills, tools, and materials, and is simple, effective, affordable, and acceptable to its users.
- *Augmentative and alternative communication:* Methods of communicating that supplement or replace speech and handwriting; for example, facial expressions, symbols, pictures, gestures, and signing.
- *Assistive devices; also assistive technology:* Any device designed, made, or adapted to help a person perform a particular task. Products may be specially produced or generally available for people with a disability.
- *Barriers:* Factors in a person's environment that, through their absence or presence, limit functioning and create

disability; for example, inaccessible physical environments, a lack of appropriate assistive technology, and negative attitudes toward disability.

- *Capacity:* A construct within the International Classification of Functioning, Disability and Health (ICF) that indicates the highest probable level of functioning that a person may achieve, measured in a uniform or standard environment: reflects the environmentally adjusted ability of the individual.
- *Communication:* Includes languages, text displays, Braille, tactile communication, large print, and accessible multimedia as well as written, audio, plain-language, human-reader, and augmentative and alternative modes, means, and formats of communication, including accessible information and communication technology. These formats, modes, and means of communication may be physical but are increasingly electronic.
- *Condition—primary:* A person's main health condition that may be associated with impairment and disability.
- *Condition—secondary:* An additional health condition that arises from the increased susceptibility to a condition caused by the primary condition, although it may not occur in every individual with that primary condition.
- *Condition—comorbid:* An additional health condition that is independent of and unrelated to the primary health condition.
- *Disability:* An umbrella term for impairments, activity limitations, and participation restrictions, denoting the negative aspects of the interaction between an individual (with a health condition) and that individual's contextual factors (environmental and personal factors).
- *Disability discrimination:* Any distinction, exclusion, or restriction on the basis of disability that has the purpose or effect of impairing or nullifying the recognition, enjoyment, or exercise on an equal basis with others, of all human rights and fundamental freedoms: includes denial of reasonable accommodation.
- *Disability management:* Interventions and case management strategies used to address the needs of people with disabilities who had the experience of work before the onset of disability. The key elements are often effective case management, supervisor education, workplace accommodation, and early return to work with appropriate supports.
- *Early intervention:* Involves strategies that aim to intervene early in the life of a problem and provide individually tailored solutions. It typically focuses on populations at a higher risk of developing problems or on families that are experiencing problems that have not yet become well established or entrenched.
- *Frail elderly:* Older people (usually over 85 years old) who have a health condition that may interfere with the ability to independently perform activities of daily living.
- *Health:* A state of well-being, achieved through the interaction of an individual's physical, mental, emotional, and social states.
- *Health condition:* Term for disease (acute or chronic), disorder, injury, or trauma. A health condition may also include other circumstances such as pregnancy, ageing, stress, congenital anomaly, or genetic predisposition.
- *Health promotion:* The process of enabling people to increase control over and improve their health.
- *Impairment:* Loss or abnormality in body structure or physiological function (including mental functions), in which abnormality means significant variation from established statistical norms.
- *Inclusive society:* One that freely accommodates any person with a disability without restrictions or limitations.
- *Independent living:* Independent living is a philosophy and a movement of people with disabilities, based on the right to live in the community but including self-determination, equal opportunities, and self-respect.
- *Intellectual impairment:* A state of arrested or incomplete development of mind, which means that the person can have difficulties understanding, learning, and remembering new things, and in applying that learning to new situations. Also known as intellectual disabilities, learning disabilities, and learning difficulties, and formerly known as mental retardation or mental handicap.
- *International Classification of Functioning, Disability and Health (ICF):* The classification that provides a unified and standard language and framework for the description of health and health-related states. ICF is part of the "family" of international classifications developed by WHO.
- *Mental health condition:* A health condition characterized by alterations in thinking, mood, or behavior associated with distress or interference with personal functions. Also known as mental illness, mental disorders, and psychosocial disability.
- *Neurodiversity:* Acceptance and inclusion of all people while embracing neurological differences. People experience and interact with the world around them in many different ways and differences are not viewed as deficits.
- *Physical and rehabilitative medicine doctors:* Conduct services to diagnose health conditions, assess functioning, and prescribe medical and technological interventions that treat health conditions and optimize functional capacity. Also known as physiatrists.
- *Prosthetist, orthotist:* Provides prosthetic and orthotic care and other mobility devices aimed at improving functioning in people with physical impairments. Orthotic care involves external appliances designed to support, straighten, or improve the functioning of a body part; prosthetic interventions involve an artificial external replacement for a body part.
- *Psychologist:* A professional specializing in diagnosing and treating diseases of the brain, emotional disturbance, and behavior problems, more often through therapy than medication.
- *Quality of life:* An individual's perception of their position in life in the context of the culture and value systems in which they live and in relation to their goals, expectations, standards, and concerns. It is a broad-ranging concept, incorporating in a complex way the person's physical health, psychological state, level of independence, social relationships, personal beliefs, and relationship to environmental factors that affect them.
- *Reasonable accommodation:* Necessary and appropriate modification and adjustment not imposing a disproportion-

ate or undue burden, where needed in a particular case, to ensure that persons with disabilities enjoy or exercise, on an equal basis with others, all human rights and fundamental freedoms.

- *Rehabilitation:* A set of measures that assists individuals who experience or are likely to experience disability to achieve and maintain optimal functioning in interaction with their environment.
- *Sign language interpreter:* A person trained to interpret information from sign language into speech and vice versa. Sign languages vary across the world.
- *Specific learning disability:* Impairments in information processing resulting in difficulties in listening, reasoning, speaking, reading, writing, spelling, or doing mathematical calculations—for example, dyslexia.
- *Speech and language therapy:* Aimed at restoring people's capacity to communicate effectively and to swallow safely and efficiently.
- *Universal design:* The design of products, environments, programs, and services to be usable by all people, to the greatest extent possible, without the need for adaptation or specialized design.

Information in this section adapted from World Health Organization: *World report on disability 2011.* Retrieved from: https://www.who.int/docs/default-source/gho-documents/world-health-statistic-reports/en-whs2011-full.pdf.

MENTORING TIP

We commonly are uncomfortable in situations that are new to us. We don't know what to do or what to say. Fortunately, most people are kind and willing to help us understand cultural differences or what it may be like to adapt to some sort of disability. It is helpful to ask others to explain the unfamiliar situation to us. This could be some sort of cultural dress or custom, use of some sort of assistive device or adaptation needed because of size or mobility issues. Practice asking questions that can help you better understand respectful communication and interaction. For example, if someone uses a cane for additional stability when walking, you might say, "I am curious about how the cane helps you move about. I have never used a cane, and I do not know anyone who does. Is there anything specific I may need to understand?"

MEDICAL TERMINOLOGY

SECTION OBJECTIVES

Chapter objective covered in this section:

6. Use medical terminology to identify the three-word elements used in medical terms and to comprehend unfamiliar medical terms.

Using the information presented in this section, the student will be able to:

- Define words by breaking them down into their word elements.
- Use Appendix A to identify indications for and contraindications to massage.
- List and define anatomical and physiological terms by body system.
- Identify pertinent abbreviations used in health care and their meanings.
- List and identify common abbreviations.
- Use relevant anatomical and physiological terminology correctly.

Fundamental Word Elements

Medical terms are made up of a combination of word elements. A word can be interpreted easily by separating it into its elements: *prefix, root word,* and *suffix.*

Prefixes

A **prefix** is a word element placed at the beginning of a word to alter its meaning (Table 4.1). A prefix cannot stand alone; it must be combined with a root word.

Root Words

The **root word** provides the fundamental meaning of a term (Table 4.2). Combinations of root words, prefixes, and suffixes form medical and scientific terms. A vowel, called a *combining vowel,* is often added when two root words are combined or when a suffix is added to a root word; the combining vowel usually is *o* and occasionally is *i.*

Table 4.1 Common Prefixes

Prefix	Meaning	Prefix	Meaning
a-, an-	Without or not	intro-	Into, within
ab-	Away from	leuk-	White
ad-	Toward	macro-	Large
ante-	Before, forward	mal-	Bad, illness, disease
anti-	Against	mega-	Large
auto-	Self	micro-	Small
bi-	Double, two	mono-	One, single
circum-	Around	neo-	New
contra-	Against, opposite	non-	Not
de-	Down, from, away from, not	para-	Abnormal
dia-	Across, through, apart	per-	By, through
dis-	Separation, away from	peri-	Around
dys-	Bad, difficult, abnormal	poly-	Many, much
ecto-	Outer, outside	post-	After, behind
en-	In, into, within	pre-	Before, in front of, prior to
endo-	Inner, inside	pro-	Before, in front of
epi-	Over, on	re-	Again
eryth-	Red	retro-	Backward
ex	Out, out of, from, away from	semi-	Half
hemi-	Half	sub-	Under
hyper-	Excessive, too much, high	super-	Above, over, excess
hypo-	Under, decreased, less than normal	supra-	Above, over
In-	In, into, within, not	trans-	Across
inter-	Between	uni-	One
intra-	Within		

Suffixes

A suffix is a word element placed at the end of a root word to alter the meaning of the word (Table 4.3). Suffixes cannot stand alone; like prefixes, they must accompany a root word. The suffix should be the starting point for interpreting medical terms.

Table 4.2 Common Root Words

Root (Combining Vowel)	Meaning	Root (Combining Vowel)	Meaning
abdomin (o)	Abdomen	neur (o)	Nerve
aden (o)	Gland	ocul (o)	Eye
adren (o)	Adrenal gland	orth (o)	Straight, normal, correct
angi (o)	Vessel	oste (o)	Bone
arterio (o)	Artery	ot (o)	Ear
arthr (o)	Joint	ped (o)	Child, foot
broncho (o)	Bronchus, bronchi	pharyng (o)	Pharynx
card, cardi (o)	Heart	phleb (o)	Vein
cephal (o)	Head	pnea	Breathing, respiration
chondr (o)	Cartilage	pneum (o)	Lung, air, gas
col (o)	Colon	proct (o)	Rectum
cost (o)	Rib	psych (o)	Mind
crani (o)	Skull	pulm (o)	Lung
cyan (o)	Blue	py (o)	Pus
cyst (o)	Bladder, cyst	rect (o)	Rectum
cyt (o)	Cell	rhin (o)	Nose
derma	Skin	sten (o)	Narrow, constriction
duoden (o)	Duodenum	stern (o)	Sternum
encephal (o)	Brain	stomat (o)	Mouth
enter (o)	Intestines	therm (o)	Heat
fibro (o)	Fiber, fibrous	thorac (o)	Chest
gastr (o)	Stomach	thromb (o)	Clot, thrombus
gyn, gyne, gyneco	Female	thyr (o)	Thyroid
hem, hema, hemo, hemat (o)	Blood	toxic (o)	Poison, poisonous
hepat (o)	Liver	trache (o)	Trachea
hydr (o)	Water	ur (o)	Urine, urinary tract, urination
hyster (o)	Uterus	urethr (o)	Urethra
ile (o), ili (o)	Ileum	urin (o)	Urine
laryng (o)	Larynx	uter (o)	Uterus
mamm (o)	Breast, mammary gland	vas (o)	Blood vessel, vas deferens
my (o)	Muscle	ven (o)	Vein
myel (o)	Spinal cord, bone marrow	vertebr (o)	Spine, vertebrae
nephr (o)	Kidney		

Root words that end in a consonant require a combining vowel. If the root word ends in a vowel and the suffix begins with a vowel, the vowel at the end of the root word is deleted.

Combining Word Elements

Word elements are the building blocks that are combined to create medical and scientific terms. Prefixes always precede root words, and suffixes always follow root words (Proficiency Exercise 4.1).

Abbreviations

Abbreviations are shortened forms of words or phrases (Table 4.4). They are used primarily in written communication to save

Table 4.3 Common Suffixes

Suffix	Meaning
-algia	Pain
-asis	Condition, usually abnormal
-cele	Hernia, herniation, pouching
-cyte	Cell
-ectasis	Dilation, stretching
-ectomy	Excision, removal of
-emia	Blood condition
-genesis	Development, production, creation
-genic	Producing, causing
-gram	Record
-graph	Diagram, recording instrument
-graphy	Making a recording
-iasis	Condition of
-ism	Condition
-itis	Inflammation
-logy	Study of
-lysis	Destruction of, decomposition
-megaly	Enlargement
-oma	Tumor
-osis	Condition
-pathy	Disease
-penia	Lack, deficiency
-phasia	Speaking
-phobia	Exaggerated fear
-plasty	Surgical repair or reshaping
-plegia	Paralysis
-rrhage, -rrhagia	Excessive flow
-rrhea	Profuse flow, discharge
-scope	Examination instrument
-scopy	Examination using a scope
-stasis	Maintenance, maintaining a constant level
-stomy, -ostomy	Creation of an opening
-tomy, -otomy	Incision, cutting into
-uria	Condition of the urine

PROFICIENCY EXERCISE 4.1

On a separate piece of paper, combine five words using the prefixes, root words, and suffixes listed in Tables 4.1 to 4.3. Define the words created. Then look up each word in a medical dictionary to verify that it exists and that you have the correct meaning and spelling.

Example

Term: Fibromyalgia

Divided into elements: *Fibro-*, fiber; *my-*, muscle; *algia-*, pain

My definition: pain in muscle fibers

Dictionary definition: diffuse muscle pain

Log onto YouTube and use the search term *medical terminology*. Watch a few videos.

Log onto MedlinePlus and locate the medical encyclopedia. Then view the Videos & Tools tab and explore resources to enhance you learning.

time and space. An extensive list of acceptable medical abbreviations can be found in most medical dictionaries.

When you use abbreviations in any type of record, including charting, provide an abbreviation key either on the forms or in a conspicuous place in the file. This is especially important if you generate a specialized list of abbreviations, such as *SWM* for Swedish massage or *CTM* for connective tissue method.

Abbreviations should not be used excessively. An overabundance of abbreviations results in a passage that is difficult to read and that requires interpretation. If you are unsure whether an abbreviation is acceptable, write out the term to communicate accurately.

Do not use jargon. Jargon consists of word forms specially developed within a system or the use of existing words that have other definitions besides the dictionary meaning. For example, the word *mouse* is computer jargon for a manual device that controls a cursor. Many forms of jargon are used in the bodywork world, a problem that continues to confuse communication. In general, the words used in record keeping should be found in either a standard comprehensive dictionary or in a medical dictionary, and they should represent the definition as listed.

Sometimes jargon becomes understandable within the general community. For the previous example, *mouse,* many readers immediately thought of the computer device rather than a brown, furry creature. This is an example of the way language can change. As massage becomes more generally accepted, much of our language will be standardized and lose its jargon quality. Until then, clarity and concise expression are crucial when choosing the words used for written records.

Terms Related to Diagnosis and Diseases

The massage practitioner must be able to understand medical terms related to diagnosis and various diseases. Two terms related to the diagnosis of a disease that massage professionals often encounter are *indication* and *contraindication.*

- An **indication** is a condition for which an approach would be beneficial for health enhancement, treatment of a particular condition, or support of a treatment modality other than massage.

Table 4.4 Common Abbreviations

Abbreviation	Meaning	Abbreviation	Meaning
Abd	Abdomen	IBW	Ideal body weight
ADL	Activities of daily living	ICT	Inflammation of connective tissue
ad lib	As desired	id	The same
alt dieb	Every other day	L	Left, length, lumbar
alt hor	Alternate hours	lig	Ligament
alt noct	Alternate nights	M	Muscle, meter, myopia
AM (AM, a.m.)	Morning	ML	Midline
AMA	Against medical advice	meds	Medications
ANS	Autonomic nervous system	n	Normal
approx	Approximately	NA	Nonapplicable
as tol	As tolerated	OB	Obstetrics
BM	Bowel movement	OTC	Over the counter
BP	Blood pressure	P	Pulse
Ca	Cancer	PA	Postural analysis
CC	Chief complaint	PM (PM, p.m.)	Afternoon
c/o	Complains of	PT	Physical therapy
CPR	Cardiopulmonary resuscitation	Px	Prognosis
CSF	Cerebrospinal fluid	R	Respiration, right
CVA	Cerebrovascular accident, stroke	R/O	Rule out
DM	Diabetes mellitus	ROM	Range of motion
DJD	Degenerative joint disease	Rx	Prescription
Dx	Diagnosis	SOB	Shortness of breath
Ext	Extract	SP, spir	Spirit
Ft	Foot or feet	Sym	Symmetric
Fx	Fracture	T	Temperature
GI	Gastrointestinal	TLC	Tender loving care
GU	Genitourinary	Tx	Treatment
h (hr)	Hour	URI	Upper respiratory infection
H_2O	Water	WD	Well developed
Hx	History	WN	Well nourished

- A contraindication is a condition or factor that may make an approach harmful. Contraindications may be further subdivided by severity:
- General/absolute avoidance of application: do not massage.
- Regional/local avoidance of application: perform massage but avoid a particular area.
- Application with caution and adaptation, usually requiring supervision from appropriate medical or supervising personnel: perform massage but carefully select the methods to be used, the duration of application, the frequency, and the intensity of the massage.

Terminology of Location and Position

Directional Terms

Directional terms are used to describe the way one body part relates to another. Massage professionals must be able to use directional terminology to describe the location of an area of the body accurately. The directional terms in Fig. 4.2 are used most often.

The abdomen is divided into four quadrants, and the locations of abdominal organs and the abdominal contents are described in terms of the quadrants in which they are found (Fig. 4.3).

Positional Terms

Positional terms are used to describe the relationship of the body to the different planes (Proficiency Exercise 4.2):

PROFICIENCY EXERCISE 4.2

1. Act out each directional and positional term by creating a movement or a pantomime or by assuming the position.
2. With a partner, place each other in the five positions listed in the text. Say each term as you position your partner.

Log onto YouTube and use search terms anatomical directional and positional terms. Watch a few videos.

- *Anatomical position*—The body is erect with the arms hanging at the sides and the palms facing forward.
- *Erect position*—The body is in a standing position.
- *Supine position*—The body is lying in a horizontal position, face up.
- *Prone position*—The body is lying in a horizontal position, face down.
- *Lateral recumbent position*—The body is lying horizontally on either the right or the left side.

BODY STRUCTURE AND BONES, JOINTS, AND MUSCLES

NOTE: This section is supported by comprehensive animations and videos with links found on the Evolve site.

SECTION OBJECTIVES

Chapter objective covered in this section:

7. Define anatomical and physiological terminology for bones, joints, and muscles.

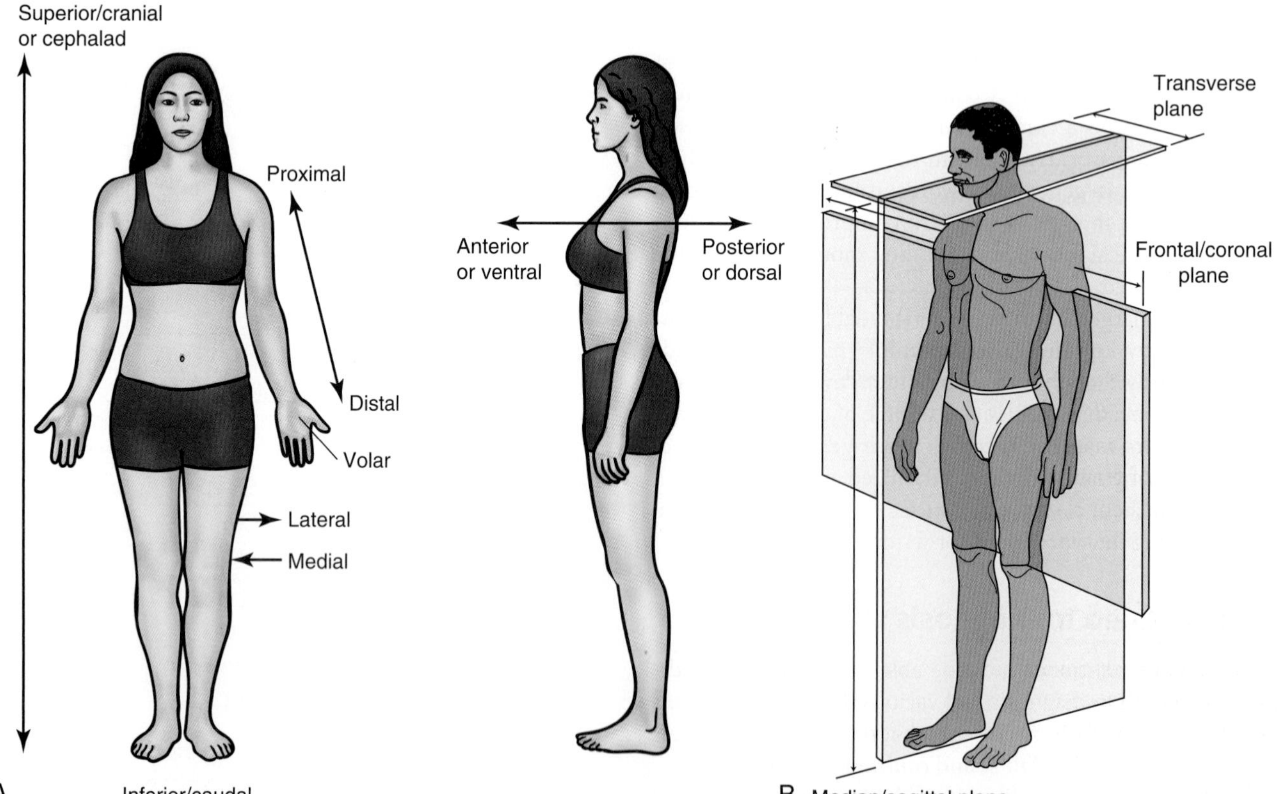

FIG. 4.2 A, Anatomical position as a reference point for directional terms. **B,** Anatomical planes. (From Fritz S. [2020]. *Mosby's Essential Sciences for Therapeutic Massage: Anatomy, Physiology, Biomechanics, and Pathology*. 6th ed. St. Louis: Mosby.)

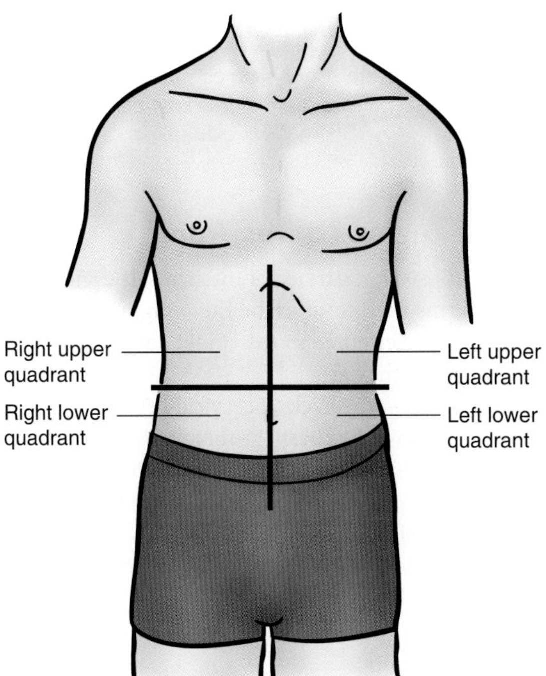

FIG. 4.3 The quadrants of the abdomen. (From Fritz S. [2020]. *Mosby's Essential Sciences for Therapeutic Massage: Anatomy, Physiology, Biomechanics, And Pathology*. 6th ed. Mosby.)

Using the information presented in this section, the student will be able to:

- Define and list the tissues of the body.
- Define the organs and systems of the body.
- Locate the body cavities and regions of the trunk.
- Describe the tissues and structures of the skeletal system.
- Describe the joint structure and function.
- Perform synovial joint movement.
- Identify the structures of skeletal muscle.
- Describe the functions of skeletal muscle.
- Define the actions of skeletal muscles.

Tissues

The structure of the body is composed of tissues. A *tissue* is a collection of specialized cells that perform a special function. *Histo* is a root word meaning "tissue." *Histology* is the study of tissue. The primary tissues of the body are the epithelial, connective, muscular, and nervous tissues (Proficiency Exercise 4.3).

PROFICIENCY EXERCISE 4.3

Using an internet-based medical dictionary/terminology site, medical terminology text, anatomy and physiology textbook, or medical dictionary, look up each of the following tissue types and list its function:
connective:
epithelial:
muscular:
nervous:

Organs and Systems

An *organ* is a collection of specialized tissues. An organ has specific functions, but it does not act independently of other organs.

Organs make up systems. The body as a whole is made up of several systems. Some of the systems are concentrated in a particular part of the body (e.g., the urinary system), whereas others involve all parts of the body (e.g., the circulatory system). The body has 10 general systems (Table 4.5). Each system is made up of organs that collectively perform specific functions. (A more extensive description of these systems can be found in any good anatomy and physiology textbook.)

Body Cavities

The body cavities, which contain the organs, are divided into ventral and dorsal regions (Fig. 4.4). The two dorsal cavities are the cranial cavity and the vertebral cavity. The three ventral cavities are the thoracic, abdominal, and pelvic cavities. Sometimes the abdominal and pelvic cavities are considered one cavity (Proficiency Exercise 4.4).

Table 4.5 Systems of the Body and Their Important Organs

System	Important Organs
Musculoskeletal (can be classified separately as the skeletal, articular [joints], and muscular systems)	Bones, ligaments, skeletal muscles, tendons, joints
Nervous	Brain, spinal cord, nerves, special sense organs
Cardiovascular	Heart, arteries, veins, capillaries
Lymphatic	Lymphatic vessels, lymph nodes, spleen, tonsils, thymus gland
Digestive	Mouth, tongue, teeth, salivary glands, esophagus, stomach, small and large intestines, liver, gallbladder, pancreas
Respiratory	Nasal cavity, larynx, trachea, bronchi, lungs, diaphragm, pharynx
Urinary	Kidneys, ureters, urinary bladder, urethra
Endocrine	Endocrine glands: hypothalamus, hypophysis (pituitary), thyroid, thymus, parathyroid, pineal, adrenal, pancreas, gonads (ovary or testis)
Reproductive	*Female:* ovaries, uterine tubes (oviducts), uterus, vagina *Male:* testes, penis, prostate gland, seminal vesicles, spermatic ducts
Integumentary	Skin: hair, nails, sebaceous glands, sweat glands, breasts

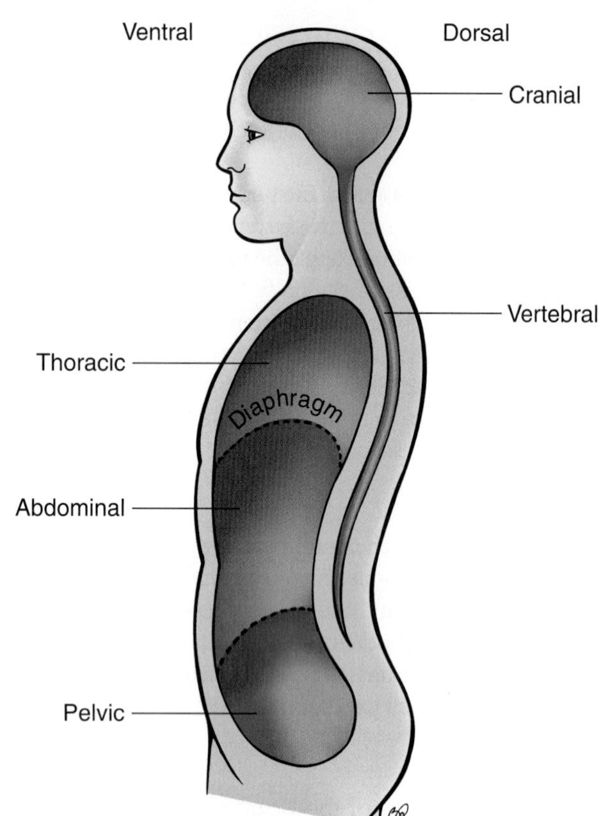

FIG. 4.4 The body cavities.

PROFICIENCY EXERCISE 4.4

Using clay or some other modeling compound, form the body cavities and the organs and structures they contain.

Posterior Regions of the Trunk

The back, or posterior, surface of the trunk is divided into regions. The terms used to describe these regions are related to the names of the vertebrae in the spinal column (Fig. 4.5). In descending order, they are:

- Cervical region—the neck (7 cervical vertebrae)
- Thoracic region—the chest (12 thoracic vertebrae)
- Lumbar region—the loin (5 lumbar vertebrae)
- Sacral region—the sacrum (5 sacral vertebrae, which are fused into one bone)
- Coccyx—the tailbone (4 coccygeal vertebrae, which are fused into one bone)

Skeletal System

The skeletal system is composed of three types of tissue: bone, cartilage, and ligaments.

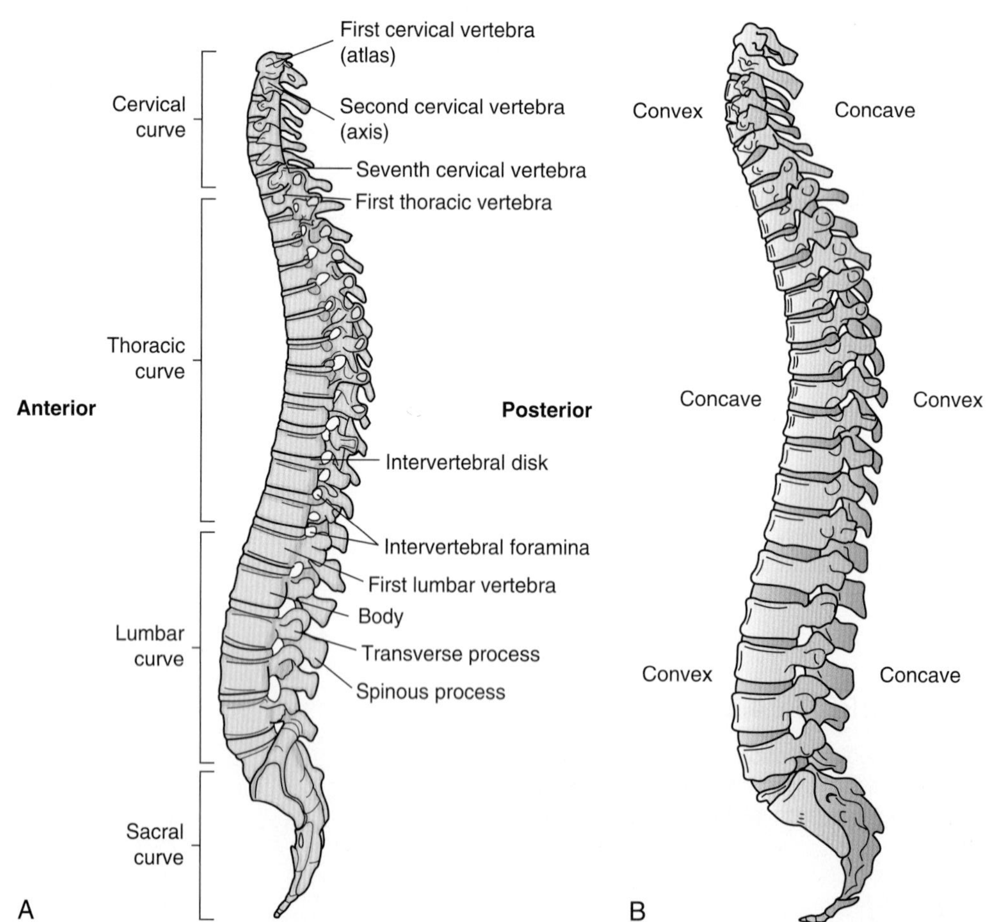

FIG. 4.5 **A,** Vertebral column. **B,** The convex and concave curves of the vertebral column. (From Fritz S. [2020]. *Mosby's Essential Sciences for Therapeutic Massage: Anatomy, Physiology, Biomechanics, and Pathology*. 6th ed. St. Louis: Mosby.)

Bone

Bone is a dense connective tissue composed primarily of calcium and phosphate; *os-*, *ossa-*, *oste-*, and *osteo-* are all combining forms that mean "bone."

The human skeleton is composed of approximately 206 bones, and massage professionals must be familiar with most of them. Terms commonly used for some of these bones include *skull* or *cranium*, *cervical vertebrae*, *thoracic vertebrae*, *lumbar vertebrae*, *sacral vertebrae*, *coccygeal vertebrae*, *ribs*, *sternum*, *manubrium*, *body*, *xiphoid process*, *clavicle*, *scapula*, *humerus*, *ulna*, *radius*, *carpal bones*, *metacarpal bones*, *phalanges*, *pelvis*, *ilium*, *ischium*, *pubis*, *femur*, *patella*, *tibia*, *fibula*, *tarsal bones*, and *metatarsal bones* (see Fig. 4.5; also Fig. 4.6). Other terms related to bones and landmarks on bones are *malleolus*, *process*, *crest*, *insertion*, *joint*, *olecranon*, *origin*, *spine*, *trochanter*, and *tuberosity*.

Cartilage

The skeletal system includes two types of cartilage. *Hyaline cartilage*, which is very elastic, cushiony, and slippery, makes up the articular surfaces at the joints; the cartilage between the ribs and at the nose, larynx, and trachea; and the fetal skeleton. It has a pearly, bluish color. The term *hyaline* means "glass." *White fibrocartilage*, which is elastic, flexible, and tough, is interarticular fibrocartilage found in joints such as the knee. The connecting fibrocartilage is cartilage that is only slightly mobile. It is found between the vertebrae (referred to as *disks*) and between the pubic bones (the symphysis pubis).

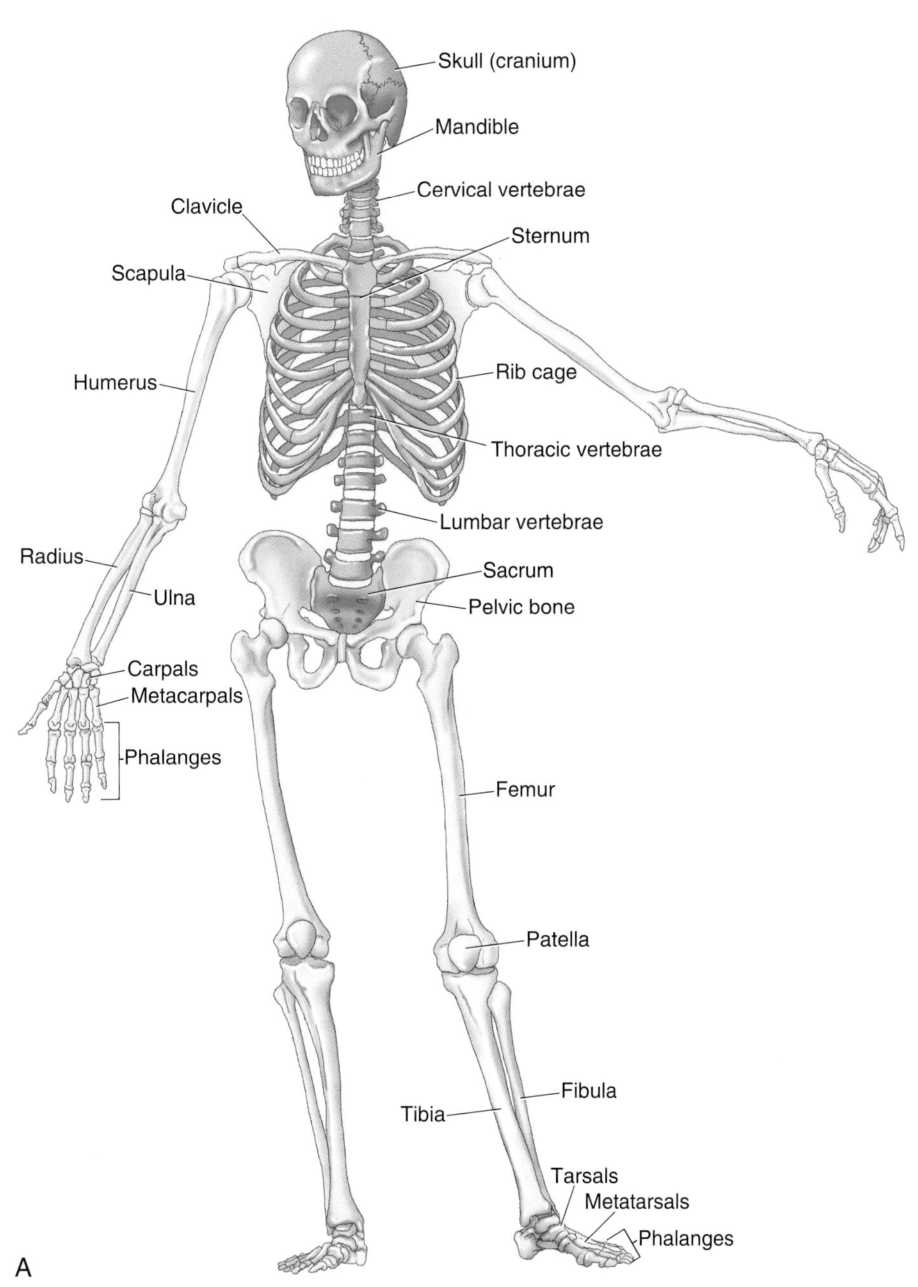

FIG. 4.6 The skeleton. A, Anterior view: axial skeleton *(green)*, appendicular skeleton *(beige)*. **B,** Posterior view: axial skeleton *(green)*, appendicular skeleton *(beige)*. (From Muscolino JE: *Kinesiology: the skeletal system and muscle function, enhanced edition*, St. Louis, 2007, Mosby.)

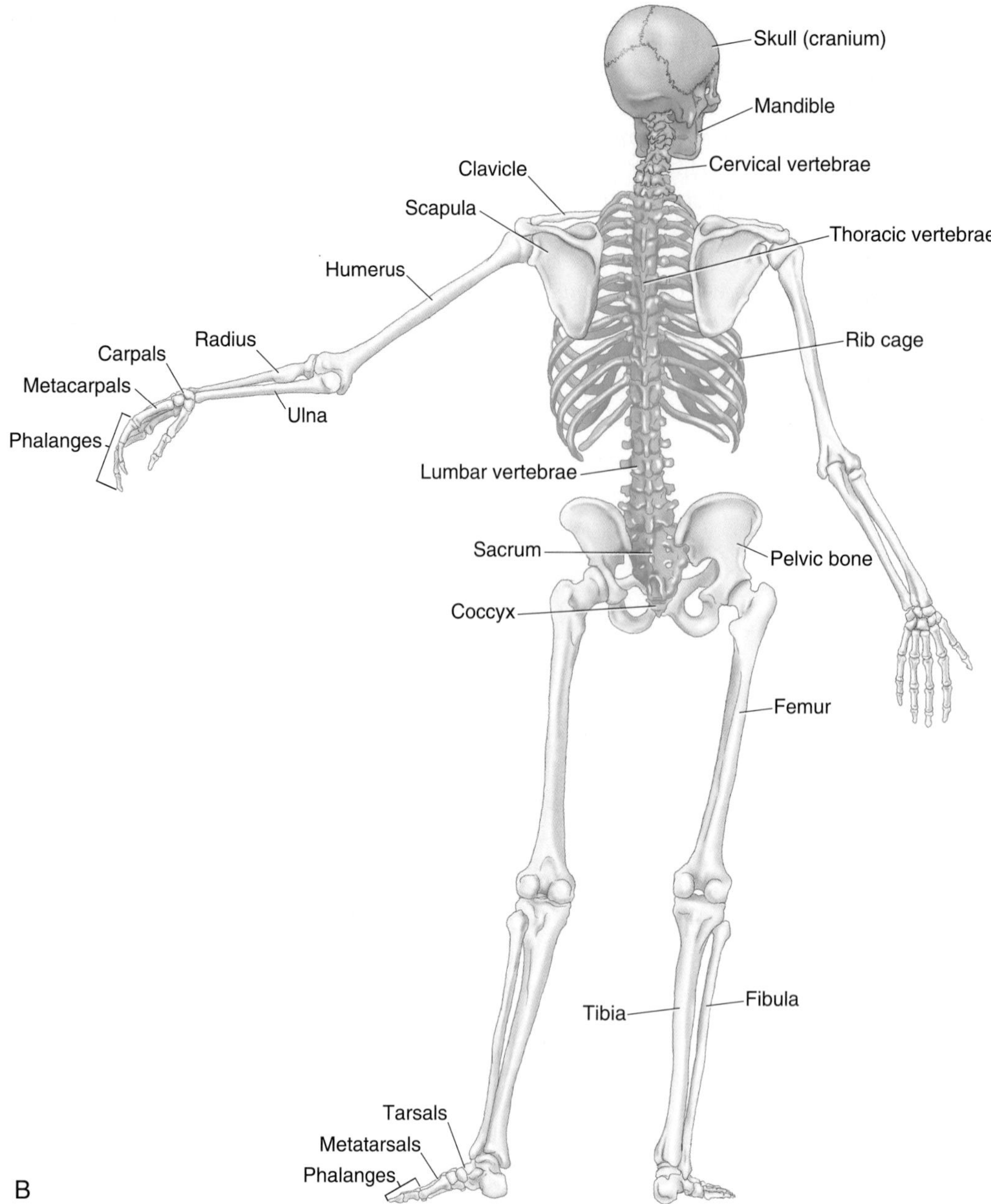

FIG. 4.6, cont'd

Ligaments

A *joint* or an *articulation* is a point where the bones of the skeleton meet. Movable joints are covered by cartilage and are held together by ligaments. Ligaments are made of white fibrous tissue. They are pliant, flexible, strong, and tough (Proficiency Exercise 4.5).

Articular System

As mentioned, articulations are joints where two or more bones meet. The articular system concerns all of the anatomical and functional aspects of the joints.

Joints

Joints are places where bones come together, where limbs are attached, and where the motion of the skeletal system occurs.

PROFICIENCY EXERCISE 4.5

1. Using your medical dictionary or medical terminology text, find the definitions of the following terms:
   ankylosing
   spondylitis
   fracture
   osteoarthritis
   osteochondritis
   osteochondrosis
   osteoporosis
2. Choose one condition from your list and, using Appendix A, note any indications or contraindications for massage.
3. Palpate each bone listed in Fig. 4.5 and say its name.
4. With a group of classmates, assign each person to be a particular bone. By lying on the floor, build the skeleton by having each person assume the proper bone position.

Some joints are rigid, and some allow a great degree of flexibility. The joints allow motion of the musculoskeletal system, bear weight, and hold the skeleton together.

Terms related to the articular system include articulation, flexibility, synarthrodial, amphiarthrodial, diarthrodial, symphysis pubis, sacroiliac, symphysis, articular cartilage, articular disks, ligaments, synovial fluid, and tendon.

Types of Movement Permitted by Diarthrodial Joints

Movement related to joints is described from the standard anatomical position. The types of movement permitted by diarthrodial/synovial (freely movable) joints (Fig. 4.7) include:

- Flexion: movement that reduces the angle of a joint
- Extension: movement that increases the angle of a joint
- Abduction: movement away from *(ab-)* the midline
- Adduction: movement toward *(ad-)* the midline
- Pronation: turning of the palm downward
- Supination: turning of the palm upward (you can hold a bowl of soup in a supinated hand)
- Eversion: turning *(-version)* of the sole of the foot away from *(e-)* the midline (when you evert your foot, you move your little toe toward your ear)
- Inversion: turning *(-version)* of the sole of the foot inward *(in-)*
- Plantar flexion: movement of the plantar surface of the sole of the foot downward (plant your toes in the ground)
- Dorsiflexion: movement of the top or dorsal surface of the foot toward the shin
- Rotation: rolling to the side (internal/medial rotation is rolling toward the midline; external/lateral rotation is rolling away from the midline)
- Circumduction: making a cone; the ability to move the limb in a circular manner
- Protraction: thrusting a part of the body forward *(pro-)*
- Retraction: pulling a part of the body backward *(re-)*
- Elevation: raising a part of the body
- Depression: lowering a part of the body
- Opposition: placing one part of the body opposite another, as in placing the tip of the thumb opposite the tips of the fingers

Bursae

A *bursa* is a closed sac or saclike structure. *Bursae* usually are found close to joint cavities. The lining of bursae often is similar to the synovial membrane lining of a true joint. Some bursae are continuous with the lining of a joint. The function of a bursa is to lubricate an area between skin, tendons, ligaments, or other structures and bones where friction otherwise would develop (Proficiency Exercise 4.6).

Muscular System

The muscular system is made up of contractile tissues. The three types of muscle tissue are cardiac muscle, smooth muscle, and skeletal muscle.

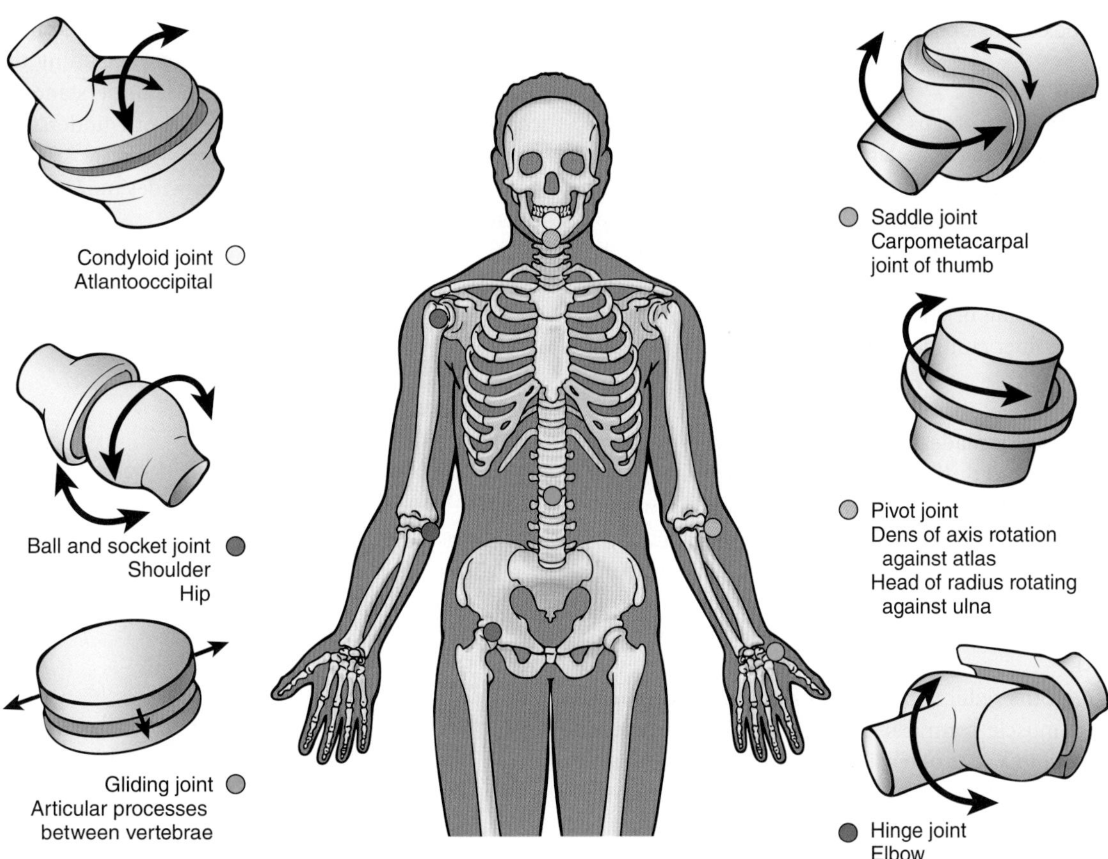

FIG. 4.7 Types of diarthrodial/synovial joints.

PROFICIENCY EXERCISE 4.6

1. Using your medical dictionary or medical terminology text, find the definitions of the following terms and write them down on a separate sheet of paper:
   ankylosis
   arthritis
   bursitis
   degenerative joint disease
   diastasis
   dislocation
   ganglion
   cyst
   genu valgum
   genu varum
   gout
   hallux
   malleus
   kyphosis
   lordosis
   rheumatoid arthritis
   osteoarthritis
   scoliosis
   slipped disk
   bulging disk
   herniate disk
   spinal curvature
   spondylolisthesis
   sprain
   subluxation
   tendinitis
   tenosynovitis
2. Choose one condition from your list and, using Appendix A, note any indications or contraindications for massage.

Many of the body's organs contain muscle tissue. Muscle tissue also makes up the muscles, which are themselves organs. Muscles give the body shape and produce movement. Muscle function is determined by the shape and location of the muscle and by the density and pliability of all the fluid, fibers, and connective tissue of the muscles. The nervous system also controls how long or short a muscle is by regulating the degree of muscle fiber contraction; this is called **muscle tone**.

Skeletal Muscle

Each skeletal muscle is made up of sections. Most muscles have two ends (proximal and distal), which are attached to other structures, and a belly. Muscles create the potential for motion by creating a pulling force. Joints allow motion to occur.

Muscles cause and permit motion by the actions of contraction and relaxation. Table 4.6 presents a list of terms used to describe the movements of different types of muscles (Fig. 4.8).

Contraction is the reduction in size or shortening of a muscle. When one muscle contracts, another, opposite muscle is stretched and put in a state of tension. *Relaxation* occurs when tension is reduced, which allows the muscle to return to its resting length.

Muscles work in pairs of agonists and antagonists. *Agonists* are muscles responsible for the primary desired movement.

Table 4.6 Terms for Describing Muscle Movement

Term	Definition
Adductor	Muscle that moves a part toward the midline
Abductor	Muscle that moves a part away from the midline
Flexor	Muscle that bends a part
Extensor	Muscle that straightens a part
Levator	Muscle that raises a part
Depressor	Muscle that lowers a part
Tensor	Muscle that tightens a part

The agonist is the prime mover, which shortens to produce movement. *Antagonists* are the muscles that oppose the action of the agonist and lengthen and control the movement produced by the agonist.

Synergists are muscles that assist the agonists by holding a part of the body steady, thereby providing leverage. In some cases, synergists also produce the same action as the prime mover.

The agonist-antagonist-synergist relationship permits the skeletal muscles to work in a purposeful manner and gives fluidity to motion. This fluid movement is called *coordination.*

Terms related to the muscular system include aponeurosis, asthenia, atrophy, belly, clonus, contracture, cramp, concentric, eccentric, fascia, fascicle, fasciculation, hyperkinesia, hypertrophy, insertion, isometric contraction, musculotendinous junction, myalgia, origin, proximal attachment, distal attachment, spasm, tendon, and tone.

The names of muscles can be broken down into the word elements of medical terminology (Table 4.7). The name of a muscle can reflect a variety of factors, including the muscle's location, function, and shape. A basic understanding of medical terminology can help learners both understand and remember muscle names (Proficiency Exercise 4.7). Appendix B Muscle Quick Reference Guide provides more information on muscles.

BODY SYSTEMS: NERVOUS, CARDIOVASCULAR, LYMPHATIC, AND IMMUNE SYSTEMS

SECTION OBJECTIVES

Chapter objective covered in this section:

8. Define anatomical and physiological terminology for the nervous, cardiovascular, lymphatic, and immune systems.

Using the information presented in this section, the student will be able to:

- Define the three basic divisions of the nervous system.
- Describe proprioception and list proprioceptors.
- Define reflexes.
- Describe the function of the nervous system.
- List and define the structures of the cardiovascular system.
- Explain blood pressure.
- Describe the functions of the lymphatic system.
- List and describe the structures of the lymphatic system.
- Locate the lymph plexuses.
- Explain the main function of the immune system.
- Define immunity.

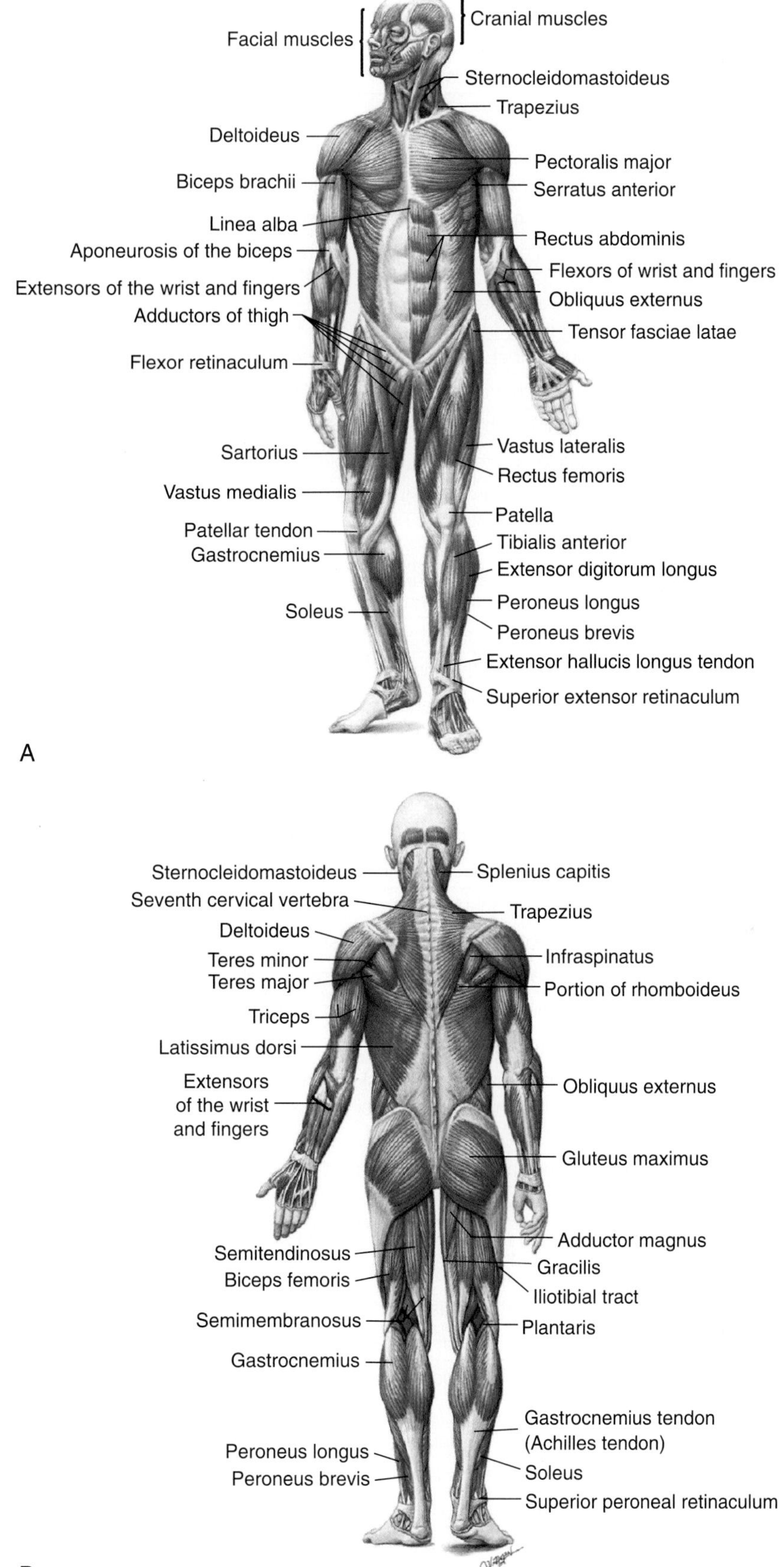

FIG. 4.8 The muscular system. A, Anterior view. **B,** Posterior view. (From LaFleur Brooks M. [2002]. *Exploring Medical Language: a Learner-Directed Approach.* 5th ed. St. Louis: Mosby.)

Table 4.7 Muscle Descriptions Using Medical Word Elements

The muscles listed have been chosen because their names are made up of common word elements. After learning this list, the learner should be able to figure out the meaning of muscle names not listed.

Muscle	Description
Abductor digiti minimi pedis	Little (minimi) muscle that moves the little toe (digit) away from (abductor) the midline of the foot (pedis)
Adductor longus	Long muscle that moves the leg toward (adductor) the midline
Adductor magnus	Large (magnus) muscle that moves the leg toward (adductor) the midline
Biceps brachii	Muscle with two (bi-) heads (ceps) in the arm (brachii)
Deltoid	Triangular (deltoid) muscle of the shoulder
Dilatator naris posterior	Muscle of the nose (naris) that opens (dilator) the back (posterior) portion of the nostril
Extensor hallucis longus	Long (longus) muscle that extends (extensor) the great toe (hallucis)
Extensor pollicis brevis	Short (brevis) muscle that extends (extensor) the thumb (pollicis)
External oblique	Outermost (external) muscle that extends at an angle (oblique) from the ribs to the pelvis at the iliac crest
Flexor carpi radialis	Muscle that flexes (flexor) the wrist (carpi) toward the radius (radialis)
Flexor carpi ulnaris	Muscle attached to the ulna (ulnaris) that flexes (flexor) the wrist (carpi) and hand
Frontalis	Muscle over the frontal bone
Gastrocnemius	Muscle that makes up the belly (gastroc) of the lower leg (nemius)
Gluteus maximus	Largest (maximus) muscle of the buttocks (gluteus)
Gluteus medius	Muscle of the buttocks (gluteus) that lies in the middle (medius) between the other gluteal muscles
Gracilis	Slender (gracilis) muscle of the thigh
Iliopsoas	Muscle that is formed from the iliacus and psoas major muscles; the iliacus extends from the iliac bone (iliacus), and the psoas major is the large (major) muscle of the loin (psoas)
Latissimus dorsi	Broadest (latissimus) muscle of the back (dorsi)
Masseter	Muscle of chewing (masseter) or mastication
Orbicularis oculi and oris	Muscles circling (orbicularis) the eye (oculi) or mouth (oris)
Palmaris longus	Long (longus) muscle of the palm (palmaris)
Pectineus	Muscle of the pubic (pectineus) bone
Pectoralis major	Large (major) muscle of the chest (pectoralis)
Peroneus longus	Long (longus) muscle attached to the fibula (peroneus)
Plantaris	Muscle that flexes the foot (plantaris) and leg
Pronator teres	Long round (teres) muscle that turns the palm downward into a prone (pronator) position
Rectus abdominis	Muscle that extends in a straight (rectus) line upward across the abdomen (abdominis); the center border of the left and right rectus abdominis muscles in the linea alba or the white (alba) line (linea) at the midline of the abdomen
Rectus femoris	Part of the quadriceps muscle that is straight (rectus) and lies near the femur (femoris)
Sartorius	Muscle of the leg that enables a person to sit in a cross-legged tailor's (sartorial) position
Semimembranosus	Muscle made up partly (semi-) of membranous tissue; part of the hamstring group
Semitendinosus	Muscle made up partly (semi-) of tendinous tissue; this is one of the hamstring muscles
Serratus anterior	Sawtooth-shaped (serratus) muscle in front of (anterior) the shoulder and rib cage
Soleus	Muscle that resembles a flat fish (sole) located in the calf of the leg
Sternocleidomastoid	Muscle attached to the breastbone (sterno), the collarbone (cleido), and the mastoid (mastoid) process of the temporal bone
Temporalis	Muscle over the temporal (temporalis) bone
Tensor fascia lata	Muscle that tenses (tensor) the fascia of the thigh (lata)
Teres minor	Small (minor) round (teres) muscle that moves the arm
Tibialis anterior	Muscle in front (anterior) of the tibia (tibialis)
Trapezius	Four-sided, trapezoid-shaped (trapezius) muscle of the shoulder
Triceps brachii	Three- (tri-) headed (ceps) muscle of the arm (brachii)
Vastus lateralis, medialis, intermedialis	Large (vastus) lateral (lateralis), toward the midline (medialis), and middle (intermedialis) muscles of the quadriceps muscle group; the quadriceps has four (quadri-) heads (ceps)

PROFICIENCY EXERCISE 4.7

1. Use Appendix B or locate a more complete list of muscles in your anatomy and physiology textbook or medical dictionary. Break down five muscle names not listed in this section into their word elements. (You will need a medical terminology book or medical dictionary or both to complete this exercise.)
2. Example: Auricularis superior: Aur- means ear; ar- means pertaining to; superior means above or upward.
   a.
   b.
   c.
   d.
   e.
3. An excellent way to remember the names of muscles is to make up ridiculous sentences that explain listed muscle names. The crazier these sentences are, the better you will remember them. Use this memory aid as you study muscles in your anatomy and physiology classes.

Examples

Rectus femoris: Part of the quadriceps muscle that is straight (rectus) and lies near the femur (femoris)

Memory aid: Attention rectus! Straighten up, and the other three of you in the quads head out to the femur.

Flexor carpi ulnaris: Muscle that flexes (flexor) the wrist (carpi) and hand and is attached to the ulna (ulnaris).

Memory aid: Help! There is a big carp pulling my wrist into flexion. It has my ulna in its mouth and my hand has it around the gills.

Log on to YouTube and, using search terms anatomy and physiology, identify videos you can use to study about the body.

Nervous System

The nervous system is the most complex system in the body. The information presented here on the workings of this system is very general, although the text expands on it where needed. Study of the nervous system is important for the massage professional. Serious learners of massage challenge themselves to study the nervous system in depth.

For purposes of study, terms related to the nervous system are presented in three groups:

- The central nervous system (CNS)
- The peripheral nervous system (PNS)
- The autonomic nervous system (ANS)

Central Nervous System

The CNS is the center *(central)* of all nervous control. It consists of the brain and spinal cord, which are located in the dorsal cavity (cranial and vertebral).

Peripheral Nervous System

The PNS is composed of cranial and spinal nerves. The term *nerve* refers to a bundle of nerve fibers consisting of individual nerve cells outside the spinal cord or brain. The PNS consists of the nerves that carry impulses between the CNS and muscles, glands, skin, and other organs located outside (peripheral) the CNS. The ANS is the part of the peripheral nervous system that exerts nervous control over smooth muscle, heart muscle, and glands. Individual nerve cells are called neurons. The two types of nerve cells are the sensory neurons and the motor neurons.

Spinal Nerves

The 31 pairs of spinal nerves are attached to the spinal cord along almost its entire length. They are named for the region of the spinal column through which they exit. Many of the spinal nerves are located in groups called *somatic nerve plexuses.* The term *somatic* refers to the body wall; these nerve plexuses contain nerves that are involved with the wall of the body rather than the organs in the body. A *plexus* is a network of intertwined (plexus) nerves. The major plexuses of spinal nerves are the cervical plexus, brachial plexus, lumbar plexus, and sacral plexus.

Autonomic Nervous System

The ANS is an automatic, or self-governing (self *[auto],* governing *[nomic]*), system. It also is called the *involuntary system* because the effects of the ANS are not usually under voluntary control. The ANS is divided in two parts: the sympathetic division and the parasympathetic division.

The sympathetic division controls the body's response to feelings *(sympath).* Because the nerves in this division come off the thoracic and lumbar segments of the spinal cord, the sympathetic division sometimes is called the *thoracolumbar division.* Actions resulting from these nerves include the fight-or-flight and fear responses. The reaction of some organs includes an increase in the heart rate, dilation of the pupils, and an increase in adrenaline secretion. A person may sometimes exhibit great strength as a result of a sympathetic response.

The nerves in the parasympathetic division come off the cranial and sacral segments of the spinal cord; therefore this division sometimes is called the *craniosacral division.* The parasympathetic division generally causes effects opposite *(para-)* those caused by the sympathetic system. These effects include constriction of the pupils, the return of the heart rate to normal, and stimulation of the lacrimal glands to produce tears.

The intertwined *(plexus)* nerves of the ANS are called the *autonomic plexuses.* Examples of these are the cardiac plexus (the intertwined nerves of the heart *[cardiac]*) and the celiac plexus (the intertwined nerves of the organs of the abdomen *[celiac]*). The celiac plexus sometimes is called the *solar plexus* because of the sunray *(solar)* fashion in which the nerves exit the plexus.

Proprioception

Proprioception is the kinesthetic sense. Sensory receptors receive information about position, rate of movement, contraction, tension, and stretch of tissues through distortion of and pressure on the sensory receptor. After proprioceptive sensory information is processed in the CNS, motor impulses carry the response message back to the muscles. The muscles then contract or relax to restore or change posture, movement, or position. Proprioception helps maintain tone in muscle.

Terms related to proprioception include *mechanoreceptor, Golgi tendon organ, joint kinesthetic receptors, kinesthetic,* and *muscle spindle cells.*

Reflex

A *reflex* is an involuntary body response to a stimulus. Important reflexes stimulated by massage are crossed-extension, extensor thrust, flexor withdrawal, gait, intersegmental, monosynaptic, nociceptive, optical righting, ocular pelvic, pilomotor, psychogalvanic, postural, proprioceptive, righting, startle, stretch, tendon, tonic neck, vasomotor, and visceromotor reflexes.

Function of the Nervous System

The function of the nervous system is to receive impressions from the external environment, organize the information, and provide appropriate responses. In other words, the nervous system allows the body to react to outside influences (environment). Outside information enters the nervous system through nerve endings in the skin and in special sense organs. These nerve endings are referred to as *receptors.*

Nerve endings in the skin are sensitive to touch, pressure, vibration, and temperature. Special sense nerve endings are responsible for taste, smell, vision, hearing, and sense of position and movement. Sensations from the environment are picked up by these receptors and sent to the CNS by way of the PNS. The CNS sorts out the information and sends back a message, again by way of the PNS. Information is transferred from one nerve to another by chemicals called *neurotransmitters.*

The nervous system and neurotransmitters, along with the endocrine system, also maintain the internal environment, or the balance of the many activities in the body (homeostasis). Although the divisions of the nervous system may be treated independently, they do not function independently (Fig. 4.9).

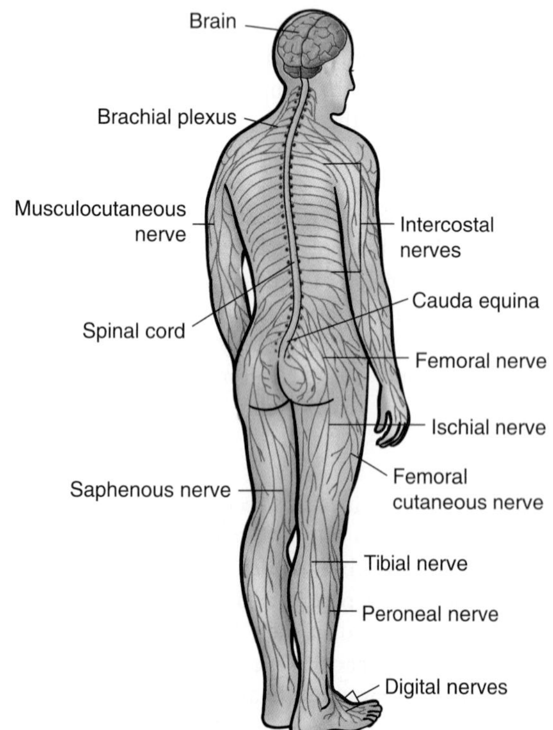

FIG. 4.9 A simplified view of the nervous system. (Modified from LaFleur Brooks M. [2002]. *Exploring Medical Language: A Learner-Directed Approach.* 5th ed. St. Louis: Mosby.)

Terms Related to Nerves

Afferent nerves are nerves that carry *(ferent)* messages to (*af-*, variation of *ad-*) the CNS; they also are known as *sensory nerves* because they pick up and transmit sensation *(sen)* (Proficiency Exercise 4.8).

Efferent nerves are nerves that carry *(ferent)* messages away from (*ef-*, variation of *ex-*) the brain, resulting in motion *(motor).* They also are known as *motor nerves.*

Cranial nerves are the 12 pairs of nerves that arise from the brainstem in the cranium or skull *(cranial).*

Spinal nerves are the 31 pairs of nerves that branch off the spinal cord.

A *ganglion* is a mass of nerve cell bodies located outside the CNS (the plural form is *ganglia*). *Neuro* is the root word meaning "nerve."

Neuroglial cells, also called *glial cells,* or *glia* (glia means glue). Different types of neuroglia in the CNS and PNS play roles in supporting the activity of neurons.

Cardiovascular System

The cardiovascular system consists of two parts, the heart, and the blood vessels (Fig. 4.10). The *heart* is a four-chambered pump. *Arteries* are tubes (vessels) that deliver oxygenated blood to the body. They carry blood under pressure and are located relatively deep in the body. *Veins* are vessels that return the blood to the heart. They are located in more superficial areas and therefore are easier to palpate. Veins have a valve system that prevents the backflow of blood. Breakdown of a valve may result in a varicose vein. *Capillaries* are very small, thin vessels (usually one cell thick) that allow the exchange of blood gasses and nutrients. Blood vessels *vasoconstrict* (become smaller inside) and *vasodilate* (become larger inside).

Blood pressure is a measurement of the pressure exerted by the circulating volume of blood on the walls of the arteries, veins, and heart chambers. Blood pressure is maintained by the complex interaction of the homeostatic mechanisms of the body. Normal blood pressure varies according to age, size,

PROFICIENCY EXERCISE **4.8**

1. On a separate piece of paper, list five of the disease conditions of the nervous system described in the indications and contraindications section in Appendix A.
2. Choose one condition from your list and, using Appendix A, note any indications or contraindications for massage.
3. Choose one of the reflexes and look it up in a medical dictionary. Define the term and then write down how you think that reflex is implicated during massage.

Example

Reflex: Psychogalvanic

Definition: *Psycho-* relates to the mind and *galvanic* pertains to electricity.

Implication: This reflex involves changes in electrical activity in the body connected with mind processes or thoughts. In the galvanic skin response, changes in electrical activity are related to the activity of the sweat glands. Massage stimulates both the skin and electrical activity in the body, which in turn may influence the mind.

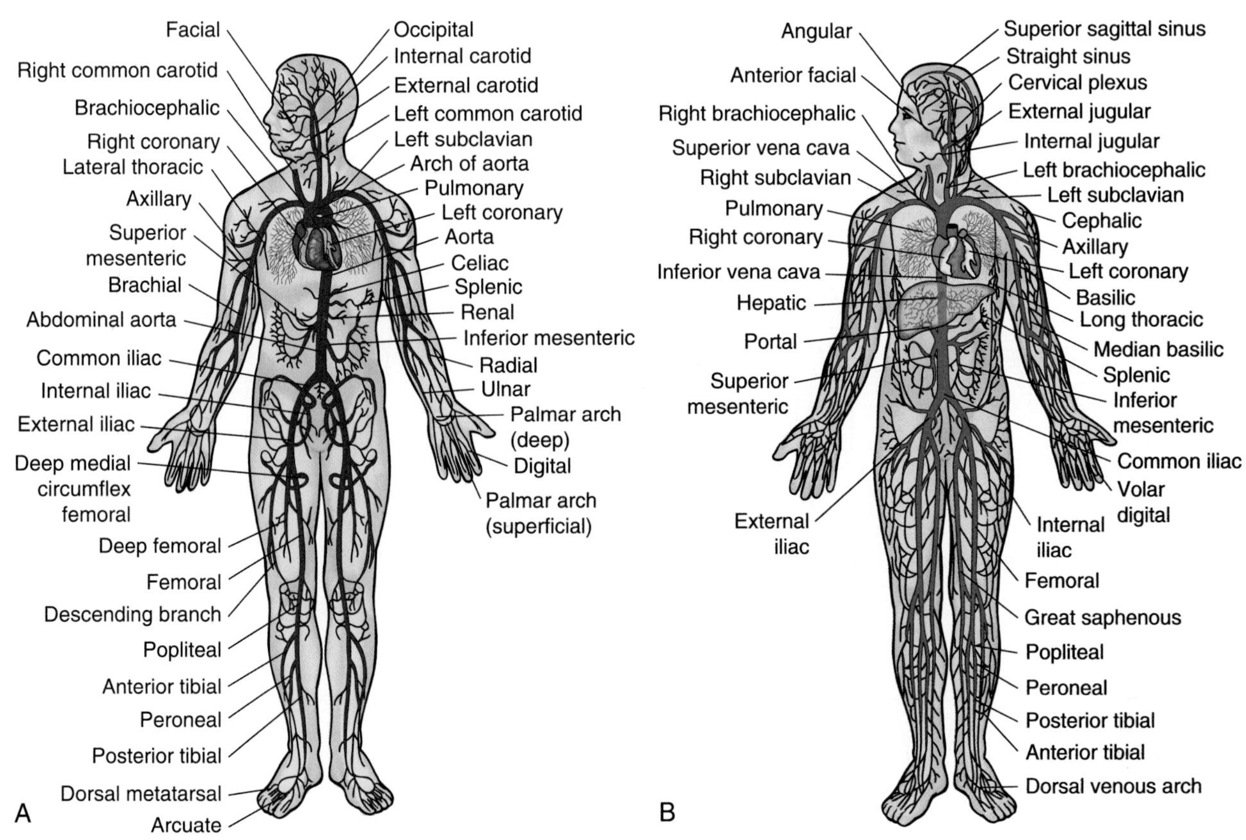

FIG. 4.10 The systemic circulation. A, Arteries. **B,** Veins. (Modified from Seidel HM, et al. [2003]. *Mosby's Guide to Physical Examination.* 5th ed. St. Louis: Mosby.)

and gender, but the average is approximately 120 mm Hg during systole and 70 mm Hg in diastole. High blood pressure is called *hypertension*, and low blood pressure is called *hypotension*.

Blood is composed of blood cells, platelets, and a clear, yellow fluid called *plasma*. The main functions of blood are to transport oxygen and nutrients to the cells and to remove carbon dioxide and other waste products. The amount of blood in muscle tissue influences the muscle tone. If muscle tissue contains too much blood, it is said to be *congested,* and methods to encourage blood flow are used.

Terms and combining forms that relate to the cardiovascular system include *angio-*, *artery*, *arteriole*, *blood pressure*, *bruise*, *capillary*, *edema*, *phleb-*, *vasoconstriction*, *vasodilation*, *vein*, and *venule* (Proficiency Exercise 4.9).

PROFICIENCY EXERCISE 4.9

1. List five of the disease conditions of the cardiovascular system described in the indications and contraindications section in Appendix A.
2. Choose one condition from your list and, using Appendix A, note any indications or contraindications for massage.
3. Look up the medication classification *anticoagulant* in a pharmacology reference text or online. List the contraindications and side effects of these medications. Also describe possible contraindications to massage for a client or patient taking an anticoagulant medication.
4. Choose a partner and draw the major arteries and veins on the body with washable markers. Target those on the arms and legs. Use red for arteries and blue for veins. Note that you can almost trace the veins because they are located near the surface of the body.

Lymphatic System

The lymphatic system is responsible for several functions; for example, it:

- Returns vital substances, such as plasma protein, to the bloodstream from the tissues of the body. The fluid around the cells in tissues is called *interstitial fluid*
- Helps maintain fluid balance by draining fluid from body tissues
- Aids the body's defense against disease-producing substances
- Aids the absorption of fats from the digestive system

The lymphatic system is a network of channels and nodes in which a substance called *lymph* travels (Fig. 4.11). Lymph is a clear, watery fluid similar to plasma. The system collects and drains fluid from around tissue cells from different areas of the body and carries it through the lymphatic channels back to the venous system. There it is deposited, mixed with venous blood, and recirculated.

Lymphatic capillaries are found near and parallel to the veins that carry blood to the heart. The ends of the lymphatic capillaries meet to form larger lymph vessels. The lymph vessels in the right chest, head, and right arm join the right

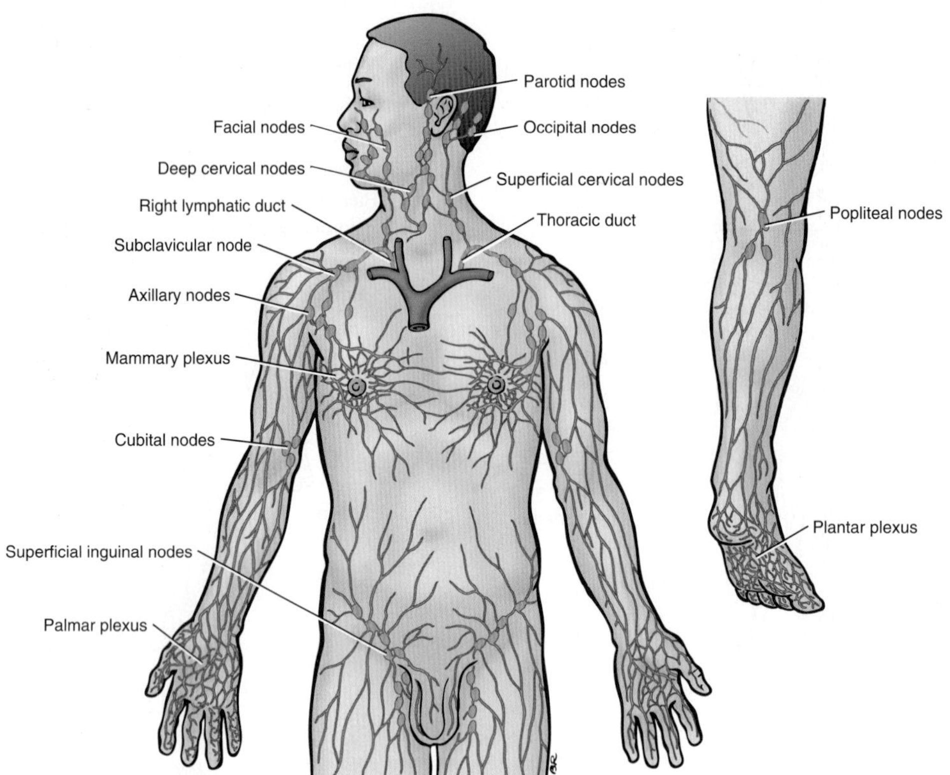

FIG. 4.11 The principal lymph vessels and nodes.

lymphatic duct, which drains into the right subclavian vein. The lymph vessels from all other parts of the body join to meet the thoracic duct, which drains into the left subclavian vein.

Lymph nodes are distributed throughout the lymphatic system (Table 4.8). Lymph nodes are small bodies present in the path of the lymph channels that function as filters for lymph before it returns to the bloodstream. The main locations of the more superficial lymph nodes are the cervical area, axillary region, and groin or inguinal area.

Plexuses of lymph channels are found throughout the body. They include the:

- Mammary plexus (lymphatic vessels around the breasts)
- Palmar plexus (lymphatic vessels in the palm *[palmar]* of the hand)
- Plantar plexus (lymphatic vessels in the sole *[plantar]* of the foot)

If soft tissue has too much interstitial fluid around the cells or if the lymph vessels are full of fluid that is moving slowly or is stagnant, the tissue is said to be *infused* or *edematous.* Excess fluid in muscle tissue contributes to problems with muscle tone.

Immune System

The human body is able to resist organisms or toxins that tend to damage its tissues and organs. This ability is called *immunity* (Table 4.9). As a massage professional, you should explore the immune system in much greater depth. Use your anatomy and physiology textbook as a place to begin, but do not stop there. Exciting new research is being published in professional journals and is available on PubMed (Proficiency Exercise 4.10).

Table 4.8 Types of Lymph Nodes

Nodes	Description
Parotid	Nodes around (para-) or in front of the ear (otid)
Occipital	Nodes over the occipital bone at the back of the head
Superficial cervical	Nodes close to the surface (superficial) of the neck (cervic)
Subclavicular	Nodes under (sub-) the collarbone (clavicular)
Hypogastric	Nodes in the area beneath (hypo-) the stomach (gastric)
Facial	Nodes draining the tissue in the face
Deep cervical	Deeply (deep) situated nodes in the neck (cervic)
Axillary (superficial)	Nodes in the armpit (axilla)
Mediastinal	Nodes in the mediastinal section of the thoracic cavity
Cubital	Nodes of the elbow (cubit)
Para-aortic	Nodes around (para-) the aorta (aortic)
Deep inguinal	Deeply (deep) situated nodes in the groin (inguin)
Superficial inguinal	Nodes in the groin (inguin) close to the surface (superficial)
Popliteal	Nodes in back of the knee (popliteal)

Table 4.9 Selected Terms Related to Immunity

Term	Meaning
Acquired immunity	Resistance (immunity) to a particular disease developed by people who have acquired the disease
Acquired immunodeficiency	A group of symptoms (syndrome) caused by the transmission (acquired) of a virus that causes a breakdown (deficiency) of the immune system (AIDS)
Active immunity	Resistance (immunity) in which the antibodies produced by the body currently exist
Allergy	A state of hypersensitivity to a particular substance; the immune system overreacts (over [hyper-], reacts [sensitive]) to foreign substances, and physical changes occur
Antigen	A substance that stimulates the immune response
Susceptible	An individual who is capable (-ible) of acquiring (suscept) a particular disease

PROFICIENCY EXERCISE 4.10

1. List five of the disease conditions of the lymphatic and immune systems described in the indications and contraindications section in Appendix A.
   a.
   b.
   c.
   d.
   e.
2. Choose one condition from your list and, using Appendix A, note any indications or contraindications for massage.
   Condition:
   Indications or contraindications:

BODY SYSTEMS: RESPIRATORY, DIGESTIVE, ENDOCRINE, AND INTEGUMENTARY SYSTEMS

Note: This section is supported by comprehensive video animations found on the Evolve site.

SECTION OBJECTIVES

Chapter objective covered in this section:

9. Define anatomical and physiological terminology for the respiratory, digestive, endocrine, and integumentary systems.

Using the information presented in this section, the student will be able to:

- Describe the function of the respiratory system.
- Explain the phases of respiration.
- Describe the structures and functions of the digestive system.
- Define the endocrine system.
- List the structures of the integumentary system.
- Describe each of the three tissue layers of the skin.
- Define sebaceous and sweat glands.
- Explain the importance of studying medical terminology.

Respiratory System

The respiratory system supplies oxygen to and removes carbon dioxide from the cells of the body (Fig. 4.12). Respiration is divided into two phases, external respiration, and internal respiration. *External respiration* involves the absorption of oxygen from the air by the lungs and the transport of carbon dioxide from the lungs back into the air. *Internal respiration* involves the exchange of oxygen and carbon dioxide in the cells of the body. The mechanisms of breathing and their relationship to massage are discussed in later chapters.

Terms and combining forms related to the respiratory system include *alveoli*, *lungs*, *nares*, *nostrils*, *olfactory cells*, *pneumo-*, *rhino-*, and *trachea* (Proficiency Exercise 4.11).

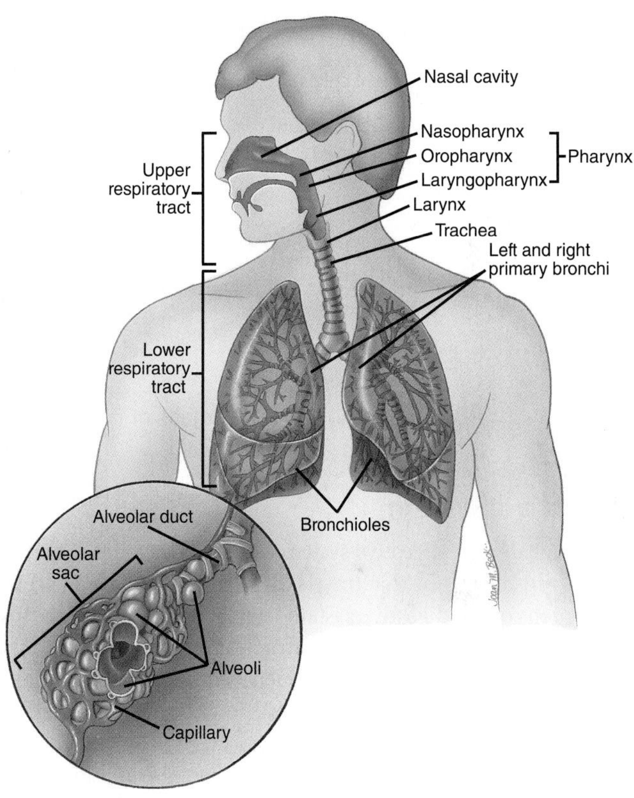

FIG. 4.12 The structural plan of the respiratory system. *Inset,* The alveolar sacs, where oxygen and carbon dioxide are exchanged through the walls of the grapelike alveoli. Capillaries surround the alveoli. (From Thibodeau GA, Patton KT. [2009]. *Anatomy and Physiology.* 6th ed. St. Louis: Mosby.)

PROFICIENCY EXERCISE 4.11

1. List five of the disease conditions of the respiratory system described in the indications and contraindications section in Appendix A.
   a.
   b.
   c.
   d.
   e.
2. Choose one condition from your list and, using Appendix A, note any indications or contraindications for massage.
   Condition:
   Indications or contraindications:

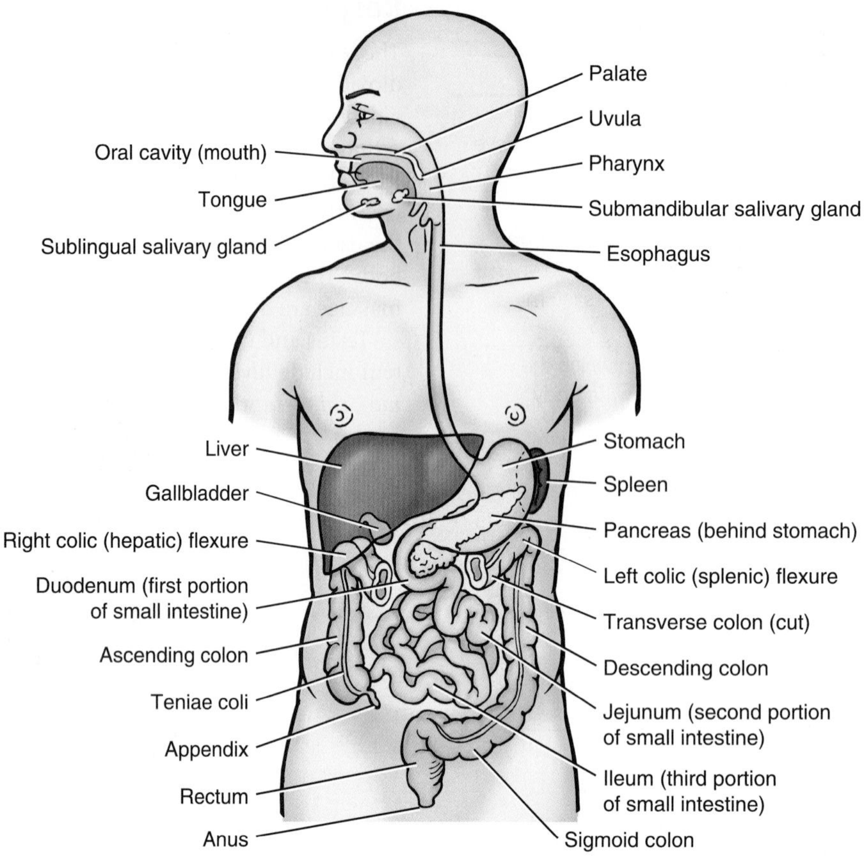

FIG. 4.13 The organs of the digestive system and some associated structures.

Digestive System

Anatomically, the digestive system can be loosely described as a long, muscular tube that travels through the body (Fig. 4.13). The organs of the digestive system transport food through this muscular tube. The wavelike contraction of the smooth muscles of the digestive tube is called *peristalsis.* Accessory organs carry out functions related to digestion and are connected to the system by means of ducts. It is important for massage professionals to understand the flow of contents through the large intestine, because methods of massage can be used to enhance this process. Refer to your anatomy and physiology textbook to learn more about the digestive process (Proficiency Exercise 4.12).

PROFICIENCY EXERCISE 4.12

1. List five of the disease conditions of the digestive system described in the indications and contraindications section in Appendix A.
   a.
   b.
   c.
   d.
   e.
2. Choose one condition from your list and, using Appendix A, note any indications or contraindications for massage.
   Condition:
   Indications or contraindications:

Endocrine System

The endocrine system is composed of glands that produce hormones, which are secreted directly into the bloodstream to stimulate cells in a specific way or to set a body function into action (Fig. 4.14). The endocrine system is complex and important because it serves as a control and regulation system for the body. As with the nervous system, the massage professional should commit to an in-depth study of the endocrine system, its relationship to the nervous system, and the connection to mind/body processes. Information from research on the mind/body phenomenon is being released too quickly to remain current in any textbook. The massage professional must read medical and scientific research reports to keep up-to-date. The implications for massage are important because the effects of massage are related to the nervous system and endocrine body control functions (Proficiency Exercise 4.13).

Integumentary System

The integumentary system consists of the skin and its appendages, including the hair and nails.

Skin

The skin is the largest organ of the body. It is composed of three layers of tissue: the epidermis, the dermis, and the subcutaneous tissue (Fig. 4.15). The *epidermis* is the outer layer of skin, which contains many layers of tissue and melanocytes, the cells that give skin color. The *dermis,* or dermal layer, lies

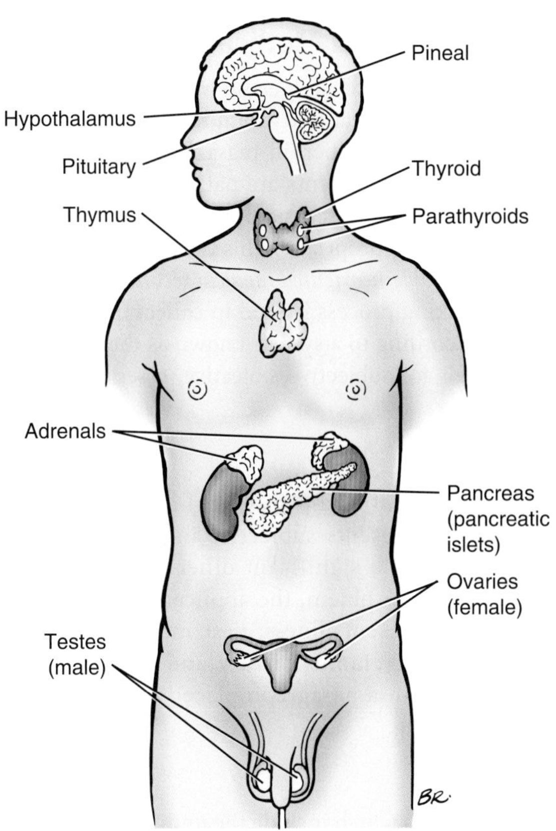

FIG. 4.14 The locations of the major endocrine glands.

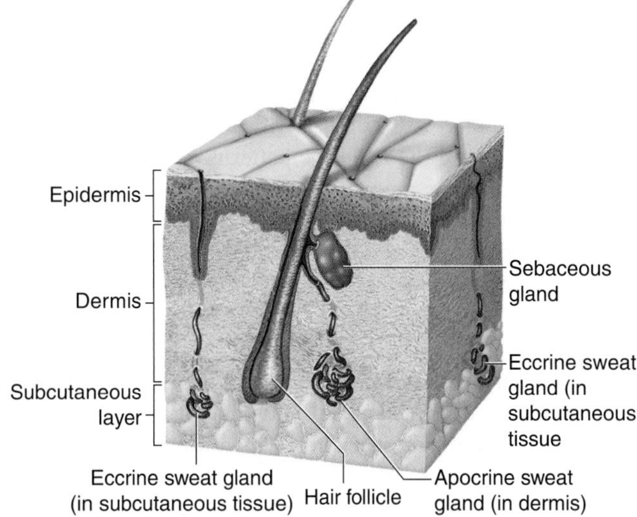

FIG. 4.15 The structure of the skin. (From Jarvis C. [1992]. *Physical Examination and Health Assessment.* Philadelphia: WB Saunders.)

PROFICIENCY EXERCISE 4.13

1. List three of the disease conditions of the endocrine system described in the indications and contraindications section in Appendix A.
   a.
   b.
   c.
2. Choose one condition from your list and, using Appendix A, note any indications or contraindications for massage.
   Condition:
   Indications or contraindications:

PROFICIENCY EXERCISE 4.14

1. Using Appendix A, list at least three skin conditions that could be contagious.
   a.
   b.
   c.
2. Choose one condition from your list and, using Appendix A, note any indications or contraindications for massage.
   Condition:
   Indications or contraindications:

directly under the epidermis and is often called the *true skin.* It is composed of connective tissue. Embedded in the dermis are the blood vessels, lymphatic vessels, hair follicles, and sweat glands. *Subcutaneous tissue* attaches the dermis to the underlying structures. This fatty tissue contains varying amounts of adipose tissue and acts as insulation for the body.

The functions of the fascial network of the skin are protection; control and maintenance of body temperature; detection of the sensations of touch, temperature, pain, and pressure; secretion of sweat and sebum; and production of vitamin D when the skin is exposed to the sun.

Many disease signs (particularly color changes) may first be noticed in the skin. Terms relating to skin color changes include *cyanosis* (bluish), *erythema* (red), *jaundice* (yellow-orange), and *pallor* (a decrease in color) (Proficiency Exercise 4.14).

Sebaceous Glands

Sebaceous glands are located in the skin. They secrete an oily substance, called *sebum,* that gives the skin and hair a glossy appearance. Most of these glands open into the walls of hair follicles. Other sebaceous glands are located at the corners of the mouth and around the external sex organs that open directly on the surface of the skin.

Sweat Glands

The function of sweat glands, which are found in most areas of the body, is to cool the body. The most abundant type of sweat gland is the eccrine sweat gland. The palms of the hands and soles of the feet contain large numbers of eccrine sweat glands. Sweat from these glands is odorless. Another type of sweat gland is the apocrine sweat gland, which is connected to hair follicles in the armpits and the pubic area and is found at the navel and nipples. Secretions from these sweat glands increase in response to sexual stimulation. These secretions lubricate the genital area, and their mild odor plays a part in sexual arousal.

Terminology as a Continuing Study

The study of medical terminology, anatomy, physiology, and pathology must be an ongoing process for the massage professional, who needs this base to understand the research, books, and journal articles that relate to massage, record keeping, and charting. This base is also required if the massage professional is to communicate effectively with other health care professionals.

Many clients are not familiar with medical terms; thus it is important to use the language patterns of the people with whom you speak. In many cases, using technical terms with a client is not appropriate; using big words and technical language is not necessary when presenting yourself to the general public. The massage professional must speak two languages and must be able to translate effectively back and forth between them.

When you speak with health care professionals and researchers who use this special language of the sciences, it is important that you ask questions about any term you do not understand. Acting as though you understand what is being said when you do not will not help you increase your knowledge and skills, and it is unprofessional. The development of this language base has prepared the learner to begin the process of maintaining records and charting.

DOCUMENTATION

SECTION OBJECTIVES

Chapter objective covered in this section:

10. Use the information in this chapter for effective professional communication and documentation.

Using the information presented in this section, the student will be able to:

- Implement the clinical reasoning/problem-solving/decision-making model for charting purposes.
- Use a problem- or goal-oriented charting process.
- Complete a client intake process using sample forms.
- Chart using the SOAP note format.
- Compare computerized/electronic record and paper records.

Accurate, comprehensive documentation is becoming increasingly important for massage professionals. Massage has adopted and adapted documentation methods used by the medical profession (Box 4.5).

Terminology describing client records can be confusing. The following terms are used in this textbook.

- **Client records** contain all information related to the client. This includes business records (e.g., payment and appointment schedules); complaints and actions taken; health care records (e.g., information obtained during the initial visit, relevant insurance information, contact information in case of an emergency, physician's name, and so forth); needs assessment records, including the client history and initial assessment; referral records; treatment plan; informed consent; release of information consent; and all session notes.
- **Documentation** is the process of creating and maintaining client records.
- **Charting** is a systematic form of documentation.
- **Progress** or **session notes** are produced by using a charting process to record each massage with the client.

Problem-Oriented Medical Record

In the 1960s, Dr. Lawrence Weed developed a method of record keeping that is organized around the problems of the client or **patient**. (Remember, in massage therapy, all patients are clients, but not all clients are patients. This text uses the term *client* for general discussion purposes and *patient* where that term is more appropriate.) This type of documentation is known as the *problem-oriented medical record (POMR) system.* A critical thinking process is used to collect information and organize it according to a system known as the *SOAP format.* "SOAP" stands for *s*ubjective, *o*bjective, *a*ssessment/analysis, and *p*lan.

Subjective Data

The chief complaint (main problem) and history portion of the record represents subjective information collected from the client or a significant other and from previous records. For each problem, the applicable parts of a traditional history (present illness, past medical history, personal/social history, family history, and review of systems) are summarized in a paragraph placed directly under the subjective heading.

Objective Data

The objective data, which include the findings from the physical examination and the results of any tests, follow the list of problems. The physical examination usually is recorded in the traditional format; that is, the results are listed by the parts of the body. After the initial assessment, this section includes any changes in the physical findings and the results of any tests or treatment.

Assessment/Analysis

The assessment/analysis section presents the conclusions reached based on the subjective and objective data. During the process of reaching conclusions, critical thinking becomes clinical reasoning.

Plan

The next section is the plan for that particular problem. A plan consists of three parts: the diagnosis (Dx), the treatment (Rx), and patient education.

- In this case, *diagnosis* means the diagnostic tests needed to identify the cause or to follow the case.
- Treatment can include special therapy, drugs, radiation, chemotherapy, and other modalities, including massage.
- Patient education is the information the patient is given about the problem.

Organizing patient data in this way shows exactly what the medical caregiver is thinking. Each problem can be followed easily through the record. This saves valuable time for the caregiver and enables others to take over the patient's care if necessary. The documentation process is based on a clinical reasoning pattern.

The massage profession began informally using the SOAP format in the 1980s. In 1993, the book *The Hands Heal: Documentation for Massage Therapy: A Guide to S.O.A.P. Charting,* by Diana L. Thompson, was published. Since then, the SOAP charting process has become the most used documentation method for therapeutic massage. Because diagnosing and prescribing are out of the scope of practice for massage therapy, the SOAP process has been modified over time to better fit the practice of therapeutic massage; however, it retains its roots in the POMR.

Progress/Session Notes

Progress (or session) notes chart each visit by the client. These notes should follow a systematic method of organizing the information for decision making (e.g., the SOAP method). This helps massage therapists organize their thinking and justify their actions. The basic plan of SOAP is easily modified to other charting styles. Computer-based electronic record keeping is becoming the norm. It is required in medical environments. There are many different electronic record keeping programs for massage therapy.

Regardless of the format of the documentation process, paper or electronic, the principles remain the same. Following the documentation rules in Box 4.5 will result in a record that is accurate, timely, specific, objective, concise, comprehensive, logical, and legible. All entries must be consistent with one another. The assessment must agree with the diagnostic testing, or the discrepancy must be explained. Records created in this way reflect the thought processes of the health care providers (including massage therapists). Not only is such a record the best defense in case of a lawsuit, but it also results in the best care for the client or patient.

Good record-keeping skills equip the massage therapist to communicate with other health care personnel. They also help create an accurate record of specified treatment goals, the methods of massage, and the effectiveness of treatment.

Box 4.5 Documentation Rules for Medical Records and Health Care Professionals

Medical records must be maintained in a specific way:

- Each page of the record must identify the patient by name and by the clinical record number of the hospital, clinic, or private physician.
- Each entry in the record must include the date and time the entry was made and the signature and credential of the individual making the entry.
- No blank spaces should be left between entries.
- All entries should be written in ink or produced on a printer or typewriter or recorded appropriately in electronic format.
- The record must not be altered in any way. Erasures, use of correction fluid, and marked-out areas are not appropriate. Errors should be corrected in a manner that allows the reader to see and understand the error. Errors are corrected as follows:

Paper

- A single line is drawn through the error, and the legibility of the previous entry is checked.
- The correct information is inserted.
- The correction is dated and initialed by the person recording the data.
- If space is inadequate to allow the correction to be made legibly at the error, a note should be made indicating where the corrected entry can be found; this cross-reference should be dated and initialed. The correct information is entered in the proper chronological order for the date the error was discovered and corrected.
- If something is spilled on the pages of a chart, they should not be discarded. The pages should be copied, and the original and copied sheets then should be put together in the chart. "COPIED" is written on the copied pages.

Electronic

- The system must have the ability to track corrections or changes once the original entry has been entered or authenticated.
- When an entry is corrected or changed, the original entry should be viewable, the current date and time should be entered, the person making the change should be identified, and the reason should be noted.
- When a hard copy is printed from the electronic record, the hard copy must also be corrected.
- The process should permit the author of the error to identify and time/date stamp whether it is an error.
- The process should offer the ability to suppress viewing of the actual error but ensure that a flag exists to notify other users of the newly corrected error.
- A practice policy should be developed to ensure that the facility corrects and reports errors in a consistent and timely manner.
- All information should be recorded as soon as possible. Memories can fade, and important facts can be omitted.
- Abbreviations should be used sparingly, and only those approved by the organization are appropriate. The same abbreviation can have different meanings, which can be misleading. Writing out the information is always better than using abbreviations that can be misinterpreted.
- All writing must be legible. Because the record is used by so many other clinicians and practitioners in providing care, it is important to the quality of care that the record be legible. An electronic format can be helpful with this issue.
- All entries must be consistent with one another. The assessment must agree with the diagnostic testing, or an explanation must be given as to the reason it does not.
- Entries should be factual accounts.
- All information given to the client before any procedure should be recorded. This ensures and verifies that the client was properly informed of the benefits and risks before they gave consent for the procedure.
- Telephone contacts with the clients should be entered into the record immediately.
- Some method of organizing entries (e.g., the SOAP or DFAR format) must be used to ensure that the entries are comprehensive and reflect the thought processes involved when decisions were made about the client's care.

Confidentiality of Medical Records

A patient's right to privacy traditionally has imposed an ethical responsibility on the people involved in the patient's care. Many different people may see and treat a patient during the provision of health care, and each of them needs particular information. Protecting the patient's right to privacy while keeping all caregivers informed can present a dilemma. Passage of the Health Insurance Portability and Accountability Act (HIPAA) in 1996 substantially strengthened the patient's right to privacy.

HIPAA's Privacy Rule includes standards that protect a patient's individually identifiable data; this type of data is considered protected health information (PHI). Generally speaking, PHI covers information that identifies a patient and their health status. The Privacy Rule applies to health plans, health care clearinghouses, and other health care providers. It covers a broad range of information. Protections apply to the information in many different formats, including electronic files (internet, intranet, private networks, and data moved from one location to another by disk, magnetic tape, or compact disk), paper records, and verbal information.

Most health care providers, and certainly hospitals, have policies and procedures governing the release of any information about a patient. Massage therapists must be aware of those policies. Policies on the release of information generally include provisions such as these:

- A requirement for the patient's consent to the release of any information to any outside entity; any exceptions are outlined.
- Special considerations for the release of information on sensitive conditions, such as alcohol, drug, or psychiatric diagnoses, and conditions related to infection with the human immunodeficiency virus (HIV).
- Required data elements for a proper consent form and specification of how long the form is valid.
- Identification of those who can release information to outside parties.
- Appropriate fees or charges for copies that may be requested.

Other issues should be addressed in separate policies. For example, individuals by title who may release information to the media could be the subject of one such policy. Another policy could indicate what information hospital employees may disclose to telephone callers regarding the condition of the patient during hospitalization.

To ensure compliance, health care providers have implemented policies and procedures that adhere to HIPAA regulations. The massage therapist in the medical environment should be specifically trained in the HIPAA procedures. This must be in-house training. If it is not offered as part of the orientation training, massage therapists should request specific information on the ways in which they are expected to comply with these regulations.

All states have laws about which diseases, conditions, and events must be reported to appropriate agencies. Such incidents include births, deaths, gunshot wounds, communicable diseases, and evidence of child and elder abuse. When reporting is required by law, confidentiality is no longer an issue. Reporting such incidents to anyone other than the responsible agency, however, is a breach of confidentiality.

Documentation in the Massage Therapy Practice

Maintenance of a written record (electronic or paper) of the professional relationship with massage therapy clients is essential. The informed consent procedure and the legal implications of documentation were presented in Chapter 2. The decision-making skills that also were introduced in that chapter will continue to be developed throughout the text. Ethical decisions are only one type of decision made in professional practice. Clinical decisions using clinical reasoning involve the client's concerns and the methods to use to achieve clients' goals, as well as business decisions. This discussion focuses on clinical decision making and the records necessary for maintaining a written account of the professional interaction. Clinical decision making is discussed in further detail in other chapters. Chapter 3 more thoroughly discussed business records, and Chapter 16 provides examples of case studies.

Client record keeping involves the creation of a handwritten or an electronic record of intake procedures, including informed consent and needs assessments (including the history and physical assessment); obtaining permission for the release of information (if communication among health professionals is anticipated); and the ongoing process of recording each session, which is called *charting*. Clients have the right to see their file, receive a copy of the file, and have any information contained in the file explained to them.

At this point you, as students, will find it difficult to complete a needs assessment and to devise an initial treatment plan, because you are still developing the assessment and technical skills required to perform these procedures. The same is true of charting. Even so, it is important that you understand the mechanics of the record keeping and charting process so that as your technical skills improve, your ability to perform record-keeping procedures also develops (Box 4.6).

Box 4.6 SOAP in the Massage Practice

The SOAP note has four parts:

Subjective data: The client's explanation of their goals for massage and information about the current and past conditions, pain, complaints, reactions, and so forth.

Objective data: The information obtained through physical assessment and observations and also the massage techniques used.

Assessment: (Think of this as an analysis.) Evaluation of the condition, based on the subjective and objective information, using clinical reasoning skills. It involves thinking about the data gathered and deciding on the main issues, the contributing factors, and possible courses of action. It also includes the information from a postmassage evaluation of the results of the massage interventions.

Plan: The details of implementation of the course of treatment chosen, including the frequency of the massage sessions, methods, client education, referrals, need for additional information, and so forth.

Clinical Reasoning and Charting

As the volume of knowledge increases and as soft tissue methods, such as massage, are integrated into health care systems, the ability to think or reason through an intervention process and justify the effectiveness of a therapeutic intervention is becoming increasingly important. Therapeutic massage practitioners must be able to gather information effectively, analyze that information to make decisions about the type and appropriateness of a therapeutic intervention, and evaluate and justify the benefits derived from the intervention. Charting is the process of keeping a written record of these professional interactions. Effective charting is more than writing down what happens during a session; it is a clinical reasoning methodology that emphasizes a problem-solving approach to client care. As noted at the beginning of this chapter, you must have a comprehensive knowledge base of massage terms, medical terms, abbreviations, and anatomy and physiology in both normal and diseased states to be able to reason clinically and chart effectively.

Effective assessment, analysis, and decision making are essential to meeting the needs of each client. Routines or recipe-type applications of therapeutic massage are often limited and ineffective because each person's circumstances and outcome goals are so varied. Effective clinical reasoning skills are the mark of an experienced professional. As with all skills, clinical reasoning can be learned (Box 4.7).

Goals: Outcomes and Problem Solving

Massage sessions are goal oriented. **Goals** describe desired outcomes. Decisions must be made regarding which goals are obtainable and the way the goals will be achieved. Problems indicate limits in functions. Goals support desired function. Consider this example:

- Description of the problem: Client has disturbed sleep pattern because of multiple physical and emotional stressors.
- Goal: Reduce physical stress symptoms to support more effective sleep.

Two primary reasons for developing treatment and care plans are to set achievable goals and to outline a general plan for the way the goals will be reached. Achievable goals often relate to day-to-day activities (functional goals), either personal or work related.

It is important to develop measurable, activity-based goals that are meaningful to the client, such as improvement in the ability to perform activities of daily living.

Quantifiable and Qualifiable Goals

Goals must be **quantifiable**; that is, they must be measurable in terms of objective criteria, such as time, frequency, rating on a 1–10 scale, a measurable increase or decrease in the ability to perform an activity, or a measurable increase or decrease in a sensation, such as relaxation or pain.

Goals also must be **qualifiable**. Massage therapists must determine measures by which they will know when a goal has been achieved. One such measure might be an activity that the client will be able to do that they are unable to do now.

These are examples of quantifiable and qualifiable goals (Proficiency Exercise 4.15):

Box 4.7 Methods of Organized Thinking

Organized thinking is based on four primary elements:

Database: The client's past and present health status.

Goals/problems list: The list of massage-related health goals and current and past problems.

Initial plan: The massage therapy plan devised to help achieve goals and overcome health problems.

Progress notes: The ongoing description of each massage session using a logical method (style) of charting.

Charting Methods

Three commonly used charting methods are SOAP, SOAPIER, and PIE.

SOAP Method

The SOAP method is used for problem-oriented charts.

S—Subjective (what the client tells you)
O—Objective (what you observe, see, assess, and measure)
A—Assessment/analyze (what you think is going on based on your data)
P—Plan (what you are going to do)

SOAPIER Method

The SOAPIER method is an expansion of SOAP.

S—Subjective (what the client tells you)
O—Objective (what you observe, see, assess, and measure)
A—Assessment/analyze (what you think is going on based on your data)
P—Plan (what you are going to do)
I—Intervention (specific methods used)
E—Evaluation (response to interventions)
R—Revision (changes in treatment)

PIE Method

The PIE method is similar to SOAP charting and also is a problem-oriented method.

P—Problem (what is bothering the client or what is the intended outcome for massage)
I—Intervention (what type and how massage was used)
E—Evaluation (what worked and what did not work)

DAR Method

In the DAR format, the progress note is based on data–action–response.

Data: Subjective and/or objective information that supports the stated focus
Action: What was done
Response: What happened related to what was done

FDAR is an expansion of DAR charting and stands for focus (F), data (D), action (A), and response (R). The addition of the (F) describes the goal.

PROFICIENCY EXERCISE 4.15

Following the examples given in this section of the text, write three quantifiable and qualifiable goals you might set for yourself in therapeutic massage.

1.
2.
3.

- Client will be able to manage independently (qualified) daily hygiene activities of bathing and dressing with a pain level of 5 on a scale of 1–10 (quantified), with 10 being unable to function without severe pain.
- Client will be able to work at the computer for 1 hour (quantified) without pain (qualified).
- Client will be able to incorporate a 30-minute walking program (quantified) without stiffness in left knee (qualified).
- Client will be able to fall asleep within 15 minutes (quantified) and sleep uninterrupted for 7 hours (qualified).
- Client will be able to increase duration of breath exhale to reduce sympathetic arousal (quantified), allowing them to drive a car to and from the market (qualified).
- Client will be able to meditate for 15 minutes (quantified) without racing thoughts (qualified).
- Client will be able to use massage to relax for 1 hour each week (quantified) to enjoy family more by being able to participate in a family outing after each massage (qualified).

Intake Procedures

Before massage therapists begin working with a client, it is important that they gather information on which to build the professional interaction, establish client goals, and develop a plan for achieving those goals. This is called a *database.*

Database

A database consists of all the information available that contributes to therapeutic interaction. It is created with information obtained from a history-taking interview with the client and other people who may have pertinent information, a physical assessment, previous records, and health care treatment orders. Information obtained during the history and assessment process becomes the needs assessment and provides the basis for the development of a treatment or care plan, identification of contraindications to therapy, and assessment of the need for referral.

To gather the information, the professional must have effective communication skills. The same communication skills learned for ethical decision making in Chapter 2 are applied in this process. The I-message pattern can be altered slightly to develop effective, open-ended questions that support data collection. The four basic questions are:

- Will you please explain the situation or tell me what happened?
- How did/do you feel about the situation?
- What has been the result of the situation in terms of costs, limitations, and changes in activity or performance?
- How would you prefer the situation to be or what would you like to occur?

Note: The answer to the last question can easily become the basis for the functionally oriented treatment goal.

History

The history interview provides information about the client's health history, the reason for contact, a descriptive profile of the person, a history of the current condition, a history of past illness and health, and a history of any family illnesses. It is important to gather information about any prescription medication, herbs, or vitamins the client may be using (see Appendix C for more information on pharmacology). The history also contains an account of the client's current health practices (Fig. 4.16).

Physical Assessment

The physical assessment findings make up the second part of the database. Assessment procedures identify both effective functioning and deviations from the norm. The extent and depth of this assessment vary from setting to setting, practitioner to practitioner, and client to client. Practitioners of therapeutic massage generally use some sort of visual assessment process that looks for bilateral symmetry and deviations. Functional assessment looks for restricted, exaggerated, painful, or otherwise altered movement patterns. Palpation is used to identify changes in tissue texture and temperature and identify areas of tenderness. Various manual tests may be used to differentiate soft tissue problems from such other problems as joint dysfunction and muscle function (Fig. 4.17).

Analysis of Data

After the information has been collected, it is analyzed. The analysis is a critical thinking and clinical reasoning process. It is an important process that follows the same model as that for decision making. Effective decision making depends on both thorough collection and effective analysis of data. The analysis process follows these steps:

1. Review the facts and information collected.
   Questions that help with this process include:
   - What are the facts?
   - What is considered normal or balanced function?
   - What has happened? (Spell out events.)
   - What caused the imbalance? (Can it be identified?)
   - What was done or is being done?
   - What has worked or not worked?
2. Brainstorm the possibilities.
   Questions that help with this process include:
   - What are the possibilities? (What could it all mean?)
   - What does my intuition suggest?
   - What are the possible patterns of dysfunction?
   - What are the possible contributing factors?
   - What are possible interventions?
   - What might work?
   - What are other ways to look at the situation?
   - What do the data suggest?
3. Consider the logical outcome of each possibility.
   Questions that help with this process include:
   - What is the logical progression of the symptom pattern, contributing factors, and current behaviors?
   - What is the logical cause and effect of each intervention identified?
   - What are the pros and cons of each intervention suggested?
   - What are the consequences of not acting?
   - What are the consequences of acting?
4. Consider how the people involved would be affected by each possibility.
   Questions that help identify these effects include:
   - In terms of each intervention considered, what is the impact on the people involved (i.e., client, practitioner, and other professionals working with the client)?

CLIENT INTAKE AND HEALTH HISTORY FORM

Name: ______________________ Date: ______________

Address: ______________ City: ________ State: ______ Zip: ________

Phone: ____________ Preferred Pronouns ________ Date of Birth: __________

Occupation: ______________________ Employer: ______________

Referred by: ______________________ Physician: ______________

Previous experience with massage:

____

Primary reason for appointment / areas of pain or tension:

____

Emergency contact—name and number: ______________________

Please mark (X) for all conditions that apply now. Put a (P) for past conditions, an (F) for family history of illness.

Pain Scale: minor-1 2 3 4 5 6 7 8 9 severe-10

_____ headaches, migraines	_____ chronic pain	_____ fatigue
_____ vision problems, contact lenses	_____ muscle or joint pain	_____ tension, stress
_____ hearing problems, deafness	_____ muscle, bone injuries	_____ depression
_____ injuries to face or head	_____ numbness or tingling	_____ sleep difficulties
_____ sinus problems	_____ sprains, strains	_____ allergies, sensitivities
_____ dental bridges, braces	_____ arthritis, tendinitis	_____ rashes, athlete's foot
_____ jaw pain, TMJ problems	_____ cancer, tumors	_____ infectious diseases
_____ asthma or lung conditions	_____ spinal column disorders	_____ blood clots
_____ constipation, diarrhea	_____ diabetes	_____ varicose veins
_____ hernia	_____ pregnancy	_____ high/low blood pressure
_____ birth control, IUD	_____ heart, circulatory problems	
_____ abdominal or digestive problems	_____ other medical conditions not listed	

Explain any areas noted above:

____

____

Current medications, including aspirin, ibuprofen, herbs, supplements, etc.:

____

____

Surgeries: ______________________________________

Accidents: ______________________________________

Please list all forms and frequency of stress reduction activities, hobbies, exercise, or sports participation:

____

____

FIG. 4.16 Sample history form. The client provides this information. To complete the form correctly, ask relevant questions to gather data.

MASSAGE ASSESSMENT/PHYSICAL OBSERVATION/PALPATION AND GAIT

PRE ⁄
POST ⊘

Client Name:____________________ **Preferred Pronouns:**________ **Date:** ______

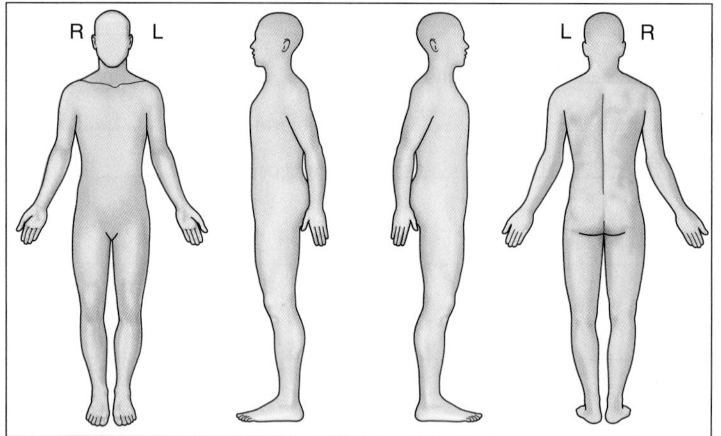

OBSERVATION & PALPATION		
ALIGNMENT	**RIBS**	**SCAPULA**
Chin in line with nose, sternal notch, navel	Even	Even
Other:	Springy	Move freely
HEAD	Other:	Other:
Tilted (L)	**ABDOMEN**	**CLAVICLES**
Tilted (R)	Firm and pliable	Level
Rotated (L)	Hard areas	Other:
Rotated (R)	Other:	**ARMS**
EYES	**WAIST**	Hang evenly (internal) (external)
Level	Level	(L) rotated ☐ medial ☐ lateral
Equally set in socket	Other:	(R) rotated ☐ medial ☐ lateral
Other:	**SPINE CURVES**	**ELBOWS**
EARS	Normal	Even
Level	Other:	Other:
Other:	**GLUTEAL MUSCLE MASS**	**WRISTS**
SHOULDERS	Even	Even
Level	Other:	Other:
(R) high / (L) low	**ILIAC CREST**	**FINGERTIPS**
(L) high / (R) low	Level	Even
(L) rounded forward	Other:	Other:
(R) rounded forward	**KNEES**	**PATELLA**
Muscle development even	Even/symmetrical	(L) ☐ movable ☐ rigid
Other:	Other:	(R) ☐ movable ☐ rigid

FIG. 4.17 Sample physical assessment form. This information is obtained by observing (looking and feeling) and measuring. To complete the form correctly, you should identify what is the same on the two sides of the body and what is different. Have the client color symptoms on the figures.

- How does each person involved feel about the possible interventions?
- Is the practitioner within their scope of practice to work with such situations?
- Is the practitioner qualified to work with such situations?
- Does the practitioner feel qualified to work with such situations?
- Does a feeling of cooperation and agreement exist among all parties involved?

Identification of Problems, Outcomes, and Goals

Problems are identified based on a conclusion or decision resulting from examination, investigation, and analysis of the data collected. A problem is defined as anything that causes concern to the client or caregiver, including physical abnormalities, physiological disturbances, and socioeconomic or spiritually based problems. Realistic and attainable massage-based outcome goals are established. A decision is then made about an intervention or care or treatment plan.

ANKLES	TRUNK	LEGS
Even	Remains vertical	Swing freely at hip
Other:	Other:	Other:
FEET	**SHOULDERS**	**KNEES**
Mobile	Remain level	Flex and extend freely through stance and swing phase
Other:	Rotate during walking	Other:
ARCHES	Other:	**FEET**
Even	**ARMS**	Heel strikes first at start of stance
Other:	Motion is opposite leg swing	Plantar flexed at push-off
TOES	Motion is even (L) and (R)	Foot clears floor during swing phase
Straight	Other:	Other:
Other:	(L) swings freely	**STEP**
SKIN	(R) swings freely	Length is even
Moves freely and resilient	Other:	Timing is even
Pulls/restricted	**HIPS**	Other:
Puffy/baggy	Remain level	**OVERALL**
Other:	Other:	Rhythmic
HEAD	Rotate during walking	Other:
Remains steady/eyes forward	Other:	
Other:		

FIG. 4.17, cont'd

Not all therapeutic goals target problems; some are related to a health-oriented outcome. Clients commonly use massage for health maintenance, stress management, and fulfillment of pleasure needs. The same analysis process is used to best determine the methods and approach to meet the goals of these clients.

Care or Treatment Plan

After the analysis is complete and problems and goals have been identified, a decision must be made about the **care** or **treatment plan**. Anytime a decision must be made about the care plan, the massage practitioner should return to the problem-solving model, which includes consideration of the facts, possibilities, logical outcomes, and effect on others involved.

The care or treatment plan is not an exact protocol set in stone but rather a flexible guide (the professional's best educated guess). The plan may evolve over the first three or four sessions, alterations including changes in the therapeutic goals. The development of the care or treatment plan is the end of the intake process (Fig. 4.18).

As the plan is implemented, it is recorded sequentially, session by session, in some form of charting process, such as **SOAP notes**. The plan is reevaluated and adjusted as necessary.

SOAP Notes and Other Documentation Styles

Charting is the process of producing an ongoing record of each client session. As was mentioned previously, commonly used methods of charting are based on the problem-oriented medical record system. The POMR system involves a problem-solving and clinical reasoning analysis process. After learning one method, adapting to any of the other charting methods is relatively easy. The most important skill involved is the ability to reason logically and comprehensively through a therapeutic interaction. A charting process can provide the structure necessary to think through a process effectively and develop a written record of the process.

The charting process includes recording any therapeutic action taken, its effectiveness, and its outcome progressively from session to session. Effective charting requires an organized approach to recording the information that relates to the facts, possibilities, logical consequences of cause and effect, and effect on involved people, an approach similar to that used for the development of the initial care or treatment plan. This process again is a direct application of the decision-making model. While charting, a practitioner gathers and records subjective and objective information, records the methods used, and analyzes the effectiveness of the process. The plan for further sessions is then indicated and noted.

Although many charting processes exist, massage professionals seem to be using the standardized SOAP model. This is a helpful choice in terms of learning because the four-part model correlates with the clinical-reasoning/decision-making model.

SOAP notes or similar charting methods are used to document all massage sessions. After the initial intake and care/treatment plan development, subsequent visits require a modified and shortened subjective and objective assessment process to determine goals for each individual massage session. When a massage is given to the client after the intake session, specific treatment goals for the particular session are developed. Information from the history pertinent to the first session is transferred to *S* in SOAP notes. Physical assessment information pertinent to this session is transferred to *O* in SOAP notes.

When using SOAP note charting, the massage practitioner should use the following format:

CARE/TREATMENT PLAN

Client Name:____________________

Choose One: ☐ Original plan ☐ Reassessment date____________________

Short-term client goals:
Quantitative:____________________
Qualitative:____________________

Long-term client goals:
Quantitative:____________________
Qualitative:____________________

Therapist objectives:

1) Frequency, 2) length, and 3) duration of visits:
1) ________ 2) ________ 3) ________

Progress measurements to be used: (Ex.— pain scale, range of motion, increased ability to perform function)

Dates of reassessment:

Categories of massage methods to be used: (Ex.— general constitutional, stress reduction, circulatory, lymphatic, neuromuscular, connective tissue, neurochemical, etc.)

Additional notes:

Client Signature:____________________ Date:________

Therapist Signature:____________________ Date:________

FIG. 4.18 Sample form for a care or treatment plan.

S – stands for subjective data, recorded from the client's point of view. Subjective information usually includes:
- Key goals that are quantified and qualified
- Activities that are affected by the situation; often stated as what can no longer be done or what increase in performance is desired
- The methods or activities currently used in adjunctive treatment

O – stands for objective data, acquired from inspection and palpation. A list of assessment procedures and interventions used during the session is recorded. Objective information usually includes:
- Significant physical assessment findings
- Intervention modalities and locations used (limit specifics to interventions used to work toward treatment goals)
- General approach used, such as general massage focus, connective tissue focus, Swedish massage focus, neuromuscular focus, or circulatory focus
- If not recorded elsewhere, the duration of the session

A – stands for analysis or assessment of the subjective and objective data. It includes an analysis of the effectiveness of the intervention and action taken, with a summary of the most pertinent data recorded.

Note: Traditionally in SOAP charting, the *A* stands for assessment. However, observation of many learners indicates that they confuse physical assessment information recorded in the objective data with assessment in the SOAP model, which is actually an analysis of the data and effectiveness of the interventions. Therefore this text uses the idea of analysis for the *A* section of SOAP charting.

Analysis of information includes:

- Changes, whether subjective (i.e., related to the client's experience, such as "pain reduced" or "feels relaxed") or objective (i.e., measurable, such as "flexion of elbow increased by 15 degrees"). If no change occurs or if the condition worsens, record this also.
- Analysis of which methods were effective or not effective, such as "Trigger point methods most effective in increase of flexion of elbow," "Client indicated she responded best to rhythmic rocking for relaxation," or "Tense-and-relax methods not effective in reducing pain in shoulder." Also indicate whether it is unclear which methods were effective: "Range of motion in neck increased 25%, but it is unclear which methods brought about the change."

The *A* (analysis/assessment) section of the SOAP charting process is important. It is, in fact, the most important area in terms of determining future intervention procedures and communicating process information to other caregivers and insurance companies.

The *A* portion of the SOAP note is where the actual process of decision making is recorded. Decision making occurs during every step of the charting process; however, in the other areas of charting, only the decision is recorded, not the way the decision was made. Obviously, a condensed version of the more detailed process is written down in the chart, but the components of the process (facts, possibilities, logical outcomes, effects on people) are evident in the *A* portion of the SOAP note.

P – stands for plan, including the methodology for future intervention. The progress of the sessions is developed and recorded. Plan information usually includes:

- Frequency of appointments
- Continuation of a step-by-step process as it unfolds session by session to achieve treatment plan goals
- Client self-care
- Referrals

A sample SOAP charting form is presented in Fig. 4.19; it has been modified for use by the beginning learner. An example of SOAP charting is presented in Box 4.8.

SESSION NOTES
SOAP CHARTING FORM

Client Name: ______________________ Preferred Pronouns: __________ Date: ______
Massage Therapist Name: ______________________

Subjective

CLIENT STATUS

- **Information from client, referral source, or reference books:**

1) Current conditions/changes from last session: ______________________

Objective

2) Information from assessment (physical, gait, palpation, muscle testing):

CONTENT OF SESSION

- **Generate goal (possibilities) from analysis of information in client status.**

1) Goals worked on this session. (Base information on client status this session and goals previously established in Treatment Plan):

What was done this session:

nalysis

RESULTS

- **Analyze results of session in relationship to what was done and how this relates to the session goals. (This is based on cause and effect of methods used and the effects on the persons involved.)**

1) What worked/what didn't: (Based on measurable and objective postassessment)

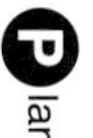
lan

PLAN

Plans for next session, what client will work on, what next massage will reassess and continue to assess: ______________________

CLIENT COMMENTS:

Time In: ______________________ Time Out: ______________________

Therapist signature: ______________________

FIG. 4.19 SOAP charting form modified for student learning. To complete the form correctly, you should answer the questions based on what happened during the massage.

Box 4.8 Example of SOAP Charting in Therapeutic Massage

In this example, a massage therapist uses SOAP charting for a new client who complains of frequent headaches. The SOAP format has been modified slightly to help learners complete the documentation process.

S (Subjective)

Client reports tension headache and indicates with hand placement that the major concentration of pain is at the occiput and upper cervical area with a secondary pain pattern at the temples. Client reports that on a pain scale of 0–10, the headache is a 7.

O (Objective)

Both shoulders are observed to be elevated, with increased elevation on the right. Range of motion of the neck appears to be generally limited to the left. Palpation of the upper back muscles elicited some pain behaviors, including pulling away, grimacing, and verbal indications of pain. The upper trapezius muscles seem to be warm but without indications of inflammation, suggesting tension in the muscles.

Approach Used (What I Did)

1. *General massage focus:* Stress reduction with specific focus on shoulder and neck tension using positional release and elongation
2. *Basic methods used:* Gliding, compression, rocking, and passive joint movement

Postassessment

After the massage session, a postassessment is done. The client is asked how they feel and what is different from before the session. The client is asked what methods used seemed to be most beneficial. One or two of the methods identified are then modified for client self-care and are taught to the client.

After the massage and postassessment, the A (assessment/analysis) part of the chart is recorded.

A (Analysis/Assessment)

Appears as if the client may be experiencing changes in soft tissue structures, leading to the described headache. Postmassage, client indicates a reduction in headache by 50% (pain rating of 3), less tension in the shoulders, and increased range of motion of the neck to the left. Pain behaviors related to the upper back are not occurring, but the client still indicates tenderness in the area during palpation. Upper trapezius area remains warm, with exaggerated vasomotor response (reddening) and itching after massage. Client now can look over the left shoulder, which he could not do without a catch before the massage. The shoulders are observed to be level within 1 inch, indicating a change in the right shoulder tension pattern. The methods that were most effective were compression and positional release. Rocking methods were ineffective, and the client reported an increase in head pain when rocking was used.

NOTE: Make sure client's feet stay warm.

P (Plan)

Client selected self-help consisting of towel compression to the head and flexion/extension range of motion of the arms and shoulders. Client scheduled an appointment for 2 weeks and will monitor response to massage. Expect three to four sessions before beginning specific work on the shoulder area. Client was advised to contact his personal physician and report that he has begun to receive massage.

NOTE: The interventions used and the plan recorded in SOAP charting need to reflect the original treatment plan developed during the intake procedure.

Individual session goals need to be in line with the initial care/treatment plan agreed to in the informed consent process. If the goals are radically different, the client needs to sign an addendum to the informed consent form. Minor changes can be reflected in the SOAP notes or session charting procedure.

To maintain the integrity of client charts, make sure that any abbreviations used are universally understood, or write out the word. Use a black pen or type the notes. Make sure handwritten notes are readable. Never erase or white-out a correction. Draw a single line through any error and make the correction above or next to the error. Share the charting notes and explain them to the client regularly.

Computer-Based Patient Record and Electronic Health Record

Paper records are becoming outdated. They are difficult to access, often lack information, and can be available only in a single location for a single use. The paper record has changed little over the past 50 years, whereas the expectations for use of the data it contains have changed significantly.

Technology has improved over the past decades, allowing the design and implementation of electronic record-keeping systems (Box 4.9). Automated record-keeping systems have

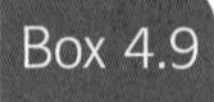

Pros and Cons of Computerized Record Keeping

Pros

- All parts of the record are legible.
- The date and time are recorded automatically.
- Abbreviations, specific terms, and formats are standardized by the facility.
- Less space is needed for record storage (computerization does not eliminate paper records, but it does significantly reduce the amount of paper needed).
- The members of a health care team are able to coordinate care.
- Searching for a particular item is quicker.

Cons

- Use of a computerized system involves a significant learning curve.
- Information and systems are not yet uniform, which makes integration difficult.
- Care must be taken to ensure that unauthorized individuals cannot see computer screens.
- A password is required, which must never be shared and must be changed frequently.

a variety of names, such as *electronic medical record (EMR), computer-based patient record (CPR), electronic patient record (EPR), computerized medical record,* and *electronic health record (EHR).* EHR is the current term used to describe computer-based systems that perform a broad range of functions related to documenting and managing patient care. Clinical documentation has grown to encompass more than just progress notes. In focus charting, progress notes are used to document progress in meeting the client's goals, and notes are written to provide documentation related to a specific focus. All electronic documentation software programs must automatically:

- Put in the date and time for all entries
- Save all entries upon the author's sign-off
- Require each user to sign off on each entry (or auto-authenticate each entry) based on the user's password identity
- Track all additions and corrections made in a record
- Print the entire record in a readable format

Many software products have been designed specifically for massage therapy. Regardless of whether the record-keeping system is electronic or on paper, high-quality client care depends on massage therapists' expertise in collecting information, their ability to interpret it, and the creation of concisely written and useful data.

Foot in the Door

The language you use and the records you keep will influence and impress both clients and employers. If you want an advantage in the career world, perfect your vocabulary, writing skills, intake skills, and critical-thinking skills. The discipline of these systems helps organize your internal and external self. An organized person stands out in the interview process. Your ability to understand terminology and maintain professional records will help you communicate and work with health and wellness and medical care professionals. If you want to practice massage therapy in the medical care setting, you will not be able to get your foot in the door without these skills. The spa and wellness industries also expect massage therapists to speak and document professionally.

SUMMARY

Record-keeping and documentation skills, in addition to a knowledge of the necessary language base for keeping records effectively, are important aspects of professional development. The ability to communicate clearly in both the written and spoken forms fosters understanding and accurate exchange of information. Consider record keeping as writing the client's professional interaction story. Realize that reflection on the healing journey provided by reading this story allows both you and your client, and any other authorized individuals, to appreciate the process and to remember and replicate the steps in achieving goals that honor the effort put forth by all concerned.

Evolve

Visit the Evolve website: http://evolve.elsevier.com/Fritz/fundamentals/

Evolve content designed for massage therapy licensing exam review and comprehension of content beyond the textbook. Evolve content includes:

- Content Updates
- Science and Pathology Animations
- Body Spectrum Coloring Book
- MBLEx exam review multiple choice questions

FOR EACH CHAPTER FIND:

- Answers and rationales for the end-of-chapter multiple-choice questions
- Electronic Workbook and Answer Key
- Chapter multiple choice question Quiz
- Quick Content Review in Question Form and Answers
- Technique Videos when applicable
- Learn More on the Web

REFERENCES

Centers for Disease Control and Prevention. Well-being concepts. Retrieved from: http://www.cdc.gov/hrqol/wellbeing.htm.

World Health Organization. World report on disability 2011. Retrieved from http://whqlibdoc.who.int/publications/2011/9789240685215_eng.pdf.

MULTIPLE-CHOICE QUESTIONS FOR DISCUSSION AND REVIEW

The answers, with rationales, can be found on the Evolve site. Use these questions to stimulate discussion and dialog. You must understand the meaning of the words in the question and possible answers. Each question provides you with the opportunity to review terminology, practice critical thinking skills, and improve your multiple-choice test-taking skills. Answers and rationales are provided on the Evolve website. Remember—it is just as important to know why the wrong answers are wrong as it is to know why the correct answer is correct.

1. Record keeping for clients involves _____.
   a. Charting each session of the ongoing process
   b. Having the client fill out a general information packet
   c. A written record of intake procedures, informed consent, assessments, recording of each session, and release of information
   d. Filing each piece of information received from physicians and insurance companies or payments received from clients
2. Charting can be defined as _____.
   a. A record of each payment made by the client
   b. A record of the time spent with each client
   c. A written record of the intake procedure
   d. The ongoing process of recording each session

3. Massage treatment goals must be quantified, meaning _____.
   a. They are achievable
   b. They are measured in terms of objective criteria
   c. How they will be done
   d. What they will cost
4. A database consists of _____.
   a. Charts on the actual session
   b. All the information available that contributes to therapeutic interaction
   c. The client's description of the problem
   d. Goals that are quantified and qualified and are functionally oriented
5. The purpose of assessment is to _____.
   a. Provide methods to correct deviations from the norm
   b. Identify effective functioning to eliminate massage to that area
   c. Do a visual and functional assessment but not a palpation assessment
   d. Identify effective functioning and deviations from the norm
6. The treatment plan _____.
   a. Is an exact protocol developed by the client and practitioner
   b. Is a fluid guideline developed by the client and practitioner
   c. Must be complete at the end of the first session and not revised
   d. Must be complete before the massage begins.
7. Problem-oriented medical records, including SOAP, require that _____.
   a. The qualified goals and the outcome of the massage be noted on the record
   b. The facts, possibilities, logical consequences of cause and effect, and impact on people involved be noted on the record
   c. The results of a palpation assessment, but not the client history, be recorded
   d. Only the interventions be noted on the record
8. The P (plan) part of SOAP should include _____.
   a. Client medication history
   b. Client self-care
   c. Key symptoms
   d. Relation of outcomes to goals
9. A client who is blind presents a physician referral that states that only general massage with light pressure is to be used because of a recent angioplasty. The suffix in angioplasty means _____.
   a. Tumor
   b. Enlargement
   c. Surgical repair
   d. Disease
10. Reading the history, the massage professional notices that the client lists myalgia. This client also uses a cane for balance related to a stroke. Which of the following defines myalgia?
    a. Muscle condition
    b. Spine pain
    c. Muscle pain
    d. Muscle paralysis
11. While reviewing a file on a client referred from another massage therapist, the massage professional finds information in the SOAP charting that indicates that applications of gliding to the legs resulted in vasodilation. Which body system was affected directly?
    a. Cardiovascular
    b. Urinary
    c. Immune
    d. Digestive
12. Where would a massage professional record this statement on a SOAP note: "Palpation identified mild scoliosis"?
    a. S
    b. O
    c. A
    d. P
13. An umbrella term for impairments, activity limitations, and participation restrictions is _____.
    a. Discrimination
    b. Reasonable accommodation
    c. Disability
    d. Standard of living
14. Which of the following is a quantified outcome goal?
    a. Client will be able to increase range of motion of the lateral flexion of the cervical area by 15 degrees.
    b. Client will be able to resume normal work activities.
    c. Client will be reassessed in 12 sessions.
    d. Client will recover ability to play golf.
15. Which of the following would be recorded in the objective data section of a SOAP note?
    a. Client states she has interrupted sleep.
    b. Client is currently taking melatonin.
    c. Observation and palpation indicate upper chest breathing.
    d. Client wishes to have weekly appointments.
16. The most important area in terms of determining future interventions based on results is _____.
    a. S: subjective—what the client states.
    b. O: objective—what was observed from the assessment and examination.
    c. A: analysis—what worked/did not work.
    d. P: plan—what the client wants to work on and what needs to be done during the next session.
17. The purpose of using a clinical reasoning model is to _____.
    a. Be able to think through an intervention process and justify the effectiveness of a therapeutic interaction.
    b. Provide a primary means of effectively supporting a diagnosis to other health care professionals.
    c. Integrate all the modalities and techniques into a user-friendly charting process for all to understand.
    d. Provide a framework for the client charting protocols and data collection

18. What needs to be done to develop a valid analysis of massage benefits in a SOAP chart?
   a. Completion of a treatment plan
   b. Preassessment and postassessment procedures
   c. Prior development of a problem-oriented medical record
   d. Dates of reassessment

19. A massage professional lists reducing neuritis as a long-term client goal in the treatment plan. Which of the following describes the outcome?
   a. Provide relief from intestinal spasm
   b. Provide a decrease in joint mobility
   c. Produce an increase in nerve conduction
   d. Provide a decrease in nerve inflammation

20. A client reports they have reduced flexion and extension in a joint. What type of joint is the client discussing?
   a. Diarthrodial
   b. Synarthrodial
   c. Amphiarthrodial
   d. Syndesmosis

UNIT II

Foundations for Massage Benefit

Research Literacy and Evidence-Informed Practice

CHAPTER 5

http://evolve.com/Fritz/fundamentals/

CHAPTER OBJECTIVES

After completing this chapter, the student will be able to:

1. Explain the meaning of evidence-informed practice.
2. Explain the meaning of research literacy.
3. Use levels of evidence guidelines to categorize research.
4. Describe the fundamentals of the Western scientific process.
5. Critically read a research paper.
6. Find and cite current research related to therapeutic massage.
7. Explain the effects of therapeutic massage in physiological terms.

CHAPTER OUTLINE

KEY TERMS

Absolute risk
Adrenaline
Adverse effect
Autonomic nervous system (ANS)
Bias
Biological plausibility
Biopsychosocial model
Breathing pattern disorder
Circulation
Compression
Connective tissue
Conservation withdrawal
Cortisol
Counterirritation
Dopamine
Dynorphins
Effectiveness
Efficacy
Endocannabinoids
Endorphins
Enkephalins
Entrapment
Epinephrine
Ethics
Evidence
Evidence-based practice (EIP)
Evidence-informed decision making
Evidence-informed practice
Experiment
Gate control theory
General adaptation syndrome
Growth hormone
Heart rate variability
Hormone
Hyperstimulation analgesia
Hypothesis
Informed consent
Intuition
Joint kinesthetic receptors
Manual therapy
Mindfulness
Muscle spindles
Neurotransmitter
Noradrenaline
Norepinephrine
Oxytocin
Parasympathetic patterns
Placebo effect
Relative risk
Research literacy
Science
Scientific method
Serotonin
Side effect
Stress
Sympathetic autonomic nervous system
Tendon organs
Tensegrity
Trigger points

Beginning students of massage may find scientific justification intimidating. However, it is important to develop an understanding of this knowledge at the beginning of the educational process because it is one of the foundations of our profession. This firm foundation in the anatomical and physiological explanations of the reasons massage may provide benefit enables us to trust our intuition while designing a massage based on information received from the client during assessment procedures. Therefore the purpose of this chapter is to help you understand the physiological basis for the effectiveness of therapeutic massage so that you can feel confident about the beneficial outcomes massage can provide.

The primary goal for massage therapists is to provide safe, beneficial massage care for clients. We need to make valid decisions and justify the decisions to achieve those goals. When something is *valid,* it is based on truth or logical reasoning. *Justification* is the process of showing something accurate and reasonable through verbal explanation or by writing to communicate the justification process. Client care/treatment planning and documentation involve justification. When we make decisions on how to work with a massage therapy client, we need to make sure that the information we use is factual and reliable and the decision-making process is rational. Critical thinking is how we make rational decisions. Critical thinking involves the evaluation of sources such as data, facts, observable phenomena, and research findings, which allows us to draw conclusions to make workable decisions.

As discussed in Chapter 2, claims made for massage benefits must be based on valid evidence. An important source of this evidence is scientific research. The *American Heritage Dictionary* defines **science** as "the intellectual process of using all mental and physical resources available to better understand, explain, and predict both normal and unusual natural phenomena." The scientific approach to understanding anything involves observation, measurement of things that can be tested, accumulation of data, and analysis of the findings. The scientific approach, therefore is different from an intuitive approach. Other terms for intuition are *feelings, inspiration, instinct, revelation, impulse,* and *idea.* Research and intuition are both important and work together to help us understand the benefits of therapeutic massage. As massage therapy becomes integrated into multidisciplinary teams that focus both on the client's well-being and health, in addition to medical care, we must be able to communicate and justify our recommendations and approaches to care.

Effectiveness refers to a result acquired in an average clinical or a real-world environment whereas **efficacy** refers to a result acquired under ideal or controlled conditions. A growing body of research supports the effectiveness and safety of massage therapy. Increasingly massage therapy is being incorporated into medical environments. (Mallory et al., 2018; Dusek et al., 2021; Dingding et al., 2022).

MASSAGE AS ART AND SCIENCE

SECTION OBJECTIVES

Chapter objective covered in this section:

1. Explain the meaning of evidence-informed practice.

Using the information presented in this section, the student will be able to:

- Define intuition.
- Describe evidence-based practice.
- Describe evidence-informed practice.
- Define biological plausibility.
- List types of bias in research.
- Explain correlation and causation.

Intuition is knowing something without using a conscious process of thinking. You may wonder why a chapter about research begins with a seemingly abstract concept; however, intuition is one of the foundations of evidence-informed decision making. Scientific and intuitive approaches are equally important. In his lecture, "Stress without Distress: Evolution of the Concept," renowned researcher Hans Selye emphasized the importance of both science and intuition. Unless there is first an idea (intuition), Dr. Selye said, there is nothing to research, and without research (science), an idea does not develop form and usefulness. One does not function without the other.

Intuition is the ability to bring subconscious information into conscious awareness. Developing intuitive skills assists the massage therapist in the assessment process and in adapting massage for each client. Through experience, massage therapists just "know" when a certain area of the client's body needs to be worked, and they can sense when the area is complete and needs no more work. This is not mystical, but a function of developed sensory awareness. Intuition is a skill that can be practiced and refined. We can all be more purposeful and conscious of intuitive information.

Biofeedback works on a similar principle. Using equipment that detects the heart rate, blood pressure, and skin temperature, a person can monitor and adjust involuntary, or subconscious, responses.

Mindfulness is the basic human ability to be fully present, aware of where we are and what we're doing, and not overly reactive or overwhelmed by what's going on around us. It takes practice to learn to pay attention to quiet, subtle information amid all the loud, exaggerated stimulation that can blast our sensory receptors every day. When we are mindful, intuition is more apparent.

Massage therapy is both an art and a science. An *art* is craft, skill, technique, and talent. Perfecting your artistic approach to massage involves disciplined and ongoing practice. As you begin learning about massage application, you must spend considerable time practicing before the art of massage application becomes evident. *Talent* is defined as a natural, innate ability. Although some may have a talent for massage, massage therapy is a learned art. Diligent practice, along with desire, passion, and compassion, will help you become an excellent massage therapist.

Recognizing how important intuition is in the art of the massage profession is important. However, realizing how scientific research validates massage therapy is equally important. This validation distinguishes massage as a biologically plausible, effective therapeutic approach from mere speculation, myths, and misinformation about massage and related bodywork methods.

Biological plausibility is the existence of a physiological mechanism that may explain a cause-and-effect relationship. For example, it is biologically plausible that mechanical force applied during massage may support movement of interstitial fluid into lymphatic capillaries. However, the claim that extremely light touch with one finger on the bottom of the feet can change thyroid function is not biologically plausible.

Massage therapy as defined in this textbook fits the model of biological plausibility and is supported by scientific research. It is the relationship of other bodywork methods to massage that creates confusion. Many of the bodywork methods, such as no-touch approaches (often called energy-based methods), and other approaches based only on the opinions of one or two individuals who claim to have the found the "secret answer," do not fit the concept of biological plausibility. When associated with massage, these types of bodywork methods undermine and weaken the clarity of massage as an evidence-informed system.

Later, in Chapter 12, a variety of bodywork methods are explored. Some, such as connective tissue methods and hydrotherapy, easily blend into the evidence-informed and biologically plausible foundation of massage. Most of the methods described in Chapter 12 are actually standard massage methods adapted to target a specific tissue type or physiological function. This is the case with the connective tissue, neuromuscular/trigger point, and fluid movement approaches. Unfortunately, these methods have been separated enough from massage therapy to be considered somewhat unique approaches. Other methods that currently do not meet the criteria for biological plausibility are also briefly described. These are included to prepare the reader to make informed decisions about whether and when to learn more about the approach or to consider how the methods may influence the development of a justifiable massage therapy treatment plan for an individual client who uses these types of bodywork. This is not a judgment about the usefulness of certain methods; rather, the intent is to clarify what can be combined with massage as adjunct bodywork methods and maintain an evidence-informed and biologically plausible approach to massage.

Evidence-Informed Massage Therapy Practice

Massage therapy is an evidence-based and evidence-informed practice. **Evidence** includes everything that is used to determine or demonstrate the validity of a claim. The evidence needs to be unbiased and valid. The term *evidence* does not necessarily mean that something is a *fact*. All a research study can do is capture a specific information set based on the **experiment**. However, as continuing research supports the findings, it becomes more likely that the application is valid. For example, if we are going to state that massage therapy is beneficial, then we need to support that assertion, and we can do that in a few areas in which systematic reviews and meta-analyses have been conducted on massage-related research studies. Systematic reviews and meta-analyses combine and review many individual research studies and are considered high-quality evidence.

When a sufficient amount of high-quality research exists, a method can be considered research based. Massage research is getting much better, but it has a long way to go before sufficient high-quality research is available to consider massage therapy a research-based system. This means that massage therapy cannot justifiably be considered an **evidence-based practice**, either. Massage therapy fits much better in an *evidence-informed* model. **Evidence-informed practice (EIP)** avoids scientific prejudices and superstitions, sometimes called *pseudoscience*. It requires that practitioners become knowledgeable about a wide range of sources (i.e., empirical studies, case studies, and clinical insights) and use them in creative ways throughout the massage therapy process, supporting a client-centered approach to care. This model supports **evidence-informed decision making**, an ongoing process involving the use of the best available evidence to provide care for clients.

As we search for evidence, we must remain objective and willing to collect all the relevant research available, not just the information that supports massage. When making informed decisions about the value and approach to massage, we need to consider all the evidence from scientific research, both supportive and nonsupportive. We also need to consider other forms of evidence, such as collective clinical experience, expert opinion consensus, historical and cultural foundations, and consistency of client experience. As the massage profession evolves and more research becomes available, it is important to search for and use interventions that have been shown by well-controlled research studies to have a statistically significant treatment effect.

As more of this type of evidence becomes available, all of us in the massage profession must examine some of the "myths" that arose before valid evidence was available. Most of the myths began as well-intentioned, educated guesses. Valid research indicates that some of those educated guesses are accurate, but many are not. For example, a few years ago, cancer was considered an absolute contraindication to massage; now, research has shown that massage therapy has many benefits for those undergoing cancer treatments.

We all need to develop an inquiring mind; therefore practice asking your instructors relevant questions. Remember, it is not the instructor's job to know all the answers. Instead, work together to find the evidence. If no systematic reviews or meta-analyses are available to address your question, begin to search for other study types, such as individual clinical multiple case reports, and consider using other types of guidance, such as the opinions of multiple experts.

A number of questions have arisen in the massage profession about the emphasis on evidence-informed practices, including:

- What should be done when there are different levels of evidence or changes in evidence?
- What are the limits of evidence?
- What should be done when no scientific evidence exists for a massage approach?
- What if an intervention, such as massage therapy, cannot be easily researched in double-blind, random, controlled studies?
- What if studies produce conflicting evidence?

Research evidence can be complicated by differences in the design, quality, and number of studies performed on any single intervention. Often the results are inconsistent. With the increase in the types and quality of research being done in massage therapy, the evidence is changing quickly, and this puts a greater demand on massage therapists to stay current. For example, this textbook is based on the most current research available at the time it was published. However, a textbook usually is revised only every 3–5 years; consequently, some of the information it contains already may be outdated. For these reasons, you must learn how to ask relevant questions and find the evidence for yourself.

As the massage profession embraces evidence-informed practices, we must be honest about the quality of the evidence for therapeutic massage (Fletcher et al., 2014). Currently the volume of research evidence is growing, but the quality of the research is less than optimal. The low quality of the research is interfering with the ability of massage therapy to take the next step toward evidence-based practice and integration into whole person care systems (Bokhour et al., 2022). As part of a health professions occupation, the massage therapy community must acknowledge this while striving to determine the best practices for massage. Often, when you are searching for research, the term *manual therapy* will yield additional results relevant to massage therapy. **Manual therapy** is defined as contact with the soft tissues, bones, and joints with the hands, arms, or elbows of the practitioners to enhance the therapeutic effect. Massage is a form of manual therapy.

Most massage therapists will not become formal researchers, but it is important for the massage community to support the individuals who have sought advanced academic degrees and are affiliated with research facilities, such as universities. The massage community also needs to develop relationships with researchers and work in conjunction with them to support high-quality research. Support for the Massage Therapy Foundation is a way to assist.

Little or no research is available on certain types of bodywork and claimed benefits. This does not mean these types of bodywork are of no value or that they are not valid. It means that we do not know, and that is okay. However, it is unethical to make claims about any approach when there is no evidence to support the claims. Instead, the client must be informed about the lack of evidence. The emphasis on evidence-informed practice should create pressure to develop and test these interventions to fill the need for informed, rather than opinion-based, massage therapy practice. When we do not know whether a massage method is valid, but the potential exists for benefit with little chance of harm, informed decision making by the massage therapist and the client together determines whether including the method in the massage session is appropriate. Mysteries will always remain, but we are professionally obligated to know the research available and to admit when we do not know the answers.

Although scientific research is not the only form of valid evidence, it is an especially important part of an evidence-informed massage practice. Most of us will not actually conduct formal research in a research laboratory. All of us, however, need to be research users and evaluators to make sure we are the most informed massage therapists possible.

Bias

Bias is a tendency toward a preconceived belief. Research bias, also called *experimenter bias,* is a process in which those performing the research influence the results in order to portray a certain outcome. Biases within research are widespread and often unintentional, but they often can be overcome by following research methods. The scientific process, with peer review and research replication, is a way to identify and correct misinformation related to bias. When critically evaluating research, we need to be aware of the potential for bias. This is why it is recommended to view multiple studies related to a topic and compare methods and results. The overlap of agreement is likely to be less influenced by bias.

If we consider the critical thinking involved with making decisions as the same process as scientific inquiry, all of us need to be aware of bias in our thinking. People tend to see patterns that do not actually exist, such as the figures in clouds. People tend to connect causal relationships between events that actually are unrelated. *Apophenia* is the tendency to perceive connections and meaning between unrelated things. *Pareidolia* is the tendency to perceive a specific, often meaningful image in a random or ambiguous visual pattern. The tendency to seek and preserve patterns make us susceptible to bias. *Cherry-picking* is the term given to the act of selecting only data that conform with what the experimenter is expecting, or hoping, to see. Cherry-picking research that supports our opinion is a form of bias. Many common types of bias can occur in research. A few of the most common are:

- Participant bias occurs when participants in the research react the way they think the researcher desires.
- Selection bias is an experimental error that occurs when the participant pool, or the subsequent data, is not representative of the target population.
- Confirmation bias occurs when a researcher forms a **hypothesis**, or belief, and uses respondents' information to confirm that belief.

Bias exists in all study designs, and researchers need to acknowledge the tendency to bias and take steps to minimize its influence. Researchers bring to each study their experiences, ideas, prejudices, and personal philosophies, just as do those reading the research. For a study to be valid, the researchers must understand the potential for bias and screen the data collection and study design. Ethics committees that review research design have an important role in considering whether the research design and methodological approaches are biased. *Peer review* is a process in which subject matter experts read, validate, and critique a research paper to make sure the research was conducted accurately, and bias was minimized. Peer review is an essential part of identifying a flawed research design and bias. The pattern of the **scientific method** helps manage the tendency toward bias. As we read research, it is important to identify whether measures have been taken to reduce bias. It is helpful to use sources that have prescreened research, such as peer-reviewed journals and the online source PubMed.

PubMed is a free search engine that provides access to bibliographical information in Medline and other life science journals. PubMed is maintained and updated by the National Library of Medicine (NLM) on a weekly basis. Medline is the National Library of Medicine's premier bibliographical database, which covers the fields of medicine, nursing, dentistry, veterinary medicine, the health care system, and the preclinical sciences. Medline collects from more than 4500 biomedical journals published in the United States and internationally. The NLM has rules for peer review, and it decides on a case-by-case basis which journals and articles are listed on PubMed. A *peer-reviewed scientific journal* is a publication that contains original articles that have been written by scientists and evaluated for technical and scientific quality and correctness by other experts in the same field.

Correlation and Causation

Science often is about measuring relationships between two or more factors. With *correlation,* two factors (or variables) are related, but one does not necessarily cause the other. With *causation,* one factor (or variable) causes the other. Without valid research, it is common to mix up correlation and causation. Correlation is different from causation; sometimes two things can share a relationship without one causing the other.

For example, we might want to know whether massage therapy promotes a reduced heart rate and blood pressure during a 30-minute, 60-minute, or 90-minute session. Let's say that massage for 30 minutes does not involve a reduction in blood pressure, but massage for 60 minutes does. We notice this relationship—correlation—but do not know if the massage actually is causing the change in blood pressure. To prove causation, you need to find a direct relationship between the variables: 60-minute massage and lower blood pressure. You need to show that one relies on the other, not just that the two appear to be related. A variety of related events occur when someone receives a massage. An *experiment* is needed to separate correlation from causation. Using the example of massage and blood pressure, an experiment may show that massage actually did cause the blood pressure change. Or the experiment might show that lying down for a certain period, not the massage, was that actual cause of the lower blood pressure readings.

We can notice many correlations, but only research conducted accurately, reviewed diligently, and repeated and compared will determine causation. When you read health-based research, it is important to remember the difference between correlation and causation.

RESEARCH LITERACY

SECTION OBJECTIVES

Chapter objectives covered in this section:

2. Explain the meaning of research literacy.
3. Use levels of evidence guidelines to categorize research.

Using the information presented in this section, the student will be able to:

- Develop a research question.
- Use search engines and databases to locate research related to massage therapy.
- Use a research question to find evidence on PubMed.
- Define forms of research.

Research literacy (or *scientific literacy*) is the knowledge and understanding of scientific concepts and processes required for personal and professional decision making. When we are research literate, we can find, read, and understand the research and use critical thinking to determine the validity of the information presented. Learning to be a critical thinker (see Chapter 2) is the first step in becoming research literate. Critical thinking and the scientific method are remarkably similar.

Developing an inquiry-based approach to life is also important. This means that we learn to ask relevant questions, such as, "Why and how does massage help reduce uncomfortable stress responses?" Relevant questions evolve from mindfulness and intuition. Only when we have relevant questions can we begin the research process. Scientifically based research methods are a way to seek answers to those questions.

A search of research literature reveals information from researchers who designed and conducted a study to look for answers to some of the same questions we might have. Because most of us will not perform complex research studies (although we can all be researchers if we do case reports), we need to find and examine other people's research on questions that are the same or similar to ours. Part of reading research articles involves making sure the research was conducted properly and that the information is scientifically valid and not just opinion. A great resource is the National Center for Complementary and Integrative Health, https://www.nccih.nih.gov/ and specifically for understanding research, view https://www.nccih.nih.gov/health/know-science and https://www.nccih.nih.gov/health/know-science/make-sense-health-research.

Literature Search and Literature Review

Every time you look for information about how to understand a client and adapt a massage session to best meet the goals of the massage, you are conducting a *literature search.* To complete a literature search, you need to:

- Define what you are searching for by identifying the topic
- Decide where to search (e.g., the internet or the library)
- Develop a search strategy by identifying search terms and key words
- Save your search results for future use

When you analyze the information found during a literature search, this is called a *literature review.* A literature review can be informal and used to guide massage application. A literature review can also be a formal scholarly paper. A literature review article discusses published information in a particular subject area. The focus of a literature review is to summarize and synthesize the arguments and ideas of others without adding new contributions. The main focus of an academic research paper is to develop a new argument, and a research paper is likely to contain a literature review as one of its parts. When you search for information, it is important to seek current information no older than 5 years. That does not mean that older information is not valuable. You can understand the progression of how information evolves by studying a historical research stream through to current time.

The focus of the literature search should be a clear, targeted statement with identified search terms. Different methods can be used to develop effective search strategies. One is the PICO strategy (Grewal et al., 2016).

PICO Strategy

Identification of the best evidence requires the construction of an appropriate research question and review of the literature. The PICO strategy (patient and problem, intervention, comparison, outcome) can be used to construct the research question and subsequent literature review. It is easily adapted to massage therapy to support a literature search.

PICO can be described in more detail:

- ***P**atient* (clients) and ***p**roblem*
  - How would I describe a group of clients similar to mine?
    Example: I have a client with ongoing stress who is not sleeping well.
- ***I**ntervention*
  - Which main intervention are you considering? What do you want to do for the client? What is the main alternative to compare with the intervention? What factor or factors may influence the prognosis for the client (e.g., age, coexisting problems)?
    Example: I am considering general, nonspecific massage for relaxation. Other options include specific work on the breathing process to reduce sympathetic arousal.
- Comparison
  - What is the main alternative to compare with the intervention? Are you trying to decide between two bodywork methods? (Your clinical question may not always have a specific comparison.)
    Example: The client has tried yoga and meditation.
- Outcome
  - What can you hope to accomplish, measure, improve, or affect? What are you trying to do for the client: relieve or eliminate the symptoms? Help the client manage stress, manage pain, or increase functional mobility?
    Example: I want to help the client manage stress and support sleep.

The question to guide the literature search would be "Can massage manage stress and support sleep?" Based on the PICO strategy, the search terms would be *massage* AND *stress* AND *sleep.*

Internet Literature Search to Obtain Evidence

Since the 1980s, the internet has permitted rapid location of relevant evidence. In the mid-1990s, PubMed and other databases that can be searched electronically became available. Research results now are available to anyone who wants to understand the underlying physiological mechanisms of therapeutic massage benefits, and they continue to support the value of therapeutic massage. Effective searching requires a series of steps to lead the massage practitioner from the clinical question "What can I do to help this client?" to informed decision making to develop a plan to help the client. Massage therapists use critical thinking to determine the validity and applicability of the evidence found through internet searches and then to decide whether the information should inform clinical decisions.

Web sites for research include PubMed, Medline, and Google Scholar. There are other sites and databases. Your local library is a great place to learn about literature searches. Begin your development of research literacy by learning to use PubMed. PubMed Central (PMC) is a free archive of biomedical and life sciences journal literature at the National Institutes of Health's National Library of Medicine (NIH/NLM). Research papers and articles published on PubMed have gone through a research screening process. These articles undergo expert assessment before publication to ensure that they are meaningful within the context of other research in the discipline and, at least in theory, have a sound methodology. The research must be published in a peer-reviewed publication approved by PubMed.

Using PubMed Central

Once you have used the PICO strategy to identify the question guiding the literature search and the search terms, log on to PubMed (https://www.ncbi.nlm.nih.gov/pubmed/). When the main page opens, find the "LEARN" tab and PubMed User Guide. This guide explains how to perform a search on PubMed. Start your search with these terms: *massage therapy, manual therapy, massage therapy systematic reviews,* and *massage therapy research.* It is exciting to see how much research exists. There are hundreds of papers and articles. It is necessary to narrow the search. Add terms or combine search terms with connector words—AND, OR, or NOT using uppercase letters (called Boolean logic):

- AND between terms returns only records that contain all of the search terms
- OR between terms returns all records that contain any of the search terms
- NOT between search terms returns only records that contain the first term and not the second

For example: massage therapy OR manual therapy AND diabetes NOT type 1 diabetes.

Another recommended site for a literature search is Cochrane (https://www.cochrane.org/). Cochrane Reviews are internationally recognized as the highest standard in evidence-based health care. They are published online in the Cochrane Library (https://www.cochranelibrary.com/), a collection of databases that contain different types of high-quality, independent evidence to inform health care decision making. Cochrane Complementary Medicine (https://cam.cochrane.org) is based at the University of Maryland Center for Integrative Medicine, where it has been in place since the establishment of the field in 1996. An international group of collaborators has contributed to systematic reviews of controlled clinical trials in areas such as acupuncture, massage, herbal medicine, and mind/body therapy, among others, and disseminated the results of these systematic reviews. The goal is to promote an evidence-based approach to health care in the area of complementary and alternative care medicine (CAM) therapies (Box 5.1).

Forms of Research

Research is an investigation to learn more about a topic and to find answers to questions. Research can be informal or formal. When you are searching for information about a client's condition to make informed decisions about adapting massage for safety and benefit, you are conducting an informal type of research. Formal research is a careful and detailed investigation

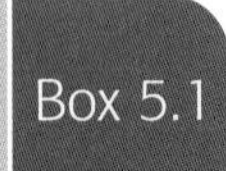

Box 5.1 Stages in the Process of Developing a Research Question and Review of the Literature

1. **Define:** Clearly define the issue using the PICO strategy (*p*roblem, *i*ntervention, *c*omparison, *o*utcome).
2. **Search:** Efficiently search for information on the issues in the research question using MedlinePlus; then research science-based evidence beginning with PubMed as an internet search. Also use Google Scholar. Your local library and librarian are other great resources.
3. **Appraise:** Critically and efficiently appraise the research sources using recommendations in this chapter.
4. **Synthesize:** Interpret information and evidence related to an issue using critical thinking skills. Relate the factual content to possible massage strategies and analysis application based on logistics and clients' feelings about the massage strategies proposed.
5. **Adapt:** Adapt the information to a specific situation based on previous critical thinking processes.
6. **Implement:** Decide whether and how to implement the adapted evidence into practice as a specific treatment or care plan for each client.
7. **Evaluate:** Evaluate the effectiveness of the implementation efforts.

into a specific problem, concern, or issue using the scientific method. Research may be applied or basic. *Applied research* seeks to solve a practical problem. *Basic research* seeks information for the sake of knowing but doesn't necessarily provide results of immediate, practical use.

Quantitative and Qualitative Designs

The two main approaches to a research problem are quantitative methods and qualitative methods. Quantitative methods are used to examine the relationship between variables, with the primary goal of analyzing and representing that relationship mathematically through statistical analysis. This is the type of research approach most commonly used in scientific research problems. Qualitative methods are chosen when the goal of the research problem is to examine, understand, and describe a phenomenon. These methods are a common choice in social science research problems and are often used to study ideas, beliefs, human behaviors, and other research questions that do not involve studying the relationship between variables.

A mixed research design involves both a quantitative design and a qualitative design. Mixed design studies take significantly more time, more resources, and require the researcher to develop expertise in qualitative and quantitative analysis techniques.

Several types of experiments are performed in research.

- *Randomized controlled trials* involve a randomization procedure in which each subject has an equal chance of being assigned to an intervention group that actually receives the treatment or a control group that receives a fake treatment. Randomization helps prevent researchers from knowingly or unknowingly creating bias in the outcomes. Randomized controlled trials are the gold standard for establishing the effects of a treatment.
- *Clinical trials* are research studies that explore whether a medical strategy, treatment, or device is safe and effective for humans.
- *Cohort studies,* also called *prospective* or *longitudinal studies,* use observation as the research method. The interventions are not manipulated; rather, the researchers select and follow a large population of people who have the same condition and/or are receiving a specific intervention over a period of time. The progression and results of treatment are compared with a group not affected by the condition.
- *Outcomes research* involves a larger group of individuals who receive the same intervention. They are evaluated for outcomes after the intervention is complete. Outcomes research seeks to understand the end results of particular health care practices and interventions. End results include effects that people experience and care about, such as a change in the ability to function. Unlike clinical trials or other highly regulated scientific studies that consider only concrete, measurable data (e.g., mortality rates), health outcomes research broadens the scope to also incorporate clinical outcomes, financial impact, and a range of functional measures, including patients' reported quality of life and satisfaction. The data gathered can come from a number of avenues and methodologies, including medical records, insurance databases, patient questionnaires, and more. By looking at a greater range of measures, health outcomes studies can provide guidance on a broader set of interventions and decisions than can clinical trials.
- A *case series* is a collection of comprehensive reports that follow the research method on a series of clients with the same condition who are receiving the same intervention.
- A *case report* involves a report on the intervention and outcome for a single client.

The best evidence to determine whether an intervention, such as massage, actually causes the outcome is the double-blind, random, controlled clinical trial. It consists of the randomized assignment of subjects or participants in a *double-blind design,* in which neither the investigators nor the study subjects know the actual treatment group in which the subjects are placed. This type of trial also uses a *control group,* in which no intervention is used, and a *sham group,* in which a fictional treatment is provided. This type of trial is difficult to design for massage therapy research; one of the biggest challenges is devising fake or fictional massage. However, progress is being made, and more quality research should be forthcoming.

Evidence can be classified into various levels. Professional journals that publish research are introducing guidelines and instructing authors to label the strength of evidence of their research in terms of rating scales. In addition multiple methods are used to categorize research. The simplest method is the ABC method (Box 5.2).

Systematic Review and Meta-Analysis

Systematic reviews and meta-analyses combine multiple research studies that are similar in design. A systematic review usually is restricted to random, controlled studies, which are considered valid evidence if they are well done. A group of

Box 5.2 Guidelines for Levels of Evidence

ABC System

Level A: Well-conducted random controlled studies (RCT) with 100 or more subjects

Level B: Well-conducted case-control studies; poorly controlled or uncontrolled observation studies with high potential for bias; or RCT with one or more major—or three or more minor—methodological flaws or case series or case reports

Level C: Expert opinion

Quality of Evidence

The quality of the overall evidence is graded on a three-point scale:

Good: Evidence includes consistent results from well-designed, well-conducted studies, in representative populations, that directly assess effects on health outcomes.

Fair: Evidence is sufficient to determine effects on health outcomes, but the strength of the evidence is limited by the number, quality, or consistency of the individual studies; the generalizability to routine practice; or the indirect nature of the evidence on health outcomes.

Poor: Evidence is insufficient to assess the effects on health outcomes because of limited number or power of studies; important flaws in their design or conduct; gaps in the chain of evidence; or lack of information on important health outcomes.

Tricoci P, Allen JM, Kramer JM, Califf RM, Smith SC. Scientific evidence underlying the ACC/AHA clinical practice guidelines. *JAMA.* 2009;301(8):831–841.

reviewers searches the available literature databases by entering common terminologies into the databases and retrieving copies of all the articles written on a specific topic. After all the research has been collected, the reviewers use critical thinking methods to evaluate the validity of each study and then synthesize the results. The final product reports on properly completed, meaningful research that is relevant to practitioners and clinicians.

A meta-analysis is a type of systematic review that uses statistical methods to combine and analyze multiple investigations. Massage therapy research has expanded enough for systematic reviews and meta-analysis research to be complete. This is an exciting development and will be the primary information focus in this chapter. The Cochrane Database of Systematic Reviews (CDSR) is a great resource for looking up health care reviews.

THE RESEARCH PROCESS

SECTION OBJECTIVES

Chapter objectives covered in this section:

4. Describe the fundamentals of the Western scientific process.
5. Critically read a research paper.

Using the information presented in this section, the student will be able to:

- List the components of the scientific method.
- Describe basic types of research.
- Critically read a research paper.

Box 5.3 We Can All Be Researchers

All massage therapists can serve as researchers and contributors to the massage body of evidence by collecting information and writing case reports. Case reports are professional narratives that outline the assessment, treatment, and outcomes of the massage benefit for individual clients. Information from case reports provides feedback on clinical practice guidelines and offers a framework for early signals of effectiveness, adverse events, and cost.

The Massage Therapy Foundation supports the massage profession in writing case reports and provides information on how to author these reports. The foundation's website is http://www.massagetherapyfoundation.org/.

The Massage Therapy Foundation supports the *International Journal of Therapeutic Massage & Bodywork: Research, Education, & Practice* (IJTMB). This journal is an open-access, peer-reviewed publication intended to accommodate the diverse needs of the rapidly expanding therapeutic massage and bodywork community. Principal sections of the journal span the areas of research, education, and clinical practice. The journal's website is http://www.ijtmb.org/index.php/ijtmb.

The IJTMB recommends the use of the CARE framework (www.care-statement.org) for writing, reviewing, and publishing case reports. The CARE guidelines provide a framework that helps ensure transparency and accuracy in the publication of case reports and in the reporting of information from patient/client encounters. The acronym CARE was created by combining CA (the first two letters in "case") and RE (the first two letters in "reports"). The CARE tools are the CARE checklist and the templates for writing a case report. These tools facilitate the writing of case reports and provide data that informs clinical practice guidelines and provides early signals of effectiveness, harm, and cost.

From Gagnier J, Kienle G, Altman DG, et al. The CARE guidelines: consensus-based clinical case report guideline development, *J Clin Epidemiol.* 2014;67(1):46–51. Available at: http://www.care-statement.org/.

This section focuses on preparing you to become a consumer of research. It provides a brief survey of the process of conducting research. In addition it teaches you how to read research papers critically so that you can make two important determinations: whether the research is valid and how the research influences massage application.

The scientific method is an excellent model for logical thinking. As a massage professional, logical thinking is a skill you use every day, whether you are designing a treatment plan or determining what information from a research paper is valid and useful and what is not. Understanding the research process can help you make successful decisions in many aspects of your life. You may even become interested in writing a case report for the Massage Therapy Foundation case report contest (Box 5.3).

Definition and Origin of Research

At its most basic, research can be defined as a process in which researchers explore one or more areas of interest (called *factors* or *variablesd*) by analyzing numerical and/or verbal data (collected information) to advance the understanding of that subject. For example, a researcher might undertake the task of characterizing the percentage of adults surveyed nationwide who have used therapeutic massage as a form of complementary and integrative health care. Researchers might also explore massage as an intervention for chronic low back pain. They might develop a detailed interview process to document a client's individual experience and perception of therapeutic massage over a designated period as an intervention for chronic low back pain. Research could explore the relationship, if any, between aquatic massage therapy and increased range of motion for clients recovering from bilateral hip replacement surgery. In another case, a massage therapist could complete an exhaustive review and synthesis of what the professional literature has to say about therapeutic massage as a viable intervention for clients with fibromyalgia. All of these examples describe different types of research processes.

Basically, two types of research are used for scientific studies: observational research and experimental research.

Observational Research

Although observational research may be used in the laboratory, it is primarily conducted in a natural setting to study the relationship between a specific factor and some aspect of health or illness. For this reason, observational research may suggest an association, but it cannot be used to determine cause and effect. An example of observational research would be a study focusing on whether males or females receive massage more frequently.

Compared to experimental studies, observational research designs are quite simple. Fundamentally, the research team simply observes the target groups or processes and uses statistical methods to determine whether an association exists. However, this approach gives rise to many problems. The results of the research may confuse the true effect of a variable and the possible effects of other factors in the environment. For example, an observational study may indicate that women receive massage 50% more often than men, but it cannot determine the reasons for this difference. Observational research is therefore often followed by experimental studies to validate cause and effect.

The most frequently used type of observational research is the epidemiological study, which is considered the basic science of public health. Usually focused on the study of large groups (sometimes tens of thousands or hundreds of thousands of people), epidemiology attempts to identify possible factors that increase the risk or probability of a disease or behavior in groups of people. Through one type of epidemiologic research, the analytic study, scientists observe certain behaviors (e.g., receiving massage) and track whether certain outcomes occur (e.g., the gender differences in massage frequency). Another type of epidemiological research, the descriptive study, involves the collection of information to characterize and summarize a behavior, health event, or problem. For example, a descriptive study may examine the massage frequency associated with such factors as the time of day, the gender of the massage therapist, or the age of the client.

Scientists also use several other methods to conduct epidemiological studies, and all of these methods have a number of significant limitations. One type of study design, the cross-sectional study, is basically the same as a survey. In this type of study, the researcher defines the population to be studied and then collects information from members of the group about their behavior. Because the data represent a point in time, this is like taking a snapshot of the population. Cross-sectional studies are good for examining the relationship between a variable and a behavior (e.g., receiving massage) or a disease (e.g., the flu) but not for determining cause and effect, which requires the collection of data over time.

In a cohort study researchers select the study population according to the group members' exposure, regardless of the health outcome being studied or whether the group has the disease. The researchers then determine the outcomes of interest and compare the results on the basis of the individuals' exposures. Cohort studies often are referred to as prospective studies because they follow the study population forward in time, from suspected cause to effect. An example of a cohort study would be defining a group of people on the basis of massage received weekly and following them for 5 years to see whether they showed a reduced tendency for muscle tension headache.

Another option is the case-control study, in which the research team works backward, from the effect to the suspected cause; for this reason, case-control studies often are referred to as retrospective studies. Participants are selected on the basis of the presence or absence of the disease or outcome in question; therefore the study involves one group of people who have the behavior or problem (case subjects) and one group of people who do not (controls). These groups are compared to determine the presence of specific exposures or risk factors. An example of a case-control study would involve forming a group of people with tension headache and another group without it and then comparing the two groups for their history of receiving massage.

Regardless of the method used, the key point to understand about the results of observational studies is that they are observations of associations and nothing more. They can tell us what but not why. By conducting observational studies, researchers can add valuable information to the existing literature on a particular topic, which helps them design future research studies, including clinical trials.

Experimental Research

Basic research generates data by investigating biochemical substances or biological processes. It often is conducted to confirm observations or to determine the way a particular process works. For example, an experiment might be conducted to examine how massage for 20 minutes on the head, hands, and feet helps promote falling asleep in less than 15 minutes after going to bed.

Basic research is often conducted in test tubes (in vitro) or with animals (in vivo). Research with animals is an important tool for determining how humans may react when exposed to particular substances. However, it is important to note that, because of differences in physiology and the fact that animals are routinely exposed to levels of compounds far higher than those humans typically encounter, one cannot assume that results from animal studies can be generalized to humans. Therapeutic massage is extremely difficult to test in vitro, although various studies based on fascia tissue samples may be possible.

For experimental research, study subjects—whether human or animal—are selected according to relevant characteristics and are randomly assigned to an experimental group (i.e., the group that will receive the treatment or intervention) or a control group (i.e., the group that does not receive the treatment). Random assignment ensures that factors that may affect the outcome of the study (variables) are distributed equally among the groups and therefore cannot lead to differences in the effect of a treatment. As a result, any differences in results between the groups can be attributed to the treatment. However, controlled experimental research can be flawed; therefore it is important to know how the study was designed and conducted.

The most significant type of experimental research is the clinical trial, which uses human subjects to evaluate the effectiveness and safety of a treatment by monitoring its effect on large groups of people. Clinical trials generally are conducted by independent researchers or by researchers affiliated with a hospital or university medical program or private industry. These studies may be small, involving a limited number of participants, or they may be large intervention trials that attempt to discover the outcome of treatments on entire populations. The more participants in the study, the greater the likelihood that the results can be replicated in the general population.

Besides the size of the study, another critical factor is the way the research was designed. As mentioned previously, scientists place the most value on the double-blind, placebo-controlled study that uses random assignment of subjects to experimental and control groups. Considered the gold standard of clinical research studies, the double-blind, placebo-controlled study provides dependable findings that are free of bias introduced by either the subject or the researcher. In this type of study, neither the subject nor the researcher knows whether the test substance or a placebo has been administered. For the results to be valid and to ensure that the subject cannot violate the blinding, the placebo and the test substance must be virtually identical (i.e., look, smell, and taste similar). Blinding for massage is difficult; what can be used as a placebo for massage? A possible blinding approach might be a study in which all participants received the same massage routine but some received trigger point therapy on four specific points related to low back pain and other participants did not. Blinding is one of the hurdles researchers must overcome in conducting massage-based research.

Ethics in Research

Research involves several important concerns related to ethics and the ethical conduct of research. Informed consent, confidentiality, the ability to exit the study at any time without prejudice, and debriefing are some of the ethical issues researchers must face. The advancement of science must not occur at the expense of the safety and well-being of research participants. Those conducting research with human subjects must get an approval. An institutional review board (IRB), also known a research ethics review committee (ERC) or an ethical review board (ERB), is a committee or board that reviews the methods proposed for research to ensure that they comply with ethical standards as laid out by the Office of Human Research Protections (OHRP). The OHRP provides leadership in the protection of the rights, welfare, and well-being of human subjects involved in research conducted or supported by the US Department of Health and Human Services (HHS).

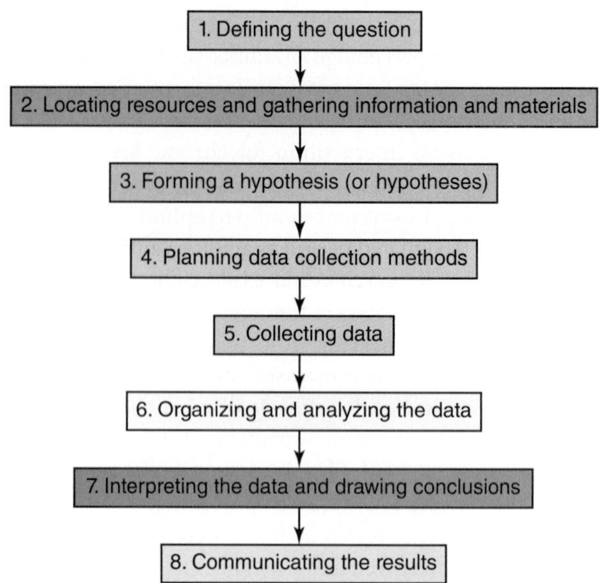

FIG. 5.1 The research process.

Research in Plain Language

The scientific method is a model for conducting scientific research. A specific vocabulary is used during the research process. The scientific method has eight primary steps (Fig. 5.1).

Step 1: Defining the Question

All research begins with a basic question: What do I want to know? Examples of research questions might include the following:

- Does using essential oils in combination with massage increase arterial circulation to the extremities better than massage alone?
- How long should a hamstring stretch be maintained during massage to affect the pliability of the associated connective tissue?
- How much pressure (compressive load) is required to influence lymphatic flow in a healthy subject?

This first step of the scientific method involves narrowing down possible topics and then choosing the question that will be the focus of the research. The research question must be specific. For example, in the preceding example question 1, the topics of essentials oils, massage, and arterial circulation are too broad. A better question would be: Does using lavender essential oil in combination with massage based on compression loading to the soles of the feet increase arterial circulation to the feet better that the same massage protocol to the soles of the feet without lavender essential oil?

To develop a research question, researchers must identify five specific goals:

1. What they want to know
2. The reason for asking the question

3. What the answer will tell them
4. How the information can be beneficial
5. Whether the question can be answered through research

Continuing with our previous example, the researchers want to know whether combining lavender oil with massage is better than massage alone for increasing circulation to the feet (goal 1). The reason for asking the question is to determine whether better results can be obtained in supporting circulation to the feet if lavender oil is used with massage (goal 2). The results (answer) will determine whether including lavender oil in compression-based massage of the feet is worth the expense and effort (goal 3). If using lavender oil with compression-based massage does increase arterial circulation better than massage alone, then clients with circulation problems in the feet would get better results (goal 4). An experiment could be conducted in which one group receives the massage protocol with lavender oil and another group receives the same massage protocol without lavender oil; or a group of people could be massaged one day without lavender oil and 2 days later with lavender oil. In both types of experiments, measurement tools are available for determining any changes in circulation; therefore research could answer the question (goal 5).

Step 2: Locating Resources and Gathering Information and Materials

After defining the research question, researchers must educate themselves on the topic to be studied by reading the existing literature and talking to experts. With regard to the question about using lavender oil with massage, the researchers would learn about essential oils in general and lavender oil specifically, in addition to cardiovascular functioning specifically, arterial functioning in the extremities, massage in general, and compression methods specifically. They also would search through any pertinent research that has already been done. They would talk to an aroma therapist, a person who combines massage and essential oils, and other professionals who would be able to provide information. Having learned as much as possible about the various aspects of the research question, the researchers then would develop a hypothesis.

Step 3: Forming a Hypothesis

Based on their knowledge of the topic, the researchers should be able to make an educated guess as to what may happen at the end of the experiment. The hypothesis is important because it will be compared to the factual information gained from the experiment. The researchers then can determine whether the hypothesis was correct. *Note that the research is still valuable even if the hypothesis is inaccurate at the conclusion of the research process.*

An example of a hypothesis might be: Using lavender essential oil during foot massage that produces compression loading increases peripheral circulation.

Step 4: Planning Data Collection Methods

The fourth step of the scientific method involves drawing up a specific, detailed plan for conducting the research. The procedure should be clear enough that other researchers could follow it exactly. During this planning phase, the following must be determined:

- What steps are necessary to find the answer to the research question (i.e., to test the hypothesis)?
- What data need to be collected?
- How will the data be collected?
- What equipment, supplies, facilities, assistants, test subjects, and support people will be required?
- What is the reference point (control) with which the data will be compared?
- How many samples, sites, and tests are required?
- What variables will be manipulated and in what ways?
- What record-keeping techniques will be used (e.g., data sheet, journal)?
- How will data collection techniques be organized?
- What are the sequential steps to the research?
- What are the schedule, timeline, and time expenditure?
- What are the financial obligations?

To complete this fourth step, the researchers must decide on the type of research design to use, such as an observation design or an experimental design.

Step 5: Collecting Data

Researchers must collect all the information (data) that could affect the answer to the research question. The criteria useful in this process are:

- All relevant data must be recorded.
- Researchers must keep track of the step-by-step process.
- Objectivity must be maintained in the data collection.

Step 6: Organizing and Analyzing the Data

In the sixth step of the scientific method, the researchers pull together the data collected and examine it more closely. The information is compared and contrasted. The data are:

1. Organized and summarized
2. Presented graphically (e.g., bar graphs, tables, pie charts, line graphs) so that others can see the results clearly
3. Tested to determine whether the results are significant

Step 7: Interpreting the Data and Drawing Conclusions

The researchers analyze the data and determine their conclusions, such as:

1. What alternative hypotheses might explain these results?
2. Were all relevant data, including extremes, or "oddball" data, analyzed?
3. How might the sampling or data collection methods have affected these results?
4. What answer do the results provide to the original question?
5. How do the results compare to what was expected to happen (the hypothesis)?
6. What can be concluded from the results? How do the conclusions affect the community or the "big picture" (implications)?

Step 8: Communicating the Results

In the final step of the scientific method, the research and its findings are presented to the public. Important questions that must be considered in this process include:

1. Who is the audience? (Who wants to read the research?)
2. What is the best way to communicate the information (e.g., written report, oral or poster presentation, video)?
3. What visual aids will help the audience clearly understand this research?

All of the following components of the research must be addressed:

- An introduction to the research question, the purpose of the research, and why it matters
- A description of methods used to collect data
- The results
- The conclusion

Reading and Interpreting a Research Paper

Research findings need to be accurate to be useful. The scientific method and its use in conducting research reduces the possibility that research findings are inaccurate and flawed. An accepted research design reduces the potential for bias that can occur if the researchers conduct the experiment and interpret the findings based on what they expect or want the results to show. The reader (consumer) of research must review the methodology of a study to make sure the objective of the analysis is clearly stated and that the researchers explain the limitations of their findings; this allows the results to be put into context. Besides knowing the limitations of the different types of studies, those who read research papers also must understand the way the study was conducted. Some important factors are:

- The setting of the study (e.g., clinic, laboratory, or population)
- How variables were controlled (How did the researchers adjust for specific subject qualities or outside influences that could affect the results?)
- The sample size
- The number of study groups
- The treatment or variables observed (e.g., a vitamin supplement, a specific diet, massage)
- The length of the study
- How the data were collected
- How and by what statistical procedures the data were analyzed

One of the most significant factors in the evaluation of a study's findings is the study design, especially the randomness of the selection of the study's participants. If the subjects were selected randomly, the study results are more predictive of the population. If the only participants in the study were volunteers who belonged to an interest group or a media organization, greater potential exists for bias in the study.

Another important factor is the sample size. Although a small sample does not mean that the study is flawed, the conclusions that can be drawn clearly have limitations. For this reason, federal agencies, such as the US Food and Drug Administration (FDA), require multiple studies involving large numbers of subjects before approving a new treatment or intervention.

In interpreting a study's findings, the reader also must understand the statistical significance. When conducting both observational and experimental research, scientists use statistical measures to convey the existence and strength of relationships. However, although statistics present the findings in an organized fashion, they do not provide information about cause and effect. Moreover, a statistically significant finding does not guarantee that the research is without bias or confounding factors that could make the statistical value irrelevant. Statistical significance is only part of the picture; to get the whole picture, the reader must consider the context of the study and the findings of other research on the subject.

A primary challenge in interpreting the findings of a research study for the public is communicating the potential risk. Those who use research must understand the difference between relative risk and absolute risk and must use these distinctions in explaining the findings of a study.

Absolute risk is the chance a person will develop a specific disease or potential injury over a specified period. For example, a female's lifetime absolute risk of breast cancer is 1 in 8; that is, one female in eight will develop breast cancer at some point in her life.

Relative risk puts the chance in comparative terms; it describes the outcome rate for people exposed to a particular factor compared with the outcome rate for those not exposed to the factor.

In most cases, the absolute risk is a far more relevant statistic for the public. For example, suppose a study shows that people who get a massage once a week are 50% less likely to develop sacroiliac (SI) joint dysfunction in the next 3 years than are people who get a massage only once a month. The relative risk is that a person who does not get a massage once a week will face a 50% greater likelihood of developing SI joint dysfunction. Yet the absolute risk for an individual who does not get a massage once a week may be only 1%. In this case, the relative risk makes the massage intervention seem more important than it really is. Therefore it is important to consider both the relative risk and the absolute risk when discussing study results.

As the research on massage increases and as current literature is interpreted, it is important for massage therapists to acquire adequate information on a study's original purpose, research design, and methods of data collection and analysis. Massage therapists also must understand the limitations of specific types of research and must recognize when a study is preliminary or when the findings differ from previous research.

Most important, proper interpretation of a new study's findings requires that the potential risk/benefit be put into perspective. It also requires clarification of cause and effect, which can be demonstrated only through rigorous experimental studies, not observational epidemiological research.

Framework for Reading a Research Article: Structure, Function, and Implied Criteria for Evaluation

The structure, or "anatomy," of an empirical research article is a rather standard feature of this form of scientific or technical writing. Because the intent is to enhance communication among professionals across various disciplines and professions, a research report has six major sections (with subsections) that serve specific purposes; they are analogous to the "physiology" of the research report:

1. Preliminary section
2. Introduction
3. Method
4. Results
5. Discussion
6. Conclusion

Examining the structure and function of a research article can help the reader identify several criteria or standards that might be used to determine whether the report provides appropriate information. The availability of appropriate information in the report allows the reader to evaluate the research effort's potential for advancing the knowledge base and thus the evidence-based practice of massage therapists. It is helpful to log on to PubMed (https://pubmed.ncbi.nlm.nih.gov/) and then use the search term *massage therapy*. Use the filters to choose a free full text article and then identify the following sections in the article.

Preliminary Section (Title and Abstract)

The first section of a research article contains the title and an abstract of the study. Although fairly self-explanatory, the title of a study must be formulated so that a potential reader (e.g., a person scanning a list of studies by bibliographic citation only) can accurately determine the type of study, the major variables involved, and the participants who were the focal point of the researchers' efforts.

In the abstract, or summary, the author synthesizes as efficiently as possible the main body of the report (i.e., the introduction, method, results, and discussion sections). A well-written abstract gives the reader a precise idea of what the study found, allowing the person to decide whether to read the entire report.

Introduction

The introduction provides the context for the rest of the report. It has five subsections: (1) a general review of the literature; (2) a specific review of the literature; (3) a purpose statement, which identifies the research question; (4) the rationale for the study's research hypothesis; and (5) a statement of the research hypothesis.

The first subsection, the general review of the literature, identifies the broader context of the study's major research problem area. This addresses at a general level earlier researchers and authors who have contributed to the research problem area.

The second subsection, the specific review of the literature, provides a more detailed treatment of related sources in the professional literature. This subsection allows the reader to become considerably more familiar with earlier literature that informs the current study.

The two literature review subsections serve a dual purpose:

1. They establish in the reader's mind the researchers' familiarity with the existing sources of information in the research problem area.
2. They inform the reader of the information and insight needed to better comprehend the current research report.

The third subsection, the purpose statement, must have the research question either implied or, preferably, stated. It represents the reason the study was performed. This subsection communicates to the reader what is truly the starting point in the study, because in any research endeavor, the many decisions are based precisely on the research question. The research question is never formulated in a vacuum. The researchers must have read relevant literature to identify the question they are asking. At the same time, the researchers must have had at least the beginnings of a research question to know exactly where in the literature they must search.

The fourth subsection, the rationale for the research hypothesis, relies on and may even extend the preceding literature review subsections. The authors of a research report must rely on the available research literature in a given problem area to justify what becomes their study's research hypothesis. The research hypothesis is basically the predicted answer to the study's research question. It is not an "educated guess," but rather a predicted answer to the research question based on concepts, theories, and/or existing empirical research from the professional literature. The rationale for the research hypothesis, then, should be presented immediately before the actual statement of the hypothesis. In this way, a context is already in place that clarifies the reasons the researchers predict a certain answer to the study's question. The rationale is usually only implied, but the preferred approach is to clearly identify it for the reader's benefit.

The final subsection of the introduction is the statement of the research hypothesis. Sometimes authors fail to provide a clear statement of what they anticipate, with justification, will be the outcome of the study (i.e., the answer to the study's research question). Many authors tend to allow the research hypothesis simply to be implied. The major advantage of a clear statement of the hypothesis is that it alerts the reader to several critical features of the study, including the research category, strategy, and method used; the variables investigated and their predicted relationship; the participants studied; and the context or setting of the study. Knowledge of a study's research hypothesis sets the stage for the study's methodology, the next major section in the research article.

Method

Just as the name suggests, the method section of the research report provides a detailed account of the methodology used to conduct the study. It identifies the various research procedures used at various stages and explains them in such detail that the study can be replicated by others. This section also gives the reader as complete a basis as possible for determining whether the implementation of the study justifies (or in any way compromises) the results and conclusions reached.

To accomplish these tasks, the method section must describe how the participants were chosen, the instruments used to measure variables, and the procedures by which the study was actually implemented. Standard subsections that constitute the method section are (1) participants and sampling procedures; (2) research method and design; (3) variables investigated; and (4) instrumentation. These four subsections allow the authors to specify precisely how the study was conducted.

Readers should keep in mind that the labeling of these subsections can vary slightly across different studies; the key point is to make sure the method section addresses the issues of participants, measuring instruments, and procedures.

The first subsection, typically labeled participants and sampling procedures, describes the characteristics of the study participants and the activities used to select and assign them. The researchers identify and justify the inclusion and exclusion criteria used to determine who did and who did not qualify as study participants. In addition the researchers must state the extent to which they used random selection of sample participants from an accessible population and random assignment of subjects to comparison groups. If the researchers used procedures other than random selection and random assignment, they must specify the alternatives chosen. These issues are critical when determining whether a study is valid. The participants and sampling procedures subsection also should specify the ethical provisions of the study that ensured the protection of participants, the overall integrity of the study, and prior approval from the appropriate IRB. As mentioned, an IRB is a federally mandated committee that provides oversight for all research activities with the aim to protect the rights and welfare of the human subjects recruited to participate in research.

The second subsection focuses on the research method and design.

The third subsection addresses the variables investigated in the study. Although this is not the first time the variables are mentioned in the report, this is where the researchers describe the variables as specifically as possible. In this subsection the reader can learn all the details of how the researchers identified, defined, characterized, controlled, manipulated, and measured the study's variables.

The final subsection of the methods section is instrumentation. Although this refers primarily to measuring instruments used to generate numerical or verbal data or both, this subsection also may specify the type or model of equipment or apparatuses that played a role in the study. Technical factors, such as the validity and reliability of instruments, are crucial and therefore prominent features of the information provided in this subsection.

Results

The results section provides the reader with a full accounting of the outcomes or results of the data analysis performed in the study.

Discussion

The final section of the report's main body is the discussion of the study's findings. This section provides the researchers with the opportunity to do the following:

- Reflect on the manner in which the study was conducted, including its limitations and delimitations (boundaries)
- Elaborate on the interpretation of the study's findings introduced in the results section
- Acknowledge the significance of the study's results and their relationship to earlier research findings in the problem area investigated
- Theorize as to the reason or reasons the results were obtained (i.e., which intervening variables may have come into play)
- Suggest areas of further research that would be a logical sequence to the current study

Conclusion (References and Other Material)

The concluding section of the research report begins with a list of the bibliographical citations for each of the sources cited in the research report. This list constitutes the references, and it is important not only because it gives detailed credit to sources used in the study but also because it provides the reader with the information necessary to access the sources cited. In addition to this list, research reports often include information in appendices, authors' notes, and footnotes.

Criteria for Critiquing a Research Article

The sections and subsections of a research report provide the foundation for identifying certain criteria that can be used to evaluate the merits of a report. They also provide an organizational framework for systematically working through the process of reflecting on the contents of a report. The following lists of specific questions can help you evaluate the designated sections and subsections of a research article (Proficiency Exercise 5.1).

Preliminary Section

1. Does the title of the study provide a basis for identifying the type of study, major variables, and participants?
2. Does the abstract summarize the main body of the report (i.e., the introduction, method, results, and discussion sections)? Does it focus on the research question, research hypothesis, participants, research method and design, major variables, instruments, statistical techniques, principal findings, and conclusions?

Introduction

1. Does the introduction contain professional literature that has bearing on the study reported? Does it provide an overview of the research problem area and more specific coverage of individual studies?
2. Is the purpose of the study clearly identified by the research question?
3. Is a rationale or justification, based on various features of the professional literature, presented as a context or framework for the study's research hypothesis?
4. Do the authors state the study's research hypothesis in such a way that the predicted answer to the study's research question is clear and unambiguous?

PROFICIENCY EXERCISE 5.1

Think about massage therapy using the PICO strategy and develop a research question that interests you on this topic. Find a free full text article on PubMed. Then use the information from Dr. Hymel's "Criteria for Critiquing a Research Article" to assess the quality of the research.

Method

1. Are the study's participants clearly characterized, along with the inclusion and exclusion criteria used to choose them?
2. Did the researchers justify the number of participants constituting the sample size?
3. Was an accessible population of potential participants acknowledged, along with an indication of how the sample was derived from such a population, whether through random selection or some other procedure?
4. Did the authors specify the manner in which the participants were assigned to the two or more comparison groups, whether through random assignment or some other means?
5. Was any clarification provided as to how the ethical aspects of the study were governed, particularly with regard to protection of the participants, the overall integrity of the research, and prior approval of the study by an IRB or ERC?
6. Were the study's variables detailed in a comprehensive fashion so that their manipulation and measurement could be replicated?
7. Did the authors clearly specify the equipment and instruments used to manipulate and measure the variables, and did they provide documentation of the technical factors?

Results

1. Were the data analysis techniques used identified and justified?
2. Were the results of the study communicated?
3. Were tables and figures used appropriately to present the data analyses in a comprehensible manner?

Discussion

1. Did the researchers reflect on the manner in which the study was designed and conducted with regard to any limitations and/or delimitations (i.e., intentional or unintentional boundaries)?
2. Did the authors elaborate on the interpretation of the study's findings beyond the interpretation that was introduced in the results section?
3. Did the researchers address the significance of the study and its findings, particularly as they relate to earlier studies in the problem area investigated?
4. Were possible intervening variables addressed that might explain the reason or reasons the results were obtained?
5. Were recommendations made regarding follow-up studies that might fully or partly replicate, or at least augment, the current study?

Conclusion

1. Does the list of references accurately reflect each of the sources cited in the research report, and is the list presented in a consistent bibliographic citation style?
2. Does the research report contain any appendices that provide more detailed information than that given earlier in the article?
3. Is any information provided, in the form of authors' notes, which gives insight into the funding support for the study?
4. Are any footnotes provided that elaborate on one or more aspects of the study and that would have been misplaced or distracting if embedded in the main body of the report?

CURRENT RESEARCH OVERVIEW

SECTION OBJECTIVES

Chapter objective covered in this section:

6. Find and cite current research related to therapeutic massage.

Using the information presented in this section, the student will be able to:

- Categorize and review current research related to massage therapy.
- Justify the outcomes of relaxation/well-being, stress management, pain management, and functional mobility.

Now that you have an idea of the importance of research to support an evidence-based and evidence-informed massage practice, we can explore the current research specific to massage therapy. As a result of growing interest and through funding provided by the National Center for Complementary and Integrative Health (NCCIH) in support of a shift in the understanding of health maintenance and the importance of methods such as massage therapy as a part of a health program.

Research on the benefits of massage is increasing in the United States. Similar research is under way in other parts of the world, such as Canada, Europe, Australia, New Zealand, Japan, and China. These studies continue to validate the benefits of therapeutic massage applications based on the four basic massage therapy outcomes (relaxation, stress management, pain management, and functional mobility) and the four approaches to care (well-being/palliative, restorative, condition management, and therapeutic change). The data are beginning to identify patterns of the underlying physiological mechanisms that massage addresses. However, at this time the way massage interacts with physiology is based primarily on theories and not supported by high-quality research. Whenever a statement is made about how massage influences physiology, resulting in beneficial outcomes, the current situation is that *we do not know specifically how massage works but the understanding is increasing*. That is okay, so long as the massage therapy community continues to attempt to find out. You too can be a researcher in your own massage practice by developing case reports (see Box 5.3).

This chapter does not attempt to list individual research results, but rather consolidates the research into categories based on safety and the four general outcomes supported by research evidence: relaxation, stress management, pain management, and functional mobility. (Chapter 6 expands on this content with more specific information about indications and approaches to care, in addition to cautions, contraindications, and recommendations for adapting massage.)

The summary of massage research that follows is based on an internet search using the terms *massage, massage therapy, manual therapy,* and *manual lymph drainage*. The search process for this text involved mainly internet sources, such as ScienceDirect, PubMed, and Google Scholar.

Studies dating from 2000 are included, and research conducted from 2015 to the present was the main focus. Systematic reviews and meta-analyses have been targeted to support evidence-informed practice for massage therapy. Because research is an evolving process, the studies and conclusions presented can be either confirmed or questioned based on the results of future research. Therefore the massage professional must remain current on advances in the understanding of the benefits of massage.

MENTORING TIP

Every textbook revision requires a critical analysis of the research cited. For the textbook authors, this analysis involves an important and sometimes tedious updated literature search and review. Often, the most current research challenges the authors beliefs about massage therapy mechanisms of action, benefits, and professional practice. There have been occasions when entire sections of the textbook have had to be rewritten based on current research findings. Remaining current with research findings involves unlearning as much as learning. Being open to changes in understanding is part of ethical professional practice. It takes motivation, commitment, time, and effort to compare and contrast research findings from the past to the present.

Massage Safety

For any treatment, safety (i.e., "do no harm") is a primary concern. If harm is possible, the benefits of receiving massage must exceed the potential for harm. Massage is not entirely risk-free, and massage therapists need to be aware of the possibility of harm. Massage can have both *side effects* and *adverse effects*. The main difference between the two is that a side effect can be either harmful or beneficial while an adverse effect is typically harmful and undesirable. A side effect is generally considered to be an adverse or harmful effect. Adverse effects are more severe and life-threatening than side effects.

Serious adverse effects have most commonly been associated with massage techniques applied to the neck area. Most adverse effects have been associated with aggressive types of massage, such as deep tissue and excessive pressure applications (Koren and Kalichman, 2018); cross-fiber friction; muscle stripping; aggressive stretching; implement-assisted massage, such as cupping and scraping methods; and massage delivered by untrained individuals. Inappropriate use of hot adjunct methods, such as hot stone massage, is a major concern with regard to adverse reactions. In addition adverse effects have been associated mostly with massage techniques other than general, moderate-pressure, nonspecific massage (Carnes et al., 2010; Posadzki and Ernst, 2013; Paanalahti et al., 2014; Yin et al., 2014; Karkhaneh et al., 2020). Adverse effects also may result when massage interferes with various types of implants, such as stents, ports, and prostheses. Overall, general, moderate-pressure, nonspecific massage therapy is safe with few adverse events that usually resolve.

Justifying the Outcomes of Relaxation, Stress Management, Pain Management, and Functional Mobility

Massage Outcome: Relaxation

- *Relaxation:* A general, all-over feeling of well-being involving mental and physical relief after effort; the massage is tranquil, soothing, and comforting.

The goal of relaxation is the foundation for almost all massage therapy interventions. Relaxation is a normal, general, and physiologically inclusive process, involving functions of the parasympathetic autonomic nervous system, which supports recovery from daily life activities. A relaxation outcome is not pathology based; therefore specific massage-related interventions are minimal, and the results occur in response to pleasurable sensation. Relaxation is a function of wellness and promotes well-being.

Research-Based Evidence for Massage Supporting Relaxation

Multiple studies identified the relationship of comfort care and general relaxation related to massage therapy. Important research related to comforting (palliative) massage for returning military veterans indicates the importance of the relaxation outcome (Mitchinson et al., 2014; Trumble et al., 2014; Mitchinson et al., 2022). Similar results related to relaxation-based massage application were found in other populations, especially with ongoing access to massage on a weekly basis (Babaee et al., 2012; Finch and Bessonnette, 2014; Mustika et al., 2021). A study on the effects of manual lymph drainage, a type of light pressure massage, on cardiac autonomic tone in healthy subjects identified increased cardiac parasympathetic activity, which led to decreased sympathetic activity in the neuromuscular system; thus it can cause relaxation (Shim and Kim, 2014; Río-González et al., 2020; Honguten et al., 2021). Massage therapy shows a positive effect on blood pressure that persists over time (Givi, 2013; Prajayanti et al., 2022). Normal blood pressure is an indicator of an appropriate response to stress. Massage's enhancement of relaxation in acute care situations (e.g., after cardiac surgery) has implications for supporting recovery (Braun et al., 2012a, 2012b; Shafiei et al., 2014; Peng et al., 2015; Wang et al., 2022; Cates et al., 2022)). In other studies, Diego et al. (2004), Diego and Field (2009), and Field (2014) found that massage must be applied with sufficient pain-free, broad-based pressure to stimulate the antiarousal response and that light massage tends to stimulate the **sympathetic autonomic nervous system** response.

The hormone oxytocin is involved in pair bonding and parental bonding, both of which support positive health states. Serotonin is another important neurochemical related to stress levels. A study conducted in The Netherlands by Bakermans-Kranenburg and van Ijzendoorn (2008) explored the relationship of oxytocin and serotonin to "sensitive parenting." Evidence indicates that serotonin may be important because of its influence on mood and the release of oxytocin. A study by Henoch et al. (2010) investigated the relational and behavioral effect of soft skin massage (affective touch) on children with severe developmental disabilities. Soft skin massage was found to contribute to greater closeness and social interaction, which fostered a sense of well-being (Moberg et al., 2022; Moberg and Petersson, 2022). Touch deprivation leads to negative health status and the positive effects of affective touch are health enhancing. Several studies have suggested that affective touch stimulates pressure receptors under the skin which, in turn, leads to increased vagal activity, reduced stress hormones and increased natural killer cells supporting immunity (Field et al., 2020). Although most studies on oxytocin involve touch, massage therapists can intelligently speculate that massage would elicit similar responses because massage is a pleasurable touch. Studies have now shown that massage does increase oxytocin levels and reduces stress hormones (Rapaport et al., 2012; Li et al., 2019).

Based on this evidence, massage therapists can confidently state that massage supports relaxation and promotes well-being in individuals who find massage therapy pleasurable.

Systematic Reviews and Meta-Analyses That Support Massage Benefits for Relaxation

Barreto DM, Batista MVA. Swedish massage: a systematic review of its physical and psychological benefits. *Adv Mind Body Med.* 2017;31(2):16–20.

Coelho A, Parola V, Cardoso D, Bravo ME, Apóstolo J. Use of non-pharmacological interventions for comforting patients in palliative care: a scoping review. *JBI Database System Rev Implement Rep.* 2017;15(7):1867–1904.

Hilfiker R, Meichtry A, Eicher M, Nilsson BL, Knols RH, Verra ML, et al. Exercise and other non-pharmaceutical interventions for cancer-related fatigue in patients during or after cancer treatment: a systematic review incorporating an indirect-comparisons meta-analysis. *Br J Sports Med.* 2018;52(10):651–658.

McFeeters S, Pront L, Cuthbertson L, King L. Massage, a complementary therapy effectively promoting the health and well-being of older people in residential care settings: a review of the literature. *Int J Older People Nurs.* 2016;11(4):266–283.

Zhang, Michael, Brittany Murphy, Abegail Cabanilla, and Christina Yidi. Physical relaxation for occupational stress in healthcare workers: a systematic review and network meta-analysis of randomized controlled trials." *J Occup Health.* 2021;63(1):e12243.

Zeng YS, Wang C, Ward KE, Hume AL. Complementary and alternative medicine in hospice and palliative care: a systematic review. *J Pain Symptom Manage.* 2018;56(5):781–794.

Massage Outcome: Stress Management

- *Stress management:* Stress is the emotional and physical way in which we respond to pressure and a demand to respond. Stress is a physiological response that enables people to cope with strain and anxiety. Stress management strategies support a normal stress response and prevent, control, or reverse stress-related pathology. Many people use massage to manage stress-related symptoms, including irritability, inability to concentrate, fatigue, and trouble sleeping. As the stress increases, pathology can develop, resulting in anxiety and depression. The physical symptoms of stress include a rapid heart rate; muscle tension, including headache and low back pain; digestive upset; and many other symptoms related to changes in breathing and regulation of the ANS and the endocrine system. Many addictive behaviors, such as overeating, smoking, drinking, and drug abuse, are linked to a stressful lifestyle. Ongoing stress can increase blood pressure and the risk for stroke, and it contributes to many diseases, such as heart disease, diabetes, and multiple autoimmune conditions. Hans Selye called the body's response to stress the general adaptation syndrome, which he suggested can be divided into three stages:
  - Stage 1: Alarm reaction—also called the fight-or-flight response, this is the body's initial reaction to a perceived stressor.
  - Stage 2: Resistance reaction—through the secretion of regulating hormones, this reaction allows the body to continue fighting a stressor long after the effects of the alarm reaction have dissipated.
  - Stage 3: Exhaustion reaction—this reaction occurs if the stress response continues without relief.

The body has various mechanisms for maintenance of homeostasis. Reversing the stress response can be divided into *reactive* (the stress response begins using feedback loops for counter-regulations), and *predictive* (anticipatory processes for future potential stress).

Once a future stressor is perceived as unavoidable, anticipatory coping processes may be initiated. Anticipatory coping involves efforts to prepare for the stressful consequence of an upcoming event that is likely to happen. Flight/fight/fear is the response to reactive stress while vigilance/anxiety can occur in response to predictive stress. The stress response to both situations may involve a wide range of mechanisms, including changes in genetic, metabolic, energetic, immune, endocrine, neural, and behavioral processes aiming to overcome and compensate for the imbalances produced by the stressor. Anticipating near-future events is fundamental to adaptive behavior (Hamel et al., 2021). Anticipatory anxiety develops when the mind attempts to predict, process, and adapt to future events. It helps individuals prepare for future events, but an overabundance of anxiety can be unhealthy. It often manifests as fear, worry, increased threat attention, and hypervigilance (Goldstein, 2021). Massage therapy can be indicated in both reactive and predictive stress responses.

There is a difference in homeostasis regulation for eustress ("good stress") versus distress ("bad stress"). An important factor in regulation is oxidative stress which involves maintaining the balance of free radicals and antioxidants in the body. Oxidative stress can perpetuate nonproductive inflammation responsible for many chronic diseases. Stress is not necessarily bad. Recall that stress involves a demand on us to adapt. It is not necessarily the type of event causing the stress response that is good or bad, but the amount and duration of the stress, and the resulting management of oxidative stress. Stress management techniques (including massage) seem to share similar neurobiological mechanisms that involve autoregulation, an adaptive mechanism of the body that responds to stimuli to restore homeostasis (Sies, 2021; Feelisch et al., 2022).

Research-Based Evidence for Massage Therapy as a Stress Management Strategy

Massage focused to manage inappropriate stress responses is an important outcome. Recall that the relaxation outcome is the foundation for massage benefit, and relaxation is necessary for wellness. As people become stressed, pathology begins to occur. The massage application focuses not only on the restoration of well-being but also on the control and reversal of stress symptoms, including anxiety and depression, and many physical symptoms that are stress related.

The evidence for massage as a stress management approach is extensive. Strong evidence has been available for over 15 years. Peng et al. (2015) and Müller-Oerlinghausen et al. (2007) concluded that slow-stroke massage is a suitable intervention for depression, along with other treatments, and is readily accepted by ill patients. The same study found that massage reduced distress in oncology patients regardless of gender, age, ethnicity, or cancer type. Based on a meta-analysis and a study by Hou et al. (2010) and Peng et al. (2015), massage therapy is significantly associated with alleviation of depressive symptoms. However, standardized protocols of massage therapy, various depression rating scales, and target populations in further studies have been suggested (Hou et al., 2010; Rapaport et al., 2018). The beneficial influence of massage therapy on the stress response, including anxiety and depression, has been shown to persist, and the cumulative effect is evident with massage on a regular basis (Imanishi, 2013; Poland et al., 2013; Shafiei et al., 2013a; Khalilian, 2014 Rapaport et al., 2018). Disrupted sleep is a common symptom of stress, and massage may help support restorative sleep (Arun, 2014; Ko and Lee, 2014; Shinde and Anjum, 2014; Whatley et al., 2022). Massage has also shown potential to manage oxidative stress (Luo et al., 2018; Simatupang et al., 2020; Skubisz et al., 2021).

The therapeutic relationship established between the massage therapist and the client (see Chapter 2) is similar to the developments that occur in psychotherapy. Some researchers believe that the effects of massage on anxiety and depression may stem from a positive therapeutic relationship (Moyer et al., 2004). Hymel and Rich (2014) suggested that massage benefits are related to health psychology as a context for massage therapy. Although most massage therapists consider massage a biomechanical intervention, process-oriented clinical reasoning used in actual massage practice mirrored models found in psychotherapy and was informed by experience, intuition, and training, which resulted in an intentionally holistic approach (Fortune and Hymel, 2015; Kelemen et al., 2020).

Correlation of stress, anxiety, depression, and pain is common. Therefore although stress, anxiety, depression, and pain often are found together, whether any one of them causes any of the others is unclear. Regardless, the four conditions often respond to the same applications of massage. For example, using a massage-like intervention, Lund et al. (2002) found a relationship between pain perception and oxytocin levels. Oxytocin is related to feelings of well-being, connectedness, and bonding. Massage, as a mode of touch, increases oxytocin and reduces adrenocorticotropin, a stress-related hormone in humans (Morhenn et al., 2012; Rapaport, 2012; Chen et al., 2020).

Massage is not always the best way to manage stress symptoms (Hanley et al., 2003; Majewska-Pulsakowska and Martyna, 2021). These researchers found that although massage was effective for managing pain and anxiety, it was no more effective than other relaxation interventions. An important point, however, is that people liked massage; this is a crucial factor in compliance with treatment.

Other studies have shown that massage therapy enhances the treatment course of hospitalized oncology patients. Currin and Meister (2008) and Billhult et al. (2007) found that therapeutic massage showed potential benefits for reducing the chemotherapy and radiation side effects of breast cancer treatment and for improving perceived quality of life and overall functioning. These findings were supported in more recent studies (Collinge et al., 2012; Jacobs, 2014; Alhamdoun et al., 2020; Gentile et al., 2021). Anxiety is also reduced in acute cardiac care (Boitor et al., 2019).

The research evidence is sufficient to support the use of massage therapy as a stress management approach. However, because ongoing stress leads to a variety of pathological conditions, the massage therapist needs more supporting evidence to devise a comprehensive assessment process; to use massage interventions purposefully and cautiously to manage stress-related symptoms; and to recognize when clients need to be referred for proper health care should anxiety or depressive symptoms increase.

Systematic Reviews and Meta-Analyses That Support Massage Benefits for Stress Management

Adams AMN, Chamberlain D, Grønkjær M, Charlotte Thorup CB, Conroy T. Nonpharmacological interventions for agitation in the adult intensive care unit: a systematic review. *Aust Crit Care.* 2023;36(3):385–400.

Chandrababu R, Rathinasamy EL, Suresh C, Ramesh J. Effectiveness of reflexology on anxiety of patients undergoing cardiovascular interventional procedures: a systematic review and meta-analysis of randomized controlled trials. *J Adv Nurs.* 2019;75(1):43–53.

Greenlee H, DuPont-Reyes MJ, Balneaves LG, Carlson LE, Cohen MR, Deng G, et al. Clinical practice guidelines on the evidence-based use of integrative therapies during and after breast cancer treatment. *CA Cancer J Clin.* 2017;67(3):194–232.

Heidari Z, Shahrbanian S, Chiu C. Massage therapy as a complementary and alternative approach for people with multiple sclerosis: a systematic review. *Disabil Rehabil.* 2021:1–12.

Lin TR, Chou F-H, Wang H-H, Wang R-H. Effects of scar massage on burn scars: a systematic review and meta-analysis. *J Clin Nurs.* 2023;23(13–14):3144–3154.

Lyman GH, Greenlee H, Bohlke K, Bao T, DeMichele AM, Deng GE, et al. Integrative therapies during and after breast cancer treatment: ASCO endorsement of the SIO clinical practice guideline. *J Clin Oncol.* 2018;36(25):2647–2655.

Maghalian M, Kamalifard M, Hassanzadeh R, Mirghafourvand M. The effect of massage on childbirth satisfaction: A systematic review and meta-analysis. *Adv Integr Med.* 2022;9(3):151–158.

Mueller SM, Grunwald M. Effects, side effects and contraindications of relaxation massage during pregnancy: a systematic review of randomized controlled trials. *J Clin Med.* 2021;10(16):3485.

Nurpadila N, Mulhaeriah M, Sangkala Moh. S. Effects of massage therapy on cancer related fatigue: a systematic review. *Enferm Clín.* 2021;31(5):S692–S696.

Owais S, Chow CH, Furtado M, Frey BN, Van Lieshout RJ. 2018. Non-pharmacological interventions for improving postpartum maternal sleep: a systematic review and meta-analysis. *Sleep Med Rev.* 2018;41:87–100.

Scales K, Zimmerman S, Miller SJ. evidence-based nonpharmacological practices to address behavioral and psychological symptoms of dementia. *Gerontologist.* 2018;58(suppl 1): S88–S102.

Tian L, Li M, Yan L. Effect of foot reflexology on pain and physiological indicators in postoperative patients: a systematic review and meta-analysis. *TMR Integ Nur* 2021;5(1):8–20.

Wang T, Zhai J, Liu X-L, Yao L-Q, Benjamin Tan J-Y. Massage therapy for fatigue management in breast cancer survivors: a systematic review and descriptive analysis of randomized controlled trials. *Evid Based Complement Alternat Med.* 2021:9967574.

Wu J, Yang XW, Zhang M. Massage therapy in children with asthma: a systematic review and meta-analysis. *J Evid Based Complementary Altern Med.* 2017;2017:5620568. Published online 2017 May 21. 10.1155/2017/5620568. PMCID: PMC5457772.

Zeng YS, Wang C, Ward KE, Hume AL. Complementary and alternative medicine in hospice and palliative care: a systematic review. *J Pain Symptom Manage.* 2018;56(5):781–794.

Massage Outcome: Pain Management

- *Pain management:* Pain is a complex topic. Pain theories are evolving to help us better understand the different types of pain sensations. Two basic types of pain are acute pain and chronic/persistent pain. Acute pain is a natural outcome of tissue damage; it warns us we have been harmed. Chronic pain is persistent pain without tissue damage; it is a serious health care problem. The biopsychosocial model of pain presents physical symptoms as a dynamic interaction between biological, psychological, and social factors. Factors promoting resilience, such as emotional support systems and good health, can promote healing and reduce potential for chronic pain development. Quality-of-life indicators and neuroplastic changes might also be reversible with adequate pain management. This approach to pain management is especially relevant to massage therapy practice.
- Pain can be categorized as nociceptive (from tissue injury), neuropathic (from nerve injury), or nociplastic (from a sensitized nervous system). While these three categories of pain can be defined, clients often experience overlap in the different types of pain. Of particular interest to massage therapists is nociplastic pain, a complex long-term pain condition. Nociplastic pain arises from altered nociception despite no clear evidence of actual or threatened tissue damage. The symptoms observed in nociplastic pain include nonproductive pain that is more widespread or intense, as well as other CNS-derived symptoms, such as fatigue, sleep, memory, and mood problems. This type of pain can occur in isolation, as often occurs in conditions such as fibromyalgia or tension-type headache, or as part of a mixed-pain state in combination with ongoing nociceptive or neuropathic pain, as might occur in chronic low back pain. It is now understood that a personalized multimodal, interdisciplinary treatment approach is needed to effectively manage this type of pain. Integrated interventions include pharmacotherapy, psychotherapy, massage therapy, and in rare instances invasive procedures such as surgery (Cohen et al., 2021). Nociplastic pain will respond to therapy differently than nociceptive pain, with a decreased responsiveness to peripherally directed therapies such as antiinflammatory drugs and opioids, surgery, or injections. (Fitzcharles et al., 2021). Repeated injury or illness involving acute inflammatory responses play a significant role in the development and progression of long-term nociplastic pain. Strategies to manage pain, such as medication, can lead to even more problems from side effects and abuse. For this reason, non-medication-based interventions, such as massage, are important (Steinmetz, 2022).

Research-Based Evidence for Massage Therapy as a Pain Management Strategy

Pain is a subjective experience, and pain perception can be modified by massage to help individuals better cope with sensations interpreted as pain (Karlson et al., 2014). Nonpharmacological approaches, including massage, are recommended as the first interventions (Utli et al., 2022; Mannes et al., 2022; Gebke et al., 2023). Gentle, moderate-pressure, nonspecific, general massage therapy has been shown to soothe and comfort individuals experiencing acute pain (Shafiei et al., 2013b; Nordness et al., 2021; Dusek et al., 2021). Controlled pain sensation applied during massage may affect pain modulation as long as tissue damage does not occur. Clients often report a "good hurt" sensation (Wilson et al., 2021). The use of massage therapy to ease the side effects of cancer treatment, including pain, has been investigated and supported (Pan et al., 2013; Somani et al., 2013; Lee et al., 2015; Pilkington 2021). Headache and low back pain have been the focus of multiple studies using massage as a pain management strategy (Fahey, 2018; De Pauw et al., 2021; Dingding et al., 2022).

The soft tissues targeted during massage are viscoelastic, can be described as that of both a solid (elastic) and a liquid (viscous) A fundamental concept of the elastic component is the relationship among stress (applied force), strain (deformation resulting from an applied force), and stiffness (Langevin, 2021). Soft tissue stiffness and pain sensations are moderated by massage if the massage is provided for about an hour on a regular basis (at least weekly) over a period of at least 12 weeks. The best results were obtained when massage therapy was ongoing for an extended time (Moraska and Chandler, 2008; Kong et al., 2013; Kumar et al., 2013; Shengelia et al., 2013; and Sherman et al., 2014). The massage approach used was a general, nonspecific, moderate-pressure, full body massage that included cautious use of more specific methods to address muscle tone and connective tissue changes, such as myofascial trigger points (Schmiege et al., 2014; Falsiroli et al., 2018). Interestingly, the researchers found no significant difference between relaxation-based (general nonspecific) massage and structural intervention-based (specific) massage in terms of relieving disability or symptoms (Furlan et al., 2008; Cherkin, 2011).

Modest preliminary support has been found for the use of massage in the treatment of mixed chronic pain conditions, headache pain, shoulder pain, neck pain, and carpal tunnel syndrome (Miake-Lye et al., 2019). Research by Kong et al. (2013) and support by Wang et al. (2022) supports massage therapy as an effective intervention that may provide immediate effects for neck and shoulder pain. However, massage does not show better effects than other active therapies for pain relief. Additionally, massage showed only short-term effects for shoulder pain in follow-up analysis.

Currently the evidence is stronger for massage management of low back pain than for neck and shoulder pain. Low back pain with massage intervention has been the source of multiple studies, including systematic reviews and meta-analyses (Cherkin, 2011; Ellythy, 2012; Kumar et al., 2013; Arun, 2014).

Another manifestation of pain sensation and perception is the more general, body-wide systemic presentation, as seen in fibromyalgia and rheumatoid arthritis, which can be classified as nociplastic pain (Sahraei et al., 2022; Antunes and Marques, 2022). Massage that engaged the superficial fascia, in which little or no lubricant was used (to support drag on the tissue), was found to be effective. Classical (Swedish) massage, in which lubricant was used (to reduce friction on the skin and support long, gliding methods), was effective as well. A manual lymphatic drainage-style application that targets gentle movement of the superficial fascia may be superior to more aggressive connective tissue massage methods, such as transverse friction. Overall, there is modest evidence for most styles of massage therapy in integrated models of palliative care for improved quality of life for people experiencing systemic pain syndromes (Castro-Sánchez et al., 2014; Li et al., 2014; Marchand et al., 2021; Mascarenhas et al., 2021).

The demand for nonpharmacological treatment of pain has resulted in an increase in massage and pain management research. Based on the research paper "Evidence-Based Nonpharmacologic Strategies for Comprehensive Pain Care: The Consortium Pain Task Force" (Tick et al., 2018), massage therapy for pain management has advanced from evidence-informed to evidence-based practice.

Research evidence supports massage therapy as a pain management strategy. Because pain may be related to pathology, it is important to make evidence-informed decisions on adapting massage for each client and to support other professionals involved with the client's care.

Systematic Reviews and Meta-Analyses That Support Massage Benefits for Pain Management

Anderson AR, Deng J, Anthony RS, Atalla SA, Monroe TB. Using complementary and alternative medicine to treat pain and agitation in dementia: a review of randomized controlled trials from long-term care with potential use in critical care. *Crit Care Nurs Clin.* 2017;29(4):519–537.

Boitor M, Gélinas C, Richard-Lalonde M, Thombs BD. The effect of massage on acute postoperative pain in critically and acutely ill adults post-thoracic surgery: systematic review and meta-analysis of randomized controlled trials. *Heart Lung.* 2017;46(5):339–346.

Boyd C, Crawford C, Paat CF, Price A, Xenakis L, Zhang W, Evidence for Massage Therapy (EMT) Working Group. The impact of massage therapy on function in pain populations: a systematic review and meta-analysis of randomized controlled trials. Part II, Cancer pain populations. *Pain Med.* 2016;17(8):1553–1568.

Boyd C, Crawford C, Paat CF, Price A, Xenakis L, Zhang W, Evidence for Massage Therapy (EMT) Working Group. The impact of massage therapy on function in pain populations: a systematic review and meta-analysis of randomized controlled trials. Part III, Surgical pain populations. *Pain Med.* 2016;17(9):1757–1772.

Calixtre LB, Moreira RFC, Franchini GH, Alburquerque-Sendín F, Oliveira AB. Manual therapy for the management of pain and limited range of motion in subjects with signs and symptoms of temporomandibular disorder: a systematic review of randomised controlled trials. *J Oral Rehabil.* 2015;42(11):847–861.

Chou R, Deyo R, Friedly J, Skelly A, Hashimoto R, Weimer M, et al. Nonpharmacologic therapies for low back pain: a systematic review for an American College of Physicians clinical practice guideline. *Ann Intern Med.* 2017;166(7):493–505.

Crawford C, Boyd C, Paat CF, Price A, Xenakis L, Yang E, et al. The impact of massage therapy on function in pain populations: a systematic review and meta-analysis of randomized controlled trials. Part I, patients experiencing pain in the general population. *Pain Med.* 2016;17(7):1353–1375.

Field T. Pain and massage therapy: a narrative review. *Curr Res Complement Altern Med: CRCAM-125.* 2018; https://10.29011/CRCAM-125/100025.

Hu J, Brettle A, Jiang Z, Zeng Y. A systematic review and meta-analysis of the effect of massage therapy in pain relief during labor. *J Nurs.* 2018;6(4).

Kukimoto Y, Ooe N, Ideguchi N. The effects of massage therapy on pain and anxiety after surgery: a systematic review and meta-analysis. *Pain Manage Nurs.* 2017;18(6):378–390.

Miake-Lye IM, Mak S, Lee J, Luger T, Taylor SL, Shanman R, Beroes-Severin JM, Shekelle, PG. Massage for pain: an evidence map. *J Altern Complement Med.* 2019;25(5):475–502.

Miri S, Hosseini SJ, Vajargah PG, Firooz M, Takasi P, Mollaei A, Ramezani S, et al. Effects of massage therapy on pain and anxiety intensity in patients with burns: a systematic review and meta-analysis. *Int Wound J.* 2023;20(6):2440–2458.

Nelson NL, Churilla JR. Massage therapy for pain and function in patients with arthritis: a systematic review of randomized controlled trials. *Am J Phys Med Rehabil.* 2017;6(9):665–672.

Pelletier R, Bourbonnais D, Higgins J. Nociception, pain, neuroplasticity and the practice of osteopathic manipulative medicine. *Int J Osteopath Med.* 2018;27:34–44.

Posadzki P, Fernández-de-las-Peñas C, Kuźdżał A, Ernst E. Massage for pain: an overview of systematic reviews. *Physiotherapy Review.* 2019;23(2). doi:10.5114/phr.2019.102953.

Qaseem A, Wilt TJ, McLean RM, Forciea MA. Noninvasive treatments for acute, subacute, and chronic low back pain: a clinical practice guideline from the American College of Physicians. *Ann Intern Med.* 2017;166(7):514–530.

Saracutu M, Rance J, Davies H, Edwards DJ. The effects of osteopathic treatment on psychosocial factors in people with persistent pain: a systematic review. *Int J Osteopath Med.* 2018;27:23–33.

Skelly AC, Chou R, Dettori JR, Turner JA, Friedly JL, Rundell SD, et al. Noninvasive nonpharmacological treatment for chronic pain: a systematic review. 2018.

Smith CA, Levett KM, Collins CT, Dahlen HG, Ee CC, Suganuma M. Massage, reflexology and other manual methods for pain management in labour. *Cochrane Database Syst Rev.* 2018;(3).

Wang Si-Qi, Jiang A-Y, Gao Q. Effect of manual soft tissue therapy on the pain in patients with chronic neck pain: a systematic review and meta-analysis. *Complement Ther Clin Pract.* 2022:101619.

Massage Outcome: Functional Mobility

- *Functional mobility:* Functional mobility means that people can accomplish the movements that allow them to take care of activities of daily life, engage in occupational pursuits, and participate in play and exercise, which contribute to health and well-being. We typically connect quality of life with the ability to move around easily in our environment. However, as a result of a variety of factors, such as injury and aging, movement can become difficult and limiting. The most common concerns are stiffness and pain sensation. Developing and maintaining control of posture and movement are often attributed primarily to the muscle system; however, recent evidence has suggested that the intricate relationship between the nervous, muscular, and fascial systems is vital for developing and maintaining control of posture and movement.

Research-Based Evidence for Massage Therapy as a Functional Mobility Management Strategy

Most individuals who seek massage are experiencing some sort of movement limitation. As previously described, low back and neck and shoulder pain can be helped with massage; however, research is still of a moderate to poor quality (Patel et al., 2012; Elibol et al., 2019). Massage therapy to support mobility is often combined with exercise in a multidisciplinary approach (Yuniana et al., 2022; Joshi and Poojary, 2022).

Much recent research related to manual therapy, including massage, involves effecting the connective tissue structures in the body, especially fascia. The fascial system is an aspect of the connective tissues of the body. Fascia tends to form interconnected sheets to form a three-dimensional continuum of solid and fluid elements. The continuum constantly transmits and receives mechano-metabolic information that can influence the shape and function of the entire body (Zugel et al., 2018; Bordoni et al., 2022). Simply described, fascia is fluid and fibers. Embedded in the fluid (a gelatin-like structure called *ground substance*) are crimped/wavy collagen fibers and elastic fibers arranged in distinct layers; the fibers are aligned in a different direction in each layer. Fascia forms as a sheet, or any other dissectible aggregation of connective tissue located beneath the skin, functioning to attach, enclose, and separate muscles and other internal organs (Adstrun et al., 2017).

Superficial fascia, sometimes called *subcutaneous fascia* (tissue containing body fat that is located under the skin but on top of muscle), forms a very elastic, sliding layer that is essential for thermal regulation, metabolic exchanges, and protection of vessels and nerves. Deep fascia is stiffer and thinner (resembling duct tape) than subcutaneous fascia. Deep fascia surrounds and compartmentalizes the muscles and forms the structures that attach soft tissues to bone. This type of fascia also forms a complex latticework of connective tissue, resembling struts, crossbeams, and guy-wires, which helps maintain the structural integrity and function of the body. Deep fascia cannot be stretched, but the tautness of the tissue can be affected by muscle shortening/lengthening. The muscle system is part of the fascial continuum and can be considered *myofascia*.

Massage may promote sliding in the fascial layers. Mechanical forces applied into fascia during massage may influence the body-wide movement capacity by normalizing the amount of pull muscles place on fascia (Coban et al., 2022). Extracellular matrix in muscle is relevant in tissue structural support and the transmission of mechanical signals between fibers and tendons and soft tissue (Simmonds et al., 2012). Manual therapy, such as massage, may aid in the treatment of muscle/myofascial-based injury, especially in obtaining a mobile scar capable of transmitting mechanical information and maintaining tissue sliding (Martínez Rodríguez and Galán del Río, 2013; Cho et al., 2014). Mechanical force application, such as massage, using moderate amplitude, duration, and frequency, are indicated in scar tissue management (Van Daele et al., 2022). Burn scar pain reduction with some effect on mobility supports symptom management (Deflorin et al., 2020). Massage therapy can influence hypertrophic scar physical characteristics but only in the short term (Nedelec et al., 2019). Limited evidence supports massage application for long-term effectiveness (Scott et al., 2022).

In 2007, Langevin and Sherman identified that pain-related fear about movement leads to a cycle of connective tissue remodeling, inflammation, and nervous system sensitization, all of which result in further decreased mobility. Current research reinforces this finding (Michalak et al., 2022). The mechanisms

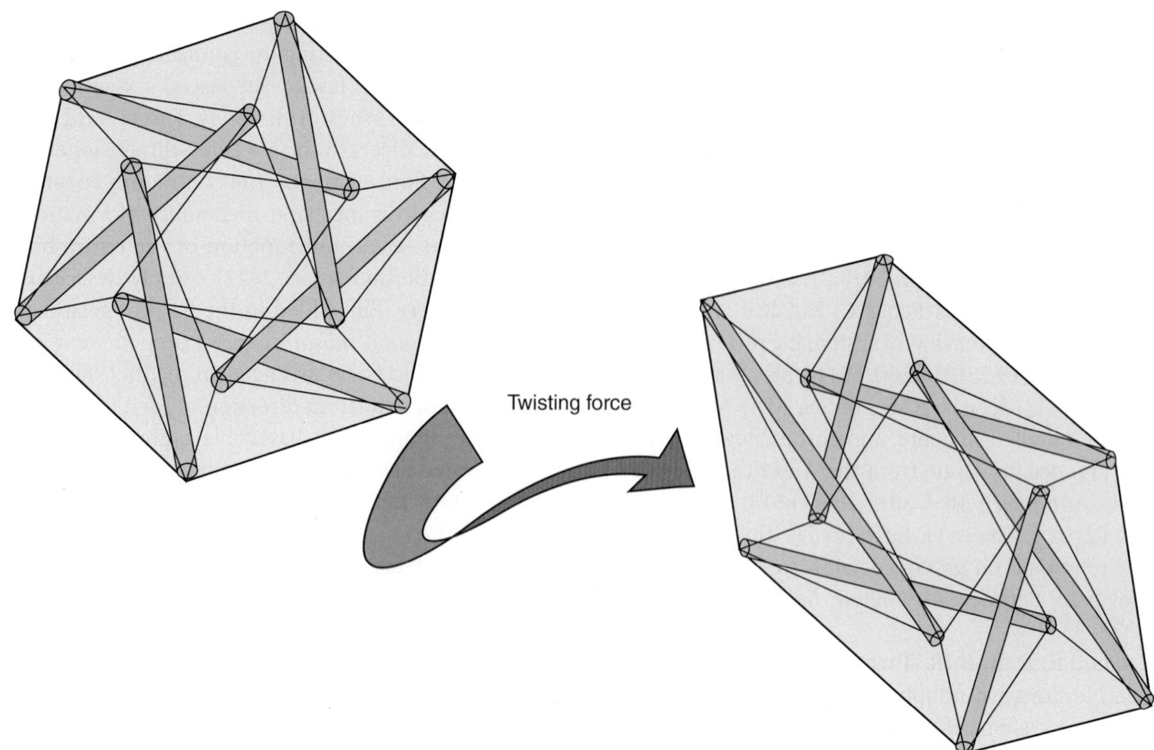

FIG. 5.2 Forces acting on a tensegrity system.

of a variety of treatments, including massage, may reverse these abnormalities by applying mechanical forces to soft tissues and altering biochemical signaling. Based on the tensegrity principle (everything is connected, as in a spider web), direct or indirect connections between fasciae seem to allow the transfer of mechanical forces over long distances. Massage applied to *deform* (change the shape of) soft tissues affects the electrical and mechanical activities of muscles that are not being massaged. Massage therapy appears to influence muscle tone not only through direct application but also through indirect effects on the entire interconnected myofascial system (Kassolik et al., 2009).

Tensegrity is an architectural principle developed in 1948 by R. Buckminster Fuller. A tensegrity system is characterized by a continuous tensional network (e.g., tendons, ligaments, and fascial structures) that is connected by a discontinuous set of compressive elements, or struts (e.g., bones). A tensegrity structure forms a stable yet dynamic system that interacts efficiently and resiliently with forces acting upon it (Fig. 5.2). Attaching tendons and muscles to the bones results in a three-dimensional tensegrity network that supports and moves the body. Bio engineering is advancing the understanding of the characteristics of cell and tissue tensegrity that provide biological tissues with remarkable mechanical properties and behaviors. Biological systems exhibit linking with each other but retaining the flexibility to shift and move around in response to pressure. Tensegrity is seen in folded proteins, cells, and tissues, responding to loading from mechanical forces and the interplay between tension and compression. Mechanotransduction is the process by which cells convert mechanical changes to biochemical signals, activating cellular pathways and influencing their function. There is increasing understanding that tensegrity plays an important role in dynamic biological processes (Boghdady et al., 2021).

Tensegrity of the body explains how inflexibility or shortening in one tissue influences the structure and movement of other parts of the body, even cellular structures (DuFort et al., 2011; Kassolik et al., 2013; Tadeo et al., 2014; Bordini et al., 2018). Sensory nerve receptors embedded in the fascia are stimulated, producing accurate directional information that is sent to the central nervous system (CNS) (Suarez-Rodriguez et al., 2022). Changes in the gliding of the fascia (e.g., too loose, too tight, or twisted) cause altered movement and thus tissue adaptation. Everything moves in the body, and parts must slide over and around other parts. A slippery fluid secreted by the body, called *hyaluronan*, allows structures to slide (Fede et al., 2018; Pratt, 2021). In muscle fascia or myofascia, part of the fascia is anchored to bone (or another structure), and part is free to slide. Tissues unable to slide efficiently can result in weakness, inflammation, and reduced range of motion (Stecco et al., 2011, 2013). Massage that drags the superficial fascia and moves individual tissue layers (including muscle layers) supports soft tissue sliding.

According to Day et al. (2009), the myofascial system is a three-dimensional continuum; this means that we cannot truly separate muscle or any other type of tissue from the surrounding fascia or the body as a whole (i.e., there is no such thing as an individual muscle). Dr. Carla Stecco and Dr. Antonio Stecco have done extensive research into the anatomy and histology of the fascia through dissection of un-embalmed cadavers (Stecco et al., 2006, 2007a, 2007b). Their ongoing

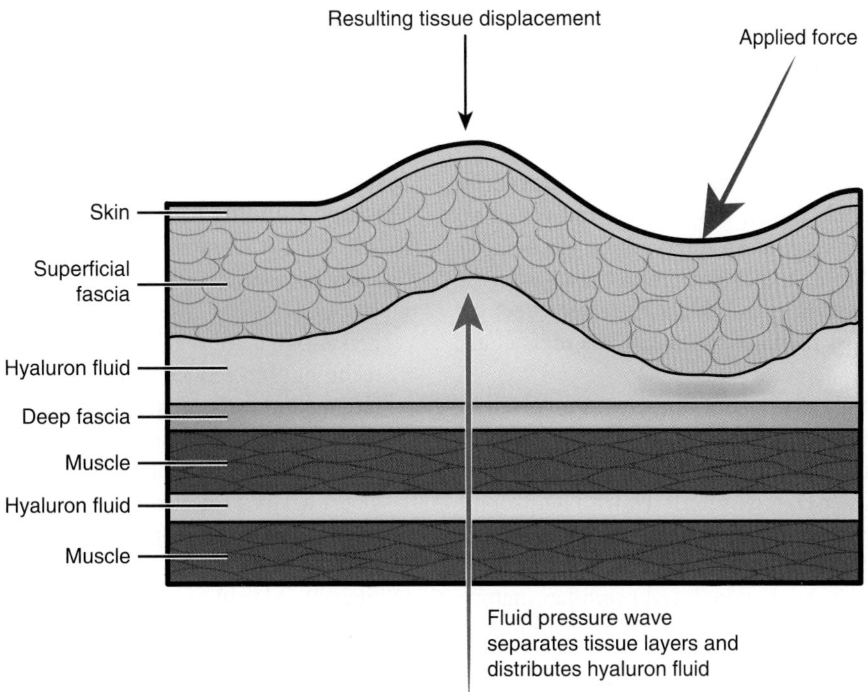

FIG. 5.3 Example of how applied force from massage can displace tissue and fluid between tissue layers to create a fluid pressure wave; this both separates tissue layers and distributes hyaluron-based fluid to restore sliding among tissue layers.

work has provided a biomechanical model that helps decipher the role of fascia in musculoskeletal disorders (Arumugam and Harikesavan, 2021).

Researchers think that the richly innervated fascia may be maintained in a taut resting state, called *fascial tone,* as a result of the different muscular fibers that pull on it (somewhat like a trampoline). This resting state enables the free nerve endings and receptors in the fascial tissue to sense any variation in the shape of the fascia (and therefore any movement of the body) (Schleip et al., 2005; Stecco et al., 2007a; Ganjaei et al., 2020). Deep fascia is designed to sense and assist in organizing movements. When body parts move in any direction, a myofascial tensional rearrangement occurs in the corresponding fascia (Schoenrock et al., 2018).

The mechanical forces generated by massage and other forms of manual therapy may stimulate fascial mechanoreceptors, which in turn may trigger tonus changes in connected skeletal muscle fibers (Chaudhry et al., 2008; Frey et al., 2009).

It is likely that the stiffness felt after periods of inactivity is related to the fascial system. If the amount of hyaluronan is reduced or if hyaluronan is not equally distributed, the tissue sticks or slides less efficiently (Bordoni and Zanier, 2014). Mechanical force applied by massage may separate tissue layers and allow for even hyaluronan distribution (Fig. 5.3).

Interestingly, reduced sliding of the various layers limits the functionality of the endocannabinoid system (McPartland et al., 2014; Buscemi et al., 2021). There is a close relationship between the endocannabinoid and endorphin system and fibroblasts. This relationship is believed to manage inflammation and pain information originating in the fascial tissue. This is a complex interaction because fascia continuously remodels daily.

If defective sliding results from a scar, the fascial continuum enables pain symptoms (Zugel et al., 2018). *Densification,* or a thickening of the ground substance, can develop into fibrosis (Pavan, 2014). Fibrosis or fibromatosis results from a disorder of connective tissue that is affected by hyperplasia and hypertrophy of the fibroblasts; this can occur as a result of a chronic inflammatory environment or nonphysiological mechanical stress and immobility; calcification phenomena can also be observed (Cao et al., 2013). The systemic effects associated with mechanical-load responses of the soft tissue remain difficult to isolate but suggest that anatomical areas with low pain can be selected for manual treatment, potentially causing body-wide benefit.

Another research focus related to functional mobility is postexercise stiffness, known as *delayed-onset muscle soreness* (DOMS). After unaccustomed exercise, which results in DOMS, the levels of the enzyme creatine kinase increase, indicating that muscle damage has occurred. Olszewski et al. (2009) and Zainuddin et al. (2005) found that massage was effective at alleviating DOMS by approximately 30% through the effect of reduced swelling. They also found that massage treatment had important effects on plasma creatine kinase activity, citing a significantly lower peak value at 4 days after exercise. Despite these changes, massage application had no effect on muscle function.

In a different study, Bakowski et al. (2008) found that massage administered 30 minutes after exercise could have a beneficial influence on DOMS by reducing soreness, but that it did not affect muscle swelling or range of motion.

Haas et al. (2013a, 2013b) investigated the effect of massage-like compressive loading on the recovery of active muscle properties after eccentric exercise in rabbits. Additional research found that massage carried out immediately after a bout of intense eccentric exercise favored a quicker recovery of muscle and joint function than massage delayed by 48 hours (Crawford et al., 2014). Research by Imtiyaz et al. (2014) also supports massage as an intervention for delayed muscle soreness. Multiple studies over many years suggest that massage after eccentric exercise has a greater effect on reducing muscle stiffness than no treatment (Bervoets et al., 2015).

Research suggests the inflammatory process is involved in DOMS. Massage has an effect on inflammation and DOMS in humans. Study results indicate that a 30-minute massage protocol applied 2 hours after exercise interfered with neutrophil emigration into the tissue, a marker for inflammation. Crane et al. (2012) found that a 10-minute massage after a controlled bout of upright cycling in humans reduced proinflammatory cytokine expression while promoting mitochondrial biogenesis, which supports tissue healing. Soft tissue manipulation may help attenuate inflammation, promote pain modulation, and improve gait function (Loghmani et al., 2021).

Massage applied too aggressively actually can interfere with the recovery process because it may cause more tissue damage, which triggers an inflammatory response and more swelling. Evidence suggests that massage may work by affecting multiple mechanisms that cause DOMS, and it may be a combination of these factors that allows for the beneficial effect of this modality. Overall, low-quality evidence suggests that massage has beneficial effects in the management of DOMS-related pain (Nahon et al., 2021).

Massage may also support soft tissue healing by increasing blood flow to the area. Cross-fiber massage increases tissue perfusion and alters microvascular function in the vicinity of healing knee ligaments (Loghmani and Warden, 2013; Zaki, 2014). It has been suggested that the effect of massage on the immune response (including inflammation) may be a factor in massage's support of tissue healing (Tejero-Fernández et al., 2015; Waters-Banker et al., 2014).

Another factor affecting the healing process is circulation, and massage has been shown to restore peripheral vascular function after exertion. Franklin et al. (2014) identified that a single massage treatment improves brachial artery endothelium-dependent, flow-mediated dilation (widening of blood vessels) for up to 48 hours, even when the massage was performed on the lower limbs. Support for circulatory changes indicates that massage promotes the local release of vasodilator mediators such as nitric oxide and histamine, and/or reduces sympathetic activity (Monteiro et al., 2020; Matsuda et al., 2021).

Research supporting massage for functional mobility is less robust. Massage appears to improve soft tissue function, supporting improved mobility, but the evidence is limited (Bervoets et al., 2015; Monteiro et al., 2018). More research supports massage for relaxation, stress management, and pain management. Compared to no treatment, massage therapy may provide short-term benefits for people with common musculoskeletal disorders. However, improvements in mobility seem more related to alternations in pain perception and a general influence on the nervous system rather than precise massage methods.

Systematic Reviews and Meta-Analyses That Support Massage Benefits for Functional Mobility

Ault P, Plaza A, Paratz J. Scar massage for hypertrophic burns scarring: a systematic review. *Burns.* 2017;44(1):24–38.

Dupuy O, Douzi W, Theurot D, Bosquet L, Dugué B. An evidence-based approach for choosing post-exercise recovery techniques to reduce markers of muscle damage, soreness, fatigue and inflammation: a systematic review with meta-analysis. *Front Physiol.* 2018;9:403.

Guo J, Li L, Gong Y, Zhu R, Xu J, Zou J, et al. Massage alleviates delayed onset muscle soreness after strenuous exercise: a systematic review and meta-analysis. *Front Physiol.* 2017;8:747.

Hilfiker R, Meichtry A, Eicher M, Nilsson BL, Knols RH, Verra ML, et al. Exercise and other non-pharmaceutical interventions for cancer-related fatigue in patients during or after cancer treatment: a systematic review incorporating an indirect-comparisons meta-analysis. *Br J Sports Med.* 2017;XX:bjsports-2016.

Lew J, Kim J, Nair P. Comparison of dry needling and trigger point manual therapy in patients with neck and upper back myofascial pain syndrome: a systematic review and meta-analysis. *J Man Manip Ther.* 2021;29(3):136–146.

Nahon RL, Lopes JSS, de Magalhães Neto AM. Physical therapy interventions for the treatment of delayed onset muscle soreness (DOMS): systematic review and meta-analysis. *Phys Ther Sport.* 2021;52:1–12.

Nelson NL, Churilla JR. 2017. Massage therapy for pain and function in patients with arthritis: a systematic review of randomized controlled trials. *Am J Phys Med Rehabil.* 2017;96(9):665–672.

Paleg G, Romness M, Livingstone R. Interventions to improve sensory and motor outcomes for young children with central hypotonia: a systematic review. *J Pediatr Rehabil Med.* 2018;11(1):57–70.

Paniagua-Collado M, Cauli O. 2018. Non-pharmacological interventions in patients with spinal cord compression: a systematic review. *J Neurooncol.* 2018;136(3):423–434.

Poppendieck W, Wegmann M, Ferrauti A, Kellmann M, Pfeiffer M, Meyer T. Massage and performance recovery: a meta-analytical review. *Sports Med.* 2016;46(2):183–204.

Wu Q, Zhao J, Guo W. Efficacy of massage therapy in improving outcomes in knee osteoarthritis: a systematic review and meta-analysis. *Complement Ther Clin Pract.* 2022;46:101522.

Xu Qinguang, Chen Bei, Wang Yueyi, Wang Xuezong, Han Dapeng. 2017. The effectiveness of manual therapy for relieving pain, stiffness, and dysfunction in knee osteoarthritis: a systematic review and meta-analysis. *Pain Physician.* 2017;20:229–243.

Yeun YR. Effectiveness of massage therapy on the range of motion of the shoulder: a systematic review and meta-analysis. *J Phys Ther Sci.* 2017;29(2):365–369.

Summary

In short, increased relaxation and reduced stress tend to correlate with reduced pain and increased mobility. This is why a general full body massage using moderate/pleasurable pressure to move multiple layers of tissue can have such a variety of benefits.

We may not be able to identify the results of specific individual applications because massage encompasses many different elements. Overall, it appears that a general full body massage can directly and indirectly influence many structures and functions to help a person adapt and cope, as well as help restore function (Clar et al., 2014).

Benefits can be derived from the quiet, nurturing presence of the massage therapist, the duration of the massage, the massage environment, and the unlimited variations in methods, pressure, speed, and so forth. A well-performed full body massage is somewhat like a tasty cookie; the ingredients are all mixed together in the right proportions, baked at the correct temperature for the right amount of time, and served in a relaxing environment.

WHY MASSAGE IS EFFECTIVE: TRANSLATING EVIDENCE INTO PRACTICAL APPLICATION

SECTION OBJECTIVES

Chapter objective covered in this section:

7. Explain the effects of therapeutic massage in physiological terms.

Using the information presented in this section, the student will be able to:

- Explain the biologically plausible anatomical and physiological influences of massage.

We have discussed the importance of valid evidence and the relationship between science and art. We also have learned about the research process, summarized current research applicable to massage therapy outcomes, and learned how to read a research paper to determine whether it is relevant and accurate. Your "inquiring mind" may be overwhelmed by now, especially if all this information is new to you. The crucial point, though, is to be able to apply the information to the actual massage process. These latter sections of the chapter consolidate the known and suspected biologically plausible benefits of massage and the mechanisms of action into a format that is usable in the practical application of massage. To really appreciate these sections, we first had to understand the process of finding and evaluating research to determine whether the evidence is relevant and justifiable. Now we can proceed with the practical application of the evidence in massage therapy practice.

The manual techniques of massage are physiologically specific and well defined by these parameters:

- Four main outcomes for massage:
  - Relaxation
  - Stress management
  - Pain management
  - Functional mobility
- Four main approaches to care (specifically described in Chapter 6):
  - Well-being/palliative
  - Restorative
  - Condition management
  - Therapeutic change
- Two actions that generate mechanical force:
  - Pushing
  - Pulling
- Nine primary massage methods that are used to create mechanical force (described in Chapter 10):
  - Static methods/holding
  - Compression
  - Gliding
  - Torsion twisting (kneading)
  - Shearing (friction)
  - Elongation
  - Oscillation
  - Percussion
  - Movement
- Twelve modifiers for adapting massage methods:
  - Pressure
  - Point of application (location and broadness of contact)
  - Magnitude (intensity)
  - Direction
  - Drag
  - Speed
  - Pacing
  - Rhythm
  - Sequencing and transitioning
  - Frequency
  - Duration
  - Intention for outcome

Adapted methods generate appropriate force to load the body tissue in order to create five stresses to which the physiology must adapt:

- Compression stress
- Tension stress
- Shear stress
- Torsion stress
- Bending stress

The techniques of therapeutic massage and other types and styles of bodywork are merely variations of the fundamental application of manual manipulations. The benefits of the techniques are simply the result of basic physiological effects. It is helpful to have a method for categorizing information into similar bundles. By doing this, we can take many large pieces of information and sort them into manageable sizes. This process helps with the clinical reasoning process used to make sense of information and to make decisions about what to do with the data. The problem with this method is that most things do not clearly fit into one category or another, and often the result is not entirely accurate. However, as long as we understand this, we can make use of the process.

Physiological Effects

Solid evidence supports massage therapy for the four main outcomes; relaxation, stress management, pain management, and functional mobility. It is important to note that research primarily supports massage therapy benefit based on biopsychosocial influences, especially the therapeutic alliance and client centered care (Chapter 2). The methods used during massage therapy touch the client directly and indirectly to interface with the nervous/neuroendocrine system, especially the central nervous system and the autonomic nervous system.

This section of the chapter will investigate the practical application of massage therapy with a focus on the:

- Biopsychosocial model
- Neuroendocrine influences
- Circulation
- Connective tissue

Although the quality of the research supporting massage therapy benefit is low to moderate, the increase in systematic reviews and meta-analyses is encouraging. However, the words, "maybe, might, plausible" are commonly linked to statements on how massage influences the body. A premise of massage application is to mimic and support normal function.

To understand the basis of research findings, we must understand the biologically plausible mechanisms by which massage applications achieve benefits. This understanding is grounded in the study of functional anatomy and physiology as they relate to therapeutic massage. The recommended text for this purpose is *Mosby's Essential Sciences for Therapeutic Massage: Anatomy, Physiology, Biomechanics, and Pathology*, by Sandy Fritz and Luke Fritz.

Three overlapping themes are foundational in massage therapy practice: the biopsychosocial model, the person-centered approach, and whole person care.

The biopsychosocial model was described by George Engel in the late 1970s and emerged from dissatisfaction with the biomedical model of illness. Often discounted in the 1980s, the biopsychosocial model still is not widely implemented into complex health care interventions, such as multidisciplinary teams and integrated health care. However, it is the basis of the World Health Organization's International Classification of Functioning (WHO ICF). The premise of the biopsychosocial model is a continuum of health and illness as a result of an interaction of biological, psychological, and social factors. Massage therapy as a body-based approach acts in all the same areas as a client-centered practice, focusing on the quality of life and well-being of the clients we serve. The biopsychosocial approach focuses on positive health and functioning, in addition to relieving psychological distress and reducing physical symptoms people experience (Wade and Halligan, 2017; Rosignoli et al., 2022).

Common in chronic conditions are depression, anxiety, and a diminished sense of control over life circumstances. People become fearful and begin to identify only with the "bad"; this is called catastrophizing. Various forms of manual therapy, including massage, can reduce fear avoidance behavior and enhance a person's health status and quality of life. The National Institute for Health and Care Excellence in the United Kingdom and the Institute of Medicine in the United States have acknowledged the need to address the psychosocial dimension of patients' health concerns, through the implementation of more and improved multidisciplinary support that understands the totality of the human experience (Farre and Rapley, 2017) (Proficiency Exercise 5.2).

PROFICIENCY EXERCISE 5.2

Review the chapter outline and reflect on the content of this chapter. Pretend you have graduated and are developing a concise informational piece about the benefits of massage. What information from this chapter would you include? In about 100 words, summarize your thoughts in a draft for that informational piece. Share it with classmates to find similarities and differences.

Massage therapy affects multiple physiological and psychological mechanisms previously discussed, which combine in the four evidence-informed outcomes of relaxation, stress management, pain management, and functional mobility and the four approaches to care: well-being/palliative, restorative, condition management and therapeutic change. It is unrealistic to separate the benefits of massage for an individual into specific biological mechanisms when massage therapy acts generally on homeostasis and self-regulation combined with compassion, focused attention, and various other components of the therapeutic alliance and therapeutic relationship described in Chapter 2 (Alves et al., 2017; de Oliveira et al., 2018).

Nociplastic pain (long-term complex pai), has been recently introduced as a third mechanistic descriptor of pain arising primarily from alterations of neural processing, in contrast to pain due to tissue damage leading to nociceptor activation (nociceptive) or due to lesion or disease of the somatosensory nervous system (neuropathic). It is characterized by hyperalgesia and allodynia, inconsistency, and reversibility, as well as dynamic cross-system interactions with biological and psycho-behavioral factors. Along with this renewed understanding, functional pain disorders, also classified as chronic primary pain, are being reframed as biopsychosocial conditions that benefit from multimodal treatment (Popkirov et al., 2020). The biopsychosocial model supports the concept personalized medicine which aims to deliver the right intervention, for the right individual, at the right time (Cormack et al., 2023).

A massage therapist works from person/client-centered approach by acknowledging the dynamic relationship of biological, psychological, and social factors affecting each client every session. This helps massage therapists understand the complexity of the client's experience, The distinguishing marker of person-centered care is that it nurtures a supportive relationship, emphasizes two-way communication, and empowers client participation in health decisions. Shared decision-making care involves three key actions: recognizing and acknowledging that a decision is required; knowing and understanding the best available evidence; and incorporating the client's values and preferences into the decision (Lebert et al., 2022).

Whole person health involves looking at the whole person—not just separate organs or body systems—and considering multiple factors that promote either health or disease. It means helping and empowering individuals, families, communities, and populations to improve their health in multiple interconnected biological, behavioral, social, and environmental areas. Instead of treating a specific disease, whole person health focuses on restoring health, promoting resilience, and preventing diseases across a lifespan (Langevin, 2021).

Consistent with its long history of innovation, the Veterans Health Administration (VA) has recently committed to a massive expansion of the provision of complementary and integrative health approaches as part of standard care, and to an even more massive transformation to a Whole Health system of care (Whitehead and Kligler, 2020).

The National Center for Complementary and Integrative Health's new strategic plan defines whole person research as including three components:

- Exploring the fundamental science of interconnected systems
- Investigating multicomponent interventions or therapeutic systems
- Examining the impact of these interventions on multisystem or multiorgan outcomes
- The NCCIH strategic-plan is built around whole person health: https://www.nccih.nih.gov/about/nccih-strategic-plan-2021-2025.

The framework of whole person health places health and disease on a spectrum. Many factors, including one's biological makeup; some unhealthy behaviors, such as poor diet, sedentary lifestyle, chronic stress, and poor sleep; as well as social aspects of life—the conditions in which people are born, grow, live, work and age—can lead to chronic diseases. On the other hand, self-care, lifestyle, and behavioral interventions may promote "salutogenesis," or the process by which an individual moves from a less healthy to a healthier state, involving the whole person.

Massage therapy practice embodies the foundation of the person as the center of focus, the therapeutic relationship and alliance (Chapter 2) and compassionate and nurturing professional touch. Massage therapy communicates these important healing elements primarily through mechanical forces applied to soft tissue and the interface with the intertwined network of the neuroendocrine systems.

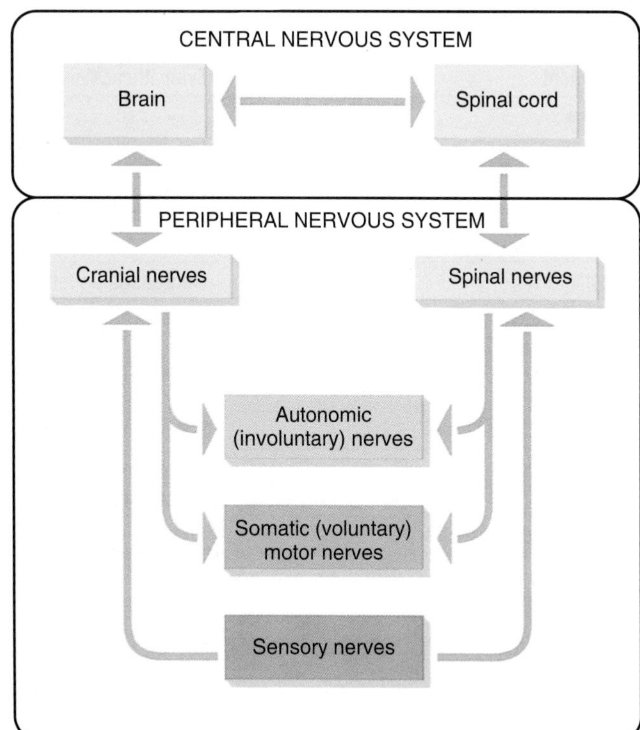

FIG. 5.4 Divisions of the nervous system. From Thibodeau GA, Patton KT. (2002). *The Human Body in Health and Disease.* 3rd ed. St. Louis: Mosby.

TRANSLATING EVIDENCE INTO PRACTICAL APPLICATION: NERVOUS/NEUROENDOCRINE SYSTEM

SECTION OBJECTIVES

Chapter objective covered in this section:

7. Explain the effects of therapeutic massage in physiological terms.

Using the information presented in this section, the student will be able to:

- Explain the possible anatomical and physiological influences of massage on the neuroendocrine system.

Effects of Massage on the Nervous/Neuroendocrine System

The body's responses to massage and its effects on the nervous system are related to sensory stimulation, motor responses, and the interface between the hypothalamus and autonomic nervous system. Massage stimulates somatosensory neurons of the body causing a cascade of signals and multisystem responses.

Briefly, the nervous system is divided into the central nervous system (CNS), which consists of the brain, the spinal cord and its coverings, and the peripheral nervous system (PNS), which consists of nerves and ganglions (Fig. 5.4). The PNS is further divided into the autonomic and somatic divisions. The **autonomic nervous system (ANS)** division is subdivided into the sympathetic, parasympathetic, and enteric systems. The sympathetic system is responsible for functions that expend energy in response to emergency or arousal situations. The parasympathetic system is restorative and normalizing and returns the body to a nonalarm state. The enteric nervous system (ENS) consists of neurons and supporting cells throughout the gastrointestinal tract, from the esophagus to the anus. The somatic division of the PNS is made up of the peripheral nerve fiber innervations of the body wall (e.g., muscles, joints, and other structures).

The ANS is best known for regulating the sympathetic fight-flight-fear and excitation response, and the parasympathetic relaxation and restorative response (Table 5.1). The sympathetic and parasympathetic systems work together to maintain homeostasis through a feedback loop system. These systems both affect and are affected by the endocrine glands (Fig. 5.5). Excessive sympathetic output causes most stress-related conditions such as headaches, gastrointestinal difficulties, high blood pressure, anxiety, muscle tension and aches, and sexual dysfunction.

The nervous system responds to therapeutic massage methods through stimulation of sensory receptors. Feedback loops are activated that intervene and adjust various homeostatic processes. The sensory stimulation from massage disrupts the existing pattern in the CNS control centers; this results in a shift of motor impulses, most often in the PNS, that reestablishes

Table 5.1 Functions of the Autonomic Nervous System

Component	Sympathetic Control	Parasympathetic Control
Viscera		
Heart	Accelerates heartbeat	Slows heartbeat
Smooth Muscle		
Most blood vessels	Constricts blood vessels	None
Blood vessels of skeletal muscle	None	Dilates blood vessels
Digestive tract	Decreases peristalsis; inhibits defecation	Increases peristalsis
Anal sphincter	Stimulates (closes sphincter)	Inhibits (opens sphincter for defecation)
Urinary bladder	Inhibits (relaxes bladder)	Stimulates (contracts bladder)
Urinary sphincters	Stimulates (closes sphincters)	Inhibits (opens sphincters for urination)
Iris	Stimulates radial fibers (dilation of pupil)	Stimulates circular fibers (constriction of pupil)
Ciliary muscles	Inhibits (accommodates for far vision; flattening of lens)	Stimulates (accommodates for near vision; bulging of lens)
Hair (pilomotor muscles)	Stimulates (goose bumps)	None
Glands		
Adrenal medulla	Increases secretion of epinephrine	None
Sweat glands	Increases secretion of sweat	None
Digestive glands	Decreases secretion of digestive juices	Increases secretion of digestive juices

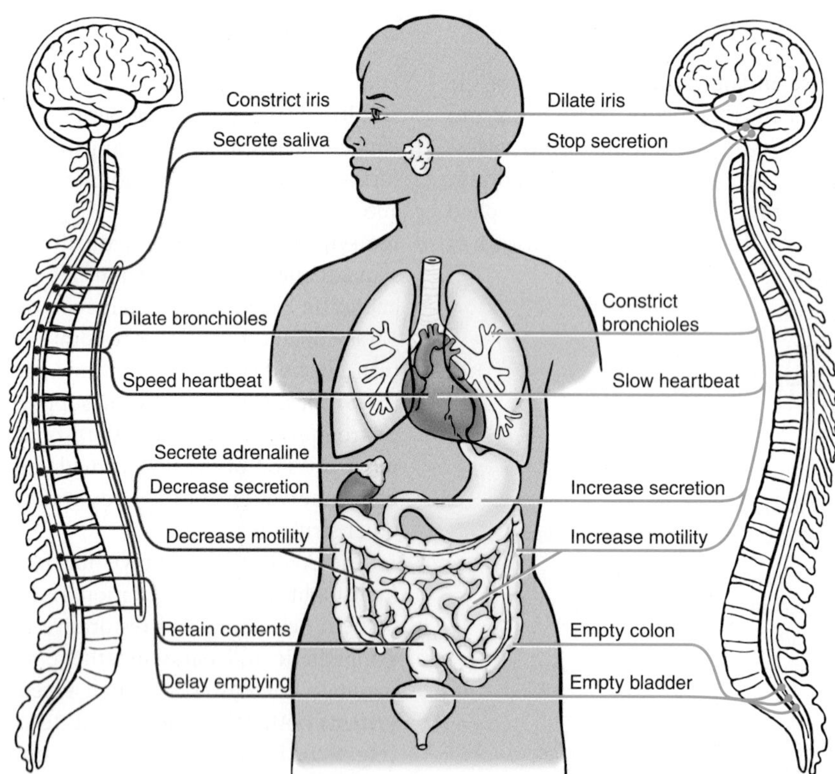

FIG. 5.5 Innervation of the major target organs by the autonomic nervous system.

homeostasis. Usually both the somatic and autonomic divisions of the PNS are influenced as balance is restored.

Manual therapy, such as massage, results in the discharge of muscle spindle afferents, Golgi tendon organs, and low- and high-threshold mechanoreceptors, as well as cutaneous, muscular, and articular receptors. The neurophysiological effects of the mechanical stimuli are hypothesized to help renormalize neural sensory input that has been altered by injury or illness. The therapeutic intent is alteration of the processing of stimuli in the sensorimotor cortical areas of the brain. Studies on animal and human subjects suggest that to generate changes in the sensorimotor cortical areas requires repetition. Neuroplastic changes to behavioral and sensory stimuli require several sessions over many weeks to result in long-term and sustainable results.

Variations in pressure applied during the massage session stimulate a variety of responses. Firm pressure massage is associated with an increase in vagal activity which reduces levels of cortisol which, in turn, leads to a reduction in pain (Field, 2014). Moderate pressure massage reduces depression, anxiety, heart rate, and altered EEG patterns, as in a relaxation response. Functional magnetic resonance imaging data have suggested that moderate pressure massage was represented in several brain regions including the amygdala, the hypothalamus and the anterior cingulate cortex, all areas involved in stress and emotion regulation. Massage therapy may facilitate information integration by restoring the activity of somatosensory cortex to restore the sensory functions (Xing et al., 2021). Light stroking is processed by C-tactile (CT) afferent nerve fibers. CT-fibers are activated by slow gentle stroking of the hairy skin, providing a pleasant sensation. Slow gentle stroking is known as affective touch and is linked to the experience of pleasure by effecting the insular cortex. This results in perceptions of well-being, stimulation of restorative processes, pain inhibition, and reduction of stress and inflammation (Meijer et al., 2022).

The endocrine system is regulated through the influence of the nervous system, and the endocrine system in turn influences the nervous system; this is a feedback loop, similar to the thermostat on a furnace. The feedback system and autoregulation (maintenance of internal homeostasis) are interlinked with all body functions. The hypothalamus links the endocrine and nervous systems together, and the pituitary gland receives signals from the hypothalamus. The hypothalamus and pituitary gland are connected by both nervous and chemical pathways. The hypothalamus produces and secretes neurotransmitters and neuropeptides along with several neurohormones that affect anterior pituitary gland function, becoming the main central regulators of the hypothalamo-pituitary-adrenal (HPA) axis and the autonomic nervous system. CT fibers connect to the oxytocin system. Oxytocin is also connected to serotonin and dopamine. Oxytocin is produced in the hypothalamus and released by the posterior pituitary. Oxytocin is involved in the decrease of sympathetic nerve activity and the increase of parasympathetic nerve activity, as well as reduction of pain and anxiety induced by gentle touch which affects C-tactile (CT) afferent nerve fibers (Schirmer and McGlone, 2022). Other vital hormones produced in the hypothalamus include corticotropin-releasing hormone, dopamine, growth hormone-releasing hormone, somatostatin, gonadotropin-releasing hormone, and thyrotropin-releasing hormone (Caria and Dall'Ò, 2022).

The endocannabinoid system modulates anxiety-like behaviors and stress adaptation (Crowe et al., 2014; Fitzgibbon et al., 2019). Researchers at the University of Georgia Neuroscience and Behavior Program demonstrated that brains in rats release endocannabinoids as a response to painful stimuli (Rahn and Hohmann, 2009). The researchers reported an increase in the concentration of endocannabinoids two minutes after the introduction of painful stimuli and again 15 minutes later. Endogenous opioids are well known to suppress pain. A strong interaction seems to occur among endorphins, dopamine, and endocannabinoids, but research has not clarified the nature of this relationship.

Massage therapy can be applied to stimulate the "good hurt" sensation that triggers endorphin action and also, possibly, endocannabinoids. Research has shown that endogenous cannabinoids also function as stress-induced analgesics (Hohmann et al., 2005). Self-regulatory homeostatic mechanisms involve opioids, cannabinoids, and dopamine. Increased levels of endocannabinoids are associated with relaxation and pain reduction. Whether massage works in a similar way would be an interesting research topic. Massage therapy has the potential to support endocannabinoid function (McPartland, 2008; McPartland et al., 2014).

Neuroendocrine chemicals are the communication transmitters of these control systems. A neuroendocrine chemical in the synapse of the nerve is called a **neurotransmitter.** A neuroendocrine chemical carried in the bloodstream is called a **hormone.** *Neuropeptide* is another term used to describe some of these substances.

Neuroendocrine substances carry messages that regulate physiological functions. Neuroendocrine regulation is a continuous, ever-changing chemical mix that fluctuates with each external and internal demand on the body to respond, adapt, or maintain a functional degree of homeostasis. The immune system also produces and responds to these communication substances. The substances that make up this "chemical soup" remain the same, but the proportion and ratio change with each regulating function or message transmission. The "flavor" of the soup, which is determined by the ratio of the chemical mix, affects such factors as mood, attentiveness, arousal, passiveness, vigilance, calmness, ability to sleep, receptivity to touch, response to touch, anger, pessimism, optimism, connectedness, loneliness, depression, desire, hunger, love, and commitment.

We now understand that most problems in behavior, mood, and perception of stress and pain, in addition to other so-called mental and emotional disorders, are caused by dysregulation or failure of the biochemicals. Problematic behaviors, symptoms, and emotional and physical states often are normal chemical mixes that occur at inappropriate times (Quattrocki and Friston, 2014). For example, anxiety, as indicated by increased, irresolvable stress, is an appropriate chemical soup to have on the mental burner in a hostage situation, because the hypervigilance accompanying such a state may allow the hostage to see an opportunity for escape. However, this same chemical soup is not productive when it is bubbling away while a person is stuck in traffic.

Breathing is a powerful way to interact with the ANS. Chest breathing and hyperventilation are common components of increased sympathetic stimulation. For the body to deal with stress, the muscular patterns of breathing must be normalized (see Chapter 15). Most meditation breathing patterns, singing, and chanting are ways to normalize those patterns through entrainment.

Breathing is an established biological rhythm. The pre-Bötzinger complex (preBötC), a cluster of interneurons in the medulla of the brainstem, is essential to the generation of respiratory rhythm in mammals (Feldman et al., 2013). There is a clear link between respiration and anxiety, and key theories of the psychopathology of anxiety, including panic disorders, and how regulation of breathing supports the relaxation response (Kinkead et al., 2014; Noble and Hochman, 2019; Van Diest et al., 2014).

Subclinical overbreathing—called breathing pattern disorder—often occurs, causing many physical symptoms (Box 5.4).

All massage approaches that restore mobility to the thorax and the muscles of respiration may positively affect the ability to breathe. Particularly with breathing pattern disorder, breathing retraining often is ineffective because the mobility of the respiratory mechanism has been disrupted. Often, massage can restore the normal function of the soft tissue involved with breathing, which enables breathing retraining to become effective.

Altering the muscle tone or changing the consistency of the connective tissue affects the ANS through the feedback loop, which in turn affects the powerful body/mind phenomenon (Seifert et al., 2018).

Massage supports balanced blood levels of serotonin, dopamine, endorphins, and endocannabinoids; this in turn facilitates the production of natural killer cells in the immune system and regulates mood. This response indicates that including massage in the treatment program for viral conditions, some forms of cancer, and mood disturbances would be beneficial. Oxytocin tends to increase feelings of connectedness. At the same time, massage might reduce cortisol and regulates epinephrine and norepinephrine, facilitating the action of growth hormone.

We may never fully understand the effects of massage on the integrated neuroendocrine mechanism; however, we do know that people who enjoy massage feel better.

The effects of massage can be processed through the somatic division of the PNS. The somatic division controls movement and muscle contraction and relaxation patterns, in addition to the motor tone of muscles.

Somatic effects are produced by means of the following:
- Neuromuscular mechanisms
- Hyperstimulation analgesia
- Counterirritation
- Reduction of impingement (entrapment and compression)

Neuromuscular Mechanisms

Nerve cells stimulate muscles to contract or to relax (release a contraction). Specialized nerve receptors called *proprioceptors* (or *mechanoreceptors*) provide a constant monitoring and protective function. Proprioceptors receive and transmit information about body position, muscle tension, static tone, degree of stretch, joint position and activity, and speed and direction of movement and equilibrium.

Dysfunction of soft tissue (muscle and connective tissue) usually occurs as a result of proprioceptive hyperactivity or hypoactivity. Proprioceptive hyperactivity causes tense or spastic muscles and hypoactivity of opposing muscle groups. Put simply, a tight muscle area results in (or from) an inhibited (weakened) muscle area and vice versa.

The three main types of proprioceptors are muscle spindles, tendon organs, and joint kinesthetic receptors.
- **Muscle spindles** are found primarily in the belly of the muscle; they respond to both sudden and prolonged stretches.
- **Tendon organs** are found in the tendon and musculotendinous junction; they respond to tension at the tendon. Articular (joint) ligaments, which have receptors similar to tendon organs, adjust reflex inhibition of the adjacent muscle when excessive strain is placed on the joints.
- **Joint kinesthetic receptors** are found in the capsules of joints; they respond to pressure and to acceleration and deceleration of joint movement. The two main types of joint kinesthetic receptors are type II cutaneous mechanoreceptors and Pacinian (lamellated) corpuscles.

Somatic Reflexes

Stimulation of nervous system receptors is interpreted and processed through the somatic reflex arcs. *Reflexes* are fast, predictable, automatic responses to a change in the environment that help maintain homeostasis. The stimulation of therapeutic massage constitutes a change in the environment, and the body is called on to restore homeostasis. The reflexes most often stimulated are the stretch reflex, tendon reflex, flexor reflex, and crossed-extensor reflex.

Stretch Reflex

The stretch reflex operates as a feedback mechanism to control muscle length by causing muscle contraction. It is activated by the muscle spindles, which sense muscle stretching. In response to massage methods that stretch muscles, a muscle spindle produces nerve impulses that stimulate a somatic sensory neuron in the posterior root of the spinal nerve. When the motor nerve impulse reaches the stretched muscle, a muscle action potential is generated, which causes the muscle to contract. Muscle contraction stops spindle cell discharge. The muscle stretch stimulates the stretch reflex, resulting in shortening of the muscle. The sensitivity of the muscle spindle in response to stretching influences the level of muscle tone throughout the body.

Therapeutic massage methods can make use of this reflex to stimulate inhibited muscle patterns by stretching the muscles and initiating the stretch reflex. An awareness of this reflex response is important in all stretches that are intended to lengthen and relax the muscles; in these circumstances the reflex must be avoided. Often this system of reflexes becomes hyperactive, resulting in an increase in muscle tension. Massage techniques that use isometric and isotonic muscle contraction to relax and lengthen muscles are helpful for normalizing short muscles and associated soft tissue.

Box 5.4 Breathing Pattern Disorder

Breathing pattern disorder is a complex set of behaviors that leads to overbreathing despite the absence of a pathologic condition. It is considered a *functional syndrome* because all the parts are working effectively, and a specific pathologic condition therefore does not exist. Instead, the breathing pattern is inappropriate for the situation, producing confused signals to the central nervous system and resulting in a chain of events.

Increased ventilation is a common component of the fight-or-flight response. However, when the breathing rate increases but the body's actions and movements are restricted or do not increase accordingly, the person is breathing in excess of the metabolic need. Blood levels of carbon dioxide (CO2) fall, and symptoms may occur. Because the person exhales too much CO2 too quickly, the blood becomes more acidic. These biochemical changes can cause many of the following signs and symptoms.

- *Cardiovascular effects:* Palpitations, missed beats, tachycardia, sharp or dull atypical chest pain, "angina," vasomotor instability, cold extremities, Raynaud's phenomenon, blotchy flushing of the blush area, and capillary vasoconstriction (face, arms, hands)
- *Neurological effects:* Dizziness; unsteadiness or instability; a sensation of faintness or giddiness (in rare cases, actual fainting); visual disturbance (blurred or tunnel vision); headache (often migraine); paresthesia (numbness, uselessness, heaviness, pins and needles, burning, limbs feeling out of proportion or as if they "don't belong"), commonly of the hands, feet, or face but sometimes of the scalp or whole body; intolerance of light or noise; and enlarged pupils (needing to wear dark glasses on a dull day)
- *Respiratory effects:* Shortness of breath, typically after exertion; irritable cough; tightness or oppression of chest; difficulty breathing; "asthma"; air hunger; inability to take a satisfying breath; excessive sighing, yawning, and sniffing
- *Gastrointestinal effects:* Difficulty swallowing, dry mouth and throat, acid regurgitation, heartburn, hiatal hernia, nausea, flatulence, belching, air swallowing, abdominal discomfort, and bloating
- *Muscular effects:* Cramps, muscle pain (particularly in the occipital area, neck, shoulders, and between the scapulae; less commonly in the lower back and limbs), tremors, twitching, weakness, stiffness, or tetany (seizing up)
- *Psychological effects:* Tension, anxiety, "unreal" feelings, depersonalization, feeling "out of body," hallucinations, fear of insanity, panic, phobias, and agoraphobia
- *General effects:* Feelings of weakness; exhaustion; impaired concentration, memory, and performance; disturbed sleep, including nightmares; emotional sweating (axillae, palms, and sometimes the whole body); and confused mental state
- *Cerebrovascular constriction:* A primary response to breathing pattern disorder, this condition can reduce the oxygen available to the brain by about one-half. Among the resulting symptoms are dizziness, blurring of consciousness, and, possibly, because of a decrease in cortical inhibition, tearfulness, and emotional instability.

Other effects of breathing pattern disorder for which massage therapists should watch are generalized body tension and chronic inability to relax. In addition individuals with a tendency for breathing pattern disorder are particularly prone to spasm (tetany) in muscles involved in the "attack posture"; they hunch the shoulders, thrust the head and neck forward, scowl, and clench the teeth.

Tendon Reflex

The tendon reflex operates as a feedback mechanism to control muscle tension by causing muscle relaxation. This reflex is mediated by the tendon organs, which detect and respond to changes in muscle tension caused by the pull of muscular contraction.

The most common massage technique used to stimulate the tendon reflex is post isometric relaxation (see Chapter 10). This technique increases tension at the tendon. The tendon organ is stimulated, which sends a signal along a sensory neuron. In the spinal cord the sensory neuron synapses with an inhibitory association neuron, which inhibits motor neurons that innervate the muscle associated with the tendon organ. This inhibition causes the muscle to relax. The sensory neuron from the tendon organ also stimulates an association neuron in the spinal cord. The association neuron synapses with a motor neuron, controlling antagonistic muscles and causing them to contract. To simplify, when one muscle contracts, its antagonist, or opposing muscle group, inhibits. This is called *reciprocal innervation*. Ballantyne and colleagues (2003) questioned the validity of the effects of proprioceptive neuromuscular facilitation (PNF) and muscle energy techniques (MET) based on the tendon reflex. They found that these methods are effective, but a different physiology appears to be involved; specifically, strong research evidence indicates that increased tolerance to the sensation of stretch is the main mechanism. MET stretching methods have been shown to bring about greater improvement in joint range of motion (ROM) and muscle extensibility than passive, static stretching, both in the short and long terms (Ellythy, 2012).

Flexor Reflex and Crossed-Extensor Reflex

The flexor (withdrawal) reflex and crossed-extensor reflex are polysynaptic reflex arcs. Stimulation of these reflexes affects both sides of the body through a series of intersegmental reflex arcs, which usually are linked in a pattern that includes postural muscles and muscle action in the limbs. A single sensory neuron can activate several motor neurons. The flexor reflex is involved in movement away from a stimulus, such as pulling away from a hot stove burner. The crossed-extensor reflex is involved in maintaining balance, such as staying upright when tripping over something. Synchronized control over the muscles that are contracting and those that are inhibited is achieved through contralateral reflex arcs, or reflex arcs on both sides of the body. Similar reflex patterns interact to coordinate movement; these are called *gait reflexes*. Others are involved with posture, such as the ocular pelvic reflex, related to how the eyes help balance and righting reflexes, which involve the ears.

By creating a noxious signal (an unpleasant sensation), therapeutic massage can stimulate a withdrawal response to stimulate opposite-side patterns of tension or weakness. This is a powerful response because withdrawal reflexes take priority over all other reflex activity occurring at the moment. If the massage application is so painful that the body tightens to guard against the noxious sensation, the effectiveness of the massage is lost. These reflex patterns also explain why tension patterns seldom occur only on one side of the body. The linked patterns of the various reflexes explain why dysfunctional patterns of groups of muscles often are identified on both sides of the body and not just where the dysfunction exists.

When working with neuromuscular mechanisms in massage, the massage therapist must keep in mind that the basic premises are to substitute a different neurological signal stimulation to support a normal resting muscle and fascial tone, and to reeducate the muscles involved (e.g., take the joint through its increased range of motion).

Movement, elongation, and pressure methods of massage focus on the activities of the muscles, tendons, joints, and ligaments to stimulate the proprioceptors. It is necessary to move the soft tissue structures in multiple directions and at multiple tissue depths. An efficient way to accomplish this is by applying mechanical forces in the direction of fibers and then across the fiber direction. Another way to think about this is making X patterns. The bending and shear strain stimulate the mechanoreceptors efficiently.

The effects of therapeutic massage appear to depend heavily on the nervous system. The effectiveness of the techniques depends on how efficiently the receptors for these reflexes are stimulated. The targeted receptor must be accessed with the appropriate technique and intensity so that the stimulated reflex can function appropriately.

Various neurological laws come into play to help explain the effects of therapeutic massage on the somatic nervous system (Box 5.5). A **law** is a scientific statement that is uniformly true for a whole class of natural occurrences. A degree of controversy exists about the validity of some of these laws, primarily Pflüger's laws; however, the neurological laws are worth considering as we attempt to understand the physiological effects of massage.

Soft tissue deformation produced during massage also influences the interstitial receptors, which may alter the nociceptive firing and alter pain perceptions. Inflammation is also an issue in increasing interstitial receptor sensitivity. Caution is necessary to avoid massage applications that cause tissue damage and inflammation.

Vestibular Apparatus and Cerebellum

The vestibular apparatus is a complex system composed of sensors in the inner ear (vestibular labyrinth), upper neck (cervical proprioception), eyes (visual motion and three-dimensional orientation), and body (somatic proprioception). These sensors send messages to several areas of the brain (brainstem, cerebellum, and parietal and temporal cortices), where they are analyzed. The messages affect the eyes (vestibulo-ocular reflexes), neck (vestibulocollic reflexes), and balance (vestibulospinal reflexes); at the same time, they keep individuals aware of where they are and how they are moving through the world (visuospatial orientation).

The vestibular apparatus and the cerebellum are interrelated. The output from the cerebellum goes to the motor cortex and brainstem. Stimulating the cerebellum by altering muscle tone, position, and vestibular balance stimulates the hypothalamus to adjust ANS functions to restore homeostasis.

The techniques that most strongly affect the vestibular apparatus and therefore the cerebellum are those that incorporate rhythmic rocking into the application of massage. Rocking produces movement at the neck and head that influences the sense of equilibrium. Rocking stimulates the inner ear balance mechanisms, including the vestibular nuclear complex and the labyrinthine righting reflexes, to keep the head level. Pressure on the sides of the body may stimulate the body righting reflex. Stimulation of these reflexes produces a body-wide effect involving stimulation of muscle contraction patterns, which pass throughout the body. Side-lying positioning during massage application allows for pressure application to the lateral aspects of the body with the pressure from the table on one side and the pressure from massage on the other side.

Massage alters the body's positional sense and the position of the eyes in response to postural change; it also initiates specific movement patterns that change sensory input from muscles, tendons, joints, and the skin and stimulates various vestibular reflexes. This feedback information, which adjusts and coordinates movement, is relayed directly to the motor cortex and the cerebellum, allowing the body to integrate the sensory data and adjust to a more efficient homeostatic balance.

Hyperstimulation Analgesia

In 1965, Melzack and Wall proposed the **gate control theory** of pain transmission (see Chapter 6). Over the past 50 years, some aspects of the original theory have been modified into what is now called the *neuromatrix theory,* but the basic premise remains the same. According to the gate control theory, a gating mechanism functions at the level of the spinal cord; that is, pain impulses pass through a "gate" to reach the lateral spinothalamic system. Painful impulses are transmitted by large-diameter and small-diameter nerve fibers. Stimulation of large-diameter fibers prevents the small-diameter fibers from transmitting signals. Stimulation (e.g., rubbing, massaging) of large-diameter fibers helps suppress the sensation of pain, especially sharp pain.

The skin over the entire body is supplied by spinal nerves that carry somatic sensory nerve impulses to the spinal cord. Each spinal nerve serves a specific segment of the skin, called a *dermatome.* Dermatomes, which can be affected by massage techniques that stimulate the skin, may account for **hyperstimulation analgesia,** which is the reduction of pain through stimulation. Hyperstimulation analgesia produced by massage and acupuncture has been used for many years (Gunn, 1992; Dorsher, 2008; Dorsher, 2009). In recent years transcutaneous electrical nerve stimulation (TENS) has become a popular method of producing hyperstimulation analgesia.

Box 5.5 Laws of Neurology and Their Implications for Massage

Arndt-Schulz's Law

Weak stimuli activate physiological processes; strong stimuli inhibit them (St. John, 1990).

Implication for massage: To encourage a specific response, use gentler methods. To shut off a response, use deeper methods.

Bell's Law

Anterior spinal nerve roots are motor roots, and posterior spinal nerve roots are sensory roots (Thomas, 2006).

Implication for massage: Massage along the spine is a strong sensory stimulation.

Bowditch's (All or None) Law

The weakest stimulus capable of producing a response produces the maximum response contraction in cardiac and skeletal muscle and nerves (Anderson et al., 2005).

Implication for massage: Techniques need not be extremely intense to produce a response; all that is needed is enough sensory stimulation to begin the process.

Cannon's Law of Denervation

When autonomic effectors are partly or completely separated from their normal nerve connections, they become more sensitive to the action of chemical substances (DeGroot and Chusid, 2002).

This denervation supersensitivity involves injured nerves, which respond to all sensory stimulation regardless of whether the stimulation is specific to that nerve. Denervation supersensitivity is a universal phenomenon that affects muscles, nerves, salivary glands, sudorific glands, autonomic ganglion cells, spinal neurons, and even neurons in the cortex. Changes in muscle structure and biochemistry also occur, as does progressive destruction of the contractile elements of fibers. Furthermore, unlike normal muscle fibers, which resist innervation from foreign nerves, degenerated muscle fibers accept contacts from other motor nerves, preganglionic autonomic fibers, and even sensory nerves.

Implication for massage: An injured area may hyperreact to all sensory stimulation, even after healing. If a person has a cold or is stressed at work or cannot sleep, previously injured areas may flare up.

Hilton's Law

A nerve trunk that supplies a joint also supplies the muscles of the joint and the skin over the insertions of such muscles (Thomas, 2006; Hebert-Blouin, 2014.).

Implication for massage: Determining whether pain originates from the joint itself, the muscles around the joint, or the skin over the joint can be difficult; stimulation of each area affects all parts.

Hooke's Law

The stress used to stretch or compress a body is proportional to the strain experienced, as long as the elastic limits of the body have not been exceeded (DeGroot and Chusid, 2002).

Implication for massage: Methods that lengthen the tissue must be intense enough to match the existing shortening but must not exceed it.

Law of Facilitation

When an impulse has passed through a certain set of neurons to the exclusion of others one time, it will tend to take the same course on a future occasion, and each time it traverses this path, the resistance will be reduced (St. John, 1990).

Implication for massage: The body likes sameness, which produces habitual patterns. After a pattern has been established, less stimulation is required to activate the response.

Law of Specificity of Nervous Energy

Excitation of a receptor always gives rise to the same sensation, regardless of the nature of the stimulus (Thomas, 2006).

Implication for massage: Whatever the method used, if a sensory receptor is activated, it will respond in a specific way.

Newton's Law

When two bodies interact, the force exerted by the first on the second is equal in magnitude and opposite in direction to the force exerted by the second on the first.

Implication for massage: This law explains various aspects of pressure delivery during massage. When two bodies interact (the massage therapist and the client), the force extended by the first (the massage therapist) on the second (the client) is equal in magnitude and opposite in direction (i.e., the client's body will push back). The point where they meet is a point of balance. This is especially important in body mechanics and how tissue binds in response to pressure.

Law of Generalization

When an irritation becomes very intense, it is propagated in the medulla oblongata, which becomes a focus from which stimuli radiate to all parts of the cord, causing a general contraction of all muscles in the body

Implication for massage: This response must be avoided if possible. It is important to keep invasive massage measures (e.g., frictioning) below the intensity level that causes a general body response.

Law of Intensity

Reflex movements usually are more intense on the side of irritation; at times, the movements of the opposite side equal the movements in intensity, but they usually are less pronounced (St. John, 1990).

Implication for massage: See Law of Symmetry.

Law of Radiation

If excitation continues to increase, it is propagated upward, and reactions take place through centrifugal nerves coming from the higher cord segments (St. John, 1990).

Implication for massage: See Law of Symmetry.

Law of Symmetry

If stimulation is increased sufficiently, a motor reaction is manifested not only on the irritated side but also in similar muscles on the opposite side of the body (St. John, 1990).

Implication for massage: By using increasing levels of massage intensity, a bilateral effect can be created, even if only one side of the body is massaged. This is especially useful for massage applications to painful areas. By massaging the unaffected side, the massage therapist can address the painful areas without performing direct massage work on those areas.

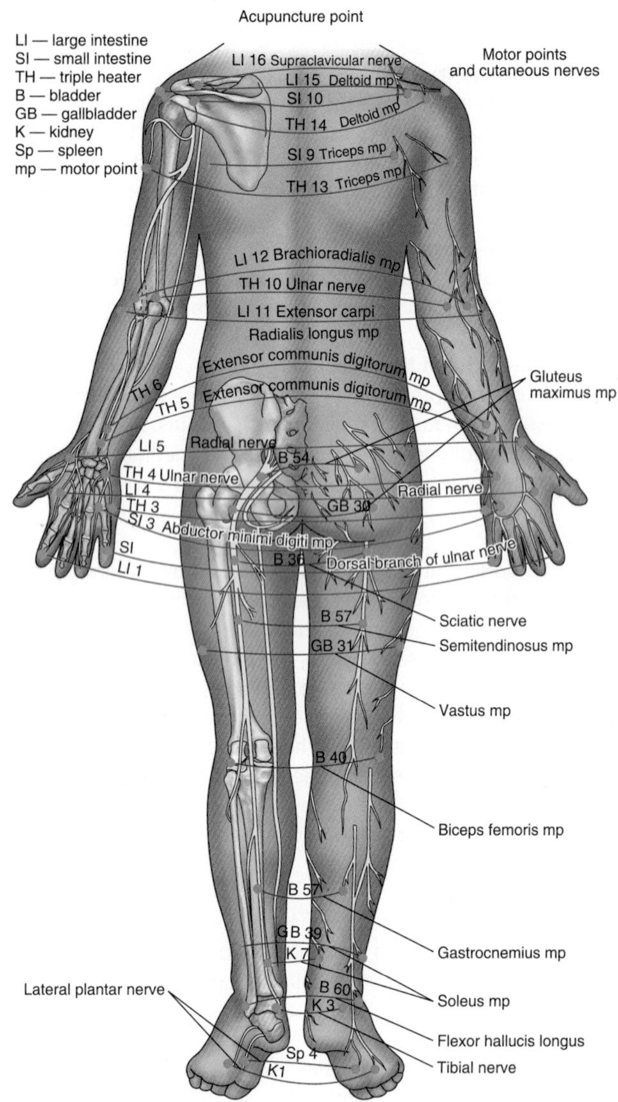

FIG. 5.6 A comparison of traditional acupuncture points, motor points, and cutaneous nerves of the arms and legs.

Stimulation of the PNS may produce analgesia by using some type of stimulation to mask pain sensation. Evidence suggests that the development of analgesia depends on the stimulation of specific points in the muscle that correspond to certain types of muscle receptors. These same points correspond with many traditional acupuncture points (Fig. 5.6). If massage targets these points with sufficient intensity, the large-diameter fibers stimulate the gating mechanism at the spinal cord and may result in hyperstimulation analgesia.

Tactile stimulation produced by massage travels through the large-diameter fibers. These fibers also carry a faster signal. In essence, massage sensations win the race to the brain, and the pain sensations are blocked because the gate is closed. Many parents and small children seem to know this instinctively. They rub an injured spot, thus activating large-diameter fibers. Stimulating techniques, such as percussion or vibration of painful areas to activate stimulation-produced analgesia (hyperstimulation analgesia), also are effective.

Counterirritation

Taber's Cyclopedic Medical Dictionary defines counterirritation as superficial irritation that relieves some irritation of deeper structures (Thomas, 2006). Counterirritation may be explained by the gate control theory. Inhibition in central sensory pathways, produced by rubbing or shaking an area, may explain counterirritation. Noxious stimuli suppress nociceptive (tissue damage potential) impulses. Changing the perception of pain by introducing a different sensory signal is akin to stepping on a person's foot to relieve the pain in the thumb just hit by a hammer.

Inhibition of central sensory pathways may explain the effect of counterirritants. Stimulation of the skin over an area of pain or dysfunction produces some relief from the pain. Various analgesic rubs and creams contain chemicals (e.g., capsaicin) that are intended to produce this kind of counterirritation.

All methods of massage can be used to produce counterirritation. Many people have learned from practical experience that touching or shaking an injured area diminishes the pain of the injury. Any massage method that introduces a controlled sensory stimulation intense enough to be interpreted by the client as recreating the symptom can create counterirritation. Massage therapy in many forms stimulates the skin over an area of discomfort. Techniques that result in reddening of the skin and underlying tissue (histamine response) are effective. Compression and movement methods require the body to deal with a different signal and temporarily ignore the original discomfort.

Nerve Impingement (Entrapment, Compression)

Soft tissue often impinges upon a nerve, a condition commonly called *pinched nerve*. Tissues that can bind include skin, fascia, muscles, ligaments, joint structures, and bones. Short muscles and stiff/dense connective tissue (fascia) often impinge upon major and minor nerves, causing discomfort (Fig. 5.7).

Entrapment and compression are technically different dysfunctions. Entrapment results when soft tissue (e.g., muscles and ligaments) exerts inappropriate pressure on nerves. Compression occurs when hard tissue (e.g., bone) exerts inappropriate pressure on nerves.

Regardless of the source of impingement, the symptoms are similar. However, the therapeutic interventions are different. Soft tissue approaches are beneficial for entrapment but less so for compression.

Because of the structural arrangement of the body, impingement often occurs at major nerve plexuses. The specific nerve root, trunk, or division affected determines the condition, such as thoracic outlet syndrome, sciatica, or carpal tunnel syndrome. Therapeutic massage techniques work in many ways to reduce pressure on nerves. The main ways are to (1) reflexively change the motor tone pattern and lengthen the muscles, (2) reduce stiffness and improve pliability of connective tissue, and (3) interrupt the pain–spasm–pain

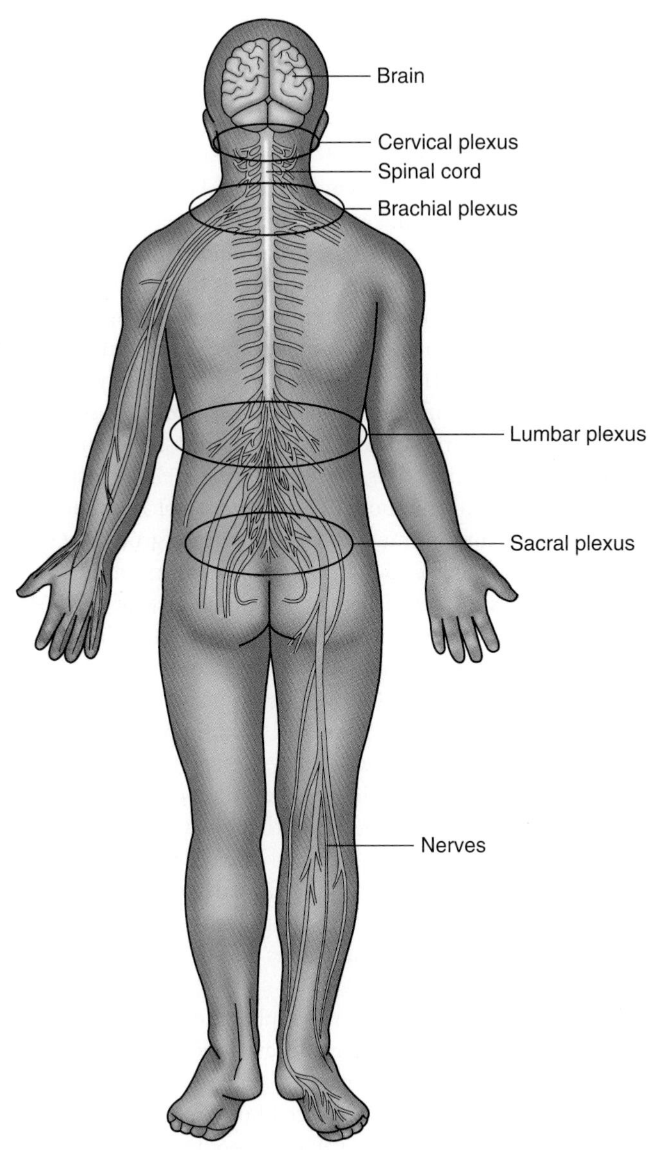

FIG. 5.7 Major nerve plexuses.

cycle caused by protective muscle spasm that occurs in response to pain.

TRANSLATING EVIDENCE INTO PRACTICAL APPLICATION: CIRCULATION

SECTION OBJECTIVES

Chapter objective covered in this section:

7. Explain the effects of therapeutic massage in physiological terms.

Using the information presented in this section, the student will be able to:

- Explain the possible anatomical and physiological influences of massage on the circulation.

Circulation involves fluid movement in tubes and tissues. Fluid as blood is found in the cardiovascular system. Fluid as lymph is in the lymphatic system which collects and filters tissue fluid. Cerebral spinal fluid (CSF) circulates in the nervous system. Connective tissues are fluid based. Fluids move by a variety of pumping actions including the pumping action of the skeletal muscles as they contract and relax. Arterial flow has the additional pumping action provided by the heart and smooth muscle tissue in the arteries. The lymphatic system has its own rhythmic pumping action. The implication is that some of the benefits of massage may be a result of its influence on this rhythm (Lancaster and Crow, 2006; Liu et al., 2015).

These circulatory functions are both linked and interdependent. For example, the carbon dioxide level of the CSF affects the respiratory center in the medulla, helping control breathing. Application of a mechanical device that produces a rhythmic massage in a proximal direction reduces edema, increases lymphatic movement from the tissues to the blood, and improves blood circulation. The massage practitioner must know the anatomy and physiology of the blood and lymph circulations to understand the effect of massage on these systems.

Circulation enhancement is fairly straightforward. More body fluids are moved by a 5-minute walk than by a 50-minute massage; however, for those unable to walk or even get out of bed, manual facilitation of the movement of body fluids can be a significant therapeutic option.

Research on massage and circulation is sparse but supportive. Castro-Sánchez and colleagues (2010) found that connective tissue massage improved blood circulation in the lower limbs of people with stage I or stage II type 2 diabetes and that it may be useful for slowing the progression of peripheral artery disease. A different study by Castro-Sánchez and colleagues (2010) indicated that a combined program of exercise and massage improved arterial blood pressure in individuals with type 2 diabetes who had peripheral arterial disease.

Massage may reduce blood flow in tissues. Wiltshire and colleagues (2010) found that massage may impair tissue recovery after strenuous exercise by mechanically impeding blood flow. There is increasing evidence of the ability of massage to influence blood flow (Franklin et al., 2014). Nelson (2015) found that massage therapy has systemic effects on endothelial function. Massage therapy lessens impairment of upper extremity endothelial function resulting from lower extremity exercise-induced muscle injury in sedentary young adults. The endothelium (the inner lining of blood vessels) contains cells that secrete substances that influence vasodilation or constriction. Franklin and colleagues also suggested that massage-induced improvements in endothelial function may help protect against vascular responses to other physical stressors, such as acute hypertension, hypoxemia, and wound healing.

Research has been done related to fluid movements for which an external compression device was used; a limb was inserted into a sleeve that mimicked a massage pattern starting in the foot, hand, or lower hip and moved upward, zone-by-zone massaging the limb and mobilizing fluid out of the extremities. This type of external pneumatic compression device using a peristaltic compression pattern affected circulation not only in the treated limb but also in the untreated limb (Martin et al., 2018). Implications for massage therapy exist showing that rhythmic, long-duration compression (30 minutes) has a body-wide effect. However, a massage therapist is unlikely to be able to perform the same level of compression, and the device is more efficient.

Arterial Flow

Arteries carry blood under pressure from the heart as a result of the pumping action of the heart muscle. The arteries themselves also have a muscular component that contracts rhythmically, facilitating arterial flow. An increase in arterial flow is beneficial in any situation in which an increase in oxygenated blood is desirable. Such situations include sluggish circulation in a sedentary person or increased demand in an athlete (see Chapter 12).

Massage application that creates direct compression into the area of an artery effectively crimps the artery, much like crimping a hose, and allows some back pressure to build up. When the pressure is released, the blood rushes through like water released from a dam. Arteries are accessible to compressive pressure on the soft medial areas of the arms and legs. Compressions should begin proximal to the heart, to take advantage of the force of the heart's pumping and move in a distal direction. Heavy pressure or sustained compression is not necessary; rather, moderate pressure is used in the right location to pump rhythmically at the client's current heart rate as the practitioner moves distally toward the fingers or toes.

Venous Return Flow

Venous return flow largely depends on contraction of the muscles against the veins. Back flow of blood is prevented by valves. Veins usually run more superficially than arteries. Because of the valve system in the veins and the fact that the blood is intended to flow back toward the heart, strokes to encourage venous flow move toward the heart.

Massage applications using short, pumping, gliding strokes are most effective in enhancing this flow. Passive and active joint movements also encourage the muscles to contract against the deeper vessels, assisting venous blood flow. If this is not possible for the client, slow, meticulous mechanical work is required to drain the area. Placing the limb above the heart, allowing gravity to assist, is beneficial (see Chapter 12). A similar massage application, which is used in lymphatic drainage massage methods, also increases the venous blood flow in the lower extremity. This research finding indicates that massage may have benefit in the prevention of venous stasis complications in chronic venous disease (dos Santos Crisóstomo et al., 2014).

Lymphatic Drainage

Two-thirds of the body is composed of water, and most of this liquid volume is contained within cells. However, the remainder that exists outside cells continuously circulates through the lymphatic system then back to the circulatory system. As described in Chapter 4, the lymphatic system consists of the tissues and organs that produce, store, and carry white blood cells that fight infection and other diseases. This system includes the bone marrow, spleen, thymus, lymph nodes, and lymphatic vessels. The lymphatic vessels are a network of thin tubes that carry white blood cells and lymph, a colorless fluid containing oxygen, proteins, glucose, and lymphocytes. As do blood vessels, lymphatic vessels branch into all the tissues of the body. The lymphatic system plays a vital role in controlling the movement of fluid throughout the body.

Lymph is derived from interstitial fluid or fluid that surrounds cells. Once interstitial fluid enters the lymphatic capillaries, it is called *lymph*. Lymphatic capillaries collect the tissue fluid by lymphangion contractions, generated by lymphatic muscle cells. The capillaries merge into small lymphatic vessels, which then merge into larger ones; along these larger lymphatic vessels are situated the lymph nodes. Lymph nodes are kidney bean-shaped tissues found in grapelike clusters in several locations in the body. They are sites of immune system activation and immune cell proliferation (growth). Once the lymph nodes have filtered lymph, the lymph drains into even larger vessels called *trunks*. All the trunks of the body drain into one of two ducts, the left lymphatic (thoracic) duct and the right lymphatic duct; these ducts return lymph to the bloodstream. The fluid in this extensive network flows throughout the body, much like the blood supply.

It is biologically plausible that massage application supports movement of interstitial fluid into the lymph capillaries which are connected to the surrounding tissue via little anchoring filaments attached outside the lymphatic cells. Some of these fibers attach all the way to the superficial dermis (skin). When the massage therapist moves the skin, the filaments pull on the openings of the lymph capillaries and the interstitial fluid moves into the vessels.

The massage procedures for lymphatic drainage are similar to those for venous return. Because lymph vessels open into tissue space, surface work that pulls gently on the skin is performed over the entire affected body region rather than focused over only the major veins. Pumping of jointed areas with passive joint movement seems to assist the movement of lymph through the areas of lymph node filtration. Deep breathing assists lymph movement in the thorax and abdomen. Unless the massage therapist is using manual lymphatic drainage as a specific therapeutic intervention (i.e., in cases of a pathological condition of the lymphatic system), precision in the specific flow patterns does not seem necessary. It is important to note that the lower abdomen (from the umbilicus down) drains into the inguinal area and eventually into the thoracic duct and that the right side (right arm and head) drains into the right lymphatic duct. Both major vessels dump into the vena cava (see Chapter 12).

Key Points on Massage's Effect on Body Fluids

- Based on current research, it is difficult to state confidently that massage influences the movement of body fluids.
- The main component of body fluid is water. It seems reasonable to expect that the mechanical forces applied during massage at least affect the fluid in a particular area while the tissue is massaged.
- Squeezing and compressing fluid in tissue (massage) should help the body move and process the various body

fluids. However, more research is needed before a specific massage effect on blood and lymphatic movement can be stated with confidence.

- The use of methods thought to influence blood and lymph movement is appropriate. However, massage professionals must explain to clients that although the methods appear to be clinically effective, research as yet is unable to prove the outcomes.

Cerebrospinal Fluid Circulation

CSF cools, nourishes, and protects the brain and nerves and influences breathing through carbon dioxide levels. The movement of CSF involves a pumping rhythm that some contend can be palpated. More research must be done before the anatomical and physiological mechanisms of this phenomenon can be understood scientifically. Recent identification of lymphatic type vessels in the brain (Abbott et al., 2018), the interstitium body wide (Benias et al., 2018), and vascular channels from skull bone marrow into the brain (Herisson et al., 2018) is questioning the past ideas related to fluid movement in the brain. As technology becomes more sophisticated, it is exciting to think what discoveries about our bodies will occur. Currently little research is available to support claims that manual methods such as craniosacral therapy can influence cranial bone movement and CSF flow. The protocol often used in cranial sacral approaches may affect pain in migraine headage (Muñoz-Gómez et al., 2022). It is likely that these types of methods are helpful in supporting relaxation and a nurturing therapist–client interaction (Downey et al., 2006). Ernst (2012) concluded that craniosacral therapy is associated with nonspecific effects and that other mechanisms are not supported by evidence.

Craniosacral treatment may have a favorable effect on autonomic nervous activity. Some studies indicate an influence on **heart rate variability** and parasympathetic response consistent with general relaxation (Bayo-Tallón et al., 2019; Henley et al., 2008; Armeni et al., 2014; Girsberger et al., 2014). This in itself is an interesting finding, but further research is needed to distinguish specific effects of the craniosacral therapy technique from less specific therapist–client interaction effects.

Massage approaches that support relaxation appear to create outcomes similar to those of more specific methods that are claimed to interact with the cranial bones and fluid movement rhythm. The typical craniosacral method involves gentle touch in the areas of the skull, face, spine, and pelvis. Further research is needed to distinguish specific effects of craniosacral technique from other noninvasive, gentle, rhythmic, compassionate touch methods.

The goal of massage to influence fluid circulation involves mimicking normal function. Increased blood flow on a local level is achieved by the compression of tissues, which empties capillary beds, lowers venous pressure, and increases capillary blood flow; this is quickly counteracted by autoregulation. Massage stimulates the release of vasodilators, especially histamine. Blood flow changes also may be induced through the autonomic vascular reflexes. This type of increase in blood flow has a body-wide effect. Compression against arteries mechanically influences internal blood pressure receptors in the arteries. As discussed previously, local blood and lymph circulation are logically affected by massage. In addition massage and other forms of bodywork mimic and assist the pumping action of the muscles and respiration. It is biologically plausible that massage influences breathing and breathing influences circulation (Atchison et al., 2021).

TRANSLATING EVIDENCE INTO PRACTICAL APPLICATION: CONNECTIVE TISSUE

SECTION OBJECTIVES

Chapter objective covered in this section:

7. Explain the effects of therapeutic massage in physiological terms.

Using the information presented in this section, the student will be able to:

- Explain the possible anatomical and physiological influences of massage on connective tissue.

Connective tissue, the structural component of the body, is the most abundant body tissue. Its functions include support, structure, space, stabilization, and scar formation. It assumes many forms and shapes, from fluid blood to dense bone. The pliability of connective tissue, which is based on its water-binding components, is significant in effective connective tissue support and function. Connective tissue is adaptive and responsive to a variety of influences, such as injury, immobilization, overuse (increased demand), and underuse (decreased demand).

Connective tissue is made up of various fibers and cells in a gelatinous ground substance. In bone this ground substance is impregnated with minerals that harden the bone. The combination of the fibers and the cells that produce the fibers and the ground substance is called the *connective tissue matrix* (Fig. 5.8).

During ANS sympathetic arousal, the ground substance thickens to provide protection from impact trauma (like a protective shell). This thickening response is called *densification.* Enzyme action reverses this process during parasympathetic dominance.

Healing of damaged body tissues requires the formation of connective tissue. The inflammatory response is one process that generates the healing mechanisms. Sometimes more tissue than is needed forms, and fibrotic tissue and adhesions can develop. An *adhesion* forms when connective tissue binds to structures not directly involved with the area of injury. When this occurs, the normal gliding of tissue layers becomes limited.

Fascia is a type of connective tissue that forms in sheets. It is embedded with smooth muscle bundles that contribute to fascial tone (tautness). The literature supports defining fascia as an innervated, continuous, functional organ of stability and motion that is formed by three-dimensional collagen matrices. Fascia can be classified into the following four categories (Kumka and Bonar, 2012):

- *Linking fascia:* Dense, regular, parallel connective tissue with a significant amount of collagen; this type includes fascia of muscles and tendons, aponeuroses, and neurovascular sheaths.

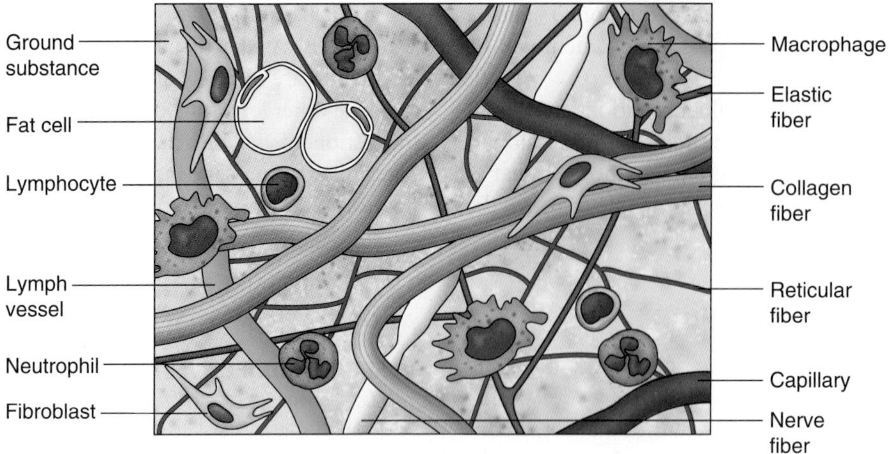

FIG. 5.8 Components of connective tissue.

- *Fascicular fascia:* Organized as a mixture of both loose and dense regular, multidirectional connective tissues that form tunnels; these tunnels bundle vessels and fascicles (small, slender bundles) within muscle, tendon, bone, and nerves. Fascicular fascia plays a significant role in organization, transport, strength, and locomotion.
- *Compression fascia:* Combination of dense, regular, woven, and multidirectional parallel-ordered connective tissue layers that cover whole limbs like a stocking. Compression fascia plays a significant role in movement and venous return because of its influence on compartmental pressure, muscle contraction, and force distribution.
- *Separating fascia:* Combination of loose connective tissue and dense, irregular tissue. Separating fascia divides the body in visible sheets and layers of varying fibers, allowing it to take up forces and friction in all directions. The major function of separating fascia is to allow more efficient sliding of tissues over one another.

The term *myofascia* refers to the muscle fibers organized as an interconnected three-dimensional network that surrounds and connects the musculoskeletal system. Many massage and bodywork systems use the term *myofascia* either in the name of the method or as the target tissue. This is somewhat confusing because many of the myofascia-based methods actually target the superficial fascia and not muscle.

Further confusing the issue is the myofascial trigger point phenomenon. **Trigger points** are tender, nodular points, but they remain somewhat of a mystery. Myofascial pain syndrome is described as the sensory, motor, and autonomic symptoms caused by trigger points, which typically develop after muscle overuse. The pain sensation from trigger points is experienced as dull and aching and is associated with muscle and soft tissue tenderness. Several theories have been proposed to explain trigger points:

- Trigger points result from nerve entrapment syndrome, in which nerve irritation or compression might cause secondary hyperalgesia in the muscles supplied by the entrapped nerve (Choi, 2014).
- Concentrations of immune system histochemical are found in the trigger point locations; these are called *proinflammatory mediators,* which are related to inflammation and pain. These chemicals create an acidic fluid around the trigger point location that acts as an irritant, causing localized pain not resulting from muscle tissue damage. Localized shortening of tissue in the area (taut band) seems to occur, which in turn can reduce circulation to the area, either causing the problem or perpetuating it. Local ischemia contributes to the lowered pH of tissue fluid, resulting in acidic tissue fluid in the area and a subsequent release of several inflammatory mediators in muscle tissue (Bron and Dommerholt, 2012; Minerbi and Vulfsons, 2018).
- Spontaneous electrical activity is involved. Some evidence indicates that spontaneous electrical activity occurs at myofascial trigger points, and that this electrical activity originates from the extrafusal motor endplate (the location where the nerve stimulates muscle contraction). Myofascial trigger points are one of the major peripheral pain generators for regional and generalized musculoskeletal pain conditions. The spontaneous electrical activity represents focal muscle fiber contraction and/or muscle cramp potentials, depending on trigger point sensitivity. Local pain and tenderness at myofascial trigger points seem to be related to nociceptor and non-nociceptor sensitization. Referred pain may depend on the sensitivity of the myofascial trigger points. Active pain-referring myofascial trigger points may play an important role in the transition from localized pain to the generalized pain conditions involved in central pain sensitization syndromes (Ge et al., 2011).

We still have no clear understanding of what a myofascial trigger point is (Isaikin and Nasonova, 2022). However, various methods, from pressure to dry needling (e.g., acupuncture) seem to help reduce the pain and dysfunction caused by these tender nodules (Ribeiro et al., 2018). One plausible physiological basis for the observation is that weak or overloaded muscles are involved in myofascial pain syndrome more often than other muscles (Minerbi and Vulfsons, 2018). The model proposed by Amir Minerb and Simon Vulfsons describes a possible causal relationship between muscle load, muscle strength, and the evolution of an energy crisis, as well as providing a logical mechanism for the threshold properties of the energy crisis phenomenon and, consequently, of the myofascial pain syndrome. The bottom line is, no one knows what a trigger point is, yet some sort of point phenomenon persists.

In areas of acute (active) dysfunction, connective tissue initially may not play a role in the dysfunctional pattern, and changes in the connective tissues are part of the healing process. Connective tissue dysfunction usually is suspected as a factor in disorders that last longer than 12 weeks, especially if nonproductive inflammation is present.

With overuse, additional connective tissue forms to provide stabilization to the musculoskeletal areas involved. When the soft tissue problem is chronic, the connective tissue ground substance can become dense and eventually fibrotic and may affect surrounding areas. Ligaments and tendons may fail to support joint stabilization, resulting in hypermobility, a major problem in somatic dysfunction that is difficult to manage. It is important not to increase flexibility in areas that are hypermobile (This is a major mistake that some massage therapists make; the most common method used inappropriately is stretching). In addition, connective tissue may thicken, bind, and stick, restricting movement and function. These types of connective tissue dysfunctions are more effectively addressed with massage that pulls and drags the tissues.

As discussed earlier, our understanding of the function of fascia in the body is increasing as more information becomes available about smooth muscle-type structures, innervation, mechanotransduction (the process by which cells convert mechanical stimulus into chemical activity), water movement, and tensegrity (Cai et al., 2010). Fascia plays a significant role in the support and function of our bodies because it surrounds and attaches to all structures. In the normal, healthy state, fascia is relaxed, wavy, and slippery, which gives it the ability to stretch and move without restriction. If fascia loses its pliability (through densification) or is not slippery, it becomes tight, restricted, and a source of tension to the rest of the body. Fascial restrictions pull, twist, and create pressure, causing all kinds of symptoms that produce pain, stiffness, aching, and/or restriction of motion. Fascial restrictions affect our flexibility and stability and are a determining factor in our ability to withstand stress and perform daily activities.

Connective Tissue Methods

Connective tissue massage was formalized in 1929 by Elizabeth Dicke, a German physiotherapist. Dr. James Cyriax contributed extensively to this methodology through his research and teaching on deep transverse friction massage. Dense tissue responds well to methods that lift, pull, and twist the tissues. Fibrotic tissue responds to the specific approaches of connective tissue massage (see Chapter 12). Similar approaches for the fascial or connective tissue component of muscles are called *myofascial technique,* although a better name would be *superficial (subcutaneous) fascia technique*. The application involves slow, sustained holding of tissues at bind, allowing for small shifts in tissue extensibility. These tiny movements can actually be felt because human tactile discrimination extends to the nano scale (Skedung et al., 2013). Myofascial tissue is specifically addressed by using pressure sufficient to deform the tissue. The direction of the force application is usually applied against the grain of the muscle fibers.

Connective tissue methods primarily affect the body structure. Methods that directly address the connective tissue do so by mechanically changing the consistency and pliability of the connective tissue (Kanazawa et al., 2009; Hernández-Hernández et al., 2014). Mechanical dysfunctions call for more direct methods and depend on an actual physiological change in the area. Cross-fiber frictioning (see Chapters 10 and 12) and inhibitory (direct) pressure approaches (see Chapter 10) are examples of mechanical massage methods. Mechanical force influences the smooth muscle bundles in the fascia (Schleip et al., 2005; Stecco et al., 2011). Changes in connective tissue, especially fascial tone, also occur through the nervous system because the tissue is densely innervated.

Massage methods most often affect the superficial fascial, the ligaments, and the tendons. The following five basic approaches are used:

- Methods that address the ground substance, which is *thixotropic* (i.e., the substance liquefies on agitation and reverts to gel when standing). Ground substance is also a *colloid.* A colloid is a system of solids in a liquid medium that resists abrupt pressure but yields to slow, sustained pressure.
- Methods that address the fibers within the ground substance; the fibers are collagenous (ropelike), elastic (rubber band-like), or reticular (mesh-like).
- Methods that influence fascial tone through direct stimulation of muscle bundles in the fascia and indirectly through influence on the nervous system.
- Concentrated massage at fascial anchoring points where multidirectional fascial connections converge (Fig. 5.9).
- Methods that support tissue sliding by interacting with the distribution of hyaluronan.

Methods that primarily affect the ground substance have a quality of slow, sustained pressure and agitation. The shearing, bending, and torsion stress and tensile stretch applied during massage to the matrix softens it, reducing density. Most massage methods can soften the ground substance, as long as the application is not abrupt, and it drags and elongates the tissue. Abrupt tapotement and compression (see Chapter 10) are less effective than slow, gliding methods that have a drag quality. Kneading and skin rolling (see Chapter 10) that incorporate a slow pulling action also are effective, especially to support distribution of hyaluronan. Parasympathetic activation helps create connective tissue pliability by causing smooth muscle contraction and chemical responses. Transverse friction (see Chapter 12) also creates therapeutic inflammation.

Fascia focal anchoring points are areas where fascia interconnects and transmission in the body is concentrated. It is logical to focus massage mechanical force application and drag in these areas. Key fascial focal anchoring points include aponeuroses, such as the lumbar dorsal fascia, plantar and palmar fascia, above and below joints where tendons weave into joint ligaments and the joint capsule, muscle investments in the scalp, and raphes (seam-like unions), such as the lateral raphe, where the abdominal fascia converges with the lumbar fascia, the linea alba of the abdomen, and the nuchal ligament.

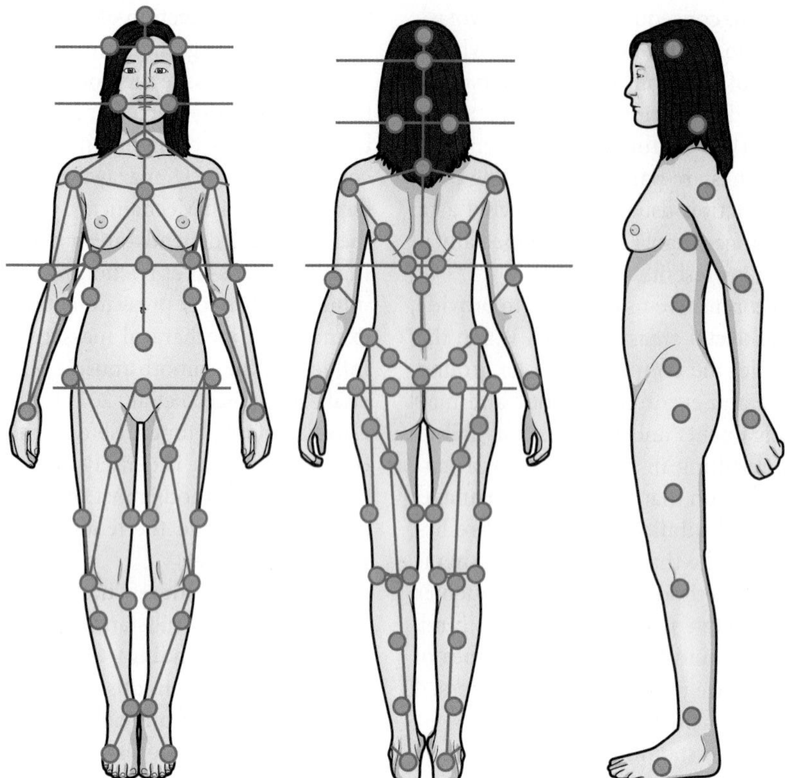

FIG. 5.9 Target areas for massage to influence fascial function.

Connective tissue applications using massage methods are addressed specifically in Chapter 12. Ongoing investigations seem to indicate that the influence of massage therapy on fascia could be clarified based on distribution of the slippery substance hyaluronan (hyaluronic acid); managing densification and fibrotic changes, including scar tissue; and, specifically, working with myofascial trigger points (Bordoni and Zanier, 2013; Stecco et al., 2013; Pavan et al., 2014; Fernández-de-las-Peñas and Dommerholt, 2014; Hughes et al., 2019). Even if we do not totally understand how the benefits occur, we can be confident that massage can be adapted to therapeutically affect these tissues.

Foot in the Door

The trend in massage therapy toward evidence-informed professional practice means that massage students must become *research literate;* that is, they must be able to translate research findings into practical applications. To remain current you must read research reports regularly. Even after your massage therapy career is well under way, you must review your information often to make sure it is up-to-date on current trends and that you understand the new and emerging evidence of massage therapy benefits and practice. Research is continually revealing new evidence of ways massage benefits the body. If you do not stay current, you could find yourself providing inaccurate information during an interview or a discussion with a client, or when documenting in clients' records. Providing inaccurate information will keep your foot out of the door for sure. Maintain your creditability by remaining accurate and informed.

SUMMARY

Massage in many forms is systematic mechanical stimulus followed by varying degrees of signaling cascades to induce a positive effect. Sufficient evidence supports the practice of massage in achieving its four main goals: relaxation, stress management, pain management, and maintaining functional mobility. Therapeutic massage methods are simple and appear to be effective in producing responses mediated through the nervous system, the interaction with the endocrine system, the connective tissue, and the circulatory system. Massage is beneficial for anxiety, depression, and chronic pain as part of an overall treatment protocol. Most forms of musculoskeletal pain and discomfort respond to massage at least temporarily. General daily stress responds well to massage. Armed with an understanding of the physiological effects of massage, massage professionals hopefully will be able to collaborate with medical, scientific, and trained personnel in the use of these old and effective methods. When provided by trained professionals, therapeutic massage can be beneficial in conservative treatment plans for chronic pain and stress-induced disease before more invasive measures are attempted.

Therapeutic massage can play an important role in prevention programs by providing a natural mechanism for stimulating the body to adjust to the stress of daily life and to restore the natural homeostatic balance. Additional information can be obtained by locating and studying the references in this chapter. Application of the techniques that bring about physiological effects is discussed in detail in Chapters 10, 11, and 12.

Most clients say they get a massage because it feels good and helps them feel better. Researching "good" and "better" scientifically is difficult. Massage professionals can provide the services of this art, confident that the reasons massage works and feels good are grounded in sound scientific research. Intuition and intent are necessary aspects of the professional application of massage. Clients care about how much you know, but they care more about how much you care and about how good they feel after a massage.

The massage profession needs more research. Therefore the massage profession needs to cooperate with researchers and appreciate the work involved in doing research. The scientific community and the public need quality research studies to strengthen their belief in massage so that they can justify receiving or recommending it. The massage profession needs the public and the scientific community to support massage. Whatever the massage or bodywork system used, the beneficial effects are elicited from the client's physiology; this occurs as the body adjusts to the external sensory information supplied by massage and responds to the mechanical forces generated by massage, and to the nurturing, confident, compassionate, mindful, and centered presence of the massage therapist involved in a productive therapeutic alliance with the client.

LEARN MORE ON THE WEB

Research sources: PubMed, The Cochrane, Agency for Healthcare Research and Quality, World Health Organization.

Evolve

Visit the Evolve website: http://evolve.elsevier.com/Fritz/fundamentals/.

Evolve content designed for massage therapy licensing exam review and comprehension of content beyond the textbook. Evolve content includes:

- Content Updates
- Science and Pathology Animations
- Body Spectrum Coloring Book
- MBLEx exam review multiple choice questions

FOR EACH CHAPTER FIND:

- Answers and rationales for the end-of-chapter multiple-choice questions
- Electronic Workbook and Answer Key
- Chapter multiple choice question Quiz
- Quick Content Review in Question Form and Answers
- Technique Videos when applicable
- Learn More on the Web

REFERENCES

Abbott NJ, Pizzo ME, Preston JE, Janigro D, Thorne RG. The role of brain barriers in fluid movement in the CNS: is there a 'glymphatic'system? *Acta Neuropathol.* 2018;135(3):387–407. doi:10.1007/s00401-018-1812-4.

Adstrum S, Hedley G, Schleip R, Stecco C, Yucesoy CA. Defining the fascial system. *J Bodyw Mov Ther.* 2017;21(1):173–177.

Alhamdoun A, Alomari K, Qadire MA. The effects of massage therapy on symptom management among patients with cancer: a systematic review. *Int Res J Oncol.* 2020;3(2):38–45.

Alves MLSD, Jardim MHDAG, Gomes BP. The effect of massage therapy on the cancer patient: mental health. *Int J Recent Sci Res.* 2018;7(3):111–121.

Anderson K, Anderson LE, Glanze WD, eds. *Mosby's Medical, Nursing, and Allied Health Dictionary.* 6th ed. Mosby; 2005.

Antunes MD, Marques AP. The role of physiotherapy in fibromyalgia: current and future perspectives. *Front Physiol.* 2022;13:968292. doi:10.3389/fphys.2022.968292. Published 2022 Aug 16.

Armeni M, Bravi V, D'Emidio S, et al. Craniosacral approach to the cardiovascular physiology: characteristics, mechanism and therapeutic perspectives. *J Cardiol Ther.* 2014;1:165.

Arumugam K, Harikesavan K. Effectiveness of fascial manipulation on pain and disability in musculoskeletal conditions. A systematic review. *J Bodyw Mov Ther.* 2021;25:230–239.

Atchison JW, Tolchin RB, Ross BS, Eubanks JE. Manipulation, traction, and massage. *Braddom's Physical Medicine and Rehabilitation.* 7th ed. Elsevier; 2021:316–337.

Arun B. Effects of myofascial release therapy on pain related disability, quality of sleep and depression in older adults with chronic low back pain. *Int J Physiother Res.* 2014;2(1):318–323.

Babaee S, Shafiei Z, Sadeghi MM, Nik AY, Valiani M. Effectiveness of massage therapy on the mood of patients after open-heart surgery. *Iran J Nurs Midwifery Res.* 2012;17(2 Suppl 1):S120–S124.

Bakermans-Kranenburg MJ, Van Ijzendoorn MH. Oxytocin receptor (OXTR) and serotonin transporter (5-HTT) genes associated with observed parenting. *Soc Cogn Affect Neurosci.* Published online 2008.

Bakowski P, Musielak B, Sip P, et al. Effects of massage on delayed-onset muscle soreness. *Chir Narzadow Ruchu Ortop Pol.* 2008;73(4):261–265.

Ballantyne B, Fryer G, McLaughlin P. The effect of muscle energy technique on hamstring extensibility: the mechanism of altered flexibility. *J Osteopath Med.* 2003;6(2):59–63.

Bayo-Tallón V, Esquirol-Caussa J, Pàmias-Massana M, Planells-Keller K, DJ Palao-Vidal. Effects of manual cranial therapy on heart rate variability in children without associated disorders: translation to clinical practice. *Complement Ther Clin Pract.* 2019;36:125–141.

Benias PC, Wells RG, Sackey-Aboagye Z, et al. Structure and distribution of an unrecognized interstitium in human tissues. *Sci Rep.* 2018;8(1):4947.

Bervoets DC, Luijsterburg PA, Alessie JJ, et al. Massage therapy has short-term benefits for people with common musculoskeletal disorders compared to no treatment: a systematic review. *J Physiother.* 2015;61(3):106–116.

Billhult A, Bergbom I, Stener-Victorin E. Massage relieves nausea in women with breast cancer who are undergoing chemotherapy. *J Altern Complement Med.* 2007;13:53. Online at: www.liebertonline.com/doi/abs/10.1089/acm.2006.6049.

Boghdady CM, Kalashnikov N, Mok S, McCaffrey L, Moraes C. Revisiting tissue tensegrity: biomaterial-based approaches to measure forces across length scales. *APL Bioeng.* 2021;5(4):041501.

Boitor M, Martorella G, Maheu C, Laizner AM, Gélinas C. Does hand massage have sustained effects on pain intensity and pain-related interference in the cardiac surgery critically ill? A randomized controlled trial. *Pain Manag Nurs.* 2019;20(6):572–579.

Bokhour BG, Hyde J, Kligler B, et al. From patient outcomes to system change: evaluating the impact of VHA's implementation of the Whole Health System of Care. *Health Serv Res.* 2022;57(Suppl 1(S1)):53–65.

Bordoni B, Zanier E. Skin, fascias, and scars: symptoms and systemic connections. *J Multidiscip Healthc.* 2013;7:11–24. doi:10.2147/JMDH.S52870. Published 2013 Dec 28.

Bordoni B, Zanier E. Clinical and symptomatological reflections: the fascial system. *J Multidiscip Healthc.* 2014;7:401.

Bordoni, B, Escher AR, Tobbi F, Pianese L, Ciardo A, Yamahata J, Hernandez S, Sanchez O. Fascial Nomenclature: Update 2022. *Cureus.* 2022;14(6).

Braun LA, Stanguts C, Casanelia L, et al. Massage therapy for cardiac surgery patients—a randomized trial. *J Thorac Cardiovasc Surg.* 2012;144(6):1453–1459.e1.

Braun L, Stanguts C, Casanelia L. 03. Stress reduction using massage in cardiac surgery patients. *BMC Complement Altern Med.* 2011;12(1):1–9.

Bron C, Dommerholt JD. Etiology of myofascial trigger points. *Curr Pain Headache Rep.* 2012;16(5):439–444.

Buscemi A, Martino S, Scirè Campisi S, Rapisarda A, Coco M. Endocannabinoids release after Osteopathic Manipulative Treatment. A brief review. *J Complement Integr Med.* 2021;18(1):1–7.

Cai Y, Rossier O, Gauthier NC, et al. Cytoskeletal coherence requires myosin-IIA contractility. *J Cell Sci.* 2010;123(3):413–423.

Cao TV, Hicks MR, Campbell D, et al. Dosed myofascial release in three-dimensional bioengineered tendons: effects on human fibroblast hyperplasia, hypertrophy, and cytokine secretion. *J Manipulative Physiol Ther.* 2013;36:513.

Caria A, Dall'Ò GM. Functional neuroimaging of human hypothalamus in socioemotional behavior: a systematic review. *Brain Sci.* 2022;12(6):707.

Carnes D, Mars TS, Mullinger B, Froud R, Underwood M. Adverse events and manual therapy: a systematic review. *Man Ther.* 2010;15(4):355–363.

Castro-Sánchez AM, Aguilar-Ferrándiz ME, Matarán-Peñarrocha GA, et al. Short-term effects of a manual therapy protocol on pain, physical function, quality of sleep, depressive symptoms, and pressure sensitivity in women and men with fibromyalgia syndrome: a randomized controlled trial. *Clin J Pain.* 2014;30(7):589–597.

Castro-Sánchez AM, Moreno-Lorenzo C, Matarán-Peñarrocha GA, et al. Efficacy of a massage and exercise programme on the ankle-brachial index and blood pressure in patients with diabetes mellitus type 2 and peripheral arterial disease: a randomized clinical trial. *Med Clin (Barc).* 2010;134(3):107–110.

Cates C, Munk N, Nemati D, Jordan K, Kelemen A, Groninger H. Comparative effectiveness study of massage therapy to improve quality of life in hospitalized patients receiving palliative care (S549). *J Pain Symptom Manage.* 2022;63(5):933.

Chaudhry H, Schleip R, Ji Z, et al. Three-dimensional mathematical model for deformation of human fasciae in manual therapy. *J Am Osteopath Assoc.* 2008;108(8):379–390.

Chen Y, Becker B, Zhang Y, et al. Oxytocin increases the pleasantness of affective touch and orbitofrontal cortex activity independent of valence. *Eur Neuropsychopharmacol.* 2020;39:99–110.

Cherkin DC. A comparison of the effects of two types of massage and usual care on chronic low back pain: a randomized controlled trial. *Ann Intern Med.* 2011;155(1):1–9.

Cho YS, Jeon JH, Hong A, et al. The effect of burn rehabilitation massage therapy on hypertrophic scar after burn: a randomized controlled trial. *Burns.* 2014;40(8):1513–1520.

Choi JI. Chicken and egg: peripheral nerve entrapment or myofascial trigger point? *Korean J Pain.* 2014;27:186.

Clar C, Tsertsvadze A, Hundt GL, et al. Clinical effectiveness of manual therapy for the management of musculoskeletal and non-musculoskeletal conditions: systematic review and update of UK evidence report. *Chiropr Man Therap.* 2014;22:12.

Coban T, Demirdel E, Yildirim NU, Deveci A. The investigation of acute effects of fascial release technique in patients with arthroscopic rotator cuff repair: a randomized controlled trial. *Complement Ther Clin Pract.* 2022;48(101573):101573.

Cohen SP, Vase L, Hooten WM. Chronic pain: an update on burden, best practices, and new advances. *Lancet.* 2021;397(10289):2082–2097.

Collinge W, MacDonald G, Walton T. Massage in supportive cancer care. *Semin Oncol Nurs.* 2012;28:45.

Cormack B, Stilwell P, Coninx S, Gibson J. The biopsychosocial model is lost in translation: from misrepresentation to an enactive modernization. *Physiother Theory Pract.* 2023;39(11):2273–2288.

Crane JD, Ogborn DI, Cupido C, et al. Massage therapy attenuates inflammatory signaling after exercise-induced muscle damage. *Sci Transl Med.* 2012;4(119):119ra13.

Crawford SK, Haas C, Butterfield TA, et al. Effects of immediate vs delayed massage-like loading on skeletal muscle viscoelastic properties following eccentric exercise. *Clin Biomech.* 2014;29(6):671–678.

Crowe MS, Nass SR, Gabella KM, et al. The endocannabinoid system modulates stress, emotionality, and inflammation. *Brain Behav Immun.* 2014;42:1–5.

Currin J, Meister EA. A hospital-based intervention using massage to reduce distress among oncology patients. *Cancer Nurs.* 2008;31(3):214–221.

Day JA, Stecco C, Stecco A. Application of fascial manipulation technique in chronic shoulder pain: anatomical basis and clinical implications. *J Bodyw Mov Ther.* 2009;13:128.

Deflorin C, Hohenauer E, Stoop R, van Daele U, Clijsen R, Taeymans J. Physical management of scar tissue: a systematic review and meta-analysis. *J Altern Complement Med.* 2020;26(10):854–886.

DeGroot J, Chusid JG. *Correlative Neuroanatomy.* 25th ed. McGraw-Hill; 2002.

De Oliveira FR, Gonçalves LCV, Borghi F, et al. Massage therapy in cortisol circadian rhythm, pain intensity, perceived stress index and quality of life of fibromyalgia syndrome patients. *Complement Ther Clin Pract.* 2018;30:85–90.

De Pauw R, Dewitte V, de Hertogh W, Cnockaert E, Chys M, Cagnie B. Consensus among musculoskeletal experts for the management of patients with headache by physiotherapists? A delphi study. *Musculoskelet Sci Pract.* 2021;52:102325. doi:10.1016/j.msksp.2021.102325.

Diego MA, Field T. Moderate pressure massage elicits a parasympathetic nervous system response. *Int J Neurosci.* 2009;119(5):630–638. doi:10.1080/00207450802329605.

Diego MA, Field T, Sanders C, et al. Massage therapy of moderate and light pressure and vibrator effects on EEG and heart rate. *Int J Neurosci.* 2004;114:31.

Dingding SO, Valdez SAD, Ong NWR, et al. A review on the effectiveness of massage therapy in pain management and treatment. *Int J Res Pub Rev.* 2022;3(6):445–455.

Dorsher PT. Can classical acupuncture points and trigger points be compared in the treatment of pain disorders? Birch's analysis revisited. *J Altern Complement Med.* 2008;14:353.

Dorsher PT. Myofascial referred-pain data provide physiologic evidence of acupuncture meridians. *J Pain.* 2009;10:723.

dos Santos Crisóstomo RS, Candeias MS, Ribeiro AMM, da Luz Belo Martins C, Armada-da-Silva PAS. Manual lymphatic drainage in chronic venous disease: a duplex ultrasound study. *Phlebology.* 2014;29(10):667–676.

Downey PA, Barbano T, Kapur-Wadhwa R, et al. Craniosacral therapy: the effects of cranial manipulation on intracranial pressure and cranial bone movement. *J Orthop Sports Phys Ther.* 2006;36:845.

DuFort CC, Paszek MJ, Weaver VM. Balancing forces: architectural control of mechanotransduction. *Nat Rev Mol Cell Biol.* 2011;12:308.

Dusek JA, Rivard RL, Griffin KH, Finch MD. Significant pain reduction in hospitalized patients receiving integrative medicine interventions by clinical population and accounting for pain medication. *J Altern Complement Med.* 2021;27(S1):S28–S36.

Elibol N, Cavlak U. Massage therapy in chronic musculoskeletal pain management: a scoping review of the literature. *Medicina Sportiva: Journal of Romanian Sports Medicine Society.* 2019;15(1):3067–3073.

Ellythy MA. Efficacy of muscle energy technique versus myofascial release on function outcome measures in patients with chronic low back pain. *Bull Fac Ph Th Cairo Univ.* 2012;17(1):51.

Ernst E. Craniosacral therapy: a systematic review of the clinical evidence. *Focus Altern Complement Ther.* 2012;17:197.

Fede C, Angelini A, Stern R, et al. Quantification of hyaluronan in human fasciae: variations with function and anatomical site. *J Anat.* 2018;233(4):552–556.

Fahey R. Integrative medicine for chronic pain: acupuncture and massage. *Integr Med Alert.* 2018;21(1):7–10.

Falsiroli Maistrello L, Geri T, Gianola S, Zaninetti M, Testa M. Effectiveness of trigger point manual treatment on the frequency, intensity, and duration of attacks in primary headaches: a systematic review and meta-analysis of randomized controlled trials. *Front Neurol.* 2018;9:254. doi:10.3389/fneur.2018.00254. Published 2018 Apr 24.

Farre A, Rapley T. The new old (and old new) medical model: four decades navigating the biomedical and psychosocial understandings of health and illness. *Healthcare (Basel).* 2017;5(4):88. MDPI.

Feelisch M, Cortese-Krott MM, Santolini J, Wootton SA, Jackson AA. Systems redox biology in health and disease. *EXCLI J.* 2022;21:623–646. doi:10.17179/excli2022-4793. Published 2022 Mar 21.

Feldman JL, Del Negro CA, Gray PA. Understanding the rhythm of breathing: so near yet so far. *Annu Rev Physiol.* 2013;75:423.

Fernández-de-las-Peñas C, Dommerholt J. Myofascial trigger points: peripheral or central phenomenon? *Curr Rheumatol Rep.* 2014;16:395.

Field T. Massage therapy research review. *Complement Ther Clin Pract.* 2014;20(4):224–229.

Field T, Poling S, Mines S, Bendell D, Veazey C. Touching and touch deprivation during a COVID-19 lockdown. *Int J Res Rev.* 2020;3:42.

Finch P, Bessonnette S. A pragmatic investigation into the effects of massage therapy on the self efficacy of multiple sclerosis clients. *J Bodyw Mov Ther.* 2014;18(1):11–16.

Fitzcharles MA, Cohen SP, Clauw DJ, Littlejohn G, Usui C, Häuser W. Nociplastic pain: towards an understanding of prevalent pain conditions. *Lancet.* 2021;397(10289):2098–2110.

Fitzgibbon M, Kerr DM, Henry RJ, Finn DP, Roche M. Endocannabinoid modulation of inflammatory hyperalgesia in the IFN-α mouse model of depression. *Brain Behav Immun.* 2019;82:372–381.

Fletcher CE, Mitchinson AR, Trumble EL, et al. Perceptions of providers and administrators in the veterans health administration regarding complementary and alternative medicine. *Med Care.* 2014;52:S91.

Fortune LD, Hymel GM. Creating integrative work: a qualitative study of how massage therapists work with existing clients. *J Bodyw Mov Ther.* 2015;19(1):25–34.

Franklin NC, Ali MM, Robinson AT, et al. Massage therapy restores peripheral vascular function after exertion. *Arch Phys Med Rehabil.* 2014;95:1127.

Frey JW, Farley EE, O'Neil TK, et al. Evidence that mechanosensors with distinct biomechanical properties allow for specificity in mechanotransduction. *Biophys J.* 2009;97:347.

Furlan AD, Imamura M, Dryden T, et al. Massage for low back pain. *Cochrane Database Syst Rev.* 2008(4):CD001929.

Ganjaei KG, Ray JW, Waite B, Burnham KJ. The fascial system in musculoskeletal function and myofascial pain. *Curr Phys Med Rehabil Rep.* 2020;8(4):364–372.

Ge HY, Fernandez-de-las-Penas C, Yue SW. Myofascial trigger points: spontaneous electrical activity and its consequences for pain induction and propagation. *Chin Med.* 2011;6(1):13.

Gebke KB, McCarberg B, Shaw E, Turk DC, Wright WL, Semel D. A practical guide to recognize, assess, treat and evaluate (RATE) primary care patients with chronic pain. *Postgrad Med.* 2023;135(3):244–253.

Gentile D, Boselli D, Yaguda S, Greiner R, Bailey-Dorton C. Pain Improvement After Healing Touch and Massage in Breast Cancer: an Observational Retrospective Study. *Int J Ther Massage Bodywork.* 2021;14(1): 12–20.

Girsberger W, Bänziger U, Lingg G, et al. Heart rate variability and the influence of craniosacral therapy on autonomous nervous system regulation in persons with subjective discomforts: a pilot study. *J Integr Med.* 2014;12:156.

Givi M. Durability of effect of massage therapy on blood pressure. *Int J Prev Med.* 2013;4:511.

Goldstein DS. Stress and the "extended" autonomic system. *Auton Neurosci.* 2021;236:102889. doi:10.1016/j.autneu.2021.102889.

Grewal A, Kataria H, Dhawan I. Literature search for research planning and identification of research problem. *Indian J Anesth.* 2016;60(9):635.

Gunn CC. *Reprints on Pain, Acupuncture and Related Subjects.* Seattle: University of Washington; 1992.

Haas C, Butterfield TA, Abshire S, et al. Massage timing affects postexercise muscle recovery and inflammation in a rabbit model. *Med Sci Sports Exerc.* 2013a;45:1105.

Haas C, Butterfield TA, Zhao Y, et al. Dose-dependency of massage-like compressive loading on recovery of active muscle properties following eccentric exercise: rabbit study with clinical relevance. *Br J Sports Med.* 2013b;47:83.

Hamel JF, Jobson S, Caulier G, Mercier A. Evidence of anticipatory immune and hormonal responses to predation risk in an echinoderm. *Sci Rep.* 2021;11(1):1–10.

Hanley J, Stirling P, Brown C. Randomised controlled trial of therapeutic massage in the management of stress. *Br J Gen Pract.* 2003;53:20.

Hébert-Blouin M-N, Tubbs RS, Carmichael SW, Spinner RJ. Hilton's law revisited. *Clin Anat.* 2014;274:548–555.

Henley CE, Ivins D, Mills M, et al. Osteopathic manipulative treatment and its relationship to autonomic nervous system activity as demonstrated by heart rate variability: a repeated measures study. *Osteopath Med Prim Care.* 2008;2:7.

Henoch I, et al. Soft skin massage for children with severe developmental disabilities: caregivers' experiences. *Scand J Disability Res.* 2010;12:221.

Hernández-Hernández V, Rueda D, Caballero L, et al. Mechanical forces as information: an integrated approach to plant and animal development. *Front Plant Sci.* 2014;5:265.

Herisson F, Frodermann V, Courties G, et al. Direct vascular channels connect skull bone marrow and the brain surface enabling myeloid cell migration. *Nat Neurosci.* 2018;21(9):1209–1217. doi:10.1038/s41593-018-0213-2.

Hohmann AG, et al. An endocannabinoid mechanism for stress-induced analgesia. *Nature.* 2005;435:1108.

Honguten A, Mekhora K, Pichaiyongwongdee S, Somprasong S. Effects of lymphatic drainage therapy on autonomic nervous system responses in healthy subjects: a single blind randomized controlled trial. *J Bodyw Mov Ther.* 2021;27:169–175. doi:10.1016/j.jbmt.2021.03.019.

Hou WH, Chiang PT, Hsu TY, et al. Treatment effects of massage therapy in depressed people: a meta-analysis. *J Clin Psychiatry.* 2010;71(7):894–901.

Hughes EJ, McDermott K, Funk MF. Evaluation of hyaluronan content in areas of densification compared to adjacent areas of fascia. *J Bodyw Mov Ther.* 2019;23(2):324–328.

Hymel GM, Rich GJ. Health psychology as a context for massage therapy: a conceptual model with CAM as mediator. *J Bodyw Mov Ther.* 2014;18:174.

Imanishi J. Effect of massage therapy on anxiety and depression in cancer patients. *Evidence-Based Non-Pharmacological Therapies for Palliative Cancer Care.* Amsterdam: Springer; 2013:35–51.

Imtiyaz S, Veqar Z, Shareef MY. To compare the effect of vibration therapy and massage in prevention of delayed onset muscle soreness (DOMS). *J Clin Diagn Res.* 2014;8:133.

Isaikin AI, Nasonova TI. Muscular factor in the development of musculoskeletal pain. Treatment options. *Neurol Neuropsychiatry Psychosom.* 2022;14(2):98–104.

Isomi M, Mak S, Lee J, et al. Massage for pain: an evidence map. *J Integr Complement Med.* 2019;25(5):475–502.

Jacobs SS. Integrative therapy use for management of side effects and toxicities experienced by pediatric oncology patients. *Children.* 2014;1:424.

Joshi MPTR, Poojary BPTN. The effect of muscle energy technique and posture correction exercises on pain and function in patients with non-specific chronic neck pain having forward head posture—a randomized controlled trail. *Int J Ther Massage Bodywork.* 2022;15(2):14–21.

Kanazawa Y, et al. Cyclical cell stretching of skin-derived fibroblasts downregulates connective tissue growth factor (CTGF). *Connect Tissue Res.* 2009;50:323.

Karkhaneh M, Zorzela L, Jou H, et al. Adverse events associated with paediatric massage therapy: a systematic review. *BMJ Paediatrics Open.* 2020;4:e000584. doi:10.1136/ bmjpo-2019-000584.

Karlson CW, Hamilton NA, Rapoff MA. Massage on experimental pain in healthy females: a randomized controlled trial. *J Health Psychol.* 2014;19:427.

Kassolik K, et al. Tensegrity principle in massage demonstrated by electro- and mechanomyography. *J Bodyw Mov Ther.* 2009;13:164.

Kassolik K, Andrzejewski W, Brzozowski M, et al. Comparison of massage based on the tensegrity principle and classic massage in treating chronic shoulder pain. *J Manipulative Physiol Ther.* 2013;36:418.

Kelemen A, Anderson E, Jordan K, Cates LC, Shipp G, Groninger H. "I Didn't Know Massages Could Do That:" a qualitative analysis of the perception of hospitalized patients receiving massage therapy from specially trained massage therapists. *Complement Ther Med.* 2020;52:102509. doi:10.1016/j.ctim.2020.102509.

Khalilian A. The effects of foot reflexology massage on anxiety in patients following coronary artery bypass graft surgery: a randomized controlled trial. *Complement Ther Clin Pract.* 2014;20:42.

Kinkead R, Tenorio L, Drolet G, et al. Respiratory manifestations of panic disorder in animals and humans: a unique opportunity to understand how supramedullary structures regulate breathing. *Respir Physiol Neurobiol.* 2014;204:3–13.

Ko YL, Lee HJ. Randomised controlled trial of the effectiveness of using back massage to improve sleep quality among Taiwanese insomnia postpartum women. *Midwifery.* 2014;30:60.

Kong LJ, Zhan HS, Cheng YW, et al. Massage therapy for neck and shoulder pain: a systematic review and meta-analysis. *Evid Based Complement Alternat Med.* 2013;2013:613279.

Koren Y, Kalichman L. Deep tissue massage: what are we talking about? *J Bodyw Mov Ther.* 2018;22(2):247–251.

Kumar S, Beaton K, Hughes T. The effectiveness of massage therapy for the treatment of nonspecific low back pain: a systematic review of systematic reviews. *Int J Gen Med.* 2013;6:733.

Kumka M, Bonar J. Fascia: a morphological description and classification system based on a literature review. *J Can Chiropr Assoc.* 2012;56:179.

Lancaster DG, Crow WT. Osteopathic manipulative treatment of a 26-year-old woman with Bell's palsy. *J Am Osteopath Assoc.* 2006;106:285.

Langevin HM, Sherman KJ. Pathophysiological model for chronic low back pain integrating connective tissue and nervous system mechanisms. *Med Hypotheses.* 2007;68:74.

Langevin HM. Fascia Mobility, Proprioception, and Myofascial Pain. *Life (Basel).* 2021;11(7):668. doi:10.3390/life11070668. Published 2021 Jul 8.

Lee SH, Kim JY, Yeo S, et al. Meta-analysis of massage therapy on cancer pain. *Integr Cancer Ther.* 2015;14(4):297–304.

Lebert R, Noy M, Purves E, Tibbett J. Massage therapy: a person-centred approach to chronic pain. *Int J Ther Massage Bodywork.* 2022;15(3):27–34. doi:10.3822/ijtmb.v15i3.713. Published 2022 Sep 1.

Li Q, Becker B, Wernicke J, Chen Y, Zhang Y, Li R, Le J, Kou J, Zhao W, Kendrick KM. Foot massage evokes oxytocin release and activation of orbitofrontal cortex and superior temporal sulcus. *Psychoneuroendocrinology.* 2019;101:193–203.

Li YH, Wang FY, Feng CQ, et al. Massage therapy for fibromyalgia: a systematic review and meta-analysis of randomized controlled trials. *PLoS ONE.* 2014;9:e89304.

Liu SL, Qi W, Li H, et al. Recent advances in massage therapy–a review. *Eur Rev Med Pharmacol Sci.* 2015;19(20):3843–3849.

Loghmani MT, Warden SJ. Instrument-assisted cross fiber massage increases tissue perfusion and alters microvascular morphology in the vicinity of healing knee ligaments. *BMC Complement Altern Med.* 2013;13:240.

Loghmani MT, Tobin C, Quigley C, Fennimore A. Soft tissue manipulation may attenuate inflammation, modulate pain, and improve gait in conscious rodents with induced low back pain. *Mil Med.* 2021;186(Suppl 1):506–514. doi:10.1093/milmed/usaa259.

Luo A, Tang C, Huang S, Zhao Da, Zhang A, Mengjia WU, Huiyu AN, Tan C. Massage relieves inflammation and oxidative stress and promotes autophagy after contusion of skeletal muscles. *Chinese Journal of Physical Medicine and Rehabilitation.* 2018:407–413.

Lund I, et al. Repeated massage-like stimulation induces long-term effects on nociception: contribution of oxytocinergic mechanisms. *Eur J Neurosci.* 2002;16:330.

Miake-Lye IM, Mak S, Lee J, Luger T, Taylor SL, Shanman R, Beroes-Severin JM, Shekelle PG. Massage for pain: an evidence map. *J Altern Complement Med.* 2019;25(5):475–502.

Majewska-Pulsakowska M, Mączka M. The influence of a relaxing massage on stress levels in women. *Aesth Cosmetol Med.* 2021;10(1):19.

Mallory MJ, Hauschulz JL, Do A, Dreyer NE, Bauer BA. Case Reports of Acupuncturists and Massage Therapists at Mayo Clinic: New Allies in Expediting Patient Diagnoses. *Explore (NY).* 2018;14(2):149–151. doi:10.1016/j.explore.2017.02.008.

Mannes ZL, Stohl M, Fink DS, et al. Non-pharmacological Treatment for Chronic Pain in US Veterans Treated Within the Veterans Health Administration: Implications for Expansion in US Healthcare Systems. *J Gen Intern Med.* 2022;37(15):3937–3946. doi:10.1007/s11606-021-07370-8.

Marchand L, Lewin D, Kozak L. Addressing Symptom Clusters with Complementary and Integrative Health Therapies in Palliative Care Populations: A Narrative Review. *OBM Integr Complement Med.* 2021;6(1).

Martin JS, Martin AM, Mumford PW, Salom LP, Moore AN, Pascoe DD. Unilateral application of an external pneumatic compression therapy improves skin blood flow and vascular reactivity bilaterally. *PeerJ.* 2018;6:e4878.

Martínez Rodríguez R, Galán del Río F. Mechanistic basis of manual therapy in myofascial injuries. Sonoelastographic evolution control. *J Bodyw Mov Ther.* 2013;17(2):221–234.

Mascarenhas RO, Souza MB, Oliveira MX, et al. Association of Therapies With Reduced Pain and Improved Quality of Life in Patients With Fibromyalgia: A Systematic Review and Meta-analysis. *JAMA Intern Med.* 2021;181(1):104–112.

Matsuda Y, Nakabayashi M, Suzuki T, Zhang S, Ichinose M, Ono Y. Evaluation of local skeletal muscle blood flow in manipulative therapy by diffuse correlation spectroscopy. *Front Bioeng Biotechnol.* 2021;9:800051.

McPartland JM. The endocannabinoid system: an osteopathic perspective. *J Am Osteopath Assoc.* 2008;108:586.

McPartland JM, Guy GW, Di Marzo V. Care and feeding of the endocannabinoid system: a systematic review of potential clinical interventions that upregulate the endocannabinoid system. *PLoS ONE.* 2014;9:e89566.

Meijer LL, Ruis C, van der Smagt MJ, Scherder EJA, Dijkerman HC. Neural basis of affective touch and pain: A novel model suggests possible targets for pain amelioration. *J Neuropsychol.* 2022;16(1):38–53.

Michalak J, Aranmolate L, Bonn A, et al. Myofascial tissue and depression. *Cognit Ther Res.* 2022;46(3):560–572.

Minerbi A, Vulfsons S. Challenging the cinderella hypothesis: a new model for the role of the motor unit recruitment pattern in the pathogenesis of myofascial pain syndrome in postural muscles. *Rambam Maimonides Med J.* 2018;9(3).

Mitchinson A, Fletcher CE, Kim HM, et al. Integrating massage therapy within the palliative care of veterans with advanced illnesses an outcome study. *J Palliat Med.* 2014;31(6):6–12.

Mitchinson A, Fletcher CE, Trumble E. Integrating Massage Therapy Into the Health Care of Female Veterans. *Fed Pract.* 2022;39(2):86–92.

Moberg KU, Petersson M. Physiological effects induced by stimulation of cutaneous sensory nerves, with a focus on oxytocin. *Curr Opin Behav Sci.* 2022;43:159–166.

Monteiro ER, Vigotsky AD, Novaes J, da S, Škarabot J. Acute effects of different anterior thigh self-massage on hip range-of-motion in trained men. *Int J Sports Phys Ther.* 2018;13(1):104–113.

Monteiro Rodrigues L, Rocha C, Ferreira HT, Silva HN. Lower limb massage in humans increases local perfusion and impacts systemic hemodynamics. *J Appl Physiol.* 2020;128(5):1217–1226.

Moraska A, Chandler C. Changes in clinical parameters in patients with tension-type headache following massage therapy: a pilot study. *J Man Manip Ther.* 2008;16:106.

Morhenn V, Beavin LE, Zak PJ. Massage increases oxytocin and reduces adrenocorticotropin hormone in humans. *Altern Ther Health Med.* 2012;18:11.

Moyer CA, Rounds J, Hannum JW. Meta-analysis of massage therapy research. *Psychol Bull.* 2004;1:30.

Müller-Oerlinghausen B, Berg C, Droll W. The efficacy of slow stroke massage in depression. *Psychiatr Prax.* 2007;34(3):S305.

Muñoz-Gómez E, Inglés M, Aguilar-Rodríguez M, et al. Effect of a craniosacral therapy protocol in people with migraine: A randomized controlled trial. *J Clin Med.* 2022;11(3):759.

Mustika IW, Sudiantara K, Lestari AS. Health education with audiovisual media and Relaxation Massage in lowering blood pressure and improved sleep quality for the elderly. *Open Access Maced J Med Sci.* 2021;9(G):118–123.

Nahon RL, Silva Lopes JS, Monteiro de Magalhães Neto A. Physical therapy interventions for the treatment of delayed onset muscle soreness (DOMS): Systematic review and meta-analysis. *Phys Ther Sport.* 2021;52:1–12.

Nedelec B, Couture MA, Calva V, et al. Randomized controlled trial of the immediate and long-term effect of massage on adult postburn scar. *Burns.* 2019;45(1):128–139.

Nelson NL. Massage therapy: understanding the mechanisms of action on blood pressure. A scoping review. *J Am Soc Hypertens.* 2015;9(10): 785–793.

Noble DJ, Hochman S. Pulmonary Afferent Activity Patterns During Slow, Deep Breathing Contribute to the Neural Induction of Physiological Relaxation. *Front Physiol.* 2019;10:1176.

Nordness MF, Hayhurst CJ, Pandharipande P. Current perspectives on the assessment and management of pain in the intensive care unit. *J Pain Res.* 2021;14:1733–1744.

Olszewski WL, et al. Where do lymph and tissue fluid accumulate in lymphedema of the lower limbs caused by obliteration of lymphatic collectors? *Lymphology.* 2009;42:105.

Paanalahti K, Holm LW, Nordin M, et al. Adverse events after manual therapy among patients seeking care for neck and/or back pain: a randomized controlled trial. *BMC Musculoskelet Disord.* 2014;15:77.

Pan YQ, Yang KH, Wang YL, et al. Massage interventions and treatment-related side effects of breast cancer: a systematic review and meta-analysis. *Int J Clin Oncol.* 2013;19(5):829–841.

Patel KC, Gross A, Graham N, et al. Massage for mechanical neck disorders. *Cochrane Database Syst Rev.* 2012;9:CD004871. http://dx.doi.org/10.1002/14651858.CD004871.pub4.

Pavan PG, Stecco A, Stern R, et al. Painful connections: densification versus fibrosis of fascia. *Curr Pain Headache Rep.* 2014;18(1).

Peng S, Ying B, Chen Y, et al. Effects of massage on the anxiety of patients receiving percutaneous coronary intervention. *Psychiatr Danub.* 2015;27(1):44–49.

Pilkington K, CAM Cancer Consortium. Massage (Classical/Swedish) [online document], February 15, 2021.

Poland RE, Gertsik L, Favreau JT, et al. Open-label, randomized, parallel-group controlled clinical trial of massage for treatment of depression in HIV-infected subjects. *J Altern Complement Med.* 2013;19:334.

Popkirov S, Enax-Krumova EK, Mainka T, Hoheisel M, Hausteiner-Wiehle C. Functional pain disorders – more than nociplastic pain. *NeuroRehabilitation.* 2020;47(3):343–353.

Posadzki P, Ernst E. The safety of massage therapy: an update of a systematic review. *Focus Altern Complement Ther.* 2013;18:27.

Prajayanti ED, Irma MS. The effect of Swedish message therapy on blood pressure in primary hypertension patients. *Gaster.* 2022;20(2):144–153.

Pratt RL. Hyaluronan and the fascial frontier. *Int J Mol Sci.* 2021; 22(13):6845.

Quattrocki E, Friston K. Autism, oxytocin and interoception. *Neurosci Biobehav Rev.* 2014;47:410–430.

Rahn EJ, Hohmann AG. Cannabinoids as pharmacotherapies for neuropathic pain: from the bench to the bedside. *Neurotherapeutics.* 2009;6(4):713–737.

Rapaport MH, Schettler P, Bresee C. A preliminary study of the effects of repeated massage on hypothalamic-pituitary-adrenal and immune function in healthy individuals: a study of mechanisms of action and dosage. *J Altern Complement Med.* 2012;18:789.

Rapaport MH, Schettler PJ, Larson ER, et al. Massage therapy for psychiatric disorders. *Focus.* 2018;16(1):24–31.

Ribeiro DC, Belgrave A, Naden A, Fang H, Matthews P, Parshottam S. The prevalence of myofascial trigger points in neck and shoulder-related disorders: a systematic review of the literature. *BMC Musculoskelet Disord.* 2018;19(1):252.

Río-González Á, Cerezo-Téllez E, Gala-Guirao C, et al. Effects of different neck manual lymphatic drainage maneuvers on the nervous, cardiovascular, respiratory and musculoskeletal systems in healthy students. *J Clin Med.* 2020;9(12):4062.

Rosignoli C, Ornello R, Onofri A, et al. Applying a biopsychosocial model to migraine: rationale and clinical implications. *J Headache Pain.* 2022;23(1):1–17.

Sahraei F, Rahemi Z, Sadat Z, et al. The effect of Swedish massage on pain in rheumatoid arthritis patients: A randomized controlled trial. *Complement Ther Clin Pract.* 2022;46:101524.

Schirmer A, McGlone F. Editorial overview: Affective touch: neurobiology and function. *Curr Opin Behav Sci.* 2022;45(101129):101129.

Schleip R, Klingler W, Lehmann-Horn F. Active fascial contractility: fascia may be able to actively contract in a smooth muscle-like manner and thereby influence musculoskeletal dynamics. *Med Hypotheses.* 2005;65:273.

Schmiege SJ, Mann JD, Moraska A. Myofascial trigger point-focused head and neck massage for recurrent tension-type headache: a randomized, placebo-controlled clinical trial. *Clin J Pain.* 2014;31(2):159–168.

Schoenrock B, Zander V, Derst S, et al. Bed rest, exercise countermeasure and reconditioning effects on the human resting muscle tone system. *Front Physiol.* 2018;9:810.

Scott HC, Stockdale C, Robinson A, Robinson LS, Brown T. Is massage an effective intervention in the management of post-operative scarring? A scoping review. *J Hand Ther.* 2022;35(2):186–199.

Seifert G, Kanitz JL, Rihs C, Krause I, Witt K, Voss A. Rhythmical massage improves autonomic nervous system function: a single-blind randomised controlled trial. *J Integr Med.* 2018;16(3):172–177.

Shafiei Z, Babaee S, Nazari A. The effectiveness of massage therapy on depression, anxiety and stress of patients after coronary artery bypass graft surgery. *Iran J Surg.* 2013a;2(4):8–16.

Shafiei Z, Nourian K, Babaee S, et al. Effectiveness of massage therapy on muscular tension and relaxation of patients after coronary artery bypass graft surgery: a randomized clinical trial. *J Clin Nurs Midwifery.* 2014;2(4):8–16.

Shafiei Z, Nourian K, Babaee S, et al. Effectiveness of light pressure stroking massage on pain and fatigue of patients after coronary artery bypass graft surgery: a randomized clinical trial. *J Clin Nurs Midwifery.* 2013b;2(3):28–38.

Sherman KJ, Cook AJ, Wellman RD, Hawkes RJ, Kahn JR, Deyo RA, Cherkin DC. Five-week outcomes from a dosing trial of therapeutic massage for chronic neck pain. *Ann Fam Med.* 2014;12(2):112–120.

Shengelia R, Parker SJ, Ballin M, et al. Complementary therapies for osteoarthritis: are they effective? *Pain Manag Nurs.* 2013;14:e274.

Shim JM, Kim SJ. Effects of manual lymph drainage of the neck on EEG in subjects with psychological stress. *J Phys Ther Sci.* 2014;26:127.

Shinde MB, Anjum S. Effectiveness of slow back massage on quality of sleep among ICU patents. *Int J Sci Res.* 2014;3:292.

Sies H. Oxidative eustress: on constant alert for redox homeostasis. *Redox Biol.* 2021;41:101867. doi:10.1016/j.redox.2021.101867.

Simatupang N, Harahap NS, Ritonga DA. Effects of sport massage in preventing decreased immunity after sub-maximal physical exercise. *Proceedings of the 1st Unimed International Conference on Sport Science (UnICoSS 2019).* Atlantis Press; 2020.

Simmonds N, Miller P, Gemmell H. A theoretical framework for the role of fascia in manual therapy. *J Bodyw Mov Ther.* 2012;16:83.

Skedung L, Arvidsson M, Chung JY, et al. Feeling small: exploring the tactile perception limits. *Sci Rep.* 2013;3(1):2617.

Skubisz Z, Kupczyk D, Goch A, et al. Influence of Classical Massage on Biochemical Markers of Oxidative Stress in Humans: Pilot Study. *Biomed Res Int.* 2021;2021:6647250.

Somani S, Merchant S, Lalani S. A literature review about effectiveness of massage therapy for cancer pain. *J Pak Med Assoc.* 2013;63:1418.

St John P. Workshop Notes: Seminar I. St John Neuromuscular Therapy Seminars; 1990. Self-published.

Stecco A, Gesi M, Stecco C, et al. Fascial components of the myofascial pain syndrome. *Curr Pain Headache Rep.* 2013;17:1.

Stecco C, et al. Histological characteristics of the deep fascia of the upper limb. *Ital J Anat Embryol.* 2006;111:105.

Stecco C, et al. Anatomy of the deep fascia of the upper limb. II. Study of innervation. *Morphologie.* 2007a;91:38.

Stecco C, et al. Tendinous muscular insertions onto the deep fascia of the upper limb. I. Anatomical study. *Morphologie.* 2007b;91:29.

Stecco C, Stern R, Porzionato A, et al. Hyaluronan within fascia in the etiology of myofascial pain. *Surg Radiol Anat.* 2011;33:891.

Steinmetz A. Back pain treatment: a new perspective. *Ther Adv Musculoskelet Dis.* 2022;14:1759720X221100293. doi:10.1177/1759720X221100293. Published 2022 Jul 4.

Suarez-Rodriguez V, Fede C, Pirri C, et al. Fascial Innervation: A Systematic Review of the Literature. *Int J Mol Sci.* 2022;23(10):5674. doi:10.3390/ijms23105674. Published 2022 May 18.

Tadeo I, Berbegall AP, Escudero LM, et al. Biotensegrity of the extracellular matrix: physiology, dynamic mechanical balance, and implications in oncology and mechanotherapy. *Front Oncol.* 2014;4:39. http://dx.doi.org/10.3389/fonc.2014.00039.

Tejero-Fernández V, Membrilla-Mesa M, Galiano-Castillo N, Arroyo-Morales M. Immunological effects of massage after exercise: a systematic review. *Phys Ther Sport.* 2015;16(2):187–192.

Tick H, Nielsen A, Pelletier KR, et al. Evidence-based nonpharmacologic strategies for comprehensive pain care: the Consortium Pain Task Force White Paper. *Explore (NY).* 2018;14(3):177–211. doi:10.1016/j.explore.2018.02.001.

Thomas CL. *Taber's Cyclopedic Medical Dictionary.* 20th ed. FA Davis; 2006.

Trumble E, Baylin A, Mitchinson A, et al. Complementary and alternative medicine (CAM) therapies as a means of advancing patient-centered care for veterans receiving palliative care. *J Altern Complement Med.* 2014;20:A50.

Utli H, Department of Elderly Care, Mardin Artuklu University Vocational School of Health Services, Mardin, Turkey. Effects of massage therapy on clinical symptoms of older people. *J Educ Res Nurs.* 2022;18(1):103–107.

Uvnäs M, Kerstin, HJ, Linda H, Maria P. Sensory stimulation and oxytocin: their roles in social interaction and health promotion. *Frontiers in Psychology* 13 (2022): 929741.

Van Daele U, Meirte J, Anthonissen M, Vanhullebusch T, Maertens K, Demuynck L, Moortgat P. Mechanomodulation: physical treatment modalities employ mechanotransduction to improve scarring. *Eur Burn J.* 2022;3(2):241–255.

Van Diest I, Verstappen K, Aubert AE, et al. Inhalation/exhalation ratio modulates the effect of slow breathing on heart rate variability and relaxation. *Appl Psychophysiol Biofeedback.* 2014;39(3–4):171–180.

Wade DT, Halligan PW. The biopsychosocial model of illness: a model whose time has come. *Clin Rehabil.* 2017;31(8):995–1004. doi:10.1177/0269215517709890.

Wang R, Huang X, Wang Y, Akbari M. Non-pharmacologic Approaches in Preoperative Anxiety, a Comprehensive Review. *Front Public Health.* 2022;10:854673. doi:10.3389/fpubh.2022.854673. Published 2022 Apr 11.

Wang SQ, Jiang AY, Gao Q. Effect of manual soft tissue therapy on the pain in patients with chronic neck pain: a systematic review and meta-analysis. *Complement Ther Clin Pract.* 2022;49:101619. doi:10.1016/j.ctcp.2022.101619.

Waters-Banker C, Dupont-Versteegden EE, Kitzman PH, et al. Investigating the mechanisms of massage efficacy: the role of mechanical immunomodulation. *J Athl Train.* 2014;49:266.

Whatley J, Perkins J, Samuel C. Reflexology: exploring the mechanism of action. *Complement Ther Clin Pract.* 2022;48:101606. doi:10.1016/j.ctcp.2022.101606.

Wilson AT, Riley JL, 3rd, Bishop MD, et al. A psychophysical study comparing massage to conditioned pain modulation: a single blind randomized controlled trial in healthy participants. *J Bodyw Mov Ther.* 2021;27:426–435.

Whitehead AM, Kligler B. Innovations in care: complementary and integrative health in the veterans health administration whole health system. *Med Care.* 2020;58(Suppl 2 9S):S78–S79. doi:10.1097/MLR.0000000000001383.

Wiltshire EV, et al. Massage impairs postexercise muscle blood flow and "lactic acid" removal. *Med Sci Sports Exerc.* 2010;42:1062.

Xing XX, Zheng MX, Hua XY, Ma SJ, Ma ZZ, Xu JG. Brain plasticity after peripheral nerve injury treatment with massage therapy based on resting-state functional magnetic resonance imaging. *Neural Regen Res.* 2021;16(2):388–393. doi:10.4103/1673-5374.290912.

Yin P, Gao N, Wu J, Litscher G, Xu S. Adverse events of massage therapy in pain-related conditions: a systematic review. *Evid Based Complement Alternat Med.* 2014;2014:480956.

Yuniana R, Kushartanti BMW, Arovah NI, Nasrulloh A. Effectiveness of massage therapy continued exercise therapy against pain healing, ROM, and pelvic function in people with chronic pelvic injuries. *J Phys Educ Sport.* 2022;22(6):1433–1441.

Zainuddin Z, Newton M, Sacco P, et al. Effects of massage on delayed-onset muscle soreness, swelling, and recovery of muscle function. *J Athl Train.* 2005;40:174.

Zaki AEM. Acceleration of recovery of muscle injuries through massage based therapies. *J Am Sci.* 2014;10(5):35–39.

Zügel, M, Maganaris CN, Wilke J, et al. Fascial tissue research in sports medicine: from molecules to tissue adaptation, injury and diagnostics. *Br J Sports Med.* 2018;52(23):1497.

MULTIPLE-CHOICE QUESTIONS FOR DISCUSSION AND REVIEW

The answers, with rationales, can be found on the Evolve site. Use these questions to stimulate discussion and dialog. You must understand the meaning of the words in the question and possible answers. Each question provides you the opportunity to review terminology, practice critical thinking skills, and improve your multiple-choice test-taking skills. The answers and rationales are on the Evolve site. Remember, it is just as important to know why the wrong answers are wrong as to know why the correct answer is correct.

1. Massage can increase a person's fine motor movements, such as handwriting. Which neurotransmitter is influenced?
   a. Serotonin
   b. Oxytocin
   c. Dopamine
   d. Endocannabinoids
2. Massage has been demonstrated to reduce some individuals' craving for food and/or reduce hunger. Which neurotransmitter is responsible?
   a. Epinephrine
   b. Serotonin
   c. Dopamine
   d. Norepinephrine
3. Connectedness and intimacy in massage are most likely the results of an increased level of ________.
   a. Cortisol
   b. Endorphins
   c. Serotonin
   d. Oxytocin
4. Massage has been shown to decreases sympathetic arousal. Which of the following could be measured to confirm changes in sympathetic dominance?
   a. Cortisol
   b. Oxytocin
   c. Growth hormone
   d. Enkephalins
5. Hans Selye described body responses to stress in three stages. The middle stage is called ________.
   a. Alarm reaction
   b. Exhaustion reaction
   c. Resistance reaction
   d. Neuromatrix reaction
6. Parasympathetic patterns are ________.
   a. Restorative: adrenaline is secreted, mobility is decreased, and the bronchioles are constricted
   b. Physical activity is curtailed, digestion and elimination are increased, and the bronchioles are constricted
   c. Physical activity is increased, pupils are dilated, saliva secretion is stopped, and stomach secretion is increased
   d. Restorative: heartbeat speeds up, bladder delays emptying, and saliva secretion increases
7. The three main types of proprioceptors are muscle spindles, tendon organs, and ________.
   a. Cervical/lumbar plexus
   b. Spinal nerves
   c. Joint kinesthetic receptors
   d. Sphincter muscles
8. What reflex is involved in maintaining balance?
   a. Flexor reflex
   b. Withdrawal reflex
   c. Tendon reflex
   d. Crossed-extensor reflex
9. The gate control theory is ________.
   a. Reduction of perception of a sensation of a sensory receptor by adaptation
   b. Control of homeostasis by alteration of tissue or function
   c. A method of teaching the body to deal with stress
   d. The hypothesis that painful stimuli can be prevented from reaching higher levels of the central nervous system by stimulating lower sensory nerves
10. Which evidence-informed outcome of massage has the largest increase in research related to reducing prescription drug use?
    a. Relaxation
    b. Stress management
    c. Pain management
    d. Mobility and physical performance
11. A client states a goal of wanting to relax and complains of having headaches, gastrointestinal problems, and high blood pressure. The client is likely to be experiencing ________.
    a. An excessive parasympathetic output
    b. An excessive sympathetic output
    c. A neuroendocrine process normalization
    d. Sleep deprivation
12. A person experiencing fluid retention, muscle weakness, vertigo, hypersensitivity, fatigue, weight gain, and breakdown in connective tissue most likely has ________.
    a. Hyperstimulation analgesia
    b. Long-term high blood levels of cortisol
    c. First-stage/alarm reaction
    d. Conservation withdrawal
13. A client becomes very relaxed in response to the music and the rhythm of the strokes used during the massage session. What has occurred?
    a. Mechanical effects
    b. Circulation decrease
    c. Entrainment
    d. Client education
14. Increased massage therapy research to manage the experience of persistent pain is related to________.
    a. Justification of massage for athletes
    b. Demand for nonpharmacological treatment of pain
    c. Validation for medical insurance payment
    d. Increases in disability claims for acute injury
15. The most common massage technique that involves the tendon reflex is ________.
    a. Myofascial release
    b. Contract/relax
    c. Acupuncture
    d. Counterirritation

16. The Arndt-Schulz law states that weak stimuli activate physiological processes; strong stimuli inhibit them. What are the implications for massage?
   a. Massage is a strong sensory stimulation.
   b. Techniques have to be intense to produce responses.
   c. It is difficult to figure out whether pain originates from a joint or surrounding tissue.
   d. To encourage a specific response, use gentler methods; to shut off the response, use deeper methods.
17. The law of facilitation states that when an impulse has passed through a certain set of neurons to the exclusion of others one time, it will tend to take the same course on a future occasion, and each time it travels this path, the resistance will be smaller. What are the implications for massage?
   a. If a sensory receptor is activated, it will respond in a certain way.
   b. Methods must override a sensation to produce a response.
   c. The body likes sameness; after a pattern has been established, less stimulation is required to activate the response.
   d. For a massage method to change a sensory perception, the intensity of the method must match and then exceed the existing sensation.
18. A biologically plausible approach to affecting arterial circulation during massage is _________.
   a. A 50-minute massage using gliding, but not heavy, pressure
   b. A 45-minute compressive massage against the arteries proximal to the heart and moving in a distal direction
   c. A 50-minute massage using short pumping gliding toward the heart
   d. A 30-minute massage emphasizing gliding strokes to passive/active joint movement distal to proximal
19. A researcher is conducting an experiment in which massage is introduced to determine whether endorphin levels change. What is the massage?
   a. The hypothesis
   b. The controlled variable
   c. The independent variable
   d. The dependent variable
20. When most experts agree and some research supports massage that primarily focuses on moderate pressure, slow strokes; broad-based compression; and rocking for exhaustion and stress the approach can be considered _______.
   a. Evidence based
   b. Quantitative
   c. Evidence informed
   d. Hypothetical

Write Your Own Questions

Write at least three multiple-choice questions. Make sure to develop plausible wrong answers and be sure that the correct answer is clearly correct. Then write a rationale for each question. The more questions you write, the better you will understand the material. Exchange questions with classmates or discuss in class. The questions from all the learners can be combined to create a review quiz.

CHAPTER 6

Indications and Contraindications for Therapeutic Massage

http://evolve.elsevier.com/Fritz/fundamentals/

CHAPTER OBJECTIVES

After completing this chapter, the student will be able to perform the following:

1. Explain well-being/palliative care, restorative care, condition management, and therapeutic change as therapeutic approaches.
2. Define *pathology* and explain the causes of disease.
3. Develop a basic understanding of pathology and use the knowledge to determine indications and contraindications for massage.
4. Identify contraindications to massage and develop massage adaptations to support any cautions identified.

CHAPTER OUTLINE

KEY TERMS

Acute
Antagonistic
Anxiety and depressive disorders
Benign tumors
Caution
Chronic
Communicable diseases
Compensation
Condition management
Contraindication
Dosage
Dysfunction
Endangerment site
General adaptation syndrome (GAS)
Health
Hemostasis
Homeostasis
Illness
Impingement syndromes
Indication
Inflammatory response
Injury
Malignant tumors
Medications
Metastasis
Neuromatrix theory of pain
Pain
Pain and fatigue syndromes
Pain–spasm–pain cycle
Palliative care
Pathology
Peak performance
Post-traumatic stress disorder (PTSD)
Referral
Referred pain
Restorative care
Signs
Stress-related illness
Suffering
Symptoms
Syndrome
Synergistic
Therapeutic change
Trauma
Well-being

Massage therapy has potential value for most people in most circumstances. Massage therapists have the responsibility of providing safe and beneficial care. Safety first is important when providing massage for clients. Being educated and using critical thinking helps you make good decisions about client care. Massage therapists need to practice with confidence and not fear. Developing confidence in decision making comes with the ability to identify, understand, and research individual client conditions; evaluate massage implications; and adapt massage care plans. The MedlinePlus website is an excellent resource for information to help make these decisions.

Massage professionals must be able to identify indications and contraindications for therapeutic massage. An **indication** is a condition for which an approach would be beneficial for health enhancement, treatment of a particular disorder, or support of a treatment modality other than massage. A **contraindication** is a condition for which an approach could be harmful. In Chapter 5, four main outcomes supported by evidence were described: relaxation, stress management, pain management, and support for functional mobility. Many individual pathologies, such as anxiety, depression, autoimmune disease, headaches, low back pain, and so forth, can be safely addressed through the four main outcomes, plus specific adaptation to an individual client based on the person's condition and treatment. Indications for massage are based on the massage's objective and subjective health-enhancing benefits. Some results of massage can be measured (objective), whereas others are assumed effective based on experience (subjective). The effects of massage are both physical and psychological. Physical effects are objective and can be measured physically through some type of observation or testing. Psychological effects are subjective perceptions that are reported by the client.

APPROACHES TO CARE

SECTION OBJECTIVES

Chapter objective covered in this section:

1. Define well-being/palliative care, restorative care, condition management, and therapeutic change as therapeutic approaches.

Using the information presented in this section, the learner will be able to perform the following:

- Explain the concepts of well-being/palliative care, restorative care, condition management, and therapeutic change.
- Implement a clinical reasoning process to determine the type of care most beneficial for the client.

The care/treatment plan is how the massage is designed: well-being/palliative approach, restorative approach, condition management, and therapeutic change. This section explains each of these approaches.

Well-Being/Palliative Care

Well-being encompasses the broader holistic dimensions of a well-lived life. Wellness is an essential element of overall well-being. Wellness is a state of complete physical, mental, and social well-being. To palliate is to soothe or to relieve. This approach to care may be the most valuable aspect of massage therapy. Regardless of outcomes and client care plans, soothing, compassionate, nurturing massage application is vital. Massage can be soothing and can provide comfort, whether the client seeks relaxation to meet pleasure needs and support well-being, to cope with some type of chronic pain, or to make the transition from life to death.

In a medical care context, **palliative care** attempts to relieve or reduce the intensity of uncomfortable symptoms, but it does not try to produce a cure. Palliative care is provided when the client's condition is most likely going to worsen and degenerative processes will continue (e.g., terminal illness, dementia). It involves massage approaches that reduce suffering.

Because the term **suffering** is inherently subjective and multifaceted, completely understanding the client's experience often is difficult. Suffering can be defined as an overall impairment in quality of life. Many times suffering overshadows the client's ability to create or participate in meaningful experiences or to experience pleasure. Some say we may not have a choice whether to experience pain, be it physical, emotional, or spiritual, but we can choose to suffer or not. Often, pain management does not alleviate suffering, because dealing with only the physical aspects of pain does not consider that suffering can also be mental and spiritual. Fortunately, massage therapy clients do not need to be suffering to benefit from massage.

Palliative care focused on well-being is also appropriate when the condition should not be changed, or when the person does not desire a specific outcome other than pleasure and relaxation. Providing massage to a pregnant person during labor, delivering a massage to someone who is on vacation, supporting an athlete during training for an event, providing massage at a public event such as a health fair, giving a massage to someone just before surgery, and providing massage to a wedding party the day before the event are all examples of the appropriate use of well-being/palliative care. Massage frequency is variable. Some clients may benefit from this type of massage session multiple times a week, whereas others may have a massage once a month. The pleasure and nurturing of the massage experience is the goal. Massage approaches are effective for well-being/palliative care as a health-enhancing approach. There is little need for in-depth assessment and corrective intervention. The pleasurable experience of touch and human connection, when presented through massage, may be one of the greatest therapeutic gifts our profession offers.

Restorative Care

A **restorative care** approach to massage supports normal rest and restorative function. It helps restore the body to a state of calm and allows it to relax and repair. Daily living, work and recreational activities, and maintenance of homeostasis require energy. It is necessary to regularly replenish resources with health-promoting behaviors, nutritious food, and restorative sleep. The parasympathetic autonomic nervous system (ANS) response is responsible for maintaining the "rest and digest" homeostasis. Massage supports parasympathetic and enteric ANS function. With a restorative approach, the client is generally healthy and has adaptive capacity. A restorative care plan functions from the premise that capacity to adapt exists for a return to the current functional state after demand. This care approach can be considered preventive and part of health maintenance. Regular massage sessions are needed to best benefit from a restorative approach to care. An ongoing weekly or biweekly appointment schedule is recommended. Regular functional assessment monitors that indicate reduced adaptive capacity and minimal interventions are used to restore function.

Restoring differs from rehabilitating. Rehabilitation implies pathology or functional deficit and a process to return to a level of function. Rehabilitation is an aspect of the therapeutic change approach. A condition management approach to care relates to a reduced adaptable capacity and compensation involved with some sort of underlying strain on function that cannot be easily reversed or improved.

A restorative approach should be the main reason people seek massage therapy. Unfortunately, it is not at this time. Many people do not understand the importance of restorative/preventive care. Individuals are more motivated to seek massage when feeling distress or discomfort and can justify the expense and time if massage is focused on issues such as condition management. Hopefully, this will change in the future.

Condition Management

Condition management is beneficial when a client is dealing with a chronic health condition or a set of life circumstances that creates chronic stress, such as caring for an ailing parent or child, having a stressful work environment, dealing with strain in a relationship, or having ongoing financial strain. Condition management also is beneficial when changing a situation is not a viable possibility (e.g., amputation, diabetes, job-related repetitive strain) or when the time frame for changing a situation needs to be postponed (e.g., pregnancy, chemotherapy, graduation from school, end of season for an athlete).

On a physical level, massage can offer benefits by managing the existing physical compensation patterns and sometimes by slowing the progression of chronic conditions or preventing a situation from becoming worse. On an emotional level, massage can assist in the management of physical stress symptoms, allowing the person to cope better with life stresses that cannot be altered.

Massage needs to be provided on a regular basis (twice weekly, weekly, biweekly indefinitely) when condition management is the approach to care. Massage benefit can have a cumulative effect, and combined effect, such as when regular massage supports sleep or exercise.

Condition management accounts for the largest client base for therapeutic massage. It has the most evidence supporting benefits. Many people find themselves in undesirable or unchanging circumstances and search for ways to cope with, but not necessarily change, the existing conditions while remaining productive. Most of us can relate to the importance of being able to remain resourceful and responsive to life events. Although the ideal is to make changes when life is not as we would like it to be, we all know that sometimes this is not possible for many reasons. Therapeutic massage offers support, acceptance, compassion, and a short-term respite.

Therapeutic Change

Therapeutic change is a beneficial alteration in the client's physical or mental state that results from a therapeutic massage process. Any change process, including beneficial change, requires energy and resource expenditure on the part of the client. The decision whether to implement a therapeutic change process requires assessment of the client's ability to expend the energy required for active change (adaptive capacity) and the availability of the support and resources often necessary during a change process. A therapeutic change approach carries the expectation of a long-term effect.

To facilitate a change process, the practitioner must have the appropriate knowledge and skills (current or acquired) and often a network of support from other professionals. The client must have the motivation and resources (e.g., information, money, time, social support, and coping mechanisms) to complete a change process. Careful assessment helps identify whether a change process holds a likely chance for success. Often massage frequency is increased during a therapeutic change approach to care. For example, the client may need to receive a massage multiple times a week for a 3-month period. A treatment plan for therapeutic change has defined ending points. For example, a client is receiving massage to improve shoulder movement. The plan is massage three times a week for 45 minutes for 10 weeks. If resources are insufficient or nonexistent or if the existing situation supports some sort of coping mechanism or allows for some sort of benefit (secondary gain) for the client, the person may not be motivated to commit to the change process.

If the conditions are not suitable for active change, other interventions can be developed. Many clients lead complex lives, and although change often is indicated, it may not be realistically possible at a particular time or under a current set of circumstances. When the likelihood of a successful change outcome is not good, condition management and palliative care can be offered instead. These approaches can increase well-being, reduce suffering, and allow clients to be more effective at addressing life's demands in their current set of circumstances.

An example of therapeutic change would be addressing scar tissue texture. Methodically using methods that introduce therapeutic inflammation and encourage increased pliability in the client's tissue may be helpful (Ault et al., 2018). However, the methods used to produce these changes can be uncomfortable and require frequent massage sessions over an extended period. In addition, the results of massage therapy targeting scar tissue are likely temporary, and ongoing care would be needed for the client to experience ongoing benefit (Nedelec et al., 2019; Lin et al., 2022). If the client is unable to commit to this type of intervention, it may be better to approach the situation in a more conservative manner, such as condition management or well-being/palliative care. Although massage therapy as a part of a therapeutic change treatment plan has value, this not the primary care approach for massage therapy. Seldom does massage function as the primary intervention when the client's conditions require intensive intervention to reverse a health issue. It is more likely that massage would be used as supportive care in conjunction with other more prescriptive medical treatment.

Determining the Massage Dosage

Part of determining the approach to care is treatment/care plan development (Chapter 4). Dosage includes duration of session and when/how often to achieve benefits. Dosage studies and recommendations for massage therapy are limited but there is some evidence to guide decision making (Rapaport et al., 2012; Juberg et al., 2015; Romanowski et al., 2017; Tick et al., 2018; Genik et al., 2020). Based on the available information, the following dosage recommendations are:

- Well-being/palliative: As needed, 15- to 60-minute sessions
- Restorative: Weekly, 60-minute sessions, ongoing
- Condition management: Twice a week or weekly, 60-minute sessions, ongoing
- Therapeutic change: Daily, twice a week or weekly, 15- to 60-minute sessions, 12 weeks

Progression of Care

Client goals change. Condition management care plans may advance with the gradual restoration of energy to a restorative care plan. Eventually a therapeutic change process ends or transforms to condition management or restorative care. An ongoing health maintenance, quality-of-life care plan is a combination of well-being/palliative, restorative, and condition management approaches (Proficiency Exercise 6.1).

Developing and Adapting a Massage Therapy Care/Treatment Plan

Chapter 1 presented information about professional touch. Chapter 2 described professional behavior and introduced the clinical reasoning process. Chapter 4 presented clinical reasoning as a process for intake procedures, which include a

PROFICIENCY EXERCISE 6.1

LEARNER'S NOTE: These problem-solving activities can seem overwhelming. However, it is important to understand them, and the only way to learn is to practice. Whenever you encounter these exercises in the book, attempt to do them. Do not worry about whether or not you are correct; just practice the process.

After reading the following client case situations, decide whether you would introduce therapeutic change, condition management, restorative care, or well-being/palliative care. Explain your reasons for the decision using the clinical reasoning model. An example of a massage therapist thinking through a case study is provided. Only the result of the process would actually be communicated to the client. Read the example case study; then, for case study write down your answers to the questions on a separate piece of paper.

Example Case Study

A male client, age 47, is experiencing fatigue and neck and shoulder pain. He is a cross-country truck driver, married, has three children, and has the normal financial obligations of a house payment, car payment, and other responsibilities. One child just started college, and the client is somewhat concerned about the tuition expenses. He likes his job and is content with his family and social life. He cannot seem to understand why he is tired or why his shoulder hurts. He can think of no reason for the pain other than the strain of the driving position and the long work hours. This pain never bothered him before. He went to the doctor for a physical examination, and nothing out of the ordinary was identified. The physician thinks that an old football injury involving his shoulder, coupled with some age-related changes, is responsible. The doctor also thinks that the pain in the shoulder might be interfering with the client's sleep and might be a cause of fatigue. The doctor recommends an over-the-counter antiinflammatory agent and painkiller, such as naproxen sodium, and suggests that massage might help. The doctor also recommends that the client cut back on his work hours and relax more. Naproxen sodium helps the shoulder pain but upsets the client's stomach. He does not want to cut back on work hours. He is seeking help for shoulder pain and would like more physical energy.

Identify the facts.

Questions that can help with this process include the following:

- What is considered normal or balanced function?
- *Answer:* The ability to work pain-free with reasonable stamina at a job one enjoys.
- What has happened? (Spell out events.)
- *Answer:* Nothing substantial has occurred to account for the changes other than age-related influences and a previous football injury.
- What caused the imbalance? (Can it be identified?)
- *Answer:* A previous injury, long work hours, a static seated position with the arms elevated on the steering wheel, and repetitive looking to the left during driving.
- What was done or is being done?
- *Answer:* Treatment with Naproxen sodium.
- What has worked or not worked?
- *Answer:* Naproxen sodium has benefits but upsets the client's stomach. The client has chosen to maintain his current work schedule.

Brainstorm the possibilities

Questions that help with this process include the following:

- What are the possibilities? (What could it all mean?)
- *Answer:*
  - The fatigue and pain could be a result of age-related changes and the previous injury, coupled with repetitive use; this in turn could interfere with sleep, as suggested by the doctor.
  - The condition could be related more to emotional stress caused by financial concerns.
  - The client may have an undiagnosed health condition that is not sufficiently evident to allow a definitive diagnosis.
  - What is my intuition suggesting?
- *Answer:* I think we likely are dealing with a combination of the doctor's diagnosis and unexpressed emotional stress over financial concerns, particularly the tuition costs for the child in college.
- What are the possible patterns of dysfunction?
- *Answer:* The static driving position may be aggravating the old football injury.
- What are the possible contributing factors?
- *Answer:* Worry, postural distortion from the static position, and age-related tissue changes, because the body becomes somewhat less flexible with age and lack of exercise.
- What are possible interventions?
- *Answer:* A job change, a stretching program, massage therapy, short-term mental health support, treatment with a different medication that does not upset the client's stomach.
- What might work?
- *Answer:* Massage and a stretching program.
- What are other ways to look at the situation?
- *Answer:* The client does not seem to want to use medications, does not want to change his job, and does not seem to think that there is anything wrong with his emotional or social life. Maybe if the financial situation were different, the stress load would be low enough so that his energy levels would increase and he could ignore the pain.
- What do the data suggest?
- *Answer:* Emotional stress seems to be a factor. The data seem to suggest that an age-related process and a previous injury are aggravated by repetitive job strain and a static seated position.

Consider the logical outcomes of each possibility.

Questions that can help determine outcomes include the following:

- What is the logical progression of the symptom pattern, contributing factors, and current behaviors?
- *Answer:* If the pain remains or worsens and sleep continues to be interrupted so that fatigue worsens, the immune system could be compromised, and other disease processes might develop. The client eventually may be unable to work. His mood would be altered, which would affect family and social relationships.
- What are the pros and cons and the logical effect of each intervention suggested?
- *Answer:*
  - Job change: would remove repetitive strain on the shoulder and eliminate static seated position, resulting

PROFICIENCY EXERCISE 6.1—cont'd

in drastic changes in lifestyle, finances, and work environment.

- Stretching program—would increase flexibility and counterbalance the static seated position; could make the situation worse if the stretching is too aggressive, not progressive, and intermittent instead of used daily; program is self-initiated and once learned would not incur any ongoing costs; does not require a regular appointment schedule (helpful because client is frequently on the road); requires discipline to do the stretches.
- Massage therapy: would help alleviate pain symptoms and support better sleep; does not require extensive self-discipline other than making regular appointments; would create a financial obligation; would support a daily stretching program; would reduce the use of medication.
- Short-term mental health support: would not require extensive self-discipline other than making regular appointments; would create a financial obligation; does not address the physical condition but does address emotional strain.
- Requesting that the physician consider treatment with a medication that does not upset the client's stomach: would help alleviate pain symptoms and support better sleep; does not require extensive self-discipline; would create a small financial obligation; does not need a regular appointment schedule (helpful because client frequently is on the road); possible side effects and development of dependency on the medication.

- What are the consequences of not acting?
- *Answer:* The situation could stabilize and resolve itself, or the condition could become more problematic, requiring more drastic intervention measures in the future.
- What are the consequences of acting?
- *Answer:* The problem would remain stable or improve. The client would be better able to cope with the current situation.

Identify the effect of each possibility on the people involved.

Questions that can help identify possible effects include the following:

- For each intervention considered, what would be the impact on the people involved: client, practitioner, and other professionals working with the client?
- *Answer:*
  - Job change: Client is not supportive; wife may or may not like idea.
  - Stretching program: Client does not like to fuss with himself and avoids activities having to do with self-care.
  - Massage therapy: Client is open to idea but nervous; wife, doctor, and massage practitioner are supportive.
  - Short-term mental health support: Client and wife are not open to this possibility at this time; they do not think that this is an emotional problem. Massage practitioner is hesitant about the client being unwilling to seek mental health services and does think emotion is involved (worry over finances) and would like client to remain open to this possibility.
  - Treatment with a medication that does not upset the client's stomach: Client does not like to take medication, and the doctor is unwilling to prescribe at this time until other measures have been explored.
- How does each person involved feel about the possible interventions?
- *Answer:*
  - Job change: None are supportive.
  - Stretching program: Client is ambivalent; massage practitioner and wife are supportive.
  - Massage therapy: All are supportive.
  - Short-term mental health support: Massage therapist is supportive; client and wife are not supportive.
  - Treatment with a medication that does not upset the client's stomach: Doctor and client are not supportive.
- Is the practitioner within their scope of practice to work with such situations?
- *Answer*: Yes.
- Is the practitioner qualified to work with such situations?
- *Answer*: Yes.
- Does the *practitioner* feel qualified to work with such situations?
- *Answer:* The *practitioner* is concerned about the client's ambivalence about a stretching program and his lack of interest in a mental health referral. These concerns raise questions for the practitioner about the ability to work effectively with the client's physical problems when other causal factors may exist.
- Does a feeling of *cooperation* and agreement exist among all parties involved?
- *Answer:* A degree of cooperation exists, as does some resistance. All agree on the benefit of massage therapy.

Result of the process.

Based on this analysis of the information provided, the massage practitioner would recommend a condition management program rather than a therapeutic change process, for the following reasons:

- Causal factors are involved that the client may not be able to address during a change process.
- The client is *resistant* to the idea of an exercise or a stretching program that would interfere with his driving schedule.

Your Turn

Case Study

The client is an 81-year-old female who is in good health for her age. Her lifelong partner died 18 months ago after a prolonged illness. She is active in the local food pantry and works in her garden. She fell 6 months ago but recovered nicely. Lately age-related aches and pains are bothering her more, especially in her knees. This is interfering with her activities. She has mild hypertension, for which she is taking medication. Currently the hypertension is under control. She takes aspirin for arthritis as needed. No problems were detected during her last physical. What are the indications for massage?

1. Identify the facts.
2. Brainstorm the possibilities.
3. Consider the logical outcomes of each possibility.
4. Identify the effect of each possibility on the people involved.
5. Result of the process.

Based on this analysis of the information provided, the massage practitioner would recommend __________ for the following reasons:

client history, physical assessment, documentation, and methods to develop this information into a care or treatment plan. Chapter 5 described the importance of research and compared the scientific method to the process of clinical reasoning and logical thinking. In this chapter, the clinical reasoning model provides a decision-making process for analyzing whether therapeutic changes or methods to maintain or support an existing state are the best approach.

The ability to analyze data collected during assessment procedures is crucial for making informed decisions about the following:

- Which massage therapy goals to pursue: relaxation, stress management, pain management, support for functional mobility
- How to gather assessment information as part of the general, nonspecific massage
- What specific intervention to use in addition to the general, nonspecific massage
- Whether the approach to care is based on a therapeutic change process, condition management, restorative care, or well-being/palliative care

The massage therapist considers these factors to develop a plan that best serves the client based on the following elements.

Determine the goals and approaches of the plan:

- Four main outcomes for massage
  - Relaxation
  - Stress management
  - Pain management
  - Functional mobility
- Four main approaches to care
  - Well-being/palliative
  - Restorative
  - Condition management
  - Therapeutic change

Determine the massage application based on outcomes and approaches to care

- Two actions that generate mechanical force
  - Pushing
  - Pulling
- Nine primary massage methods used to create mechanical force
  - Static methods/holding
  - Compression
  - Gliding
  - Torsion/twisting (kneading)
  - Shearing
  - Elongation
  - Oscillation
  - Percussion
  - Movement
- Twelve modifiers for adapting methods
  - Pressure
  - Point of application (location and breadth of contact)
  - Magnitude (intensity)
  - Direction
  - Drag
  - Speed
  - Pacing
  - Rhythm
  - Sequencing and transitioning
  - Frequency
  - Duration
  - Intention for outcome
- Five stresses to which the physiology must adapt, created by adaptive methods that produce appropriate force to load the body tissue and generate these stresses
  - Compression stress
  - Tension stress
  - Shear stress
  - Torsion stress
  - Bending stress

How these elements are organized provides the specifics of a care plan.

Examples

A client is seeking massage therapy for general health maintenance. They occasionally experience low back stiffness.

Outcomes: Relaxation, functional mobility

Approach: Well-being, restorative, condition management

Massage Application Based on Outcomes and Approaches to Care: Mechanical force delivery creating multiple stress loads using all 9 massage methods adapted as needed using the 12 modifiers.

Dosage: Weekly, 60-minute session

A new massage client is visiting family and seeking a massage therapist for occasional massage when in the area. The client is older and somewhat frail.

Outcomes: Relaxation

Approach: Well-being/palliative

Massage Application Based on Outcomes and Approaches to Care: Mechanical force delivery creating low level compression and tension stress loads using static methods/holding, compression, gliding, torsion/twisting (kneading) adapted to modify pressure, point of application (location and breadth of contact) and magnitude (intensity) based on client adaptive capacity, especially related to pressure and drag.

Dosage: 60-minute session as needed.

PATHOLOGY

SECTION OBJECTIVES

Chapter objective covered in this section:

2. Define *pathology* and explain the causes of disease.

Using the information presented in this section, the learner will be able to perform the following:

- Define the terms health, dysfunction, and pathology.
- Explain the disease process, including risk factors for the development of pathological conditions.
- Recognize a client condition that should be evaluated by a primary medical care provider.
- List the mechanisms and risk factors that predispose people to disease processes.
- Explain the stress response, inflammatory response, and pain response.
- Explain the mechanisms of pain and evaluate pain for referral purposes.
- Identify indications for massage therapy and justify those indications.

NOTE: SEE APPENDIX A–DISEASES/CONDITIONS AND INDICATIONS/CONTRAINDICATION FOR MASSAGE THERAPY.

Pathology is the study of disease. To practice safely, massage practitioners need a basic understanding of pathological processes. The body is designed for health. A sequence of events must occur for disease to develop. Trauma is an abrupt shock or injury to the body or psyche; like disease, trauma requires the body to heal.

The diagnosis of disorders is not a function of a massage professional. However, to refer clients appropriately to a medical care professional, the massage practitioner must be able to recognize when the client's condition represents an irregularity that should be evaluated by the person's primary medical/health care provider. When working with a referral and under proper supervision, the massage professional also uses clinical reasoning to adapt the application of massage if any disease process or trauma is present so that the client receives the benefits of massage without harm.

Massage therapists should have both a general awareness of the types of disorders that occur in each major body system and more specific knowledge of the signs and symptoms of selected disorders that could endanger the health of either the client or the practitioner (see Appendix A for specific contraindications to massage). The massage professional also needs a basic understanding of pharmacology and the possible interactions between medications and massage (see Appendix C for specific information on these interactions).

A massage therapist is not a physician or a mental health professional and is not expected to know the symptoms of all diseases; however, resources for locating specific information must be available. The massage practitioner also should have a current medical dictionary and comprehensive pathology reference available to research unfamiliar terms and pathological conditions. Internet search programs are helpful, especially MedlinePlus. Use the case studies in Chapter 16 as examples of how this process is conducted.

To understand disease, we first must understand the definition of health. Health is optimal functioning with freedom from disease or abnormal processes. Health is influenced by many factors, including inherited (genetic) and acquired conditions. Lifestyle, activity level, rest, loving relationships, exercise, a balanced diet, empowering beliefs and attitudes, self-esteem, authentic personality, and freedom from self-hindering patterns all support health. A healthy individual has the capacity to respond and adapt to daily life events, maintain mental clarity, and sustain function when ongoing stress occurs. When a state of health no longer exists or is interrupted, adaptive capacity diminishes, and dysfunction begins.

Dysfunction is the in-between state of "not healthy" but also "not sick" (i.e., experiencing disease). Unfortunately, many people experience dysfunctional states with reduced ability to respond and adapt to daily demands. Western medicine does not easily identify and deal with dysfunctions because these are prepathological states that often are not revealed by current diagnostic methods. An actual pathological condition usually needs to exist before medical tests and diagnostic methods can detect a disease state.

Prevention methods, many modeled after more "Eastern" or "holistic" approaches, are beginning to address the states of dysfunction. Many ancient healing methods are more focused on the process of dysfunction, introducing restorative methods before a system breaks down into a disease process. When used in the prepathological state of dysfunction, these methods of mind/body medicine, stress management, and prevention are effective. They are less effective when applied to an active pathological process, although they remain an important part of the total healing program. Often more targeted approaches are required to reverse the pathological condition and allow healing to begin.

Peak performance is defined as maximum conditioning and functioning in a particular action. Although most associated with athletes or entertainers such as dancers, peak performance also can occur in more mental actions, such as studying for school or dealing with a demanding workload or with family issues. Peak performance also can pertain to massage professionals who keep themselves in the best shape possible for performing treatments in their massage practices. Maximum use of body functions and resources becomes energy consuming and stressful to the body. During peak performance, the body does not hold back energy expenditure, and all available resources are used. If the person's lifestyle does not support recuperation time or if anatomical or physiological limits are exceeded, injury or depletion commonly occurs, and illness results (Goodman and Fuller, 2021).

Disease

Homeostasis is the relative constancy of the body's internal environment. If homeostasis is disturbed, as occurs in a disease process, a variety of feedback mechanisms usually attempt to return the body to normal. A disease condition exists when homeostasis cannot be restored easily. The ability to respond and adapt to daily demands is significantly limited. In acute conditions, the body recovers its homeostatic balance quickly. In chronic diseases, a normal state of balance may never be restored, and compensation develops with reduced adaptive capacity. Compensation is the process of counterbalancing a defect in body structure or function. Initially compensation is functional. However, within a reasonable time, compensation patterns should either reverse or stabilize resulting in a "new normal" function.

For example, a client has had a knee joint replacement. Prior to the surgery, the client modified (compensation) how they walked because of the joint discomfort. In the first couple of weeks after surgery, the area around the knee was stiff and the surgical site tender (also normal compensation). The knee joint pain was gone. The client began to move more normally (reversing compensation). Over time the client's walking improved but the client remained cautious of falling and learned to tolerate a bit of stiffness in the knee supporting stability (new normal).

A pathological condition is seldom caused by one thing; rather, a series of events usually occurs. For example, the flu is caused by the influenza virus, but not everyone exposed to the virus gets the flu. Suppose that one person gets the flu, and another does not. The person who has the flu smokes, had a minor car accident 2 weeks ago, is experiencing a short-term financial setback, and got into an argument with a coworker 3 days before the onset of the flu. The person who does not have the flu has not experienced anything out of the ordinary for the past 3 months, exercises moderately, and follows a fairly supportive dietary plan with lots of fruits and vegetables; stress and lifestyle habits are therefore contributing factors in the breakdown of the body's healing mechanisms.

Functioning Limits

The body has anatomical and physiological functioning limits. The heart can beat only so fast, the endocrine glands can secrete only a maximum amount of hormones, and the skeletal muscles can lift only so much weight or jump so high. However, extraordinary events push the body's limits of functioning. Athletes and new parents, for example, often function at maximum body limits or peak performance.

Under normal conditions the body functions within a margin of safety. Normal physiological mechanisms inhibit the tendency to function at the body's limits. We usually do not run as fast as we can, work as long as we could, or exert all of our energy to complete a task. Instead, the body signals fatigue, pain, or strain before the anatomical or physiological limits are reached, and we back off. This important protective mechanism allows us to live within a healthy range of energy expenditure while keeping reserves in place in case of an emergency or extraordinary demand (Fig. 6.1). Each time we tap into this reserve, the body tends to work to restore what was used and, if possible, to add a little more to the reserve.

Dysfunction occurs when the reserve runs low because restorative mechanisms are unable to function effectively or when the body begins to limit function in an attempt to maintain higher energy reserves.

Massage professionals serve many people at the beginning of dysfunctional patterns (when the client does not feel their best but is not yet sick). Monitoring clients to make sure the dysfunctional patterns do not progress is important. Early intervention and referral to appropriate health care professionals are important for identifying potential problems; this gives clients the opportunity to act appropriately to prevent these problems from developing.

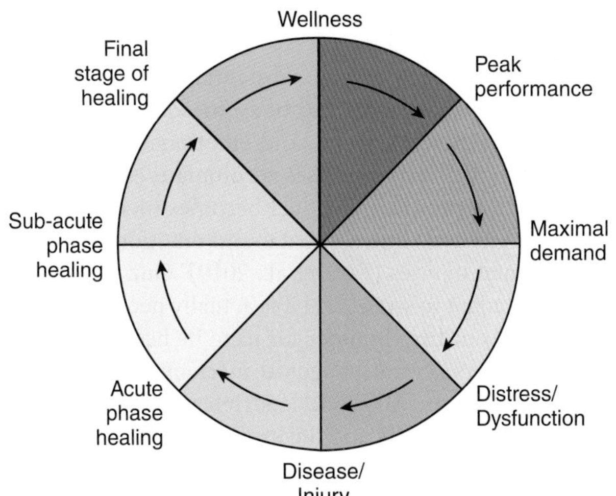

FIG. 6.1 The health–wellness–injury–illness continuum.

Massage also can support the restorative process to help maintain peak performance for short periods of time. No one can maintain peak performance for long periods. Attempts to do so will eventually result in physical and emotion strain and breakdown. The benefits of massage are most effectively focused on helping people stay within healthy ranges of functioning.

Development of Pathological Conditions

As mentioned previously, homeostasis is the relative constancy of the body's internal environment. Therapeutic massage has widespread effects on the physiological functions of the body. Therefore the massage professional must learn about pathological conditions, contraindications, and endangerment sites.

Communicable diseases can be transmitted from one person to another. The study of communicable diseases is an important process for the massage professional (see Chapter 7), and a variety of safely and sanitation procedures are required. Obtaining a consensus on such information is difficult, however, because all sources do not agree on all points. This textbook provides recommendations based on clinical experience, expert opinion, and research-based evidence targeted to entry-level practice. The client's safety is the primary concern; therefore these recommendations are conservative because entry-level practitioners have minimal experience. As you gain experience and learn more in professional practice, it is likely that you will be able to provide massage therapy for more complex client conditions. This does not mean that the massage application becomes more complex and specific. Actually, the more complex the client, the more basic the massage approach. Recall from Chapter 5 that the foundation of massage therapy benefits is the full body, nonspecific, general, moderate pressure, pleasurable massage that lasts about an hour and is provided about once a week.

Illness and Injury

There are two general pathology classifications: illness and injury. Therapeutic massage is indicated for both illness and injury. Inflammation is a factor in both illness and injury because healing for both involves appropriate activation of the inflammatory response system. Healing an illness or injury is taxing on the body and strains its restorative abilities. If an ill or injured person is not in a state of health to begin with, the stress of the illness or injury frequently compromises the immune system, and the person becomes susceptible to more serious illness and has an increased potential for injury.

Illness

Illness occurs when a body's protective and restorative processes break down. A person whose immune system did not effectively fight off a cold virus becomes ill with a cold. Chronic fatigue syndrome, ulcers, cancer, diabetes, and multiple sclerosis are all examples of illnesses. Illness tends to indicate general cautions and contraindications targeted to support recovery and restore adaptive capacity. Especially during acute illness, body resources are used for healing, and other forms of demand to adapt, including massage, may not be beneficial. Certainly, in these situations, the goal of massage is relaxation, and the approach to care is palliative. Massage approaches for illness involve a very general application of massage to support the body's healing responses (e.g., relaxation, stress management, pain management, restorative sleep). This approach to massage, sometimes called a *general constitutional application,* is used to reduce the stress load so that the body can heal. Remember, the massage approach is a general, nonspecific massage using moderate, pleasurable pressure for about 45–60 minutes and adapted to any specific cautions for the client, such as the need for an alternate position for comfort.

Injury

Injury occurs when tissue is damaged. Cuts, bruises, burns, contusions, fractured bones, sprains, and strains are examples of injuries. Injury more often creates regional cautions and contraindications. Typically the injured area is avoided, and the massage is adapted so that the healing tissues are not disturbed. Massage for injury incorporates aspects of general massage because healing is necessary for tissue repair. In addition, interstitial and lymphatic fluid movement focus can be used to control edema. Gliding methods are used to approximate (bring close together) the ends of some types of tissue injuries, such as minor muscle tears and strains. Hyperstimulation analgesia and counterirritation reduce acute pain (see Chapter 5). Methods to increase circulation to the area support tissue formation. Connective tissue applications are used to manage scar tissue formation.

Signs and Symptoms

Disease or injury conditions usually are diagnosed or identified by signs and symptoms. **Signs** are objective abnormalities that can be seen or measured by someone other than the patient. **Symptoms** are the subjective abnormalities felt only by the patient. A **syndrome** is a group of different signs and symptoms, usually arising from a common cause. A disease is classified as acute when signs and symptoms develop quickly, last a short time, and then disappear. Diseases that develop slowly and last for a long time (sometimes for life) are classified as chronic. Because many diseases and injuries have similar symptoms, determining the specific underlying causes of a pathology can be difficult. The massage professional must refer clients to qualified, licensed health care providers for a specific diagnosis.

Risk Factors

Certain predisposing conditions may make the development of a disease or some types of injury more likely. Usually called *risk factors,* these conditions may put an individual at risk for developing a disease, but they do not actually cause the disease. Based on information from Chapter 5, evidence suggests that massage therapy may modulate risk factors decreasing potential for disease development. Examples of risk factors include genetic factors, age, lifestyle, environmental factors, preexisting conditions, and stress.

Genetic Factors

Several types of genetic risk factors can play a role in illness. An inherited trait may put a person at a greater than normal risk for developing a specific disease. For example, a genetic link has been established to a specific form of breast cancer. A family history of disease processes and causes of death usually can reveal possible genetic traits. Steps can be taken to support the body against the genetic tendency for a disease process. Careful monitoring by the physician allows early detection and treatment. In addition, the individual can make beneficial changes in diet and lifestyle to reduce risk.

Age

Biological and behavioral factors increase the risk of developing certain diseases or injuries at certain ages. For example, musculoskeletal problems are common between the ages of 30 and 50.

Lifestyle

The way we live, work, and play can put us at risk for some diseases or injuries. Some researchers believe that the high-fat, low-fiber diet common among people in developed nations increases their risk of developing certain types of cancer and cardiovascular diseases. Smoking cigarettes, drinking excessive alcohol, and not getting enough exercise are all lifestyle risks. Some athletes face an increased risk; playing hockey, for example, predisposes one to bruises, sprains, and broken bones. Chapter 15 explores a healthy lifestyle.

Environmental Factors

Some environmental conditions put people at greater risk of contracting certain diseases. For example living in an area with high concentrations of air pollution may increase a person's risk of developing respiratory problems. Snow and ice predispose people to injury from falls.

Preexisting Conditions

A primary (preexisting) condition can put a person at risk of developing a secondary condition. For example, a viral infection can compromise the immune system, making the person more susceptible to bacterial infection.

Stress

Stress can be defined as any substantial change in routine or any activity that forces the body to adapt. Stress places demands on physical, mental, and emotional resources. Research has shown that as stresses accumulate, especially if the stress is long term, the individual becomes increasingly susceptible to physical illness, mental and emotional problems, and accidental injuries (Fava et al., 2019). Our physiology is designed to adapt to stress, and it is actually necessary to have challenges in our lives in order for us to be healthy. Exposure to stress triggers several biological mechanisms in the body known as allostasis. Allostatic load refers to the cumulative burden of chronic stress and life events. When challenges exceed the ability to cope, then allostatic overload occurs. Allostatic load and overload are associated with poorer health outcomes (Guidi et al., 2021; Lenart-Bugla et al., 2022). This type of stress is a factor in stress-related pathology. Stress has been cited as an indirect cause or an important risk factor for many conditions. Stress and stress management are important topics and will be discussed more later in the chapter.

COMMON PATHOLOGICAL CONDITIONS AND INDICATIONS FOR MASSAGE

SECTION OBJECTIVES

Chapter objective covered in this section:

3. Develop a basic understanding of pathology and use the knowledge to determine the indications and contraindications for massage.

Using the information presented in this section, the learner will be able to perform the following:

- Define stress and explain the three stages of the stress response.
- Describe the relationship between resilience and stress management.
- Justify massage therapy as a stress management intervention.
- Describe the inflammatory response.
- Explain adaptation of massage application during the three healing stages.
- Explain the mechanisms of pain and evaluate pain for referral purposes.
- Define acute and chronic/persistent pain.
- Define and provide examples of nociceptive, neuropathic, neuroplastic, and mixed pain.
- Describe five common pain sensations.
- Identify viscerally referred pain patterns.
- List common types of cancer-related pain.
- List factors that influence pain threshold and tolerance.
- List various pain management strategies.
- Justify massage therapy as a pain management strategy.
- Identify and justify indications for massage therapy regarding impingement syndromes and psychological dysfunctions.

Massage has been shown to be beneficial for managing the stress response and psychological manifestations related to stress, chronic inflammation, pain management, and impingement syndromes. It is especially effective for anxiety disorders related to the autonomic nervous system (ANS) that manifest with physical symptoms (called *somatization*). Inflammation and pain are signs and symptoms of many pathological conditions. A common source of soft tissue pain is impingement syndrome, in which nerves are compressed, causing pain to radiate. A common response to pain is an increase in anxiety. The indications for massage often are based on the beneficial effects of massage that target the body's ability to soothe anxiety, resolve inflammation, manage pain, and reduce pressure on nerves. Chapter 5 provided research support for massage therapy as an evidence informed intervention for stress and pain management.

What Is Stress? General Adaptation Syndrome

Dr. Hans Selye, a pioneer in stress research, labeled the body's response to stress the **general adaptation syndrome (GAS)**. The GAS describes the way the body mobilizes different defense mechanisms when threatened by harmful stimuli (actual or perceived). In generalized stress conditions, the hypothalamus acts on the anterior pituitary gland to cause the release of adrenocorticotropic hormone (ACTH), which stimulates the adrenal cortex to secrete glucocorticoid. In addition, the sympathetic division of the autonomic nervous system (ANS) is stimulated by the adrenal medulla, resulting in the release of epinephrine and norepinephrine to assist the body in responding to the stressful stimulus. Unfortunately, during periods of prolonged stress, glucocorticosteroids (cortisol) may have harmful side effects, including a diminished immune response, altered blood glucose levels, altered protein and fat metabolism, and decreased resistance to stress.

Oxidative stress occurs when there is an imbalance between the production of free radicals and the body's ability to counteract their damaging effects through neutralization with antioxidants. Inflammation triggered by oxidative stress causes many chronic diseases. Oxidative damage is harm sustained by cells and tissues unable to keep up with free radical production.

Considering the variety and number of organs and glands innervated by the ANS, it is no wonder that autonomic disorders have varied and broad consequences. This is especially true of stress-induced diseases. A prolonged or excessive physiological response to stress, the fight-or-flight response, can disrupt normal functioning throughout the body.

The autonomic nervous system is responsible for monitoring, regulating, and coordinating almost all systems of the body including temperature, pH, oxygen levels, volume of blood, blood pressure, intake of food, digestion and absorption of food and water, and excretion of waste products. The response of the autonomic nervous system to a stressor is the fight–flight–freeze response. Whenever we perceive we are physically or psychologically threatened, an inbuilt reflex alarm system in our brain triggers the release of electrical impulses and a variety of hormones. The alarm reaction is designed for short-term use to deal with physical threats in which the emergency resolves quickly, in a few seconds or minutes. Many of the stressors today are psychological in origin, and they are chronic, lasting days, weeks, months, and even years in some cases.

Modern stressful events (such as job security, financial problems, health worries, difficult neighbors, relationship problems, etc.) cannot be resolved by fighting or running away. Regardless, these psychological stressors still trigger the fight–flight–freeze response. This is then complicated by the fact that we do not get enough physical exercise. Exercise can help counter the stress response by reducing blood clotting, boosting immune function, reducing blood pressure, relaxing muscles, increasing metabolism (which burns up stress hormones), and making the sympathetic nervous system (which triggers the stress response) less sensitive.

Simply, there are two functions and parts of the autonomic nervous system:

1. The sympathetic nervous system triggers the biochemical and physiological changes brought about by the fight–flight–freeze response. Think of it as the accelerator on a car.
2. The parasympathetic nervous system reverses the fight–flight–freeze response and returns all hormones, organs, and systems back to pre-stress levels. Think of it as the brake on a car.

There are three stages of the fight–flight–freeze response. This response exists to keep people safe, preparing them to face, escape, or hide from danger and involves a number of physiological changes that help someone prepare to:

- Fight: take action to eliminate the danger
- Flee: escape the danger
- Freeze: become immobile

The freeze response involves a different physiological process than fight or flight. While the person who is "frozen" is extremely alert, they are also unable to move or act against the danger. Consider the car example again. Freeze can be pushing on the accelerator and the brake at the same time.

The brain cannot distinguish between a real or potential threat. It does not matter if you are really chasing someone who threatened you or if you are playing a video game where you are chasing someone who is a threat. The brain responds to both by triggering the fight–flight–freeze response. Stress is not simply a case of cause and effect. Numerous factors influence whether the fight–flight–freeze response is triggered, how long it remains switched on, and the degree to which it has a negative effect on us. Factors that influence the fight–flight–freeze response, some of which we can influence to reduce our stress, include the following:

- Perception of the event
- Social support
- Beliefs
- Diet
- Cumulative stressors
- Degree of control over stressor
- Unpredictability of the stress
- Duration of the stressor

Some manifestations of arousal of the sympathetic nervous system are dilation of the pupils, increased heart rate and blood pressure, increased respiratory rate, dry mouth, and sweating hands. Gastrointestinal tract activity is diminished. Muscles tense, particularly in the neck, shoulders, and torso. Prolonged tension causes responses such as neck stiffness, backache, headache, and teeth clenching. Also, stress inhibits the production of thyroid, reproductive, and growth hormones to conserve energy. Therapeutic massage is particularly helpful in managing this aspect of stress.

Perception of Stress

An individual's perception of stress is significant. Anything that is perceived as a threat—whether real or imagined—arouses fear or anxiety. How a person responds is influenced by other conditions; some are under conscious control, and some are not. Physical and mental health, hereditary predisposition and genetics, past experiences, current coping habits (learned and inborn), diet, environment, and social support all determine which stimuli are interpreted as stressors. Most stress management methods support the functions of the parasympathetic autonomic nervous system (rest and restore).

Persons who experience excessive or ongoing stress often say they feel overwhelmed by tension, anger, fear, and frustration and the resulting anxiety. This causes adrenaline levels to rise, blood pressure and heart rate to increase, and breathing to change. Stressed individuals often experience one or more of the following:

- Overbreathing often results in over-oxygenation of the blood, which reduces carbon dioxide levels and leads to breathing-pattern disorders. This is discussed in more detail in Chapter 15. This response can mark the beginning of panic attacks.
- Sleep disorders and depression commonly accompany long-term stress. A decrease in memory and the ability to concentrate and solve problems are also common, as are complaints of stomach pain, heart palpitation, fatigue, and muscle aches.
- Blood levels of glucose and fatty acids rise, and the combination eventually causes plaque to be laid down in the arteries, which causes the development of coronary artery disease.
- Immune function becomes less effective, and the body is less capable of dealing with pathogens and cancer cells. Susceptibility to infection increases.
- Water retention caused by certain hormones increases blood volume, which can cause high blood pressure.
- Mood and behavior are affected by stress as well. There is an ongoing interplay between physiological and psychological stress that is best described by the chicken-and-egg question, "Which came first?" Certainly, psychological stress can result in physiological response, and the physiological stress response alters perception, mood, thought processes, and behavior, thus creating psychological stress. Another consequence of chronic stress is stress-induced disease, although the exact cause-and-effect relationship is often unclear.

Adaptation

One of the remarkable effects of change, internal and external, is the body's ability to adapt. The body is better able to adapt if changes occur gradually. Sudden changes, along with a diminished physiological reserve, can have dramatically negative effects on the body.

Genetic makeup contributes to the effects of stress on the body. It is responsible for how well the organs adapt and respond to stressful situations. With age, the ability to adapt diminishes. Individuals who are fit mentally and physically are able to adapt to stress more easily than others. Those who are strongly motivated to live are well known to be capable of surviving the worst onslaughts made on their minds and bodies.

Restorative and optimal amounts of sleep are important for restoring energy, regenerating tissue, and coping with stress. Irregular cycles of sleep and wakefulness can reduce immunity and physical and psychological functioning. Proper nutrition protects us from detrimental effects of stress. Poor nutrition is itself a stress-causing agent.

Resilience

Resilience is the process of adapting well in the face of adversity, trauma, tragedy, threats, or significant sources of stress, such as family and relationship problems, serious health problems, or workplace and financial stressors. It means bouncing back from difficult experiences. Resilience involves maintaining flexibility and balance in your life as you deal with stressful circumstances and traumatic events. This happens in several ways, which people can develop in themselves. To develop resilience, you do the following:

- Identify productive ways to alter difficult situations and learn to control reactions to adversity even if unable to alter the situation. Discover ways to grow and learn by dealing with difficult situations.
- Develop realistic plans and steps to carry them out to deal with your problems and meet the demands of daily living, and step back to rest and reenergize yourself. Cultivate a positive view of yourself and confidence in your strengths and abilities, including skills in communication and problem solving.
- Allow yourself to experience strong emotions but have the capacity to manage strong feelings and impulses and realize when you may need to avoid experiencing them at times in order to continue functioning. Actively seek ways to replace the losses encountered in life.
- Rely on yourself and others. Spend time with loved ones to gain support and encouragement, while also nurturing yourself. Relationships that create love and trust provide role models and offer encouragement and reassurance to bolster resilience.
- Realize and nurture your physical, mental, and spiritual health, and pursue your sense of purpose and aspirations with persistence and patience while adapting to change.

Stress-Related Disorders

The primary cause of the stress may require a multidisciplinary approach for resolution or effective long-term management, and massage therapy can play a part. A person's perception of stressful events combined with the amount of stress, not the type of stress, determines the response. Anything that can change the perception of threat to a perception of safety or that can reduce the intensity of the physical stress response will promote mechanisms of good health. These supportive changes include allowing for effective sleep, reducing pain, and establishing a sense of affiliation that supports effective social contact and enhances the restorative and self-regulating processes of the body.

Usually, when people feel well physically, they also feel well mentally. The reverse, too, is often the case; feeling bad mentally results in physical dysfunctions. Neurochemicals such as serotonin and dopamine exert a strong influence on a person's mental state.

The major mental health dysfunctions that affect Western society are trauma and post-traumatic stress disorder, pain and fatigue syndromes, anxiety and depressive disorders, and stress-related illness.

Trauma

There is no universal definition of trauma. However, the Substance Abuse and Mental Health Services Administration describes **trauma** as resulting from: "an event, series of events, or set of circumstances experienced by an individual as physically or emotionally harmful or life-threatening with lasting adverse effects on the individual's functioning and mental, physical, social, emotional, or spiritual well-being." (Substance Abuse and Mental Health Services Administration-Health Resources and Services Administration Center for Integrated Health Solutions. "Trauma." Available at: http://www.integration.samhsa.gov/clinical-practice/trauma.)

Following are definitions of stress-based terms related to trauma:

Toxic Stress: Strong, frequent, and/or prolonged adversity that stimulates the body's natural protections against stress and can have a long-term negative impact on neurobiology, psychology, and physical health.

Allostatic Load: Wear-and-tear on the body from toxic stress that can lead to poor health and health risk behaviors.

Protective Factors: Social conditions or personal attributes that help lessen the risks of trauma for an individual, family, or community.

Post-traumatic stress disorder (PTSD), as described by the *Diagnostic and Statistical Manual of Mental Disorders (DSM-5-TR [2022])* is a trauma and stressor-related disorder. PTSD symptoms cluster into four factors: reexperiencing, avoidance, numbing, and hyperarousal. The person diagnosed with PTSD was exposed to death, threatened death, actual or threatened serious injury, or actual or threatened sexual violence. The traumatic event is persistently reexperienced, there is avoidance of trauma-related stimuli after the trauma, and the person experiences negative thoughts or feelings that began or worsened after the trauma. Certain triggers can bring back strong memories. Triggers can include sights, sounds, smells, or thoughts that remind of the traumatic event in some way. Triggers don't necessarily have to be accurate, just accurate enough for the brain to form a connection back to the trauma.

Those with PTSD may experience the following:

Irritability or aggression
Risky or destructive behavior
Hypervigilance
Heightened startle reaction
Difficulty concentrating
Difficulty sleeping

Symptoms last for more than 1 month and create distress or functional impairment. The symptoms are not due to medication, substance use, or other illness. PTSD is a serious multidimensional condition requiring a multidisciplinary treatment. Post-traumatic stress disorder can have long-term effects. Massage therapists should not attempt to manage PTSD symptoms without support from a dedicated care team. Referral is needed to determine appropriate care.

Pain and fatigue syndromes are defined as multicausal and often chronic nonproductive patterns that interfere with well-being, activities of daily living, and productivity. Some conditions currently included in this category are fibromyalgia, chronic fatigue syndrome, headache, arthritis, chronic cancer pain, neuropathy, low back syndrome, idiopathic pain, somatization disorder, and intractable pain syndrome. Acute pain can be a factor, as can acute "episodes" of chronic conditions.

Anxiety and depressive disorders are characterized by anxiety and depression. *Anxiety* is an uneasy feeling usually connected with increased sympathetic arousal responses. *Depression* is characterized by a decrease of vital functional activity and mood disturbances of exaggerated emptiness, hopelessness, and melancholy, or by unbridled periods of high energy with no purpose or outcome. Anxiety and depressive disorders commonly are seen with fatigue and pain syndromes. Panic behavior, phobias, and a sense of impending doom, along with the sense of being overwhelmed and hopeless, are common with these disorders. Mood swings, breathing pattern disorder, sleep disturbance, concentration difficulties, memory disturbances, outbursts of anger, fatigue, and changes in habits of daily living, appetite, and activity levels are symptoms of these disorders.

Stress-related illness is defined as an increased stress load or reduced ability to adapt that depletes the reserve capacity of individuals, increasing their vulnerability to health problems. Stress-related illness can encompass the previously mentioned conditions as the primary cause of dysfunction or as the result of the stress of the dysfunction. Excessive stress sometimes manifests as cardiovascular problems, including hypertension; digestive difficulties, including heartburn, ulcer, and bowel syndromes; respiratory illness and susceptibility to bacterial and viral illness; endocrine dysfunction, particularly adrenal or thyroid dysfunction and delayed or reduced cellular repair; sleep disorders; and breathing pattern disorder.

Medical Assistance

More individuals are seeking medical assistance to help sort out and identify stress-related symptoms. Because each person responds to stress differently, accurate diagnoses become difficult. This lack of specificity has led to frustration in clients and health care providers, but as more research is done in the area of coping and adaptive capacities, the situation is continuing to improve. In contemporary health care, excessive and long-term stress is now recognized as an important and widespread cause of disease.

Psychophysiology is the study of the interplay between psychological and physiological stressors and neuroimmunology; it is sometimes referred to as psychoneuroimmunology, or the study of the mind-immunity link within the larger field of the mind/body connection. Increased openness to, respect for, and understanding of approaches, such as massage and other forms of bodywork, along with acupuncture, meditation, and relaxation methods using breathing, biofeedback, music therapy, hypnosis, exercise, and other forms of movement therapy, allow for additional ways of managing stress as well as pain.

Indications for Massage

Massage intervention has a strong physiological effect through the comfort of compassionate touch, in addition to a physical influence on mental state through the effect on the ANS and neurochemicals. Therefore people experiencing mental health problems may benefit from massage. Management of pain is an important factor if the client is experiencing pain. Because therapeutic massage often can offer symptomatic relief from chronic pain, the helplessness that accompanies these difficulties may dissipate as the person realizes that management methods exist. Soothing of any ANS hyperactivity or hypoactivity provides a sense of inner balance. Normalization of the breathing mechanism allows the client to breathe without restriction and can reduce the tendency for breathing pattern disorder, which feeds anxiety and panic.

Therapeutic massage can provide intervention on a physical level to restore a more normal function to the body, thereby supporting appropriate interventions by qualified mental health professionals. Strong and appropriate indications exist for the use of massage therapy in the restoration of mental health, but caution is needed regarding dual roles and maintenance of professional boundaries. It is important to work with mental health providers in these situations.

Trauma-Informed Care

Trauma-informed care principles are important for the massage therapist. Awareness begins as part of the ongoing assessment process. Focus is shifted from "What's wrong with you?" to "What happened to you?" Support for individuals who have experienced traumatic events is a complex, multidisciplinary, integrative approach. A trauma-informed care approach aligns with the biopsychosocial, whole person, client-centered approaches described in Chapter 5 and reflect ethical behavior presented in Chapter 2.

Briefly, Trauma-informed care seeks to:

- Realize the widespread impact of trauma and understand paths for recovery
- Recognize the signs and symptoms of trauma in patients, families, and staff
- Integrate knowledge about trauma into policies, procedures, and practices
- Actively avoid retraumatization.

Key principles include:

- Empowerment: Using individuals' strengths to empower them in the development of their care
- Choice: Informing people regarding treatment options so they can choose the options they prefer
- Collaboration: Maximizing collaboration among the individual, care staff, and their families during treatment planning
- Safety: Developing health care settings and activities that ensure physical and emotional safety
- Trustworthiness: Creating clear expectations with individuals about what proposed treatments involve, who will provide services, and how care will be provided.

Massage therapy can be an effective aspect of a care plan but additional education in trauma-informed care is necessary. Building foundational awareness of trauma-informed approaches should begin at entry level education and be reinforced through continuing education. This education needs to be provided by experts in the field and these experts do not need to be massage therapists.

Begin a search for this type of education at: Center for Health Care Strategies (CHCS). https://www.chcs.org/.

For more information, visit CHCS' Trauma-Informed Care Implementation Resource Center at: TraumaInformedCare.chcs.org, and https://www.chcs.org/topics/trauma-informed-care/.

The Substance Abuse and Mental Health Services Administration (SAMHSA) is the overseeing agency within the US Department of Health and Human Services: https://www.samhsa.gov/resource/dbhis/samhsas-concept-trauma-guidance-trauma-informed-approach.

Inflammatory Response

Inflammation may occur as a response to any tissue injury, and the inflammatory response is an active and important part of the healing process. The **inflammatory response** is a combination of processes, which attempts to minimize injury to tissues and promote healing, thus maintaining homeostasis. Inflammation also may accompany specific immune system reactions. Acute inflammation occurs during the onset of injury or illness and is an essential aspect of the healing process. Chronic inflammation is an inflammatory process that occurs or persists without a beneficial outcome and thus becomes a disease-producing process. The signs and symptoms of inflammation include heat, redness, swelling, and loss of function/movement brought on by swelling and pain.

- *Heat* and *redness:* When tissue cells are damaged, they release inflammatory mediators, such as histamine, prostaglandins, and compounds called *kinins.* Some inflammatory mediators cause the blood vessels to dilate, increasing the blood volume available to the tissue. The increased blood volume produces the redness and heat of inflammation. This response is important, because it allows immune system cells (white blood cells) in the blood to travel quickly and easily to the site of injury.
- *Swelling* and *pain:* Some inflammatory mediators increase the permeability of blood vessel walls. When water (plasma fluid) leaks out of the vessel, tissue swelling (edema) results. The pressure caused by edema triggers pain receptors. The fluid that accumulates in inflamed tissue (inflammatory exudate) has the beneficial effect of diluting the irritant. Inflammatory exudate is removed slowly by the lymphatic system. Bacteria and damaged cells are held in the lymph nodes and are destroyed by white blood cells. Occasionally lymph nodes enlarge when they process a large amount of infectious material.

Sometimes the inflammatory response is more intense or prolonged than desirable. Inflammation can be suppressed by antihistamines, which block the action of histamine, and by antiinflammatories, such as aspirin, which disrupts the body's synthesis of prostaglandins.

Tissue Repair

When tissue is injured, a process occurs to repair the tissue. This can be called tissue healing response. The first response is to control any bleeding called *hemostasis.* Within minutes or even seconds, blood cells start to clump together and clot, protecting the wound and preventing further blood loss. The next phase is inflammation. The process of inflammation triggers tissue repair. Tissue repair is the replacement of dead cells with living cells. In a type of tissue repair called *regeneration,* the new cells are similar to those they replace. Another type of tissue repair is *replacement.* In replacement, the new cells are formed from connective tissue and are different from those they replace, resulting in a scar. Often, fibrous connective tissue replaces the damaged tissue, resulting in a condition called *fibrosis.* Most tissue repairs are a combination of regeneration and replacement. A goal in the healing process is to promote regeneration and minimize replacement. Massage has been shown to slow the formation of scar tissue and to keep scar tissue pliable when it does form.

Inflammatory Disease

Productive local inflammation occurs in a limited area, such as in a small cut that becomes infected. Productive systemic inflammation occurs when the irritant spreads throughout the body or when inflammatory mediators cause changes throughout the body.

As mentioned earlier, inflammation that is persistent without benefit is considered chronic inflammation. Conditions involving chronic inflammation are classified as inflammatory diseases (Table 6.1). Among the most common inflammatory

Table 6.1 Diseases Related to Chronic Inflammation

Many seemingly unrelated diseases have a common link: inflammation. This is a partial list of common medical problems associated with chronic inflammation.

Disease or Disorder	Mechanism
Allergy	Mediators induce autoimmune reactions
Alzheimer's disease	Chronic inflammation destroys brain cells
Anemia	Mediators disrupt erythropoietin production
Aortic valve stenosis	Chronic inflammation damages heart valves
Arthritis	Inflammatory mediators destroy joint cartilage and synovial fluid
Asthma	Mediators close the airways
Cancer	Chronic inflammation causes most cancers
Cardiovascular disease	Inflammation contributes to the formation of plaque in blood vessels
Congestive heart failure	Chronic inflammation causes wasting of the heart muscle
Fibromyalgia	Mediators are elevated
Fibrosis	Mediators attack traumatized tissue
Heart attack	Chronic inflammation contributes to coronary atherosclerosis
Kidney failure	Mediators restrict circulation and damage nephrons
Lupus	Mediators induce an autoimmune attack
Pancreatitis	Mediators induce pancreatic cell injury
Psoriasis	Mediators induce dermatitis
Stroke	Chronic inflammation promotes thromboembolic events
Surgical complications	Mediators prevent healing

conditions are arthritis, inflammatory bowel disease, asthma, eczema, and chronic bronchitis. Autoimmune conditions overall have an inflammatory component. There is increasing evidence of chronic inflammation being a factor in mental health status, including depression (Arteaga-Henríquez et al., 2019).

Indications for Massage

Generally, acute inflammatory conditions indicate cautions for massage application. Local areas of inflammation typically are avoided during the acute inflammatory phase, especially if infection is present. A systemic acute inflammatory response related to infection typically involves fever, although not always. Productive fever supports healing and indicates that adaptive capacity is strained. Massage typically (but not always) is avoided during the acute phase of disease.

Massage is indicated with cautions when local acute inflammation is present. The area of inflammation is avoided, and if the area is related to injury and susceptible to infection, diligence about sanitation and infection control is necessary. An example is massage application after surgery.

If the acute inflammation is systemic, the individual is ill. Palliative massage may support restorative sleep. However, it is important to avoid any approach that adds more adaptive strain than the client can manage. When in doubt, do not massage. Wait until the illness has resolved.

Therapeutic massage seems to be beneficial in cases of prolonged chronic inflammation. Current theories suggest that massage helps resolve tissue level inflammatory signaling and/or stimulates antiinflammatory signaling. Mechanotransduction (cellular activity stimulated by mechanical forces) may activate the body's own antiinflammatory agents (White et al., 2020; Gao et al., 2022; Krol et al., 2022).

Pain

Massage professionals especially need to understand the mechanisms of pain (Box 6.1). Chapter 5 presents evidence supporting massage as beneficial for the symptomatic reduction of pain perception. In this section, we consider the types of pain, and the ways massage may be indicated or contraindicated for pain. Understanding the distinct types of pain sensation helps the massage practitioner recognize when to refer the client to a physician. Pain is a complex, private, abstract experience that is difficult to explain or describe. It is the main symptom or complaint that causes people to seek health care.

Box 6.1 National Pain Strategy, Federal Pain Research Strategy, CDC Clinical Practice Guideline for Prescribing Opioids for Pain (United States, 2022)

Opportunities for Integration of Massage Therapy:

- Integrative health care incorporates complementary approaches into mainstream health care to achieve health and wellness.
- Interdisciplinary care is provided by a team of health professionals from diverse fields who coordinate their skills and resources to meet patient goals.
- Multimodal pain treatment addresses the full range of an individual patient's biopsychosocial challenges by providing a range of distinct types of therapies that may include medical, surgical, psychological, behavioral, and integrative approaches as needed.

The Interagency Pain Research Coordinating Committee (IPRCC) is a Federal advisory committee created by the Department of Health and Human Services to enhance pain research efforts and promote collaboration across the government, with the ultimate goals of advancing the fundamental understanding of pain and improving pain-related treatment strategies.

Learn more at: https://www.iprcc.nih.gov/.

The US health care system is evolving toward a care model that is patient-centered, evidence and outcomes-guided yet personalized, and provided through high-performing, interdisciplinary care. The National Pain Strategy endorses a population-based, disease management approach to pain care that is delivered by integrated, interdisciplinary, patient-centered teams and is consistent with real world experience. Massage therapists could be included in these teams.

The Federal Pain Research Strategy (FPRS) is a long-term strategic plan to guide the federal agencies and departments that support pain research and to advance the science to better understand pain and improve pain care. The strategy identifies a set of research priorities that align with the missions of numerous agencies within the Department of Health and Human Services, the Department of Defense, and the Department of Veterans Affairs. Overall, the priorities cover basic through clinical, dissemination, and implementation research to support the translation of scientific discoveries into clinical practice and improve the lives of people with pain.

As a massage therapist, it is crucial that you have current and accurate information about pain. Pain is a major health issue. The National Center for Complementary and Integrative Health (NCCIH) reports that massage therapy is recommended as a pain management strategy (NIH).

The Centers for Disease Control (CDC) updated Clinical Practice Guideline for Prescribing Opioids for Pain in 2022 in the United States. The guidelines recommend a variety of nonpharmaceutical subacute and chronic pain treatments which include massage therapy.

The CDC considers acute pain duration of less than 1 month, subacute pain duration of 1–3 months, and chronic pain duration more than 3 months. Medical care staff are encouraged to educate and recommend pain management strategies that do not involve prescription medication including opioids. Evidence suggests therapies that don't involve medications may actually work better for some conditions and have fewer risks and side effects. https://www.cdc.gov/mmwr/volumes/71/rr/rr7103a1.htm. Dowell D, Ragan KR, Jones CM, Baldwin GT, Chou R. CDC Clinical Practice Guideline for Prescribing Opioids for Pain — United States, 2022. MMWR Recomm Rep 2022;71(No. RR-3):1–95. DOI: http://dx.doi.org/10.15585/mmwr.rr7103a1.

https://www.cdc.gov/opioids/patients/guideline.html.

Massage therapists need to be able to adapt the massage application to pain-based conditions and also work with other health and medical care professionals in an informed and professional manner.

Pain provides information about situations that can damage tissue; it therefore often enables us to protect ourselves from greater damage. The individual's subjective description and indication of the location of the pain help pinpoint the underlying cause of trauma or disease. Pain is an important predictive signal to alert to potential threat. The nervous, endocrine, and immune systems function together in a complex, adaptive manner responding to internal and external stressors to avoid homeostatic breakdown.

Pain neuroscience education typically decreases the threat value of pain, diminishes catastrophic thinking about pain, and facilitates a more active coping strategy. A combination of tissue-based interventions such as massage therapy (bottom-up techniques) should be combined with neuroscience pain education (top-down techniques). The neuromatrix theory of pain is an explanatory model of how pain is produced and therapeutically managed. The neuromatrix theory of pain provides a framework that may explain why selected nonpharmacological methods of pain relief, like massage, are effective and supports the biopsychosocial model of care.

The theory was developed by Ronald Melzack and Patrick David Wall and is an expansion of their original "gate theory" of pain, first proposed in 1965. The gate control theory of pain says that nonpainful sensory input closes the "gates" to painful input, which prevents pain sensation from traveling to the central nervous system. This theory suggests that the spinal cord contains a neurological "gate" that either blocks pain signals or allows them through to the brain. The neuromatrix theory of pain addresses the complex nature of pain as follows:

- Pain is an output of the brain that is produced whenever the brain concludes that the body is in danger and action is required. Each person's brain has developed an individual neural network referred to as the body-self neuromatrix. Pain is a multisystem output that is produced when an individual's pain neuromatrix is activated.
- An individual's neuromatrix consists of genetic neural programs, individual experience, and behavior. The intensity and location of sensory inputs from skin, organs, and other somatic receptors influence the perception of danger, triggering activity of the body's stress regulation systems.
- Pain becomes chronic as the pain neuromatrix is strengthened via nociceptive and non-nociceptive mechanisms, which means that less input, both nociceptive and non-nociceptive, is required to produce pain. This is called *sensitization.*

Acute Pain

Acute pain is a symptom of a disease condition or a temporary aspect of medical treatment. Acute pain acts as a warning signal because it can activate the sympathetic (fight–flight–freeze response) nervous system. Acute pain is usually temporary, of sudden onset, easily localized, can be described, and often subsides with or without treatment.

Chronic/Persistent Pain

Chronic pain is identified as a major health problem. Acute pain has a purpose. Chronic pain is nonproductive and no longer has any value. Approximately 25% of the population is affected. Chronic pain is a symptom that persists or recurs for indefinite periods, usually for longer than 6 months. Chronic pain frequently has an obscure onset, and the character and quality of the pain change over time. The pain usually is diffuse and poorly localized and often requires the efforts of a multidisciplinary health care team for its effective management.

Pain can also be classified as nociceptive, neuropathic, and neuroplastic.

Nociceptive Pain

Nociceptive pain occurs when actual or threatened tissue damage occurs and is due to activation of nociceptors. Nociceptive pain typically starts as acute pain which lessons with time/tissue healing. This protective and productive response is a normal and appropriate function of the nervous system.

Neuropathic Pain

Neuropathic pain refers to pain that is generated or sustained by the nervous system. It is the result of nerve damage or a malfunctioning nervous system and involves problems with signals from the nerves. Neuropathic pain is commonly associated with a variety of neurodegenerative, metabolic, and autoimmune diseases. Neuropathic pain is, by definition, chronic and may escalate with time. There are two categories of neuropathic pain:

- Central neuropathic pain results directly from central nervous system (CNS) injury such as a stroke.
- Peripheral neuropathic pain is related to injury or disease of the peripheral somatosensory nervous system.

These conditions often begin with productive, normal nociceptive pain. However, in chronic neuropathic pain, the nervous system responds inappropriately to the damage through multiple mechanisms misreading sensory inputs and generating nonproductive painful sensations. Secondary symptoms that commonly accompany neuropathic pain include depression, sleep disturbance, fatigue, and decreased physical and mental functioning.

Mixed Pain

Mixed pain is a combination of nociceptive and neuropathic pain. Nociceptive pain can be somatic or visceral and is usually localized–often described as achy, throbbing, or dull, deep, and pulling. Neuropathic pain is typically described as burning, shooting, tingling, and radiating. With mixed pain, elements of both neuropathic and nociceptive pain are described. The causes of the pain sensations can also be mixed.

Neuroplastic Pain

Pain can modify the way the central nervous system processes sensory signals. Structural and functional changes can occur at every level of the nervous system including the periphery, the spinal cord, and in higher brain centers following injury, inflammation, and other events. These changes may increase the magnitude of the perceived pain and may contribute to the development of chronic pain syndromes and increased pain sensitivity. Neuroplasticity is the brain and nervous system's ability to form new pathways or synapses and adapt to change.

Neuroplastic changes may be responsible for persistent pain as a nonbeneficial neuroplastic adaptation. Sometimes a person becomes more sensitive to stimuli and experiences more pain with less sensory stimulation. Rather than the nervous system functioning properly to sound alarm regarding tissue injury, in neuropathic pain the peripheral or central nervous systems are malfunctioning and become the cause of the pain. It is common for neuroplastic changes to occur with neuropathic pain. Following a peripheral nerve injury, anatomical and neurochemical changes can occur within the central nervous system that can persist long after the injury has healed. When the problem begins in the peripheral nerves, it is called *peripheral sensitization*. The increased responsiveness in the central nervous system is called *central sensitization*. Central sensitization is a factor in chronic pain in which peripheral stimuli are interpreted as more painful than they would normally be. Central sensitization results in amplification of peripheral signals and is not an independent pain generator in peripheral neuropathic pain conditions. There are three main dysfunctions:

- Allodynia is pain, generally on the skin, caused by something that would not normally cause pain. Allodynia is believed to be a hypersensitive reaction that may result from central sensation.
- Hyperalgesia is an increased pain response—basically, pain being more painful than it should be.
- Paresthesia is the experience of unpleasant or painful feelings even when there is nothing touching you and no stimulus.

Chronic/persistent pain is now considered a separate condition from acute pain. This is why current affective treatments for acute pain do not work for chronic/persistent pain. For example opiate medications are appropriate for the short-term treatment of acute pain. However, you cannot treat chronic pain using acute pain measures. Attempting this was a factor leading to the opiate addiction crisis (Smith, 2018; Tick et al., 2018; Elibol and Cavlak, 2019).

Pain Sensations

An understanding of the pain pathways is important because massage application can modulate pain transmission. Nociception is the sensing of danger through stimulus of the nervous system. Pain and itch are both forms of nociception. Pain tells the body either that there has been an injury or that one is imminent. Itch (pruritus) signals that there is an irritant or potential toxin around. In both cases, the skin is vital to signaling. The nerve endings transmit the signal through circuits of multiple nerve cells toward the brain.

The receptors for tissue damage, called *nociceptors*, are the branching ends of the dendrites of certain sensory neurons. These receptors are found in almost every tissue of the body and respond to noxious (unpleasant/harmful) mechanical stimuli, temperature, and chemical substances. In situations of trauma or inflammation, inflammatory chemicals stimulate the nociceptors. Injured tissue releases bradykinin, which causes the release of inflammation-producing chemicals such as histamine and prostaglandins. Inflammatory mediators make nociceptors more sensitive to the normal pain response. This is why pain and inflammation are interconnected (Gerdle et al., 2014).

Four distinct processes are involved in pain sensation: transduction, transmission, modulation, and perception. *Transduction* is the process by which noxious stimuli lead to electrical activity in the nociceptors. *Transmission* involves the process of transmitting impulses from the site of transduction over peripheral sensory nerves to the spinal cord and the brain. *Modulation* involves neural activity through descending neural pathways from the brain that can influence transmission at the level of the spinal cord. *Perception* is the subjective experience of pain by the person; it is somehow produced by the neural activity of nociceptor transmission over multiple brain areas and the response to the neurochemicals (e.g., endorphins and endocannabinoids) that modify the experience of pain (Benedetti et al., 2013). When stimuli for other sensations, such as touch, pressure, heat, and cold, reach a certain intensity, they also transmit danger signals to the central nervous system. This process connects pain sensation with danger and remembered experiences.

Nociceptor signals are carried on two types of nerve fibers: large, myelinated A fibers and small, nonmyelinated C fibers. A and C nerve fibers can be distinguished by the two speeds of transmission. Fast signals are transmitted to the spinal cord by the A nerve fibers and are felt within 0.1 second. Fast signals are typically experienced as pain sensation that is local and specific and has a prickling, sharp, or electrical quality. Fast nociceptor transduction is elicited in response to mechanical or thermal stimuli on the skin surface but is not felt in deeper tissues of the body. Slow nociceptor signals are transmitted by the C fibers and felt 1 second after a noxious stimulus. Slow transmission sensation is less well localized and has a burning, throbbing, or aching quality. Slow nociceptor transduction may be elicited by mechanical, thermal, or chemical stimuli in the skin or most deep tissues or organs and usually is associated with tissue damage. Because of this double system of innervation, tissue injury often occurs as two distinct pain sensations: an early, sharp pain (transmitted by A nerve fibers), followed by a dull, burning, somewhat prolonged pain (transmitted by C nerve fibers).

Sensory impulses related to noxious stimuli are conducted by the CNS along spinal and cranial nerves to the thalamus. From there the impulses may be relayed primarily to the parietal lobe of the brain. Recognition of the type and intensity of most nociceptor-transmitted sensation is perceived as pain in the cerebral cortex of the brain. Pain is called a *thalamic sense* because it is probably brought to the consciousness in the thalamus. Neurons in the thalamus carry the impulses to the primary somatosensory cortex, where the sensory aspects of pain are identified by location, nature, and intensity.

This system of nociceptive transmission through the thalamus influences the expression of pain in terms of tolerance, behavior, and sympathetic autonomic responses; this is especially true in relation to chronic pain because of the associated autonomic responses, emotional behavior, and lowered pain thresholds that often occur.

The point where a stimulus is perceived as painful, known as the *pain threshold*, varies somewhat from person to person. One factor that affects the pain threshold is perceptual dominance, in which the pain felt in one area of the body diminishes or obliterates the pain felt in another area. Not until the most severe pain is diminished does the person perceive or acknowledge the other pain. *Pain tolerance* is the duration or intensity of noxious stimuli that a person can endure before acknowledging the pain and seeking relief. Pain tolerance is more variable from one person to another than is the pain threshold. A person's tolerance to pain is influenced by a variety of factors, including personality type, psychological state at the onset of pain, previous experiences, sociocultural background, and the meaning of the pain to that person (e.g., the ways in which it affects the person's lifestyle). Factors that reduce pain tolerance include repeated exposure to pain, fatigue, sleep deprivation, and stress (Simpson et al., 2018).

Warmth, cold, distraction, alcohol consumption, hypnosis, strong religious beliefs/faith, and nonpainful massage increase pain tolerance (Price and Wilson, 2002; Mohammed et al., 2018; Staveski et al., 2018).

Somatic and Visceral Pain

There are two other ways to look at pain: somatic and visceral. Somatic pain arises from the stimulation of receptors in the skin (superficial somatic pain) or from stimulation of receptors in skeletal muscles, joints, tendons, and fasciae (deep somatic pain). Visceral pain results from the stimulation of receptors in the viscera (internal organs).

Superficial somatic pain is transmitted along finely myelinated (a fatty insulation) A delta nerve fibers at a fast rate (an analogy for this is a highway or expressway). Deep somatic pain and most visceral pain are transmitted slowly by unmyelinated (no insulation) C nerve fibers (an analogy for this is a dirt road).

This difference in the transmission of pain signals explains why superficial somatic stimulation transmitted on A delta fibers can block or mask deep somatic or visceral pain. Stimulation of more A fibers than C fibers blocks the C fiber transmission from entering the spinal cord. If the signal does not enter the spinal cord, it cannot be felt as pain.

Methods of touch and pressure and most methods of movement are transmitted on A fibers; any stimulus of this type increases A-fiber transmission, blocking pain signals. Treating pain in this way is called *counterirritation*.

Referred Pain

The ability of the cerebral cortex of the brain (the thinking part of the brain) to locate the origin of pain is related to past experience. In most instances of somatic pain and in some instances of visceral pain, the brain accurately projects the pain back to the stimulated area.

The visceral pain also may be felt in a surface area far from the stimulated organ. This phenomenon is called **referred pain**. In general, the area to which the pain is referred and the visceral organ that is stimulated receive their nerves from the same section of the spinal cord. Because of this association, the brain may misinterpret the source. For example, the pain of a heart attack is typically felt in the skin over the heart and along the left arm. The same factor is at work in the referred pain in the shoulder caused by gallstones. Fig. 6.2 illustrates cutaneous

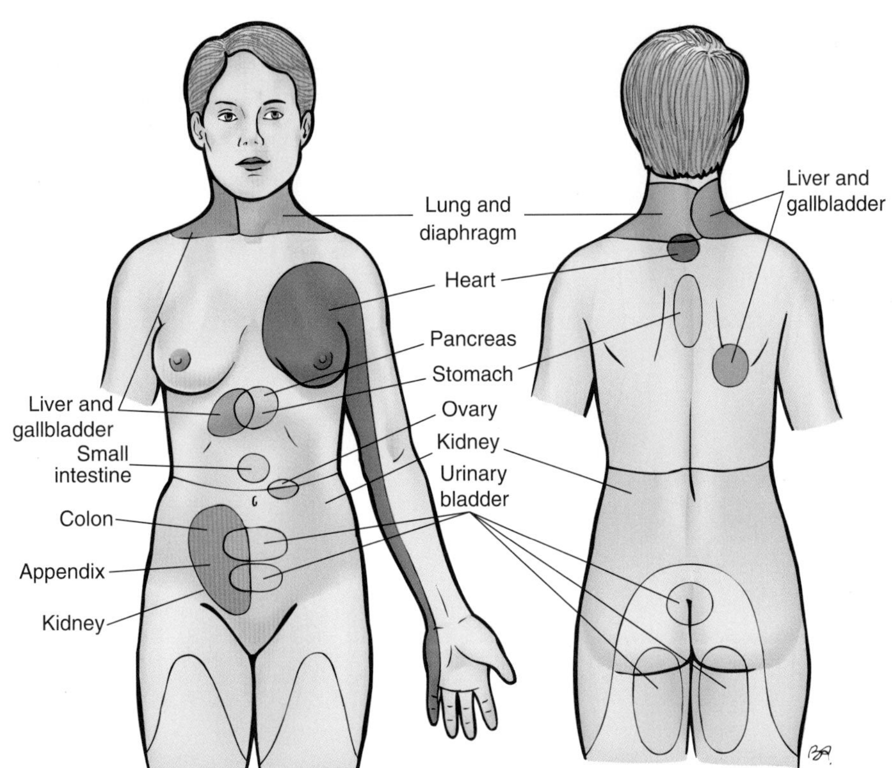

FIG. 6.2 Referred pain. The diagram indicates cutaneous areas to which visceral pain may be referred. If pain is encountered in these areas during a massage, the massage practitioner should refer the client to a physician for diagnosis to rule out visceral dysfunction.

(skin) regions to which visceral pain may be referred. If the client has a recurring pain pattern that resembles the patterns on the chart, the client should be referred to a physician for an accurate diagnosis.

Irritation of the viscera frequently produces pain that is felt not in the viscera but in some somatic structure that may be a considerable distance from the viscera. Such pain is said to be referred to the somatic structure. Deep somatic pain also may be referred, but superficial pain is not. When visceral pain is local and referred, it sometimes seems to radiate from the local to the distant site.

Visceral pain, like deep somatic pain, initiates reflex contraction of nearby skeletal muscle. Because somatic pain is much more common than visceral pain, the brain has learned to project the pain to the somatic area and initiate the reflex contraction there.

Obviously, knowledge about referred pain and the common sites of pain referral from each of the viscera is important to massage practitioners and other health care professionals. The most common example of referred pain is that of a heart attack, which is commonly experienced as chest pain. Another example is pain in the tip of the shoulder, which may be due to irritation in the central portion of the diaphragm.

However, remember that sites of reference are not stereotyped, and unusual reference sites occur with considerable frequency. Heart pain, for instance, may be experienced as purely abdominal, may be referred to the right arm, and may even be referred to the neck.

As previously noted, experience plays a key role in referred pain. Although pain originating in an inflamed abdominal organ usually is referred to the midline, in clients who have had previous abdominal surgery, the pain of an inflamed abdominal organ is commonly referred to their surgical scars. Pain originating in the maxillary sinus usually is referred to nearby teeth, but in clients with a history of traumatic dental work, such pain is regularly referred to the previously traumatized teeth. This is true even if the teeth are distant from the sinus.

When pain is referred, the reference is usually to a structure that developed from the same embryonic segment or is located in the same dermatome (nerve map) as the structure in which the pain originates (Fig. 6.3). For example during embryonic development, the diaphragm moves from the neck to its adult location in the abdomen and takes its nerve supply, the phrenic nerve, with it. One-third of the fibers in the phrenic nerve are afferent, and they enter the spinal cord at the level of the second to fourth cervical segments, the same location at which

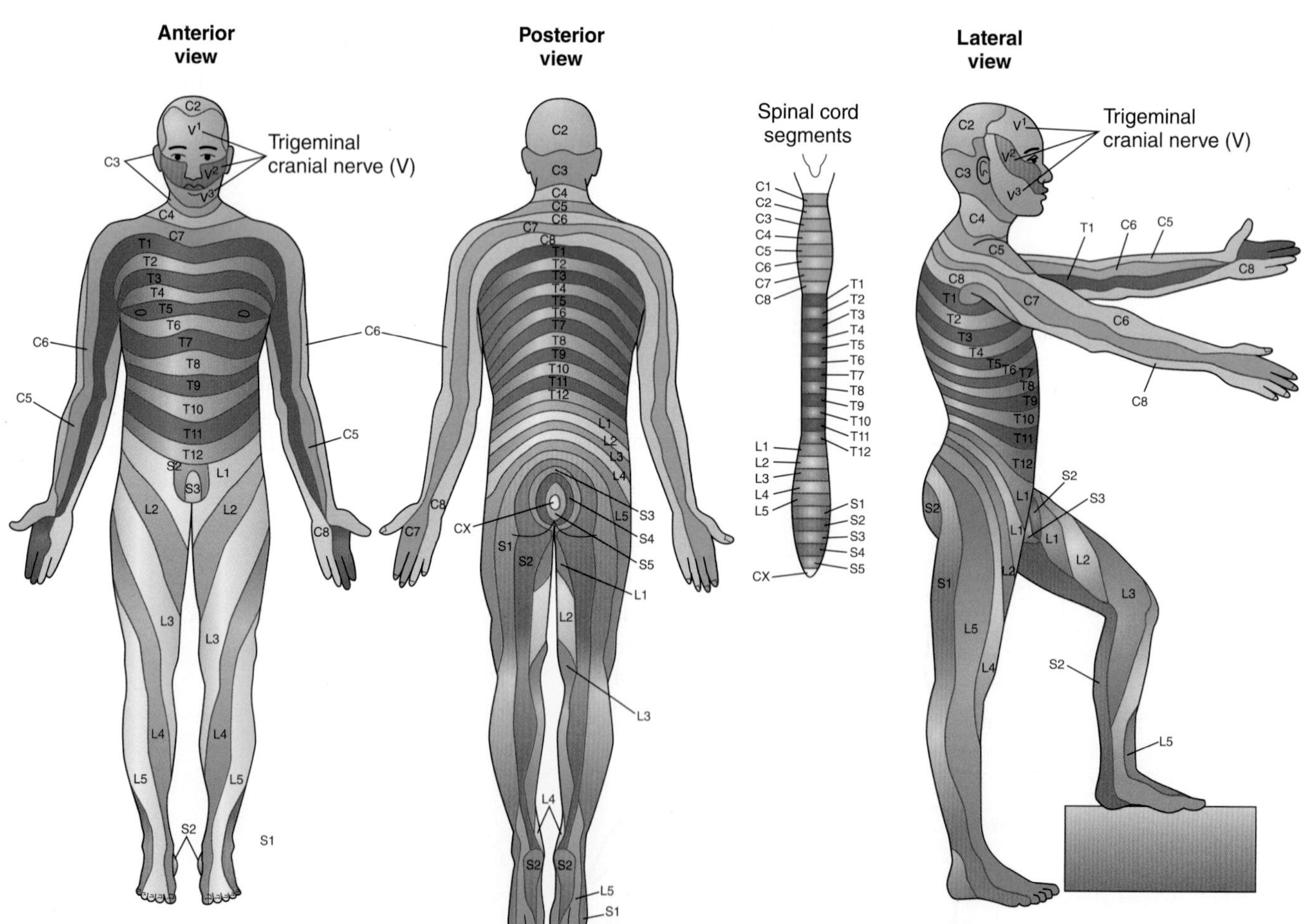

FIG. 6.3 Dermatomes. Segmental dermatome distribution of spinal nerves to the front, back, and side of the body. *C,* Cervical segments; *T,* thoracic segments; *L,* lumbar segments; *S,* sacral segments; *CX,* coccygeal segments. (From Thibodeau GA, Patton KT: *The human body in health and disease,* ed 4, St. Louis, 2010, Mosby.)

afferent nerves from the tip of the shoulder enter. Similarly, the heart and the arm have the same embryonic segmental origin.

Phantom Pain

A kind of pain commonly experienced by persons who have undergone limb amputation is called *phantom pain*. They experience pain or other sensations in the extremity as though the limb were still there. Phantom pain is believed to occur because the remaining proximal portions of the sensory nerves that previously received impulses from the limb are being stimulated by the trauma of the amputation. Stimuli from these nerves are interpreted by the brain as coming from the nonexistent (phantom) limb. New research about phantom pain indicates connection to established patterns in the brain as a cause.

Cancer-Related Pain

The two most common causes of cancer pain are the cancer itself and the treatments used to treat cancer. An example of pain related to the cancer itself would be tumor formations putting pressure on organs, bones, nerves, and/or blood vessels.

Some examples of treatment-related pain include the following:

- Chemotherapy: peripheral neuropathy, bone/joint pain
- Surgical treatments/procedures

Most types of cancer pain can be managed with drug and nondrug therapies. How much pain is experienced depends on where the cancer is located, what kind of damage it is causing, and the various medications and other treatments that are being used to treat the cancer (Box 6.2).

Common types of cancer-related pain include the following:

- Acute pain lasting a brief time. The intensity of the pain experienced can range from mild to severe.
- Chronic/persistent pain that will not go away or comes back often. The intensity of the pain experienced can range from mild to severe.
- Breakthrough pain is an intense pain experience. It may occur as pain medication affects begin to diminish. It may be triggered by a specific activity or for no observable reason.
- Neuropathic pain may occur if treatment damages the nerves. The pain is often burning, sharp, or shooting (Box 6.3).

Pain Management

Pain management is a catchall phrase used to describe multiple types of health care services for pain. Pain management can include the following types of services:

- Acute care for injuries and illness
- Postsurgical pain care
- End-of-life, or palliative, care
- Burn unit services
- Wound care
- Chronic pain management

These different types of care are usually considered to fall into three broad categories:

- Acute pain management
- Terminal, or palliative, care
- Chronic pain management

Box 6.2 Warning Signs of Cancer

- Sores that do not heal
- Unusual bleeding
- A change in the appearance or size of a wart or mole
- A lump or thickening in any tissue
- Persistent hoarseness or cough
- Chronic indigestion
- A change in bowel or bladder function

Box 6.3 How Cancer Pain Differs

Cancer pain is different from other forms of acute or chronic pain. Pain is often of the mixed type. The psychosocial aspects of pain may involve worries about an uncertain future and loss of control, with the potential of disfigurement from surgery and even the possibility of death.

When cancer invades tissue, neuroimmune interactions excrete cellular and neuroinflammatory substances that promote new nerve growth that increase sensitivity to pain. Cancer pain syndromes, from both the cancer and the medical treatment, remain a challenge. Neuropathy, inflammation, and ulceration of the mucous membranes and pathological fractures because of reduced bone density all are a source of pain. For those and other cancer pain syndromes, complementary and integrative health (CIH) approaches combined with multimodal therapies are considered a best practice. Analgesic medications, including opiates, may be necessary to manage cancer pain. Adding nondrug therapies to the treatment plan is also indicated. There has been extensive research indicating the benefits of massage therapy as a pain management strategy.

From Arnstein P: 2018. Adult cancer pain: an evidence-based update, *J Radiol Nurs* 37(1):15-20, 2018; https://www.sciencedirect.com/science/article/pii/S1546084317301165#bib35

Acute Pain Management

Acute pain usually is caused by tissue injury. Inflammation is commonly present (Box 6.4). Management of acute pain involves short-term interventions best monitored by the physician using multimodal treatments.

Medication

Over the counter analgesics, including NSAIDs and acetaminophen, are effective for treating acute pain because they target the natural inflammation that occurs with an injury. Opioids are a key part of pharmacotherapy for acute pain. They are quite effective, particularly when used in combination with other analgesics, and are essential for both planned and unplanned severe acute pain situations. However, opioids must be used judiciously, for the shortest duration possible, and while giving proper respect to the risks of adverse effects, misuse, and abuse.

Topical Analgesics

Topical analgesics that contain menthol, camphor, methyl salicylate, or a combination of these counterirritants can be useful in managing localized musculoskeletal injuries, particularly when they can be massaged into the painful area...

Box 6.4 Guide to Acute Injury Care

Recommendations for acute care management of soft tissue injury has evolved over the years. As recommendations change it can be confusing. The main changes are related use of ice and other antiinflammatory treatment including medication in the acute injury healing phase. The acute injury phase occurs within the first 3 days after the injury. Massage therapy is considered a local contraindication at the injury site during the acute phase. During the subacute phase use of ice to manage pain and massage around the injury site can begin.

The PEACE and LOVE acronym was proposed in 2019 (Dubois, Blaise, and Jean-Francois Esculier. "Soft-tissue injuries simply need PEACE and LOVE." British journal of sports medicine 54, no. 2 (2020): 72-73.).

The current guidelines for immediate management of mild to moderate soft tissue and transition to subacute care are:

PEACE immediately after the injury.

P for Protect: Immobilize and avoid all movements that can cause pain 1–3 days postinjury.

E for Elevate: The injured area should be elevated above the level of the heart.

A for Avoid antiinflammatory modalities of treatment: The inflammatory process is a natural part of the healing process and data are emerging to show that use of antiinflammatory treatments can in fact hinder long-term healing of damaged tissues. Ice, which is the mainstay of all the earlier approaches for managing acute injuries, is included for its analgesic effect and a possible antiinflammatory effect. In this new approach ice and antiinflammatory medication is not included in injury management.

C for Compression: Using compression bandages immediately after injury has been shown to reduce swelling and aid recovery.

E for Educate: It is well known that an educated client will be far more compliant and active in their recovery process than someone who does not understand their injury and its management.

Subacute care involves LOVE to the tissues.

L for Load: Mechanical stresses should be added with attention paid to the loading not exacerbating pain while promoting repair, remodeling, and building tissue strength.

O for Optimism: The psychological impact of injury should not be ignored. Focus must be placed on ensuring injured persons remain optimistic. Persons who catastrophize injuries and become depressed will have poorer outcomes than those who remain optimistic.

V for Vascularization: Pain-free aerobic activity should be started as soon as the person can tolerate it. This aids with increasing blood flow to the damaged tissues and motivates the injured person.

E for Exercise: Exercises focused on strength, mobility, and proprioception of the injured area will lead to better functional outcomes

CARE for moderate to severe injury: a proposed strategy for the management of techniques that will limit further damage and create conditions to accelerate healing.

C for Cryotherapy and Compression: Apply ice in combination with compression as soon as possible after injury and several times during the first 48 hours after injury to reduce pain, secondary hypoxic injury, and extent of edema-hematoma.

A for Avoid: Avoid harmful and painful loading of the injured area. Gentle pain-free movement is ok.

R for Rehabilitation: Apply early weight-bearing exercises with support, manual therapy, and progressive therapeutic exercises.

E for Elevation: Elevate the injured area in combination with cryotherapy and compression to reduce the accumulation of edema.

Fousekis, Konstantinos, and Elias Tsepis. "Minor Soft Tissue Injuries may need PEACE in the Acute Phase, but Moderate and Severe Injuries Require CARE." Journal of Sports Science & Medicine 20, no. 4 (2021): 799.

What about ICE, PRICE, POLICE?

Localized cold therapy (ice) has long been an accepted part of initial treatment of acute soft tissue injury, but it is now recognized that inflammation is necessary to promote healing and ice is no longer recommended except in the CARE process for moderate to severe injury.

I—Ice. Ice or cryotherapy is the application of cold, typically with an ice pack applied to the injured area. Ice lowers skin and tissue temperature, which decreases nociceptive signaling and can lead to reduced pain sensation. There is some controversy over the use of ice because it can reduce the productive acute inflammatory response. To prevent frostbite, do not apply it directly to skin when applying ice to a local area. Ten-minute ice application is sufficient for pain management, then removed to allow tissue to warm. The treatment can be repeated. Ice should not be applied for more than 20 minutes.

C—Compression. Compression after an injury helps in the prevention of further swelling and a bit of immobilization. Compression to a local area is usually applied using an elastic bandage wrap. The bandage should not be so tight that it causes discomfort or interferes with blood flow.

E—Elevation. Elevating the injured area results in a decrease in hydrostatic pressure, which, in turn, reduces the accumulation of interstitial fluid and manages edema.

Next, "R" and "P" were added.

R—Rest. The intention of rest is to support the healing process. Not excessive rest but taking it easy for 24 hours may be prudent.

P—Protection. Protection prevents further injury and involves some type of immobilization such as the compression bandage or reduced weight bearing or demand such as crutches or a sling.

The result is PRICE. However, overtime best practices indicated that PRICE needed updating, and POLICE came into being. The "R" was removed, and the "O" and "L" were added.

OL—Optimal Loading. Optimal loading uses movement, weight bearing, and resistance to stimulate the healing process of bone, tendon, ligament, and muscle. The intensity of the loading increases as the healing progresses. The right amount of activity can help manage swelling.

MEAT—The acronym stands for movement, exercise, analgesics, therapy; and the MCE acronym stands for move–compress–elevate. Movement is within a pain-free range.

The MEAT protocol has elements of Optimal Loading by recommending movement, exercise, and therapy such as physical therapy. MEAT and MCE suggests gentle movement without exceeding pain tolerance improves blood flow.

Cryotherapy continues to be recommended for pain management, management of chronic inflammation, and a recovery strategy from exercise. In humans, the primary benefit of traditional cryotherapy is reduced pain following injury or soreness following exercise. Thomas, Kathryn. "IS COLD THERAPY Still Applicable Today?" Co-Kinetic Journal 92 (2022).

Thermotherapy

Thermotherapy consists of application of heat or cold (cryotherapy) for the purpose of changing the cutaneous, intra-articular and core temperature of soft tissue with the intention of improving the symptoms of certain conditions. Using ice or heat as a therapeutic intervention decreases pain (see Chapter 12).

Massage therapy can be a method for managing acute pain. Massage is adapted to target outcomes of relaxation and stress management. The approach to care is palliative. Critical thinking for care plan development involves understanding affects and side effects of all methods being used, such as medication, to manage acute pain and adapt appropriately. Typically a massage approach is 15–60 minutes, provided as needed, is general and pleasurable with potential local contraindications. Massage application should not strain the client's adaptive capacity. Remember that the acute pain will resolve–there is no need to attempt to "fix" the condition (Hsu et al., 2019).

Terminal (Palliative) Care

Management of pain related to terminal illness is best coordinated by the medical team. The persistence of the pain is a result of the terminal illness itself, or of the therapeutic approach, such as chemotherapy, neuropathic, or from other conditions such as osteoarthritis. Pharmacological management of pain includes nonopiate analgesics, opiates, and antianxiety medications. Massage is adapted to target outcomes of relaxation and stress management. The approach to care is palliative and focused on comfort and compassion. Critical thinking for care plan development involves understanding affects and side effects of all pain management methods being used and adapting appropriately. Typically a massage approach is 15–30 minutes, provided as needed, is pleasurable, often focuses on hands and feet, and may involve local contraindications. Typically, massage is done in the client's bed or chair. Massage application should not strain the client's adaptive capacity. Remember the goal is comfort, connection, and compassion.

Chronic Pain Management

Management of chronic pain is difficult. Massage therapy has strong evidence for chronic pain management especially when provided as part of an interdisciplinary, integrated, multimodal approach. Multimodal treatments incorporate both pharmacologic and nonpharmacologic strategies. Nonpharmacologic approaches including therapeutic exercise, manual therapy (including massage), cognitive behavioral therapy, thermotherapy (e.g., both heat and cold) are delivered by clinicians across the rehabilitative spectrum, including acupuncturists, chiropractors, nurses, osteopaths, physical therapists, psychologists, and massage therapists. Options work for some and not for others. Many of these strategies come under the heading of "neuromodulation," or distracting the brain from signals it is getting from the body's "periphery." *Placebo response* involves the use of any treatment process creating a positive response. Because of a person's belief that the treatment will be effective, rather than the painkilling properties of the method, 20–40% of persons in whom pain has been induced by stimuli have reported pain relief with the use of placebos. The following pain management strategies can be used alone or in combination for both acute and chronic pain (Eucker et al., 2022).

Transcutaneous Electric Nerve Stimulation

Electrodes attached to a small portable unit are used to stimulate the skin surface over the area of pain. Transcutaneous electric nerve stimulation stimulates large A delta fibers in the skin and, according to the gate-control theory, the fibers inhibit pain-conducting fibers in the spinal cord. Research has shown that low-voltage doses of electricity increase the levels of endogenous (made in the body) opioids (such as endorphins, enkephalins, and dynorphins).

Acupuncture/Acupressure

Acupuncture is performed by inserting thin needles into the skin along acupuncture meridians. One of the ways acupuncture works is that it releases endogenous opioids (Nielsen et al., 2022). Acupressure stimulates acupuncture points without using needles. Pressure is applied to the points with the thumb, a finger, or a blunt instrument. The physiological explanations are the same as for acupuncture.

Distraction and Imagery

Distraction is focusing the attention on stimuli other than pain. Imagery consists of using the imagination to create or remember a mental picture that is relaxing and relieves pain.

Biofeedback

Biofeedback is a technique in which a person is made aware of body functions by means of external measuring equipment, such as a computer-generated image of blood pressure. It allows control of the function at the conscious level. Likewise, nerve fibers in the cerebral cortex that can inhibit the impulses ascending in the pain pathways can be controlled to relieve pain. This kind of treatment is especially useful in treating migraines, tension headaches, and other forms of pain in which muscle tension is involved.

Aromatherapy

Essential oils are lipid extracts from various parts of plants. They can penetrate the skin quickly or be inhaled to stimulate the olfactory nerve. Olfaction refers to sense of smell. The olfactory nerve links parts of the brain that involve emotions and endocrine function. Therefore aromas can have profound effects on the mind and emotions. Essential oils can be used as compresses, for inhalation, in baths, and with massage oils.

Music Therapy

Music has been used to reduce pain. The pain relief may result from a reduction in anxiety, the inhibition of pain pathways, distraction, or an increase in endorphins that is produced by the music. However, music therapy can also aggravate pain, so preferences in music must be considered before using music during massage.

Hypnosis

Hypnotic techniques alter the focus of attention and enhance imagery by using suggestions. Individuals vary widely in their ability to be hypnotized.

Heat

Heat can be used to reduce pain. Heat dilates local blood vessels and increases blood flow. The increase in blood flow can reduce pain by washing away pain-producing chemicals. Temperature receptors are stimulated by heat, and the impulses are carried by large, myelinated nerve fibers that may inhibit the pain fibers. Heat softens collagen fibers, making them more pliable, which allows joints, tendons, and ligaments to be stretched farther before pain receptors are stimulated.

Cold

Cold relieves pain by decreasing swelling through vasoconstriction, by decreasing the stimulation of pain nerve endings, and by stimulating the release of endogenous opioids. Cold application is especially effective for nerve-related pain because cold slows neurotransmission.

Massage

Massage can have an analgesic effect. Various methods may help speed up the drainage of pain-producing substances from the area. Release of histamine and direct stimulation cause local blood vessels to dilate and bring oxygen to the area. Massage can temporality reduce muscle spasms, improve blood flow, and remove pressure on pain receptors. The touch and pressure sensations carried by large, myelinated fibers can inhibit nociceptive signaling. Massage can be used for distraction and often includes relaxing music.

Other Forms of Therapy

Art, prayer, meditation, and laughter are other forms of therapy that are being used effectively for pain management.

Medical Treatment

Painkilling medications are called *analgesics*. Oral analgesics (such as aspirin) reduce inflammation and inhibit transmission of pain impulses. They are nonaddictive. Narcotic analgesics (such as morphine) are addictive, and tolerance may develop. Narcotics (opioids) are used in individuals in whom relief cannot be obtained by other means, especially those suffering from cancer pain and those whose life expectancy is limited.

Surgical techniques are used to remove the cause or block the transmission of pain. Because damage to nerve cell bodies produces irreversible changes, surgery is used as a last resort.

It is helpful to have a reference text of pathology and pharmaceuticals. Texts written for nurses are likely the most useful (Box 6.5).

Common Pain Conditions

Generalized Stiffness and Fascia Densification and Fibrosis

The sensations experienced as "stiff" and "stuck" are often perceived as pain. Feeling stiff and stuck is likely related to changes in the extracellular matrix of the fascia and the fascial layers' ability to produce a lubricant called *hyaluronan* (or *hyaluronic acid*), which allows sliding between the fascia and muscle layers. The ground substance in the extracellular matrix absorbs water, which increases pressure, making the tissue stiffer. In addition, various chemicals in the fascia can make the fluid thicken (think gelatin).

The water content of fascia partly determines its stiffness. Stretching or compression of fascia causes water to be extruded from the tissue (like water from a sponge); as a result, the

Box 6.5 Opiate Crisis

The misuse of and addiction to opioids—including prescription pain relievers, heroin, and synthetic opioids such as fentanyl—have developed into a serious national crisis affecting public health.

It is hard to predict one's tendency to become addicted to opiate medications. Addiction is a disease that affects brain function and behavior. People who are addicted feel that they cannot function without the drug. Addiction causes a person to obsessively seek out the drug, even when the drug use causes behavior, health, or relationship problems.

Misuse of opioids has been a been a problem for centuries, but the current situation is different. Opioids are a type of medicine often used to help relieve acute pain from toothaches and dental procedures, injuries, surgeries, and cancer. Opioids are safe when used correctly for a short time (a few days) for acute pain or appropriately for longer periods for cancer pain or end-of-life pain. People who do not follow doctor's instructions and those who misuse opioids can become addicted.

It is likely that opiate abuse and misuse can be related more to distress than to pain. Signs and symptoms of distress include the following:

- Poor self-care and personal hygiene
- Being demanding of others
- Loss of motivation
- Perspiring excessively
- Having breathing difficulties
- Muscular spasms
- Obvious intense pain
- Extreme fatigue
- Complaints of sleep problems
- Anxiety and panic attacks
- Irritability and displaying agitation

Opioid drugs include the following:

- Opium
- Codeine
- Fentanyl
- Heroin
- Hydrocodone
- Hydromorphone
- Methadone
- Morphine
- Oxycodone
- Oxymorphone
- Paregoric
- Sufentanil
- Tramadol

From https://medlineplus.gov/opioidabuseandaddiction.html.

tissues become more pliable and supple. Eventually the water is taken up again and stiffness returns, but temporarily structures can move more effectively than when densely packed with water (Schleip et al., 2012). The sensation of being stuck likely relates to fibrosis, in which fibers in the matrix become matted and adherent. Fibrosis can be beneficial when tissues are too loose.

Vascular Disease or Injury

Vascular disease or injury, such as vasculitis (inflammation of blood vessels), coronary artery disease, and peripheral circulatory problems, all have the potential to cause pain. Vascular pain occurs when communication between blood vessels and nerves is interrupted. Ruptures, spasms, constriction, or obstruction of blood vessels also can result in pain, as can a condition called *ischemia,* in which the blood supply to organs, tissues, or limbs is cut off.

Neuropathic Pain

Neuropathic pain is a type of pain that can result from injury to nerves, either in the peripheral or central nervous system. Neuropathic pain can occur in any part of the body and is frequently described as a hot, burning sensation. It can result from diseases that affect nerves (e.g., diabetes) or from trauma and pressure on nerves. Neuropathic pain can occur as a result of cancer treatment because chemotherapy drugs affect nerves. There are many neuropathic pain conditions, such as diabetic neuropathy; complex regional pain syndrome, which can follow injury; and postherpetic neuralgia, which can occur after an outbreak of shingles. Some who have had an injury to the spinal cord experience intense pain ranging from tingling to burning and are sensitive to hot and cold temperatures and touch. This condition is called *central pain syndrome* or, if the damage is in the thalamus (the brain's center for processing bodily sensations), *thalamic pain syndrome.*

Impingement syndromes are compression or entrapment neuropathies. As explained in Chapter 5, *compression* is pressure on a nerve by a bony structure, and *entrapment* is pressure on a nerve from soft tissue. Massage is beneficial for entrapment and can manage some symptoms of nerve compression, even though the direct causal factor is not addressed.

Cervical Plexus

The cervical plexus is formed by the upper four cervical nerves. The phrenic nerve is part of this plexus. It innervates the diaphragm, and any disruption to this nerve affects breathing. Many cutaneous (skin) branches of the cervical plexus transmit sensory impulses from the skin of the neck, ear, and shoulder. The motor branches innervate muscles of the anterior neck.

If the impingement is on the cervical plexus, the person experiences headaches, neck pain, and breathing difficulties. The muscles most responsible for pressure on the cervical plexus are the suboccipital and sternocleidomastoid muscles. Shortened connective tissues at the cranial base also can press on these nerves.

Brachial Plexus

The brachial plexus is situated partly in the neck and partly in nerves that innervate the upper limb. Any imbalance that brings pressure on this complex of nerves results in shoulder pain, chest pain, arm pain, wrist pain, or hand pain.

The muscles most often responsible for impingement on the brachial plexus are the scalenes, pectoralis minor, and subclavius. Muscles of the arm occasionally impinge on branches of the brachial plexus. Brachial plexus impingement is responsible for thoracic outlet symptoms, which often are misdiagnosed as carpal tunnel syndrome. Whiplash injury involves the brachial plexus.

Lumbar Plexus

Impingement on the lumbar plexus may give rise to low back discomfort with a belt-like distribution of pain, in addition to pain in the lower abdomen, genitals, thigh, and medial lower leg. The main soft tissue structures that impinge on the lumbar plexus are the quadratus lumborum muscles and associated fascia.

Sacral Plexus

The sacral plexus has approximately a dozen named branches. Almost half of these serve the buttock and lower limb; the others innervate pelvic structures. The main branch is the sciatic nerve. Impingement of this nerve by the piriformis muscle gives rise to sciatica. Ligaments that stabilize the sacroiliac joint can affect the sacral plexus. Pressure on the sacral plexus can cause gluteal pain, leg pain, genital pain, and foot pain.

Pain Assessment

Because pain is a primary indicator in many disease processes, massage practitioners must have a basic evaluation protocol for pain so that they can determine when to refer their clients to the appropriate health care provider. Massage professionals gather subjective information by asking the client about symptoms associated with the pain. Practitioners should provide time to discuss with the client what the pain means to them by asking its impact on the client's lifestyle. They also should document pain treatment methods the client has used in the past and the effectiveness of those methods. Direct observation of nonverbal and verbal behavior may provide additional clues to the client's pain experience. Nonverbal behaviors such as grimacing, flinching, tearing, abnormal gait or posture, muscle tension, and guarding of the body are common indicators of pain. Verbal and emotional signals indicating pain may include crying, moaning, groaning, irritability, sadness, and changes in voice tone.

Gender and cultural differences affect the types of displays people use to express pain. As described previously, acute pain often activates a sympathetic response, resulting in increases in heart and respiratory rates, blood pressure, pallor, flushing, sweating, and pupil dilation. Very brief, intense pain may be followed by a rebound parasympathetic response, such as nausea and dizziness.

The massage practitioner should cautiously and carefully inspect and palpate the painful area to evaluate the range of motion of involved joints, to determine whether muscle guarding is present, and to identify tender points and areas of decreased sensation or increased sensitivity. When interacting with the massage client, avoid overfocusing on the pain experience and maintain a neutral conversation regarding the pain.

The following guidelines for evaluating pain can help in this process.

Evaluation of Pain

Location of Pain

- Localized pain is confined to the site of origin of the pain.
- Projected pain typically is a result of proximal nerve compression. This pain is perceived in the tissue supplied by the nerve.
- Radiating pain is diffuse pain around the site of origin that is not well localized.
- Referred pain is felt in an area distant from the site of the painful stimulus.

Types of Pain Sensation

- Pricking or bright pain: This type of pain is experienced when the skin is cut or jabbed with a sharp object. It is short-lived but intense and easily localized.
- Burning pain: This type is slower to develop, lasts longer, and is less accurately localized. It is experienced when the skin is burned, and it often stimulates cardiac and respiratory activity.
- Aching pain: Aching pain occurs when the visceral organs are stimulated. It is constant, not well localized, and often is referred to areas of the body far from where the damage is occurring. This type of pain is important, because it may be a sign of a life-threatening disorder of a vital organ.
- Deep pain: The main difference between superficial and deep sensibility is the different nature of the pain evoked by noxious stimuli. Unlike superficial pain, deep pain is poorly localized, nauseating, and frequently associated with sweating and changes in blood pressure. This type of pain initiates reflex contraction of nearby skeletal muscles. This reflex contraction is similar to the muscle spasm associated with injuries to bones, tendons, and joints. The steadily contracting muscles become ischemic, and ischemia stimulates the pain receptors in the muscles. The pain, in turn, initiates more spasms, creating a vicious cycle called the **pain–spasm–pain** cycle (Fig. 6.4).
- Muscle pain: If a muscle with an adequate blood supply contracts rhythmically, pain does not usually result. However, if the blood supply to a muscle is occluded (cut off), contraction soon causes pain. The pain persists after the contraction until blood flow is reestablished. If a muscle with a normal blood supply is made to contract continuously without periods of relaxation, it also begins to ache, because the maintained contraction compresses the blood vessels supplying the muscle.

Indications for Massage

Pain is a complex problem with physical, psychological, social, and financial components. Subjective measurements of pain intensity (what the client says) are more reliable than observable ones. Pain scales, such as a 1-to-10 scale, are helpful for measuring pain perception. Only the client can determine the degree of severity. Pain is rarely the same at all times. It is felt and perceived differently over time and differs with various precipitating and aggravating factors. Pain can range from excruciating to mild and may be difficult for the client to verbalize.

Pain can be alleviated in many ways. The massage professional, as part of a health care team, can contribute valuable manual therapy in various pain conditions using direct tissue manipulation and reflex stimulation to affect the nervous system and circulation. Obviously, for clients in extreme pain, the massage therapy must be monitored by a physician or other appropriate health care professional. Most people experience pain in less severe forms occasionally throughout life. Massage may provide temporary symptomatic relief of moderate pain brought on by daily stress (Box 6.6).

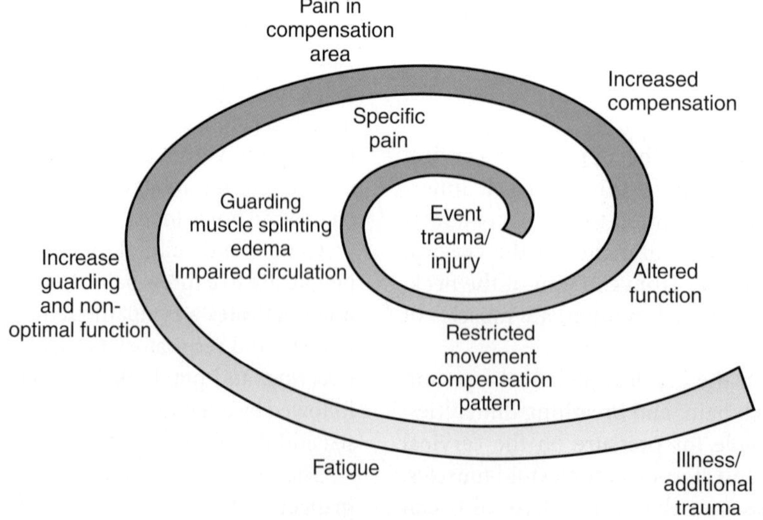

FIG. 6.4 Pain–spasm–pain cycle.

Box 6.6 Reacting to a Medical Emergency

Stay calm

Call 911

- Tell the operator there is an emergency.
- Say your name and where you are (the exact address if you know it).
- Explain what happened. The operator will need all the information you can provide, so give as many details as you can.)
- Follow all of the operator's instructions carefully.
- Stay on the line until the operator says it's okay to hang up.

Assess the person

- Check to see if they are alert, coherent, and breathing, and also confirm that you're able to find their pulse. If they are breathing and have a pulse, keep them as comfortable as possible and stay with them until emergency professionals arrive.
- Do not move a person unless absolutely necessary.
- Be prepared to administer CPR until professionals arrive.

Assist professionals once they arrive

- Follow instructions closely and provide as much information as possible so they're equipped to respond appropriately.

Notify the person's emergency contacts

Make a record

- Once the emergency is over, write down as accurately as possible your memory of the events that transpired.

Adult Medical Emergency Symptoms

Difficulty breathing, shortness of breath

Chest or upper abdominal pain or pressure lasting 2 minutes or more

Fainting, sudden dizziness, weakness

Changes in vision

Choking

Head or spine injury

Injury due to a serious accident

Ingestion of a poisonous substance

Difficulty speaking

Confusion or changes in mental status, unusual behavior, difficulty waking

Any sudden or severe pain

Uncontrolled bleeding

Severe or persistent vomiting or diarrhea

Coughing or vomiting blood

Suicidal or homicidal feelings

Unusual abdominal pain

CONTRAINDICATIONS TO MASSAGE THERAPY

SECTION OBJECTIVES

Chapter objective covered in this section:

4. Identify contraindications to massage and develop massage adaptations to support any cautions identified.

Using the information presented in this section, the learner will be able to perform the following:

- Evaluate a client's status to determine whether massage is contraindicated.
- Interpret the reference list of indications and contraindications in Appendix A.
- Interpret the basic pharmacology information.
- Recognize the warning signs of cancer.
- List the endangerment sites for massage.
- Effectively refer a client to a primary health care provider.

As mentioned earlier in this chapter, a contraindication is any condition that renders a particular treatment improper or undesirable or that raises cautions concerning treatment, requiring caution, adaptation, and possible supervision by a health care professional, such as a nurse.

Contraindications to massage are the responsibility of both physicians and massage practitioners. The massage professional is not expected to diagnose any condition but should learn about the client's particular condition by taking a thorough history and completing a physical assessment. The massage professional must be able to recognize indications and contraindications for therapeutic massage based on this information.

As previously described, massage therapy is indicated for musculoskeletal discomfort, relaxation, stress reduction, and pain control–and also for situations in which analgesics, anti-inflammatory drugs, muscle relaxants, and blood pressure, antianxiety, and antidepressant medications may be prescribed. The general effects of relaxation, such as reduced stress and pain and the physical comfort derived from therapeutic massage, complement most other medical and mental health treatment modalities (Chapter 5). However, when other therapies, including medication, are used, the physician must be able to evaluate accurately the effectiveness of each treatment the client is receiving. If the physician is unaware that the client is receiving massage, the effects of other therapies may be misinterpreted.

Clients with any vague or unexplainable symptoms of fatigue, muscle weakness, and general aches and pains should be referred to a physician. Many disease processes share these symptoms. This recommendation may seem overly cautious, but in the early stages of some serious illnesses, the symptoms are not well defined. If the physician is able to detect a disease process early in its development, often a more successful outcome is possible. A specific diagnosis is essential for effective treatment. Massage should be avoided in all infectious diseases suggested by fever, nausea, and lethargy until a diagnosis is made and the infection has resolved.

MENTORING TIP

Massage practitioners should not rely on lists of specific contraindications, but rather should use a set of medical and therapeutic guidelines pertinent to clinical applications and research developments. Unfortunately, such guidelines are not consistent in current literature. You will have to learn to make appropriate, informed decisions for each client. As mentioned earlier, this text is targeted to the entry-level massage therapist; therefore the recommendations are conservative. With increased experience and education, the massage therapist develops the ability to work with more complex client situations.

Contraindications are unique to each client and to each region of the body. The ability to reason clinically is essential to making appropriate decisions about the advisability of, modifications to, or avoidance of massage interventions. It is important to understand when to refer a client for diagnosis and when to obtain assistance in modifying the approach to the massage session so that it will best serve the client. Remember—when in doubt, refer!

Contraindication Terminology and Types

There are multiple terms used to categorized contraindications. Contraindications can be divided into regional and general types, and each type can involve avoidance or application with caution and appropriate massage adaptations.

Terms used to describe contraindications include:

- *Absolute/total contraindication*: When a particular treatment or procedure should not be used under any circumstance because of the severe and potentially life-threatening risks involved and the reason for not performing a particular diagnostic or therapeutic procedure is so compelling that performing the procedure would constitute malpractice. An absolute/total contraindication suggests that massage must be avoided. Although there are few absolute contraindications to massage, so long as proper cautions and adaptations are used, it is important to be aware of situations in which a client could be harmed more than helped by massage. Appendix A describes conditions that may present absolute/total contraindications.
- *General contraindications*: This term can be used to mean absolute/total contraindication or be considered as a unique category where the intervention is delayed for a period of time or modified extensively. General contraindications exist for acute infections in which fever is present. Other reasons for general avoidance of massage include a significant decline in a client's health status and adaptive capacity. Additionally, a pattern of changes in a client's health requires a physician's evaluation to rule out serious underlying conditions, and referral is indicated. Mental health dysfunctions can fall into this category.
- *Relative Contraindication*: This term can be used when a particular treatment or procedure should be used with caution. The risk of using the treatment or procedure is acceptable because the benefits outweigh the risks. Precautions and cautions relate to relative contraindications.
- *Regional/local contraindications*: relate to a specific area of the body. For our purposes, a regional contraindication means that massage may be provided but not to the problematic area. The client should be referred to a physician, who can make a diagnosis and rule out underlying conditions.
- *Precaution*: A precaution exists when the risk of adverse reactions becomes more likely. However, the risk for this happening is less than the risk expected with a contraindication. Precautions are also measures taken in advance to prevent something dangerous, unpleasant, or inconvenient from happening. Precautions relate to risk assessment based on the idea that the potential for benefit is more than the potential for harm and potential harm can be reduced with adaptive measures. Example: A massage therapy–related precaution would be scheduling of massage sessions after an athletic competition instead of before to limit any potential that massage might alter performance.
- *Caution*: can be used interchangeably with precaution or relative contraindication or to indicate that some sort of situation requires more thoughtful planning and adaption. Common adaptations required by cautions include the type of massage lubricant used, depth of pressure, duration of the massage, client positioning, avoidance of a type of massage application etc.

Examples

- An elderly client has osteoporosis and thinning skin. Both of these conditions are cautions for massage application. Adaptation of the massage to benefit this client would include careful monitoring of depth of pressure and using enough lubricant to reduce friction on the skin.
- A middle-aged client has plantar fasciitis. Two days prior they received a cortisone injection at the site of inflammation. The caution is the site of the injection; the area needs to be avoided.

Appendix A provides guidelines to help you make decisions about the safety of massage.

Medications

The massage professional needs to be aware of any medications the client takes. Internet resources are available, such as MedlinePlus for researching medications. In addition, clients may be able to provide information about each medication they take.

In general, a medication is prescribed to do one of the following:

- Stimulate a body process.
- Inhibit a body process.
- Replace a chemical in the body.

Therapeutic massage also can stimulate, inhibit, and replace body functions. When the medication and massage stimulate the same process, the effects are **synergistic**, and the result can be too much stimulation. If the medication and massage inhibit the same process, the result again is synergistic, but this time with too much inhibition. If the medication stimulates an effect and massage inhibits the same effect, massage can be **antagonistic** to the medication. Although massage seldom interacts substantially with a medication that replaces a body chemical, it is important to be aware of possible synergistic or inhibitory effects.

Massage often can be used to manage undesirable side effects of medications. In particular, medications that stimulate sympathetic ANS function can cause uncomfortable side effects, such as digestive upset, constipation, anxiety or restlessness, and sleep disruption. The mild inhibitory effects of massage resulting from stimulation of parasympathetic activity sometimes can provide short-term relief of the undesirable effects of the medication without interfering with its desired action. Especially in these instances, caution is required, as is close monitoring by the primary care physician. For example, a side effect of some medications is anxiety. Massage may help by reducing anxiety, or it may be the cause of an adverse reaction. If the physician is using the client's level of anxiety to monitor the correct medication dosage and if anxiety levels are lowered through massage, the medication dosage may appear too high.

Massage professionals should be able to assess the effects of medications and should be aware of the ways massage may influence these effects. Massage practitioners need to be especially knowledgeable about antiinflammatory drugs, muscle relaxants, anticoagulants (blood thinners), analgesics (pain modulators), and other medications that alter sensation, muscle tone, standard reflex reactions, cardiovascular function, kidney or liver function, or personality. They also should be aware of the effects of over-the-counter (OTC) medications, herbs, and vitamins. Additional information on basic pharmacology and a list of common medications and possible interactions with massage can be found on the Evolve site.

Medical Emergencies

Although such situations are rare, a massage therapist may have a client who experiences a medical emergency. All massage therapists should have current first aid training. First aid training is primarily received through the American Heart Association, American Red Cross, and National Safety Council (NSC), all of which offer standard and advanced first aid courses via their local chapter/training centers (Box 6.6).

Massage practitioners should be especially aware of the conditions discussed in the following sections.

Venous Thromboembolism (Deep Vein Thrombosis and Pulmonary Embolism)

Venous thromboembolism (VTE) is a disease that includes both deep vein thrombosis (DVT) and pulmonary embolism (PE). DVT is an underdiagnosed, serious, potentially preventable medical condition that occurs when a blood clot forms in a deep vein, such as in the lower leg, the thigh, or the pelvis. A PE occurs when part of the clot, or the entire clot, breaks off and travels through the bloodstream to the lungs. Without appropriate diagnosis and treatment, PE can be fatal. Blood clots may form when the flow of blood in the veins is slowed or changed. Risk factors include hypertension, diabetes mellitus, cigarette smoking, a high cholesterol level, immobility, sitting for extended periods, air travel, surgery, cancer treatment, giving birth within the previous 6 months, pregnancy, obesity, fractures in the pelvis or legs, and some medications, including hormone replacement, birth control, and some types of nonsteroidal antiinflammatory drugs (NSAIDs). The lower extremities are the most common site for DVT. Symptoms of DVT include pain or tenderness and swelling. Signs include increased warmth, edema, and erythema (reddening of skin). *Because of the seriousness of this condition, refer the client immediately if it is suspected.*

Stroke

Strokes happen when blood flow to the brain stops. Within minutes, brain cells begin to die. There are two kinds of stroke. The more common kind, called an *ischemic stroke,* is caused by a blood clot that blocks or plugs a blood vessel in the brain. The other kind, called a *hemorrhagic stroke,* is caused by a blood vessel that breaks and bleeds into the brain. "Mini-strokes," or transient ischemic attacks (TIAs), occur when the blood supply to the brain is briefly interrupted. A stroke happens quickly, and most people show two or more signs. The most common signs of a stroke are as follows:

- Sudden numbness or weakness of the face, arm, or leg (mainly on one side of the body)
- Sudden trouble seeing in one or both eyes
- Sudden trouble walking, dizziness, or loss of balance
- Sudden confusion or trouble talking or understanding speech
- Sudden bad headache with no known cause

Females may have unique symptoms:

- Sudden face and arm or leg pain
- Sudden hiccups
- Sudden nausea
- Sudden tiredness
- Sudden chest pain
- Sudden shortness of breath
- Sudden pounding or racing heartbeat

Stroke Warning Signs:

A good memory aid to help you recognize the signs of a stroke is "Spot a stroke FAST."

- **F**acial drooping: Does one side of the face droop or is it numb? Ask the person to smile.
- **A**rm weakness: Is one arm weak or numb? Ask the person to raise both arms. Does one arm drift downward?
- **S**peech difficulty: Is the person's speech slurred? Is the personunable to speak or difficult to understand? Ask the person to repeat a simple sentence, such as "The sky is blue." Is the sentence repeated correctly?
- **T**ime to call 911: If the person shows any of these symptoms, even if the symptoms go away, call 911 and get the person to the hospital immediately.

Concussion

Concussion is a brain injury. All concussions are serious and should be evaluated by a physician Although usually not life threatening, a delayed response to this type of brain injury may lead to bleeding in or around the brain which can be life threatening. The medical emergency issue is that the bleeding may slowly occur over days before becoming potentially fatal. In rare cases, a dangerous blood clot may form on the brain in a person with a concussion and crowd the brain against the skull. Second impact syndrome occurs when a second concussion occurs before signs and symptoms of a first concussion have resolved and may result in rapid and usually fatal brain swelling. Persons taking blood thinners are at increased risk of bleeding. Clients who have had a head trauma may think they are fine and may seek massage for stiffness and headache at the point that the bleeding and swelling is becoming serious and life threatening. Signs of medical emergency include the following:

- Headache that gets worse and does not go away
- Weakness, numbness, or decreased coordination
- Repeated vomiting or nausea
- Slurred speech
- Increasing drowsiness or the client cannot be awakened
- One pupil larger than the other
- Convulsions or seizures
- Inability to recognize people or places
- Growing confusion, restlessness, or agitation
- Unusual behavior
- Loss of consciousness (a brief loss of consciousness should be taken seriously, and the person should be carefully monitored)

Refer immediately to the emergency room and call 911 if necessary. Educate clients that even minor head trauma is serious and head trauma events need medical evaluation and monitoring.

Heart Attack

A heart attack occurs when the blood flow that brings oxygen to the heart muscle is severely reduced or cut off completely. This happens because coronary arteries that supply the heart muscle with blood flow can slowly become narrow from a buildup of fat, cholesterol, and other substances that together are called *plaque.* This slow process is known as *atherosclerosis.* When plaque in a heart artery breaks, a blood clot forms around the plaque. This blood clot can block the blood flow through the heart muscle. When the heart muscle is starved for oxygen and nutrients, the condition is called *ischemia.* When damage or death of part of the heart muscle occurs as a result of ischemia, this is called a *heart attack* or *myocardial infarction* (MI). Symptoms of heart disease that may lead to a heart attack include the following:

- Undue fatigue
- Palpitations: The sensation that the heart is skipping a beat or beating too rapidly
- Dyspnea: Difficult or labored breathing
- Chest pain: Pain or discomfort in the chest from increased activity; this is known as *angina pectoris* (also called *stable angina* or *chronic stable angina*)

The following are signs that can mean a heart attack is happening:

- Chest discomfort. Most heart attacks involve discomfort in the center of the chest that lasts more than a few minutes or that goes away and comes back. It can feel like uncomfortable pressure, squeezing, fullness, or pain.
- Discomfort in other areas of the upper body. Symptoms can include pain or discomfort in one or both arms or the back, neck, jaw, or stomach.
- Shortness of breath with or without chest discomfort.
- Breaking out in a cold sweat, nausea, or lightheadedness.
- Females are somewhat more likely than males to experience some of the other common symptoms, particularly shortness of breath, nausea/vomiting, and back or jaw pain. Learn about the warning signs of a heart attack in females.

If the client shows any of these symptoms, even if the symptoms go away, call 911 and get the person to the hospital immediately.

Sepsis

Sepsis is a life-threatening condition caused by an overwhelming response by the body to infection which begins to cause injury to the body's own tissues and organs. Any infection minor or major can trigger sepsis. The infection can be bacterial, viral, fungal, or parasitic. People who have recently been hospitalized are at greater risk, as are those with an overall increased risk for infection such as the very young or very old and those with chronic diseases or a compromised immune system. The symptoms come on gradually. When there is an infection, sepsis can occur. Sepsis symptoms start off subtly and may mimic a flu or virus. It is important to look for the warning signs of sepsis. Spotting these symptoms early could prevent the body from entering septic shock and could save a life.

Symptoms include the following:

S—Shiver, fever, or extreme cold
E—Extreme pain or general discomfort ("worst ever")
P—Pale or discolored skin
S—Sleepiness, difficulty rousing, confusion
I—Statements such as "I feel like I might die"
S—Short of breath

Mortality from sepsis increases by as much as 8% for every hour that treatment is delayed. As many as 80% of sepsis deaths could be prevented with rapid diagnosis and treatment. Approximately 6% of all hospitalizations are due to sepsis, and 35% of all deaths in hospitals are due to sepsis.

Remember, sepsis is a medical emergency. If sepsis is suspected, refer the client immediately for medical attention.

Anaphylaxis

Anaphylaxis is a life-threatening type of allergic reaction. The condition is severe and involves the whole body. Tissues in different parts of the body release histamine and other substances. This causes the airways to tighten and leads to other symptoms. Anaphylaxis can occur in response to any allergen. Common causes include the following:

- Drug allergies
- Food allergies
- Insect bites or stings

Symptoms develop quickly, often within seconds or minutes, and may include any of the following:

- Abdominal pain
- Abnormal (high-pitched) breathing sounds
- Anxiety
- Chest discomfort or tightness
- Cough
- Diarrhea
- Difficulty breathing
- Difficulty swallowing
- Dizziness or lightheadedness
- Hives, itchiness
- Loss of consciousness
- Nasal congestion
- Nausea or vomiting
- Palpitations
- Skin redness
- Slurred speech
- Swelling of the face, eyes, or tongue
- Wheezing

If the client shows any of these symptoms, even if the symptoms go away, call 911 and get the person to the hospital immediately. A person with a known allergy often carries an epinephrine autoinjector, or EpiPen, with instructions on how to inject into the middle of the outer thigh.

Diabetic Emergencies

It is estimated that more than 20 million people in the United States have diabetes, and an estimated 6 million people are unaware that they have it. People with diabetes may experience life-threatening emergencies as a result of too much or too little insulin in their bodies. Too much insulin can cause a low sugar level (hypoglycemia), which can lead to insulin shock. Insufficient insulin can cause a high level of sugar (hyperglycemia), which can cause a diabetic coma.

Symptoms of insulin shock include the following:

- Weakness, drowsiness
- Rapid pulse
- Fast breathing
- Pale, sweaty skin
- Headache, trembling
- Odorless breath
- Numbness in the hands or feet
- Hunger

Symptoms of diabetic coma, or impending diabetic coma, include the following:

- Weak, rapid pulse
- Nausea
- Deep, sighing breaths
- Unsteady gait
- Confusion
- Flushed, warm, dry skin
- Breath odor of nail polish or sweet apple
- Drowsiness, gradual loss of consciousness

If the client shows any of these symptoms, even if the symptoms go away, call 911 and get the person to the hospital immediately.

Rhabdomyolysis

Rhabdomyolysis is a serious syndrome due to a direct or indirect muscle injury. It results from the death of muscle fibers and release of their contents into the bloodstream. These substances are harmful to the kidneys and often cause kidney damage. Rhabdomyolysis has many causes. Some of the common ones a massage therapist may encounter include the following:

- Muscle trauma or crush injury
- Severe muscle contractions from prolonged seizures
- Extreme physical activity (running a marathon, extreme workouts)
- Drug and alcohol use
- Low electrolytes
- Medications: most notably statins used to treat high cholesterol
- Variety of viruses and some bacteria
- Lack of blood perfusion to a limb

The following are common signs and symptoms of rhabdomyolysis:

- Muscle pain, especially in the shoulders, thighs, or lower back
- Muscle weakness or trouble moving arms or legs
- Abdominal pain
- Nausea or vomiting
- Fever, rapid heart rate
- Confusion, dehydration, fever, or lack of consciousness
- Dark red or brown urine; reduced or no urine output

There have been reports of aggressive, heavy-pressure, friction-based massage causing mild cases of rhabdomyolysis. This type of massage application for an individual with risk factors for rhabdomyolysis, such as extreme exercise, may increase the seriousness of the condition.

Seizure

A seizure is a sudden, uncontrolled electrical disturbance in the brain. Nerve cells in the brain create, send, and receive electrical impulses, which allow the brain's nerve cells to communicate. Anything that disrupts these communication pathways can lead to a seizure. The most common cause of seizures is epilepsy. But not every person who has a seizure has epilepsy. Sometimes seizures may be caused or triggered by:

- High fever, which can be associated with an infection such as meningitis
- Lack of sleep
- Flashing lights, moving patterns or other visual stimulants
- Low blood sodium (hyponatremia), which can happen with diuretic therapy
- Medications, such as certain pain relievers, antidepressants, or smoking cessation therapies, which lower the seizure threshold
- Head trauma that causes an area of bleeding in the brain
- Abnormalities of the blood vessels in the brain
- Autoimmune disorders, including systemic lupus erythematosus and multiple sclerosis
- Stroke
- Brain tumor
- Use of illegal or recreational drugs, such as amphetamines or cocaine
- Alcohol misuse, during times of withdrawal or extreme intoxication
- COVID-19 virus infection

Most seizures last from 30 seconds to 2 minutes. A seizure that lasts longer than 5 minutes is a medical emergency.

Signs and symptoms of a seizure can range from mild to severe and vary depending on the type of seizure. Seizure signs and symptoms may include:

- Temporary confusion
- A staring spell
- Uncontrollable jerking movements of the arms and legs
- Loss of consciousness or awareness
- Cognitive or emotional symptoms, such as fear, anxiety, or deja vu

Endangerment Sites

An endangerment site or *cautionary site* is an area on the body where it is possible to do damage with the application of mechanical force. When the massage therapist is working over an endangerment site, avoidance or lighter pressure is indicated to prevent damage. Endangerment sites include areas in which nerves and blood vessels surface close to the skin and are not well protected by muscle or connective tissue. Deep, sustained pressure in these areas can damage the vessels and nerves; however, surface gliding with lighter pressure is appropriate. Areas containing fragile bony projections that could be broken off also are considered endangerment sites; surface gliding with light pressure also is appropriate in these areas. The kidney area is considered an endangerment site because the kidneys are loosely suspended in

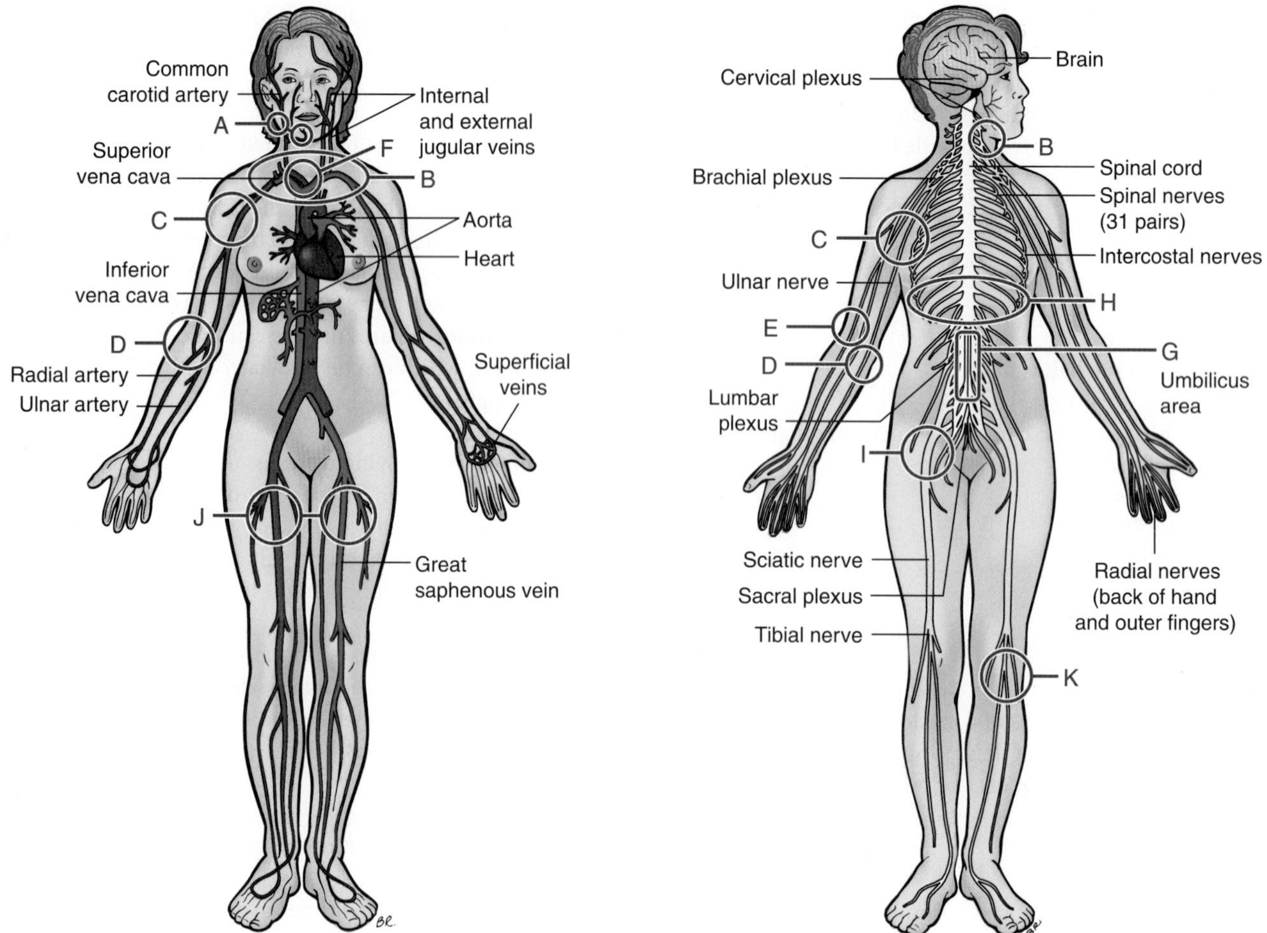

FIG. 6.5 Endangerment and cautionary sites of the nervous system and the cardiovascular system. **A,** Anterior triangle of the neck—carotid artery, jugular vein, and vagus nerve, which are located deep to the sternocleidomastoid muscle. **B,** Posterior triangle of the neck—specifically the nerves of the brachial plexus, the brachiocephalic artery and vein superior to the clavicle, and the subclavian arteries and vein. **C,** Axillary area—brachial artery, axillary vein and artery, cephalic vein, and nerves of the brachial plexus. **D,** Medial epicondyle of the humerus—ulnar nerve; also the radial and ulnar arteries. **E,** Lateral epicondyle—radial nerve. **F,** Area of the sternal notch and anterior throat—nerves and vessels to the thyroid gland and the vagus nerve. **G,** Umbilicus area—to either side; descending aorta and abdominal aorta. **H,** Twelfth rib, dorsal body—location of the kidney. **I**, Sciatic notch—sciatic nerve (the sciatic nerve passes out of the pelvis through the greater sciatic foramen, under cover of the piriformis muscle). **J,** Inguinal triangle located lateral and inferior to the pubis—medial to the sartorius, external iliac artery, femoral artery, great saphenous vein, femoral vein, and femoral nerve. **K,** Popliteal fossa—popliteal artery and vein and tibial nerve.

fat and connective tissue. Heavy pounding is contraindicated in that area; however, other massage methods are appropriate. The areas shown in Fig. 6.5 are commonly considered endangerment sites for the massage therapist (Proficiency Exercise 6.2). Other endangerment sites include the following:

- Eyes
- Area inferior to the ear (fascial nerve, styloid process, external carotid artery)
- Posterior cervical area (spinous processes, cervical plexus)
- Lymph nodes
- Medial brachium (between the biceps and triceps)
- Musculocutaneous, median, and ulnar nerves

Referral

Referral is a method by which a client is sent to a health care professional for diagnosis and treatment of a disease.

PROFICIENCY EXERCISE 6.2

Locate all of the following endangerment sites on a fellow learner:

- Carotid artery
- Brachial artery
- Basilic vein
- Cubital (anterior) area of the median nerve, radial and ulnar arteries, and median cubital vein
- Inguinal triangle
- Axillary area
- Popliteal fossa

Massage professionals may pick up subtle changes in the tissue before the client consciously recognizes that something is out of balance. When this happens, the client should be referred to a qualified professional for a specific diagnosis.

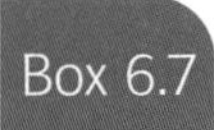

Box 6.7 Example of a Referral by a Massage Therapist

A veteran massage practitioner has been seeing a client every other week for massage for about 1 year. The client has a mole on their left shoulder. At the previous two visits, the massage practitioner noticed that the mole had started to change shape and looked different and thinks these signs should be evaluated by a health/medical care professional with more specific training. The massage practitioner says to the client, "The mole you have on your left shoulder looks a little different to me. Have you noticed any change? It's important to have your doctor look at any changes in a mole. Will you please make an appointment with your personal physician to have the mole examined?"

If the client does not have a personal physician, the massage practitioner could say, "I have talked with various health/medical care professionals in our area and have developed a referral list. I am sure one of the doctors listed will be able to help you, or you can ask a family member or friend for a recommendation."

The client says, "What do you think the change in the mole means?" The massage practitioner replies, "I'm trained to notice changes in the body and indicators that I should refer a client. However, I'm not trained to diagnose any specific condition; that's the role of a physician. You need to have the mole checked by someone with much more training in this area."

Massage therapists should become familiar with the health professionals in their area, including medical doctors, osteopathic doctors, podiatrists, chiropractors, physical therapists, occupational therapists, psychologists, licensed counselors, athletic trainers, exercise physiologists, and dentists. Because clients trust the massage practitioner, the practitioner should take the time to get to know a health professional before referring a client to them. This can be done by calling the professional's office and making an appointment for a short visit, during which the professional's feelings about massage could be discussed. Information about massage should be left for reference.

Clients must always be referred to their personal health care professionals. The massage therapist should make no attempt to direct them to different health care professionals. If the client does not have a physician, nurse practitioner, chiropractor, or counselor, a list of professionals who have been contacted and educated about therapeutic massage should be provided.

When referral is indicated, the massage therapist should simply tell the client the reason for recommending referral to a health care professional, explaining that the observed set of signs or symptoms should be evaluated by someone with more specialized training (Box 6.7). No specific condition should be named. The client should be given the massage professional's business card or brochure to give to the health care professional to facilitate contact. The client must sign a release of information before information can be exchanged between professionals.

FOCUS ON PROFESSIONALISM

Massage therapy must never interfere with or contradict the physician's care plan, nor should the massage therapist assume the role of counselor. If the health care professional must be contacted directly, the massage professional should always work through the receptionist. Leave whatever information is needed with the front desk; if the doctor believes that speaking with the massage therapist directly is important, they will call. Ongoing interaction with the physician follows guidelines for consultations described in Chapter 2.

The reason for referral and the date of referral must be noted on the client's record, along with the signs and symptoms. If the client responds in any unusual way, such as by panicking or refusing to go to the doctor, this must be indicated in the client's record.

As mentioned, most disease processes present with a few basic symptoms (see Appendix A). A client should always be referred for diagnosis if the symptoms listed in Box 6.8 do not have a logical explanation (e.g., if the client has been up late or working long hours, they will show symptoms of fatigue). Massage practitioners should use common sense tempered with accurate information and caution (Proficiency Exercise 6.3).

Box 6.8 Indications for Referral

If any of the following conditions are present and cannot be explained logically, the client should be referred to a health care professional:

- Pain (local, sharp, dull, achy, deep, superficial)
- Fatigue
- Inflammation
- Lumps and tissue changes
- Rashes and changes in the skin
- Edema
- Mood alterations (e.g., depression or anxiety)
- Infection (local or general)
- Changes in habits (e.g., appetite, elimination, or sleep)
- Bleeding and bruising
- Nausea, vomiting, and diarrhea
- Temperature (hot [fever] or cold)

PROFICIENCY EXERCISE 6.3

1. Using the reference section in Appendix A, list five regional/local contraindications to massage that you have encountered (or that you think you may encounter) with clients.
   a.
   b.
   c.
   d.
   e.
2. List the five general or relative contraindications. you think you will encounter most often.
   a.
   b.
   c.
   d.
   e.

Foot in the Door

If you want to get your foot in the door and boost your chances of career success, you must learn how to think and justify the results of massage applications. Clients, employers, and health care professionals who refer clients expect you to know when massage can help or harm and why. Results that meet goals ensure career success. No recipes or checklists are used for massage application. Each client requires individualized and adaptive treatment. You can get your foot in the door by looking and acting professionally, being business savvy, using medical terminology correctly, having good documentation skills, and being able to look up and analyze research. Most important is the ability to identify cautions/contraindications and develop and implement appropriate effective massage care.

SUMMARY

Indications for massage are based on the physiological effects that provide the benefits of massage. Massage is beneficial for most people; however, contraindications do exist. Responsible massage professionals always refer a client for diagnosis and treatment by a qualified health care professional without delay as soon as any condition is noticed that may suggest an underlying physical or mental health problem. After the condition has been diagnosed and appropriate treatment has been established, the massage professional may provide massage under medical supervision. Massage may prove beneficial and supportive to the interventions of the health care professional and may enhance the healing process by temporarily reducing pain, relaxing the client, reducing stress responses, increasing circulation, and much more. In addition, the one-on-one contact given by the massage professional may provide support and compassionate touch during a difficult time, thereby reducing the feelings of frustration, isolation, anxiety, and depression that often accompany illness or periods of stress.

LEARN MORE ON THE WEB

Access to journals: BioMed Central
Information: MedlinePlus, American Chronic Pain Association, National Fibromyalgia and Chronic Pain Association, National Institute of Neurological Disorders and Stroke, National Institute of Arthritis and Musculoskeletal and Skin Diseases, National Center for Complementary and Integrative Health; links and more information are available on the Evolve website

Evolve

Visit the Evolve website: http://evolve.elsevier.com/Fritz/fundamentals/.

Evolve content designed for massage therapy licensing exam review and comprehension of content beyond the textbook. Evolve content includes:

- Content Updates
- Science and Pathology Animations
- Body Spectrum Coloring Book
- MBLEx exam review multiple choice questions

FOR EACH CHAPTER FIND:

- Answers and rationales for the end-of-chapter multiple-choice questions
- Electronic Workbook and Answer Key
- Chapter multiple choice question Quiz
- Quick Content Review in Question Form and Answers
- Technique Videos when applicable
- Learn More on the Web

REFERENCES

Arteaga-Henríquez G, Simon MS, Burger B, Weidinger E, Wijkhuijs A, Arolt V, Birkenhager TK, Musil R, Müller N, Drexhage HA. Low-grade inflammation as a predictor of antidepressant and anti-inflammatory therapy response in MDD patients: a systematic review of the literature in combination with an analysis of experimental data collected in the EU-MOODINFLAME consortium. *Front Psychiatry*. 2019;10:458.

Asim MW, Athanasios P, Dinkar S. Effect of mindfulness based stress reduction (MBSR) in increasing pain tolerance and improving the mental health of injured athletes. *Front Psychol*. 2018;9:722.

Ault P, Plaza A, Paratz J. Scar massage for hypertrophic burns scarring—a systematic review. *Burns*. 2018;44(1):24–38.

Benedetti F, Thoen W, Blanchard C, et al. Pain as a reward: changing the meaning of pain from negative to positive co-activates opioid and cannabinoid systems. *Pain*. 2013;154:361.

Elibol N, Cavlak U. Massage therapy in chronic musculoskeletal pain management: a scoping review of the literature. *Sports Medicine Journal/Medicina Sportivâ*. 2019;15(1).

Eucker Stephanie A, Knisely Mitchell R, Simon Corey. Nonopioid treatments for chronic pain—integrating multimodal biopsychosocial approaches to pain management. *JAMA Network Open*. 2022;5(6):e2216482.

Fava GA, McEwen BS, Guidi J, Gostoli S, Offidani E, Sonino N. Clinical characterization of allostatic overload. *Psychoneuroendocrinology*. 2019.

Gao T, Chen S, Han Y, Tan Y, Zhang D, He Y, Liu M. Abdominal massage regulates the SIRT1/NF-κB signaling pathway to ameliorate inflammation in the adipose tissue of insulin-resistant rats. 2022.

Genik LM, McMurtry CM, Marshall S, Rapoport A, Stinson J. Massage therapy for symptom reduction and improved quality of life in children with cancer in palliative care: a pilot study. *Complement Ther Med*. 2020;48:102263.

Gerdle B, Ghafouri B, Ernberg M, et al. Chronic musculoskeletal pain: review of mechanisms and biochemical biomarkers as assessed by the microdialysis technique. *J Pain Res*. 2014;7:313.

Goodman C, Fuller K. *Pathology: Implications for the Physical Therapist*. 5th ed. St Louis: Elsevier; 2021.

Guidi J, Lucente M, Sonino N, Fava GA. Allostatic load and its impact on health: a systematic review. *Psychothe Psychosom*. 2021;90(1):11–27.

Hsu JR, Mir H, Wally MK, Seymour RB. The orthopaedic trauma association musculoskeletal pain task force. Clinical practice guidelines for pain management in acute musculoskeletal injury. *J Orthop Trauma*. 2019;33(5):e158–e182. doi:10.1097/BOT.0000000000001430.

Juberg M, Jerger KK, Allen KD, Dmitrieva NO, Keever T, Perlman AI. Pilot study of massage in veterans with knee osteoarthritis. *J Altern Complement Med*. 2015;21(6):333–338.

Król M, Kupnicka P, Bosiacki M, Chlubek D. Mechanisms underlying anti-inflammatory and anti-cancer properties of stretching—a review. *Int J Mol Sci*. 2022;23(17):10127.

Lenart-Bugla M, Szcześniak D, Bugla B, Kowalski K, Niwa S, Rymaszewska J, Misiak B. The association between allostatic load and brain: a systematic review. *Psychoneuroendocrinology*. 2022:105917.

Lin TR, Chou F-H, Wang H-H, Wang R-H. Effects of scar massage on burn scars: a systematic review and meta-analysis. *J Clin Nurs*. 2022.

Marazziti D, Arone A, Palermo S, Annuzzi E, Cappellato G, Chiarantini I, Prete LD, Dell'Osso L. The wicked relationship between depression and metabolic syndrome. *Clin Neuropsychiatry*. 2023;20(2):100.

Nedelec B, Couture MA, Calva V, et al. Randomized controlled trial of the immediate and long-term effect of massage on adult postburn scar. *Burns*. 2019;45(1):128–139.

Nielsen A, Dusek JA, Taylor-Swanson L, Tick H. Acupuncture therapy as an evidence-based nonpharmacologic strategy for comprehensive acute pain care: the academic consortium pain task force white paper update. *Pain Med*. 2022;23(9):1582–1612.

Price SA, Wilson LM. *Pathophysiology: Clinical Concepts of Disease Processes*. 6th ed. St Louis: Mosby; 2002.

Rapaport MH, Schettler P, Bresee C. A preliminary study of the effects of repeated massage on hypothalamic–pituitary–adrenal and immune function in healthy individuals: a study of mechanisms of action and dosage. *J Altern Complement Med.* 2012;18(8):789–797.
Romanowski MW, Špiritović M, Rutkowski R, Dudek A, Samborski W, Straburzyńska-Lupa A. Comparison of deep tissue massage and therapeutic massage for lower back pain, disease activity, and functional capacity of ankylosing spondylitis patients: a randomized clinical pilot study. *Evid Based Complement Alternat Med.* 2017;2017.
Schleip R, Duerselen L, Vleeming A, et al. Strain hardening of fascia: static stretching of dense fibrous connective tissues can induce a temporary stiffness increase accompanied by enhanced matrix hydration. *J Bodyw Mov Ther.* 2012;16(1):94–100. http://dx.doi.org/10.1016/j.jbmt.2011.09.003.
Simpson NS, Scott-Sutherland J, Gautam S, Sethna N, Haack M. Chronic exposure to insufficient sleep alters processes of pain habituation and sensitization. *Pain.* 2018;159(1):33–40.
Smith BH. *SP0073 Opioid Prescribing: What's the Problem?* 2018.
Staveski SL, Karen B, Erman L, et al. The impact of massage and reading on children's pain and anxiety after cardiovascular surgery: a pilot study. *Pediatr Crit Care Med.* 2018;19(8):725–732.
Tick H, Nielsen A, Pelletier KR, Bonakdar R, Simmons S, Glick R, Ratner E, Lemmon RL, Wayne P, Zador V. Evidence-based nonpharmacologic strategies for comprehensive pain care: the consortium pain task force white paper. *Explore.* 2018;14(3):177–211.
White GE, West SL, Caterini JE, Di Battista AP, Rhind SG, Wells GD. Massage therapy modulates inflammatory mediators following sprint exercise in healthy male athletes. *J Funct Morphol Kinesiol.* 2020;5(1):9.

MULTIPLE-CHOICE QUESTIONS FOR DISCUSSION AND REVIEW

The answers, with rationales, can be found on the Evolve site. Use these questions to stimulate discussion and dialogue. You must understand the meaning of the words in the question and possible answers. Each question provides you with the ability to review terminology, practice critical thinking skills, and improve multiple choice test taking skills. Answers and rationales are on the Evolve site. It is just as important to know why the wrong answers are wrong as it is to know why the correct answer is correct.

1. If a client is experiencing pain in a surface area away from the stimulated organ, this is termed ______.
a. Muscle pain
b. Referred pain
c. Deep pain
d. Acute pain

2. Neck pain on the right side can be indicative of referred pain from what organs?
a. Appendix and kidney
b. Colon and bladder
c. Heart and lungs
d. Liver and gallbladder

3. Lung and diaphragm pain may be referred to which cutaneous area?
a. Right side of the neck
b. Right side of the chest
c. Left side of the neck
d. In the hip girdle area

4. Facial drooping could be a sign of which medical emergency?
a. Rhabdomyolysis
b. Stroke
c. Anaphylaxis
d. Venous thromboembolism

5. What occurs when medication and massage stimulate the same process?
a. Antagonism
b. Synergism
c. Metastasis
d. Impingement

6. Intractable pain is ______.
a. Cutaneous distribution of spinal nerve sensations
b. A diffuse, localized discomfort that persists for indefinite periods
c. Chronic pain that persists even when treatment is provided
d. An abnormality in a body function that threatens well-being

7. Predisposing conditions that may make the development of disease more likely by the client than by another person are called ______.
a. Metastasis
b. Pathology
c. Signs
d. Risk factors

8. What is the major reason that massage practitioners need to be aware of endangerment sites?
a. These are soft areas that are unable to tolerate any pressure or movement.
b. They may be a sign of a life-threatening disorder.
c. The remaining proximal portions of sensory nerves are exposed here.
d. These areas are not well protected by muscle or connective tissue.

9. A client is complaining of a stiff back from working at the computer for 2 days. There are no stated contraindications. The client wants to reverse the condition. Which approach is the best process?
a. Referral
b. Therapeutic change
c. Condition management
d. Palliative care

10. Which of the following persons may request restorative care from a massage therapist?
a. An athlete with a sprained ankle
b. A 48-year-old individual with a broken arm
c. A person with normal function and adaptive capacity
d. A pregnant person in the first trimester

11. A client is taking an anticoagulant. Which of the following would be contraindicated?
a. Resting stroke
b. Friction
c. Muscle energy
d. Rocking

12. Which of the following is contraindicated for application of deep sustained compression?
a. Lymph nodes
b. Trigger points
c. Dermatomes
d. Ground substance

13. A doctor referral is indicated if the ______.
    a. Client has mild edema in the lower legs after a plane flight
    b. Client complains about care at the local outpatient clinic
    c. Client bruises easily
    d. Client is beginning a new medication
14. A massage client has a history of car accidents. During one of the accidents, they were seriously burned. What additional education would benefit the massage therapist?
    a. Trauma-informed care
    b. Whole person care
    c. Biopsychosocial care
    d. PEACE and LOVE care
15. A massage therapist is developing a care plan for a client scheduled to have knee replacement surgery in the next month. What would be the best approach to care sequence?
    a. Current: relaxation. Immediately after surgery: functional mobility. Six weeks post-surgery: acute pain management. Twenty-four months post-surgery: stress management.
    b. Current: well-being/palliative. Immediately after surgery: restorative. Six weeks post-surgery: stress management. Twenty-four months post-surgery: therapeutic change.
    c. Current: condition management. Immediately after surgery: well-being/palliative. Six weeks post-surgery: therapeutic change. Twenty-four months post-surgery: restorative.
    d. Current: pain management. Immediately after surgery: functional mobility. Six weeks post-surgery: therapeutic change. Twenty-four months post-surgery: well-being/palliative.
16. A massage client is requesting pain management for shoulder arthrosis, stress management to support restorative sleep, and reduced migraine headache frequency. Which type of contraindication is most likely to require the massage therapist to adapt to provide the best care for this client?
    a. Relative
    b. Absolute
    c. Total
    d. Local
17. What would be the most common suggestion for a massage dosage when the approach to care is condition management related to nonspecific low back stiffness?
    a. As needed, 15- to 60-minute sessions
    b. Weekly, 60-minute sessions, ongoing
    c. Twice a week or weekly, 60-minute sessions, ongoing
    d. Daily, twice a week or weekly, 15- to 60-minute sessions, 12 weeks
18. A massage therapist is justifying a massage therapy care plan recommending ongoing weekly massage sessions for an individual with an autoimmune condition. What would be the best indication for massage?
    a. Support productive allodynia
    b. Manage chronic inflammation
    c. Reverse joint pain
    d. Reduce tendency to hyperalgesia
19. A client recently completed a successful course of chemotherapy and radiation therapy, and cancer is in remission. They are experiencing ongoing discomfort related to the treatment. What is most likely occurring?
    a. Brachial plexus impingement
    b. Phantom pain
    c. Viscerally referred pain
    d. Neuropathic pain
20. Which of the following people would primarily seek a massage therapy outcome of relaxation, a well-being approach to care, and have a regional contraindication?
    a. A client with resilience and with contact dermatitis on their arm
    b. A client taking antianxiety medication and is hypermobile
    c. A client who has had multiple right shoulder dislocations and is a competitive athlete
    d. A client taking an anticoagulant medication and is otherwise healthy

Write Your Own Questions

Write at least three multiple choice questions. Make sure to develop plausible wrong answers and be sure that the correct answer is clearly correct. Then write a rationale for each question. The more questions you write, the better you will understand the material. Exchange questions with classmates or discuss in class. The questions from all the learners can be combined to create a review quiz.

Hygiene, Sanitation, and Safety

CHAPTER 7

http://evolve.elsevier.com/Fritz/fundamentals/

CHAPTER OBJECTIVES

After completing this chapter, the student will be able to perform the following:

1. Identify and implement effective health and personal hygiene practices.
2. Explain the major disease-causing agents and implement Standard Precautions.
3. Provide information about human immunodeficiency virus infection, hepatitis, tuberculosis, and other contagious conditions.
4. Describe measures for ensuring a clean, hazard-free massage and a safe environment.

CHAPTER OUTLINE

KEY TERMS

Acquired immunodeficiency syndrome (AIDS)
Aseptic technique
Bacteria
Centers for Disease Control and Prevention (CDC)
Common respiratory virus
Coronaviruses
Environmental contact
Fungi
Harassment
Hazard
Hepatitis
Human immunodeficiency virus (HIV)
Methicillin-resistant *Staphylococcus aureus* (MRSA)
Opportunistic diseases
Opportunistic invasion
Pathogenic animals
Person-to-person contact
Personal protective equipment (PPE)
Protozoa
Sanitation
Standard Precautions
Transmission-Based Precautions
Tuberculosis (TB)
Viruses

This chapter discusses hygiene, sanitation, and safety practices in a professional setting. The information may seem mere common sense, but specific skills are needed to practice massage in a way that protects the safety of both the client and the massage professional. We will also learn about safety in the workplace and how to recognize and avoid harassment and violence.

The primary importance of **sanitation** is prevention of the spread of contagious diseases through practices that contain and dispose of contaminated materials. Worldwide, the major sanitation issues include clean drinking water and proper sewage disposal. For the massage therapist, the term is broadened to mean professional practices that ensure a clean, safe environment, including proper implementation of safety standards established by the **Centers for Disease Control and Prevention (CDC)**. The CDC is the government agency in the United States that is responsible for protecting Americans' health and medical safety. Other countries have similar agencies.

The CDC fights disease and supports communities' and citizens' efforts to do the same. Massage professionals should become familiar with the CDC website (www.cdc.gov) and check it often for health and disease-prevention updates.

Currently, concern is rising about the global spread of infectious diseases caused by several viruses, including the various forms of the influenza virus and coronavirus. Respiratory syncytial virus, or RSV, is a **common respiratory virus**. RSV can be serious for infants and older adults. Once a rare disease in humans, monkeypox cases continue to grow globally, and the World Health Organization and the United States recently declared monkeypox a public health emergency. Although monkeypox spreads primarily through direct skin-to-skin contact, it can also spread by touching environmental surfaces. Multidrug-resistant microbes (MDROs) are on the rise, infecting millions globally. Misuse and overuse of antimicrobials is one of the world's most pressing public health problems. Infectious organisms adapt to the antimicrobials designed to kill them, making the drugs ineffective. People infected with

PROFICIENCY EXERCISE 7.1

Visit and explore the following websites:
Centers for Disease Control and Prevention: www.cdc.gov.
MedlinePlus: http://www.nlm.nih.gov/medlineplus.
American Red Cross: http://www.redcross.org.

List above at least one topic on each site relevant to sanitation or safety.

antimicrobial-resistant organisms are more likely to have longer, more expensive hospital stays and may be more likely to die as a result of an infection.

Human coronaviruses in general and common cold and influenza viruses constantly mutate, preventing the scientific development of any sort of consistent vaccine, and each year the flu and coronavirus vaccines must be developed. The key, then, is prevention. Contagious diseases are best controlled by sanitary practices before infection occurs. Because new information about the spread and control of contagious diseases becomes available almost daily, it is important that massage practitioners keep themselves well informed. As information develops, the CDC adjusts its standards and guidelines for prevention of the transmission of communicable diseases. Massage practitioners are responsible for updating themselves at the very least semiannually on changes in the CDC's recommendations and for following the most recent standards and guidelines.

In addition to a sanitary environment, the massage professional must provide a safe environment. The prevention of accidents and fire for both the client and the professional is an important consideration. The massage professional should be certified in first aid procedures taught by the Red Cross (or a similar agency), cardiopulmonary resuscitation (CPR), and the use of an automated external defibrillator (AED) (Proficiency Exercise 7.1).

Let's begin with the personal care of the massage practitioner. As wellness and health professionals, it is important that we take care of ourselves not only to function at our best but also to set an example for our clients. Clients notice the way we look and act, in addition to our energy and vitality levels. Clients respect professionals who care for themselves. The ethical principle of respect (see Chapter 2) is reflected in the way we care for ourselves and for our clients. Chapter 15 describes in depth the importance of sleep, nutrition, and exercise. Chapter 8 provides guidance for using your body in the most efficient way while performing massage sessions.

PERSONAL HEALTH, HYGIENE, AND APPEARANCE

SECTION OBJECTIVES

Chapter objective covered in this section:

1. Identify and implement effective health and personal hygiene practices.

Using the information presented in this section, the learner will be able to perform the following:

- Identify the basic hygiene procedures important to a professional environment.

One of the best ways to control disease is to stay healthy. If our bodies are strong and our immune systems are functioning properly, we do not become sick easily. If injured, we heal better if we are healthy. Diet, sleep, rest, body mechanics (the way we use our bodies), exercise, and lifestyle all must be considered in the overall health picture, in addition to actively practicing prevention. It also is important to keep to a schedule of regular physical checkups because early detection of disease leads to more successful treatment.

Smoking

Smoking is considered one of the leading causes of disease. It is directly linked to cardiovascular disease, and it is the leading cause of lung cancer. Exposure to secondhand smoke has been found to cause cancer and other health problems in nonsmokers. Besides its dangerous health effects, smoking is offensive to many people. Smoke odors linger in the air and on the hands, hair, and clothing. Many nonsmokers find this smell offensive, and the smell of smoke can cause reactions in sensitive individuals. Because the massage professional works physically close to the client, any smoke odors from the professional are reason for concern. Ideally, the massage practitioner should seek to quit smoking for both personal and professional reasons.

Massage professionals who smoke should inform clients, when they make appointments, that the practitioner smokes. If the client is bothered by smoke odors, referral to a different massage professional is appropriate. Massage professionals who smoke should never smoke in the massage therapy room, even when clients are not present, because the smell of smoke lingers in carpets, draperies, and furniture. If the practitioner must smoke during business hours, it should be done outside, away from any access doors or windows. After smoking, these practitioners should wash their hands carefully and brush their teeth before performing a treatment.

Alcohol and Drugs

Alcohol, cannabis, and drugs interfere with the ability to function as a massage professional. Because these substances affect thinking, feeling, behavior, and functioning, the practitioner must never be under the influence of alcohol, cannabis, or illegal drugs when working with a client; this would be extremely unethical. A massage professional should wait at least 8 hours after the last alcoholic drink or cannabis use before working with a client because it takes this long for the direct effects to wear off. The indirect effects last for the next 24 hours. Clients should be referred or rescheduled if the professional's ability to function is affected. Any prescription or over-the-counter (OTC) medications that affect mental or physical abilities must be considered carefully because use of these substances by the massage professional can place the client at risk.

Hygiene

The massage professional must pay careful attention to personal hygiene (Fig. 7.1). Preventing breath and body odor without using chemical coverups is essential. Massage professionals should not use essential oils, perfume, aftershave, or perfumed hair products during work hours because many clients are sensitive to these odors.

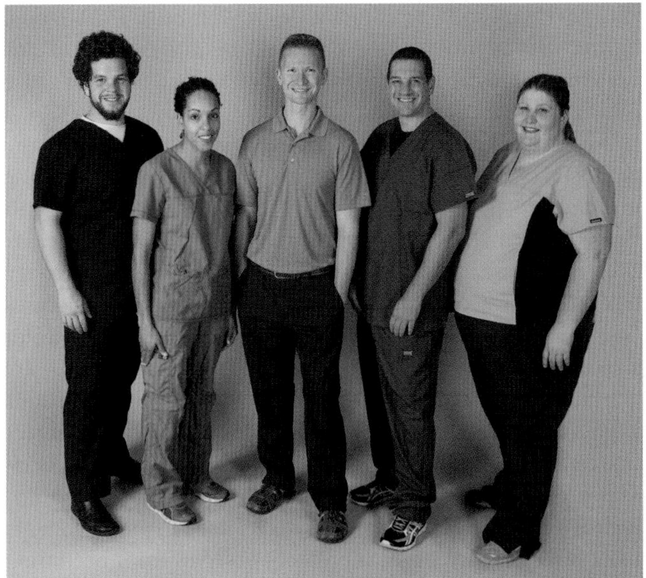

FIG. 7.1 Properly groomed massage professionals. (From Fritz S: *Mosby's massage therapy review*, ed 4, St. Louis, 2015, Elsevier.)

Massage professionals should bathe or shower at the start of each workday. The armpits, genitals, and feet should be washed carefully with soap or a similar cleaning agent. Female professionals must be especially mindful of odor during menstruation.

Because breath odor is offensive, careful brushing and flossing of the teeth and scraping of the tongue after each meal are important. Any food that may cause breath odor should be avoided during work hours. Gum chewing is unsanitary, unprofessional, and irritating to many people and is ineffective in combating breath odors. Breath mints may help, but they are no substitute for good dental hygiene.

Hair should be kept clean. Chemicals such as hair spray or gel must be avoided because they may cause an allergic reaction in chemically sensitive clients. The hair must not fall onto the professional's face or drag on the client. If it is longer than the bottom of the ears, it should be kept pulled back.

Proper care of the hands is especially important. To avoid hurting the client while performing massage, practitioners should keep their nails short and well manicured, and nails should not extend past the tips of the fingers. Fingernails can harbor bacteria and other pathogens. Care must be taken to keep the space under the nails clean, which is best accomplished with a nailbrush. Any hangnails, breaks, or cracks in the skin of the hands must be kept clean and covered during a massage. Intact, strong skin is the professional's first line of defense against infection. Nail polish, nail lacquer or enhanced nail lacquer and synthetic nails promote the growth of bacteria, obscuring a nail infection, hindering the effectiveness of hand hygiene.

Massage work clothing and uniforms should be loose and modest. Because body temperature increases while the professional gives a massage, clothing must "breathe" and absorb and evaporate perspiration. Sleeves should be above the elbow, but the uniform should not be sleeveless. All clothing should be opaque and modest. T-shirts and shorts usually are inappropriate. If skirts or shorts are worn, they should be knee length or longer; loose pants are preferable. Clothing is laundered with detergent in hot water. If clothing comes in contact with a client's bodily fluids, it needs to be laundered in detergent and a disinfectant, such as bleach. The uniform must be able to withstand this type of laundering. If perspiration is heavy or if the clothing becomes stained, the practitioner may need to change clothes. A spare uniform should be kept available. Underclothing must be changed daily, more often if perspiration is heavy. Some professionals use uniforms called *scrubs*. Scrubs meet all the previously mentioned criteria, are inexpensive, and are easy to obtain.

PROFICIENCY EXERCISE 7.2

Design your ideal uniform and ask three massage professionals their opinion of your idea.

The practitioner should wear clean, comfortable shoes while giving a massage. Going barefoot or wearing only socks is neither sanitary nor professional. Changing socks daily helps prevent foot odor (Proficiency Exercise 7.2).

If worn, makeup should be modest; heavy makeup is never appropriate. Facial hair needs to be shaved or neatly trimmed.

Jewelry of all types creates sanitation and safety hazards and should not be worn while giving a massage. Necklaces, bracelets, and hair jewelry can become tangled or can drag on the client, and all types of jewelry, including piercings, can harbor pathogens and collect debris, creating a sanitation hazard. Hand jewelry can harbor pathogens and injure clients; these should not be worn while the practitioner gives a massage. The more professional you look, the more others will treat you as a professional (Focus on Professionalism).

FOCUS ON PROFESSIONALISM

Tattoos, Piercings, Jewelry, and Body Art

Any type of piercing or jewelry, and even eyeglasses, can easily become contaminated and harbor pathogens. Jewelry, including piercings, should be removed during massage, and eyeglasses should be cleaned if touched after each massage. Tattoos do not present a clear safety or sanitation hazard for clients, and massage professionals must decide about the advisability of this type of body art in the professional setting based on different criteria. Various employers require that no tattoos be visible. In this instance, the decision to have tattoos on parts of the body that cannot be covered while giving massage may limit employment opportunities. Clients may be offended by the body art or even think tattoos are unsanitary. This chapter is about sanitation and safety. Because tattoos do not present a hazard to the client, the decision about the professionalism of this type of body art is up to you. Remember that most people are most comfortable with those who are similar in appearance to themselves. It does not matter whether this is right, wrong, fair, or socially acceptable. We all know that we should not judge others by appearance, but we all do it anyway.

SANITATION

SECTION OBJECTIVES

Chapter objective covered in this section:

2. Explain the major disease-causing agents and implement Standard Precautions.

Using the information presented in this section, the student will be able to perform the following:

- Identify the transmission routes for disease-causing pathogens.
- Describe methods for preventing and controlling disease.
- Give specific recommendations for sanitary practices for massage businesses.
- Demonstrate Standard Precautions during massage.
- Develop and implement sanitation practices with an infection control plan to prevent and control the spread of disease.

The content in this section is extremely important. Sanitary massage methods promote conditions that are conducive to health. This means that the massage area and the massage therapist must be clean, and pathogenic organisms must be eliminated or controlled. The importance of sanitation is increasing because more infectious agents are being spread and becoming resistant to treatment.

Pathogenic Organisms

Pathogenic organisms cause disease. Pathogens are spread by direct contact, through blood or other body fluids, or by airborne transmission. They include viruses, bacteria, fungi, protozoa, and pathogenic animals.

Viruses

Viruses invade cells and insert their own genetic code into the host cell's genetic code. They use the host cell's nutrients and organelles to produce more virus particles. By bursting the cell membrane, the new virus particles escape to infect other cells.

Bacteria

Bacteria are primitive cells that have no nuclei. They cause disease in one of three ways: (1) by secreting toxic substances that damage human tissues, (2) by becoming parasites inside human cells, or (3) by forming colonies in the body that disrupt normal function. Because bacteria can produce resistant forms, called *spores,* under adverse conditions, pathogenic bacteria are difficult for the human body to destroy.

Fungi

Fungi are a group of simple parasitic organisms that are similar to plants but have no chlorophyll (green pigment). Most pathogenic fungi live on the skin or mucous membranes (e.g., athlete's foot, vaginal yeast infections). Yeasts are small, single-celled fungi, and molds are large, multicellular fungi. Because fungal, or mycotic, infections can be resistant to treatment, they can become quite serious. *Candida auris* is an emerging fungus that presents a serious global health threat.

Protozoa and Pathogenic Animals

Protozoa are one-celled organisms that are larger than bacteria. They can infest human fluids and cause disease by parasitizing (living off) or directly destroying cells. **Pathogenic animals**, sometimes called *metazoa,* are large, multicellular organisms. Most are worms that feed off human tissue or cause other diseases.

Many of these pathogens cause skin diseases when the pathogen commonly is spread through direct contact. Because massage professionals spend much time working directly with skin, they would be wise to learn to recognize these various skin conditions. Most anatomy, physiology, and pathology textbooks have color plates showing different skin diseases (see Appendix A for color illustrations showing examples of skin disorders).

Intact skin (skin integrity) prevents infection and various skin diseases, whereas abrasions and cuts breach the protective layer of the skin. Therefore it is important that the massage professional obtain additional information about pathological skin conditions. Not only do we need to protect clients from infection; we need to protect ourselves from becoming infected. If the client or professional is ill and if any concern exists that the condition might be contagious, the massage professional should refer to the proper health care specialist and reschedule the client for a time after the condition has healed.

Disease Prevention and Control

The key to preventing many diseases caused by pathogenic organisms is to prevent the organisms from entering the body. This sounds simple enough, but often it is difficult to accomplish. Three primary means by which pathogens can spread are environmental contact, opportunistic invasion, and person-to-person contact.

- **Environmental contact.** Many pathogens are found in the environment—that is, in food, water, and soil and on various surfaces. Diseases caused by environmental pathogens often can be prevented by avoiding contact with certain materials and by following safe sanitation practices.
- **Opportunistic invasion.** Some potentially pathogenic organisms are found on the skin and mucous membranes of nearly everyone. These organisms do not cause disease until they have the opportunity to do so. Preventing opportunistic infection involves avoiding conditions that promote infection. Changes in pH (acidity), moisture, temperature, or other characteristics of the skin and mucous membranes often promote these infections. Aseptic treatment and cleansing of wounds can prevent them.
- **Person-to-person contact.** Small pathogens often can be transmitted in the air from one person to another. Direct contact with an infected person or with materials handled by the infected person is a familiar mode of transmission. The rhinovirus that causes the common cold often is transmitted in these ways. Some viruses, such as the hepatitis B virus (HBV), are transmitted when infected blood, semen, or other body fluids enter the bloodstream.

Precautions

Standard Precautions are used for all client care. They're based on a risk assessment and make use of common sense practices and personal protective equipment that protect health care providers from infection and prevent the spread of infection.

Transmission-Based Precautions are the second tier of basic infection control and are to be used in addition to Standard Precautions for patients who may be infected or colonized with certain infectious agents for which additional precautions are needed to prevent infection transmission. There are three different types of transmission precautions:

- Contact Precautions—used for infections, diseases, or germs that are spread by touching the patient or items in the room (examples: MRSA, VRE, diarrheal illnesses, open wounds, RSV).
- Droplet Precautions—used for diseases or germs that are spread in tiny droplets caused by coughing and sneezing (examples: pneumonia, influenza, whooping cough, bacterial meningitis).
- Airborne Precautions—used for diseases or very small germs that are spread through the air from one person to another (examples: tuberculosis, measles, chickenpox).

Aseptic Technique and Infection Control Plan

Aseptic technique kills or disables pathogens on surfaces before they can be transmitted. Most sanitation conditions for massage require cleaning and disinfection. Occasionally, protective apparel is necessary. In rare instances, use of a mask, gown, and gloves may be appropriate to protect the massage professional or the client. These cases are discussed later in the chapter.

Infection Control Plan

Massage professionals have a responsibility to provide a safe environment for clients. Controlling infection is part of this responsibility. A written infection control program helps prevent or reduce the risk of disease transmission. The plan should outline the policies, procedures, practices, technologies, and products used to clean and disinfect the massage environment. For a disease to be transmitted, a number of conditions must be met; this is referred to as the *chain of infection*:

- A pathogen must be present in sufficient numbers to cause infection. The disease-causing agent may be a virus (e.g., those that cause hepatitis B, hepatitis C, or herpes) or bacteria (e.g., staphylococci, streptococci, or *Legionella* species).
- The pathogen must have a reservoir where it can reside and multiply, such as the bloodstream, mucous membranes, or intestinal tract. This reservoir is the *source host.*
- The pathogen must have a mode of transmission from a source host. A cough or sneeze or contaminated hands that touch surfaces are examples.
- The pathogen must have a proper portal of entry into a new host. For example, for a blood-borne pathogen to cause infection in a new host, it must have a way to enter the bloodstream, such as through a break in the skin.
- The new host must be susceptible to the pathogen. If the individual has been vaccinated or has had a previous exposure to the pathogen that resulted in immunity, re-exposure will not result in disease.

An infection control plan involves breaking one or more links in the chain of infection. Infection control encompasses two main themes: managing contaminated surfaces and proper handling and disposal of contaminated items and waste. The CDC categorizes items based on the degree of contact, which suggests their risk of disease transmission; the risk of disease transmission, in turn, indicates how the items should be processed for reuse. For example, during massage, reusable materials for covering the face cradle have a greater risk of transmission than does the lamp in the room. The CDC lists several categories of items:

- *Critical items* penetrate soft tissue. These generally are not used by massage professionals, although there are some exceptions. For example, in implement-assisted massage, certain tools are used to scrape the skin, and suction cup devices may cause enough damage to the soft tissue to result in bleeding. In such cases these items would be considered critical. Clean or use germicides categorized as chemical sterilants and heat-sterilize critical instruments before each use.
- *Semicritical items* touch only mucous membranes. They have a lower risk of transmission than do critical items. The linens used during massage might touch mucous membranes of the eyes, nose, and mouth; therefore these items must be cleaned and disinfected with a high-level disinfection product before each use.
- *Noncritical items* contact only intact skin and have the lowest risk of disease transmission. These items are common in the massage environment. Linens for draping and surfaces (e.g., the massage table) are examples. These items need to be cleaned and disinfected after each use with a hospital disinfectant registered with the Environmental Protection Agency (EPA) (Box 7.1 and Mentoring Tip).

Surface Management

Environmental surfaces include surfaces of equipment, furniture, walls, and flooring. All of these are considered noncritical. Because they carry the lowest risk of disease transmission, they can be managed using methods that are less rigorous. Environmental surfaces are further categorized as either clinical contact surfaces or housekeeping surfaces. *Clinical contact surfaces* are surfaces that come in direct contact with contaminated devices, hands, or gloves. For example, after touching a client, you put the lotion container bottle on a counter; the bottle thus can be considered a device, and the counter is a clinical contact surface. The massage table is a clinical contact surface. *Housekeeping surfaces* are not directly touched (e.g., a picture on the wall).

A barrier can be used on clinical contact surfaces. Using our previous example of the lotion bottle, a disposable towel can be placed on the counter and the lotion bottle put on the towel. Clinical contact surfaces are disinfected with an intermediate- or low-level disinfection product.

The CDC offers the following general guidelines for managing environmental surfaces:

- Follow the manufacturers' instructions for correct use of cleaning and EPA-registered hospital disinfecting products.
- Never use liquid chemical sterilants/high-level disinfectants to cleanse environmental surfaces. Some of these

Box 7.1 Clean, Sanitize, and Disinfect

The Environmental Protection Agency (EPA) has defined three different functions for managing soiled items: clean, sanitize, and disinfect.

- *Cleaning* is the physical removal of surface or area debris. Cleaning removes germs, dirt, and impurities from surfaces or objects. Cleaning works through the use of soap (or detergent), water, and scrubbing to physically remove dirt and germs from surfaces. This process does not necessarily kill germs, but it removes many of them, and removal lowers their numbers and the risk of spreading infection.
- *Sanitize* means using a product that can kill 99.9% of germs identified on the product's label. In general, sanitizers are used on hard surfaces that require a reduction of microorganisms to levels that are considered safe. Sanitizers are most appropriate for use on surfaces that have not been contaminated with bodily secretions or excretions. Sanitizing lowers the number of germs on surfaces or objects to a safe level, as judged by public health standards or requirements. This process works by either cleaning or disinfecting surfaces or objects to lower the risk of spreading infection.
- *Disinfect* means using a product that destroys nearly 100% of pathogens. Disinfectants must be shown to be effective against 99.99% of bacteria in multiple tests. Disinfection works through the use of chemicals to kill germs on surfaces or objects. This process does not necessarily clean dirty surfaces or remove germs; however, by killing germs on a surface that has already been cleaned, disinfection can further lower the risk of spreading infection.

Depending on their effectiveness, disinfectants are classified into three categories: limited efficacy, general efficacy, and hospital-grade disinfectants. The label information on products registered as hospital-grade disinfectants usually indicates effectiveness against *Salmonella choleraesuis, Staphylococcus aureus*, and *Pseudomonas aeruginosa.* The EPA requires that hospital-grade disinfectants be proven effective against these three organisms. Disinfectants should be used on hard surfaces to destroy infectious bacteria and fungi. Hospital-grade disinfectants should be used on surfaces that are known to be or commonly are contaminated with bodily secretions and excretions.

An *antiseptic* is a chemical that can be safely applied over skin and mucus membranes to destroy pathogens. An ideal antiseptic or disinfectant should have the following properties:

- A wide spectrum of activity (i.e., has the ability to kill many different types of pathogens)
- The ability to destroy microbes within a practical period of time
- Stable, with a long shelf life
- Inexpensive and readily available

Bleach (sodium hypochlorite)

Bleach can be used to sanitize or disinfect, depending on the dilution or concentration prepared. Chlorine bleach kills the widest range of pathogens of any inexpensive disinfectant and breaks down quickly into harmless components (primarily table salt and oxygen). Chlorine bleach is effective against most common pathogens, including difficult organisms such as tuberculosis (Mycobacterium tuberculosis), hepatitis B and C, fungi, and antibiotic-resistant strains of staphylococci and enterococci. It even has some disinfectant action against parasitic organisms. Whether a sanitizer or disinfectant should be used depends on the type of contamination of the surface and the desired or required result. These guidelines should be followed when using bleach as a disinfectant to ensure its effectiveness.

Solution Mix

1:10 bleach solution recommended by the CDC for disinfecting 1 cup of bleach per gallon of water, or ¼ cup of bleach per 32 ounces (1 quart) of water

Never mix bleach with ammonia or any other cleaner. Only mix with water.

- Use a fresh chlorine bleach solution daily.
- Bleach solutions should be stored in opaque containers.
- Bleach solutions require a full 10 minutes of contact time to ensure complete disinfection.
- Bleach must be applied to a surface that has previously been cleaned with an appropriate detergent. Care must be taken to completely rinse all detergent residues and thoroughly dry the surface prior to applying bleach so as not to further dilute the bleach solution.
- When cleaning, sanitizing, and disinfecting with bleach, keep your work area well ventilated, and wear gloves to protect your hands.

Other Disinfectants

Choose disinfectant products that are registered with the EPA and regulated by the FDA. Read the labels carefully to determine the kind of microorganisms these products can kill, the contact time required, and how much should be used because full-strength disinfectants require dilution. The EPA registration number is listed on the product's label, along with the manufacturer's claims (e.g., "kills germs such as *E. coli*"). The EPA classifies these products based on the number and stringency of tests they are required to pass.

Look for these types of labels: EPA-registered; meets CDC and OSHA guidelines; effective against *E. coli,* HIV-1, Staph, TB, and Hepatitis A; complies with OSHA Bloodborne Pathogens standard; meets FDA guidelines for sanitizing food surfaces; NSF/USDA Class 1; and meets both Universal and Standard Precautions set by OSHA and CDC. Products will contain alcohols, chlorine and chlorine compounds, glutaraldehyde, orthophthalaldehyde, hydrogen peroxide, iodophors, peracetic acid, phenolics, and quaternary ammonium compounds (quats). The quaternaries commonly are used for the ordinary environmental sanitation of noncritical surfaces, such as floors, furniture, and walls. EPA-registered quaternary ammonium compounds are appropriate for disinfecting medical equipment that contacts intact skin (e.g., blood pressure cuffs). Disinfectants containing quats have several advantages over bleach or bleach-based compounds—namely they do not damage clothing, other fabrics, or carpets; they do not corrode metal pipes or other surfaces; and, although they require a longer contact time to work on bacteria, they are able to clean and sanitize surfaces at the same time.

Remember that how the product is used is just as important as the kind of product used:

1. Clean the areas that need disinfecting thoroughly until they are free of dirt, dust, grease, spills, and so on.
2. Apply disinfectant thoroughly and let it stand for 10 to 15 minutes to maximize its bacteria-killing properties.

Disinfectant Wipes and Sprays

Disinfectant wipes and sprays are convenient to use, but they must meet EPA standards. Disposable wet wipes clean and

Box 7.1 Clean, Sanitize, and Disinfect—cont'd

disinfect but must be wet enough to cover the area. Make sure to follow the directions on the product label.

Hand Sanitizers

If soap and water are not available, an alcohol-based hand sanitizer that contains at least 60% alcohol can be used. Antimicrobial-impregnated wipes (i.e., towelettes) may be considered as an alternative to washing the hands with nonantimicrobial soap soap and water. However, hand sanitizers are not as effective as alcohol-based hand rubs or washing the hands with soap and water for reducing bacterial counts on the hands.

Use Products Safely

Pay close attention to hazard warnings and directions on product labels. Cleaning products and disinfectants often call for the use of gloves or eye protection. For example, gloves should always be worn to protect your hands when working with bleach solutions.

Do not mix cleaners and disinfectants unless the labels indicate it is safe to do so. Combining certain products (e.g., chlorine bleach and ammonia cleaners) can result in serious injury or death.

Handle Waste Properly

Place no-touch wastebaskets where they are easy to use. Throw disposable items used to clean surfaces and items in the trash immediately after use. Avoid touching used tissues and other waste when emptying wastebaskets. Procedures for handling waste include wearing gloves. Be sure to wash your hands with soap and water after emptying wastebaskets and touching used tissues and similar waste.

Learn More and Stay Up to Date

The following websites are excellent sources of more information on cleaning, sanitizing, and disinfecting:
http://www.epa.gov/epp/pubs/products/cleaning.htm.
http://www.cdc.gov/hicpac/pdf/guidelines/disinfection_nov_2020.pdf.

agents present a respiratory hazard and should not be used outside of a closed container.

- Wear appropriate personal protective equipment when cleaning and disinfecting environmental surfaces. Such equipment may include puncture- and chemical-resistant utility gloves; a protective gown, jacket, or lab coat; and protective eyewear or face shield worn with a mask.

MENTORING TIP

The question is often asked, "Should I do massage when I am sick?" There is both an easy answer and a not-so-easy answer to this question. Certainly, if you are sick and contagious you should not work. This is the easy answer. The more difficult question concerns issues such as whether you are contagious. Typically, but not always, a fever indicates an active infection. Also, coughing, a runny nose, vomiting, and diarrhea are related to infection. Some conditions, such as tuberculosis and hepatitis, are contagious but may not show symptoms. All of us should be screened by our physician for these types of contagious conditions.

What about the question, "I am not contagious, but I don't feel good, so do I work?" Such ailments include many chronic conditions, such as low back pain, headache, and a variety of autoimmune conditions. If you cannot provide a quality massage for the client, then this becomes an ethical concern based on value. Clients want reliable service, and these conditions can interfere with quality and reliability. Each of us must make these types of decisions, and using a decision-making process such as that described in Chapter 2 may help.

The guidelines for maintaining clinical contact surfaces are as follows:

- Use surface barriers to protect clinical contact surfaces and change surface barriers between clients. Barrier protection is preferred for surfaces that are difficult to clean.
- After each client, clean and disinfect clinical contact surfaces that are not barrier protected.
- Use an EPA-registered hospital disinfectant with low- to intermediate-level activity to clean clinical contact surfaces. Use an intermediate-level disinfectant if the surface is visibly contaminated with blood (Box 7.2).

Indications for the Use of Standard Precautions by the Massage Professional

Under normal circumstances the massage professional does not come in contact with a client's blood, body fluids, or body substances (e.g., urine, feces, and vomit). However, in rare cases an accident may occur in which such contact is possible. The best recommendation is to always make Standard Precautions part of professional practice (Box 7.3). Gloves are not necessary for most massage sessions unless the skin of the massage practitioner's hands or any skin area of the client has a rash, cut, abrasion, infection, or any other condition that would allow the transmission of fluids. A mask may be appropriate if transmission of an airborne pathogen, such as the flu virus, is a concern. In most cases, use of a mask protects the client from the massage professional's pathogens; therefore a mask is used with clients who have any form of immune suppression, including excessive stress, which makes the client more susceptible to infection.

Required Use of Standard and Transmission-Based Precautions

With additional training and under medical supervision, massage professionals may work with clients who have a contagious condition. In these cases, a knowledge of Standard and Transmission-Based Precautions is essential. However, it is wise to remember the importance of the massage professional's gentle, nurturing touch. Massage therapists must always keep in mind that their normal germs can be very dangerous for any immune-suppressed client, and Standard Precautions must be used to protect the client from viral, bacterial, and fungal infection. Extra effort is required to follow Standard Precautions, but this extra effort should not hinder the safety of either the client or the practitioner. All clients must be treated with respect, dignity, and kindness. The professional must remember to touch the person and not the disease, to see and listen to the person rather than the disease. These are people who are sick—not sick people.

Box 7.2 Sanitation, Facility, and Equipment Requirements for Massage Therapy

Facilities and Sanitation

All permanent structures and mobile facilities where a massage therapist routinely conducts massage and bodywork must meet the following requirements:

- The facility must be established and maintained in accordance with all local, state, and federal laws, rules, and regulations, including building, health, and fire codes.
- A finished lavatory must be provided that is well maintained, provides a system for sanitary disposal of waste products and sewage in a manner approved by local and state law, is capable of being fully closed and locked from the inside, supplies hot and cold running water, is supplied with liquid soap and single-use towels, is supplied with toilet paper at each toilet, and has a sign prominently displayed that encourages hand washing. It must be conveniently located for use by employees and clients. Bathroom doors must be tight fitting, and the rooms must be kept clean, in good repair, and free of flies, insects, and vermin. A supply of liquid soap in a covered dispenser and single-use sanitary towels in a dispenser must be provided at each lavatory installation, in addition to a covered waste receptacle for proper disposal. Lavatory and toilet rooms must be equipped with fly-tight containers for garbage and refuse. These containers should be easily cleanable, well maintained, and in good repair. Any refuse must be disposed of in a sanitary manner.
- Financial responsibility and insurance coverage are necessary. Each establishment must maintain property damage and bodily injury liability insurance coverage. The original or a copy of such a policy must be available on the premises.
- All doors and windows opening to the outside must be tight fitting and must ensure the exclusion of flies, insects, rodents, or other vermin. All floors, walks, and furniture must be kept clean, well maintained, and in good repair.
- All rooms in which massage is practiced must meet the following requirements: (1) heating must be adequate to maintain a room air temperature of 75°F, (2) ventilation must be sufficient to remove objectionable odors, and (3) lighting fixtures must be capable of producing a minimum of 5 foot-candles of light at floor level; this level of lighting should be used during cleaning.
- All sewage and liquid waste must be disposed of in a municipal sewage system or approved septic system. All interior water distribution piping should be installed and maintained in conformity with the state plumbing code.
- The water supply must be adequate, deemed safe by the health department, and sanitary. Drinking fountains of an approved type or individual paper drinking cups should be provided for the convenience of employees and clients.
- Massage therapists shall maintain their facilities to provide for client privacy when clients disrobe; have heating, cooling, and ventilation to enhance client comfort; be lit sufficiently for safety and cleaning; be clean, sanitary, and free of mold and contaminants, clutter, garbage, and rubbish; and be free of flies, insects, rodents, and all other types of pests. The facility must be barrier free, well maintained, and free of falling, tripping, and slipping hazards.
- In any temporary location (onsite/mobile) where the massage therapist conducts massage and bodywork, the massage therapist must provide and use safe, sanitized, and well-maintained equipment, tools, and preparations, sanitary linen practices, and client privacy practices.

Safety

- Provide for safe and unobstructed human passage in the public areas of the premises.
- Ensure that the premises are barrier free.
- Eliminate all falling, tripping, and slipping hazards.
- Maintain a fire extinguisher in good working condition on the premises.
- Avoid all open flames, including candles and incense.
- Maintain adequate lighting.

Equipment

- All equipment and tools used in conjunction with a treatment on a client must be maintained on a regular basis and be cleaned after each use.
- Cushions on tables and chairs, in addition to bolsters and pillows, must be covered with impervious material that is cleaned after every use.
- Massage tables must be covered with an impervious material that is cleanable and must be kept clean and in good repair. The table must be cleaned thoroughly with soap or other suitable detergent and water, followed by an adequate sanitation procedure (10% bleach solution made daily is recommended) before use with each client.

Topical Preparations

- Topical preparations must be stored in a manner that maintains the integrity of the product and prevents spoilage and contamination.
- Massage lubricants, including but not limited to oils, lotions, powders, and alcohol, should be dispensed from suitable containers and used and stored in such a manner as to prevent contamination. Containers must be disinfected after each use.
- The bulk lubricant should be stored separately from the container used for application. The bulk lubricant should be poured, squeezed, or shaken into a separate container. Any unused lubricant that comes into contact with the client or massage professional must be discarded.

Linens

- All clean linens should be stored in compartments, shelves, or cabinets, at least 4 inches off the floor. Used linens must be stored in a closed bag or container while in the massage room or during transport.
- For each client massage therapists must furnish clean and fresh single-service materials, linens, and any other items, materials, or tools that come into contact with a client's body.
- The use of soiled linens is prohibited. All soiled linens must be immediately placed in a receptacle that closes and prevents cross-contamination. They must be handled as little as possible and laundered in a manner that eliminates the risk of spreading parasites, communicable diseases, and infections and removes all residue of topical preparations. All soiled linens should be washed in a machine at a hot water temperature of at least 140°F, with detergent and an antiviral cleaning agent (at least 10% bleach solution, or nine parts water to one part bleach).

Box 7.2 Sanitation, Facility, and Equipment Requirements for Massage Therapy—cont'd

Communicable Disease Control

- Therapists must always practice communicable disease prevention and control.
- Hands and forearms must be clean and washed thoroughly with soap before touching each client. Use an alcohol-based hand sanitizer that contains at least 60% alcohol.
- Any infected wound or open lesion on any exposed portions of the body is a contraindication to massage until the condition has healed.
- Clean clothing must be worn daily to reduce the risk of spreading any communicable disease or virus that may have come in contact with the clothing either at work or home. Clothing must be changed if contaminated.
- Floors should be considered dirty. Any object that falls on the floor should not be used for a client.
- Observe the following rules when cleaning the massage area: (1) Clean from the cleanest area to the dirtiest to prevent soiling of a clean area; (2) clean away from your body and uniform; if you dust, brush, or wipe toward yourself, microorganisms will be transmitted to your skin, hair, and uniform; (3) do not shake linen, and dust with a damp cloth to minimize the movement of dust.

Box 7.3 Standard Precautions and Transmission-Based Precautions

Standard Precautions, established by the Centers for Disease Control and Prevention (CDC), synthesize the major features of Universal Precautions (relating to blood and body fluids), which are designed to reduce the risk of transmitting blood-borne pathogens, and body substance isolation, which is designed to reduce the risk of transmitting pathogens from moist body substances.

Standard Precautions

Standard Precautions represent the minimum infection prevention measures that apply to all patient care, regardless of the suspected or confirmed infection status of the patient, in any setting where health care is delivered. These evidence-based practices are designed to both protect health care personnel and prevent the spread of infections among patients. Standard Precautions replace earlier guidance related to Universal Precautions and Body Substance Isolation. Standard Precautions include (1) hand hygiene; (2) the use of personal protective equipment (e.g., gloves, gowns, face masks), depending on the anticipated exposure; (3) respiratory hygiene and cough etiquette; (4) safe injection practices; and (5) safe handling of potentially contaminated equipment or surfaces in the patient environment.

Transmission-Based Precautions

Transmission-Based Precautions are intended to supplement Standard Precautions in patients with known or suspected colonization or infection of highly transmissible or epidemiologically important pathogens. These additional precautions are used when the route of transmission is not completely interrupted using Standard Precautions. The three categories of Transmission-Based Precautions are (1) Contact Precautions, (2) Droplet Precautions, and (3) Airborne Precautions. For diseases that have multiple routes of transmission, a combination of Transmission-Based Precautions may be used. Whether used singly or in combination, they are always used in addition to Standard Precautions.

The risk of infection transmission and the ability to implement elements of Transmission-Based Precautions may differ between outpatient and inpatient settings (e.g., facility design characteristics). However, because patients with infections are routinely encountered in outpatient settings, ambulatory care facilities need to develop specific strategies to control the spread of transmissible diseases pertinent to their setting. This includes developing and implementing systems for the early detection and management of potentially infectious patients at initial points of entry to the facility.

Standard Precautions apply to (1) blood; (2) all body fluids, secretions, and excretions except sweat, regardless of whether or not they contain visible blood; (3) nonintact skin; and (4) mucous membranes. Standard Precautions are designed to reduce the risk of transmitting microorganisms from both recognized and unrecognized sources of infection in hospitals. Standard Precautions include the following:

- Personal hygiene practices, including hand hygiene and cough etiquette
- The use of personal protective equipment (PPE)
- Aseptic technique
- Safe handling and disposal of sharps and other waste
- Environmental controls, such as design and maintenance of the clinical environment, spills management, cleaning, laundry, and waste management
- Correct reprocessing of reusable equipment and appropriate use of cleaning products

Standard Precautions must be used if it is likely you will come into contact with any of the following:

- Blood, wet or dried
- All other body fluids, except sweat, regardless of whether or not blood can be seen
- Mucous membranes
- Nonintact skin
- Items or surfaces that have come into contact with blood or body fluids

Standard Precautions assist in establishing a basic level of infection control. However, additional precautions are used to prevent the spread of infection when Standard Precautions alone are not adequate, such as when known or suspected infection could be spread (e.g., outbreaks of the flu or gastroenteritis). Often referred to as *Transmission-Based Precautions,* these additional precautions are categorized according to the three routes of infection transmission in health care settings:

- Contact Precautions
- Droplet Precautions
- Airborne Precautions

Contact in the early stage of the illness before visible signs occur. In addition to consistent use of Standard Precautions, additional precautions may be warranted in certain situations as described here. This list from the CDC has been modified for massage therapy practice recommendations:

A. Identifying Potentially Infectious Individuals

Continued

Box 7.3 Standard Precautions and Transmission-Based Precautions—cont'd

B. Facility staff are to remain alert for any patient arriving with symptoms of an active infection (e.g., rash, respiratory symptoms).
C. Clients are directed to reschedule the appointment until symptoms have resolved and the illness has run its course.
D. Contact Precautions
E. Apply to individuals with any of the following conditions or diseases:
- Presence of stool incontinence (may include patients with norovirus, rotavirus, or *Clostridium difficile*), draining wounds, uncontrolled secretions, pressure ulcers, or the presence of ostomy tubes or bags draining body fluids. *(Unlikely in the massage therapy setting, but possible.)*
- Presence of generalized rash or exanthems. An exanthem is any eruptive skin rash that may be associated with fever or other systemic symptoms. Causes include infectious pathogens, medication reactions, and, occasionally, a combination of both *(could occur as an unrecognized illness in its early stages).*

F. Individual may need to be referred and refused treatment until the condition resolves.
G. If providing massage, perform hand hygiene before touching the client and prior to wearing gloves.
H. Personal protective equipment (PPE) use:
- Wear gloves when touching the individual and the immediate environment or the individual's belongings.
- Wear a gown if substantial contact with the individual or his or her environment is anticipated.

I. Perform hand hygiene after removal of PPE. **Note:** Use soap and water when hands are visibly soiled (e.g., blood, body fluids) with known or suspected infectious diarrhea (e.g., *Clostridium difficile*, norovirus).
J. Clean/disinfect the area, including the restroom and any other high-touch points.
K. Droplet Precautions
L. Apply to individuals known or suspected to be infected with a pathogen that can be transmitted by droplet route; these include, but are not limited to, the following:
- Respiratory viruses (e.g., influenza, adenovirus)
- Bordetella pertussis (whooping cough)
- Neisseria meningitides (meningococcus, common cause of meningitis and sepsis); A Streptococcus (group A strep) is a bacterium that can cause many different infections, including strep throat, scarlet fever, impetigo, and others

M. Instruct client to reschedule when the illness passes.
N. If choosing to provide massage PPE, do the following:
- Wear a face mask, such as a procedure or surgical mask, for close contact with the individual; the face mask should be donned upon entering the room.
- If substantial spraying of respiratory fluids is anticipated, gloves and a gown as well as goggles (or a face shield in place of goggles) should be worn.

O. Perform hand hygiene before and after touching the individual and after contact with respiratory secretions and contaminated objects/materials. **Note:** Use soap and water when hands are visibly soiled (e.g., blood, body fluids).
P. Instruct the individual to wear a face mask when exiting the area, avoid coming into close contact with other people, and practice respiratory hygiene and cough etiquette.
Q. Clean and disinfect the area.
R. Airborne Precautions
S. Apply to individuals known or suspected to be infected with a pathogen that can be transmitted by the airborne route; these include, but are not limited to the following:
- Tuberculosis
- SARS-CoV-2
- Measles

T. Refer for medical treatment. Do not provide massage.
U. Perform hand hygiene.
If client is referred for diagnosis, do the following:
- Provide and instruct individual to wear a face mask, avoid coming into close contact with other people, and practice respiratory hygiene and cough etiquette.
- Once the individual leaves, the therapy room should remain vacant for generally 1 hour before anyone enters; however, adequate wait time may vary depending on the ventilation rate of the room and should be determined accordingly.
- If staff must enter the room during the wait time, they are required to use respiratory protection.

Hand Washing

Many consider hand washing the single most important measure for reducing the risk of transmitting organisms from one person to another or from one site to another on the same client. Washing your hands as promptly and thoroughly as possible between clients is important. The facility should have easy access to hand-washing sinks, hand-washing solutions, paper hand towels, and alcohol-based hand products (ABHP) when appropriate.

- Wash the hands after touching blood, body fluids, secretions, excretions, and contaminated items, regardless of whether gloves were worn. Wash the hands immediately after removing gloves, between client contacts, and when otherwise indicated to prevent the transfer of microorganisms to other clients or environments.
- It may be necessary to wash the hands between tasks and procedures on the same client to prevent cross-contamination of different body sites. Use a plain (nonantimicrobial) soap for routine hand washing; use an antimicrobial agent or a waterless antiseptic agent if hand washing is not possible.
- Alcohol-based hand rub is the preferred method for decontaminating hands, except when hands are visibly soiled (e.g., dirt, blood, body fluids). Alcohol-based hand rub means the alcohol-containing preparation designed for application to the hands for reducing the number of viable microorganisms on the hands. In the United States, such preparations usually contain 60% to 95% ethanol or isopropanol. Formulations include foams, gels and liquid rinses.
- Perform hand hygiene before and after glove removal.

Note: Massage therapists may use forearms and feet to apply massage. These areas would be managed using similar procedures for hand washing techniques.

Gloves

Gloves are worn for two important reasons: to provide a protective barrier and to reduce the likelihood that microorganisms on the massage practitioner's hands will be transmitted to clients. Wearing gloves does not eliminate the need for hand washing because gloves may have small, unapparent defects or may be torn during use, and hands can become contaminated during

Box 7.3 Standard Precautions and Transmission-Based Precautions—cont'd

the removal of gloves. Gloves must be changed and the old ones discarded after each use.

- Wear gloves (clean, nonsterile gloves are adequate) when touching blood, body fluids, secretions, excretions, and contaminated items. Put on clean gloves just before touching mucous membranes and nonintact skin.
- Change gloves between tasks and procedures on the same client after contact with material that may contain a high concentration of microorganisms.
- Remove gloves promptly after use, before touching uncontaminated items and environmental surfaces, and before going to another client; wash the hands immediately to avoid transferring microorganisms to other clients or environments.

Masks, Eye Protection, and Face Shields

Wear a mask and eye protection or a face shield to protect the mucous membranes of the eyes, nose, and mouth. A mask provides protection against the spread of infectious, large-particle droplets that are transmitted by close contact and that generally travel only short distances (up to 3 feet) from infected patients who are coughing or sneezing. Massage professionals occasionally use masks.

Gowns and Protective Apparel

Various types of gowns and protective apparel are worn to provide barrier protection and to reduce the opportunity for the transmission of microorganisms. Wear a gown (a clean, nonsterile gown is adequate) to protect the skin and to prevent soiling of clothing. Select a gown that is appropriate for the activity and the amount of fluid likely to be encountered. Remove a soiled gown as promptly as possible and wash the hands to prevent the transfer of microorganisms to other clients or environments.

Modified from the Centers for Disease Control and Prevention, National Center for Infectious Diseases: https://www.cdc.gov/infectioncontrol/basics/standard-precautions.html.

Personal protective equipment (PPE) refers to specialized clothing or equipment worn as protection against infectious materials. Personal protective equipment prevents contact with the infectious agent, or body fluid that may contain the infectious agent, by creating a barrier against the infectious substance.

Gloves protect the hands. Gowns or aprons protect the skin and clothing. Masks and respirators protect the mouth and nose. Goggles protect the eyes. Face shields protect the entire face. The work environment and the status of the client will determine the type of protection needed. The massage professional may need to wear gloves, a face mask, and possibly a gown if a client is infected with a contagious, transmittable disease or if a client is in an immunosuppressed state (such as might occur with chemotherapy) and must be protected from pathogens. Masks should fit snuggly over the nose and mouth. Most likely, the massage therapist who is working with significantly immunosuppressed individuals will be working under the supervision of a medical professional, and it is important to follow all of the medical professional's directions carefully. Proper wearing and removal and disposal of PPE is called donning and doffing.

- Don (put on) and use PPE properly to achieve the intended protection and minimize the risk of exposure.
- Doff (remove) PPE in a way that avoids self-contamination. For example, avoid skin and mucous membrane contact with potentially infectious materials and chemical/biological agents.

There are four key points related to PPE use:

1. Donning PPE: Put on the PPE before you have any contact with the individual and before entering the room.
2. Once you have the PPE on, use it carefully to prevent spreading contamination.
3. Doffing PPE: When you have completed your tasks, remove the PPE carefully and discard it in the receptacles provided.
4. Immediately perform hand hygiene.

Most massage-related activities require the use of a single pair of nonsterile gloves. Products used to manufacture gloves are nitrile rubber, latex, or vinyl. Advantages and disadvantages of each glove type include the following:

Nitrile advantages
- Latex-free
- A high level of touch sensitivity
- Close, comfortable fit
- Durable for wearing for an extended length of time
- A long shelf life

Nitrile disadvantages
- Not biodegradable

Latex advantages
- Close, comfortable fit
- A high level of touch sensitivity
- Durable for wearing for an extended length of time
- Biodegradable

Latex disadvantages
- Latex allergy

Vinyl advantages
- Latex-free
- Most economic option
- Antistatic properties
- Best for use with nonhazardous materials

Vinyl disadvantages
- Looser fit
- Less durable

Gowns

When used for Standard Precautions, gowns are worn if contact with blood/body fluids is expected. For contact precautions, gowns are worn during physical contact and when in the environment. Isolation gowns are made of either cotton or a spun synthetic material that dictates whether they can be

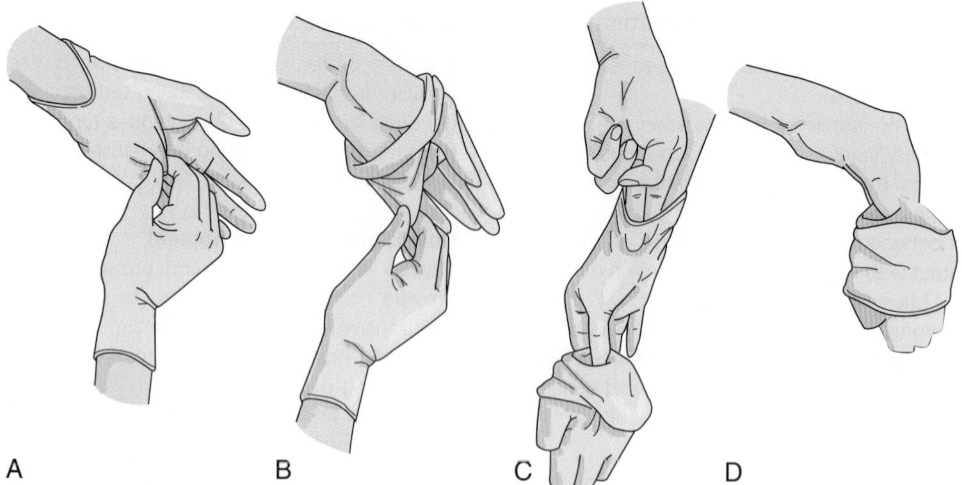

FIG. 7.2 Procedure for removing gloves. A, Grasp the glove below the cuff. **B,** Pull the glove down over the hand, turning the glove inside out. **C,** Insert the fingers of the ungloved hand into the other glove. **D,** Pull the glove down and over the hand, turning the glove inside out. (From Fritz S: *Mosby's massage therapy review*, ed 4, St. Louis, 2015, Elsevier.)

laundered and reused or must be disposed. Isolation gowns are considered clean but not sterile. Gowns are always worn in combination with gloves and with other PPE when indicated.

In general, removal of gloves and gowns involves the following techniques:

Gloves (Fig. 7.2)

- Grasp outside of glove with opposite gloved hand; peel off.
- Hold removed glove in glove hand.
- Slide ungloved fingers under the remaining glove at the wrist; peel off and discard into the proper receptacle.

Gowns

- Remove in a manner that prevents contamination of clothing or skin.
- Turn contaminated outside surface toward the inside (inside out).
- Roll or fold into a bundle, and discard into the proper receptacle.
- Always perform hand hygiene immediately after removing PPE.

Face Mask

A face mask is a loose-fitting, disposable device that creates a physical barrier between the mouth and nose of the wearer and potential contaminants in the immediate environment. It may come with or without a face shield. A face mask is meant to help block large-particle droplets, splashes, sprays, or splatter that may contain viruses and bacteria. Face masks may also reduce exposure of your saliva and respiratory secretions to others. Face masks do not provide complete protection from germs and other contaminants because of the loose fit between the surface of the face mask and your face. Face masks are single-use items and need to be disposed of in the proper receptacle. Wash your hands after handling the used mask.

If massage professionals work in a medical care setting, such as a hospital, an extended care facility, or a rehabilitation center, it is essential that they follow the posted standard precautionary procedures for that facility. Most often the facility will provide special training. If this is not the case and the massage professional is concerned in any way about the application of required sanitation procedures, they should speak directly to the supervisor.

Possible Exposure to Contaminants and Body Fluids

Any individuals whose job may cause them to come in contact with blood or other body substances (e.g., vomit, urine, or feces) should wear single-use, disposable gloves. Such contact conceivably could happen during a massage. The most common blood exposure is to menstrual blood, an incident that can occur if the client's protective product is inadequate. In rare cases, men who have a history of premature ejaculation could be stimulated indirectly by the general massage and ejaculate or leak fluid. An incontinent client could leak urine or feces, or a client could suddenly become sick and vomit. Standard Precautions should be followed during any cleanup.

An infection control kit should be available and is used when an infectious disease is suspected or confirmed. The kit should be kept in a rigid, walled container, such as a bucket; a lid is preferred but not essential. The kit should contain these items:

- Nonsterile examination gloves
- Protective masks
- Tissues, plastic rubbish bags for used tissues
- Disposable vomit bags
- Alcohol-based hand product
- Alcohol wipes or disinfectant spray for cleaning surfaces
- Yellow biohazard bags
- Disposable gown or plastic apron

Cleanup Procedures Using Standard Precautions

Cleaning Agents

Bleach is the preferred cleaning agent. A 10% bleach solution (one part bleach to nine parts water) should be used to clean up spills of body fluids. A bleach and water solution should be prepared daily, and any leftover solution should be discarded at the end of the day. If blood or body fluid seepage is excessive, a stronger mixture of bleach should be used.

The spill should be surrounded with solution and then mopped or wiped up by working slowly and carefully inward to avoid splashes or aerosols (airborne particles). Afterward, the mop head or cloth should be soaked in the bleach solution. The mop head should be agitated carefully to ensure that all its surfaces are exposed to the cleaning fluid. All linens should be rolled to contain the body fluid and double-bagged in plastic, separate from other soiled linens. The outside bag should be marked "contaminated with body fluids." The table should be washed with a strong disinfectant solution and allowed to air-dry.

If a contaminated substance comes in contact with a person's skin, the skin should be washed immediately with soap and hot water and an antiseptic agent applied. When disinfectants are used to kill microorganisms on the body, they are referred to as *antiseptics*. Commonly used antiseptics are isopropyl alcohol, hydrogen peroxide, iodine, phenol, methyl salicylate, and thymol. Most of the antiseptic products on the market contain one or more of these ingredients.

If an open wound is exposed to a contaminated substance, it should be flushed immediately with large amounts of hydrogen peroxide and then washed with hot, soapy water. Hydrogen peroxide should not be used on mucous membranes or in any body orifice (e.g., mouth, eyes).

Any massage equipment and tools that have come in contact with blood or other body substances should be soaked in 10% bleach solution before they are washed in hot, soapy water.

All surfaces, including those in bathrooms, should always be cleaned as if they were contaminated.

Environmental Cleaning

The place where massage is provided is considered the *premise* or *facility*. Local, state, and federal public health codes are the regulations that govern maintenance of a safe environment. The Department of Health and the CDC are the best resources for the most current information on maintaining facilities.

A facility's infection-prevention plan must include procedures for routine cleaning and disinfection of environmental surfaces. *Cleaning* refers to the removal of visible soil and organic contamination from a device or environmental surface using the physical action of scrubbing with a surfactant or detergent and water. Cleaning removes large numbers of microorganisms from surfaces and must always precede disinfection.

Emphasis for cleaning and disinfection should be placed on surfaces that are most likely to become contaminated (e.g., frequently touched surfaces, such as doorknobs). Facility policies and procedures should also address prompt and appropriate cleaning and decontamination of spills of blood or other potentially infectious materials.

Disinfectant products should not be used as cleaners unless the label indicates that the product is suitable for such use. Health care professionals should follow manufacturers' recommendations for use of products selected for cleaning and disinfection (e.g., amount, dilution, contact time, safe use, and disposal).

Complete guidance for the cleaning and disinfection of environmental surfaces, including for cleaning blood or body substance spills, is available in the Guidelines for Environmental Infection Control in Health-Care Facilities and the Guideline for Disinfection and Sterilization in Healthcare Facilities, which are available on the CDC website. Although these guidelines are not massage specific, the recommendations are appropriate for massage therapy facilities.

To establish policies and procedures for routine housekeeping, cleaning, and disinfection of environmental surfaces, the massage professional should do the following:

- Focus on surfaces that are frequently touched.
- Use EPA-registered disinfectants or detergents/disinfectants labeled for use in health care.
- Follow the manufacturers' recommendations for use of cleaners and EPA-registered disinfectants (e.g., amount, dilution, contact time, safe use, and disposal).

Massage therapists can use the following recommendations for low- or intermediate-level disinfection, depending on the nature and degree of contamination:

- Nonsterile items are those that may come in contact with intact skin but not mucous membranes; these should undergo low- or intermediate-level disinfection, depending on the nature and degree of contamination.
- Environmental surfaces (e.g., floors, walls) generally do not come in contact with the client during delivery of care. Cleaning may be all that is needed to manage these surfaces, but if disinfection is indicated, low-level disinfection is appropriate.
- Cleaning to remove organic material must always precede disinfection or sterilization because residual debris reduces the effectiveness of the disinfection and sterilization processes.
- Many disinfectants are used alone or in combinations in the health/medical care setting. These include alcohols, chlorine and chlorine compounds, formaldehyde, glutaraldehyde, ortho-phthalaldehyde, hydrogen peroxide, iodophors, peracetic acid, phenolics, and quaternary ammonium compounds. Commercial formulations based on these chemicals must be registered with the EPA or cleared by the U.S. Food and Drug Administration (FDA). In most instances, a given product is designed for a specific purpose and is to be used in a certain manner. Therefore users should read labels carefully to ensure that the correct product is selected for the intended use and applied efficiently (Box 7.4).
- Sterilizers (also known as sporicides) eliminate all bacteria and fungi, their spores, and viruses. These products should be used on critical instruments that come in contact with sterile body tissues.
- Disinfectants kill microorganisms, but not necessarily their spores, and should be used on hard, inanimate, nonporous surfaces and semi-critical (contact mucus membranes) and nonporous (contact intact skin, environmental surfaces) objects in health care settings.

Box 7.4 How to Clean

The following methods can be used for the periodic maintenance of housekeeping surfaces:

- Clean floors, walls, sinks, and other housekeeping surfaces with a detergent and water (or an EPA-registered hospital disinfectant/detergent) on a routine basis.
- Consider the nature of the surface, the type and degree of contamination likely, and the location of the surface in the facility to determine how frequently the area should be cleaned. For example, sinks must be cleaned more often than walls.
- Clean mops and cloths after use and allow them to dry before reuse. Alternatively, use single-use, disposable mop heads or cloths.
- Prepare fresh cleaning or EPA-registered disinfecting solutions daily and use as instructed by the manufacturer.
- Clean walls, blinds, and window curtains regularly or when visibly dusty or soiled.

Cleaning Methods

The following are some general guidelines on cleaning methods:

- Hard floors should be cleaned with a wet mop, not a broom. Brooms spread dust and bacteria in the air, aiding the spread of infection.
- For the same reason, hard surfaces should be cleaned with a damp or dust-retaining cloth. For general or routine cleaning, the use of detergent and warm water is acceptable.
- Surfaces that come in contact with the client should be cleaned with soap and water, dried, disinfected with a suitable disinfectant, and left to air-dry.
- Surfaces contaminated with oils and grime should be cleaned with detergent and water before a disinfectant is used.
- Reusable cleaning cloths and mops should be cleaned or washed after use and allowed to dry when stored. Sponges are not recommended because they do not easily dry once wet.
- Carpets and other soft furnishings should be cleaned with a vacuum cleaner fitted with a particulate-retaining filter. Carpet and cloth furnishings provide an ideal breeding ground for microorganisms. These surfaces also are more difficult to clean than nonporous surfaces. The CDC recommends avoiding carpet and cloth furnishings.
- Waiting room areas and items should be cleaned regularly with detergent and water using either a spray or wipes. It is important to note that if a disinfectant is to be used, items or surfaces should be cleaned first.
- Clean up spills of blood or other potentially infectious materials and decontaminate the surface with an EPA-registered hospital disinfectant with low-level activity (i.e., HBV and HIV label claims) or intermediate-level activity (i.e., tuberculocidal claim), depending on the size of the spill and the porosity of the surface.

In the facility, make sure an adequate supply of hand hygiene products is available and that the following criteria are met:

- Hand-washing sinks with running water are within easy access of the client treatment rooms. These sinks are used for hand washing only and not for any other purpose.
- Hand basins are fitted with taps that are not hand operated.
- Liquid hand wash or an alcohol-based hand product (ABHP) is provided, preferably in a disposable container.
- Disposable paper towels are available to dry hands completely.
- An ABHP is placed in the treatment room to encourage the practitioner to comply with hand hygiene recommendations.

Stay up to date on policies and news. Be continually aware of updates from organizations such as the CDC, the Society for Healthcare Epidemiology of America, the Association for Professionals in Infection Control and Epidemiology, the Infectious Diseases Society of America, and state and local health departments.

- Sanitizers reduce microorganisms (but do not necessarily eliminate them) to meet the levels considered safe as determined by health codes and regulations. Sanitizers should be used as labeled for food contact or nonfood contact surfaces.
- Cleaning refers to the physical removal of soil and germs by washing or wiping to lift dirt and germs off of surfaces.

Hand Hygiene

The most important disease control measure is hand washing. Hand hygiene procedures include hand washing with soap and water and the use of an alcohol-based hand product (ABHP) that is 60% to 95% alcohol. Proper hand washing is the single most effective deterrent to the spread of disease (Fig. 7.3). The CDC recommends the following steps to properly wash the hands:

1. Wet your hands with clean, running water, and apply soap.
2. Rub your hands together to make a lather, and scrub them well; be sure to scrub the backs of your hands, between your fingers, and under your nails using a nail stick.
3. Continue rubbing your hands for at least 20 seconds. As a 20-second timer, sing "Happy Birthday" or "Mary Had a Little Lamb" twice to the end.
4. Rinse your hands well under running water.
5. Dry your hands with a clean towel or allow them to air-dry.

The following are additional important tips to remember about hand hygiene:

- The hands and forearms must be washed before and after each massage and after blowing the nose or coughing into the hands, touching a contaminated surface, or using the toilet.
- The hands and forearms must be washed in warm, running water for at least 20 seconds to remove any infectious organisms. It is necessary to scrub to remove pathogens.
- Soap or another antiseptic hand-washing product must be used, and a clean towel is used to dry the hands and forearms.
- Faucets and door handles are contaminated and should not be touched after washing the hands. The towel should be used to turn off the water and open the door.
- Frequent hand washing may dry and chap the skin, and using a lotion after washing helps replace natural oils. Using

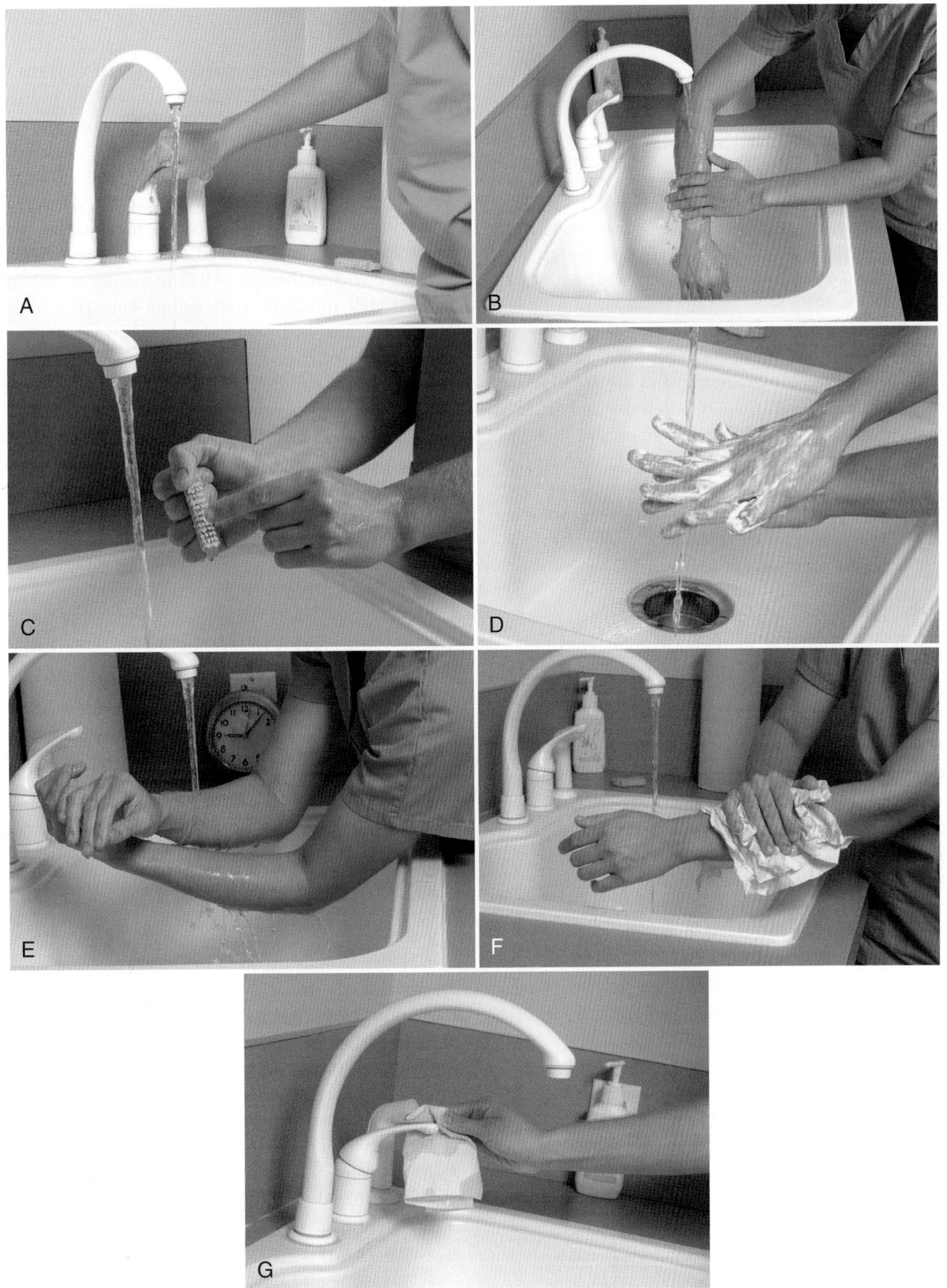

FIG. 7.3 Correct hand-washing technique. A, Turn on the water. **B,** Wet your hands, forearms, and elbows. **C,** Clean underneath your fingernails. **D,** Soap your hands. **E,** Rinse your hands thoroughly. **F,** Dry your hands. **G,** Turn off the water using a paper towel. (From Sorrentino SA, Remmert LN: *Mosby's essentials for nursing assistants*, ed 5, St. Louis, 2014, Elsevier.)

the clean towel to hold the lotion bottle helps prevent contamination of the hands.

- If you use an alcohol-based hand product, follow the manufacturer's directions. In general, apply the product to the palm of one hand. Rub the hands together, covering all surfaces of the hands, fingers, and forearms until they are dry (no rinsing is required). Alcohol-based products should contain ethanol (ethyl alcohol), isopropanol

PROFICIENCY EXERCISE 7.3

Contact your local health department for information on disease control, health practices, and sanitation requirements.

PROFICIENCY EXERCISE 7.4

Obtain a 1-quart spray bottle. Using a permanent marker, mark the bottle so that it is divided into 10 equal portions. This bottle now can be used as a dispenser for a 10% bleach solution: fill the bottle to the first line with bleach; then fill it to the top line with water. Make sure to put the cap on tightly, and then shake the bottle to mix the solution.

(isopropyl alcohol), or n-propanol (n-propyl alcohol), or a combination of these ingredients. The ideal ABHP has an ethanol content greater than 70%. Jewelry and artificial fingernails can interfere with hand hygiene and therefore should not be worn. Fingernails should be kept short (less than 5 mm/0.25 inch long). Bracelets, watches, and rings with stones or ridges should not be worn when providing clinical care (CDC, https://www.cdc.gov/handhygiene/providers/index.html#SkinandNail%20Care 2021).

Respiratory Hygiene and Cough Etiquette

Respiratory hygiene/cough etiquette is a component of Standard Precautions that highlights the need for prompt implementation of infection prevention measures to block the transmission of respiratory infections. Measures include the following:

- Cover the mouth and nose with a tissue when coughing or sneezing. If a tissue is not available, cough or sneeze into the upper sleeve by the elbow (sleeve sneeze). Think, cover the cough.
- Dispose of the used tissue in the nearest waste receptacle.
- Perform hand hygiene after contact with respiratory secretions and contaminated objects or materials.
- If you have respiratory infections, avoid direct client contact. In the rare situation where this is not possible, wear a face mask while providing massage and practice frequent hand hygiene (Proficiency Exercises 7.3 and 7.4).

PREVENTING THE TRANSMISSION OF CONTAGIOUS CONDITIONS

SECTION OBJECTIVES

Chapter objective covered in this section:

3. Provide information about human immunodeficiency virus infection, hepatitis, tuberculosis, and other contagious conditions.

Using the information presented in this section, the student will be able to perform the following:

- Define HIV and AIDS, hepatitis, tuberculosis, coronavirus severe acute respiratory syndrome (SARS and SARS-CoV-2) and methicillin-resistant *Staphylococcus aureus* (MRSA) in detail.
- Identify behavior that could result in the transmission of contagious conditions.
- Use the Centers for Disease Control website to remain current about contagious conditions.

HIV and AIDS

The **human immunodeficiency virus (HIV)** is the virus that causes HIV infection. HIV causes **acquired immunodeficiency syndrome (AIDS)**, the most advanced stage of HIV infection. HIV is spread through contact with the blood, semen, pre-seminal fluid, rectal fluids, vaginal fluids, or breast milk of a person with HIV. In the United States, HIV is spread mainly by having anal or vaginal sex or sharing injection drug equipment, such as syringes or needles, with a person who has HIV.

Antiretroviral therapy (ART) is the use of HIV medicines to treat HIV infection. ART cannot cure HIV infection, but HIV medicines help people with HIV live longer, healthier lives. HIV medicines can also reduce the risk of HIV transmission. Despite more than 30 years of documentation of the AIDS epidemic, there are no known cases of AIDS or HIV infection being transmitted by casual social contact, not even among people living in the same household. The contact between the massage professional and the client falls under this classification because we touch only the skin, which is not a transmission route.

Hepatitis

The liver is the body's largest internal organ. It performs many important jobs, including changing food into energy and cleaning alcohol and poisons from the blood. The liver also does the following:

- Makes bile, a yellowish green liquid that helps with digestion
- Produces proteins and blood-clotting factors
- Regulates glucose (sugar) in the blood, and stores extra sugar
- Works with the stomach and intestines to digest food
- Stores vitamins and minerals
- Removes toxic (poisonous) substances from the blood

Hepatitis swells the liver, preventing it from working well. The disease can lead to scarring (cirrhosis) or cancer. Viruses cause most cases of hepatitis. The various types of the disease are named for the viruses that cause them. For example, the cause of hepatitis A is the hepatitis A virus. Vaccines prevent some viral hepatitis forms. Currently, five different viruses are known to cause viral hepatitis:

- Hepatitis A (HAV): Sometimes called "infectious hepatitis," hepatitis A is spread by eating food or drinking water contaminated with human waste. Hepatitis A is rarely life threatening.
- Hepatitis B (HBV): Also called "serum hepatitis," hepatitis B spreads from mother to child at birth or soon after, and also through sexual contact and contaminated blood transfusions and needles. Hepatitis B may scar the liver (cirrhosis) and lead to liver cancer.
- Hepatitis C (HCV): Formerly known as "non-A, non-B hepatitis," hepatitis C is the most common form of viral hepatitis. It can be transmitted through contaminated blood transfusions or needles, but for a substantial number of patients the cause is unknown. Hepatitis C may scar the liver. About 25% of HIV-positive individuals have hepatitis C, and the disease affects

nearly 90% of injection drug users who have HIV. Hepatitis C tends to be more severe in patients with HIV.

- Hepatitis D (HDV): Hepatitis D most often infects intravenous (IV) drug users who are also carriers of the hepatitis B virus. HDV is spread only in the presence of the hepatitis B virus and is transmitted in the same ways. Hepatitis D is a serious health problem because it occurs in individuals with hepatitis B, increasing the severity of symptoms associated with hepatitis B disease.
- Hepatitis E (HEV): Similar to hepatitis A, hepatitis E is prevalent in countries with poor sanitation. It is rare in North America and rarely life threatening.

Hepatitis A and E are spread through contaminated food, water, and human waste. Hepatitis B, C, and D are spread through an infected person's blood or body fluids.

Acute hepatitis is the initial infection, which may be mild or severe. If the infection lasts 6 months or longer, the condition is called chronic hepatitis. HAV and HEV do not cause chronic hepatitis. HBV, HCV, and HDV can produce both acute and chronic episodes of the illness. Chronic hepatitis B and C are especially serious. Vaccines protect against hepatitis A and B. No vaccines are available for hepatitis C, D, or E. Hepatitis B, C, and D can cause long-lasting problems, including liver scarring (cirrhosis) and cancer.

Following Standard Precautions prevents the spread of hepatitis. It is important to be cautious with all behaviors in which body fluids are contacted and to ensure that no unsanitary conditions exist that may allow the transmission of HIV and the hepatitis viruses.

Coronaviruses

Coronaviruses are common throughout the world. They can infect people and animals. Most species of coronavirus do not affect humans. So far, seven coronaviruses have caused illness in humans—including severe acute respiratory syndrome coronavirus 2 (SARS-CoV-2), which causes coronavirus disease 19 (COVID-19). The COVID-19 pandemic, also known as the coronavirus pandemic, affected a generation and changed the understanding of how disease can affect a population. This virus and many other viruses are transmitted when people breathe in air contaminated by droplets and small airborne particles containing the virus. The risk of breathing these in is highest when people are in close proximity, but they can be inhaled over longer distances, particularly indoors. Transmission can also occur if contaminated fluids reach the eyes, nose or mouth, and, rarely, via contaminated surfaces. It is possible for people to be infected through contact with contaminated surfaces or objects (fomites), but the risk is generally considered to be low. Infected persons are typically contagious for 10 days and can spread the virus even if they do not develop symptoms. Mutations have produced many strains (variants) with varying degrees of infectivity and virulence.

Nonpharmaceutical interventions that may reduce spread include personal actions such as wearing face masks, self-quarantine, and hand hygiene, and community measures aimed at reducing interpersonal contacts such as closing workplaces and schools and cancelling large gatherings.

Disinfection is recommended in indoor community settings where there has been a suspected or confirmed case of COVID-19 within the last 24 hours. The risk of fomite transmission can be reduced by wearing masks consistently and correctly, practicing hand hygiene, cleaning, and taking other measures to maintain healthy facilities.

It is expected that SARS caused by a coronavirus will remain an ongoing infectious agent in the world. COVID-19 vaccines are available, as are other treatments.

Norovirus

Norovirus infection can cause the sudden onset of severe vomiting and diarrhea. The virus is highly contagious and commonly spread through food or water that is contaminated during preparation, contaminated surfaces, or contact with an infected person.

Diarrhea, abdominal pain, and vomiting typically begin 12 to 48 hours after exposure. Norovirus symptoms last 1 to 3 days, and most people recover completely without treatment. However, for some people—especially infants, older adults, and people with underlying disease—vomiting and diarrhea can be severely dehydrating and require medical attention.

Norovirus infection occurs most frequently in closed and crowded environments such as hospitals, nursing homes, childcare centers, schools, and cruise ships. Some people with norovirus infection may show no signs or symptoms. However, they are still contagious and can spread the virus. Proper hand washing and environment decontamination is essential for management.

Pseudomembranous Colitis (Also Called Antibiotic-Associated Colitis or *C. Difficile* Colitis)

Clostridium difficile (*C. difficile*) is a bacterium that causes diarrhea and more serious intestinal conditions such as colitis. Pseudomembranous (SOO-doe-mem-bruh-nus) colitis, also called antibiotic-associated colitis or *C. difficile* colitis, is inflammation of the colon associated with an overgrowth of the bacterium Clostridium difficile (C. diff). This overgrowth of *C. difficile* is most often related to recent antibiotic use. Factors that may increase the risk of pseudomembranous colitis include the following:

- Taking antibiotics
- Staying in the hospital or a nursing home
- Increasing age, especially over 65 years
- Having a weakened immune system
- Having a colon disease, such as inflammatory bowel disease or colorectal cancer
- Undergoing intestinal surgery
- Receiving chemotherapy treatment for cancer

Symptoms include the following:

- Watery diarrhea (at least three bowel movements per day for two or more days)
- Fever
- Loss of appetite
- Nausea
- Abdominal pain or tenderness

C. difficile is more common in people who need to take antibiotics for a long period of time. Elder adults have a higher risk of getting infection. The infection can spread in hospitals and nursing homes. *C. difficile* transmission is most likely a result of person-to-person spread through the fecal–oral route via the hands or, alternatively, direct exposure to the contaminated environment. Hand hygiene is considered to be one of the cornerstones of prevention of transmission of *C. difficile.*

Tuberculosis

Tuberculosis (TB) is an infection caused by a bacterium that usually affects the lungs but may invade other body systems. It is estimated that approximately 1.86 billion people, more than one-third of the world's population, are infected with TB. Transmission occurs via airborne droplets that are produced when an infected person coughs, sneezes, or talks. TB also can be spread through contaminated food.

In many infected individuals, tuberculosis is asymptomatic. In others, symptoms develop so gradually they are not noticed until the disease is advanced. However, symptoms can appear in immunosuppressed individuals within weeks of exposure to the bacillus. Symptoms include fatigue, weight loss, lethargy, anorexia (loss of appetite), and a low-grade fever that usually occurs in the afternoon. A cough that produces a mucous matter that contains pus (purulent sputum) develops slowly and becomes more frequent over several weeks or months. Night sweats and general anxiety often are present. Because these are common signs and symptoms of all chronic infections, referral is necessary for diagnosis. Difficulty breathing, chest pain, and coughing up blood or bloody sputum may also occur as the disease progresses.

Tuberculosis is diagnosed by a positive tuberculin skin test (purified protein derivative, or PPD), sputum culture, and chest x-ray film. A positive tuberculin skin test indicates that an individual has been infected and has produced antibodies against the bacillus. By itself, the positive skin test does not indicate the presence of an active disease. Treatment consists of antibiotic therapy to control active or dormant tuberculosis and to prevent transmission.

Multidrug-resistant Organisms

A multidrug-resistant organism (MDRO) are bacteria that have become resistant to certain antibiotics, and these antibiotics can no longer be used to control or kill the bacteria. Antibiotic resistance often occurs following frequent antibiotic use or frequent exposure to a health care setting. For most healthy people, these bacteria don't cause a problem.

MDRO can enter the body and cause infection. MDRO are most likely to enter the body if:

- There is an open wound in the skin
- There is an IV, catheter, or other invasive device in place
- The person has a suppressed immune system.

Candida auris (*C. auris*)

Candida auris (*C. auris*) is a type of fungus that can cause serious illness. Infections with this fungus can be difficult to treat. C. auris only recently appeared in the United States, and public health officials are researching more about how it is spread. Symptoms may not be noticeable, depending on the part of the body affected. C. auris can cause many different types of infection, such as bloodstream infection, wound infection, and ear infection. C. auris is more likely to affect people who have weakened immune systems from conditions such cancer or diabetes, receive lots of antibiotics, or have devices like tubes going into their body. Most C. auris infections are treatable with a class of antifungal medications, but the fungus is becoming treatment resistant. The primary infection control measures for prevention of C. auris transmission are hand hygiene, transmission-based precautions.

Methicillin-Resistant *Staphylococcus Aureus*

MRSA, an MDRO, is usually transmitted by direct skin-to-skin contact or by contact with shared items or surfaces. Although serious MRSA disease is still predominately related to exposures in hospital or health care settings, MRSA infections outside of health care settings are increasing. According to the CDC, most MRSA infections acquired in the community are skin infections that may appear as pustules or boils; these are often red, swollen, and painful or have pus or other drainage. Most staphylococcal (or "staph") skin infections, including MRSA, appear as a bump or an infected area on the skin. These skin infections commonly occur in cuts or abrasions and on areas of the body covered by hair. Signs may include the following:

- Redness
- Swelling
- Pain
- Warmth to the touch
- Pus or other drainage
- Accompanying fever

Treatment for MRSA skin infections may involve drainage of the lesion by a health care professional and, in some cases, antibiotic therapy.

PREMISE AND FIRE SAFETY

SECTION OBJECTIVES

Chapter objective covered in this section:

4. Describe measures for ensuring a clean, hazard-free massage and a safe environment.

Using the information presented in this section, the student will be able to perform the following:

- Define hazard and risk.
- List potential hazards.
- Recognize and avoid fire and safety hazards.
- Complete an accident report.
- Define, recognize, and report workplace violence and harassment.

Workplace Safety

For any individual to perform well and work productively, a relaxed, congenial work environment must ensure physical safety and help maintain mental balance. Because therapeutic massage promotes a sense of safety, relaxation, comfort, and support, it is necessary to make sure that the environment provides these elements. For example, burning candles can be relaxing, but the danger of a fire or of someone being burned and exposure to the chemical scent are health and safety hazards. Burning candles in the massage environment is not worth the risk. Any type of throw rug in the environment can be a tripping hazard, even if it is part of a beautiful decorating scheme. Plants in the environment are beautiful and can positively affect air quality, but some are very poisonous, and people may be allergic to the pollen. Ensuring the safety of the massage environment requires regular assessment of potential hazards. Consider what could possibly happen, and then do what you can to eliminate or reduce the risk.

Safety Measures

A **hazard** is something that may cause harm or injury. A *risk* refers to the likelihood that a hazard will cause specific harm or injury to people or may damage property. A *health hazard* is any agent, situation, or condition that can cause an occupational illness; these also are referred to as *occupational hazards.* A *safety hazard* is anything that may cause an injury. Safety hazards cause harm when workplace safety controls are not adequate.

The Occupational Safety and Health Administration (OSHA), a division of the U.S. Department of Labor, is responsible for ensuring safe and healthful working conditions. OSHA does this by establishing and enforcing standards and by providing training, outreach, education, and assistance.

OSHA's hazard communication standards require all health professionals to develop and implement a program that involves employee training, compiling a list of hazardous chemicals, maintaining safety data sheets (SDSs), and labeling all chemicals in the office. This program must apply to all activities in which an individual may be exposed to hazardous chemicals under normal working conditions. The hazardous chemicals most likely to be encountered by a massage therapist are cleaning and sanitizing chemicals and essential oils.

Workers are entitled to working conditions that do not pose a risk of serious harm. To help ensure a safe and healthful workplace, OSHA also gives workers the right to do the following:

- Ask OSHA to inspect their workplace.
- Use their rights under the law without fear of retaliation and discrimination.
- Receive information and training about hazards, methods to prevent harm, and the OSHA standards that apply to their workplace, in a language the workers can understand.
- Get copies of the results of tests performed to determine hazards in the workplace.
- Review records of work-related injuries and illnesses.
- Get copies of their medical records.

Identifying Health and Safety Hazards

Risk assessment and management is a process by which potential risks are identified, and control measures to reduce such risks are implemented. Risk assessment is an important activity to reduce risk in the workplace. Box 7.5 presents a checklist of safety measures.

Incident and Accident Documentation

If an incident occurs and there may be a misunderstanding about the intent of the action, immediately acknowledge the error (e.g., slipped draping, unfortunate comment), apologize, and inform the client that you are required to document the incident. The documentation should be placed in the client's file. This lets someone who is looking to falsely accuse know that the incident has already been acknowledged, discussed with the client, and documented. If the massage professional is an employee, the incident must be reported immediately to management. It is unfortunate that we have to be so cautious, but litigation is common, and it is important that you protect yourself.

If an accident occurs, all information about the accident must be written down. An insurance company will need the following information:

- Where and when the accident occurred
- Details about the accident
- Names and addresses of the person or people involved in the accident
- Names of any witnesses to the accident
- Names of manufacturers if equipment is involved

Be careful but not fearful. A confident demeanor combined with professional etiquette prevents most misunderstandings and creates communication channels to resolve unfortunate and unintentional issues. Remember that there is no excuse for unprofessional behavior. Your actions affect the entire massage therapy profession.

Most accidents can be prevented. Knowing the common safety hazards, recognizing which clients need extra assistance, and using common sense are all necessary to promote safety.

Ergonomic Considerations and Safety

According to OSHA, attention must be given to workplace design, which may be associated with musculoskeletal injury and injuries or illnesses caused by forceful exertion; constrained, poor postures; and long-duration or continuous work—these are referred to as *ergonomic hazards.* This issue is especially important to the massage therapist, and it is often neglected or misunderstood because the massage community has not supported an ergonomics and biomechanics assessment of how to provide massage.

Chapter 8 discusses ergonomics and biomechanics in detail. The information presented there has been researched and reviewed by experts in ergonomics and biomechanics to enable massage therapists to safeguard their own body and well-being while providing massage.

Workplace Violence

Massage therapy is based on safe, respectful, compassionate, professional human touch and interaction. Workplace violence is absolutely contrary to the principles of massage ethics, but as massage moves into a broader public arena, the massage professional is more likely to encounter individuals who do not live by the same standards of behavior. No textbook on the professional practice of massage therapy can ignore this subject.

Box 7.5 Checklist for Compliance With Safety Measures

Safety and health are everyone's responsibilities. A checklist, such as the one presented here, can help the massage therapist ensure that these important safety measures have been implemented.

General

- Emergency escape procedures and routes have been developed and communicated to all.
- An alarm emergency warning system is recognizable and perceptible above ambient conditions and is properly maintained and tested regularly.
- All workers know their responsibilities for reporting emergencies, responding to emergency warnings, performing rescue, and providing first aid.
- All work areas are clean and orderly.
- Walking surfaces inside and outside are dry or slip resistant. All floors are slip resistant and are regularly cleaned to maintain a safe surface. All outside entrances are free of clutter and hazards caused by ice, snow, or rain.
- No throw rugs or other tripping hazards (e.g., electrical cords, materials on the floor) are present in walkways.
- Caution signs are posted for doors that open onto stairways.
- Stairways have suitable handrails and are free of worn treads.
- Running on stairs or in corridors, or elsewhere, is prohibited.
- Areas inside and outside are adequately lighted.
- Spilled materials or liquids are cleaned up immediately.
- The appropriate number of toilets and washing facilities are provided, and toilets and washing facilities are sanitary.

Exits

- All exits are marked with an exit sign and illuminated by a reliable light source if used in darkness.
- Directions to exits are marked with visible signs if the exits are not immediately apparent. Doors, passageways, or stairways that are neither exits nor access to exits and that could be mistaken for exits are marked NOT AN EXIT, TO BASEMENT, STOREROOM, or otherwise clearly designated.
- Exit signs are provided with the word EXIT in lettering at least 6 inches high and at least 0.75 inch wide.
- Exit doors are side hinged, are kept free of obstructions, and are unlocked or equipped with an emergency push bar opener and open out in the exit direction.
- There are sufficient exits to permit prompt escape in emergencies. At least two exits are provided from building interiors.

Fire Safety

- No smoking is allowed in the workplace.
- No open flame of any type is allowed in the workplace.
- Windows are easy to open.
- Fire and emergency evacuation plans are posted in appropriate areas.
- All personnel are aware of the nearest emergency exit.
- A written fire prevention plan is developed that describes the types of fire protection equipment and systems available, in addition to established practices and procedures to control potential fire hazards and ignition sources.
- The workplace has a fire alarm system that is tested at least annually; portable fire extinguishers are provided in adequate numbers and types; the extinguishers are mounted in readily accessible locations, recharged regularly, and have dates noted on the inspection tags; and individuals are trained in the use of the fire extinguishers.
- Combustible scrap, debris, and other wastes are safely contained and removed promptly.
- All personnel are rehearsed in how to evacuate the building immediately in case of a fire; they are familiar with the emergency rescue plan of the building and are able to recognize the fire alarms installed in the building; and they know to crawl (not walk) to find ways to escape, to avoid elevators completely, and to stay calm (Proficiency Exercise 7.5).

Equipment

- All equipment is maintained in safe working order through inspection and preventive maintenance programs.
- All personnel are trained to switch off equipment at the power point before pulling out the plug and to not overload circuits and fuses by using too many appliances from one power point.
- Electrical cords are kept off the floor to reduce the risk of damage from drag or contact with sharp objects. A damaged electrical cord can cause a fatal electric shock.
- All electrical fans are protected with guards, which have mesh no larger than 0.5 inch.
- Photocopiers are located in well-ventilated rooms or work areas and are properly maintained to reduce the hazards of emissions, heat, noise, and toner dust.
- Adequate ventilation is maintained throughout the environment to provide fresh air.
- All equipment is used according to the instruction booklets.

Storage

- Supplies are stored so that they do not create a hazard or block lights, fire extinguishers, sprinklers, aisles, exits, or electrical control panels.
- Stored items are stacked, blocked, or interlocked so that they are stable, secure, and will not collapse.
- Storage areas are free of tripping, fire, and explosion hazards.
- Hazardous materials are stored separately from other materials and identified with appropriate warning signs.
- Heavy objects, such as boxes of documents, are placed on shelves low enough to be safe, although not so low that back strain occurs when lifting them.
- Workers use steps or a ladder to reach high objects and never stand on chairs or stacked boxes.
- No top-heavy filing cabinets are used; heavier items are placed in lower drawers. Only one filing drawer is pulled out at a time.
- Objects are not put on top of high furniture.
- First aid supplies are available in a clearly marked container that protects them from damage, deterioration, and contamination. All personnel are trained in basic first aid procedures.
- Emergency numbers, with the address of the business location, are clearly posted near all phones.

Box 7.5 Checklist for Compliance With Safety Measures—cont'd

- All guidelines on infection control from the Occupational Safety and Health Administration (OSHA) are posted in easily visible locations and followed meticulously.

Safety Measures Specific to Massage Therapy Practice

A massage professional's facility must be kept free of hazards. Some clients will need additional assistance to prevent falls or other injury. The following safety rules are guidelines for creating a hazard-free massage environment:

- Never use candles, incense, or any open flame.
- Be cautious with live plants as decoration because some are poisonous.
- Be careful using heat on clients, especially hot stones.
- Daily check and maintain all massage equipment for safety and stability.
- Follow all sanitation requirements regarding infection control for massage linens and supplies.
- Avoid nut-based products for lubricants, and be very cautious with scented products (e.g., essential oils and air fresheners) to prevent allergic reactions.
- Infants and young children should not be left unattended. Parents or guardians should always be present during massage for minors.
- People in the last trimester of a pregnancy should not be left in the massage room alone and may need assistance getting on and off the massage table; they also may need help rolling over.
- Elder adults may be less steady on their feet and should not be left in the massage room unattended.
- Any client whose mobility is impaired, including those with visual impairments, may need assistance getting on and off the massage table. People with disabilities should be asked what assistance they need, and their instructions should be followed carefully.
- When providing assistance on or off the massage table the massage therapists needs to be extremely cautious to avoid harm to themselves or the client. Do not lift the client. Instead assist the client in moving themselves. Learn more at https://www.cdc.gov/niosh/topics/safepatient/default.html.

Preventing falls is important. The massage professional should observe the following rules to prevent falls:

- Provide barrier-free access.
- Provide good lighting (never perform a massage in a dark room).
- Do not use throw rugs; they may slip or tangle around the feet.
- Do not allow clients to get off the massage table with lubricant still on their feet because the lubricant would increase the risk of slipping.

PROFICIENCY EXERCISE 7.5

1. Contact your local fire marshal and learn more about fire prevention.
2. Draw up a fire escape route and emergency plan for your massage business.
3. Contact the local building and safety inspector and find out more about accident prevention.
4. Contact a local insurance agent. Find out about the requirements for reporting accidents to the insurance company and also the insurance plan recommended for this type of protection.
5. Take basic and advanced first aid classes and learn cardiopulmonary resuscitation (CPR).
6. Contact the local or state police to find out more about protecting yourself from violent acts.

Workplace violence can be any act of physical violence, threat of physical violence, harassment, intimidation, or other threatening, disruptive behavior that occurs at the worksite. Workplace violence can affect or involve you specifically, if you are self-employed, in addition to employees and others (e.g., clients) in the environment.

Several events in the work environment can trigger workplace violence. Assault can be considered an intentional act that causes another person to fear they are about to suffer physical harm, regardless of whether actual physical violence occurs. It may even be the result of situations that are not work related, such as domestic violence or road rage that has carried over into the workplace. Workplace violence can be inflicted by an abusive employee, manager, supervisor, coworker, client, family member, or stranger. Whatever the cause or whoever the perpetrator, workplace violence cannot be accepted or tolerated.

There is no sure way to predict human behavior. Although possible warning signs may exist, there is no specific profile of a potentially dangerous individual. The best prevention comes from identifying any problems early and dealing with them. The following are indicators of potential workplace violence:

- Intimidating, harassing, bullying, belligerent, or other inappropriate and aggressive behavior
- Numerous conflicts with customers or clients, coworker, or supervisors
- Statements indicating desperation (over family, financial, or other personal problems) to the point of contemplating suicide
- Direct or veiled threats of harm
- Substance abuse
- Extreme changes in normal behavior

If you notice any of these signs, you should take the following steps:

- If the person is a coworker, notify management immediately about your observations.
- If the person is a customer or client, notify management immediately.
- If the person is your supervisor, notify that person's manager.
- If the person is the owner or manager, there will be no avenues to pursue within the business, making this a difficult situation. Possible avenues include a group intervention with the owner or notifying one of the owner's trusted

peers. However, be sure to take care not to spread unfounded rumors.

Risks for Workplace Assault

Be extra cautious in these situations:
- Poorly lit parking areas
- Delivery of passengers, goods, or services
- Having a mobile workplace
- Working with unstable or volatile individuals
- Working alone or in small numbers
- Working late at night or during early morning hours
- Working in high-crime areas

Bullying

Bullying is a form of aggressive behavior in which someone intentionally and repeatedly causes another person injury or discomfort. Bullying can take the form of physical contact, words, or more subtle actions. Bullying includes actions such as making threats, spreading rumors, attacking a person physically or verbally, and deliberately excluding someone from a group. Bullying in the workplace can lead to increased absenteeism, employee turnover, and even lawsuits.

There is no universally accepted definition of bullying, but most agree that it involves these core elements: (1) intentional aggression, (2) repetition, and (3) the existence of a power difference between the people involved.

The four main types of bullying are verbal, social, physical, and cyber bullying. Cyber bullying is verbal or social aggression conducted through technology. The bullied individual typically has trouble defending themselves and does nothing to "cause" the bullying. Some bullying actions can fall into criminal categories, such as harassment, hazing, and assault.

There should be a zero-tolerance policy to bullying in the professional practice of massage therapy. You must not bully, and you must not allow others to be bullied. Avoid forming exclusive groups and leaving others out. Do not tolerate or participate in any form of gossip. Instead, encourage inclusive team building and communication. Even if you are self-employed, bullying can occur. If you find yourself bullied, it is helpful to increase your communication skills and learn how to become more assertive in a positive and productive manner.

Prevent Violence and Be Prepared

Guidelines and procedures should be established to prevent violence and ensure safety. State clearly to clients and coworkers that violence is not permitted or tolerated:
- Post the antiviolence policy in multiple, easily visible locations.
- Establish a liaison with local police and state prosecutors and report all incidents of violence. Provide physical layouts of facilities to the police to expedite investigations.
- Report all assaults or threats and keep logbooks and reports of such incidents.
- Institute a sign-in procedure for everyone.
- Avoid working alone.
- Do not wear necklaces, to prevent the possibility of strangulation.
- Use the buddy system, especially when personal safety may be threatened.
- Wear identification badges or an embroidered uniform name tag.

Develop a policy that you can implement should a threat occur. Include steps for contacting emergency services, evacuation, and harboring in place. The facility should have a "safe room." This room needs a door that locks and a place to take cover. A bathroom, especially with metal stalls, is a common option. The safe room should be equipped with an emergency mobile phone. Emergency cell phones are affordable and often run on batteries so no charging is necessary. Assemble a crisis kit containing the following items:
- Emergency phone and extra batteries
- Floor plans
- Staff roster and staff emergency contact numbers
- First aid kits
- Flashlights

Be prepared. Invite local police to visit and make recommendations for a safer workplace. Use resources such as Department of Homeland Security (https://www.dhs.gov/xlibrary/assets/active_shooter_booklet.pdf).

Use these guidelines to help you plan a strategy for survival should a threat occur:
- If you hear what sounds like gunshots or popping, immediately assume they are gunshots and do not investigate. Secure yourself and, if it is safe, immediately call 911.
- Proceed to a room that can be locked if possible, close and lock all the windows and doors, and turn off all the lights; if possible, have everyone get down on the floor and ensure that no one is visible from outside the room. If the room cannot be locked, barricade the door with heavy furniture such as desks, tables, and bookcases if possible.
- One person in the room should call 911; you may hear multiple rings but stay on the line until it is answered. Tell the dispatcher what is taking place and state your location; remain in place until the police say "all clear."
- If you determine that escape is possible, run and attempt to alert others as you exit the area/building. As you exit, warn others not to enter the area/building of danger. Do not attempt to carry anything while fleeing; move quickly, keep your hands visible, follow the instructions of any police officer you may encounter, and remain calm.
- Do not attempt to remove injured people; instead, leave wounded victims where they are and notify authorities of their location as soon as possible.

When Violence Occurs

After a violent incident, a person experiences three stages of crisis reaction, to some degree:
- Stage 1: Emotional reactions are characterized by shock, disbelief, denial, or numbness. Also common is a fight-or-flight survival reaction, in which the heart rate increases, perceptual senses become heightened or distorted, and adrenaline levels increase to meet a real or perceived threat.
- Stage 2: Also known as the impact stage, this phase involves a variety of intense emotions, including anger, rage, fear, terror, grief, sorrow, confusion, helplessness, guilt, depression, and withdrawal. This stage may last a few days, a few weeks, or a few months.

- Stage 3: This is the reconciliation stage, in which victims attempt to make sense of the event, understand its impact, and, through trial and error, reach closure. Working through this stage may be a long-term process.

Although it is difficult to predict how an incident will affect a particular individual, several factors influence the intensity of trauma: the duration of the event, the degree of terror or horror the victim experienced, the sense of personal control (or lack thereof) the individual had during the incident, and the extent of injury or loss the victim experienced (e.g., loss of property, self-esteem, physical well-being). Other variables include the person's previous victimization experiences, recent losses (e.g., death of a family member), and other intense stresses. Professional counseling and a supportive social support system help individuals through the reconciliation process.

Sexual Harassment

Sexual harassment is a form of sex discrimination that violates Title VII of the Civil Rights Act of 1964. It includes any unwelcome sexual advances, requests for sexual favors, and other verbal or physical conduct of a sexual nature. Important facts about sexual harassment include the following:

- The victim and the harasser may be any gender. The victim does not have to be of the opposite sex.
- The harasser can be the victim's supervisor, an agent of the employer, a supervisor in another area, a coworker, or a client.
- The victim does not have to be the person harassed but may be anyone affected by the offensive conduct.
- The harasser's conduct must be unwelcome.
- Sexual harassment can occur off business premises if the activity is related to employment (e.g., company picnic, dinner).

Sexual harassment includes a broad spectrum of conduct, including harassment based on sex, gender, gender transition, gender identity or expression, and sexual orientation. According to the federal Equal Employment Opportunity Commission (EEOC) guidelines, sexual harassment is defined as "unwelcome sexual advances, requests for sexual favors, and other verbal or physical conduct of a sexual nature" when the following occurs:

- Submission to such conduct is made explicitly or implicitly a term or condition of employment.
- Submission to or rejection of such conduct by an individual is used as the basis for employment decisions affecting the individual.
- Such conduct has the purpose or effect of unreasonably interfering with an individual's work performance or creating an intimidating, hostile, or offensive working environment.

Sexual harassment can include the following:

- Verbal abuse (e.g., propositions, lewd comments, sexual insults)
- Visual abuse (e.g., leering or display of pornographic material designed to embarrass or intimidate an employee)
- Physical abuse (e.g., touching, pinching, cornering)
- Rape

Box 7.6 Preemptively Protect Yourself

Please respond to each item by placing an X after either Y or N. Protect yourself from false allegations of sexually inappropriate activity. Use written permission any time the following areas are included in the massage session. The following permissions statements are examples:

- Permission to address lower lumbar/ hip region with appropriate draping and total avoidance of gluteal cleft and groin region. Y__N__
- Permission to address abdomen with appropriate draping and total avoidance of pubic and groin region. Y__N__
- Permission to address anterior thorax (chest) with appropriate draping and total avoidance of breast tissue. Y__N__

Prevent sexual solicitation. Clearly inform clients in written documents about a NO TOLERANCE POLICY related to sexualizing the massage session. Use the following illustration to clearly indicate to clients that the following areas are considered NO TOUCH ZONES related to any form of inappropriate or sexualized requests or behaviors. This includes clients touching themselves for sexual purposes.

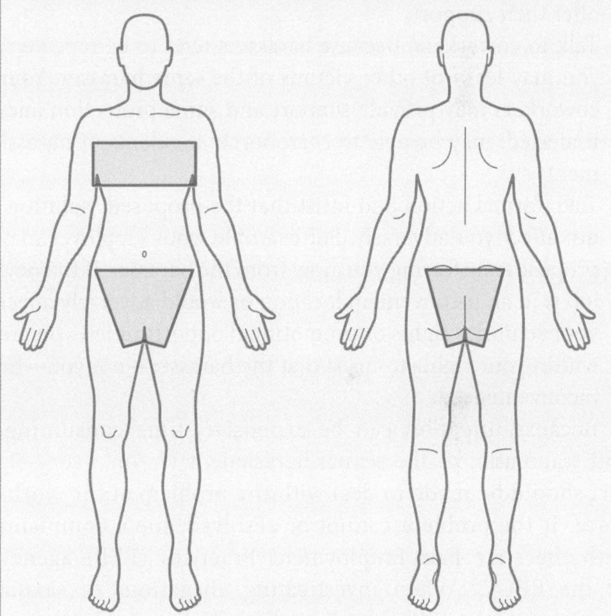

No Touch Figure.

NOTE: There are valid therapeutic reasons for massage in the indicated regions to avoid. However, these areas should only be included in the massage to address specific therapeutic outcomes, always with written permission to protect the massage therapist from misconduct allegations. The genitals or anal area are NOT target areas for massage application.

Vulnerability to Sexual Harassment

Massage therapists may be the victims of sexual harassment by clients because modern society is still confused about the nature and purpose of touch (Box 7.6). Other health professionals also experience sexual harassment. Nurses, for example, often must deal with inappropriate behavior by clients/ patients. If sexual harassment occurs among coworker, do the following:

- Say "Stop" immediately. Directly inform the harasser that the conduct is unwelcome and must stop.
- Object! Make it clear to the harasser that his or her behavior is unwelcome. You may prefer to object verbally in the beginning, but if the harassment continues, object in writing, and keep a copy of the letter. Be specific about what behavior you find objectionable.
- Document the incident.
- Get witnesses' support.
- Make a report using any complaint mechanism or grievance system available.
- Keep a log or diary of incidents, including the date, time, place, behavior, what was said, and names of witnesses. Keep the log in a safe place at home, not at work.
- Do not suffer in silence. The harasser is counting on you to keep it a secret.
- Do not blame yourself. Do not assume that you are doing something to provoke the harassment. Sexual harassment usually is about power rather than sex.
- Talk to friends and family. Let people who care about you offer their support.
- Talk to coworkers. Because harassers tend to be repeaters, you may learn of other victims of the same harasser. Your coworkers may provide support and some protection and, if alerted, may be able to corroborate incidents of harassment.
- Take formal action and insist that the proposed "solution" not affect you adversely. For example, your employer may propose transferring you away from the harasser. If the new job is in an inconvenient location or would adversely affect your seniority rights or promotional opportunities, you are within your rights to insist that the harasser—not you—be inconvenienced.

Because litigation can be expensive, time consuming, and traumatic for the sexual harassment victim, every effort should be made to deal with the problem at the workplace. If the problem cannot be resolved, file a complaint with the state Fair Employment Practices (FEP) agency or the EEOC. When investigating allegations of sexual harassment, the EEOC looks at the whole record: the circumstances, such as the nature of the sexual advances, and the context in which the alleged incidents occurred. A determination on the allegations is made from the facts on a case-by-case basis. You can also consult an attorney experienced in sexual harassment cases. If the harasser's behavior included assault and battery or rape, file criminal charges with the police.

If a massage therapist is sexually harassed by a client and is working where reception services are provided:

- Leave the room immediately.
- Immediately report the incident to the front desk and go to the breakroom or other safe location.
- Write down every detail of the incident, including your behavior and the behavior of the client.
- Ask the front desk staff to tell the harasser to leave. If only one person is at front desk, and this individual could be vulnerable to harassment or assault, they should leave the area and place a note for the client on the counter telling the individual to leave. If you suspect any possibility of aggressive behavior, call 911.

If a massage therapist who works alone is sexually harassed by a client:

- Leave the room.
- Go to a safe room or leave the facility.
- Call 911.

Solicitation for sexual services is a crime. Report the incident to the police. Clearly post in a visible place that there is *zero tolerance* for any type of sexual behavior/harassment from anyone: clients, massage therapists, or other staff.

If a client believes a massage therapist sexually harassed them, the client should be informed that there is a zero-tolerance policy for inappropriate touch and sexual harassment. Clients and staff should have clear policies in place for what is safe touch in massage and what is inappropriate touch. Policies need to be clear and describe how to manage accidents such as a slipped drape or in inadvertent, unintentional touch in a no-touch area. All reports should be acknowledged respectfully and be thoroughly documented.

Prevention

Prevention is the best tool to eliminate sexual harassment in the workplace (see Box 7.6). If you are self-employed, clearly explain to clients what constitutes assault and sexual harassment and the result of inappropriate behavior. Also clearly post rules for behavior, including the reporting process for clients if a massage therapist behaves inappropriately. Employers are encouraged to take the necessary steps to prevent sexual harassment. They should clearly communicate to employees, customers, clients, and anyone who enters the environment that sexual harassment is not tolerated. They can do so by posting the business policy against sexual harassment in a prominent, highly visible place; establishing an effective complaint or grievance process; and taking immediate and appropriate action when an employee complains. The number of sexual harassment incidents in the massage business setting can be decreased by employing the following measures:

- Draft, publicize, and prominently post a zero-tolerance sexual harassment policy. The policy should be posted at the reception desk and in all treatment rooms.
- Implement a procedure for massage therapists and other employees to follow if they feel they have been the victim of sexual harassment.
- Conduct organization-wide sexual harassment–prevention training.
- Have all clients sign an agreement to comply with the business's zero-tolerance policy on sexual harassment.
- Develop positive relationships with local law enforcement.

Appropriate Behavior for All Massage Therapists

Always inform new clients that sexualizing the massage in any way, by the client or the massage therapist, is inappropriate. Inform the client that you will end the session immediately if you consider any behavior to be inappropriate. Should this occur, the client is expected to exit the massage area and leave the premises. You will leave the massage session and report the behavior immediately to your supervisor. Taking this sort of action is more difficult if you are self-employed, and one of the advantages of working with others is protection in these instances. It may be advantageous for the receptionist or some individual other than the massage therapist to discuss all office policies with new clients and coworkers; this indicates agreement among all employees about what constitutes appropriate and inappropriate behavior. Harassment of any type should *never* be tolerated.

When working with clients, follow these guidelines to prevent accusations of or commitment of sexual misconduct:

- Never lock the door. The door remains unlocked for the client's protection and yours to make it easier for the person who feels violated to exit if something inappropriate occurs.
- Inform clients that they can have another person in the room with them. It is acceptable for a family member or friend to accompany them while they receive a massage.
- Clearly inform clients of no-touch zones. Copy and use Box 7.6.
- Assure clients that meticulous draping procedures will provide privacy.
- Require clients to wear undergarments that cover the pelvic and buttock region.
- Use additional draping to make sure breast tissue is not touched, especially when clients are in the prone position when breast tissue can bulge to the side.
- If a draping accident happens or inadvertent touch occurs, acknowledge it immediately, apologize, and correct the situation. Document the incident and the action taken.
- Always avoid pressing the groin area against the client.
- Do not lean over the client in such a way that the therapist's groin is near the client's head.
- Make sure that client's hands are tucked under their body or located so that it cannot seem as if the massage therapist has leaned his or her groin into the client's hands.
- Never make exceptions to the rules.
- If a client makes sexual advances, even minor innuendos, leave the room immediately and report the incident to the front desk. If front desk staff is unavailable, leave a note stating that the client's behavior was inappropriate and that the client should be told to leave the premises. This notice should be created ahead of time and placed in a convenient location in the reception area where the client will see it. Leave the area, and do not interact with the client. Immediately write down all details of the session. Add the description of the incident to the client's file. If direct solicitation for sexual services occurred, this is a crime and should be reported to the police.

Likewise, prior to the massage session, clients should be educated about what constitutes inappropriate behavior by a massage therapist and what actions to take if they believe inappropriate behavior occurred. Guidelines for client education and reporting actions include the following:

- Create a document that describes appropriate behavior expected of massage therapists and clients.
- Review this document with clients prior to their first session.
- Keep a signed copy of this document in the client's file. (Box 7.7.)

Fraudulent Accusations of Sexual Harassment

The rights of sexual harassment victims are clear and protected. The rights of those accused of sexual harassment are less well defined. After millions of dollars in lawsuits filed by victims, it is much less risky for employers to quickly err on the side of the accuser, even if this means that there is an increased risk of someone being accused unjustly.

There are many reasons a person may make false accusations. For most, it is the potential for a monetary settlement. False accusations also occur as a form of retribution, as these examples illustrate:

- A client attempts to engage a massage therapist in a personal relationship but is told that it is not possible. The client may then attempt to retaliate by claiming misconduct on the part of the massage therapist.
- A massage therapist may be envious of the retention business success of another massage therapist working in the same location. One way to remove the more successful massage therapist is through allegations of sexual harassment.

Although it is not common for someone to falsely accuse another of this type of behavior, it does occur, and it most often is directed against men. Male massage therapists must be extremely cautious about their behavior and continuously assess their actions to prevent career-ending allegations.

Individuals accused of sexual harassment have privacy rights that prohibit others from divulging information about the complaint except as part of the resolution process. The accused is informed of the allegations, the identity of the complainant, and the facts surrounding the allegation. Individuals accused of sexual harassment have due process rights that prohibit them from being disciplined without adequate notice and an opportunity to be heard.

If you are ever unjustly accused, you need to get an attorney, and make sure the attorney contacts everyone who currently works or has worked with you to establish that you are not in the habit of sexually harassing anyone. If a client accuses you of sexual misconduct, the same process applies. The attorney should also investigate the accuser to see whether the person has a history of suing; the attorney also may be able to find prior lawsuits filed by the accuser.

Do not speak to the accuser at all—not by phone, e-mail, or through any other contact. Absolutely do not talk about the accuser or the sexual harassment incident with anyone except your attorney or a government agency representative who is investigating the alleged incident.

It is difficult to prove sexual harassment if there is no proof because it is their word against yours. This is why actual victims of sexual harassment have such a difficult time receiving help and why the laws and rules are more favorable for the victim. However, if there is any prior misconduct with others or if you have been accused before, this history can be considered as proof of a pattern of sexual harassment behavior.

You must protect yourself from accusations that are unfounded, and you must constantly be aware of how your conduct can be interpreted as sexual harassment. It is advantageous to take sexual harassment training courses to learn how to prevent sexual harassment behavior. Document that you

Box 7.7 Safe Therapeutic Touch Policy

Clients should expect massage therapists to behave as follows:

- Engage in respectful, nonsexual, and gender-neutral conversation.
- Secure modest draping with specific permission to work in the hip, lower back, abdomen, and anterior thorax area.
- Immediately acknowledge any inadvertent accidental touch or draping mishap with an apology. This type of mistake should not happen again and be truly accidental.
  Massage therapists should expect clients to behave as follows:
- Feel free to engage in respectful, nonsexual, and gender-neutral conversation.
- Abide by disrobing rules, and wear under garments that covers the gluteal/genital region.
- Ensure that there is no casual touching of the massage therapist and no physical contact in any no-touch zone. Review Box 7.6
- Maintain secure draping of no-touch zones with no attempt to shift or remove draping in these areas.
- Immediately acknowledge any inadvertent accidental touch or draping mishap with an apology. This type of mistake should not happen again and be truly accidental.

Actions and Consequences Should Violations Occur

Inappropriate Behavior of Massage Therapist: Client Actions

- As the client, you should say "Stop" immediately, end the session by telling massage therapist to leave the massage area, then redress and leave the massage area.
- Immediately report the incident to the front desk staff and complete an incident report form provided by reception staff. It is your right to talk directly with the manager or business owner.
- If you were touched in any of the no-touch zones or feel that any part of the massage application was hostile or aggressive, you have the right to file assault charges with the police. Front desk staff will assist you in making this call.
- It is best to disclose inappropriate behavior immediately. However, if upon reflection you determine that the massage therapist behaved inappropriately, it is your right to call or visit the facility and make an incident report. If you feel you were physically assaulted, it is your right to contact the police.
- If no desk/reception staff is available, you can contact the police if you feel you were assaulted.
- A massage therapist who behaves inappropriately and unethically for any reason should be reported to the state's massage licensing board.

Inappropriate Behavior of the Client: Massage Therapist Actions

- The massage therapist has the right to end the massage session at any time if they feel uncomfortable with a client's behavior.
- The massage therapist will leave the room and be unavailable for discussion.
- The incident will be carefully documented.
- The client is expected to leave the massage area and the premises.
- The client will not be rescheduled for any massage sessions.
- If the client purposely exposes any no-touch zone areas, inappropriately touches the massage therapist, or themselves, or attempts to solicit sexual services of any type, *this is a crime and the police will be called.* The following template can be used to report to law enforcement and inform the offending person of the consequences of their behavior.

have taken these classes. Most important, always be professional and think before speaking or acting. Do not put yourself in situations in which you could be accused.

Specifically for Massage Therapists Identifying as Male

Male massage therapists must be more careful than female massage therapists.. Although this is unjust, it is the reality. For example, a male massage therapist should never go to the home of a female client alone; never work alone in the office with a female client; never lock the door of the treatment room while giving a massage; always have another individual (e.g., another massage therapist or receptionist) in the office within hearing range; never work on the breast area of a female client (even if the work is justified for scar tissue management); never massage into the upper thigh region of a female client (always refer female clients to female massage therapists for this type of work); always meet female coworkers or employees only in a public area; and never invite female clients, coworkers, or employees to his home if he is alone.

Men must be careful about how they treat female coworkers and clients. Do not call them "honey," "babe," or other offensive terms of endearment. Do not make sexist comments, even if kidding. Do not allow anyone else to speak this way. No massage professional should allow anyone to speak in an offensive way or to post or display sexist and offensive jokes, comics, cartoons, calendars, or anything else that is sexual in nature.

All massage therapists must be aware of behavior that others may consider offensive, even if you do not. Before acting or speaking, ask yourself the following questions:

- Would I do or say this if I knew it were going to be shown on TV or presented on social media?
- Would I want anyone to say or do this to my parent, spouse, or child?
- In what ways may this behavior or conversation be misinterpreted?

Foot in the Door

The foot you put in the door needs to be clean; it also needs to be wearing a nonskid shoe for safety purposes. To maintain a successful massage practice, you must be clean, scent free, well groomed, and professionally dressed. You also must meticulously follow the rules of sanitation to ensure not only your own safety but that of your clients and coworkers. Sanitation is not an option. Both your massage methods and your environment must be safe. When evaluating a possible job location, find out whether others in the practice maintain professional hygiene, sanitation, and safety. You will not be successful in an environment that is dirty and unsafe. You may not even want your foot in that door! Instead, make sure to put your foot in a door that opens to a clean, professional, neat, fresh, sanitary, and safe, harassment-free environment.

SUMMARY

The information in this chapter can help you establish a safe, professional practice. Massage professionals should review these procedures regularly to maintain the diligence that ensures a secure, sanitary massage environment for our clients. It is our responsibility to act reliably in emergencies. As massage professionals, we must understand the use of Standard Precautions and fire and premise safety measures so that we are able to serve our clients in a health-promoting and hazard-free manner. Finally, it is important to protect ourselves and our clients from sexual harassment and the violent or criminal acts of others.

LEARN MORE ON THE WEB

A textbook, even the best textbook, can cover only a portion of the information you will need and want. Practice exploring reliable information-based websites, especially those created by government agencies (those ending in .gov). The website for the Centers for Disease Control and Prevention (www.cdc.gov) has a trove of information relevant to the practice of therapeutic massage. Textbooks can become dated; therefore it is important to hang out where the information is current. It is amazing what you can find using the search boxes. MedlinePlus is one of the most helpful sites. The Occupational Safety and Health Administration (OSHA, a division of the U.S. Department of Labor) has important information on safe work practices and environments, in addition to recommendations for reducing workplace violence. The U.S. Equal Employment Opportunity Commission (EEOC) is responsible for enforcing federal laws that make it illegal to discriminate against a job applicant or an employee.

Evolve

Visit the Evolve website: http://evolve.elsevier.com/Fritz/fundamentals/.

Evolve content designed for massage therapy licensing exam review and comprehension of content beyond the textbook. Evolve content includes:

- Content Updates
- Science and Pathology Animations
- Body Spectrum Coloring Book
- MBLEx exam review multiple choice questions

FOR EACH CHAPTER FIND:

- Answers and rationales for the end-of-chapter multiple-choice questions
- Electronic workbook and answer key
- Chapter multiple choice question quiz
- Quick content review in question form and answers
- Technique videos when applicable
- Learn more on the Web

REFERENCE

Centers for Disease Control and Prevention (CDC). Clean hands count for healthcare providers. Available at www.cdc.gov/handwashing, https://www.cdc.gov/handhygiene/providers/index.html.

MULTIPLE-CHOICE QUESTIONS FOR DISCUSSION AND REVIEW

The answers, with rationales, can be found on the Evolve site. Use these questions to stimulate review and discussion and dialogue. You must understand the meaning of the words in the question and possible answers. Each question provides you with the ability to review terminology, practice critical thinking skills, and improve multiple choice test taking skills. Answers and rationales are on the Evolve site. It is just as important to know why the wrong answers are wrong as it is to know why the correct answer is correct.

1. Pathogenic disease-causing organisms include ______.
   a. Dirt, sweat, and grime
   b. Paint, tar, and dust
   c. Viruses, bacteria, and funguses
   d. Smoking, drinking, and washing
2. The three primary ways pathogens are spread are person-to-person contact, environmental contact, and ______.
   a. Hand washing
   b. Standard Precautions
   c. Shoes
   d. Opportunistic invasion
3. The simplest, most effective deterrent to the spread of disease is ______.
   a. Hand washing
   b. Sterilization technique
   c. Using a towel barrier
   d. Keeping vaccines up to date
4. Acquired immunodeficiency syndrome is a(n) ______.
   a. Inflammatory process caused by a virus
   b. Human immunodeficiency virus
   c. Group of clinical symptoms caused by a dysfunction in the immune system
   d. Disease contracted by casual contact such as shaking hands or sharing bathroom facilities
5. Which of the following is NOT a safe professional practice?
   a. Inspecting facility for tripping hazards
   b. Burning candles for atmosphere in the massage room
   c. Maintaining good lighting in massage areas
   d. Regularly checking cables of portable massage tables
6. Severe acute respiratory syndrome is _____.
   a. Noncontagious
   b. Spread by person-to-person contact
   c. Not deadly
   d. Controlled with nutrition
7. Which of the following is an example of a noncritical item used in the massage environment for sanitary purposes?
   a. A face cradle cover
   b. A massage tool with an edge
   c. Bolsters
   d. A pillowcase
8. Which of the following is an example of a clinical contact surface that requires disinfection?
   a. A waiting room chair
   b. A restroom mirror
   c. A linen cabinet
   d. A massage lubricant bottle

9. Which client would need to have the massage therapist wear a protective mask?
a. A client who is immune compromised
b. A client in the 30th week of pregnancy
c. A client who uses a wheelchair
d. A client who is an athlete

10. Which of the following is a slipping hazard?
a. A common use hand towel
b. Water on the floor
c. An uncovered water container
d. A bowl of unwrapped mints

11. What is a "safe room"?
a. A place where files are stored
b. The room where clients wait between massage sessions
c. A location equipped with an emergency cell phone
d. A location where people can express emotion

12. Which of the following is necessary for workplace fire safety?
a. An evacuation plan
b. Candles only in reception area
c. A contact number for the fire department
d. Keeping doors other than the main entrance locked

13. Which of the following would often involve workplace gossip?
a. Inappropriate touching
b. Bullying
c. Sexual harassment
d. Litigation

14. Which of the following is the appropriate action if a client inappropriately touches the massage therapist?
a. Give a warning and tell the client to stop.
b. Leave the massage room and document the details.
c. Report the incident to the manager after the session has ended.
d. Ignore the incident unless it happens again.

15. You are running behind today, and your next client has been waiting for 15 minutes. It is most important that you _______.
a. Maintain your scheduled appointments on time.
b. Have materials and activities available for clients to entertain themselves.
c. Make sure sheets and linens are changed and equipment disinfected between massages.
d. Apologize to the client for being late.

16. A massage therapist has been implicated for inappropriate touching. The client does not want to call the police but does want the business owner to address the situation. The massage therapist indicates that they did not sexually touch the client or act inappropriately. Which of the following could be mistaken for inappropriate touching?
a. Moving the bolster while the client changes position
b. Providing gliding methods on the back with the client's arm resting alongside them
c. Securing the drape under the client's leg to massage the anterior thigh
d. Guiding the client to the massage area by placing a hand on the client's shoulder

17. A coworker has been sullen and appears frustrated with the schedule prepared by the front desk. The manager has corrected them for not completing client charts in a timely manner. You know that they have financial issues related to a car that needs repair. The massage therapist just received a complaint about the massage session from a client who is often hard to please. What is the workplace concern?
a. The massage therapist is likely to be fired.
b. The massage therapist is at risk for emotional outburst.
c. The client will need to file a formal complaint with the licensing board.
d. Coworkers need to avoid the massage therapist to prevent sexual harassment.

18. A sole practitioner massage therapist with a small office located within a multidisciplinary wellness center is having difficulty with another practitioner in the facility who is constantly asking for advice and wants to become a massage client. The massage therapist does not feel comfortable with this suggestion and has told the individual that it would be inappropriate for them to have a professional relationship because they work in the same location. The individual continues to request massage sessions. Which of the follow statements is most accurate based on this scenario?
a. No harassment is taking place, but there are professional boundary issues.
b. There is an underlying sexual attraction, and this is an example of stalking.
c. The massage therapist needs to be more assertive in managing this conflict.
d. The massage therapist is being harassed by this individual, as evidenced by the unwanted attention.

19. A massage therapist who has a home-based office and also travels to clients' homes is concerned about a client who has a traumatic brain injury related to a car accident. The client has coordination issues and is concerned about navigating the stairs in the therapist's home office. A solution is for the therapist to provide massage at the client's home. The client also has difficulty managing frustration and has emotional outbursts that are typically displayed by yelling and cursing. The client has hepatitis C and currently has a MRSA infection due to a series of scrapes and cuts from a fall. Which of these issues poses the most immediate concern for the safety and health of the massage therapist?
a. Providing the massage in the client's home
b. The hepatis infection
c. The emotional instability
d. The MRSA infection

20. A massage client is taking anti-rejection medication due to a liver transplant 2 years ago. The massage therapist is taking action to reduce exposure of infection for this client. Which pathogen transmission route would be most difficult to address?
a. Airborne
b. Droplet
c. Fomite
d. Personal contact

Activity

Write at least three more multiple choice questions, one of each type: factual recall and comprehension, application and concept identification, and clinical reasoning and synthesis. Develop plausible wrong answers and be sure that the correct answer is clearly correct. Then write a rationale for each question. The more questions you write, the better you will understand the material. Exchange questions with fellow classmates or discuss in class. The questions from all the learners can be combined to create a review quiz.

UNIT III

The Massage Process

CHAPTER

8

Ergonomics, Biomechanics, and Body Mechanics

http://evolve.elsevier.com/Fritz/fundamentals/

CHAPTER OBJECTIVES

After completing this chapter, the student will be able to perform the following:

1. Interpret biomechanical research related to massage application.
2. Create an ergonomically effective massage environment.
3. Apply basic biomechanical principles to develop effective body mechanics.
4. Distinguish among appropriate pressure, drag, and duration application while applying various massage methods.
5. Recognize nonoptimal performance of massage application through the presence of pain and discomfort.
6. Adapt ergonomic and biomechanical principles based on gender, body shape, practice environment, and other factors.

CHAPTER OUTLINE

KEY TERMS

Asymmetrical standing	Ergonomics
Balance	Friction
Balance point	Leverage
Biomechanics	Pressure
Center of gravity	Therapeutic edge
Force	Traction
Drag	

STUDENT NOTE: Most models in this chapter are pictured in sportswear to enhance and clarify the various body positions. Draping materials are not used in the examples in this chapter so that positions may be seen more clearly.

This chapter is particularly important to your success as a massage therapist. You want to be able to provide an effective massage for the client without putting yourself at higher risk for injury in the process. You want to generate enough income to meet your financial goals, which directly depends on whether clients value the massage you provide and how many quality massage sessions you are able to do each day. The information in this chapter has been compiled from available research, the Massage Therapy Foundation's Ergonomics Project, standard ergonomics recommendations for service and health professions, has been reviewed by certified ergonomic professionals and a kinesiology and biomechanics professor and a massage therapy educator with expertise in ergonomics and adult education, as well as from personal observation and the author's professional and teaching experience.

IMPORTANT DEVELOPMENT

In 2019, the Massage Therapy Foundation (https://massagetherapyfoundation.org/) began a multistaged project conducted by professional ergonomists guided by subject matter experts and professionals, including two of the researchers cited in this chapter and the textbook author. The goal is to help establish safe practice parameters for the massage therapy profession. Phase one was completed in 2022. The goals of phase one were to establish foundational knowledge about the practice of massage therapy work and its related tasks, provide information that can be researched further for efficacy and application, and formulate best practices for career longevity and safety of massage therapy professionals in their work environments. Phase one content is incorporated into this chapter. Phase two is underway as of this writing.

Massage is physical, labor-intensive work. It is important to have the capacity and ability to perform full-time service work for 7 to 8 hours per day, which includes 5 to 6 hours of massage as well as non-massage work activities. Some massage therapists may choose to work fewer hours. Nevertheless, regardless of full or part-time work status, knowing the safest and most effective ways to work is beneficial. Although most performance expectations are for massage as a full-time practice, efficient body mechanics are just as important for part-time massage therapy work schedules.

Effective body mechanics involves good posture, stability, balance, leverage, and use of the strongest and largest muscles to perform the work. There is no single correct way to use the human body efficiently, and the recommendations in this chapter are effective methods that support adaptability to the individual practitioner. Three important things the massage practitioner must learn and remember are to remain relaxed, stay comfortable, and avoid straining and awkward postures when doing massage. The postures and movements used while giving a massage should be efficient, fluid, and deliberate. Movements and postures should be similar to other daily physical activities. If while performing a massage therapy session you find yourself positioned or moving in a way that differs greatly from your typical daily activity, you may need to alter your approach; likewise, if you feel as though you are working hard while giving a massage, something is wrong with your body mechanics and movement efficiency.

Think of the body as a mechanical device. The action of muscles and bones is the result of **leverage**, operating within mechanical laws of physics. As with all mechanical devices, they are subject to deterioration with extended use, especially if used improperly on a repetitive basis. However, the advantage of the human body is that it is made up of living tissue that has the ability to heal. A deeper understanding of the biomechanical principles of the body helps prevent injury and to restore function when injury occurs. Fatigue, muscle strain, and injury, including overuse and misuse syndromes, can result from poor and inefficient positioning of the massage practitioner's body while giving a massage. Efficient use of the body helps prevent repetitive strain, injury, and burnout. These topics are explored throughout this chapter and in Chapter 10 as you learn to perform a massage. In this chapter you will learn methods of working more efficiently so that providing massage in a 7- to 8-hour workday that includes 5 to 6 hours of massage application does not cause dysfunction or pain.

UNIQUE POSTURAL AND PHYSICAL DEMANDS OF MASSAGE THERAPY APPLICATION

The delivery of therapeutic massage creates unique postural and physical demands. For most physically demanding professions, body mechanics tends to focus on lifting or exerting a force in an upward direction, such as when a nurse lifts a patient from the bed to a chair. Other aspects of body mechanics are applied to dynamic movement, such as various forms of dancing, martial arts, and athletic participation. In contrast, during massage most of the effort exerted is sustained, controlled, and sometimes static movements, with pressure focused downward and forward to create mechanic force applied into the tissue, resulting in compressive and tension stress acting on tissues. The massage practitioner uses the forearms, wrists, hands, fingers, thumbs, knees, and feet extensively to deliver the push or pull of mechanical force application. Because of these differences, the standard recommendations provided to most physically demanding professions for safe body mechanics are not applicable to massage therapists in all cases. The use of ergonomic principles as they relate to massage therapy work tasks specifically is a safe and effective approach to career longevity (Anderson, 2018).

Massage professionals need to consider their individual body types and musculoskeletal limitations. The suggestions in this chapter can help most learners develop the best personal body mechanics approach for them as individual practitioners. If you use effective body mechanics, you will decrease your potential for injury and will not likely be any more fatigued than is expected after a full day of work. If your body mechanics are effective, the client will also experience a quality massage. If you do not use your body in a biomechanically efficient way, the massage pressure is uneven, too light or too deep, pokey (painful), and generally uncomfortable for both the client and you. The ultimate goal is for you as the therapist to work effectively and safely and for your client to experience a quality massage. Make sure to view the video segment on the Evolve site for this chapter and practice.

RESEARCH: EFFICACY OF BODY MECHANICS IN MASSAGE THERAPISTS

SECTION OBJECTIVES

Chapter objective covered in this section:

1. Interpret biomechanical research related to massage application.

Using the information presented in this section, the student will be able to perform the following:

- Correlate research findings to support the recommendations for safe body mechanics while applying massage.

In the past, little ergonomic or biomechanical research has been done in the area of massage therapy. Most of the skills related to how to perform a massage have been based on opinion and experience of individual teachers. A legacy is something handed down or received from a predecessor. Until recently, educators only had experience and legacy as a foundation for ergonomics and biomechanics education. This legacy-based education from the past is not based on actual ergonomics and biomechanics research. That has now changed with the Massage Therapy Foundation Ergo Project (https://massagetherapyfoundation.org/mtf-ergo-project/) (Box 8.1).

Two basic factors of body mechanics are important for the massage therapist: ergonomics and biomechanics. **Ergonomics** focuses on the application of anatomical and physiological science to design equipment and objects, work systems both from management and financial aspects, and their respective environments for human use. Ergonomics also involves the adaptation and optimization involved in matching the job tasks to the

Box 8.1 Basic Terminology and Concepts of Body Mechanics

Basic Terminology

- *Biomechanics* is the understanding of the motion and forces produced by the human body as a living machine.
- *Ergonomics* is the science and art of adapting or modifying work tasks to the individual worker. This is applicable to many industrial forms such as manufacturing work; specialty skills work like plumbing, construction, and information technology; the office work environment; or even massage therapy and its many different practice settings (Pheasant, 1991).
- *Work* is the result of a force acting through a distance. From an ergonomics standpoint, work can also be viewed as *energy expenditure*, meaning that the body uses energy in order to perform a work task (Pheasant, 1991).
- *Power* relates to the time element and the work accomplished. This can also be related to the amount of effort exerted to perform the task, which correlates to energy expenditure.
- *Applied force* is the energy or effort provided to perform work. Applied force has many forms, such as the power of an electric motor or the push from human hands.
- *Muscle contraction* is the action of the work being done by the muscles and reflects the consumption of mechanical energy. Using muscles to generate applied force during massage application is progressively fatiguing.
- *Joint structures* are the mechanisms by which movements occur within the human body that are initiated through muscle contraction. They are designed to adapt to external and internal forces of energy expenditures if these forces are not excessive and sustained.
- *Joint stress* is defined as the mechanical force that develops in a joint, which with some repetitive work tasks can be deteriorating to the joint structures over time. This is why repetitive stress injuries (RSIs) are an element of concern from an ergonomics viewpoint (see the definition offered later in the box).
- The *closed packed position* is the most stable joint position (where movement normally halts or has the most sustainable reinforcement to protect the joint structures). During massage application, some joints are placed in this stable position.

Basic Laws of Physics

Some basic laws of physics, mechanics in massage therapist work. There are three main laws:

- According to Sir Isaac Newton, the general conceptual basis for applying effective body mechanics is the law of action and reaction (for every force, an equal and opposite force is created), the law of inertia (a body at rest stays at rest or stays in motion), and the law of acceleration (more effort is needed to move objects with larger mass). Each of these laws can be applied to creating safe and effective body mechanics for massage therapy work.
- Be careful of creating too much joint stress when applying massage. A force directed against a structure so that the parts slide against each other produces a shearing stress. Both parts may be movable, with the parts sliding in opposite directions, or one part may be fixed. The incorrect application of massage causes compression and shearing stress to the massage therapist's joints, rather than supported sustainable movement.
- According to ergonomics assessment standards and safe work environments, repetitive bending or twist is a main contributor to lower back issues (Pheasant, 1991). Spinal bending involves the actions of tension, compression, and torsion (twisting). It is important that the massage therapist avoid bending over or twisting while performing massage.
- *Repetitive stress injuries or RSIs* are the cumulative effects of constant or repeated small stresses over a long period that can cause the same difficulties as the severe and sudden onset of stresses that creates injury. This means that even if you apply the same massage method at a less than optimum position every time you do it, the action might not cause pain while performed at that moment; however, performing this same action over and over incorrectly eventually leads to difficulty due to muscle fatigue from high energy expenditure or poorly protected or unstabilized joint structures.
- Through the use of safe and effective body mechanics, a massage therapist can apply force to the client's tissues using the least amount of muscular and joint effort and energy expenditure, thus promoting the potential for career longevity and daily sustained and consistent workday endurance levels with a reduction in risk factors, leading to less overall strain.

worker or use of a product to the user in the interest of ease of use for the overall health and safety of workers (Pheasant, 1991). Biomechanics, or *body mechanics,* concentrates on the body as a machine and utilizes this perspective to analyze the structures, motions, and muscular forces used to complete tasks.

For massage therapists, there are two major ergonomic issues to consider: work environment and technique delivery/application. Factors that affect the work environment are the height and width of the massage table, the type of floor covering, and the amount of space around the table, all of which must support the ease of massage application. The number of massage sessions or hours performed each workday or week also is a factor. Technique delivery involves the actual application of massage by the individual and the effective use of the massage practitioner's own body while applying any variety of skills or techniques.

The major biomechanical concern is improper use of body areas that cannot easily be sustained in a stable position (i.e., the thumb, shoulder, low back, and knee), such as overusing fine motor movements and musculature in the hands rather than applying more gross motor movements from the shoulder and trunk. The position of the massage therapist in straining and fatiguing non-neutral joint position is a major concern (Buck et al., 2007). Another important factor is the repetitive delivery of mechanical forces as the massage methods load tissues during pushing and pulling actions, which, again, supports the overuse of fine motor skills in cases where the application of gross motor skills would be a more efficient option.

Research Outcomes

Because of the past legacy-based teaching of body mechanics it is important to justify recommendations for change based on objective research and expert analysis which is now available. The most recent research indicates 85% of massage therapists had experienced or were experiencing work-related pain. The female massage practitioners aged between 21 and 30 years old reported significantly more frequent pain localized in neck, shoulders, wrist-hand, upper back, and lower back. This is important, since the massage therapy occupation is dominated by female massage therapists. Females in general are at more risk of work-related musculoskeletal injury (Rossettini et al., 2016; Anyfantis and Biska, 2017; Chow et al., 2017; Kruger et al., 2017). Work-related pain was attributed to the gradual onset of musculoskeletal conditions (Cid et al., 2019). There is a clear indication of work-related pain impacting the lives of massage therapists including activities of daily living, loss of income, and working in pain. Almost one-third of massage therapists have considered changing or have changed their profession. This research indicates that how massage therapy is provided must evolve with greater focus on efficient biomechanics, ergonomic equipment / space, and balanced work/duty cycles, with the goal being to support productivity, longevity, and happiness (Kareem et al., 2021; Barraclough et al., 2022; Friedman et al., 2022; Sirbu et al., 2022; Sung and Liu, 2022).

Even though little research is currently available about ergonomics and body mechanics related to massage therapy, there are studies that have investigated how massage therapists work and their potential for work-related injury. This information can guide recommendations for professional practice. Guruprasad and colleagues (2016) have suggested that when the work time exceeds 6 hours of hands-on massage, the injury potential increases. Although this information is relatively consistent with most workplace models for massage therapists, there is more to consider than just the length of the workday.

The study conducted at Montana State University (Page, 2012) involved massage therapists from the United States and Canada. The majority of therapists actually practiced a self-care routine regularly but were still reporting issues with work-related pain. In terms of their typical approach to massage therapy work, most used portable massage tables; performed sessions primarily in standing positions; and used moderate pressure techniques such as kneading, deep pressure approaches, and compressions with clients typically positioned either supine or prone. The average time between treatment sessions was 18+ minutes, during which time less than 5 minutes was used as an actual physical rest period before the next client session began. The observational results showed that the average to maximum number of hands-on hours per week was 12 to 21, which equated to almost 3 to 5 hours of hands-on time per day. The key factors from the study are that massage therapists are at higher risk for upper extremity injuries (particularly wrist and thumb injuries), and often do not have sufficient rest time between treatments focused on injury prevention (Page, 2012).

A study by E.G. Mohr, a certified engineer and ergonomist, found that the economic viability (ability to make money) of the manual therapy practitioner depended on the number of massages or treatments that could be given in a day or a week (Mohr, 2010). Fatigue or injuries can have a major effect on income potential.

Another study by Blau and colleagues (2013) found that both physical "wear and tear" and "mental fatigue" can lead massage therapists to reduce the number of massage sessions that they feel capable of providing. The study's authors recommend sufficient time between massages and, if possible, varying one's massage technique.

Studies clearly show that even with the best biomechanics, the thumb cannot withstand the strain placed on it during manual therapy (Snodgrass et al., 2003; Albert et al., 2006; Buckingham et al., 2007; Albert et al., 2008; Hu et al., 2009; Rossettini et al., 2016; Kruger et al., 2017; Kareem et al., 2021). We must provide massage with minimal use of the thumb and never use the thumb to generate pressure. Work-related risk factors for arm–hand elevation and shoulder hand force exertion load double the risk of specific shoulder disorders (Van der Molen et al., 2017). Neck disorders were associated with head inclination, upper arm elevation, muscle activity of the trapezius and forearm extensors, and wrist posture.

The ergonomic risk factors for injury include awkward postures such as bending and twisting of the body, raised shoulders, contact stress related to direct pressure, and stress on the fingers (Jacquier-Bret et al., 2023). Excessive force application is a concern. The typical human can only exert so much mechanical force. Demands on massage therapists to provide heavy pressure during the session is a cause of injury. The demand for so-called "deep tissue massage" and the confusion related to how much force needs to be applied to achieve client goals has contributed to injury in massage therapists.

Long excursion gliding, such as a continuous stroke from neck to low back or shoulder to hand is problematic. The cumulative effects of using these long gliding methods must be avoided.

Working in non-neutral positions is another contributing factor to work fatigue and injury. On average, during 50% of the massage, the trunk was required to be flexed away from neutral. Deviation from neutral also was required of the arms for 70% of the massage, and of the shoulders and neck for 60% of the massage. This is significant because most of the massage time was spent performing these techniques.

RECOMMENDATIONS BASED ON AVAILABLE RESEARCH

Ergonomic strategies that are used to minimize fatigue and work-related injury include:

- Stand more upright.
- Trunk flexion occurs at the hips and does not exceed 20 degrees of flexion.
- Use asymmetrical stance.
- Adjust table height. Use higher table for light to moderate pressure delivery. Higher table supports forearm use. A higher table is used for a majority of the massage application. Lower table would be used for heavy pressure delivery.
- Work close to the client and alter positioning of the client's body.
- Avoid reaching over the head of the client.
- Avoid working at the ends of the table.
- Concentrate providing massage when positioned at the sides of the table—not the ends.
- Shorten the length/excursion of gliding strokes to 12 inches or less. Longer movements cause overreaching, excessive shoulder and trunk flexion, and rotation. To glide over a longer area do not reach at the shoulder. Move feet during the gliding strokes in the direction of the stroke.
- Avoid gliding strokes that span the entire length of the spine.
- Divide neck/shoulder and low back regions and avoid crossing from one region into another without significant changes in posture that include moving the feet.

Table 8.1 Recommended Duty Schedule, Hours of Duty, and Work Shift Schedules

	LEAST COMMON	MOST COMMON	COMMON
	Full-time	¾ time	½ time
Hours worked per week	37–40	25–30	17–20
Hours of massage performed per week	25–30	20–25	12–15
Hours worked per shift	7.5–8	5.5–6	4
Hours of massage performed per shift	5.5–6	4–5	3–3.5
Non-massage hours worked per shift*	1–1.5	45 minutes	30 minutes
Work Breaks**	Two 15 minute	One 15 minute	None
Meal Break***	One 30 minute	One 30 minute	None

*Non-massage worktime: Time between sessions, room turnover, laundry or other facility management tasks, completing client documentation, or as specifically scheduled blocks and assigned tasks. Can accumulate throughout the work shift.
**Work Break: Downtime away from work duties
***Meal Break: 30-minute break approximately mid-shift as a food break.
NOTE: Federal labor laws do not require scheduled breaks, and a break over 30 minutes does not have to be paid. WHD I U.S. Department of Labor (dol.gov).

- Avoid reaching under the client especially when client is positioned supine.
- Make sure hands are visible. Do not work with hands under the client.
- Minimize use of pulling techniques and use a staggered stance.
- Optimize client positioning/bolstering.
- Minimize reaching across the client's midline. Monitor the duration of application since this technique requires active trunk extension in an unsupported position.
- When providing massage in the seated or kneeling position keep the trunk vertical (at 90 degrees to the floor).
- Use lighter-pressure techniques in a seated position. Lighter force applications may be done with more upright trunk postures when sitting rather than standing.
- Avoid using the thumbs.
- Minimize using fingertips.
- Consider using joint-saving tools.

https://massagetherapyfoundation.org/download/8654/?uid=a686e97e74.

Massage Scheduling

- Concentrate on perfecting the 50-minute massage application within a 60-minute session scheduling pattern. This time pattern is most efficient for scheduling and includes sufficient breaks between sessions to prevent injury and fatigue.
- The 90-minute massage session should be the maximum length.
- Avoid the 2-hour massage appointment. It is not necessary to work this long to achieve results for the client, and 2 hours is typically too long for the massage therapist to apply massage without a break.
- There should be sufficient time between sessions for restroom use as needed and proper hand and forearm hygiene procedures.
- If a receptionist is available for client check in and out, and if massage sessions are scheduled based on the 60-minute session with 50 minutes of actual massage application, there should be adequate time between sessions for these activities and room turnover.
- Those working in a self-employed practice or in an establishment with no receptionist support may find it prudent to space massage sessions at least 15 minutes or more apart and to include an hour mid-workday break.

The remainder of this chapter provides suggestions to minimize the potential for injury and fatigue while performing massage application and as a result support financial success by increasing the number of massage sessions you can provide. It is important to learn to work efficiently and intelligently for your own well-being (Table 8.1).

ERGONOMICS AND BIOMECHANICS

SECTION OBJECTIVES

Chapter objectives covered in this section:

2. Create an ergonomically effective massage environment.
3. Apply basic biomechanical principles to develop effective body mechanics.
4. Distinguish among appropriate pressures, drag, and duration applications while applying various massage methods.

Using the information presented in this section, the student will be able to perform the following:

- Apply principles of ergonomics and biomechanics to massage therapy.
- Adapt and utilize massage equipment that benefits the individual massage therapist ergonomically.
- Discuss how massage application directs mechanical force to the client's body.
- Demonstrate the application of pressure when providing massage.
- Execute effective body mechanics principles while doing massage.
- Apply a variety of pressure levels during massage.
- Modify massage application using drag and duration.

The practical application of ergonomics and body mechanics involves integrating the research and information discussed earlier into the actual performance of a massage. It is one thing to understand the principles and quite another to actually do what has been described. In this section, we will learn how to "do."

Applying Ergonomics

General ergonomics concepts deal with the human body's responses to the physical work environment and the physiological loads of work tasks performed. The following are primary topics that apply to massage therapists' work (Barnett and Liber, 2006):

- Manual materials handling, workstation layout, job demands, and risk factors (e.g., repetition, vibration, force, and awkward or static posture), as they relate to musculoskeletal disorders and repetitive strain injury.
- Work activities, which should allow workers to adopt several different postures, all equally healthy and safe. Muscular force should be exerted by the largest appropriate muscle groups available.
- Human push capability (weight transfer to apply force), which involves strength, weight, weight distribution, push angle, footwear/floor friction, and the friction between the upper body and the pushed object (Argubi-Wollesen et al., 2017).

Ergonomically, the workstation is a primary focus. In most cases, massage therapists have an uncomplicated work environment: a massage area and equipment such as a massage table, a massage mat or chair (or both), and a stool or chair to sit on. Improper workstation design, including the width and height of the massage table and the size of the massage room, can lead to poor posture and body mechanics, resulting in an increase in musculoskeletal injuries.

Massage Area

The massage area encompasses the open space around the massage table, mat, or chair. This space must be large enough to allow the practitioner to move easily around the equipment. The massage table dimensions for space planning are an average of 75 inches long, or just over 6 feet, and 2½ feet wide (190.5 × 76 cm). There needs to be at least 36 to 48 inches (3–4 feet /0.9/1.22 meters) of floor space all around the table (Lee, 2018). The area should not be smaller than 9 × 12 feet (2.7 × 3.4 meters). A space that is 12 × 12 feet is ideal, but other dimensions will work. For example a 10 × 10 foot room will work if the table is placed on an angle. There needs to be a narrow table or counter within easy reach of the massage table to place supplies. If the area is cluttered, too small, or an odd shape (e.g., narrow), the therapist must alter their foot placement and stance, and smooth movement around the client becomes more difficult, whether the person is on a massage table or mat or in a massage chair.

The floor of the massage area must be nonslip to ensure safety and to allow the therapist's feet to obtain a grip on the floor. The table must not slip on the floor. Massage therapists should wear nonslip shoes even when working on a nonslip floor surface. Working in stockings or bare feet is not recommended.

Proper airflow, temperature, lighting, and noise levels are other ergonomic factors that promote the well-being of both the massage therapist and the client. The ideal massage area is quiet and has windows to allow natural light and fresh air, adjustable heat and air conditioning, circulating airflow, and lighting that can be adjusted from bright to dim. Most massage therapists work in conditions that are less than ideal; however, it is important to strive for the healthiest and most ergonomically correct workspace possible.

Massage Equipment

Massage Table

Massage therapists typically work in the standing position. Therefore the width and height of the massage table determine the postures the therapist uses. Massage therapists are at higher risk of cumulative episodes of pain in the low back and upper extremities if they are required to maintain awkward, static postures for the duration of a massage treatment. The massage table can cause these awkward postures in three main ways:

- If the table is too low, the therapist may be required to slouch and bend over or have too wide of a stance at the feet. In this case the table should be raised.
- If the table is too high, the therapist may have to elevate the shoulders, use lateral flexion and twisting of the torso, and stand on the toes. The solution is to lower the table.
- If the table is too wide (or the massage stroke is too long), the therapist must reach. The solution is to use a narrower table, shorten the strokes, step forward and perpendicular to the massage table, and reposition the client.

It is recommended that the forearm be used as much as possible to provide massage to spare overuse of the hands. A higher table supports using forearms, whereas a lower table results in excessive trunk flexion and increased hand use.

Ideally, the table height can be varied according to the technique used and the client's size. However, this is seldom actually possible when using a portable table. Although electric-lift adjustable massage tables are becoming more common, they are not portable.

One common recommendation taught in training programs is that the proper working height of a table is equal to the distance from the floor to a point between the therapist's wrist and the tips of the extended fingers (or about the middle of the hand) when the arm is hanging at the side of the body. Some educators and resources suggest that the optimal height may be as low as the therapist's knees or as high as the waist (Fig. 8.1). Because massage therapy work tasks have not been extensively studied and analyzed through a professional ergonomics lens, these recommendations are opinion based and often inaccurate (Box 8.2). A way to determine table height for each massage therapist is to identify what 20 degrees of trunk flexion is when using both the forearm and palm of the hand. Factor in 6 to 12 inches for the width of the client and set the table at that height. Generally, this table height will fall at the location of the massage practitioner's hip joint.

Awkward posture is associated with an increased risk for injury, and the more a joint can deviate from the neutral position, the greater the risk of injury (Jacquier-Bret and Gorce, 2023) (Box 8.3). Every joint in the body has a neutral position, in which joint spaces are even and symmetrical (Box 8.4). The muscles around a joint in neutral position are neither short nor long, but rather at their neutral physiological resting lengths. Joint stability is provided with the least amount of muscle activity while maximizing stability provided by joint shape, joint capsule, ligaments, and normal co-contraction of the muscles around the joint. Awkward posture refers to positions of the body that deviate significantly from the neutral position while performing work activities. When you are in an awkward posture, muscles operate less efficiently and you expend more force to complete the task (Hairani et al., 2018).

Examples of awkward postures are legs and feet either too close together or too wide apart, twisting, bending, reaching, pulling, or lifting. Other examples of awkward postures are working with your hands above your head, working with your elbows above your shoulders, and working with your neck or back bent more than 20 degrees without support and without the ability to vary posture.

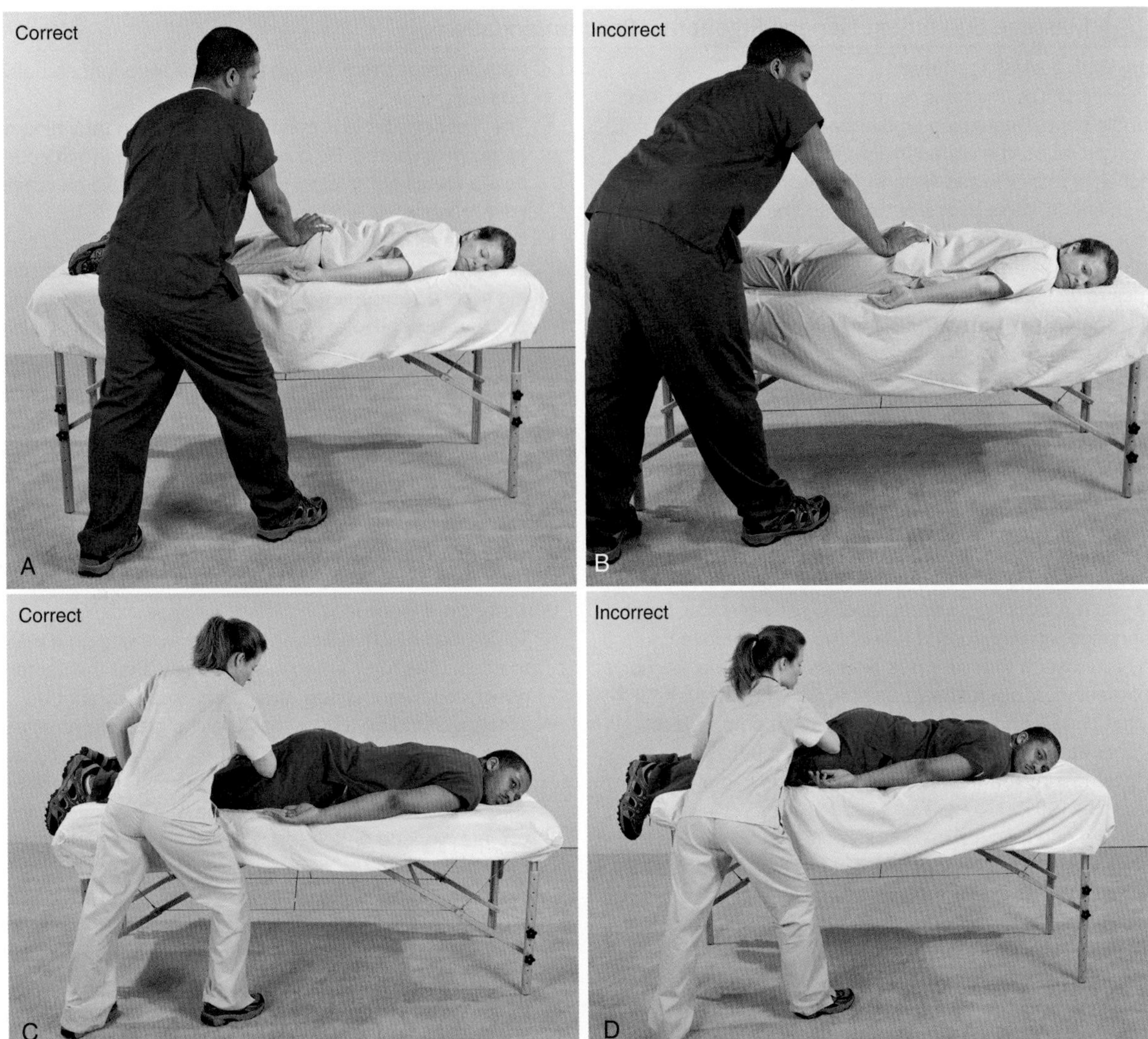

FIG. 8.1 Table height. A, Table at the correct height. **B,** Table too low. **C,** Efficient body mechanics with table at the appropriate height. **D,** Table too high.

Massage therapists need to consider all these factors to prevent injury and have a long, prosperous massage career (Mentoring Tip).

MENTORING TIP

If you experience any discomfort while doing massage, raise the table a few inches. Specific recommendations are presented later, but increasing the height of the table often reduces the strain on the massage therapist's body. Of course, the table can be too high as well, but in the author's experience, most often the table height is lower than what best supports using your forearm when applying massage. Because you want to maximize using the forearm and minimize using the hands during massage, a higher table is logical. A higher table also allows you to stand up straighter and concentrate any forward flexion at the hip joint to reduce strain on the back.

You also need enough floor space to effectively use foot placement to generate push and pull action. Ideally there should be 36 to 48 inches of floor space all around the massage table. This means that the space where massage is performed would be 10 feet wide and 12 feet long.

Biomechanics: Center of Gravity and Leaning

The basic concept of the style of body mechanics presented in this text is that force should be applied to the client's soft tissue by shifting body weight and moving the center of gravity forward. The average position of an object's weight distribution is called the center of gravity. Your center of gravity is closest to the area where most of the weight is located in your body; this usually is somewhere around the navel when you are standing upright with your feet about shoulder width apart. In biomechanics, balance is the ability to maintain the body's center of gravity within the base of support. When the center of gravity is moved outside a base of support created by your feet on the floor, the center of gravity is supported by another support structure, such as the client's body.

The point of contact between the practitioner and the client is the balance point; the practitioner would fall forward if the hand were moved off the client. The practitioner's center of gravity moves forward between the hand or forearm contact, rather than dropping between the feet, as occurs in martial arts or similar systems.

Box 8.2 Massage Equipment General Ergonomic Recommendations

Working With a Massage Table

- As a general rule, the table height should be at the hip joint or pubic bone. Depending on the therapist's torso, arm, and leg length ratios, the correct height for the table will be 2 to 3 inches higher or lower. An individual with long arms may need a shorter table than a person with short arms. A person with a short torso, short arms, and long legs often needs a taller table. There will be some variations to this when it comes to various massage techniques. The lighter the technique application, the higher the table height or it should be as close to the hip joint height as recommended earlier.
- Typically, a female needs a taller table than a male of the same height.
- A table that is 28 to 30 inches wide provides adequate space for the client to lie down comfortably, but it is not so wide that the therapist must reach for the client in the middle of the table. When moving around the table while performing massage, minimize the potential for overreaching by positioning your body as close to the client body area you are working without breaching any physical touch boundaries. An ergonomics rule of thumb is to move your body as close to the work task as possible to keep the body in its most ideal operational position. Referring to the OSHA recommendations as pictured in Box 8.4, it emphasizes this concept. When ergonomists evaluate job tasks, they are looking for the safest and best practices in movement (Pheasant, 1991).
- The knees and hips are used to lift portable tables. The therapist should not bend forward at the waist when lifting the massage table. Some tables have shoulder straps, wheel bases, and other devices to aid in transport by redistributing the weight load.
- Consistently carrying the table on only one side of the body may be harmful. Alternate carrying arms; for example, carry in with the left arm, carry out with the right. The best ergonomic solution is to use a table cart whenever possible to transport a portable table.
- For the most adaptability for massage pressure and technique application, height variability, and best body positioning for each client on your table, use an electric lift/hydraulic table whenever possible.

Sitting on a Chair or Stool at a Massage Table

- Sitting and providing massage is an option especially when lighter pressure is the focus, if there are extended periods of standing or static positioning, or if you are working on a specific finite area on a client's body.
- Sitting for part of the massage session provides posture variation and allows for a bit of a break or rest for larger muscle groups that are sustaining your upright standing position.
- The massage table is generally lower when providing massage while seated. Be sure that you are able to fit your flexed knees completely under the table while minimizing your reach when working seated.
- If using a rolling chair or stool, make sure the wheels can lock so the chair/stool does not roll back when force is applied into the client's body. Alternatively, the massage therapist's feet and legs may need to hold the chair/stool in place, which is still acceptable provided the foot and leg positioning used is similar to standing positions (e.g., transverse and longitudinal stances). Be sure that the stool or chair is an appropriate size for your use, such as making sure that you fit comfortably in the seat pan and the height is adjustable to where your knees can be in a comfortable, flexed, 90-degree position. Also, use a stool that has back support whenever possible for the best neutral seated positioning (Pheasant, 1991).

Working on a Floor Mat

- Table body mechanics also apply for working on a mat on the floor. The main notable difference is that the center of gravity is lower, necessitating greater core strength.
- When working on a floor mat, there is greater potential for torso bending and twist due to the lower center of gravity as mentioned earlier. To assume the most ideal position, be sure to position your body as close to the client body area you are working on to reduce overreach or bending when possible.
- Movement around the client is different when the person is on a floor mat rather than a massage table. The weight-bearing balance points on the floor are from the knees instead of the feet.
- Padding on the knees may be required. Kneepads are a good, available option for protective equipment for the therapist.
- The mat must be large enough so that the massage therapist can keep their knees on the mat while doing the massage.

Working With a Massage Chair

Specially designed massage chairs help with positioning the client so that compression can be applied correctly. However, due to the variations of client size in relation to the size and shape of the massage therapist, prolonged use of a massage chair to deliver massage can increase the risk of strain in the massage therapist's body. Whenever possible, utilize a stool or chair to take a seated position when performing chair massage, such as when working on the forearms or hands of a seated client.

The center of gravity is moved by "leaning" on the client, just as someone would comfortably lean against a wall or on a table. During massage application, you lean forward from the ankle as body weight is transferred to the client in the direction in which you will apply pressure, and your back leg is used for translating weight forward and the front leg for balance (Fig. 8.2 and Proficiency Exercise 8.1).

Even though a force is either a push or a pull, the practitioner seldom "pushes" against the client. Pushing requires a tense body and the use of muscle contraction to exert pressure. It is important that the practitioner use body weight. Although muscle strength is not a big factor, leverage is essential (Magee and Zachazewski, 2007). By leaning to transfer weight, the practitioner can substantially reduce muscle tension in the shoulders, neck, wrists, hand, elbows, and lower back and efficiently apply mechanical forces during the massage. When pushing, create a hinge moment with the upper body in front of the base of support (leaning in against the

Box 8.3 Causes of Muscle Injury

Information in this box is contributed by Dr. Wayne Albert, who has a Bachelor of Science in kinesiology from the University of Ottawa, a master's degree from the University of Western Ontario, and his PhD in occupational biomechanics from Queen's University. The major focus of Albert's research pertains to occupational biomechanics (ergonomics) and the prevention of musculoskeletal injuries in the workplace as well as general low back health. This has led to numerous collaborative projects with researchers from Ontario and Atlantic universities: https://www.unb.ca/faculty-staff/directory/kinesiology/albert-wayne-j.html

Four theories have been proposed to explain how people incur muscle injuries.

1. *Multivariate interaction theory:* The combined effects of an individual's genetics, body type, and psychosocial makeup, along with occupational biomechanical hazards, lead to injury.
2. *Differential fatigue theory:* Different muscles are loaded differently, depending on the motion, and this may not occur in proportion to the muscles' capacity; therefore they fatigue more quickly (e.g., the thumbs compared with the trunk or smaller muscles of the back), causing injury.
3. *Cumulative load theory:* Cumulative submaximum loads result in injury as a result of the cumulative loading of the muscle, which reduces the tolerance of the soft tissues to manage the load.
4. *Overexertion theory:* Exertion exceeds the tolerance limit, and musculoskeletal injury occurs.

In terms of providing massage, this means that the therapist engages several body parts to deliver a massage treatment, but muscles are not equal in strength and endurance capabilities. Different body parts will fatigue more quickly than others. Over a prolonged period, a change in technique may be initiated to accommodate the fatigued body segments, placing higher stress on some joints.

Box 8.4 OSHA's Ergonomics Recommendations

The Occupational Safety and Health Administration (OSHA) has performed numerous studies of body mechanics and ergonomics for various occupations. The following are some of OSHA's consistent recommendations. Later on in the chapter, applications of these guidelines for massage therapists will be applied (see Box 8.7).

- Any posture significantly different from "neutral" is considered to be at risk for musculoskeletal distress. "Neutral" is considered to be the position about halfway through the available range of motion for the joint.
- The number and severity of torso flexions should be limited. Generally, torso flexion should be limited to 6 to 10 degrees from vertical.
- The head should be vertical and should not tilt forward more than about 15 degrees.
- Awkward postures should be avoided, including torso bending, twisting, and reaching.
- The arms should hang normally at the sides of the body and should not reach forward farther than 16 to 18 inches. When reaching, the hands should be maintained vertically between the waist and mid-chest.
- Midrange working postures should be maintained by sitting or standing upright and not bending the joints into extreme positions. The neck, back, arms, and wrists should be kept within a range of neutral positions.
- When standing, the weight should be shifted from one leg to the other.
- The most stable position of the knee is extension.
- Work should not be performed at too low or too high a height.

Risk Factor Zones

There are four zones that a worker might encounter while sitting or standing while performing work tasks:

Zone 0 (Green Zone): This is the preferred or optimal zone because movement occurring in this range causes little to no stress on muscles and joints.

Zone 1 (Yellow Zone): This is the minimal zone because movement occurring in this range creates lower risk exposure to muscles and joints.

Operating within Zones 0 (green) and 1 (yellow) minimizes cumulative effects of repetitive work tasks and potential for injury.

Zone 2 (Red Zone): This range is considered risky and increases potential for injury due to continual use of awkward postures and positioning of limbs. Greater strain on muscles and joints is present. Changes in the performance of the work task is recommended to reduce injury potential.

Zone 3 (Beyond Red Zone): This is the extreme zone because this poses the greatest strain on muscles and joints leading to injury. Work tasks performed frequently in this zone should be avoided if possible, especially with heavy lifting, pushing, pulling, or other similar repetitive tasks. A change in the execution of the work task is required and necessary.

Continued

Box 8.4 **OSHA's Ergonomics Recommendations—cont'd**

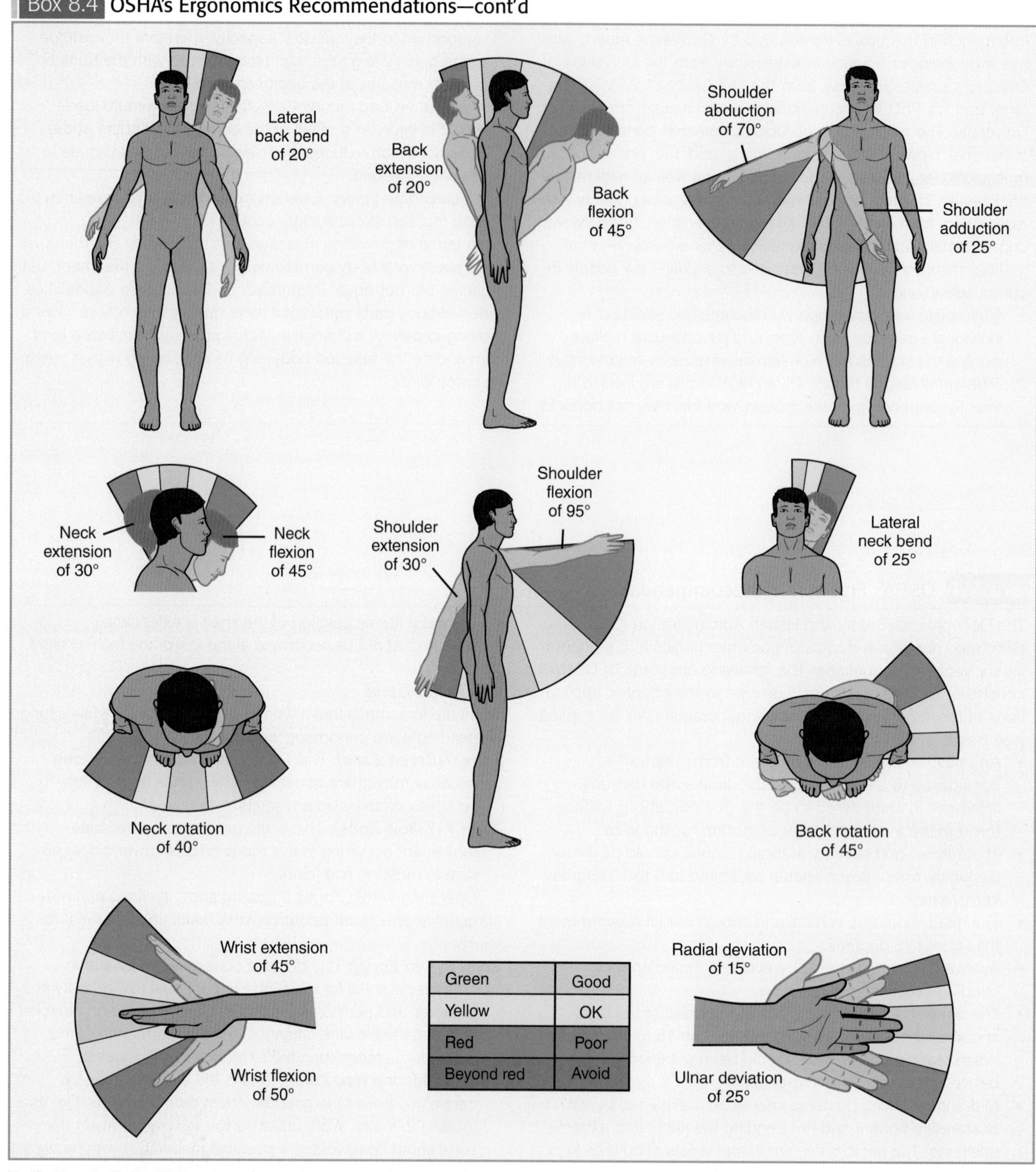

Green	Good
Yellow	OK
Red	Poor
Beyond red	Avoid

Modified from the National Institute for Occupational Safety and Health (NIOSH). Retrieved from http://www.osha.gov/ergonomics/guidelines/retailgrocery/retailgrocery.html. Accessed November 17, 2011.

weight). For pulling, the hinge moment is created with the upper body behind the base of support (leaning back against the weight) (Argubi-Wollesen et al., 2017) (Box 8.5).

When the hand is used to apply pressure during massage, the most correct position of the arm is with the elbow joint straight so that the forces produced flow directly along the bones and through the joints. This means that the elbow must be in extension (but not hyperextension) to reduce the amount of muscular effort required by the massage therapist. The other biomechanically correct position of the arm is with the arm held close to the body and the elbow flexed at 90 degrees.

The knee of the weight-bearing leg also must be in extension (not hyperextension) to transmit force from the foot pushing into the floor. Muscles fatigue; bones do not. Therefore we should maximize massage techniques that use weight

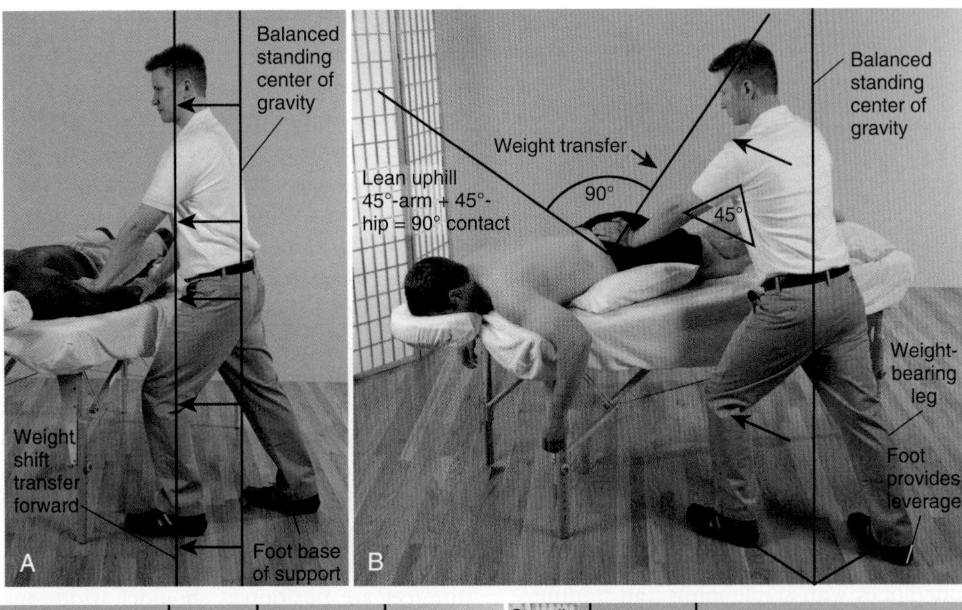

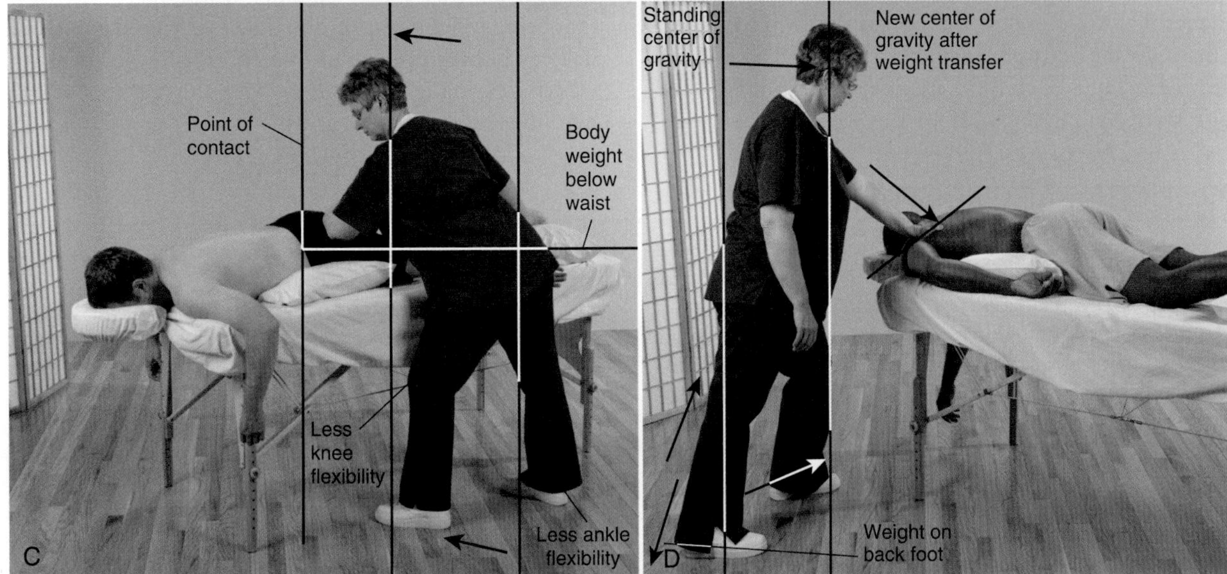

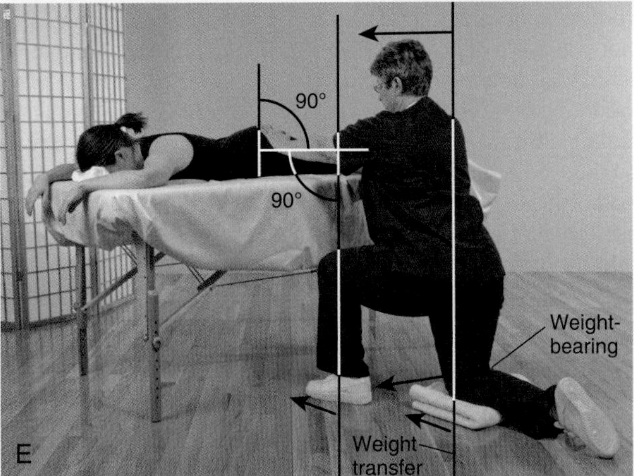

FIG. 8.2 A, Using the principles of body mechanics in a weight shift. **B,** During a weight shift, the center of gravity moves from between the feet to between the contact point and the original balanced center of gravity, allowing leaning to achieve a 90-degree contact on the body with the massage therapist's shoulder stabilized at approximately 45 degrees and the client's body sloped at 45 degrees. **C,** Gender differences, female example: The body weight is below the waist; less knee and ankle flexibility require a higher massage table than for a male. **D,** The ground reaction force from weight on the back leg during a weight shift results in the application of forces at the client contact. **E,** Weight transfer while kneeling or **F,** seated.

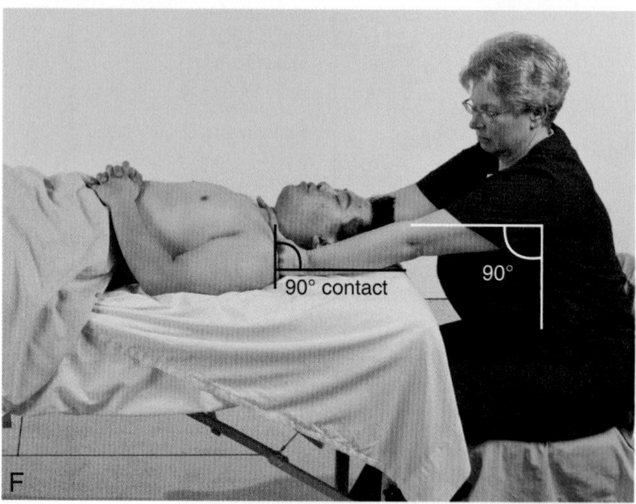

FIG. 8.2 cont'd

transfer through our bones with stable joints and minimize techniques that use muscles. This means that while performing a massage, the body positioning is subtle and should look like normal and typical body functions such as walking, standing, or relaxed leaning (Fig. 8.3).

Friction and Traction: The Importance of the Feet

Body mechanics for massage begin at the feet. Ground reaction forces at the foot and floor represent one of the most important—yet often overlooked—aspects of massage application. For our purposes, we can say that ground reaction forces occur when the body pushes into the floor and the floor pushes back, so long as no slipping occurs. **Friction** is the force that prevents slipping. Traction is required to prevent slipping. **Traction** is the maximum frictional force that can be produced between surfaces without slipping; this applies, during massage, between the foot and the floor, or in contact with the client's body. Massage should not be performed in bare or stockinged feet because this is unsafe and unsanitary. The only way to ensure adequate friction (and therefore the ability to generate force) is to wear shoes that have a nonslip sole and that can be tied or strapped around the arch (e.g., athletic shoes) (Fig. 8.4).

The massage therapist can generate the greatest force when the feet are positioned shoulder width apart and with one foot being weight bearing and the other placed approximately halfway between the point of contact with the client and the weight-bearing foot. In this posture, the rear foot will be behind the body's center of gravity.

PROFICIENCY EXERCISE 8.1

After being observed by a peer or instructor and obtaining your score from the Assessment Tool in Box 8.7, use some of these exercises to help you improve on your identified risk factors.

1. Have someone record you giving a massage using a digital video camera, smartphone, or tablet device. Do you look graceful and relaxed, or are you working too hard? Use the assessment tool in Box 8.7 and evaluate yourself or have someone evaluate you and compare the results. Sometimes seeing yourself in action can help pinpoint where you might be developing discomfort or the potential for injury.
2. Experiment with different ways of positioning of the client. Is the side-lying position the best option to achieve this client's goals and promote less work effort on your part? Does the part of the client's body that you are working on need to be moved closer to you? Match your treatment planning with the application of massage that works best with your individual body mechanics. Practice different positions and appropriate draping regularly so that you are proficient with them. This gives you many more options when treatment planning to adapt your work environment and work based on the size, shape, and treatment needs for each individual client.
3. Tie the end of a thin short rope or string around one wrist, wrap it around your waist, and then tie the other end around your other wrist. The length of the rope should allow you to reach out to about a 40- to 45-degree angle with relaxed shoulders. Perform a massage. The rope/string will prevent you from reaching too far with the stroke and will tug at your waist when it is time to shift the body by taking a step closer to the area you are working on.
4. Vary the table height. What happens when a client gets on your portable table and you have not been able to adjust the table height to suit your needs ergonomically? How do you manage this situation? Use a step stool with nearby support to increase your leverage when needed for applying compressive pressure effectively.
5. Refrain from using the anterior hand. As massage therapists, we tend to use the palms of our hands extensively when performing our work. This is a repetitive motion issue that can lead to repetitive stress injuries such as carpal tunnel syndrome, tenosynovitis, De Quervain's syndrome, and many others. So how often do you use your palms? What if you could not use them? What other tools could you use to still provide an effective quality massage session? Experiment.
6. Practice providing massage in a seated position. Using a rolling or stationary stool or chair, experiment with your table height, your stances, and your stroke delivery while in a seated position. Are there areas where you feel more relaxed performing massage in a seated position than standing? Could you incorporate this as part of your massage session to allow for microbreaks for your larger core muscle groups? Can you put the stool or chair in a safe position around the massage table that allows for you to move freely while still being able to use it for short periods during a massage session?
7. Do you stretch before and after performing a massage? Practice leaning on a wall with your back and posterior side against it. Are your shoulders more medially rotated? Head more forward? Tight pectorals? Pelvic tilt? Upper or lower crossed syndromes? Assess the postural issues that could be affecting the way you perform massage and do some stretching before and after sessions to relieve some of the strained postures that may be enabled from your massage work preferences. Make changes to limit the tendencies that lead to issues for therapists just as they do for our clients.
8. Experiment with manual support tools. Massage suppliers make many handheld tools to help us preserve our thumbs and hands. Are they effective for you? Why or why not?

Box 8.5 Force

Force is a push or pull on an object, which then causes acceleration, deceleration, or a change in shape if the object is stable. Massage application employs mechanical forces. The body can move in response to the force (joint movement), or it can change shape, as happens when the soft tissue is massaged.

Forces always occur in pairs. You cannot apply a force to the client's body without the body applying a force back. This is the reason we can lean on something (a wall, a desk, a client's body) and not fall.

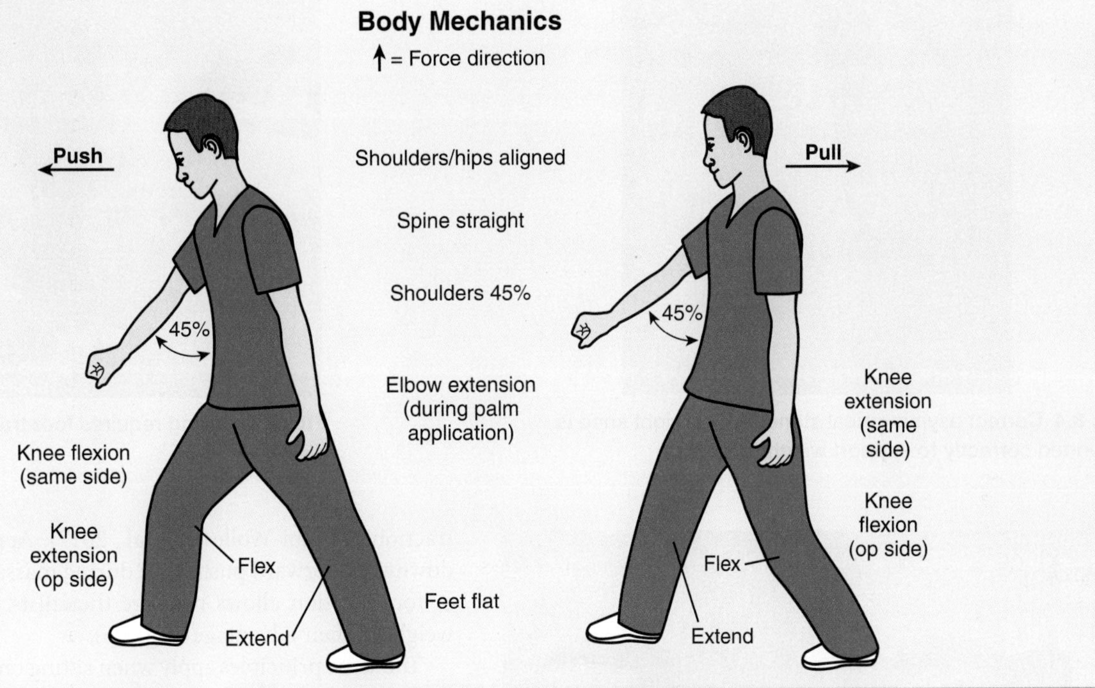

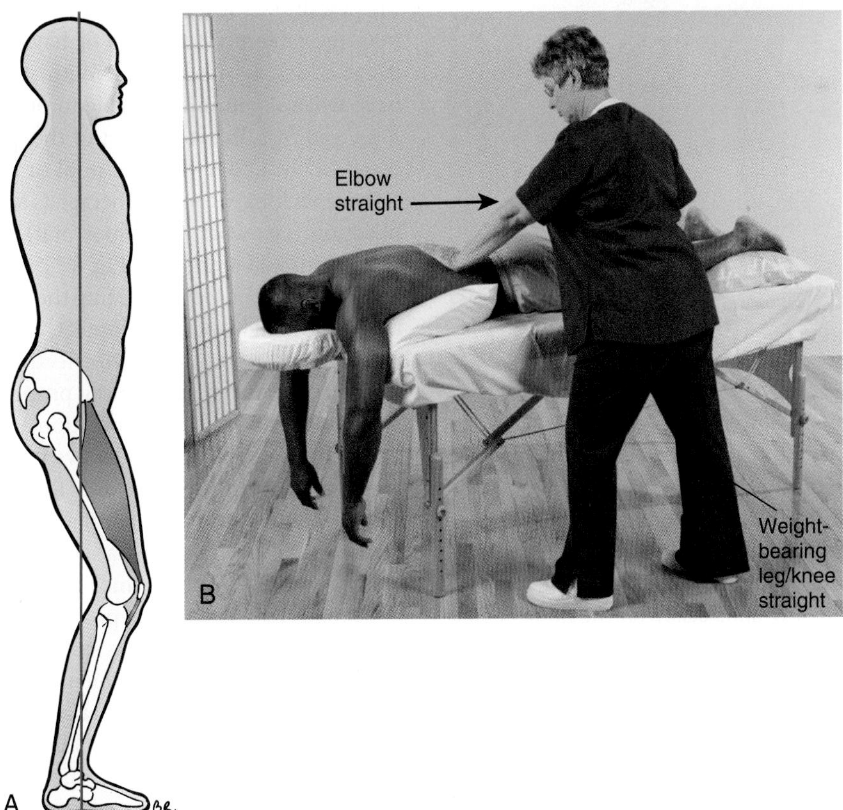

FIG. 8.3 A, Improper leg position, which puts excessive strain on the joints and requires muscle activity to maintain balance. The gravitational line improperly falls behind the knees. **B,** Stability for a weight transfer relies on an extended (but not hyperextended) knee and elbow.

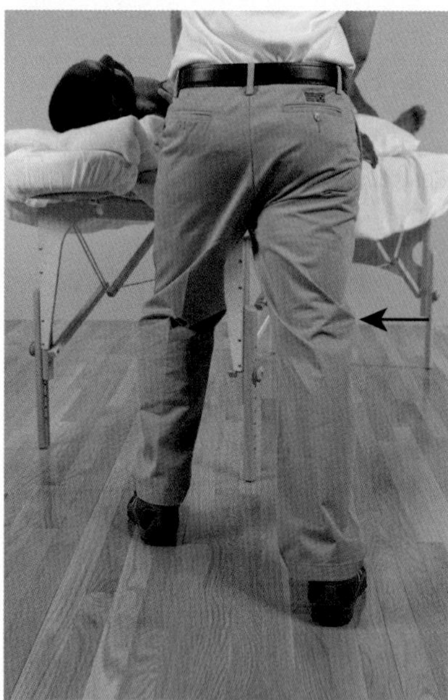

FIG. 8.4 Correct asymmetrical standing. The right knee is extended correctly to support weight bearing.

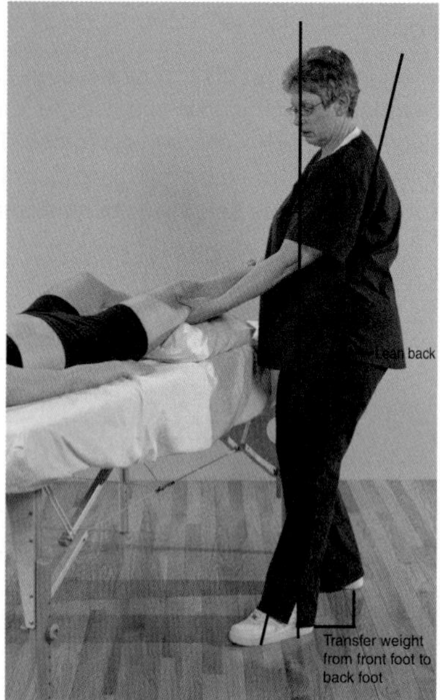

FIG. 8.6 Pulling requires foot traction.

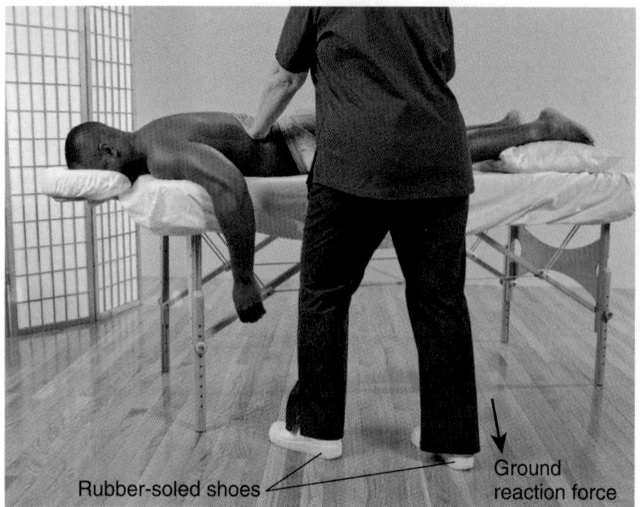

FIG. 8.5 Ground reaction forces require nonslip surfaces.

According to Newton's law, for every force on a body, an equal and opposite reaction force occurs. Therefore whatever force is applied to the client's body by the hands and forearms elicits a reaction by an equal force at the foot–floor interface. For example if you apply 15 pounds of force (moderate pressure) during massage, the friction force at your feet must be equal to 15 pounds. If the foot slips easily on the floor or in a sock, or even in ill-fitting shoes, the amount of force you can apply during massage is limited to the amount of friction force or traction at the feet. To get more pressure you must push with your muscles, which is inefficient (Fig. 8.5).

Furthermore, with limited traction at the feet, you cannot safely lean into the client's body or away as in a pulling because the feet will begin to slip. Researchers have shown that a person pushing with good traction can generate as much as 50% more force than can be obtained when pushing with poor traction (Argubi-Wollesen et al., 2017). Applying an oblique, downward-forward push force during massage with the proper foot traction allows massage therapists to use their body weight to their advantage (Fig. 8.6).

The same principles apply when sitting on a chair or stool to perform massage. The chair or stool must not slip back when the practitioner leans forward to apply pressure. For safety, the massage table must not slip or have wheels or rollers unless it has a locking mechanism. With stools or chairs, if they do have wheels, you must be able to put both feet solidly on the floor and fit fully on the seat of the stool or chair in order to use it safely. Otherwise, the stool or chair must be stationary or have locking wheels. If therapists kneel during massage application (i.e., work on a floor mat), their knees become the contact instead of the feet (Fig. 8.7). A similar approach occurs if seated with the feet stabilizing the chair or stool and the hips being the weight-bearing contact, and it is still possible for a massage therapist to perform effective strokes from this position. With the feet maintaining proper floor contact, knees in a relaxed 90-degree angle position while seated, the table at an appropriate height that allows for force to be utilized and transferred from the core, and foot positioning (e.g., transverse and longitudinal stances) as used in standing, a massage therapist can effectively use a seated position periodically. This creates moments where some of the same core and thigh muscles supporting a standing posture can be given microbreaks or micropauses. Ergonomics studies have shown in many different types of work environments that the use of microbreaks during a workday decreases fatigue compared with taking no microbreaks (Pheasant, 1991). Use Proficiency Exercise 8.1 to experiment with safely incorporating seated positions into your massage session.

When using the feet to perform a massage while the client is on a mat, massage therapists must make sure they are standing on a nonslip surface. A stable, non-skid cane (available at

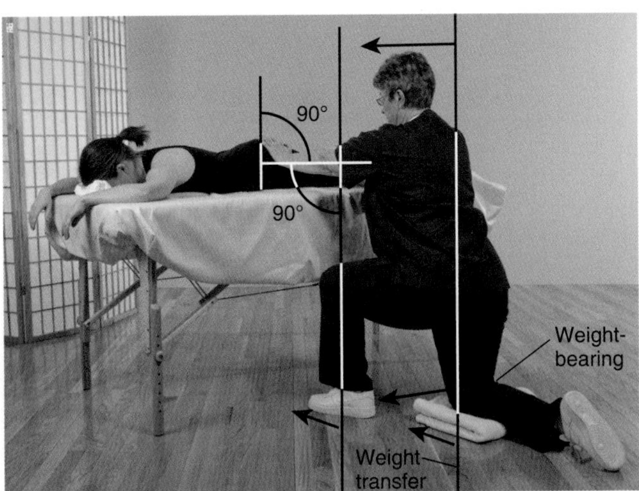

FIG. 8.7 When the practitioner kneels to provide massage, the back knee becomes weight bearing; a folded towel can be used as a cushion.

medical supply retailers) can be used to support balance in these cases (Fig. 8.8).

Massage therapists also must keep in mind that although they use lubricant to reduce friction on the client's skin, this also reduces traction. If too much lubricant is used, pressure is difficult to apply regardless of your positioning.

Basic Concepts of Body Mechanics

Four basic concepts of body mechanics are common to all techniques used to apply compressive force to the body tissues during massage:

- Keeping the back straight and maintaining core stability
- Weight transfer
- Perpendicularity
- Stacking the joints

A straight back and a straight pressure-bearing leg are essential components of body mechanics. If the back is not straight, the practitioner often ends up pushing with the upper body instead of using the more effortless feeling of transferred weight. The practitioner's weight should be held on the back leg and flat foot, concentrated toward the heel. At first this may feel uncomfortable; however, some of the biggest muscles in the body are in the legs. If you use the muscles of your upper body, fatigue sets in more quickly. The muscles of the torso, especially the abdomen, make up the body's core. Core stability is necessary for back stability (Neumann, 2010).

With weight transfer, massage practitioners transfer their body weight by shifting the center of gravity forward to achieve a pressure that is comfortable to the client. To transfer weight, the practitioner stands (or kneels) with one foot forward and the other foot (or knee) back in an asymmetrical stance. In the standing position, the front leg is in a relaxed hip and knee flexion with the foot forward enough to be in front of the knee. The flexion angle at the hip should be no more than 20 degrees. The back leg is straight, and the hips and shoulders are aligned so that the back is straight. The transfer is made by taking the weight off the front leg and moving it to whichever

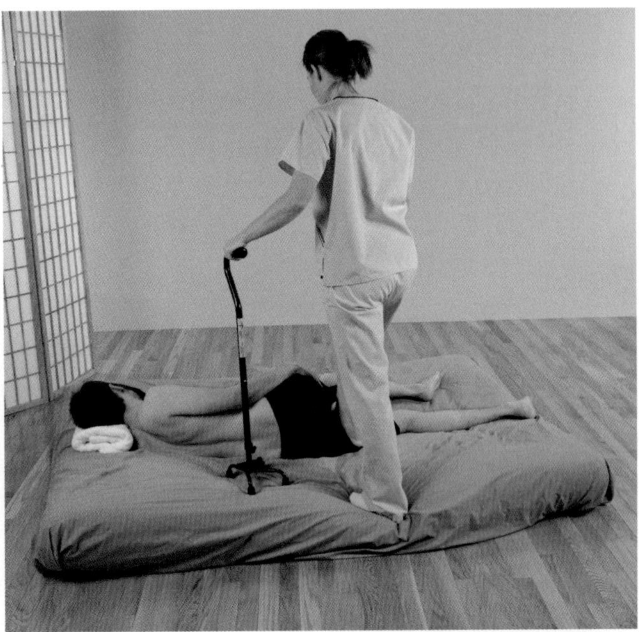

FIG. 8.8 A cane provides support when the foot is used to apply massage.

part of the arm and hand is used to apply pressure (Fig. 8.9). The massage therapist's body weight is distributed to the flat foot of the weight-bearing leg, and the weight should be directed more toward the heel. Practitioners should not stand on their toes.

Perpendicularity ensures that the pressure exerted by the massage therapist sinks straight into the client's tissues. Massage primarily uses a force generated forward and downward with a 90-degree contact against the body (Fig. 8.10). The combination of a 45-degree slant from the contours of the client's body plus the 45-degree angle of force used during appropriate body mechanics results in the 90-degree contact (Fig. 8.11).

Stacking the joints one on top of another is essential to the concepts of perpendicularity and weight transfer. The practitioner's body must be a straight line from the feet and then through the shoulder to the forearm, or through the elbow acting as an extension of the shoulder, to the palms of the hands (Fig. 8.12). The ankle, knee, hip of the back leg, and spine are stacked. The shoulder is stacked over the elbow, which in turn is stacked over the wrist. Stacking the joints in this way allows the pressure to move straight into the client's body effortlessly as the center of gravity moves forward. Stability of the shoulder girdle and elbow also is essential. Even with the best body mechanics, stabilizing the shoulder is difficult. It is important to keep the scapula fixed in place against the rib cage. The normal biomechanical position of the shoulder blade should always be resting flat against the rib cage, regardless of the position of the arm.

The two common stability problems for massage therapists are the core and the shoulder complex. The primary muscle that stabilizes the scapula to the rib cage is the serratus anterior. Other muscles that offer support in that role are the middle and lower trapezius and rhomboids. The serratus anterior fibers contract when the arm is pushing against

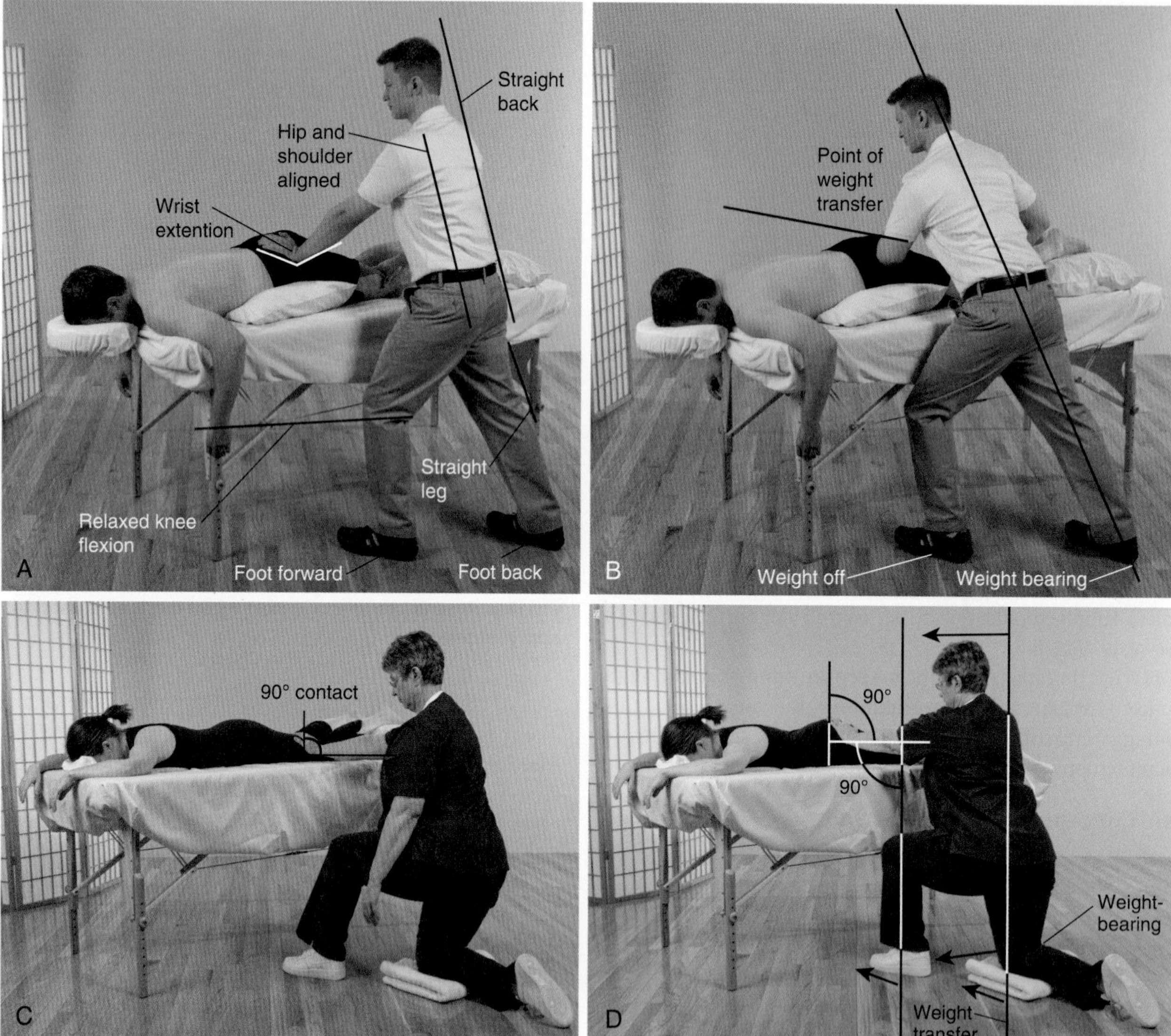

FIG. 8.9 **A,** Maintaining alignment of the shoulder and pelvic girdle is part of the stacking of the joints. **B,** To achieve the most pressure during a weight transfer, the point of contact on the client (hand or forearm) and the therapist's back foot opposite the working arm are weight bearing. The front foot on the same side as the working arm is used only for balance. **C, D,** Weight transfer while kneeling.

resistance, which is what happens in giving a massage. The client is the point of resistance. In such a situation, the middle fibers of the trapezius (an adductor) and the serratus (acting as an abductor) contract simultaneously to stabilize the scapula. The scapula slides upward, downward, forward, and backward and also rotates clockwise or counterclockwise as the arm moves; however, it should not come away from the rib cage.

If the muscles that hold the shoulder blade against the rib cage do not work properly and scapular winging occurs, inappropriate activation of other muscle groups will compensate, resulting in overuse and strain in these muscles.

When using the forearm to apply massage methods use the proximal one-third from the elbow to the mid-forearm. This position allows the scapula to remain stable. Avoid using the distal part of the forearm near the wrist, as this will allow the elbow to drop and the contact is unstable (Fig. 8.13).

Pressure

In massage we often use the word **pressure** to indicate magnitude. Light pressure = small magnitude and heavy/firm pressure = increased magnitude. Pressure is the amount of force applied into the tissue. Pressure during massage is usually applied down into the client's body at an angle of 45 to 90 degrees. Pressure applied within the 45-degree range will orient more horizontally, and pressure applied closer to the 90-degree range will be more perpendicular.

Another factor that influences the application of pressure is the size of the point of contact. Most clients appreciate moderate, even pressure that is distributed over a wide area. Pressure over a large contact area is less intense than that applied through a small contact point. More pressure can be applied safely with a broad base of contact, such as the forearm or full hand, than through a small point of contact, such as the thumb, fingertips, or point of the elbow. For example, firm pressure

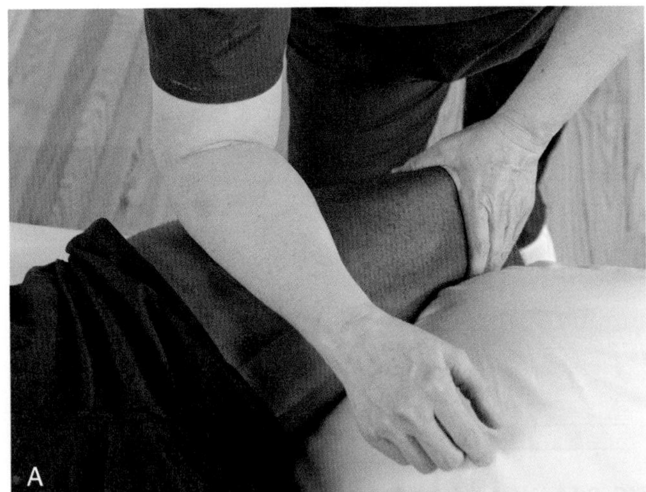

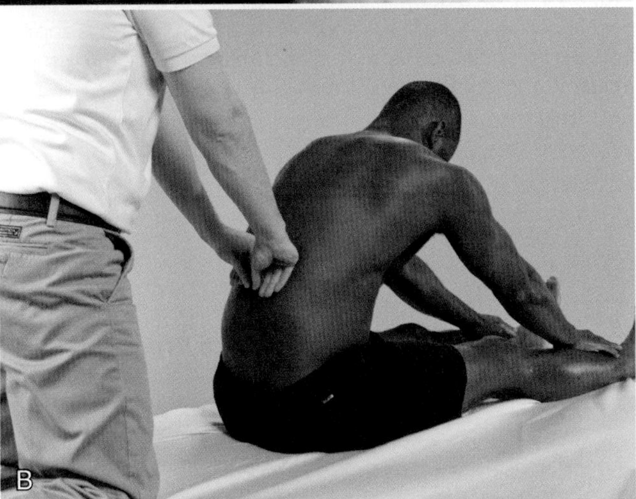

FIG. 8.10 The principle of perpendicularity means that pressure exerted by the massage therapist sinks straight into the client's tissues when the forearm **A,** and hand **B,** are used.

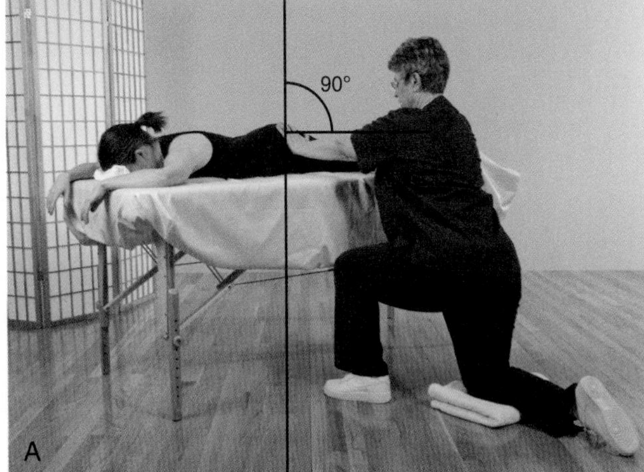

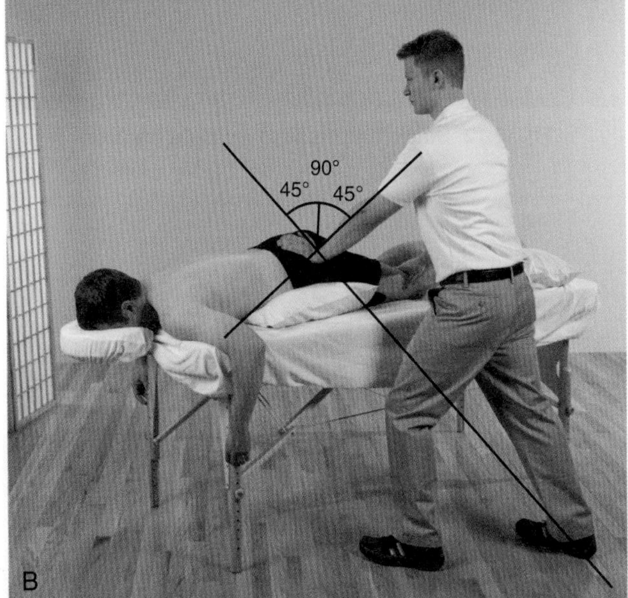

FIG. 8.11 **A,** Kneeling or seated position with transfer forward creates a 90-degree contact. **B,** In the standing position, leaning by weight shift and shoulder angle about 45 degrees plus the approximate 45-degree angle at the client contact results in a 90-degree contact.

applied to the back with the forearm is pleasant. However, the same pressure applied with the point of the elbow or the thumb would be painful because the pressure is concentrated in a small space instead of dispersed over a broad area. The tissue feels as if it is being poked, and the potential for tissue damage rises. When the practitioner's weight is maintained on the back foot and core stabilization is maintained, the pressure levels are more even; however, when the weight shifts to the front foot and core stabilization is lost, the pressure becomes more concentrated and uneven and may be uncomfortable to the client.

To apply pressure to a client, especially during a gliding stroke, moving uphill is always more efficient than moving downhill. When a force vector is applied at an angle, the force can be broken down into horizontal and vertical components. When a force is applied uphill, both the horizontal and vertical components are directed into the client's tissue. However, when a force is applied downhill, only the vertical component is directed into the tissue; the horizontal component is dissipated and thus wasted (Fig. 8.14).

The foot and arm positions can also affect pressure levels. In the asymmetrical stance, where one foot is in front of the other, which arm is used to apply the massage method can influence the pressure depth. More pressure is applied when the arm applying the method is on the same side as the forward leg—that is, if the left leg is back and weight bearing, then the right leg is forward and used for balance and the right arm is the working arm. For less pressure, the working arm is paired with the back leg instead. For example, the left leg is back and weight bearing, the right leg is forward, and the left arm is used to apply the massage method. This shift occurs because pressure delivery relates to the base of support at the feet. When the same arm and front leg are used, the arm and back foot are the points of weight transfer. When the working arm is paired with the back leg, the front leg also becomes weight bearing. To investigate this further, research more about triangles and types of angles (Fig. 8.15).

A variety of pressure depths are accessed when mechanical force is applied to tissues. More pressure involves an increase in force magnitude and less magnitude is needed for

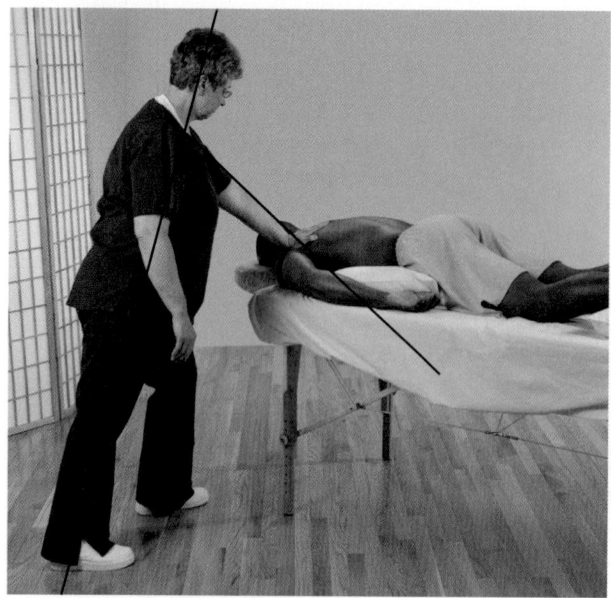

FIG. 8.12 Stacked joints with a weight transfer.

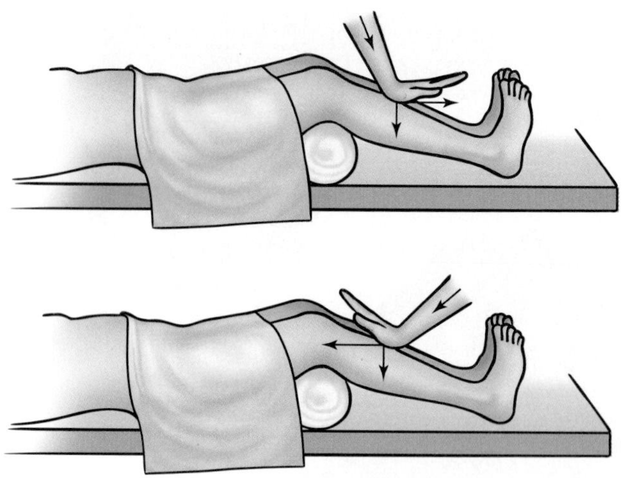

FIG. 8.14 When a downhill stoke is applied, only the vertical component penetrates the tissue *(top).* When an uphill stroke is applied, both the horizontal and vertical components penetrate the tissue *(bottom).* Therefore the uphill stroke is more efficient.

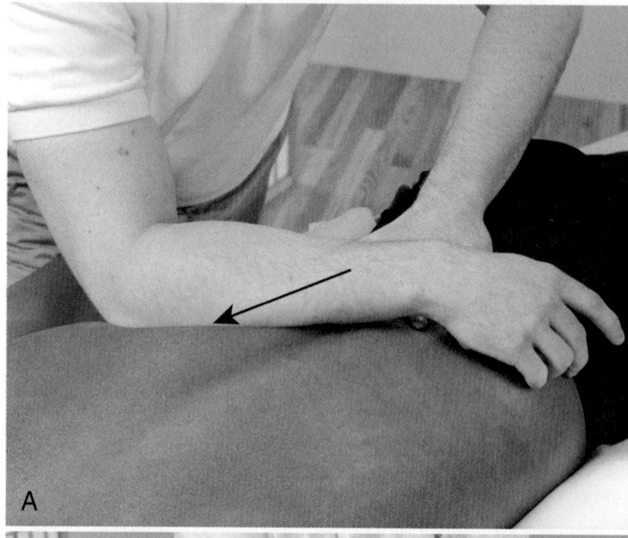

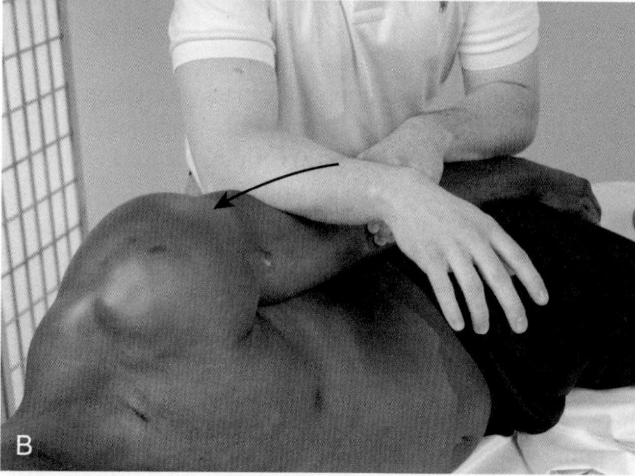

FIG. 8.13 Proper forearm technique. The proximal third aspect of the forearm from the tip of the elbow (olecranon process) to one-third of proximal the ulna contacts the client. Avoid using the tip of the elbow. Avoid using mid-forearm to wrist to apply pressure. Do not use the arm proximal to the elbow to avoid pressure on the ulnar nerve.

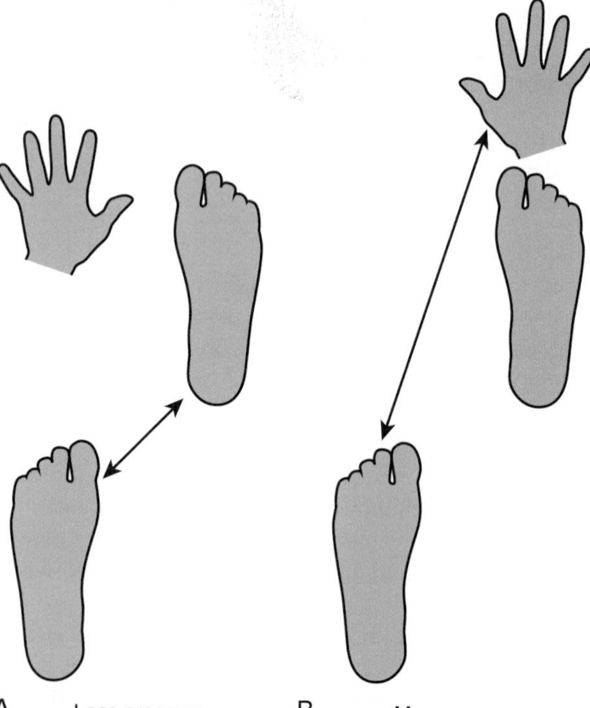

FIG. 8.15 Pressure applied during massage can be adapted based on foot and hand/forearm placement. For less pressure, see Part **A.** A three-point contact distributes weight between the two feet resulting in less weight distributed to the working arm/hand. In **B** more pressure is generated since the weight is distributed between the opposite foot and hand/forearm resulting in a three-point contact, back foot to opposite hand/arm with the front foot used primarily for balance and non-weight-bearing.

a lighter pressure. Obviously, determining the right pressure is more difficult than it appears. A variety of pressure depths will be needed to affect various layers of soft tissue. Hypothetically speaking, the tissues in the fleshy areas of the body (i.e., between the joints) can be divided into seven layers, which require seven levels of pressure depth. The seven tissue layers, surface to deep, are as follows:

Level 1—Skin surface
Level 2—Skin
Level 3—Superficial fascia
Level 4—First muscle layer
Level 5—Second muscle layer
Level 6—Third muscle layer
Level 7—Bone

The corresponding levels of pressure required to reach each of these layers are as follows (Fig. 8.16):

- *Level 1:* Pressure touches the skin but does not dent it. It slides on the skin and cannot produce drag or tension of the skin. The therapist's fingertips do not blanch (change color). A bathroom scale or other scale does not move at this pressure (Fig. 8.16A).
- *Level 2:* Pressure slightly dents the skin. It moves (drags) the skin to bind but cannot apply a tension force to stretch the skin past bind. The therapist's fingertips blanch, but the nail bed does not change color. A scale would move just 0–5 pounds, depending on the density of the person's skin (Fig. 8.16B).
- *Level 3:* Pressure magnitude should penetrate the skin but should not reach the muscle; palpation of muscle structure indicates that the force application is too intense. The therapist's fingertips and nail beds blanch. A scale would move 3–10 pounds. Body mechanics involve slight leaning into the tissue (Fig. 8.16C).
- *Level 4:* Pressure magnitude penetrates the skin and superficial fascia. The skin layer is displaced (pressed away), and the therapist should be able to palpate muscle tissue. Body mechanics require moderate leaning into the tissue. A scale would move 7–16 pounds, depending on the tissue density (Fig. 8.16D).
- *Level 5:* Pressure displaces the surface tissues (i.e., skin, fascia, and first muscle layer), and the applied force penetrates to the middle muscle layer. Point or narrow-based contact would feel "pokey." Broad-based contact with leaning body mechanics typically is used. A scale would move 12–35 pounds, depending on the tissue density and the bulk of the first layer of muscle (Fig. 8.16E).
- *Level 6:* Pressure displaces surface tissues (skin, fascia, and first and second muscle layers), and the applied force penetrates to the third muscle layer. This layer of muscle is smaller than the first and second layers and lies next to the bone. Applying force compresses the muscle against the bone; however, if bone is felt, the force is too intense. Full leaning body mechanics with simultaneous counterpressure may be required to reach this layer. Counterpressure involves pulling up against the table or the client's body while compressive force is applied. Broad-based contact must be used, or pain and protective guarding will occur in the first and second muscle layers. A scale would move 25–60 pounds (sometimes higher), depending on the recipient's muscle bulk and tissue density (Fig. 8.16F).
- *Level 7:* Pressure is slightly more intense than at level 6. The therapist feels bone pressing against the tissue except around the joints where the muscle layers are not prominent and the bone is beneath the skin and superficial fascia (Fig. 8.16G).

Counterpressure

The practitioner should not push, even if intense pressure is required. Instead, weight transfer shifting the massage therapist's center of gravity occurs as the practitioner leans on the area of the client's body that requires the intense pressure and then, using the nonworking hand, lifts at the table edge (Fig. 8.17). A variation of counterpressure involves the client. The massage therapist applies a broad application of force into the tissue area (which is braced and stabilized). Then the client is asked to push or lean back into the massage therapist's contact area, which will combine the force exerted by the massage therapist with the counterforce provided by the client to increase the pressure. These types of applications need to be monitored because force magnitude can be increased substantially and involve potential tissue damage to the client. Also, these methods need to be limited because generating force at this magnitude has the potential to cause injury to the massage therapist. Directing the client to move slowly is recommended.

Drag

Drag is the resistance to glide. Glide moves horizontally to the tissues. Drag applies tension stress to tissues to elongate them. The angle of force is directed away from the point of contact and can range from just less than 90 degrees to 180 degrees. Pressure combined with drag therefore can produce a broad range of intensities. For example, light pressure with extensive drag significantly stretches the skin and superficial fascia. If the pressure is increased slightly and significant drag is maintained, the superficial fascia is stretched as it slides over the deep fascia (tension loading is applied) (Fig. 8.18).

The following is a suggested scale for determining drag:

0—Minimal drag (Fig. 8.18A)
1—Moves tissue but not to bind
2—Moves tissue to bind
3—Maximum drag: Moves tissue past bind (Fig. 8.18B)

Duration

Duration can modify intensity. Guidelines for duration include the following:

- For a specific application, a short duration is 10 seconds, a moderate duration is 30 seconds, and a long duration is 60 seconds.
- For a whole massage session, a short duration is 5 to 15 minutes, a moderate duration is 15 to 30 minutes, and a long duration is 45 to 60 minutes.

Speed

The speed of the massage application also can influence the intensity of the massage and the outcomes. Typically, the slower

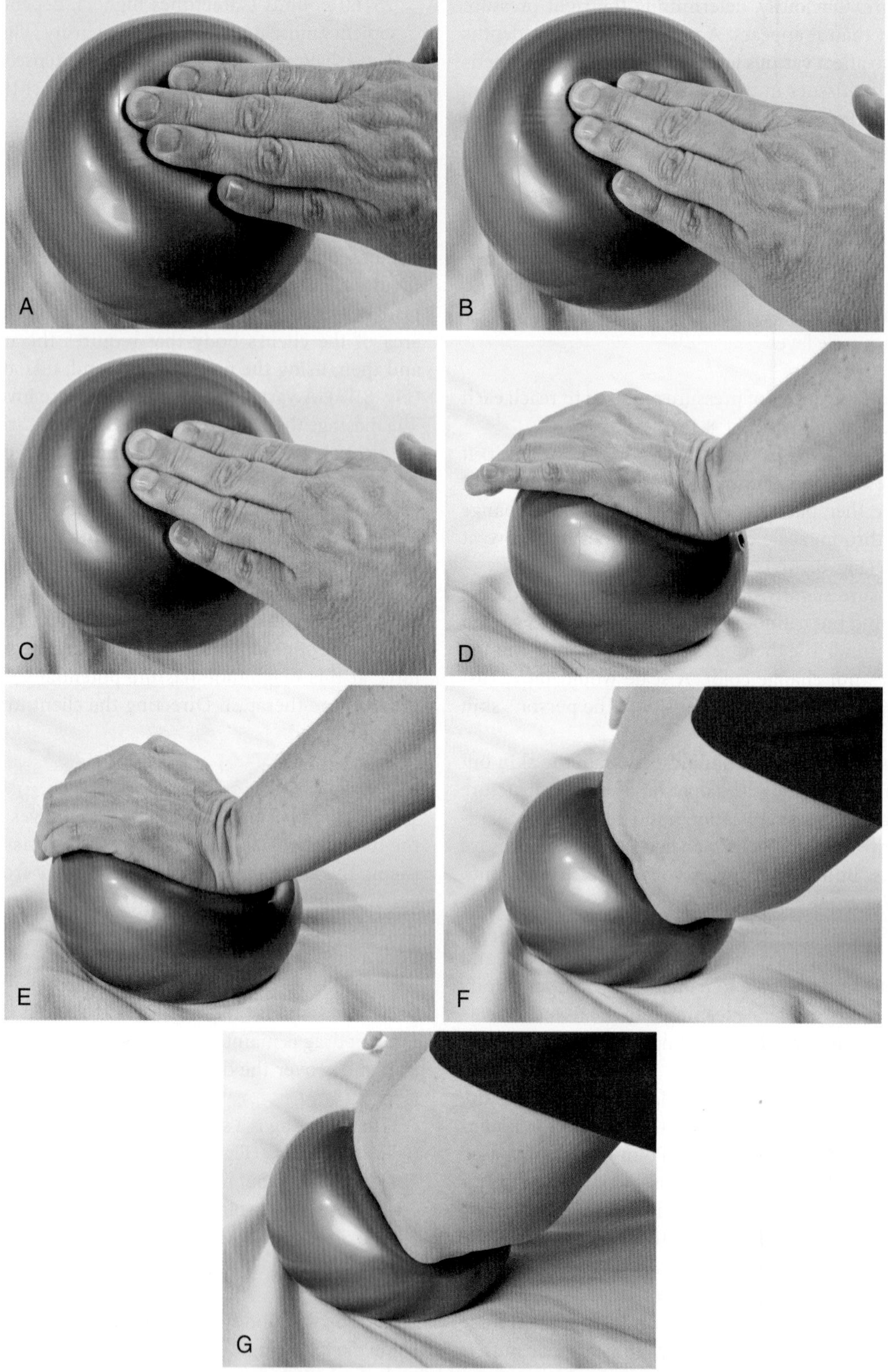

FIG. 8.16 Pressure levels. **A,** Level 1, light. The therapist's fingertips do not blanch. **B,** Level 2. **C,** Level 3. **D,** Level 4. **E,** Level 5. **F,** Level 6. **G,** Level 7.

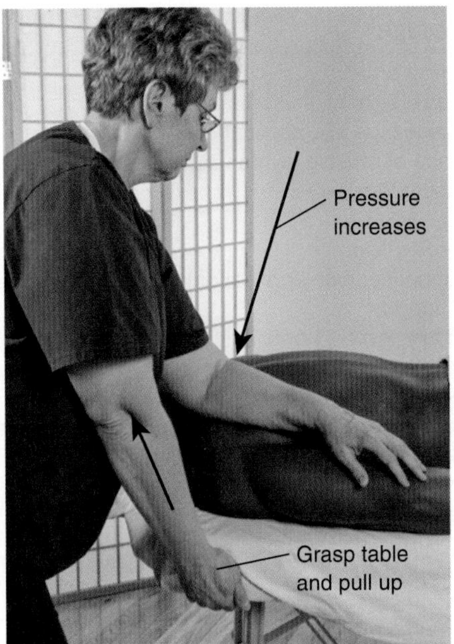

FIG. 8.17 Application of counterpressure.

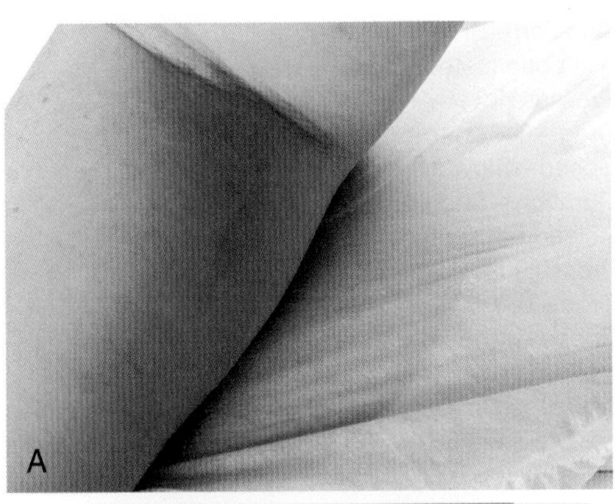

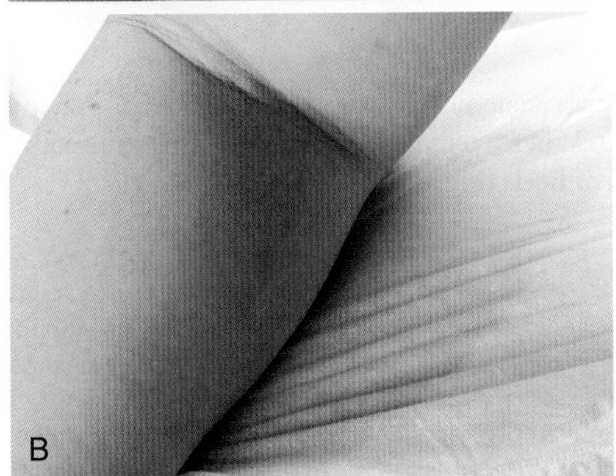

FIG. 8.18 (A) Minimal drag. (B) Maximum drag.

the speed, the more relaxing the massage. The faster the speed, the more stimulating the massage. Speed can be considered as follows:

- Slow—10 seconds from beginning to end of stroke
- Moderate—5 seconds from beginning to end of stroke
- Fast—2 seconds from beginning to end of stroke

Intensity

Describing various pressures and drag intensities is difficult because they are affected by many factors, including (1) the client's body size, tissue quality, and treatment preferences; (2) the massage therapist's strength, expertise, and technique preference; and (3) the location of the pressure and the desired outcome for the massage. The perception of the application depends extensively on the client. Pressure perceived as deep by one client may be perceived as lighter pressure by another. Massage therapists learn to gauge the most beneficial and safest pressure and drag intensity. Duration can modify intensity. In general, long duration is more intense and short duration is less intense. Speed is also a factor. A term used to describe the combination of pressure, drag, duration, and speed that is most beneficial and most satisfying to clients is **therapeutic edge**.

Client Rhythm

It is important that massage practitioners allow their bodies to rock and sway with the massage movements. Slow rocking keeps the massage manipulations slow; this is crucial for efficient adaptation or change in the client's muscle tissue or in the consistency of the connective tissue. The resulting rhythmic movement keeps the practitioner's body relaxed and is comforting to the client. Practitioners should remember to work with smooth, even movements, shifting position often.

The general guidelines presented in Box 8.6 can be used to combine the elements of pressure, drag, speed, and duration to achieve various massage outcomes (Focus on Professionalism 8.1) (Mentoring Tip).

GENDER DIFFERENCES

SECTION OBJECTIVES

Chapter objective covered in this section:

5. Alter ergonomic and biomechanical principles based on gender.

Using the information presented in this section, the student will be able to perform the following:

- Explain the necessary changes in body mechanics based on research findings in gender differences.

The differences between the male body and the female body affect proper body mechanics (Bisiacchi and Huber, 2006). Most massage therapists identify as female (American Massage Therapy Association, 2022). Generally, females have more elastic tissues than males. Also, females tend to have a slightly broader range of joint movement but less ankle flexibility. Regardless, it is important to use the most efficient body mechanics possible.

Center of Gravity

A female's center of gravity is lower and farther back than a male. Females also carry more weight below the waist. Males are broader in the chest and shoulders and carry their weight above the waist (Fig. 8.19).

Box 8.6 Guidelines for Pressure, Drag, Speed, and Duration of Massage

- Fragile patient outcomes: comforting and soothing
  - Pressure level—1 or 2/7
  - Drag—0
  - Speed—Slow
  - Duration—Short
- Palliative, pleasure-based massage (nonfragile)
  - Pressure level—2 or 3/7
  - Drag—1–2/3
  - Speed—Slow
  - Duration (full session)—Short to moderate or moderate to long
- Lymphatic drainage, surface tissues
  - Pressure level—2 or 3/7
  - Drag—2/3
  - Speed—Slow
  - Duration—Varies; moderate to long
- Lymphatic drainage, deep tissues
  - Pressure level—4 or 5/7
  - Drag—2/3
  - Speed—Slow
  - Duration—Short
- Myofascial release, superficial fascia
  - Pressure level—3/7
  - Drag—3/3
  - Speed—Slow
  - Duration (specific application)—Moderate to long
- General relaxation (inhibition of sympathetic arousal)
  - Pressure level—4 or 5/7
  - Drag—2/3
  - Speed—Slow
  - Duration—Long
- Trigger point therapy
  - Pressure level—4–6/7 (depending on location)
  - Drag—0
  - Speed—Not a factor
  - Duration (specific application)—Moderate
- Scar tissue surface (mature scar)
  - Pressure level—2 or 3/7
  - Drag—2 or 3/3
  - Speed—Slow
  - Duration (specific application)—Moderate
- Adherence of muscle layers
  - Pressure level—4–6/7
  - Drag—3/3
  - Speed—Slow
  - Duration (specific application)—Short to moderate
- Arterial support
  - Pressure level—4 or 5/7
  - Drag—0
  - Speed—Moderate to fast over arteries
  - Duration (specific application)—Short to moderate
  - Duration (entire session)—Short to moderate
- Support for venous return
  - Pressure level—3 or 4/7
  - Drag—1/3
  - Speed—Slow
  - Duration (specific application)—Moderate
  - Duration (entire session)—Short to moderate
- Client who takes anticoagulants
  - Pressure level—1 or 2/7
  - Drag—0 to start; monitor results
  - Speed—Slow
  - Duration—Short to moderate
- Fragile bone (osteoporosis)
  - Pressure level—1–3/7
  - Drag—0–3/3—monitor results
  - Speed—Slow
  - Duration—Short to moderate
- Stimulation of sympathetic autonomic nervous system tone
  - Pressure level—2–5/7
  - Drag—0–1/3
  - Speed—Moderate to fast
  - Duration—Short to moderate

Pressure scale: 0–7; 0 = no pressure, 7 = heavy/deep/firm pressure. Drag scale: 0–3; 0 = no drag, 3 = maximum drag.

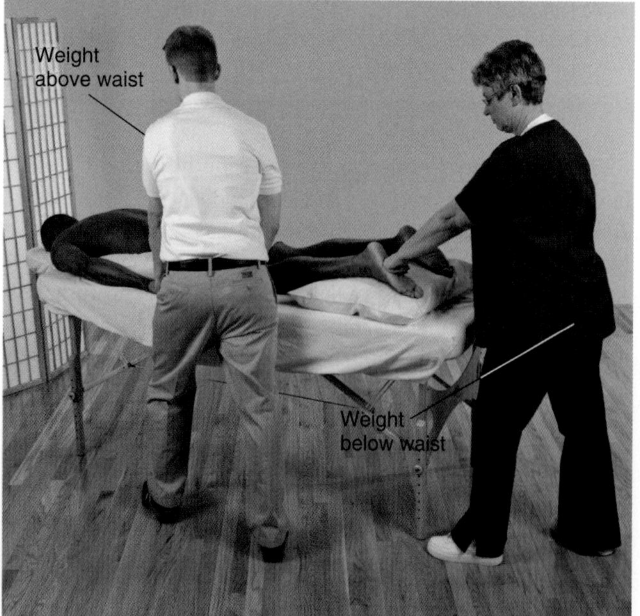

FIG. 8.19 Comparison of male and female weight distribution.

When a male flexes forward, the center of gravity is over the toes. When a female flexes forward, the center of gravity is over their heels (Fig. 8.20).

FOCUS ON PROFESSIONALISM 8.1

Most clients are not experts in massage. They depend on you to inform them about beneficial and safe massage therapy utilization. A client may request a type of massage application simply because they heard about it from others. An example is "deep tissue massage." There is an unfortunate impression that this style is more therapeutic and less pampering. Typically, the client wants an intensity level that is experienced as therapeutic and more than having oil or lotion rubbed on the skin. There is a misconception that the "Swedish massage style" is only for relaxation and therefore not intense enough to be considered therapeutic. This is inaccurate. Most clients are going to receive the most benefit with the least potential for adverse effects with a massage that uses moderate pressure and moderate drag that is generally slow and rhythmic. Besides, the experience of massage intensity is subjective. What is light pressure for one

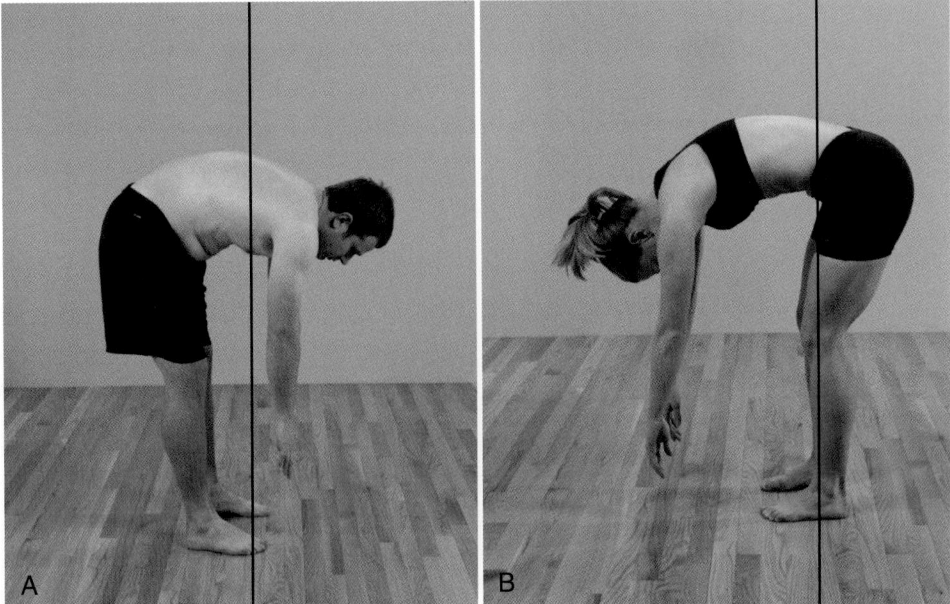

FIG. 8.20 A, In males, weight and the center of gravity are over the toes. **B,** In females, weight and the center of gravity are over the heels.

person may feel like heavy pressure for another. As a massage professional, it is your responsibility to educate clients. The three main ways to increase the intensity experience of massage is to reduce the amount of lubricant so that the massage application can push and pull the tissues; use a broad, flat surface such as the forearm or full palm of the hand to apply the mechanical force; and proceed slowly, deliberately, and mindfully. Also, if you know you are putting your own body at risk by providing a level of intensity that you cannot deliver effectively and safely, then as a professional share this with the client, but assure the client that his or her treatment goals can still be achieved with the approaches you will provide. Keep in mind that we cannot be all things to all clients, and in some cases you may not be a "good fit" for a client because of what his or her expectations are for a session. That is perfectly fine. Remember, you are the professional, this is your livelihood, and you must do what is best to minimize your work risk factors as well as provide a quality massage session for a client. These factors are all important for a successful practice.

Pelvis and Knee

A female's pelvis is wider than a male pelvis, which means that a female's femur approaches the knee at a wider angle, called the *Q angle.* A greater Q angle can result in a knock-kneed stance, which stresses the knee. The structural supports of the knee, the ligaments and tendons, are stretched on the insides and pinched on the outsides. Females have more mobile knees related to wider hips and the resulting tendency is knocked knees (Fig. 8.21).

Ankles

Females cannot bend at the ankles and knees as far forward as males. They also have less total ankle strength. Because females tend to have less flexibility at the ankle, they require a taller massage table (Fig. 8.22).

MENTORING TIP

When doing a massage, avoid exaggerated and atypical postures that create risk and potential injury. For example, think about what most of your daily movements look like. We walk, stand with one foot in front of the other and shift back and forth, and lean up against walls, tables, and so forth. During typical daily activities, we do not hunch over, stand in a semi-squat, stand on tiptoes or with our feet placed wider apart than our shoulders, sustain exaggerated reaching forward motions, twist into odd shapes, or generally look awkward. We should not look awkward when providing a massage either; we should be relatively relaxed and move as efficiently as possible. Take a look at the assessment tool provided in Box 8.7 to help you with this.

Another thing to consider is that massage is physically labor intensive, much like athletics. Therefore we should be taking care of our bodies, or "work tools," to make sure they are able to provide optimal performance. A racecar gets tune-ups and maintenance regularly as well as during a high-intensity race; you must have this mindset as well to keep yourself in good massage maintenance. The recommendations in Chapter 15 on wellness will help you create a long-term plan for your massage career. As it relates to body mechanics for this chapter, it is important as part of a workday to take small breaks, eat regularly but in small quantities to maintain your body fuel and energy, and gently stretch your muscles to help with persistent use and fatigue. These are good habits to start as you build up your skills to perform full-time massage therapy work.

Spine

In females, the spine as a whole and individual vertebrae in certain regions of a normal spine are more backwardly inclined

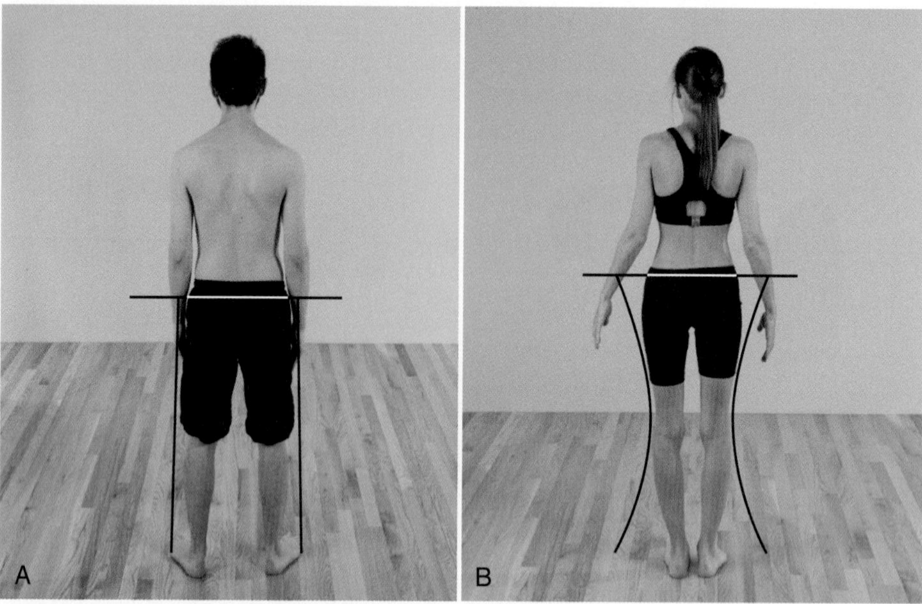

FIG. 8.21 A, In males, the narrow pelvis keeps the hip, knee, and foot in alignment. **B,** In females, the wider pelvis places the knee and foot medial to the hip.

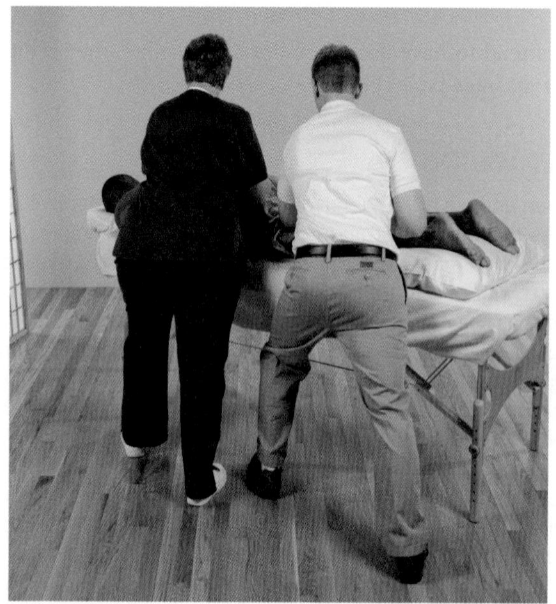

FIG. 8.22 Males and females have different stances due to differences in ankle and knee flexibility. Stance is a factor in determining the height at which the massage table is set.

than in men. These spinal regions are subjected to different biomechanical loading conditions. Females have less rotational stability than do males. Therefore females must maintain alignment of the shoulder girdle and pelvic girdle during massage to prevent torsion forces (twisting) on the spine while doing massage (Janssen et al., 2009; Kiapour et al., 2020; Maurer-Grubinger et al., 2021).

Physical Strength

Females generally are not as physically powerful as males. The average female, because of tendency to smaller size, works at a higher proportion of maximum strength than does the average male. Females have only 55% to 58% of the upper body strength of males; on average, a female is only 80% as strong as a male of identical weight. Females must use leverage by leaning their body weight to apply pressure during massage application.

Male massage therapists may be able to use a shorter table without as much strain for two reasons: when they lean forward, their center of gravity also moves forward; also, they have more upper body strength. However, just because the

Box 8.7 Determining Risk Factors for Massage Therapy Work Tasks

As discussed earlier in this chapter, there is little consistency in teaching effective body mechanics methods to help with career longevity for massage therapists. Utilizing the basic risk factor recommendations from OSHA and her expertise and educational research, R. B. Anderson (2018) created a risk assessment tool to help you identify potential risk factors included here. Here are recommendations on how to use this tool effectively:

- Have a student peer or an instructor observe you performing massage for a minimum of 20 minutes. The massage should address many body parts and ideally should utilize a variety of techniques. For example, you could perform massage on the posterior side of the body only with the client in the prone position.
- Try to perform the massage in the therapist's typical massage work environment. For students, this might be in your school's clinic stations or your lab classrooms. Use the standard equipment available to the therapist. Portable or hydraulic tables? Seated massage? Working in a hospital at bedside with patients? Stools with back support or not? Use whatever equipment or techniques are common for a typical massage workday for a typical massage client.
- If you are the person watching the therapist work, just observe, do not correct the therapist while they are working. Pay attention to how many times the therapist puts themselves in risky positions such as overreaching or head tilting

Box 8.7 Determining Risk Factors for Massage Therapy Work Tasks—cont'd

and note it on the scoring tool based on the parameters given for each body area. Use the pictures on the tool to guide you with scoring what you observe. Remember when scoring, you are looking for positioning that is repetitive. So if the therapist only does it one or two times during the session, then it should not be scored as a risk factor.

- After the massage observation session has concluded, tally the score based on what you honestly observed to determine the overall risk level for the therapist and the areas where they may have the highest risk scores. Then discuss your findings with your peer or your student. Give constructive and helpful feedback so that the therapist may become more aware of any risky positions.
- To develop some awareness of your risky positions or tendencies to overstrain, use some of the suggestions presented in Proficiency Exercise 8.1 to help you.

Ergonomics Risk Factor Assessment Tool for Massage Therapists

Instructions: Using the pictures provided as a guide, determine which color range or attributes match the actions demonstrated by the person you are observing for the majority of the observation time for each body area. Complete each body area score, and then calculate the total score to determine the therapist's total risk factor potential.

Neck:

1A.

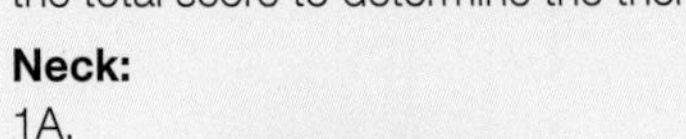

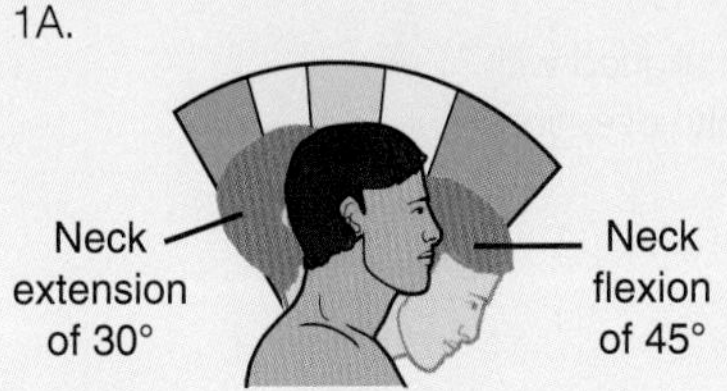

(+0 Green / +1 Yellow / +2 Red)

1B. If lateral bend present, ADD + 1.

Lateral neck bend of 25°

1C. If head turning present, ADD +1

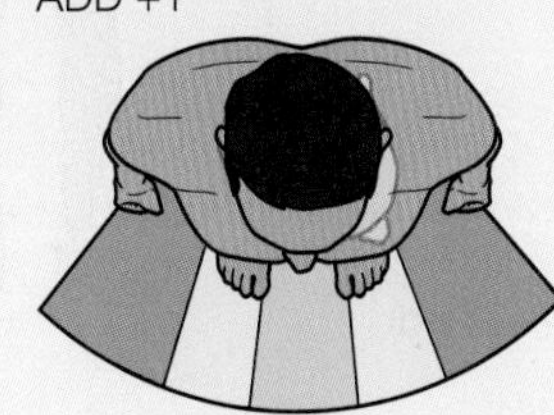

ADD
1A ________
+1B ________
+1C ________
TOTAL NECK SCORE:
____

Upper Arm:

2A.

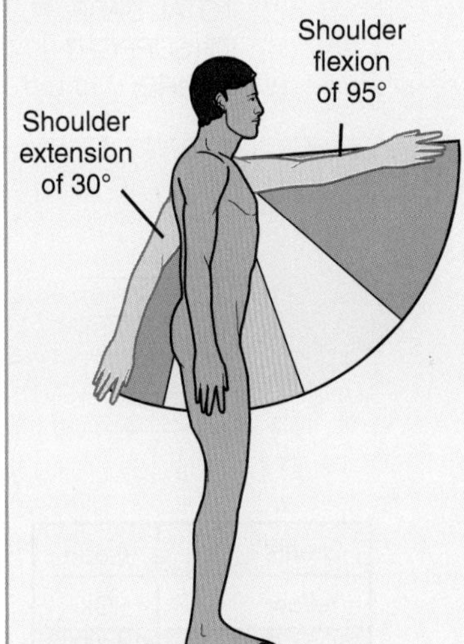

(+0 Green / +1 Yellow / +2 Red)

2B. If arms abducted from body, ADD +1

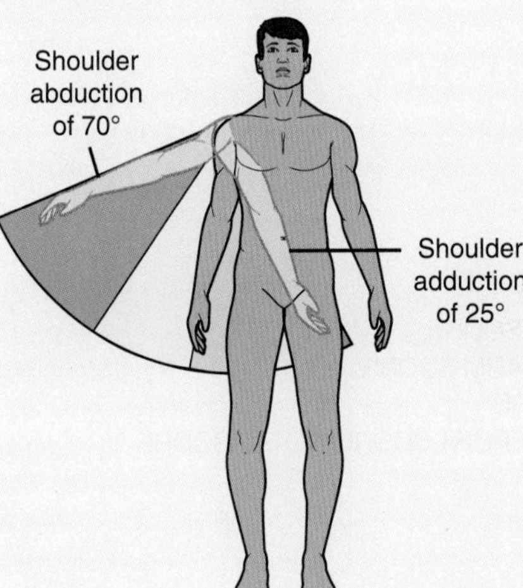

2C. If arms crossover frequently, ADD +1

2D. If shoulders elevated, ADD +1

ADD
2A ________
+ 2B ________
+ 2C ________
+ 2D ________
UPPER ARM SCORE:
____

Wrist/Forearm:

3A. Is wrist aligned with forearm? (Yes +0 / No +1)

3B. Is wrist bent? (Add +1)

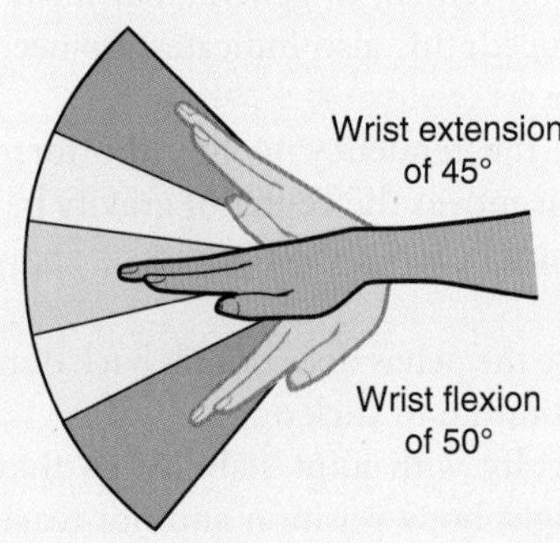

3C. Is wrist deviated? (ADD +1)

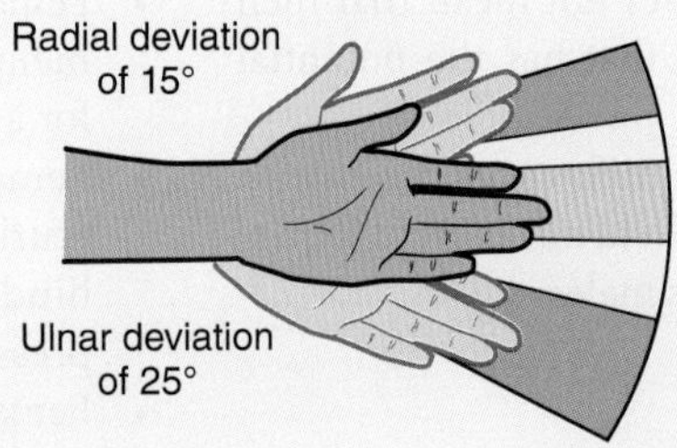

3D. Wrist twist? (ADD +1 for partial / ADD +2 for full pronation)

3E. Overusing anterior hand? (ADD +1)

ADD
3A ________
+ 3B ________
+ 3C ________
+ 3D ________
+ 3E ________
WRIST/FOREARM SCORE:
____

Continued

Box 8.7 Determining Risk Factors for Massage Therapy Work Tasks—cont'd

Trunk:
4A.

Back extension of 20°

Back flexion of 45°

(+0 Green / +1 Yellow / +2 Red)

4B. If lateral bending to the side, ADD +1

Lateral back bend of 20°

4C. If torso twist present, ADD +1

Back rotation of 45°

4D. If trunk/hips are aligned with ASIS's facing in stroke direction, SUBTRACT −1

ADD
4A ________
+ 4B ________
+ 4C ________
- 4D ________
TRUNK SCORE:
____

Base of Support:
5A. *Stances*—either transverse or longitudinal versions (+0 Normal)
(+1 Narrow)
(+2 Too Wide)

5B. ADD +1 if elevated on toes frequently for support
ADD +1 if stagnated and not moving around the table or moving from the core
SUBTRACT −1 if using a stool with good positioning or kneeling using core movement

ADD
5A ________
+
5B ________
TOTAL BASE OF SUPPORT SCORE:
____

ADD UP SECTION SCORES

NECK SCORE: ________
UPPER ARM SCORE: ________
WRIST/FOREARM SCORE: ________
TRUNK SCORE: ________
BASE OF SUPPORT SCORE: TOTAL SCORE ________

Below 6 — *Low Risk*
7—15 — *Moderate Risk*
16—22 — *High Risk*

Green	Good
Yellow	Ok
Red	Poor
Beyond red	Avoid

typical man can "get away with it" does not mean that men should perform massage in any way that has the potential for harm.

So, what do all these male–female differences mean with regard to massage therapy? Females should not attempt to perform massage in the exact same way as males.

Key Points

- Female massage practitioners generally need a higher massage table to compensate for their lower center of gravity as it shifts to the back when the torso is flexed forward.
- Females have more joint movement in general, but movement at the ankles is reduced; this also indicates the need for a higher massage table.
- Females need to curtail the tendency to flex the torso (curl/slouch), because this moves the center of gravity behind them, and more muscle force is required to apply pressure.
- Females need to make sure the pelvis does not tilt back during massage, causing the bottom to stick out.
- Females have more difficulty with joint stability, so they need to maintain an upright body position and not reach or overextend the body when doing massage.

- Females need to pay specific attention to core strength and stability to stabilize the spine and scapulae.
- Females should use their forearms more than their hands.

SELF-CARE AND THE EFFECTS OF IMPROPER BODY MECHANICS

SECTION OBJECTIVES

Chapter objective covered in this section:

6. Recognize nonoptimal performance of massage application through the presence of pain and discomfort.

Using the information presented in this section, the student will be able to perform the following:

- Identify common dysfunctions related to poor body mechanics resulting from repetitive stress injuries.
- Evaluate and improve one's own body mechanics to minimize discomfort and risk factors.

Attention to body mechanics begins before the massage even takes place. The practitioner's body should be warmed up with general light aerobic activity. Massage professionals need to be comfortable and should dress in loose, unrestrictive clothing that does not interfere with movement. A short break should be taken after each massage. The massage therapist should use the time not only to set up for the next client but also to lengthen all the short tissue areas involved in giving a massage such as the chest and hips, rehydrate, and eat a healthy snack if needed. During the massage session four to five microbreaks can be helpful. A microbreak is a rest period of less than 1 minute.

To analyze the potential risk of work-related injury, ergonomists use assessment tools to identify where adaptation or improvement can be recommended to create a safer work environment. The Massage Therapy Foundation Ergonomics projects used these types of assessments. Based on guidelines and ergonomics concepts recommended by the Occupational Safety and Health Administration (OSHA), an assessment tool has been provided to help estimate your potential risk factors when performing massage. The goal of this tool is to provide some indicators of areas where you can improve your body mechanics before they become "bad habits" and increase the potential for injury in the long term (Box 8.7). When using this tool, either have a colleague observe you performing massage or take a video of you performing massage to see how you move and what positions your body migrates to when giving a massage (Anderson, 2018).

Massage professionals who are not attentive to body mechanics commonly feel the effects in the neck and shoulder, wrist and thumb, lower back, knee, ankle, and foot. The following recommendations are methods of protecting the practitioner's body.

Neck and Shoulder

Neck and shoulder problems most often develop when the massage practitioner uses upper body strength to push and exert pressure for massage. These problems can be avoided if the student learns to use leverage and leans with the body weight to provide pressure. The practitioner's arms and hands should be relaxed while giving a massage because tension in the arms and hands translates to the shoulders and neck. Remember, the joints need to be stacked and stable so that the force is easily distributed from the body weight through the joint structure to create mechanical force. If the core is not stable, the scapula will be unstable, making maintaining shoulder stability difficult (Fig. 8.23). Avoid working at the ends of the massage table or mat to apply long gliding strokes.

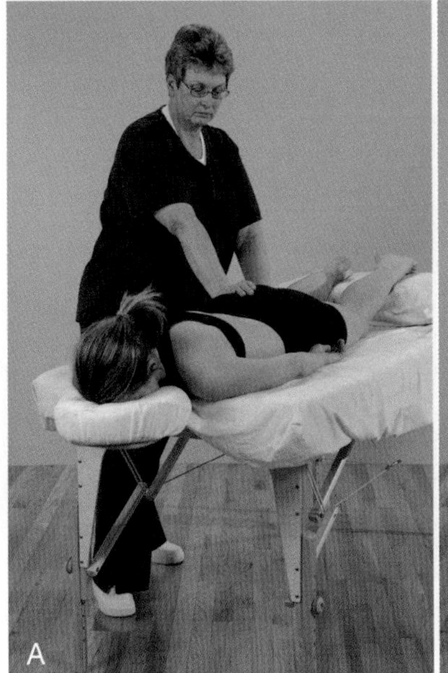

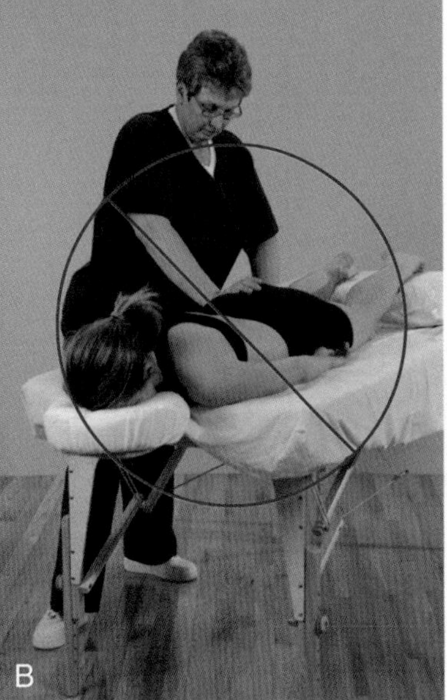

FIG. 8.23 A, When core stability is functional, scapula and shoulder stability is supported. **B,** An unstable core can affect the foot position, causing rotation and tilt at the pelvis and strain on the knee. The bent elbow interferes with weight transfer in the muscular effort to apply pressure. The shoulder becomes displaced and unstable, and the head moves into a forward position.

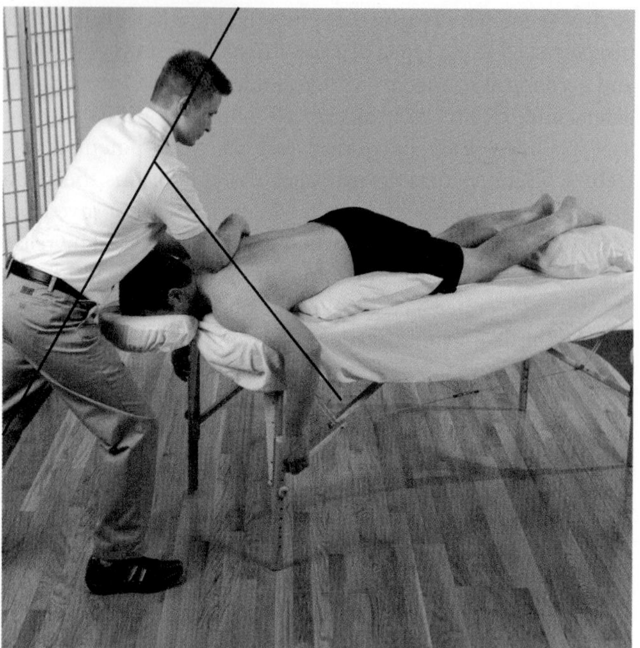

FIG. 8.24 Avoid working at the head of the table and gliding toward hips.

This results in overreaching and stains the stability of the shoulder (Fig. 8.24).

Forearm, Wrist, and Hand

Massage professionals need to protect their wrists by preventing the development of excessive compressive forces from the delivery of massage methods. Using a proper wrist angle and staying behind the massage stroke protects the wrist. Tense wrists and hands also contribute to shoulder problems. It is important always to maintain a relaxed hand and wrist while giving a massage. Avoid using the thumb when applying pressure. The design of the joints in the thumb does not allow adequate stability to protect the joint. Whenever possible, use the forearm to apply massage to spare the hands and wrists (Fig. 8.25).

Low Back

Some reasons for low back problems include core instability, inappropriate bending by curling and slouching in bent static positions, twisting, improper knee position, improper foot position, bending of the elbows, and reaching for an area instead of stepping closer to the area. Maintaining a stable spinal

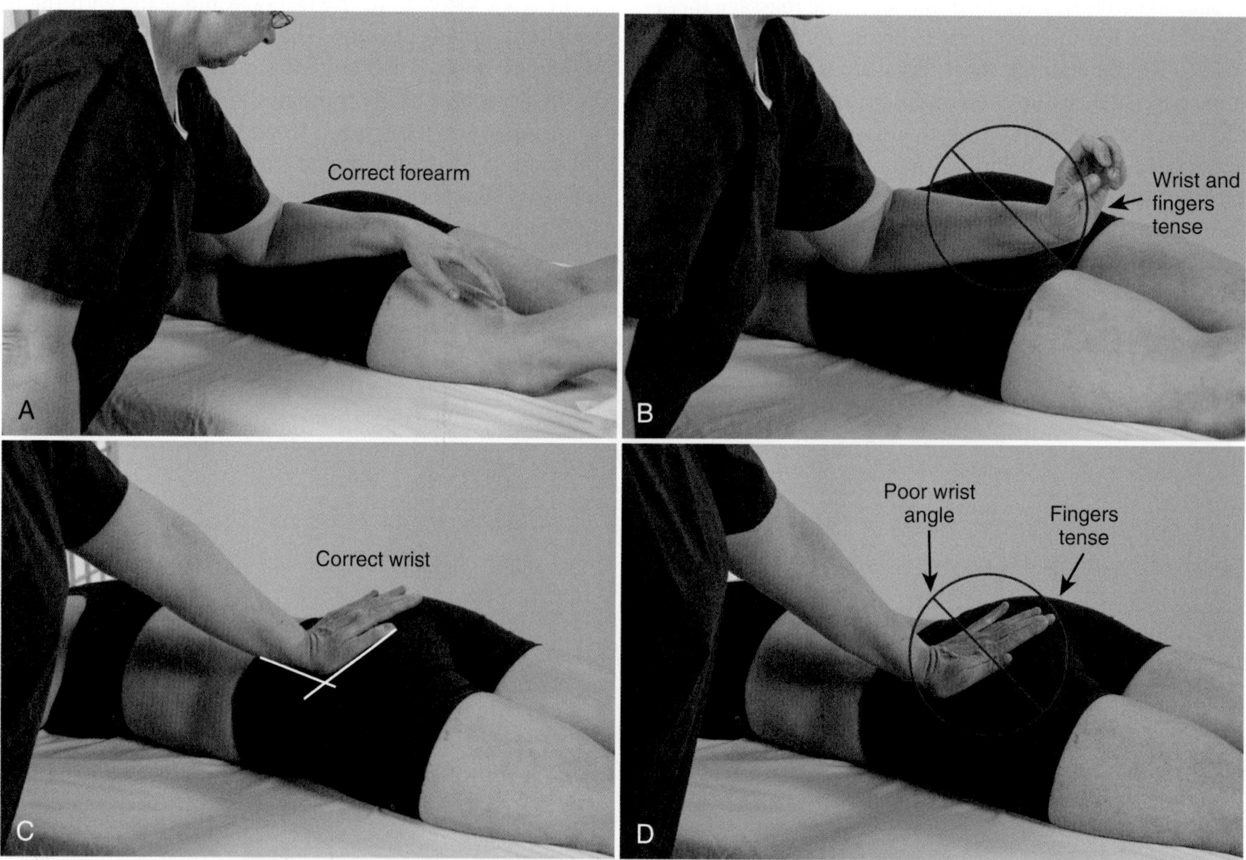

FIG. 8.25 A, Use the forearm to apply massage whenever possible to spare the wrists and hands. B, Incorrect wrist and finger position during use of forearm for massage. C, Correct wrist and hand position; note the relaxed fingers and the wrist angle greater than 90 degrees. D, Incorrect wrist and hand position; the wrist angle is close to 90 degrees, and the fingers are tense.

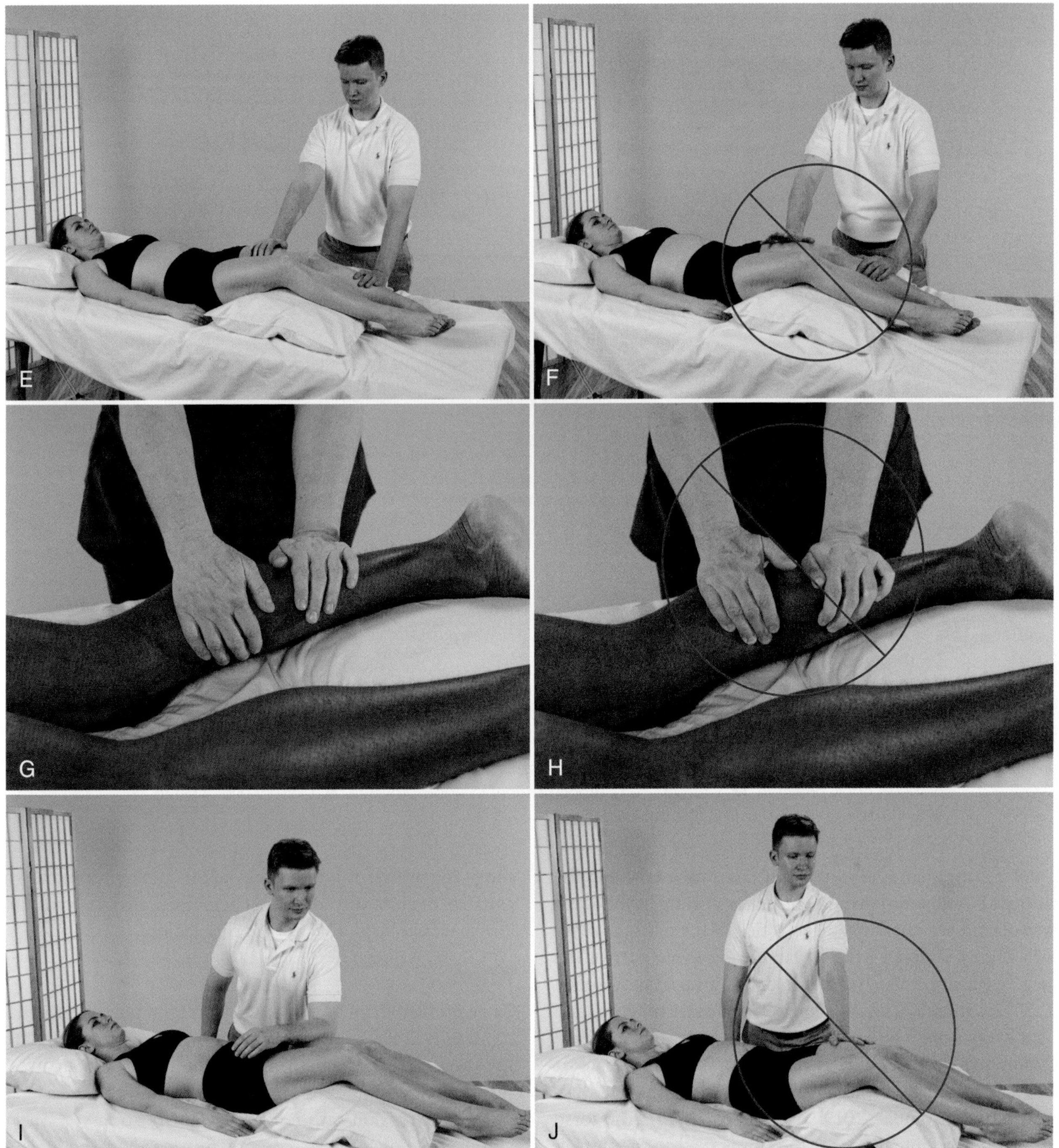

FIG. 8.25—cont'd E, Correct use of the hand during massage; note the position of the elbow and shoulder. **F**, Incorrect arm, forearm, and hand position; the shoulder is rolled forward, the elbow is bent, the angle of the wrist joint is close to 90 degrees, and the fingers are tense. **G**, Correct positioning and use of the hands during kneading. **H**, Incorrect hand position for kneading; the fingers are tense and performing most of the work. **I**, Correct arm position when using the forearm for massage. **J**, Incorrect arm position: the arm is across the body toward the midline, straining the elbow and shoulder, and the body is not lined up with the direction of the weight transfer.

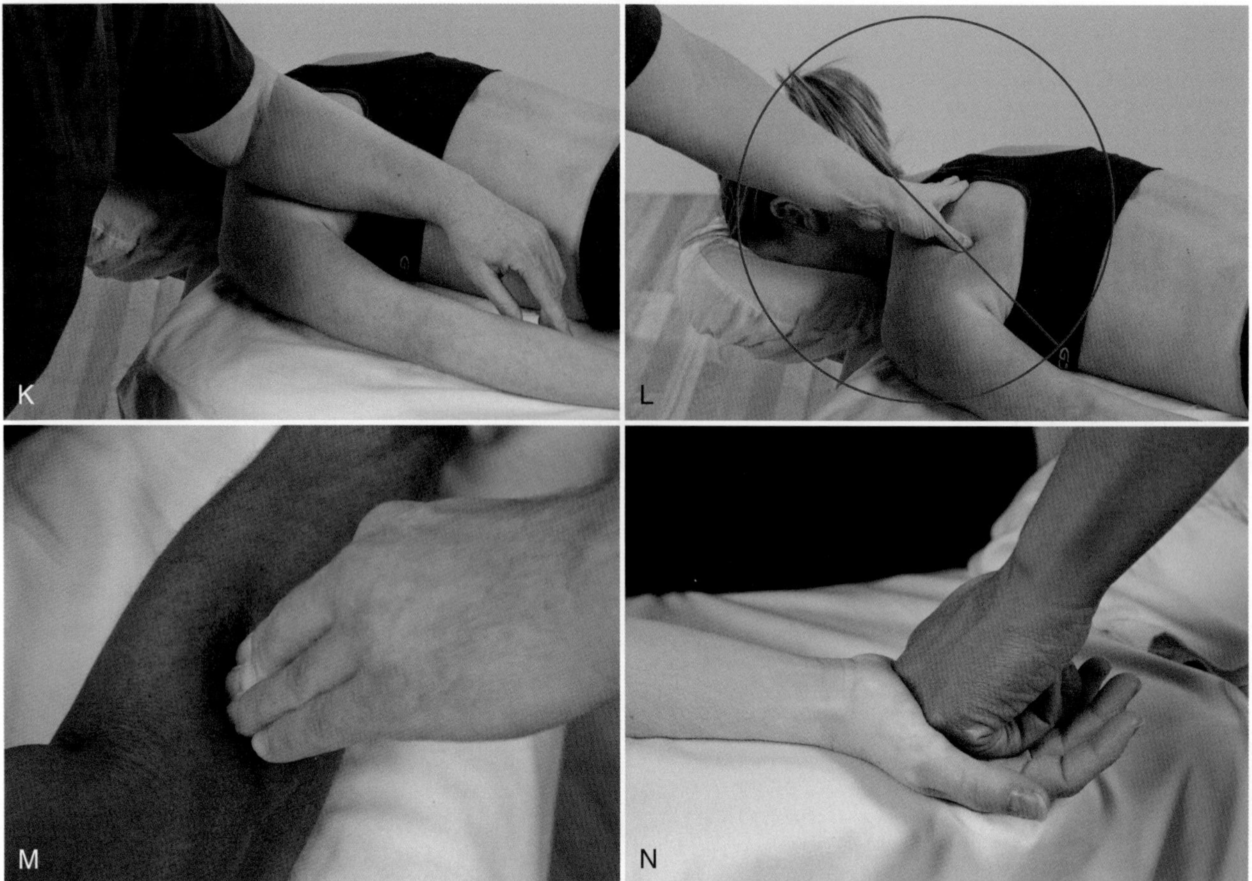

FIG. 8.25—cont'd **K**, Use the forearm whenever possible to apply pressure. **L**, Incorrect: do not use the thumb to apply pressure. **M**, Correct use of braced fingers to apply pressure. **N**, Correct use of fist to apply pressure.

line and a strong core helps prevent this problem. Keep the lower back straight and avoid bending or curling at the waist while working. Frequent posture shifting of the massage practitioner's body coupled with sitting during some part of the massage application also helps protect the lower back (Coenen et al., 2017). There is a connection between knee function and low-back function. It is logical to maintain knee stability when performing massage (Iijima et al., 2018). The lower back is further supported by avoiding twisting and reaching (Chaiklieng and Homsombat, 2019; Wami et al., 2019). The torso can move into slight flexion as the hip is flexed. The flexion occurs at the hip joint on the leg that is forward with the flexed knee. Hip flexion should not exceed 20 degrees. The joints of the arm must be kept effectively stacked, with the elbow straight if using the hand. If the elbow is bent, the body tends to curl at the waist and slouch in the lower back (Fig. 8.26).

A common ergonomic-based injury to the low back occurs during lifting. Rarely does the massage practitioner lift or reposition a client during a session. The client is responsible for moving themselves. There are times, however, when a client may require some assistance when getting on or off the massage table, mat, or chair. This assistance typically involves support related to balance. Caution is required if any lifting or pulling is involved when assisting a client. The general population of clients receiving massage does not require the massage therapists to lift the client during the session. If a client cannot move themselves it is likely they are in an environment where assistive devices and additional personnel are involved. An example would be in a long-term care facility.

Knee

Knee problems can be prevented by respecting the basic stability design of the knee and frequently shifting the weight from foot to foot. The most efficient standing position involves the normal screw-home (or knee-lock) position in the last 15 degrees of extension on the back weight-bearing leg. This position provides the least compressive force on the knee capsule and the least muscular action for stability. As the knee is flexed, compressive forces increase in the joint capsule, and muscular action for stability increases. Knee hyperextension should be avoided (Fig. 8.27).

Confusion and disagreement exist about the proper position of the knee while giving a massage. Some advise a slightly flexed knee, rather than the locked knee recommended by this text. These concerns tend to arise from information founded on movement principles, such as tai chi, forms of dance, and martial arts. Although a flexed knee is appropriate for these systems, massage requires the application of sustained pressure from a stable position with the least amount of effort, muscular activity, and compressive force to the joint.

The knee needs to be in a slightly flexed position as the massage practitioner changes position and moves around the

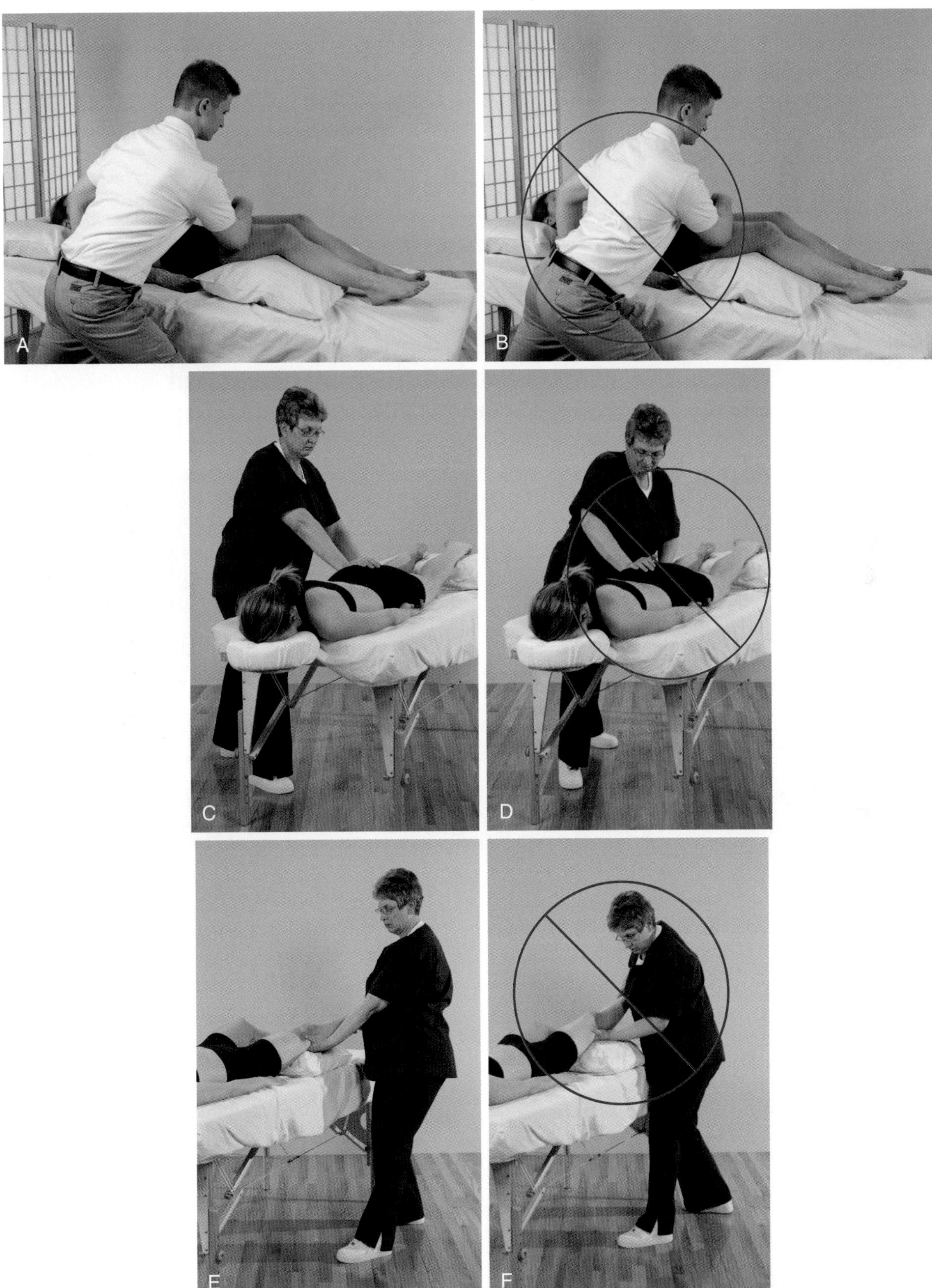

FIG. 8.26 A, Demonstration of a stable lower back. **B,** Incorrect. The table is too short and the therapist's core is unstable, as is the scapula. The arm is medially across the body, which is not lined up with the direction of the weight transfer. All of this contributes to low back strain while giving a massage. **C,** Using an asymmetrical stance and normal knee-lock position in the weight-bearing leg protects the back. **D,** Incorrect. The therapist has the weight on the front foot and is standing on the toes. The elbow is bent, and the table is too high. Muscle is used to apply pressure. **E,** Stack the joints and lean back when applying a pull to stretch an area. **F,** Incorrect. Pulling is being accomplished by using muscle strength instead of leaning back to stretch or traction the area.

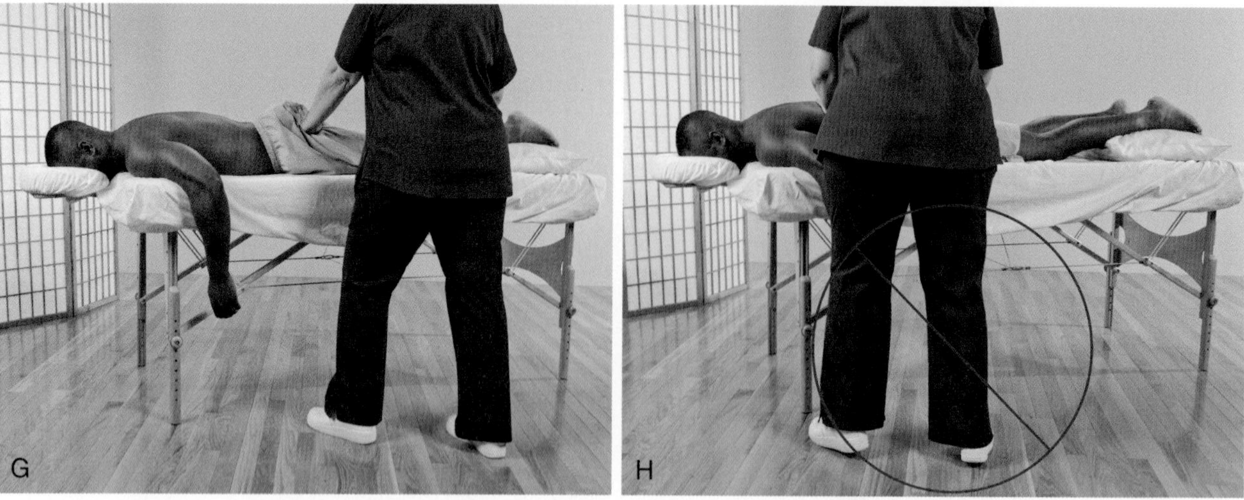

FIG. 8.26—cont'd G, Correct foot position. **H,** Incorrect. Foot position is on the toes, too close to the table.

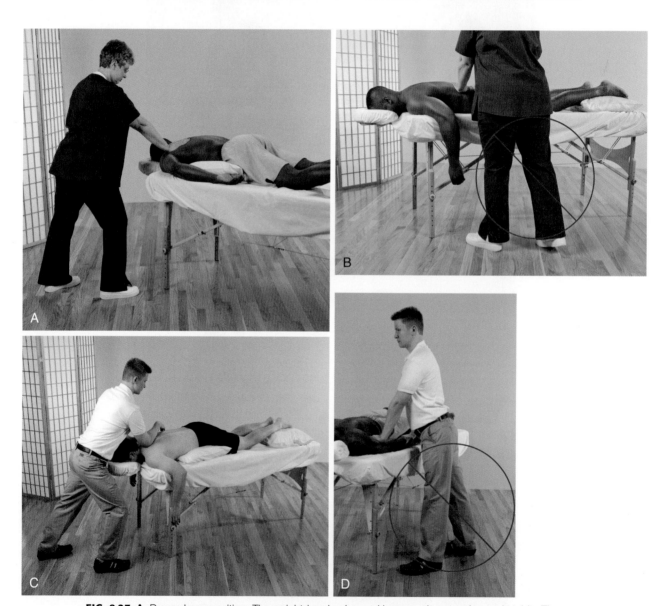

FIG. 8.27 A, Proper knee position: The weight-bearing leg and knee are in extension and stable. The knee of the front balance leg is flexed to allow forward movement during weight transfer. **B,** Incorrect. The weight is on the front leg, which is straight, and the back leg is on the toes; this increases the strain on the knees. **C,** Incorrect. The feet are in a symmetrical stance, with both knees extended.

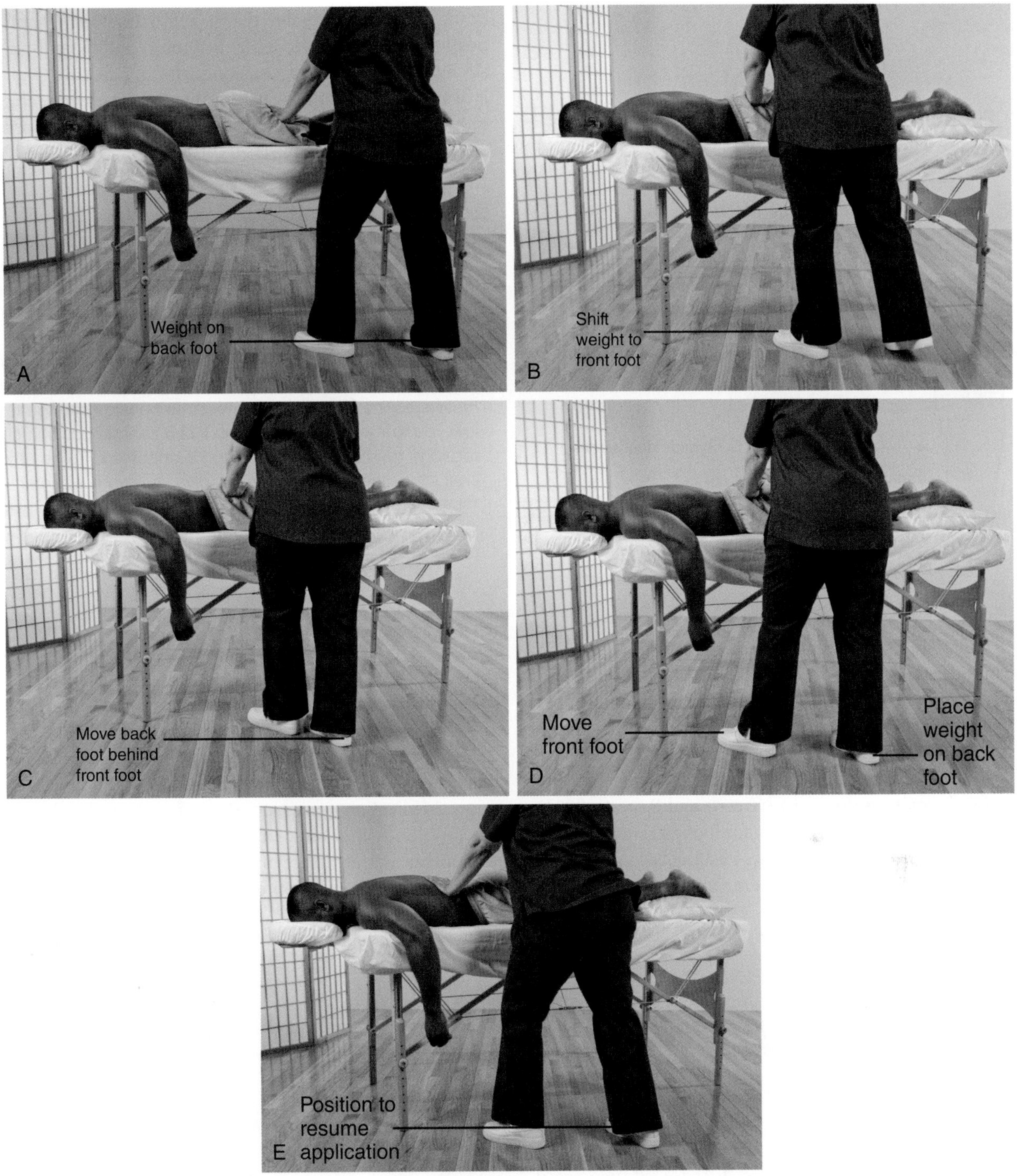

Weight on back foot
A
Shift weight to front foot
B
Move back foot behind front foot
C
Move front foot
Place weight on back foot
D
Position to resume application
E

FIG. 8.28 Moving around the massage table. **A,** Start with the correct knee position (normal knee-lock position) for stability. The moving process remains parallel to the massage table. Avoid moving closer to or farther from the table. **B,** Begin the move. Both knees are flexed; the weight is on the front foot; and the back leg is on the toes, ready to transfer the full weight to the front as the back leg is lifted off the floor. **C,** The back foot moves close to but is still behind the front foot. **D,** The weight is again shifted to the back foot, and the front foot moves to the asymmetrical stance; the feet are shoulder width apart. **E,** Correct body mechanics are resumed.

table (Fig. 8.28). However, when pressure is applied, the anatomical design of the knee provides stability in the knee-lock position in the last 15 degrees of extension. The body mechanics presented in this chapter have been developed to support the knee (Smith et al., 1996; Norkin and Levangie, 2005; Kim et al., 2015; Zhang et al., 2016).

Ankle and Foot

Asymmetrical standing (i.e., standing with one foot in front of the other) is the most efficient standing position. The weight is shifted from one foot to the other in an energy conservation mechanism. Symmetrical standing, in which the weight is equally distributed on the two feet, is fatiguing, interferes

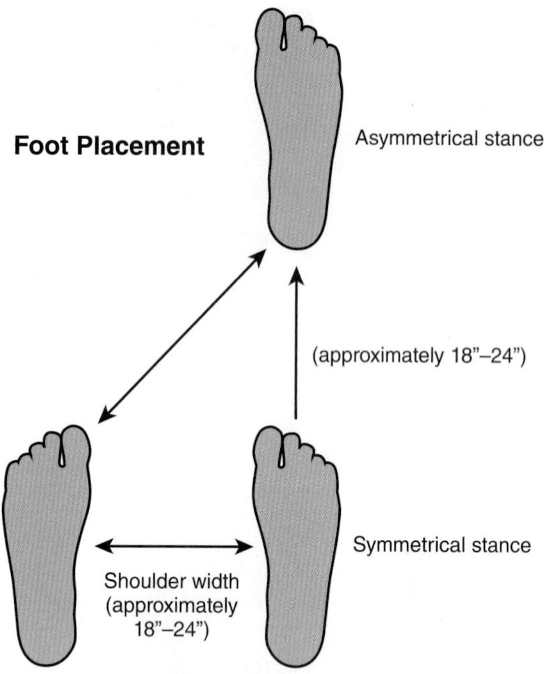

FIG. 8.29 Correct foot placement.

with circulation, and should be avoided (Smith et al., 1996; MacKinnon, 2002) (Figs. 8.29 and 8.30). The ankle and foot are protected by the asymmetrical stance and frequent position changes. The body mechanics presented in this chapter are based on the asymmetrical stance because it exerts less energy, uses the force generated more efficiently, and prevents fatigue for the massage therapist (Greene and Roberts, 2004). It is necessary to have enough room for foot placement during the push/pull application of massage. Pushing tasks need more space than pulling tasks. Practitioners should have floor space around the massage table that is approximately 70% of their height in order to exert their maximum pulling and pushing strengths. For example, someone who is 5 feet tall will need at least 3.5 feet of floor space around the massage table. An individual who is 6 feet tall will need 4 to 4.5 feet of floor space around the massage table (Lee, 2018).

Foot in the Door

Body mechanics begin at the feet. The ability to perform five or six quality massage sessions a day without hurting yourself will get your foot in the door in most work environments and keep you on the path to career success. If you can confidently demonstrate body mechanics that are efficient and effective, an employer (and your clients) will be impressed. You also need an environment that supports your ability to provide massage. The massage area needs to be large enough to allow you to move around the table and change position comfortably. You need equipment that is adaptable. To be at your best, you need fresh air and a pleasant work environment. When you evaluate a potential place of employment, imagine yourself in that massage area for 8 hours. Does it feel like a place where you would want to work?

SUMMARY

Massage therapists take care of others. To sustain a massage therapy career, we must also take care of ourselves. Chapter 15 expands on self-care. The massage professional's body is a vital, irreplaceable tool. It is crucial that massage professionals take care to use proper body mechanics when giving a massage. Application of ergonomics concepts and utilization of effective body mechanics are the essential keys to injury prevention and career longevity. If the practitioner is uncomfortable, the client will become uncomfortable and therefore the

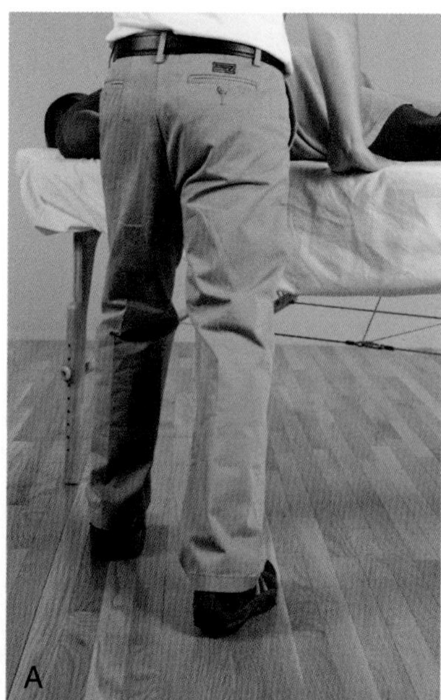

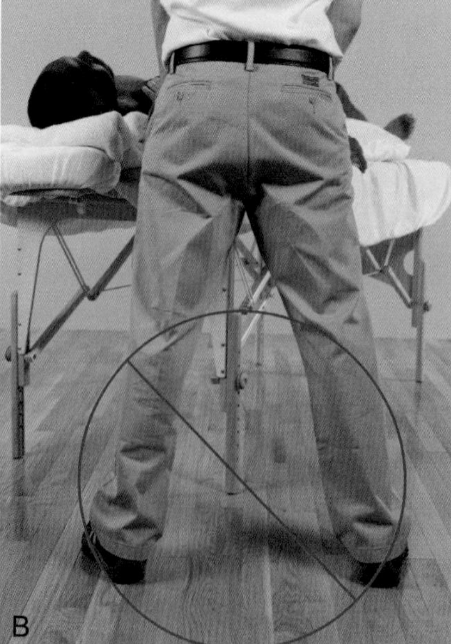

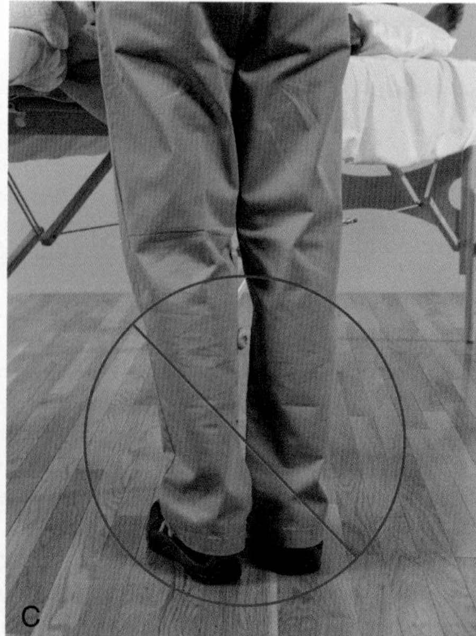

FIG. 8.30 **A,** Correct asymmetrical stance with the feet shoulder width apart. **B,** Incorrect. The feet are too far apart, the stance is symmetrical, and both knees are flexed. **C,** Incorrect. The feet are too close together, the stance is symmetrical, and both knees are flexed.

massage session delivered is ineffective. If the practitioner can give a massage in a relaxed, efficient, and energy-conserving manner, the client will be able to relax and be satisfied with the treatment received. Practice over and over until you develop graceful, efficient body mechanics. This supports your longevity and the ability to deliver the best massage for every client.

LEARN MORE ON THE WEB

The US Department of Labor's Occupational Safety and Health Administration (OSHA) is an excellent site for researching ergonomics and workplace safety.

Evolve

Visit the Evolve website: http://evolve.elsevier.com/Fritz/fundamentals/

Evolve content designed for massage therapy licensing exam review and comprehension of content beyond the textbook. Evolve content includes:

- Content Updates
- Science and Pathology Animations
- Body Spectrum Coloring Book
- MBLEx exam review multiple choice questions

FOR EACH CHAPTER FIND:

- Answers and rationales for the end-of-chapter multiple-choice questions
- Electronic workbook and answer key
- Chapter multiple choice question quiz
- Quick content review in question form and answers
- Technique videos when applicable
- Learn more on the Web

REFERENCES

Albert WJ, Currie-Jackson N, Duncan CA. A survey of musculoskeletal injuries amongst Canadian massage therapists. *J Bodywork Move Ther.* 2008;12:86.

Albert WJ, Duncan C, Currie-Jackson N, et al. Biomechanical assessment of massage therapists. *Occup Erg.* 2006;6:1.

American Massage Therapy Association. *The 2022 Massage Profession Research Report* Copyright ©2022. https://www.amtamassage.org/publications/massage-profession-research-report/. Retrieved 9/2022.

Anderson RB. Improving body mechanics using experiential learning and ergonomic tools in massage therapy education. *Int J Therap Massage Bodywrk.* 2018;11(4):4.

Anyfantis ID, Biska A. *Musculoskeletal Disorders Among Greek Physiotherapists: Traditional and Emerging Risk Factors. Safety and Health at Work.* The Low Back, Wrist and Thumbs was the Most Common Injury Site Reported by Females; 2017.

Argubi-Wollesen A, Wollesen B, Leitner M, Mattes K. Human body mechanics of pushing and pulling: analyzing the factors of task-related strain on the musculoskeletal system. *Saf Health Work.* 2017;8(1):11–18.

Barraclough W, Baskwill A, Higgs C, Neilson S, Wilcox D. A survey of Canadian massage therapists experiences of work-related pain. *Int J Ther Massage Bodywork: Res Edu Pract.* 2022;15(3):18–26.

Barnett RL, Liber T. Human push capability. *Ergonomics.* 2006;49:293.

Bisiacchi DW, Huber LL. Physical injury assessment of male versus female chiropractic students when learning and performing various adjustive techniques: a preliminary investigative study. *Chiropr Osteopat.* 2006;14(1):17.

Blau G, Monos C, Boyer E, et al. Correlates of injury-forced work reduction for massage therapists and bodywork practitioners. *J Ther Massage Bodywork.* 2013;6(3):6.

Buck FA, Kuruganti U, Albert WJ, et al. Muscular and postural demands of using a massage chair and massage table. *J Manip Physiol Ther.* 2007;30:357–364.

Buckingham G, Das R, Trott P. Position of undergraduate learners' thumbs during mobilisation is poor: an observational study. *Aust J Physiother.* 2007;53(55):55.

Chaiklieng S, Homsombat T. Incidence and postural risk factors for low back pain among informal garment female workers. *international conference on applied human factors and ergonomics.* Cham: Springer; 2019:222–230.

Chow AY, La Delfa NJ, Dickerson CR. Muscular Exposures During Standardized Two-Handed Maximal Pushing and Pulling Tasks. *IISE Trans Occup Ergon Hum Factors.* 2017;5(3-4):136–147 (Gender difference).

Cid MM, Oliveira AB, Januario LB, Côté JN, de Fátima Carreira Moreira R, Madeleine P. Are there sex differences in muscle coordination of the upper girdle during a sustained motor task? *J Electromyogr Kinesiol.* 2019.

Coenen P, Gilson N, Healy GN, Dunstan DW, Straker LM. A qualitative review of existing national and international occupational safety and health policies relating to occupational sedentary behaviour. *Appl Ergon.* 2017;60:320–333.

Friedman LS, Madigan D, Cambron JA. Barriers and facilitators of implementing injury prevention practices by massage therapists. *J Occup Environ Med.* 2022;64(5):443–449.

Greene D, Roberts S. *Kinesiology: Movement in the Context of Activity.* 2nd ed. St Louis: Mosby; 2004.

Guruprasad S, Ramakrishnan KS, Gowda H. Prevalence of musculoskeletal problems in masseuse. *Int J Ther Rehabil Res.* 2016;5(5):140–148.

Hairani IHM, Jalil SZA, Yusoff NM. Akademia baru. *J Adv Res Occup Health Saf.* 2018;1(1):1.

Hu MT, Hsu AT, Lin SW, et al. Effect of general flexibility on thumb-tip force generation: implication for mobilization and manipulation. *Man Ther.* 2009;14:490.

Iijima H, Suzuki Y, Aoyama T, Takahashi M. Interaction between low back pain and knee pain contributes to disability level in individuals with knee osteoarthritis: a cross-sectional study. *Osteoarthritis and Cartilage.* 2018;26(10):1319–1325.

Jacquier-Bret J, Gorce P, and Rouvière E. Ergonomic risk assessment during massage among physiotherapists: introduction of generic postures notion. Work Preprint. 2023;75(3):1021–1029.

Jacquier-Bret J, Gorce P. Prevalence of body area work-related musculoskeletal disorders among healthcare professionals: a systematic review. *Int J Environ Res Public Health.* 2023;20(1):841.

Janssen MM, Drevelle X, Humbert L, et al. Differences in male and female spino-pelvic alignment in asymptomatic young adults: a three-dimensional analysis using upright low-dose digital biplanar x-rays. *Spine.* 2009;34:E826.

Kareem I, Amjad F, Arif S, Batool S. Prevalence of Thumb Pain Among Physiotherapists Perform Manual Techniques During Clinical Practice. *Pakistan J Phy Ther (PJPT).* 2021:09–14.

Kiapour A, Joukar A, Elgafy H, Erbulut DU, Agarwal AK, Goel VK. Biomechanics of the sacroiliac joint: anatomy, function, biomechanics, sexual dimorphism, and causes of pain. *Int J Spine Surg.* 2020;14(Suppl 1):3–13.

Kim HY, Kim KJ, Yang DS, Jeung SW, Choi HG, Choy WS. Screw-home movement of the tibiofemoral joint during normal gait: three-dimensional analysis. *Clin Orthop Surg.* 2015;7(3):303–309.

Kruger H, Khumalo V, Houreld NN. The prevalence of osteoarthritic symptoms of the hands amongst female massage therapists. *Health Sa Gesondheid.* 2017;22(1):184–193.

Lee TH. Foot placement strategy in pushing and pulling. *Work, (Preprint).* 2018:1–5.

MacKinnon SN. Effects of standardized foot positions during the execution of a submaximal pulling task. *Ergonomics.* 2002;45(4):253–266.

Magee DJ, Zachazewski JE. *Scientific Foundations and Principles of Practice in Musculoskeletal Rehabilitation.* St Louis: Mosby; 2007.

Maurer-Grubinger C, Holzgreve F, Fraeulin L, Betz W, Erbe C, Brueggmann D, Wanke EM, Nienhaus A, Groneberg DA, Ohlendorf D. Combining ergonomic risk assessment (RULA) with inertial motion capture technology in dentistry—using the benefits from two worlds. *Sensors.* 2012;21(12):4077.

Mohr EG. Proper body mechanics from an engineering perspective. *J Bodyw Mov Ther.* 2010;14:139.

Neumann DA. *Kinesiology of the Musculoskeletal System.* 2nd ed. St Louis: Mosby; 2010.

Norkin CC, Levangie PK. *Joint Structure and Function: A Comprehensive Analysis.* 2nd ed. Philadelphia: FA Davis; 2005.

Page LT. September. Licensed Massage Therapist Strain Index Scores. In: *Proceedings of the Human Factors and Ergonomics Society Annual Meeting.* 56. Sage CA: Los Angeles, CA: SAGE Publications; 2012:1163–1167.
Pheasant S. *Ergonomics, Work and Health.* Gaithersburg, MD: Aspen Publishers, Inc.; 1991.
Rossettini G, Rondoni A, Schiavetti I, Tezza S, Testa M. Prevalence and risk factors of thumb pain in Italian manual therapists: An observational cross-sectional study. *Work.* 2016;54(1):159–169.
Sirbu E, Varga MG, Rata AL, Amaricai E, Onofrei RR. Work-related musculoskeletal complaints in massage practitioners. Work Preprint. 2022:1–7.
Smith LK, Weiss E, Lemkuhl LD. *Brunnstrom's Clinical Kinesiology.* 5th ed. Philadelphia: FA Davis; 1996.
Snodgrass SJ, Rivett DA, Chiarelli P, et al. Factors related to thumb pain in physiotherapists. *Aust J Physiother.* 2003;49:243.
Sung P-C, Liu Y-P. Assessments of forearm muscular demands and perceived exertions for different massage techniques of the Swedish-type massage. *Int J Appl Sci Eng.* 2022;19(1):1–11.
Van der Molen HF, Foresti C, Daams JG, Frings-Dresen MHW, Kuijer PPFM. Work-related risk factors for specific shoulder disorders: a systematic review and meta-analysis. *Occup Environ Med.* 2017;74(10):745–755.
Wami SD, Abere G, Dessie A, Getachew D. Work-related risk factors and the prevalence of low back pain among low wage workers: results from a cross-sectional study. *BMC Public Health.* 2019;19(1):1072.
Zhang LK, Wang XM, Niu YZ, Liu HX, Wang F. Relationship between patellar tracking and the "screw-home" mechanism of tibiofemoral joint. *Orthop Surg.* 2016;8(4):490–495.

MULTIPLE-CHOICE QUESTIONS FOR DISCUSSION AND REVIEW

The answers, with rationales, can be found on the Evolve site. Use these questions to stimulate discussion and dialogue. Each question provides you with the ability to review terminology, practice critical thinking skills, and improve multiple choice test taking skills. Answers and rationales are on the Evolve site. It is just as important to know why the wrong answers are wrong as it is to know why the correct answer is correct.

1. When a massage practitioner is in a relaxed standing posture supporting the gravitational line with the normal knee-locked position, which muscles are used for balance?
   a. Psoas
   b. Gastrocnemius
   c. Hamstrings
   d. Quadriceps
2. What is the most efficient standing position when performing a massage session?
   a. Symmetrical
   b. Wide stance (shoulder length apart)
   c. Asymmetrical
   d. Lead foot with the pressure on it
3. Most massage applications use a force generated ______.
   a. Downward
   b. Forward
   c. Downward and forward
   d. Forward and across
4. When one is applying compressive force down and forward, weight transfer is most efficient when the massage therapist puts weight ______.
   a. On the back leg and foot
   b. On the front leg and knee
   c. On the back foot and toes
   d. On the front foot and toes
5. Increasing levels of pressure delivered during massage application are achieved by ______.
   a. Moving closer to the massage table
   b. Using the arm that is on the same side as forward leg
   c. Standing on the toes
   d. Shifting the weight-bearing foot to the front
6. A client keeps complaining of discomfort at the end of the massage stroke. What is happening?
   a. The practitioner is pushing with the legs.
   b. The practitioner is off balance and using counterpressure.
   c. The skin is being pulled from lack of lubricant.
   d. The compressive force is distributed over a narrow base at the end of the stroke.
7. Observation of a fellow massage practitioner indicates that the shoulder girdle is aligned with the pelvic girdle, the pressure-bearing arm is opposite the weight-bearing leg, the fingers are relaxed, the head is up, the back is straight, trunk flexion at the hips is 35 degrees, and the stance is asymmetrical. Which of these areas needs correction?
   a. Trunk
   b. Stance
   c. Back position
   d. Shoulder position
8. When stretching the legs of a client by applying a pull against the ankle, the massage practitioner should ______.
   a. Fix the feet and pull with the shoulders.
   b. Move to a symmetrical stance and lean back.
   c. Maintain an asymmetrical stance and lean back, keeping the back straight.
   d. Bend the knees and push back.
9. The massage therapist needs to have ______ to be effective with body mechanics?
   a. Core stability
   b. Hyperflexibility
   c. Hypoflexibility
   d. Forearm strength
10. A massage professional is feeling strain in the shoulders and arms after completing four massage sessions. Which of the following is the most logical reason?
    a. The massage professional is using muscle strength in the arms to exert force.
    b. The massage professional is standing in an asymmetrical stance.
    c. The client is positioned for best mechanical advantage.
    d. The massage professional is effectively changing table height.
11. A massage practitioner with a full-time practice has been experiencing increasingly severe low back pain. The practitioner has 24 clients per week. What could the massage practitioner do to reduce back strain?
    a. Bend the knees past 15 degrees of flexion while performing massage.
    b. Raise the table height to prevent torso bending.
    c. Keep the head forward and down to change the center of gravity.
    d. Externally rotate the back foot away from the line of force.

12. A massage professional is complaining of pain in the wrist and near the elbow. Which of the following is an appropriate corrective action?
   a. Maintain the hands in a clenched fist to promote stability.
   b. Increase the movement of the stroke at the shoulder joint.
   c. Relax the hand and fingers during massage.
   d. Shift the compressive force to the fingers and thumb.

13. A massage professional is feeling strain in the knees. Which of the following is the most logical cause?
   a. Doing massage on hard floors
   b. Working with clients in the side-lying position
   c. Keeping the knees flexed and static
   d. Moving whenever the arm reach is beyond 60 degrees

14. What is the importance of the Massage Therapy Foundation's Ergonomics Project?
   a. Detailed specific guidelines for body mechanics
   b. Provided objective recommendations for massage practice
   c. Confirmed accuracy of legacy-based body mechanics instruction
   d. Determined the number of hours a massage therapist should work

15. A massage practitioner is experiencing shoulder stiffness and adjusts their massage table. What type of adaptation did the practitioner make?
   a. Ergonomics
   b. Biomechanics
   c. Weight transfer
   d. Applied force

16. A team of massage therapists work together in the same facility sharing massage rooms. One of the massage therapists is 6 feet tall. Another is 5 ft. 7 in. Two of the massage therapists are approximately the same height at 5 ft. 4 in. One therapist is male. Which ergonomic issue is likely to cause concern?
   a. Requirement of wearing nonslip shoes
   b. Width of the massage table
   c. Height of the massage table
   d. Size of the massage area

17. A fitness center is creating a massage therapy center adjacent to the workout area. The potential clients are indicating a need for moderate to heavy pressure during the massage sessions. Which published policy best protects the massage practitioner from workplace injury?
   a. Requests for firm pressure during the session require a 90-minute session appointment.
   b. Moderate-heavy pressure will be applied with the therapists forearms or a massage tool.
   c. The massage practitioner will only use hands, fingers, and thumbs when applying point pressure.
   d. Deep pressure requests for massage need to be made prior to the session with additional $20 fee.

18. A massage therapist is developing policies for a mobile practice in clients' homes. Which policy is most relevant based on reduction of work-related injury protentional?
   a. Massage will be scheduled between the hours of 10 am and 4 pm.
   b. Setup in the home does not require carrying massage equipment up or down stairs.
   c. Massage location must have nonslip floors and adjacent restroom.
   d. Clients will supply and launder massage linens.

19. A massage practitioner is choosing between two employment positions. Pay and scheduling is similar. Which of the following would most influence the best work location?
   a. Size of massage rooms
   b. Number of rooms available
   c. Access to laundry facilities
   d. Ability to work on mat or table

20. Which approach to massage application would contribute most to the practitioner's potential for developing shoulder discomfort?
   a. Seated position when applying kneading on the legs and arms while client is supine.
   b. Standing position at side of the table applying compression with forearm.
   c. Seated position with client side-lying to work on the feet using loose fist gliding.
   d. Standing position at client's head gliding on the back toward the hips.

Exercise

Write at least three more multiple choice questions—one of each type: factual recall and comprehension, application and concept identification, and clinical reasoning and synthesis. Develop plausible wrong answers and be sure that the correct answer is clearly correct. Then write a rationale for each question. The more questions you write, the better you will understand the material. Exchange questions with fellow classmates or discuss in class. The questions from all the learners can be combined to create a review quiz.

CHAPTER

9 Preparation for Massage

http://evolve.elsevier.com/Fritz/fundamentals/

CHAPTER OBJECTIVES

After completing this chapter, the student will be able to perform the following:

1. List the equipment and setup procedures required to prepare for a massage session.
2. Create a massage setting in different types of environments.
3. Explain massage procedures to a client.
4. Identify gender issues that may influence the client's expectations and respond appropriately.
5. Obtain and give relevant feedback during the massage.
6. Perform pre-massage procedures to prepare both the client and the therapist for the massage session.
7. Perform post-massage procedures to close the massage session and prepare for the next client.
8. Effectively drape and position a client.

CHAPTER OUTLINE

KEY TERMS

Body supports
Draping
Draping material
Feedback
Lubricants
Massage chair
Massage mat
Massage table
Positioning

The massage therapist makes certain preparations before beginning the massage. All necessary supplies are gathered, and the room is set up. The type of lubricant used and the way it is dispensed, the temperature of the massage room, and the warmth of the therapist's hands are additional considerations. The massage therapist uses history-taking and assessment procedures to identify client outcomes and formulate the approach for the massage. The therapist discusses the plan with the client and obtains informed consent. Other considerations include client positioning and modest, appropriate draping procedures. All sanitation procedures must be performed. Massage professionals benefit from developing a method to help them focus on the client and the session to come. This chapter is designed to help learners develop these important pre-massage procedures, which support the massage relationship and the professional environment first discussed in Chapter 2.

EQUIPMENT

SECTION OBJECTIVES

Chapter objective covered in this section:

1. List the equipment and setup procedures required to prepare for a massage session.

Using the information presented in this section, the student will be able to perform the following:

- Care for and protect hands, arms, and general health.
- Make informed decisions about the purchase of a massage table, chair, mat, body supports, draping materials, and lubricants.
- Make the most effective use of massage equipment.

Care of the Massage Therapist's Hands and Body

The most important pieces of equipment for massage professionals are their hands, arms, and body. They should make sure to protect their hands from abrasion and damage by wearing gloves when doing outdoor chores or other work in which the hands may be injured. Using the forearms during a massage protects the hands and limits their use. In some circumstances, such as when working on a floor mat, the knees and feet are used for certain massage techniques. The massage therapist has a professional responsibility to be attentive to efficient and proper body mechanics (see Chapter 8) and the maintenance of personal health. Chapter 15 expands on self-care information and strategies.

Massage Table

Another important piece of massage equipment is the surface on which the client may sit or lie while receiving the massage. The first choice of most therapists for this purpose is a massage table. The table must be sturdy and properly assembled so that there is no chance of it collapsing while a client is lying on it. The two primary types of massage tables are the portable table, which folds into a smaller unit and can be carried easily from place to place (Box 9.1), and the stationary table, which remains in one location.

Most manufacturers offer a basic model, and many have tables with all sorts of features, such as automatic height and tilt adjustments, arm supports, and face cradles. The more features a table has, the more expensive it is. Massage tables should be purchased from an experienced manufacturer. Buying a product that has been tested for safety is worth the investment. All massage tables must be checked prior to each use for structural stability. It is important to perform a complete maintenance check on all connectors, bolts, cables, and hinges every week and to repair any defects immediately.

Portable Tables

Almost all portable tables are built with a hinge in the middle that allows them to fold in half for ease of carrying (Fig. 9.1).

Box 9.1 Features of a Massage Table

A portable massage table is the most versatile type of massage table. At a minimum, it should have the following features:

- Sturdy construction, including cable support on the legs if portable
- Minimum 450 lb/204 kg weight capacity recommended
- Manual or hydraulic/pneumatic height adjustment
- A face cradle
- A washable covering (usually vinyl) that also can be cleaned with disinfectant
- Adequate padding to ensure comfort and firm support
- A width of 28–30 inches appears to be best suited to most situations. Portable tables wider than 32 inches are difficult to carry and ergonomically inefficient. Note that most tables are about 6 feet long, which can accommodate most clients.
- A stationary massage table is an option if the table will not be transported from location to location.
- There are multiple styles: fixed leg height, adjustable leg height, and hydraulic/pneumatic lift tables. The fixed-leg table is the least adaptable.
- If at all possible, make the investment in a lift table or choose to be employed at an establishment where lift tables are standard equipment.

This hinged area is a weak spot in the table, and cable supports on the legs counterbalance the weakness. Most tables are strong and can hold between 300–600 pounds (136–272 kg) if the weight is distributed evenly over the entire surface of the table. Problems occur when the client sits in the middle of the table when lying down or sitting up, which focuses all the weight in one spot. With cumulative use, the hinge weakens. It is important to check the cable tension regularly to ensure that no sag develops. Otherwise, the table may buckle, injuring the client and damaging the table. Manually adjustable legs allow the massage table to be lowered or raised to accommodate clients of various sizes while allowing the therapist to use proper body mechanics.

Many clients may be concerned about the sturdiness of the table. The lightweight, portable tables may look weak, but a quality table is well built and strong. Before the massage, demonstrate the stability of the table to the client or offer alternatives, such as a chair or massage mat.

Stationary Tables

Stationary tables (Fig. 9.2) do not have the instability problem because the table is heavier, and cross-bracing and leg supports make it even safer. However, the lack of portability is a major drawback if the massage practice involves any on-site mobile work.

Lift Tables

Two basic types of adjustable lift tables are available: hydraulic and electric. Hydraulic tables do not need electricity. With the client on the table, height adjustments are made using a hand crank or foot pump. Electric lift tables provide an electric lift

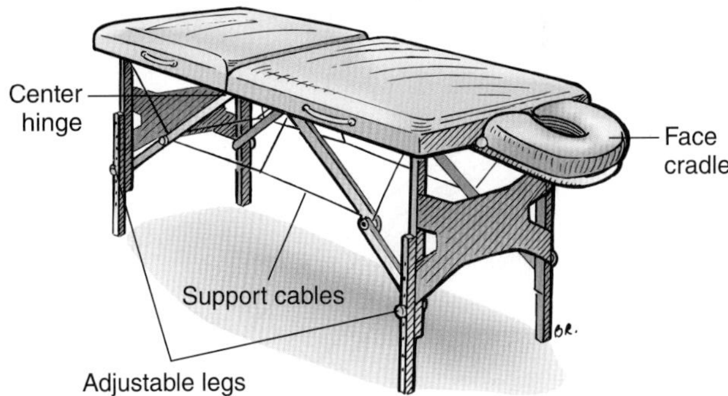

FIG. 9.1 A portable massage table with a center hinge, support cables, and a face cradle.

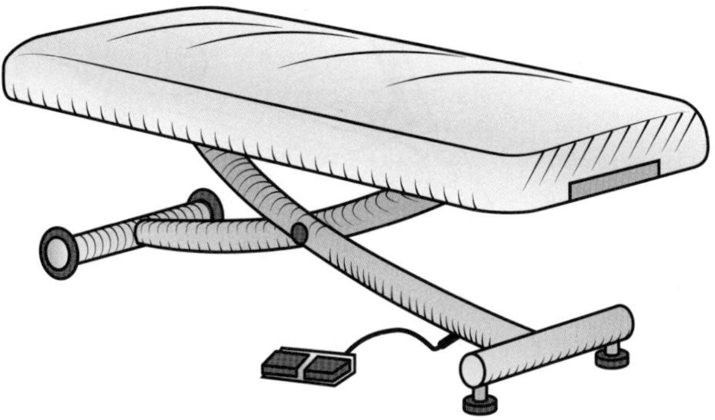

FIG. 9.2 A stationary massage table with height adjustment.

mechanism with push-button controls. A lift massage table is the most ergonomically supportive massage equipment. At a minimum, it should have the same features as portable and stationary massage tables (see Box 9.1), in addition to a hydraulic or electrical mechanism that allows height adjustment to at least 40 inches.

The only disadvantage of both types of lift tables is that they are not usually portable. However, continuing innovation by manufacturers of massage tables should address this issue. Future models may have a lift base that allows the tabletop to be removed and converted to a portable table, or a lift mechanism that is more portable may be developed. Lift tables are expensive, but they can be considered an important investment in supporting proper body mechanics.

Massage Chair

A special **massage chair** can be purchased for seated massage. These chairs are a worthwhile investment to provide options for clients (Fig. 9.3). The seated massage is typically provided in a public setting (e.g., a business location) and is done over clothing. Massage chairs also are excellent for working with clients who are more comfortable sitting upright (Box 9.2).

A straight-backed chair with no arms also can be used. The client sits facing the back of the chair and leans on the chair back, supported by pillows. A stool or chair pushed up to a table or desk is another option. The client leans forward on supporting pillows placed on the table. Special triangular or block-shaped foam forms can be purchased to provide support. A professionally manufactured desktop support, which could replace the pillows, is available (Fig. 9.4).

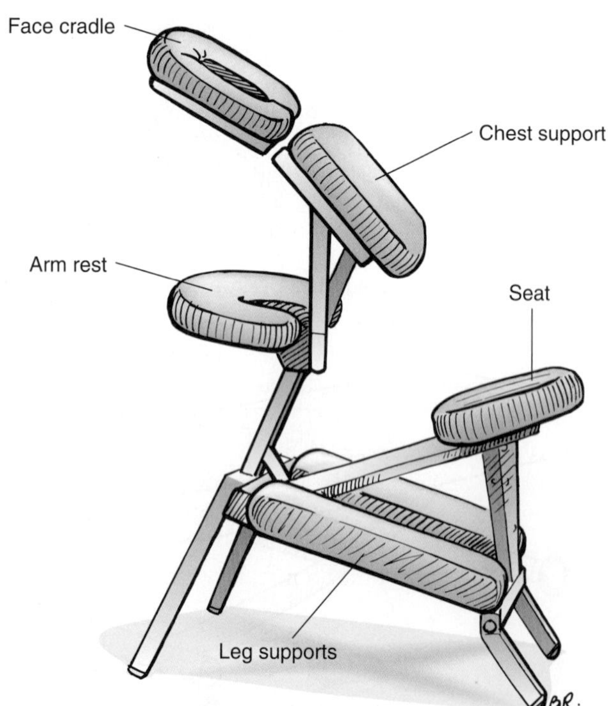

FIG. 9.3 A massage chair.

Box 9.2 Advantages and Disadvantages of a Massage Chair

Advantages

1. Massage chairs, which are specially designed for that purpose, usually are comfortable and easy to use.
2. Professionally manufactured equipment adds to the professional atmosphere of the massage setting and ensures safety through quality workmanship in construction and design.
3. Professionally manufactured massage chairs are lightweight and portable.
4. Clients with certain respiratory, vascular, and cardiac conditions are best given a massage in a seated position.

Disadvantages

1. Some people have difficulty getting into and out of the semi-kneeling position required to use the massage chair.
2. Access to certain body areas is limited.

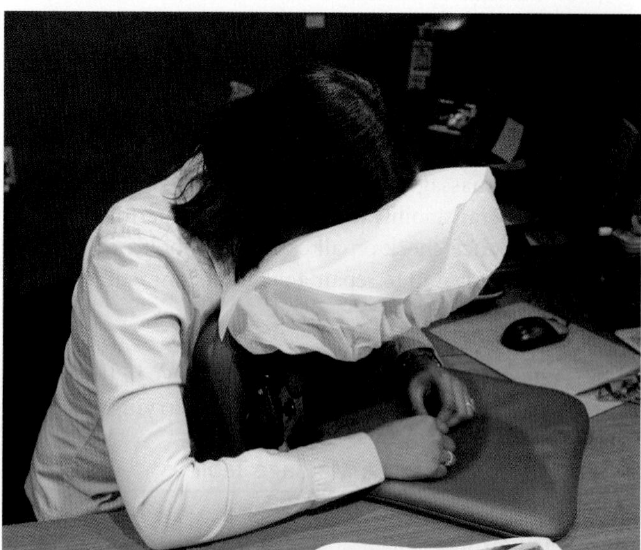

FIG. 9.4 A massage support device for working at a desk. (From Holland P, Anderson S: *Chair massage,* St. Louis, 2010, Mosby.)

Massage Mat

A mat on the floor is used for some methods of massage (Box 9.3). The **massage mat** can be a futon or an exercise mat, but it must be protected by a sanitary covering (Fig. 9.5).

Body Supports

Body supports are used to bolster the body during the massage and give contour to the flat working surface (Fig. 9.6). Commercial body support products, consisting of various shapes and sizes of pillows and foam forms, can be purchased. As an alternative, the therapist can buy assorted shapes and densities of hypoallergenic foam and make covers for them. A wedge, a round tube, and two or three square or oblong pieces will be needed, each with a different depth and density. A rectangular-shaped bolster that is 6″ high x 8″–12″ wide x 30″–36″ long, cut from dense foam is recommended for bolstering the

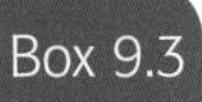

Key Features, Advantages, and Disadvantages of a Massage Mat

Key Features
1. The mat should be soft enough and provide sufficient support to ensure the client's comfort.
2. It should be large enough to allow the massage therapist to move around the client's body while staying on the cushioned surface, thereby protecting their knees and body.
3. It should be made so that it can be protected with a sanitary covering.

Advantages
1. A mat often is less expensive than a massage table.
2. It may be lighter and therefore easier to carry than a massage table.
3. Mats are particularly safe (i.e., the client has little risk of falling off).
4. A mat is a popular choice when working with infants and children.
5. Mats are portable.
6. Because a mat is so safe and comfortable, it may be the best choice for working with clients who have certain physical disabilities; a transfer from a wheelchair to a mat may be accomplished more easily.

Disadvantages
1. Proper training is needed to work effectively on the floor; many massage therapists are not familiar with this kind of work.
2. The floor may be drafty or cold for the client.
3. Physically challenged or elder adult clients may have difficulty getting down on or up from the floor.
4. Mats do not have face cradles to maintain alignment of the neck in the prone position. However, face cradles from massage tables or bolstering systems can be adapted to use on the floor. They are placed on the floor at the end of the mat or on the mat itself, depending on the client's preference.

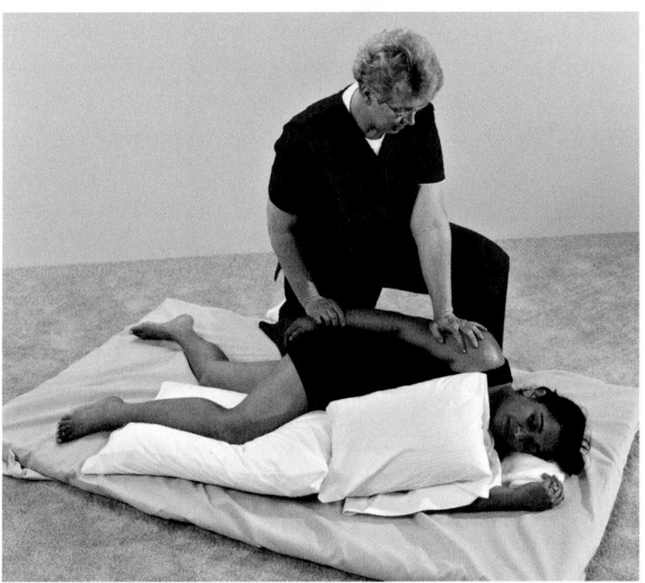

FIG. 9.5 A generic massage mat covered with a sheet.

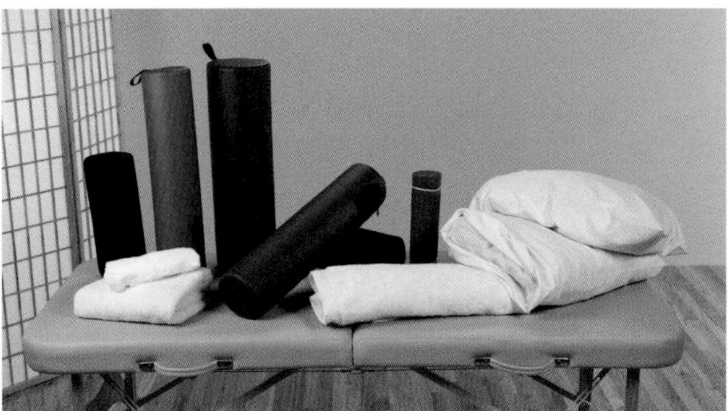

FIG. 9.6 Different types of body supports.

PROFICIENCY EXERCISE 9.1

1. Collect information from at least three manufacturers of massage tables and massage chairs. Compare the cost, quality, and construction of the equipment.
2. Research a variety of styles of body supports for clients with specific needs.
3. Locate a source of foam (an upholstery or a mattress company is a good start). See how many different body supports you can build from foam scraps.

client's top leg in the side-lying position. Rolled towels, blankets, and various sizes of pillows also can function as body supports (Proficiency Exercise 9.1).

Draping Materials

Opaque **draping material** is used to provide the client with privacy and warmth. Standard bed linens are the coverings most commonly used because they are large enough to cover the entire body and are easily used for most draping procedures. Both full and twin-size sheets fit nicely on most massage tables. The therapist can either buy these linens and launder them in a sanitary fashion or use a linen service. Sheets made of cotton or cotton blends are the best choice because they do not slip on the client. Cotton flannel sheets are a consideration for the winter months because they feel warm to the skin. Whatever linen is used, it must be able to withstand washing with bleach or other disinfecting solutions (Fig. 9.7).

Large towels may be used for draping because they are both warm and opaque. They must be at least the size of a beach towel and must have a soft texture. Be sensitive to the client's comfort and provide a choice of towels or sheets. Because towels are smaller, a client may feel more exposed and may prefer the security offered by a sheet. As an alternative, both sheets and towels can be used, with a bath-size towel used as a chest covering.

Disposable linen also is available. Some higher-quality disposable products may look and feel like cotton fabric, but they do not provide the same warmth. Disposable linens are convenient and sanitary, but they cannot be washed or recycled.

Draping Material Recommendations

A twin fitted sheet should be put over the massage tabletop to protect the table. Laundering this additional sheet is much less expensive than replacing the covering on the table. A full or twin flat

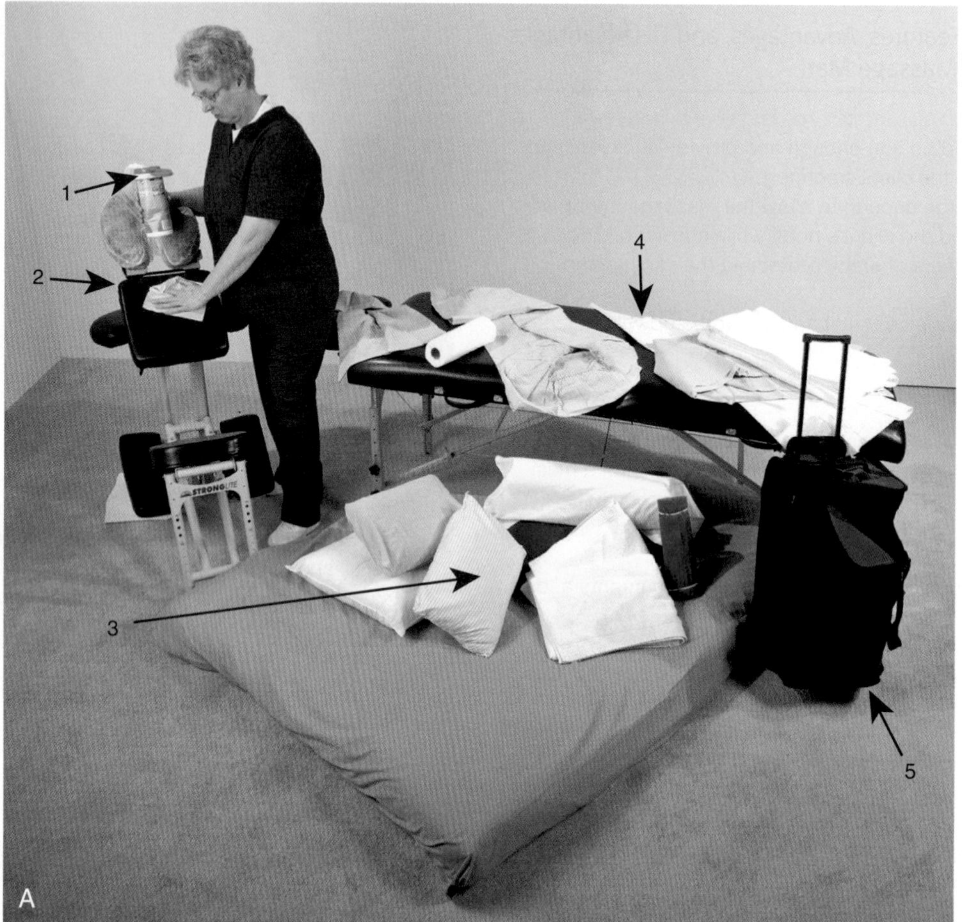

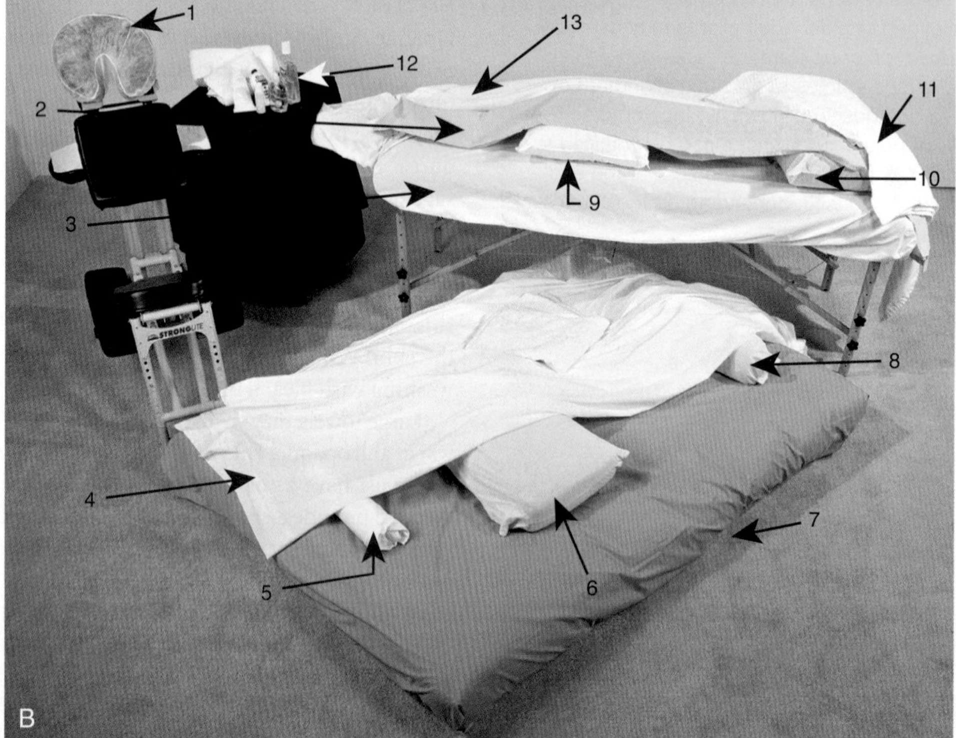

FIG. 9.7 A, Bolsters and draping material. *1,* Sanitizing wipes. *2,* Disposable face cover. *3,* Bolsters and pillows. *4,* Sheets, pillowcases, and blankets. *5,* Rolling carry bag. **B,** Massage area setup. *1,* Disposable face cover. *2,* Bottom sheet. *3,* Fitted sheet. *4,* Top sheet. *5,* Neck roll (rolled towel). *6,* Pillow for placement beneath abdomen or knees. *7,* Mat sheet. *8,* Ankle support. *9,* Bolster (knee or abdomen). *10,* Ankle bolster. *11,* Blanket. *12,* Various lubricants and hand sanitizers. *13,* Top sheet.

Box 9.4 Draping Material Required for One Client

- 1 twin fitted sheet (table protector)
- 2 full or twin flat sheets (bottom and top drapes)
- 1 pillowcase or hand towel (face cradle)
- Additional pillowcases (body supports)
- 1 bath-size towel
- 1 flannel sheet, light blanket, or beach-size towel for warmth

sheet then is placed over the protective covering. The top sheet can be either a full or a twin sheet. Both sheet sizes have advantages and disadvantages. Twin sheets fit a bit better on the table but sometimes can be inadequate for draping. Full sheets provide more material, which facilitates draping, but can be cumbersome. Also, for sanitary purposes, care must be taken that sheets do not drag on the floor. Face cradles should be draped with a hand towel, a pillowcase, or an additional piece of fabric sewn just to fit the face cradle. Inexpensive disposable face cradle covers are available. All body supports and pillows that come into direct contact with the client are covered with pillowcases.

In addition to the sheets and pillowcases, a bath-size towel is used for various draping procedures. A large beach-size towel, a flannel sheet, or a blanket should be available in case the client becomes chilled.

Keeping different colors of sheets and towels for each set of drapery material can be helpful because if all are the same color, distinguishing between the top and bottom sheets can be difficult. For example, the protective fitted sheet may be white; the bottom flat sheet, blue; the top flat sheet, green; and the towel and pillowcase, yellow. The blanket or flannel sheet for additional warmth could be a printed material. The draping materials required for one client are listed in Box 9.4.

When possible, soft pastel colors should be chosen for draping materials because they withstand bleaching, are more opaque than white linens, and tend not to show lubricant stains. If a linen service is used, access to multiple colors may be limited. Some people are allergic to cotton blends, which may irritate their skin. If the client has sensitive skin, the therapist should use white, pure cotton sheets to reduce the risk of a reaction.

At least 10 full sets of draping material are needed; this is sufficient for 2 standard business days, with laundry done every other day. Massage therapists who use a laundry service should order enough linen for 10 days to make sure they do not run out of linens if delivery is late. Whenever linens come in contact with the client, they must be laundered in an approved fashion before they are reused. (Sanitation procedures for any linens that come in contact with a client's bodily fluids are discussed in Chapter 7). Most linens must be replaced every 1–2 years if used often. Lubricants build up, and bleach wears out the fabric (Proficiency Exercise 9.2).

PROFICIENCY EXERCISE 9.2

1. Obtain a set of sheets and some towels Practice draping methods with them. Which type of material did you prefer to use?
2. Have another student or a massage therapist give you a massage using the different draping materials. Which type did you prefer to have used on you?

Lubricants

Lubricants serve only one purpose for the massage therapist: they reduce drag on the skin during gliding-type massage strokes. The medicinal or cosmetic use of lubricants is out of the scope of practice for therapeutic massage.

Scented Lubricants

Because headaches and other allergic responses to lubricants often are caused by the volatile oils in scented products, scented lubricants should not be used. This recommendation does not discount the therapeutic benefit of aromatherapy; the sense of smell is a powerful sensory mechanism, and physiological processes can be triggered by the deliberate use of aroma. However, this textbook does not cover all these applications, and additional education is required to use aromas specifically, purposefully, and therapeutically. Until receiving this training, massage therapists should not use them. (A short discussion of the use of essential oils is included in Chapter 12).

Types of Lubricants

The types of lubricants include oils, creams, lotions, and gels. Oils are fats that are liquid at room temperature. Plant-based oils are derived from one or more parts of a plant, shrub, or tree. Seeds and nuts are common sources of oil. Mineral oils are petroleum-based.

The lubricant traditionally used for massage is oil. Oils used for massage are primarily derived from plants. Oil is easy to dispense from a squeeze bottle and can be kept free of contamination. However, natural vegetable oils can become rancid quickly, and some commercial products use additives that may cause allergic reactions in clients. In addition, oils are messy, they can spill and drip, and they stain linens (although specialized laundry products are available for removing oil stains).

Creams are becoming as popular as oils for massage application. Creams are a semisolid emulsion of 50% oil and 50% water; they spread easily, absorb quickly, and wash off with water. Creams are packaged in a tub or a tube because they are too thick to be dispensed in a pump.

Lotions are also an excellent alternative to oil as a massage lubricant. Lotions are thinner than creams and are often packaged in a pump bottle. A lotion is similar to a cream but has a lighter or thinner formulation. They absorb quickly and feel light on the skin. Lotions are easier to distribute on hairy body areas.

Gels are available as a massage lubricant. Gels are emulsions that contain oil-in-water and usually have an alcohol base. Gels do not feel oily or greasy. Gels have a jelly consistency with high viscosity and can be dispensed from a pump container. Like lotions, they are easy to use on hairy body areas.

If possible, massage therapists should use the most natural products available and should avoid using petrochemicals and talc because many people are allergic to these substances. All lubricants must be dispensed from a contamination-free container. This means that the opening of the container does not come in contact with contaminants. For example, if a squeeze tube is used to dispense massage cream, the therapist should not wipe their hand over the opening to stop the

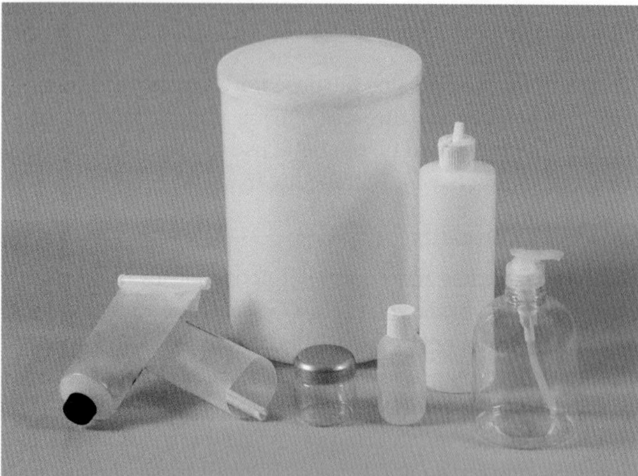

FIG. 9.8 Massage lubricant containers.

flow. A hygienic approach is to use small, sterile containers that are filled from a larger container to hold the lubricant for an individual massage (Fig. 9.8). Typically a single-use or sanitized spoon is used to remove the amount of cream needed for the massage.

Using Massage Lubricants

Only a small amount of lubricant is needed for a massage. Remember that the reason for using lubricant is to reduce drag on the skin from the massage movements. More lubricant is required to work over body hair. Sometimes the use of any type of lubricant is contraindicated; therefore it is important to be able to perform massage without a lubricant.

In Chapter 10, you will learn about different massage methods. The long, gliding methods are best for applying lubricant. Keep the application even and thin. Applying more is easy, but removing excess is difficult. Keep a clean towel available in case removal is necessary.

Do not pour the lubricant directly onto the client. Warm the lubricant in your palms first by rubbing your hands together. Apply the lubricant to one area at a time rather than to the entire body. Do not use lubricant on the face or hair because it disturbs makeup and hairstyles. For sanitary reasons, wash and dry your hands or clean your hands with a hand sanitizer before working on the face. Some therapists begin the massage with the face and head, before using any lubricant.

Some clients may appreciate having the lubricant removed after the massage. An alcohol-based product can do this, but alcohol is drying to the skin. Rubbing the skin with an absorbent towel removes most of the lubricant.

Additional Equipment

Music

Music often is used to distract the client from or to block out surrounding noise. A less recognized use is to achieve interaction and modulation of the autonomic nervous system through entrainment. Simple, soft music with a base of under 60 beats per minute tends to activate a parasympathetic response, which produces a soothing, relaxing effect. Music faster than 60 beats per minute encourages sympathetic responses, producing a stimulating, invigorating effect.

When using music, the therapist must consider the effect to be created and whether both the client and the massage therapist enjoy the music. The best course is to have available various types of music from which the client is allowed to choose. An assortment of styles, rhythms, and instruments, in addition to equipment to play music, should be available. The volume should be kept low but loud enough so that the music can be heard without straining.

The music itself can help to pace the massage because the massage therapist can gain a sense of timing/rhythm without looking at the clock (Proficiency Exercise 9.3).

PROFICIENCY EXERCISE 9.3

1. Obtain the four basic types of lubricants: oil, cream, lotion, and gel. Give a massage with each type. Which do you prefer to use?
2. Find a practice client with a hairy body, and practice using the different types of lubricants. Which one was the easiest to use? Which one did the client prefer?
3. Have a fellow learner give you a massage using all four types of lubricants on different parts of the body. After receiving the massages, compare and decide which type you prefer.
4. Practice giving a massage with as little lubricant as possible.
5. Assemble a music library consisting of different types of music. Mentally mark each 15-minute segment to assist with the timing of the massage.

MASSAGE ENVIRONMENT

SECTION OBJECTIVES

Chapter objective covered in this section:

2. Create a massage setting in different types of environments.

Using the information presented in this section, the student will be able to perform the following:

- Design an efficient therapeutic massage environment.
- Organize an office and massage room.

Clients return for regular massage because they appreciate the quality of the service and a professional personality and environment. Thoroughly plan the image you want your massage environment to convey to the public. Various wellness centers, massage therapy franchises, and spas carefully develop the business environment. To maintain the integrity of the professional relationship, the environment created for the massage setting, including decorations and the reading material provided for clients, should reflect the scope of practice of massage.

When most people think of massage, they picture a quiet, private room with low lighting and soft music. However, therapeutic massage can be provided almost anywhere and under almost any conditions. Successful massage practices have been developed in noisy public locations, such as airports, in a client's home, in the workplace, and outdoors at sporting events or retreats. Whatever the physical location of the massage environment, the most important aspect is to present and deliver the highest standard of professional care to the public.

General Conditions

General conditions for massage areas that must be considered are the room temperature, the fresh air supply, privacy, and accessibility. When considering an employment-based facility or developing a self-employed location the environment is important for both the massage practitioner and the clients.

Room Temperature

The air temperature in the massage room should be kept at 72–75°F (22–24°C). Massage produces a vasodilative effect, which brings the blood closer to the surface of the body and allows internal heat to escape, cooling the client. Clients cannot relax if they are cold. The massage therapist is active and fully dressed and can become warm while doing the massage. Some therapists put a table warmer or an electric blanket on the table to keep clients warm. A piece of lamb's wool may be used because it traps and retains body heat. Placing a hot water bottle or other form of heating device at the client's feet and another at the neck or wherever comfortable may increase body temperature. Care needs to be taken to prevent burns any time heat is applied to a client's body.

The most comfortable uniform for a massage therapist is one made of cotton or a cotton blend that will wick away moisture and perspiration from the skin. It should have short sleeves and be loose-fitting to help prevent the therapist from becoming too warm.

Fresh Air and Ventilation

Ventilation is important for controlling the spread of airborne pathogens, managing indoor pollution, ensuring adequate airflow, and cleaning/filtering the air. It is also important to control moisture and keep humidity below 60% (ideally, 30–50%). Heating, ventilation, and air conditioning (HVAC) is the use of various technologies to control the temperature, humidity, and purity of the air in an enclosed space. When used properly, air cleaners and HVAC filters can help reduce airborne contaminants including viruses in a building or small space. HEPA is a type of pleated mechanical air filter. It is an acronym for "high-efficiency particulate air [filter]" This type of air filter can theoretically remove at least 99.97% of dust, pollen, mold, bacteria, and any airborne particles.

In the massage therapy treatment area, ventilation is important. The room should have access to fresh air, but a window that opens to the outside is not always available. Room-size HEPA filters are desirable if maintained. A small fan in the room pointed at the ceiling or the wall keeps the air moving without causing a draft on the client. Learn more at the US Environmental Protection Agency https://www.epa.gov/.

Privacy

Clients need privacy to remove their clothes in preparation for the massage treatment. If the massage room is separate from other public areas, the client can be left alone to get ready for the massage. Sometimes a screen or curtained area can be used to divide one large room into two distinct areas.

Accessibility

Locating the massage practice so that it is easily accessible to clients is important. Barrier-free access and restrooms are required.

Lighting

The massage area must be lit well enough to meet the standards for proper cleaning and safety (see Chapter 7). Bright overhead lighting often is too harsh and glaring for the client. Indirect or natural light from a window filtered through a privacy shade is much better. If the massage area has overhead lights, turn them off and use a lamp in the corner of the room instead. A dimmer switch is excellent because it allows adjustment of the lighting. Never work in a dark room, to prevent accidents caused by tripping, and never work by candlelight, because an open flame is a safety hazard.

Scents, Incense, Flowers, and Plants

Massage therapists work with a variety of people during the day, each one with different ideas about what is pleasant and what is offensive. Many clients are also environmentally sensitive and react to scents, incense, and flowers. The best recommendation is to avoid using such items because the fragrance lingers and can cause problems for a client.

Non-flowering (foliage) plants usually are less of a problem. However, if the therapist serves an allergic population, the best course may be not to use them.

Hygiene, Chemicals, Perfume, and Warm Hands

Recall from Chapter 7 that it is important for the massage professional to address personal hygiene and prevent body odors because people are sensitive to these smells. Avoid the use of aftershave, perfume, scented cosmetics, hair spray, or other scented products, including essential oils. Clients usually do not comment on offensive breath or body odors; they may simply not return for further sessions. Because recognizing odors on ourselves can be difficult, ask a family member or friend who will answer truthfully if you have such a problem.

If the massage therapist is a smoker, the smell of smoke can linger in fabric, carpeting, and furniture and on the therapist. This can be distasteful to a nonsmoking client. Because removing the odor is difficult, the massage environment should be located in a nonsmoking area. Refraining from smoking during professional hours may help prevent the smell from clinging to the hands, clothes, hair, and breath.

If a massage therapist has cold hands, the hands should be heated with warm water, on a hot water bottle or other warming device, or by rubbing them together before the therapist touches the client. A towel-warming cabinet is a common piece of equipment in the massage area. A strategy for managing hand temperature is to begin the massage with hot towel application (such as on the client's neck or feet), which also then warms the massage practitioner's hands.

Typical Massage Room, Home Office, or Clinical Setting

Business and Massage Areas

A massage area separate from the business area in the massage setting is desirable. People associate behavior with locations and expect certain activities at those locations. It is important that these two activities remain separate in the client's mind. The interaction that takes place when appointments are made and money is taken is different from the one that takes place during a massage.

The business or reception area should be near the entrance. An appointment book or a computer or device for scheduling, a calendar, forms, receipts, pencils, and a telephone, in addition to a chair and a small table, should be set up in the business area. The massage area should be located farther from the door or in an adjacent area (Fig. 9.9).

In the massage area or room, make sure clients have a place to sit and place their clothes. Use an enclosed cabinet to store linens and lubricants and designate a place to keep the body supports. A covered hamper, located away from the massage table, is needed for used linens.

Hand-washing and restroom facilities must be easily accessible. If the massage room has no sink, a liquid hand cleanser must be available. If no direct access exists between the massage room and the restroom, make sure the client uses the facilities before the massage session begins. You should also have a plan for getting the client to the restroom during the massage session if necessary. This can get tricky if the only way to the facilities is down a public hall. Having a robe and slippers (laundered after each use) available and escorting the client to the bathroom are options. When considering the location of the massage area, be mindful of the restroom location and ease of access.

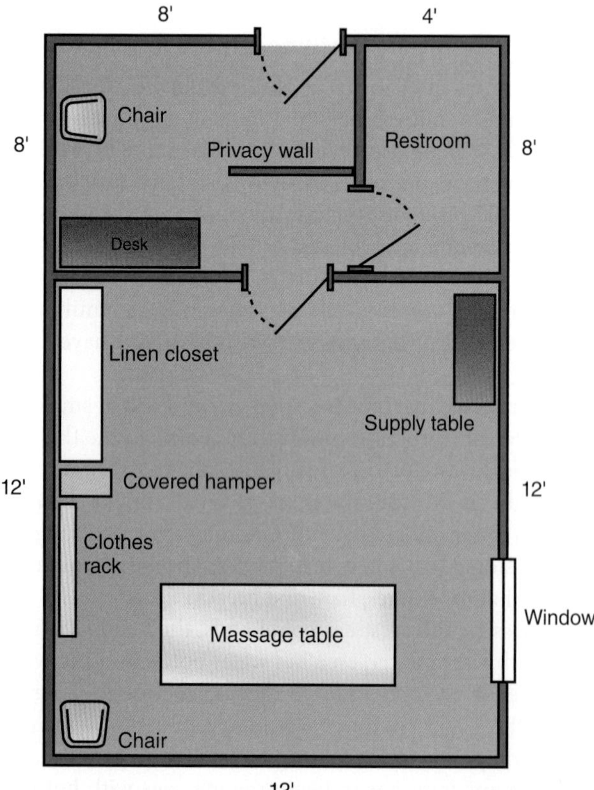

FIG. 9.9 A sample layout of a massage office in which the business office and massage area are separate.

Room Size

The following recommendations cover a variety of options. First discussed is the solo self-employed massage therapist who has a small office. The location can be self-contained or part of a larger shared space. Then described is how massage areas are designed in the massage clinic/spa setting. Finally described is a home office setting.

Independent Massage Office

The reception and business area can be small, about 8 × 8 feet (64 square feet). A room for massage should be at least 10 × 10 feet (100 square feet); this is the minimum amount of space that allows therapists to move comfortably around the client on the table and enables them to use proper body mechanics.

If the two areas are in the same room, a space of at least 12 × 12 feet (144 square feet) is needed to provide the necessary working area (Fig. 9.10). A private restroom should be easily accessible. Visualize how a hotel room is designed. There is typically a seating/desk area, a small adjacent restroom, and the sleeping area would be the massage area. There is a storage closet. This type of design is ideal for a sole self-employed massage therapist.

Office in a Shared Facility

In a shared facility, where the massage therapist rents a designated massage room, the therapist typically also shares a reception area and restrooms. The actual massage room should be no smaller than 10 × 10 feet; a better size is 12 × 10 feet or larger. It is possible to work in an area with one dimension at 9 feet, but this is not recommended if it can be avoided. A 9 × 9-foot room is the smallest area that can support proper ergonomics and the practice of body mechanics.

Preferably each area has an adjacent private restroom, but this is not common. It is best if the area is equipped with a sink for hand washing. Visualize how a hotel room is designed. There is typically a seating/desk area, a small adjacent restroom, and a sleeping area that in this case would be the massage area. There is a storage closet. Before signing a lease consider examining and measuring the space.

Massage Area in a Clinic/Spa Facility

In this situation, the massage therapist is typically an employee. There is a formal reception area with front desk staff. The massage therapy rooms are located in a separate area with access to restrooms. When considering an employment position, pay attention to the facilities and the design of the massage areas. The massage therapy rooms should be no smaller than 9 × 9 feet, and this size is barely adequate. Preferred is a room that is 10 × 10 feet with an option of 9 × 10 feet. An 8 × 11 room potentially allows enough space if cabinets, chairs, and other items are placed at one end of the room. Also pay close attention to ventilation, as most of these types of facilities do not

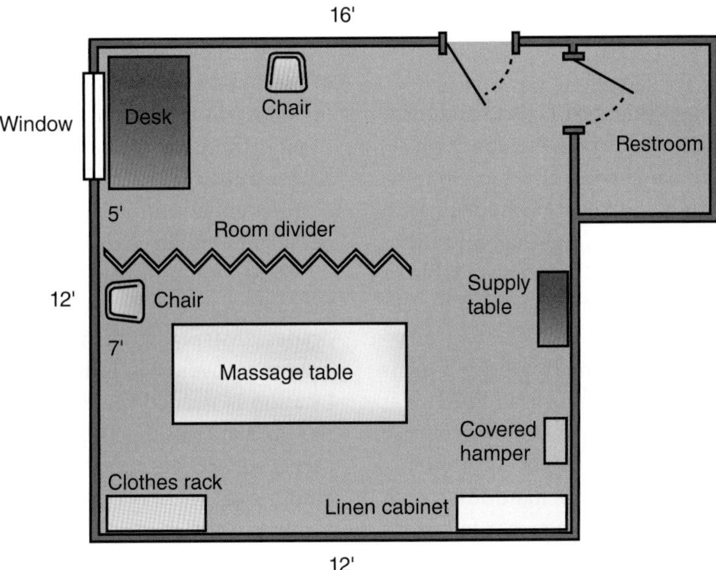

FIG. 9.10 A sample layout of a massage office with the business office and massage area in one room.

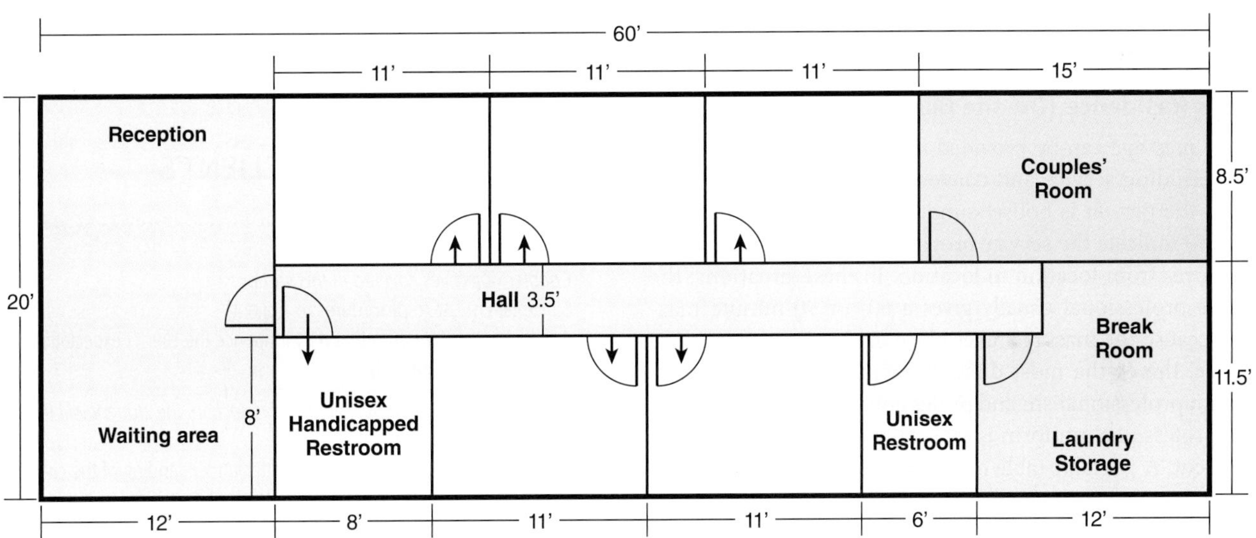

FIG. 9.11 A typical massage clinic layout.

have windows in the massage areas. The overall facility design is set up to maximize the use of office space. Often these facilities are located in commercial rentals that are 20 feet wide by 60 feet long. A reception area is typically 20 × 10 feet with door access to the treatment rooms. A minimum 3-foot-wide hall may run down the middle, with treatment rooms off to either side. Based on these dimensions the treatment rooms will be limited, barely 9 feet in depth with 8.5 feet more likely, and barely adequate with the table set up on an angle in the room. If the width is 10 feet, this is a workable massage therapy session room. There can be four treatment rooms on either side of the hall with additional space designated for restrooms and a staff break room, laundry, and storage. The temptation is to shorten the width of the rooms to 9 feet instead of 10 feet to gain space, and this is a common adaptation. The hope is that as more of these types of facilities are built, better ergonomic designs will be implemented (Fig. 9.11).

Office in the Therapist's Home

Designating a professional area in your home as an office is a business option if zoning regulations in your area allow home office businesses (see Chapter 3). Establishing a professional office in the home involves special considerations. If at all possible, the massage area should have a private entrance (zoning regulations usually require this). Barrier-free access and restrooms are a major consideration in planning a home office. Most homes are not designed with these accommodations.

If pets are in the home, potential clients must be informed in case of allergy or fear of animals. Pets should not be allowed in the business or massage areas. Family members must understand the privacy issue of the massage environment, and massage clients must understand the boundaries of the private home area. This more personal environment requires careful attention to professional boundaries.

Public Environment: Event Sports Massage, Demonstration Massage, On-site/Mobile, or Corporate Massage

In the public setting, the massage therapist goes to the location rather than having the client come to the therapist's office. These public massage sessions normally last less than 30 minutes, and the client remains fully clothed. As the therapist, you usually have little control over noise, lighting, and other conditions. Clear enough space to set up the massage table or chair. If indoors, try to locate this area in a corner, which gives two walls to provide some privacy.

Regardless of the massage location, creating both a business area and a massage area is always important. Find a flat surface and use it to set up a portable office from a briefcase or similar carrying case that contains receipts, an appointment book, an alternative scheduler, and handouts, such as cards and brochures. Set up the massage area a few steps away.

Although the use of linens and lubricants usually is limited in these circumstances, having them available is important. They should be carried in a closed bag to maintain sanitation. Make provisions for hand-washing or hand-cleaning products to maintain hygiene and sanitation.

Client's Residence (On-site Massage)

On-site massage can be provided in the home for many reasons, including service and convenience for the client, especially if the person is housebound. The term *mobile massage* is used to indicate the service provided by a massage therapist who moves from location to location. In these situations, the massage professional usually gives a 60- or 90-minute massage. Because the massage takes place in the client's residence or office, this is the most difficult environment in which to maintain professionalism and professional boundaries. Therefore a professional uniform is especially important in this environment. A portable table most often is used, but a massage chair or mat also is acceptable.

Find a private location for the massage but avoid the bedroom; opt for a family room or den. If the only room available is a bedroom, try to use the guest room or a child's room rather than the client's bedroom. Make sure it is near an area where hands can be washed. Set up a business area using a briefcase as the office and maintain a professional atmosphere. Do not sit at the kitchen table or in the living room because the professional role of the massage therapist may be obscured in these traditional conversation locations.

Linens, body supports, and lubricants are needed. Also, bringing along a small fan to keep the air moving and to drown out noise from other areas may be wise.

Never lock the door, because a locked door invites secrecy and creates an environment in which maintaining professionalism is difficult. Under rare circumstances it could constitute entrapment, or the client could perceive it as a violation of the boundaries of the therapeutic relationship. Carry a sign to hang on the door that says, "Massage in session." If music is used, it is typically provided by a mobile device.

Outdoors

Outdoor massage usually is provided at a sports massage event or promotional activity. Some massage professionals also work on ships, on the beach, and poolside at spas and resorts. Although these are casual settings, the massage therapist's behavior must reflect professional and ethical standards. Again, a professional uniform is especially important in these more casual and public environments.

Wind, sun, rain, and insects create special conditions. Picnic table clips can be used to keep the wind from blowing the drapes. Instructing clients to wear a swimsuit or loose clothing for an over-the-clothing massage also helps. A firm, level location is needed for the table because tables that sink into the sand are unsafe. This can be prevented by putting sample carpet squares on the ground and placing the table legs in large empty cans such as coffee cans. The massage should be performed in the shade to prevent sunburn. A roof or canopy is helpful in case of rain. If the area is screened in, technically it is not outdoors. True outdoor massage will likely involve insects landing or crawling on the client; just blend the brushing away of insects into your massage techniques as best you can. If an area for washing hands is not available, use a disinfectant hand cleanser. Set up the portable office in an area away from the massage setting (Fig. 9.12 and Proficiency Exercise 9.4).

DETERMINING A NEW CLIENT'S EXPECTATIONS

SECTION OBJECTIVES

Chapter objectives covered in this section:

3. Explain massage procedures to a client.
4. Identify gender issues that may influence the client's expectations and respond appropriately.

Using the information presented in this section, the student will be able to perform the following:

- Interview a new client to gain a better understanding of the client's expectations of massage in general and of the outcome of a particular massage session.
- Recognize differences based on gender in clients' expectations and interpretation of touch.

Massage therapists must carefully help the client define the outcome of the massage, explain the limitations of massage, and put the client's expectations into perspective. This must be done before the massage is started as part of the informed consent procedure.

An important consideration is how the new client thinks a massage is given. The expectations of clients who have never had a massage are determined by what they have heard, read, or observed. Because methods and applications of massage vary so much, the client may not expect the style of massage that is offered. The difference between what is expected and what is received may be confusing. The client's answer to a simple question or statement, such as "What do you think a massage is like?" or "Describe for me how you think a massage is done," gives the massage therapist an idea of the client's expectations for the session. The massage therapist should explain the different approaches used so that the client is not

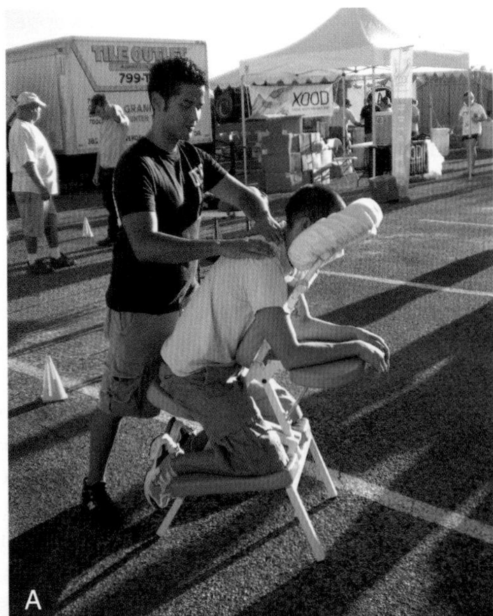

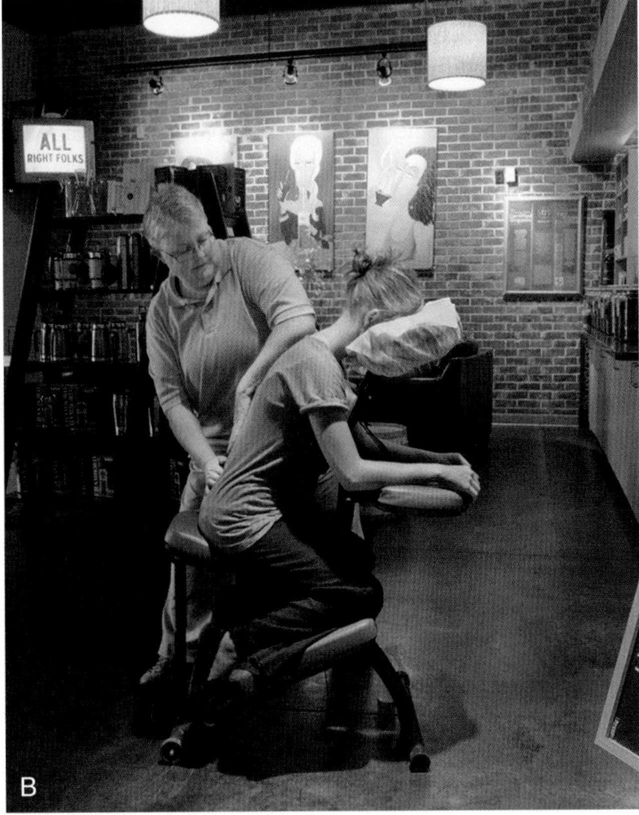

FIG. 9.12 A, An outdoor sports massage setting involving the use of a massage chair. **B,** On-site massage in a public setting. (From Holland P, Anderson S: *Chair massage,* St. Louis, 2010, Mosby.)

PROFICIENCY EXERCISE 9.4

1. Arrange to give a massage in each of the four basic environments. What was different about each experience?
2. Put together a briefcase office.
3. Identify massage practice software for your mobile device that supports your briefcase office.
4. On separate pieces of paper, design three different setups for a massage environment. Indicate the business and massage areas.

on the table wondering why this massage is so different from what they expected.

If a new client has had a massage before from someone else, it is natural to compare the different styles. The massage therapist must explain the procedures and methods used so that the client understands that massage can be done in many ways.

The outcome of massage is what the client can anticipate in response to the benefits of the proposed massage plan. Each massage manipulation has an anticipated response (discussed in Chapters 5 and 10). A client can be made aware of these responses and any risks inherent in the proposed massage interventions (see Chapter 6). Do not confuse expectations with outcomes (Focus on Professionalism 9.1).

FOCUS ON PROFESSIONALISM 9.1

Never discount another massage professional's methods or approach and say that your way is better; this is unethical behavior. The only exception is if the other therapist's massage violated professional ethics, scope of practice, or standards of practice. If a client describes an experience with another massage therapist that includes questionable behavior on the part of the therapist, explain to the client that you follow a professional code of ethics (as should everyone). The code of ethics example in this textbook or one from a professional organization can be used as a framework for the discussion (see Chapter 2).

EXAMPLE

A new client has never had a massage, but a friend in another city regularly receives therapeutic massage. The client explains that their friend receives massage for chronic headaches that seem to be related to daily stress and that the massage helps a lot (expectation). When you ask your client why they came for a massage (outcome), they indicate no real problems, although sometimes they experience headaches just as their friend does. Your client thinks a massage would feel good, and the outcome is a general massage that feels good, not the more specific approach to address headaches.

The client's expectations were based on information from their friend. A first-time client naturally considers this type of information, but the outcome may be very different. If the massage therapist does not carefully differentiate the two, the massage may not meet the client's expectations.

The therapist can ask a number of questions to help determine a new client's expectations, such as the following:

- How do you want to feel after the massage?
- What do you think massage will do for you?
- What results do you want from the massage?

After determining the client's expectations and the outcome, the therapist should carefully go over all the client policies and procedures discussed in Chapter 2. Never assume that a client understands the complexities of massage practice. Explain everything in detail in terms the client can understand.

For example, when the massage therapist explains client boundaries, the client may not understand the meaning of *boundaries* in terms of the professional relationship. Many people understand a boundary as a border, the official line that divides one area of land from another. If the massage therapist instead uses a term such as *limit,* which means a restriction on what can be done, the client may better understand the concept:

- "Certain boundaries define the professional relationship between the massage therapist and the client."
- "Certain limits define the professional relationship between the massage therapist and the client."

Another example is the term *draped,* which may make a client think of heavy curtains; *covered* may be a better word:

- "While you receive a massage, you will be draped."
- "While you receive a massage, you will be covered."

Gender and Age Concerns

Therapists may experience differences in a client's expectations and interpretation of touch. Gender identity is generally understood as one's personal experience of one's own gender. Gender identity can correlate with assigned sex at birth or can differ from it completely. The physiological, social, and biological aspects of gender are fluid. An understanding of and respect for the spectrum of gender identity is acknowledged by the textbook authors. However, a detailed exploration of this important topic is beyond the scope of this text. In the professional setting all health professionals, including massage therapists, should present as gender-neutral as possible. Clients may make judgments and be biased related to both the gender and age of the massage therapist. We all know this is wrong. However, a professional should be prepared for such situations and strive for their own behavior to be nonjudgmental and unbiased.

One vexing issue for massage therapists is the entanglement of therapeutic massage with sexually oriented business. Especially with first-time clients, it is important to establish clear boundaries concerning the inappropriateness of sexual interaction and create a safe, non-sexual, professional environment. These boundaries may need to be reinforced as the professional relationship evolves.

EXAMPLE

SCRIPT:
It is my policy to reinforce with all new clients that massage therapy is not in any way a sexually oriented business. It is unfortunate that the term "massage" has been used as a cover for prostitution. Sexually oriented businesses using that term are illegal and usually involved in human trafficking. Because of this illegal activity confusing the public, it is necessary for me to make it clear that any sexualizing of the massage session, all forms of harassment, and any type of solicitation will result in the immediate end of the session. The client is expected to leave the massage area and will not be rebooked. The incident will be recorded and reported to local law enforcement. This is why a client will not be scheduled for massage sessions unless they provide an accurate name, address, and phone number. Clients seeking therapeutic massage appreciate this strict zero-tolerance policy knowing that it assures them of a safe professional health care environment.

It is important to address societal gender bias related to massage. Put simply, people tend to be more comfortable with middle-aged (40+ years) female therapists. This appears to be based on several factors:

- Body image on the part of female clients (they may be more comfortable having another female see their bodies)
- The discomfort of the client's male partners (e.g., husbands) at having a male massage professional interact with their wives or significant others
- Concern about safe touch from males
- Male's discomfort with being touched by another male
- Social conditioning to predominately accept comfort/touch from females
- Cultural/religious influences

Massage professionals identifying as male must be aware of the possibility of encountering these preconceived ideas. They must present themselves in such a way as to alleviate concerns (with education when possible) and to respect the feelings of the individual client through referral to a female massage professional if necessary. As public awareness of massage grows, this gender difference and biased behavior will hopefully begin to dissipate.

Age is also a concern. Massage therapists under age 25 may experience bias because older clients may see them as lacking experience. In addition, younger therapists may be subjected to peer stress from clients their own age.

Regardless of whether gender or age is the issue, all massage professionals must present themselves as neutral, competent, and ethical. Preemptively addressing these issues can be effective.

EXAMPLE

A male therapist may greet a new client as follows: "Hello, my name is ______. I know it may seem unusual to have a male for a massage therapist because, currently, most massage therapists are women. However, just as is happening in nursing, more males are entering the massage profession. I'm a fully qualified health care professional, and you can be assured of competent care."

A young massage therapist (any gender) might greet a client as follows: "Hello, my name is _____. I know I look young, but I'm fully qualified, and I can assure you that I practice my professional responsibilities with a mature focus."

FEEDBACK

SECTION OBJECTIVES

Chapter objective covered in this section:

5. Obtain and give relevant feedback during the massage.

Using the information presented in this section, the student will be able to perform the following:

- Elicit feedback from the client.
- Provide the client with appropriate feedback.

Feedback is a non-invasive, continual exchange of information between the client and the professional. Feedback is not social conversation. It is common for a client to talk during the massage and appropriate for a massage professional to listen to the client while remaining focused on the massage. **NOTE:** It is inappropriate for the professional to engage in social conversation with clients, particularly about their personal lives (Mentoring Tip).

MENTORING TIP

One of the most common complaints of massage clients is a chatty therapist. It is not necessary to be absolutely silent during the massage; however, conversation initiated by the massage therapist must relate to the client's massage session. As a self-check, ask yourself whether the conversation between you and the client specifically relates to the client's massage goals, assessment procedures, comfort, and/or response to massage methods. It is important to acknowledge the client's experiences and listen attentively for information that can help you better provide a beneficial massage. However, it is inappropriate to ask for additional information and engage the client in telling a story because you want to know what happened or to disclose similar events you have experienced in an attempt to perpetuate the conversation. When you speak, be deliberate. If what you are saying is not directly massage-related, then it is best to stop and be quiet.

Client Feedback

Whether working with a new client or providing regular massage services to an existing client, encouraging feedback from the client is important. Explain the importance of feedback on comfort levels (e.g., warmth, positioning, restroom needs) and the quality of any sensations (i.e., "good pressure," such as is often experienced with some massage methods, and "undesirable pain," which the client may feel if the methods are too aggressive).

The therapist benefits from feedback about the effectiveness or ineffectiveness of the various massage methods. Session-to-session reports of progress, post-massage sensations and experiences, and the duration of effects help the therapist adjust the application of the massage. Feedback from the client about professionalism and the quality of the professional relationship also is valuable.

Some clients may find giving feedback difficult. They may not have enough body awareness to give an accurate report on sensations during the massage or the effectiveness of the methods used. With education from the therapist, this communication can improve.

Clients commonly find what they perceive as negative feedback difficult to communicate, such as what they did not enjoy about the massage, methods that were uncomfortable or ineffective, and inappropriate behavior by the therapist. People generally tend to avoid confrontational situations or don't want to hurt another's feelings. Both of these behaviors interfere with the client's ability to provide effective feedback to the therapist. The massage professional is responsible for developing a professional trusting relationship that allows the client to feel safe in giving positive, constructive feedback.

Clients should be told during pre-massage procedures about the importance of feedback. Explain to the client that all feedback is taken as constructive, that it is not personal, and that it enhances the service of massage therapy. It is important to ease the client's concerns about the therapist's possible reaction to "negative feedback." Gentle, open-ended questions before, during, and after the massage encourage feedback (Box 9.5). Reminder statements also are helpful.

Instilling the idea of "client as a teacher" is one way to encourage feedback from the client. The client teaches the massage professional about themself and guides the therapist in providing the best massage for them both. Knowledge and experience accumulate, adding depth to the knowledge base of the massage professional.

Box 9.5 Questions and Reminder Statements to Use With Clients

- Questions and reminder statements that could be used before the massage:
  - Is there a position in which you are most comfortable?
  - Does the temperature of the room feel comfortable?
  - I am going to place my forearm on the massage table; you apply pressure to it at a level you think you would like during the massage and explain how you want the massage to feel. (This is a great way to understand the client's expectations of pressure.)
  - Remember to tell me if a method is painful or if the pressure is too deep.
  - I would appreciate it if you would indicate when a method seems particularly beneficial or enjoyable.
- Questions and reminder statements that might be used during the massage:
  - I'll use three different pressure levels on your back; please tell me which you prefer.
  - Might there be a more comfortable position for you?
  - Are you comfortable with massage in this area?
  - Remember that it's okay to tell me if you are uncomfortable.
  - Remember to turn over slowly.
- Questions and reminder statements to use after the massage:
  - What methods were most effective for you today?
  - What might I improve on during the next session?
  - Remember to evaluate the aftereffects of the massage, and we'll discuss them at the next session.

Therapist Feedback

Massage therapists also provide feedback to their clients. Therapists must develop effective communication skills (see Chapter 2) to ensure that the feedback they give is not taken personally by the client but rather as valuable information to be used.

EXAMPLE

Examples of feedback the therapist can give the client include the following:

- Do you notice that your breathing is beginning to slow a bit as you relax?
- Are you aware that you have a bruise on the back of your calf?
- The muscle tension in your shoulder appears greater than last week. Can you think of a logical reason?
- You seem to tense up when I apply pressure to this area.

Client Conversation

New clients often talk quite a bit during the first massage, usually the result of nervousness. In future sessions, particularly those for relaxation and stress reduction outcomes, the talking usually diminishes.

EXAMPLE

The following example presents an appropriate dialogue:

Client: "My, it has been a very busy week. My child was in two band competitions. I was only able to attend one. It disturbs me when I miss these events. They placed second and third. I'm proud. Do you remember that last week I told you they might get a scholarship to college for music?"

Therapist: "Yes, I do remember you speaking of that possibility. If I remember correctly, it was to Mott College, right?"

Client: "Yes. You know, it's hard being a single parent. My work interferes with my ability to be with my child as much as I think is important."

Therapist (replying with feedback): "Were you aware that your shoulders became more tense just now?"

Client: "Yes, it felt as if you were applying more pressure all of a sudden. Were you?"

Therapist: "No, I didn't increase the pressure, but your muscles did tense while you were speaking about your lack of time with your child."

Client: "What would you do about this if you were me?"

Therapist: "I appreciate your feelings about your time availability with your child. I hesitate to give you my personal opinions, and this area is outside my professional expertise. However, I can use some methods to relax your shoulders and teach you some methods to keep them relaxed throughout the week."

Here is the same dialogue presented in an inappropriate way:

Client: "My, it has been a busy week. My child was in two band competitions. I was only able to attend one. It disturbs me when I miss these events. They placed second and third. I am proud. Do you remember that last week I told you they might get a scholarship to college for music?"

Therapist: "Yes, I do remember you speaking of that possibility. If I remember correctly, it was to Mott College, right? My child went to Mott College and had difficulty with the registration procedure, and it took forever to work out the snag. Make sure your child doesn't work with Blake Jones, who was very rude." (Inappropriate because the response was personalized to the therapist's experience.)

Client: "Yes, Mott College is correct, but now I wonder if they will be okay. You know, it's hard being a single parent. My work interferes with my ability to be with my child as much as I think is important."

Therapist: "I sure do understand because my sibling is a single parent, and just read a really good book about it. I told them to take a day away once a month, and so should you. By the way, were you aware that your shoulders became more tense just now?" (Inappropriate because the response was personalized and the advice given does not directly relate to massage.)

Client: "Yes, it felt as if you were applying more pressure all of a sudden. Were you?"

Therapist: "No, I didn't increase the pressure, but your muscles did tense while you were speaking about the guilt feelings you have about your lack of time with your child." (Inappropriate because of the named emotion: guilt.)

Client: "What would you do about this if you were me?"

Therapist: "Well, a social group or even a support group might help. I think I would talk with my child and see if the situation really bothers them. But you know teenagers, probably won't tell you anything. It was so hard to get any information from my child when they were that age. I can use some methods to relax your shoulders and teach you some methods to keep them relaxed throughout the week, because you seem to get more upset when you think about these issues, and I'm sure this entire situation is a big reason for this muscle tension." (Inappropriate because the massage therapist is offering personalized advice.) (Proficiency Exercise 9.5).

Clients commonly talk more during the first 15 minutes of massage as they acclimate to the environment and begin to relax. Some talk during the entire massage; this is appropriate and should be accepted. Many people seek massage not only for the therapeutic physical benefit but also, unconsciously, for social interaction. The professional respectfully listens to the client and limits conversation to appropriate feedback and necessary verbal exchanges to indicate an understanding of what the client is saying.

PROFICIENCY EXERCISE 9.5

Compare the two dialogues presented in the example above, and list three differences between them.

Example: In the first dialogue, the client did most of the talking.

Your Turn

1.
2.
3.

PRE-MASSAGE AND POST-MASSAGE PROCEDURES

SECTION OBJECTIVES

Chapter objectives covered in this section:

6. Perform pre-massage procedures to prepare the client and the therapist for the massage session.
7. Perform post-massage procedures to close the massage session and prepare for the next client.

Using the information presented in this section, the student will be able to perform the following:

- Set up an orientation process for a new client.
- Develop a personal method for focusing on the massage session.

Pre-Massage Procedures

Orientation Process

After the intake process, a new client is ready to learn about the massage process. The orientation proceeds in the following manner:

1. Take the client to the massage area.
2. Show the client where to hang or place clothes and explain that the client should remove only the clothing that is necessary and that they feel comfortable removing. These directions must be clear and direct. For example, you could say, "You can remove all your clothes except your lower body

underclothes/garments if that is comfortable for you (you will be covered modestly with a sheet at all times), or you may leave on your bra, shirt, pants, etc. if you would prefer to be more covered during your massage." Then explain what happens if the clothing is not removed, such as reduced use of gliding methods. Most clients, especially new ones, are more comfortable leaving the lower body underclothes/garments on to cover the genital area. This recommendation is also a clearer designation of no-touch zones. If you have any other special requirements about clothing, now is the time to explain them. Avoid ambiguous statements such as "undress to your comfort level." Provide clear step-by-step instructions such as "The typical procedure is for you (the client) to remove outer garments such as shirt, undershirt, pants/skirt, and socks and shoes. You will leave on your lower body underwear. Hang your clothes on the hook behind the door. You may leave on upper body undergarments if you like. Massage application can be adapted for over-clothing work if that is what you desire."

3. Demonstrate the massage table, how it is draped, and how the draping works. Explain the massage positions that will be used (prone, supine, side-lying) and the requested starting position (prone, supine, side-lying).
4. If you are using a massage chair or mat, show the client how to use the chair or mat for proper positioning.
5. Ask about the use of music and offer a few selections.
6. Show the client where the restroom is and how to get there if it is not next to the massage area.
7. Briefly explain any charts you may have on the walls.
8. Ask about a lubricant. Show the client what you have and offer a choice. For example, you could say, "I typically use a massage lotion in a pump bottle for sanitation purposes. Here are the ingredients in the lotion (show the client the ingredients list). I also have a gel-based lubricant if you prefer."
9. Explain that you will leave the room to allow the client privacy to undress and position themselves on the massage table. The exception is if a client is an elder adult or a person in an advanced stage of pregnancy who requests assistance, or any other special situation in which the client requires the therapist's assistance. If you will be staying in the room, explain how you will help the client and maintain modesty. This usually is done by holding up a sheet in front of the client or by using a screen. If direct assistance is necessary for disrobing, present yourself in a professional and matter-of-fact way while providing the help needed.
10. Explain all sanitary precautions.
11. Show the client the sign on the door stating that a massage is in session and explain why the door is not locked.
12. Give a general idea of the massage flow. For example, state that the massage will start on the back and take about 10 minutes, and then the legs and feet will be done for 15 minutes. Explain the effect of any change in a basic pattern; for example, make clear that spending more time on the neck means that less time will be available for the back.
13. Instruct the client to get on the table by sitting between the end of the table and the hinged area (if the table is a portable one) or in the middle of the table (if it is a free-standing table). Next, the client should lean on one side to position themselves side-lying or roll to the supine or prone position. To get off the table, the client reverses the procedure; that is, the client rolls to one side, pushes up to a seated position, and sits for a minute to prevent dizziness. The client then gets off the table. If any chance exists that the client may fall or may need assistance getting on or off the table, stay in the room to help. Demonstrate the procedures, if necessary, but do not use any draping materials on the table. It is unsanitary for anything or anyone to touch the drapes before the client uses them.
14. Ask the client if there are any questions.
15. Explain that you will be washing your hands and forearms and preparing for the massage while the client gets ready.
16. Tell the client how long you will be gone and that you will knock and announce yourself before entering the room.

Any modifications that need to be made because of the location and environment of the massage should be taken into consideration. People can become anxious if they do not know how to act or what they are supposed to do. Do not assume that a client remembers the instructions or knows what is expected. Explain all steps in detail.

Reminding repeat clients of the previously mentioned procedures is important. Just as the information gathered during the intake procedure is updated each week and reassessment continues as the massage sessions progress, clients must be updated about any changes in procedures, new equipment, and so forth.

Focusing on the Client

While waiting for the client to prepare for the massage, the therapist should do the same through some sort of mindfulness activity. This can be done in many ways. Slow, deep breathing combined with stretching slows the mind and focuses the attention on the body. Looking at a nature scene or a painting is another way. Listening to music or performing some sort of repetitive behavior, such as washing your hands under warm water while visualizing the water carrying away all concerns for the next hour, can become a trigger for focus. The goal is to be present in the moment for the client and not focused on lists of things that need to be done. Developing a routine sequence for focus enables the therapist to become calm and client-centered much faster (Proficiency Exercise 9.6). During the focusing moments, the massage professional

PROFICIENCY EXERCISE **9.6**

1. Develop a checklist of everything the client needs to know before preparing for the massage.
2. Role-play with two other students. One student is the first-time client, another is the massage therapist, and the third evaluates the performance. Practice using the checklist and explaining procedures to the client. Switch roles so that each student plays all three parts.
3. Develop three different ways to focus your attention before beginning a massage. Make note of your ideas for future reference.
4. Work with two other students to teach one another ways to focus. Discuss what works and what does not work.

solidifies a clear intention for the massage based on the client's desired outcomes. An important aspect of professional behavior is to be clearly focused on the client and deliver the massage with positive intention toward their desired outcomes.

Post-Massage Procedures

When the massage is finished, the client should be left alone for 5 minutes to rest and get dressed.

Remind the client how to get up from the massage table and exit the room:

1. Roll to one side.
2. Use your arms to push up to a seated position.
3. Sit for a minute before getting up.
4. Leave the sheets on the table.
5. Get dressed and return to the business area.

Helping the Client off the Massage Table

Rarely does a client need help getting off the massage table but may require some assistance if they have balance issues. Reenter the massage area to assist the client. The client should be instructed to

1. Roll to one side.
2. Use your arms to push up to a seated position.
3. Sit for a minute before standing up.
4. While the client is repositioning make sure they are not tangled in the draping material. Support the top sheet loosely around the client's shoulders and hold it so that it does not slip. Place a steadying hand on their shoulder or back.
5. In case of dizziness, stabilize the client for a moment after the client is in the seated position.
6. Still holding the sheet, help the client to a standing position.
7. Shift the position of the sheet so that the client can hold it securely.

In rare instances, the client may need help dressing. Let the client do as much as possible. Be matter-of-fact and deliberate with any assistance.

Closing the Session

Making the Next Appointment and Collecting the Fee

When the client is dressed and ready to leave, make the next appointment or provide a written reminder if it already has been made. If the fee was not collected in advance, the client should pay at this time.

Saying Good-Bye

After the massage is finished, do not linger in conversation. The attitude in the business area is one of courteous completion. Sometimes getting a client to leave can be difficult. After spending time in a comfortable, caring environment, many people want to talk. Breaking this pattern when business picks up can be a problem, so the best course is to establish a short, consistent departure routine in the beginning. People respond well to sameness. A client will get used to leaving and making the break from the massage therapist in a reasonable period more easily if the sequence is always the same.

In the post-pandemic society, common physical social behaviors have been altered. Handshaking and close face-to-face physical contact such as a social hug are examples. In some situations, a quick, friendly hug is appropriate, but only if it is initiated by the client and the therapist is comfortable with the interaction. Then say goodbye while gesturing or looking toward the door. At this point, it is important for the massage therapist to make a move to leave the area, or the client may initiate additional conversation.

EXAMPLE

The client approaches the desk, and the massage therapist or receptionist taking payment provides a receipt and confirms the next appointment. The massage therapist says, "I really enjoyed working with you today. I'm glad you continue to feel that massage is beneficial. It'll be nice to see you again in 2 weeks. I hope the flexibility activities we talked about are helpful. Keep track of any changes, and we'll discuss them next time I see you."

After the Client Has Left

Once the client has gone, the therapist should update all records (see Chapter 4), prepare the room for the next client, and attend to personal hygiene and self-care (Proficiency Exercise 9.7).

POSITIONING AND DRAPING THE CLIENT

SECTION OBJECTIVES

Chapter objective covered in this section:

8. Effectively drape and position a client.

Using the information presented in this section, the student will be able to perform the following:

- Position and drape a client and perform a massage using the four basic positions.
- Drape effectively with two basic styles.

Positioning

Positioning is placing a client into the position that best enhances the benefits of the massage. The four basic massage positions are supine (face up), prone (face down), side-lying, and seated (Fig. 9.13). This section explains the use of body supports and proper draping for these basic positions.

A client may be placed in all four positions during a massage session because remaining in one position longer than 15 minutes may become uncomfortable. The exception

PROFICIENCY EXERCISE 9.7

1. Practice helping people off the massage table. Find 10 different body shapes and sizes to work with and note the difference in leverage needed for each client.
2. Write down your departure routine and practice it with other students. What will you do to end a massage session successfully with a client who does not want to leave? Have one of the students in your practice group role-play this situation so that you can gauge the success of your routine.

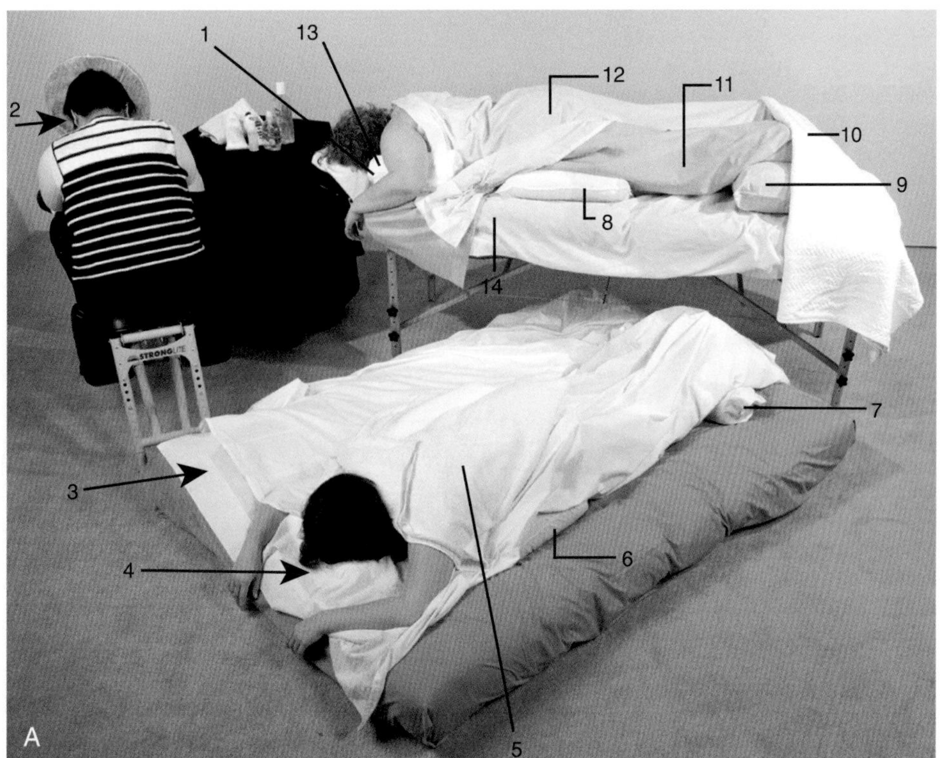

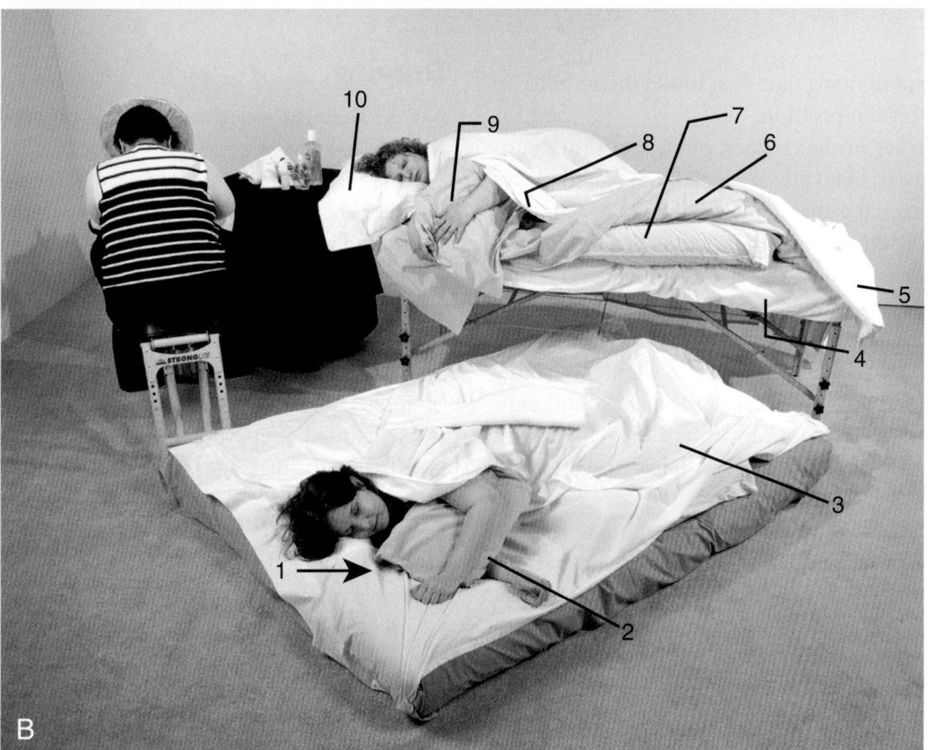

FIG. 9.13 Positioning the client in the seated, prone, side-lying, and supine positions. **A,** Prone. *1,* Rolled towel. *2,* Face cradle cover in seated position. *3,* Bottom sheet. *4,* Rolled towel at forehead. *5,* Top sheet. *6,* Support for abdomen or chest. *7,* Ankle support. *8,* Support for abdomen or chest. *9,* Ankle support. *10,* Blanket. *11,* Bottom sheet. *12,* Top sheet. *13,* Shoulder support and rolled towel to shield breast tissue. *14,* Fitted sheet. **B,** Side-lying. *1,* Towel roll or pillow. *2,* Pillow. *3,* Knee support (under sheet). *4,* Fitted sheet. *5,* Blanket. *6,* Bottom sheet. *7,* Knee/leg bolster. *8,* Top sheet. *9,* Pillow for arm and shoulder. *10,* Pillow.

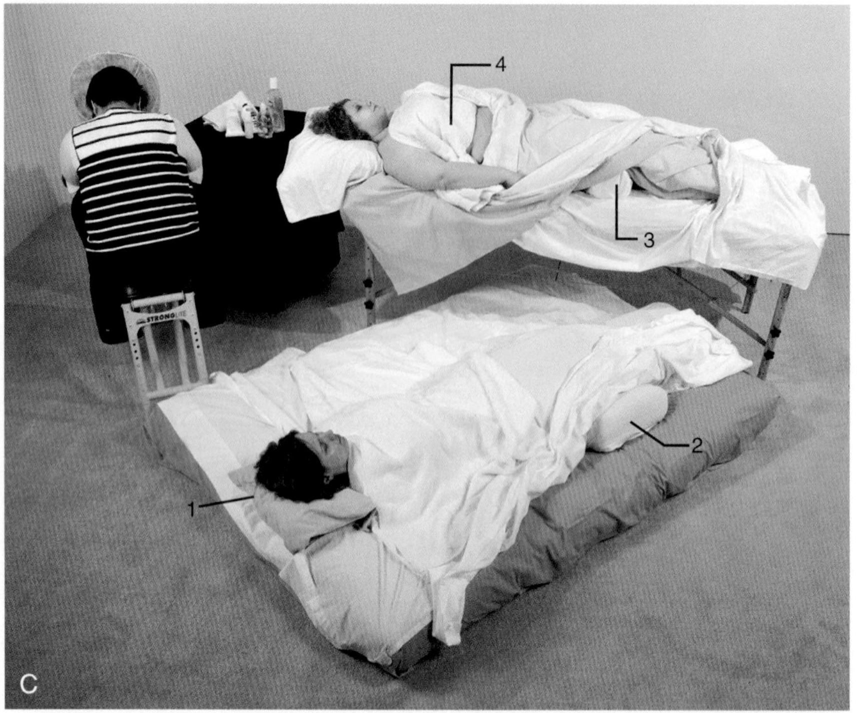

FIG. 9.13, Cont'd **C,** Supine. *1,* Pillow. *2,* Knee support. *3,* Knee support. *4,* Chest towel.

is when a client is experiencing pain that limits their ability to be comfortable in a certain position.

As mentioned earlier in the chapter, pillows or other supports (e.g., folded towels, blankets, or specially designed pieces of foam) are used to make the client comfortable. The supports fill any gaps in contour when the client is positioned and provide soft areas against which the client can lean. Supports generally are used under the knees, ankles, and neck.

After the first trimester, a pregnant person probably will be most comfortable in a side-lying position. If a client has a large abdomen, supports should be used to lift the chest and support the abdomen. This can be done by using a foam form with an area cut out for the abdomen. People with large breasts may need a chest pillow.

Side-lying positions require pillows or supports for the arms and support for the legs. The client will be most stable if this support is rectangular dense foam with dimensions of 30 inches long, 8–12 inches wide, and 5–6 inches deep. Two stacked bed pillows can be used so long as the pillows do not slide and are firm. You can secure the pillows together with a cord or large band.

Clients with lower back pain may be more comfortable with a support such as a pillow or folded large towel under the abdomen when lying prone. This prevents the lumbar spine from moving into extension and helps maintain a more neutral spine position.

Changing the client's position requires shifting the body supports. All supports must be under the sanitary drape or protected with sanitary coverings that are changed after each client. If the supports are located under the sheets, simply fold the bottom sheet over the top to expose the supports and move them.

Draping

Note: Detailed videos of draping proceedures are found on the Evolve site.

Draping has two purposes: to maintain the client's privacy and sense of security and to provide warmth. The drape becomes the boundary between the therapist and the client. It is a way to establish touch as professional. Skillfully undraping an area to be massaged and purposefully redraping the area is much more professional and less invasive than sliding the hands under the draping materials. Respect for the client's personal privacy and boundaries fosters an environment in which the client's welfare is safeguarded. Preparing the massage table with linens and bolsters before the massage is sometimes called "dressing the table."

Principles of Draping

Draping can be done in many ways, although certain primary principles apply:

- All reusable (multiple-use) draping materials must have been freshly laundered with bleach or some other approved solution for each client (see Chapter 7). Disposable (single-use) linens must be fresh for each client and then disposed of properly.
- Only the area being massaged is undraped. Avoid working under the draping material.
- The genital area is never undraped. The breast area is not undraped during routine wellness massage. Specific massage targeting the breast, which is provided under the supervision of a licensed medical professional, may require special draping procedures for the breast area. (Specific recommendations for therapeutic breast massage are provided in Chapter 13).
- Draping methods should keep the client covered in all positions, including the seated position.

- If the client uses a dressing area away from the massage table, a robe, top sheet, or wrap large enough to cover the body will be needed for the walk to the massage area. If a wrap or top sheet is used, it can become the top drape once the client is on the table.

The two basic types of draping are flat draping and contoured draping.

Flat Draping Methods

With flat draping, the top sheet is placed over the client in the same manner that a bed is made, with a bottom sheet and a top sheet. Instruct the client to lie supine, prone, or side-lying between the drapes on the massage table. The entire body is then covered. The top drape (and sometimes the bottom drape) is moved in various ways to cover and uncover the area to be massaged.

Note: To ensure the privacy of men, the massage therapist should avoid smooth, flat draping over the genitals while the client is supine. The penis may become partly erect as a result of parasympathetic activation or a reflexive response to the massage. This response is purely physiological and does not necessarily suggest sexual arousal. Loose draping that does not lie flat against the body provides a visual shield and reduces the client's embarrassment.

Contoured Draping

Contoured draping can be done with two towels or with a sheet and a towel. The drapes are wrapped and shaped around the client. This type of draping is effective for securely covering and shielding the genital and buttock areas. Positioning the drape may feel invasive to the client, but having the client assist in placing the drapes preserves a sense of modesty. For women, a separate chest towel can be used to drape the breast area.

Alternative to Draping

As an alternative to draping, the client can wear a swimsuit or shorts and a loose shirt. The table or mat must have a sanitary covering, such as a bottom drape, and a top drape must be available because the client may become chilled even if partly clothed. When working with a client who is wearing clothing or a swimsuit, the therapist must still observe all the precautions for sanitation, privacy, and respect.

PROFICIENCY EXERCISE 9.8

1. Receive three different professional massages and observe how the massage therapist drapes and uses body supports.
2. With a fellow learner or practice client, practice each draping method shown in Fig. 9.13.

Suggested Draping Procedures

Fig. 9.14 shows the sequence for draping procedures. Practice these procedures, and then combine the methods to fit the client's particular needs.

Notice how the draping material is placed so that the therapist's clothing does not come in contact with the client. This maintains sanitation and appropriate professional distance between the therapist and the client.

These draping procedures are a starting point for the modest, secure use of towels and sheets for proper and appropriate draping. Modification is encouraged. Many other methods are available and can be used instead of or combined with the procedures presented here (Proficiency Exercise 9.8).

Foot in the Door

In some work environments, you will be considered the massage therapy expert. That means you may be asked for your recommendations on setting up and managing the massage environment. Certainly, this is your responsibility if you plan to be self-employed. All the details, added together, create the massage experience you want to provide for your clients. If you can adapt to providing massage on either a table or a mat, you can serve more clients. Seated massage is a great promotional tool and an excellent way to get your foot in the door of many businesses. Once you are established in business, it is an effective marketing tool to set up the massage chair in a public area, such as the lobby or reception area, and provide sample massages. Draping makes clients feel warm, safe, secure, and respected. The way you introduce clients to the massage environment, procedures, and methods helps them acclimate once they put their foot in your door.

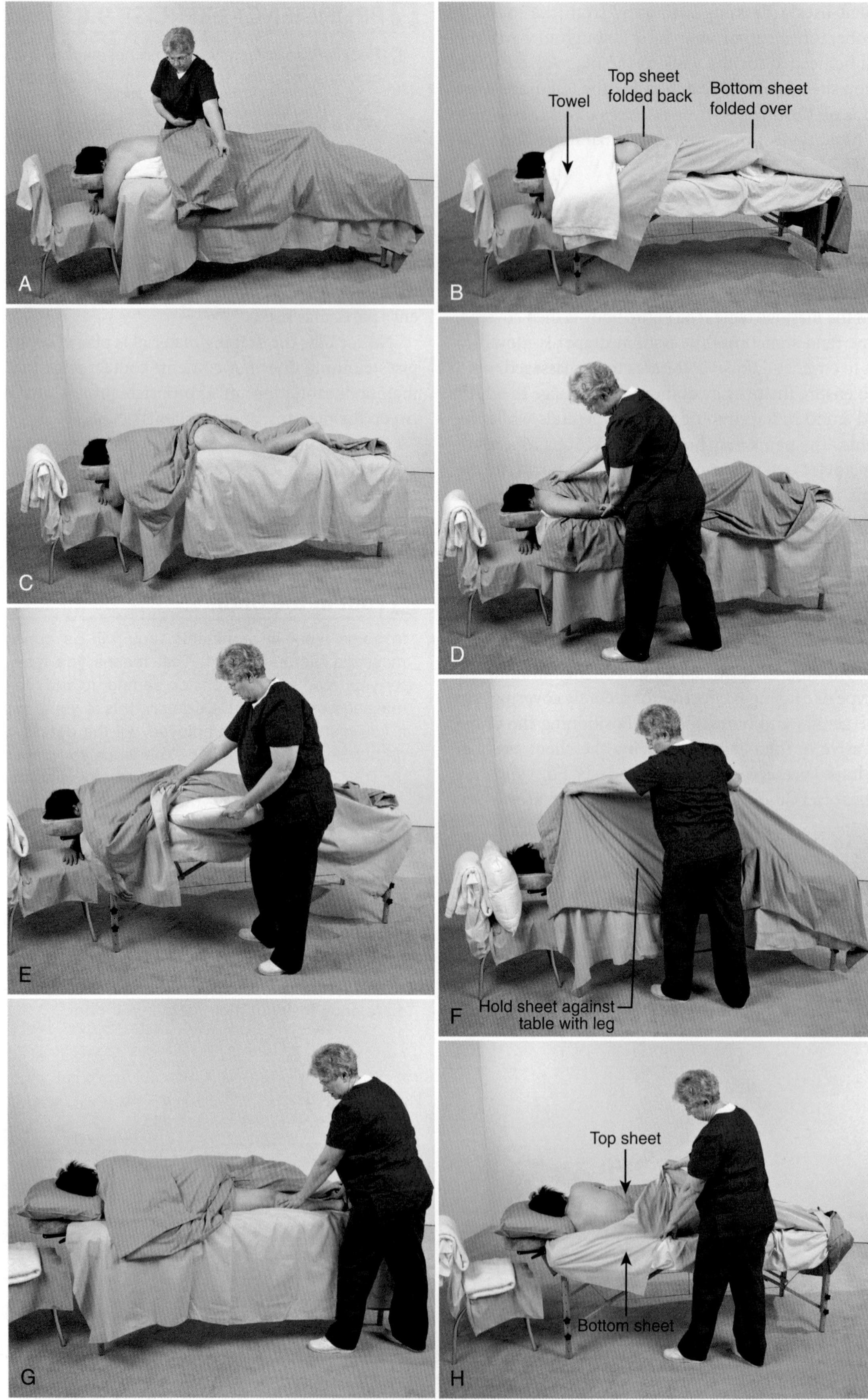

FIG. 9.14 Draping. **A,** Prone: Undraped back with rolled towel to shield breast tissue. **B,** Prone: Draping for the gluteal area. **C,** Prone: Draping for the leg. **D,** Prone: Draping for the arm. **E,** Preparing to place the client in the side-lying position; remove the bolster. **F,** Lift the top sheet in the middle to allow the client to roll. **G,** Side-lying: Draping for the leg. **H,** Side-lying: Draping for the back. Use the bottom sheet to fold over the leg and hips.

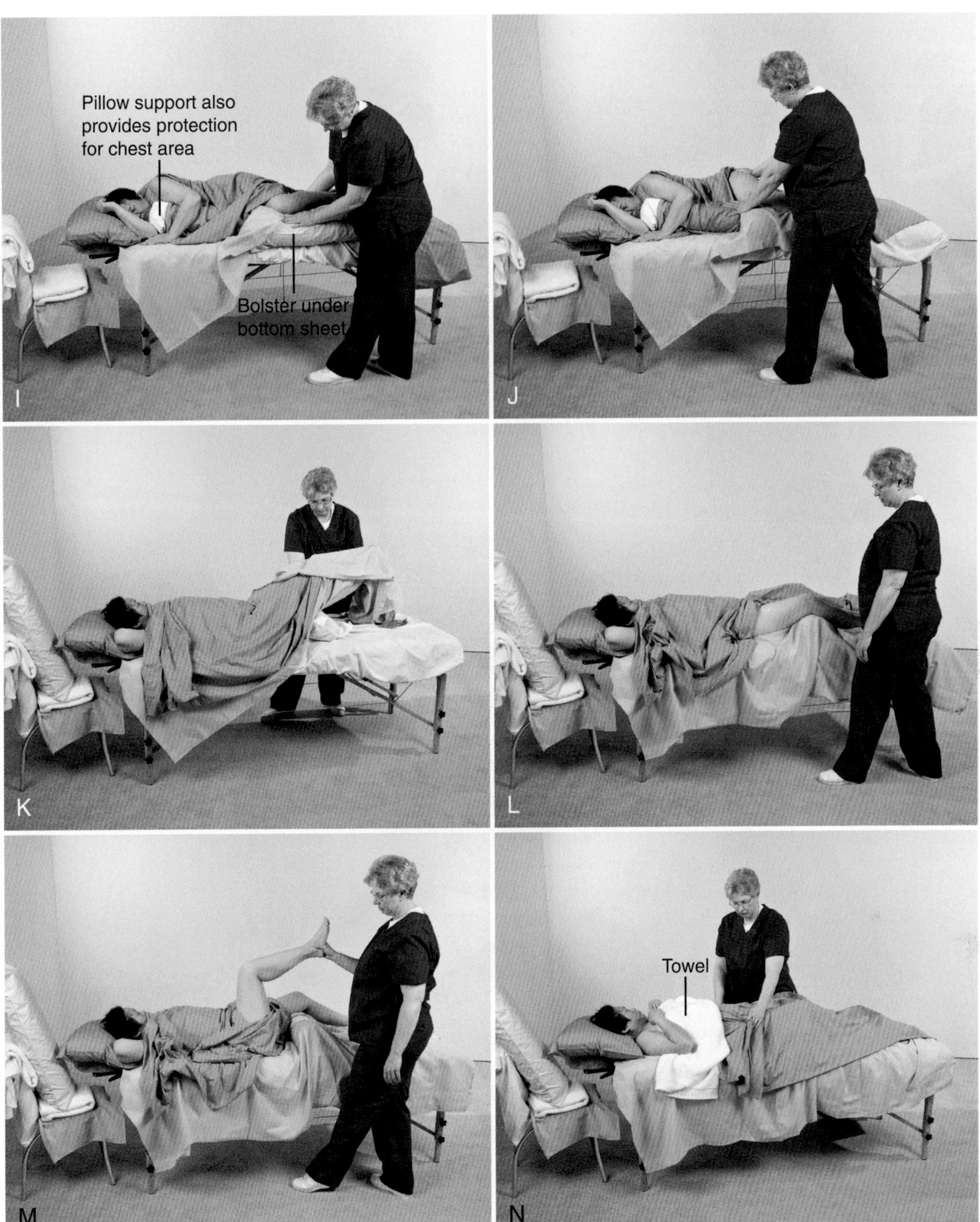

FIG. 9.14, Cont'd I, Side-lying: Draping for the leg. **J,** Move the drape to provide access to the upper thigh and gluteal area. **K,** Supine: Fold the bottom sheet over the top sheet. Lift to position the bolster. **L,** Supine: Draping for the leg. **M,** Contour the drape to prevent exposing the groin area. **N,** Towel over the top sheet: The client holds the towel while the sheet is moved.

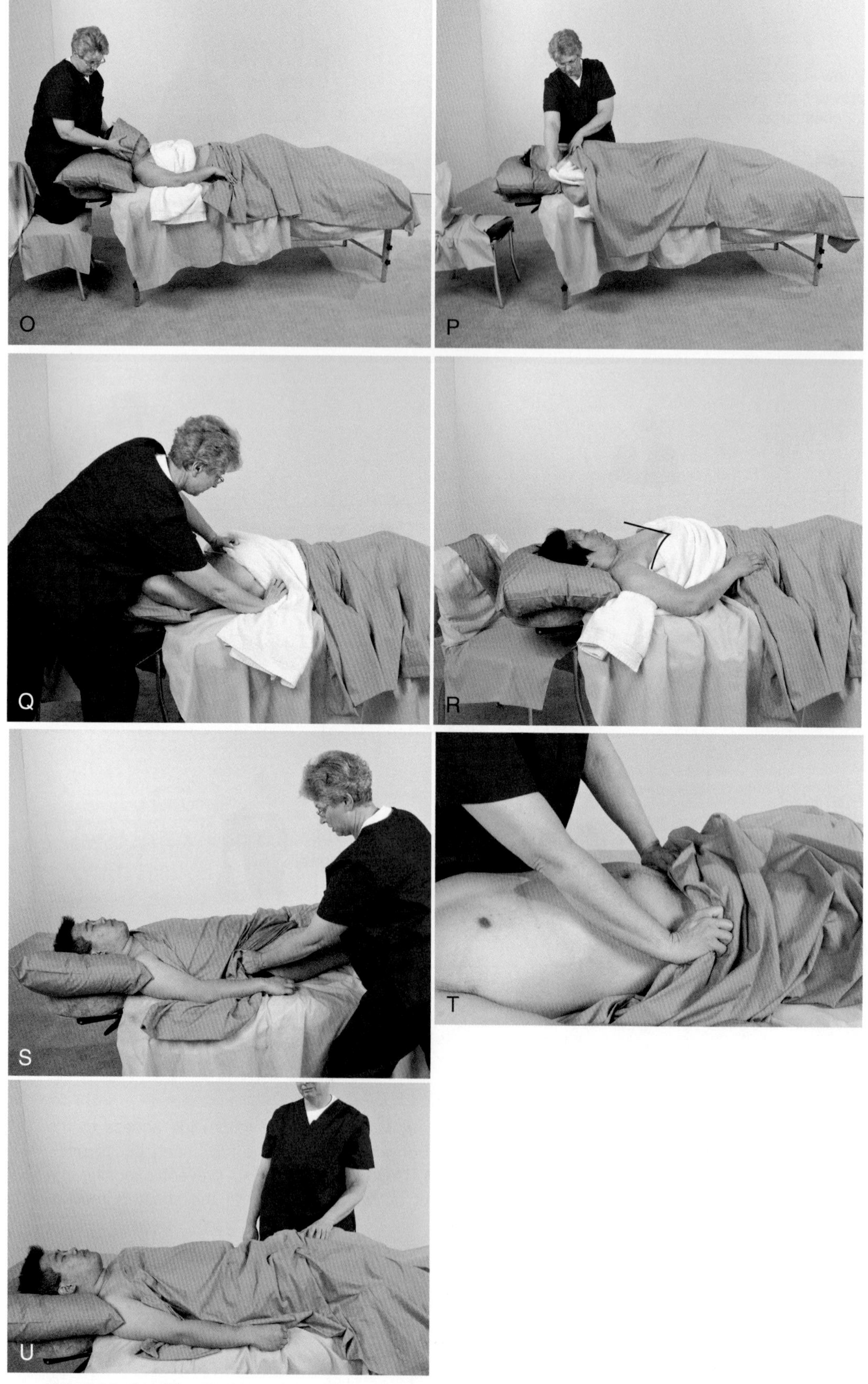

FIG. 9.14, Cont'd **O,** Draping for the abdomen. Optional use of a pillowcase to cover the eyes. **P,** Redrape and remove the towel. Secure the drape. **Q,** Working around the female breast. Use the towel to move the breast tissue. **R,** Contour the drape around the breast. **S,** Working near the groin area. Use a top sheet to slide the drape tightly into the area. For males, this moves the genitals out of the massage area. **T,** Use the drape to slide to the top of the pubic bone. For males, this moves the genitals away from the massage area. **U,** Avoid flat draping on males in the supine position. Bunched sheets disguise the genital area.

SUMMARY

The information discussed in this chapter is just as important as any other aspect of professional therapeutic massage. The different locations and environments for massage set the mood, reflect the personality of the massage therapist, and influence the client's general experience.

Careful consideration of the type of equipment (e.g., massage tables, body supports), supplies (e.g., lubricants, linens), music, and other amenities that you will use in your practice results in a professional yet personalized approach. Taking the time to explain massage procedures to a client, taking a basic history, and learning and understanding the client's expectations and desired outcome for each massage help create an approach that meets the client's needs. Providing safe, respectful touch by using careful, modest draping and positioning is important.

This chapter has described professional skills that create the confidence, respect, and trust important to the successful application of therapeutic massage. Professional massage practice requires attention to these details.

Evolve

Visit the Evolve website: http://evolve.elsevier.com/Fritz/fundamentals/

Evolve content designed for massage therapy licensing exam review and comprehension of content beyond the textbook. Evolve content includes:

- Content Updates
- Science and Pathology Animations
- Body Spectrum Coloring Book
- MBLEx exam review multiple choice questions

FOR EACH CHAPTER FIND:

- Answers and rationales for the end-of-chapter multiple-choice questions
- Electronic Workbook and Answer Key
- Chapter multiple-choice question Quiz
- Quick Content Review in Question Form and Answers
- Technique Videos when applicable
- Learn More on the Web

MULTIPLE-CHOICE QUESTIONS FOR DISCUSSION AND REVIEW

Answers, with rationales, can be found on the Evolve site.

As you discuss and review the following questions, make sure you know the definitions of all of the terms, understand what the question is asking, relate the content area to the broader topic, and be able to explain why the correct answer is correct and the wrong answers are wrong.

1. The most important stability feature of a portable massage table is the ______.
   a. Frame
   b. Cable support
   c. Adjustable legs
   d. Center hinge
2. Regardless of the type of draping material used, it must be ________.
   a. Disposable
   b. Large
   c. Opaque
   d. Cotton
3. To maintain a sanitary practice, draping material must be ______.
   a. Laundered in hot soapy water with a disinfectant such as bleach
   b. Sterilized and heat-pressed
   c. Professionally laundered
   d. Warm, large enough to cover the client, and of different colors
4. To prevent allergic reactions, all lubricants should be ______.
   a. Oil-based
   b. Water-based
   c. Dispensed in a sanitary fashion
   d. Scent-free
5. The purpose of lubricant is ______.
   a. To moisturize the skin
   b. To reduce drag on the skin
   c. To transport nutrients
   d. Counterirritation
6. Which environment is the most difficult for maintaining professional boundaries?
   a. Public events
   b. A private office in a commercial building
   c. On-site at a residence
   d. A home office
7. Which of the following would be the best-sized massage area for a clinic/spa employee?
   a. 9 × 9-foot square
   b. 7 × 11-foot rectangle
   c. 9 × 10-foot rectangle
   d. 8 × 10-foot rectangle
8. What is the most common difference between a private office space and a shared space in a multiuse facility?
   a. A shared reception area
   b. A door that exits to the outside
   c. Access to on-site laundry
   d. A break room
9. What is a common reason clients avoid providing feedback to the massage therapist?
   a. To avoid confrontation about the massage therapist's skill set
   b. Massage therapist does not ask for feedback
   c. Lack of understanding about the massage process
   d. Perception of hurting the massage therapist's feelings
10. Why do directions about disrobing for the massage session need to be clearly described?
   a. So the client does not make a policy mistake
   b. To help the client become comfortable with self-image
   c. So the client knows what to do when the massage therapist leaves the room
   d. So the massage therapist has access to the largest skin area possible
11. A client is particularly concerned with safety and is afraid of falling. Of the following massage equipment, which would make the client most comfortable?

a. A mat
b. A stationary table
c. A portable table
d. A chair

12. A massage professional has just rented office space and fully decorated the area. The massage room has a window and overhead and indirect lighting. The central thermostat is in another area, but the massage room has a fan and an electric heater to adjust the temperature. The small waiting area is bright and comfortable, with many sorts of flowering plants. A private restroom is just off the waiting room. The massage room does not have a closet but does have hooks for the clients' clothing. A closed cabinet holds supplies. The business area is small but has a locked file cabinet and a small desk. What suggestion would you make for improving the massage environment?
a. Add an aromatherapy atomizer.
b. Put a lock on the massage room door.
c. Move the file cabinet into the massage room.
d. Remove the flowering plants.

13. A massage practitioner has been seeing the same client weekly for 3 months. The client often discusses personal issues with the massage practitioner. At the last session, the massage professional provided some reading material to help the client regarding these matters and talked with the client about how the practitioner had dealt with a similar issue. The client has canceled the last two appointments. What is the most logical cause?
a. Feedback about the massage broke down.
b. Conversation with the client overshadowed the massage session.
c. Gender issues are influencing the session.
d. The orientation process needs to be repeated.

14. A massage professional is preparing an orientation process for a new client. The professional has developed the following checklist: Show the client the massage area, where to change and hang clothes, the massage table draping and positioning, how to get on and off the massage table, music choices, and restrooms. Explain charts and equipment, lubricant types, sanitary procedures, and privacy methods. What did the massage professional forget?
a. To explain the general idea of massage flow
b. To provide a centering meditation with the client
c. To provide education on self-help
d. To introduce the client to products for sale

15. A client complains of mild general low back pain. Which of the following is appropriate?
a. Use a side-lying position with knee support.
b. Work with the client prone, using no support under the ankles.
c. Work with the client supine, using support only under the neck.
d. Place the client in a seated position and avoid supports.

16. A client is shy and modest. Which of the following draping methods would be the best choice?
a. Contoured draping with towels
b. Partial body towel draping
c. Full body sheet and towel draping
d. Sheet draping with no towels

17. In which situation would you stay in the massage room and support a client as they get on and off the massage table?
a. The client is in the first trimester of pregnancy.
b. The client is 65 years old with diabetes.
c. The client is an elder adult with high blood pressure.
d. The client is an adolescent with a wrist cast.

18. An adolescent athlete, accompanied by a parent, is coming in for a massage. You have been informed that the client is uncomfortable with disrobing. Which of the following is the most logical alternative?
a. An educational session
b. A draping demonstration
c. Working only with the feet
d. Having the client wear loose shorts and a T-shirt

19. A client regularly lingers after the massage session to talk, causing the massage professional to fall behind schedule. What is the most likely cause of this problem?
a. Policies regarding promptly leaving after the massage were not addressed.
b. The client requires a longer appointment.
c. The client needs more frequent appointments.
d. The massage professional is displaying transference.

20. How do the no-touch zones relate to draping?
a. These zones are where clients leave on clothing, so they have no influence on draping
b. Opaque drapes are only required in these areas.
c. An extra blanket is needed to prevent access to no-touch areas.
d. Draping is especially meticulous in these areas, which are never undraped.

Exercise

Using the foregoing questions as examples. Develop plausible wrong answers and be sure that the correct answer is clearly correct. Then write a rationale for each question. The more questions you write, the better you will understand the material.

CHAPTER 10

Massage Manipulations and Techniques

http://evolve.com/Fritz/fundamentals/

CHAPTER OBJECTIVES

After completing this chapter, the student will be able to perform the following:

1. Evaluate and adapt massage manipulations based on 12 criteria.
2. Use massage manipulations to apply mechanical force to the soft tissue.
3. Incorporate movement of the joints as an aspect of massage application.
4. Incorporate muscle energy techniques into the massage application.
5. Incorporate elongation methods into the massage application when appropriate.
6. Perform a full-body massage using the methods and techniques presented in the chapter.

CHAPTER OUTLINE

KEY TERMS

Active assisted movement
Active joint movement
Active resistive movement
Anatomical barriers
Approximation
Arthrokinematic movements
Comfort barrier
Compression
Concentric isotonic contraction
Depth of pressure
Direction
Direction of ease
Drag
Duration
Eccentric isotonic action
Effleurage
Frequency
Friction
Gliding
Holding
Intention for outcome
Isometric contraction
Isotonic contraction
Joint end-feel
Joint movement
Joint play
Kneading (pétrissage)
Lengthening
Magnitude
Multiple isotonic contractions
Muscle energy techniques
Oscillation
Osteokinematic movements
Pacing
Passive joint movement
Pathological barrier
Percussion (tapotement)
Physiological barriers
Point of application
Positional release technique (PRT)
Postisometric relaxation (PIR)
Pressure
Pulsed muscle energy procedures
Range of motion
Reciprocal inhibition (RI)
Resting position
Rhythm
Rocking
Sequencing
Shaking
Skin rolling
Speed
Strain/counterstrain
Stretching
Target muscle
Technique
Transitioning
Vibration

LEARNER'S NOTE: Most models in this chapter are pictured in sportswear to enhance and clarify the various body positions. A properly groomed massage professional, of course, wears a professional, modest uniform. See Chapter 9 for draping procedures.

TERMINOLOGY USED TO DESCRIBE MASSAGE

The massage profession is in the process of clarifying its terminology, and anatomical terminology also is changing (Degenhardt et al., 2023). Therefore varying terms are presented together in this chapter so that the reader can identify multiple terms for the same concept. At this point, the terms **technique**, *method, soft tissue mobilization*, and *manipulation* can be used interchangeably. A technique is the way a person performs the basic physical movements or skills, procedures, and methods used in any specific field; it is also a method or manner of accomplishing something. A method is a way of doing something or a procedure that is performed. Soft tissue mobilization is a manual therapy treatment where the practitioner manipulates muscles and fascia using a variety of pressures and stretches. Manipulation means to treat or operate with the hands or by mechanical means, especially in a skillful manner. These terms are congruent with the textbook definition of massage: "Massage is a patterned and purposeful soft tissue manipulation accomplished by use of digits, hands, forearms, elbows, knees and/or feet, with or without the use of emollients, liniments, heat and cold, hand-held tools or other external apparatus, for the intent of therapeutic change."

Massage is a form of manual therapy. According to the UK National Guideline Centre (2021), manual therapy is the use of hands or a hands-on technique with therapeutic intent. Treatments are commonly described as manipulation, mobilization, soft tissue techniques, or muscle energy techniques (Beyer et al., 2022). Manual therapy is usually delivered as a therapeutic approach by a range of clinicians including physiotherapists, occupational therapists, osteopaths, chiropractors, and massage therapists.

There are many different approaches that may be used within manual therapy. Additionally there are multiple terms used interchangeably, and these include:

- Soft Tissue Techniques, Mobilization or Manipulation: Methods that use mobilization/manipulation of tissues such as muscles, tendons, or ligaments, without causing movement or change of joint position, for example, massage, muscle energy technique, myofascial/trigger point release.
- Traction: Manual distraction of a body part, for example, the neck.
- Joint Manipulation and Mobilization: Manual techniques specifically applied to joints. Manipulation is application of a high-velocity, low-amplitude force near end of range of joints. This is often, but not always, accompanied with a pop or click. Mobilization is passive movement of joints aimed to reduce pain and/or restore range.
- Mixed-Modality Manual Therapy: A combination of the above techniques.

In this textbook, the methods that specifically apply mechanical force into the tissue using the hands, forearms, legs, or feet are called manipulations. The term *technique* is used for methods that involve joint movements and muscle contractions.

This is a core technical chapter. It contains definitions, descriptions, and directions for the application and use of the most common massage manipulations and techniques. As a student of therapeutic massage, you must learn to problem solve by using clinical reasoning to devise variations of the applications of massage techniques. Because massage routines offer limited benefits, each treatment session must be designed specifically for the individual client (see Chapter 11).

FOCUS ON PROFESSIONALISM

A technician has been taught a set of skills to be applied in a safe and consistent manner. It does not take long to teach and learn a massage routine and follow the determined sequence in a generic or "one size fits all" massage.

However, to be considered a therapist, you must recognize that there is more to massage than being able to give a massage. There is an expectation of benefit from a uniquely adapted massage for each client that is based on the client's goals. To be a massage therapist, you must use assessment procedures to distinguish normal and functional anatomy and physiology from abnormal function. Then you must use critical thinking to determine whether the changes you have found are resourceful and need to be supported or not resourceful and could be altered. There is a relationship between assessment and intervention. We assess all the time during massage. Every touch, every move is assessment. We are asking each part of the client's body, "How ya doing today?" and most of the time the response is "Doing okay," or normal function. Once in a while we find areas that are not "doing okay" and that need either tender loving care or some help changing. Only when change is indicated do we use massage methods as interventions.

The general massage is assessment, and the data must be gathered and interpreted before a plan to support wellness and function can be implemented. A therapist provides massage based on a foundation of anatomy and physiology and the ability to use critical thinking to help make the client feel and function better.

It is important to understand both why and where massage methods and techniques are used and how to organize a process that uses the various therapeutic approaches efficiently. In the application of therapeutic massage, therapists use their fingers, thumbs, hands, forearms, and sometimes their knees, legs, and feet. Although this chapter focuses on methods that use the hands and forearms, applications that use the legs and feet also are presented. Remember to always stay mindful of how best to use your body when applying massage manipulations and techniques (see Chapter 8).

Although the approach presented in this text is comparable to the style currently called "classical" or "Swedish" massage, it is much more expansive and should not be limited by a label or to a specific style or form of massage. The more appropriate term is *therapeutic massage.*

All massage applications introduce mechanical force, which is a push or pull, into the soft tissues, stimulating various physiological responses. The massage methods in this textbook are explained and organized in a manner that consolidates and simplifies application. Proceeding according to the following steps is important:

1. First, learn about each individual method.
2. Then, learn how to perform the method.
3. Next, learn to use the methods in combination to create a general massage.
4. Finally, develop skill in using massage methods to assess the client's body and support efficient function with appropriate intervention while maintaining the integrated experience of a well-designed massage session.

Box 10.1 Massage by the Numbers

Recall the 4 main outcomes for massage:

- Relaxation well-being
- Stress management
- Pain management
- Functional movement support

Also remember the 4 main approaches to care:

- Palliative
- Restorative
- Condition management
- Therapeutic change

Consider the 9 primary methods:

- Static methods/holding
- Compression
- Gliding
- Torsion twisting (kneading)
- Shearing (friction)
- Elongation
- Oscillation
- Percussion
- Movement

Methods are used to generate a mechanical force by doing the following:

- Pushing
- Pulling

Methods are adjusted through use of 12 modifiers:

- Pressure
- Point of application (location and broadness of contact)
- Magnitude (intensity)
- Direction
- Drag
- Speed
- Pacing
- Rhythm
- Sequencing and transitioning
- Frequency
- Duration
- Intention for outcome

Adjusted methods generate appropriate force to load the body tissue to create the following 5 stresses, to which the physiology must adapt:

- Compression stress
- Tension stress
- Shear stress
- Torsion stress
- Bending stress

If the stress acting on the tissue is great enough, it can cause the object to change its shape or to become distorted. This is called *deformation*. One characteristic of the body's soft tissue is that it tends to be *elastic,* meaning it can be forced out of shape when a force is applied, and then return to its original shape when the force is removed. When soft tissue becomes distorted by an applied force, the tissue is strained; this is called the *stress/strain relationship.* Strain is distortion. Tissue strain (distortion) in this case is the deformation of the tissue that results from the applied forces. The strain and distortion (change in shape) of tissue trigger physiological adaptation.

The infinite variations of massage application do not come from using many different manipulations and techniques and various combinations of massage methods; rather, massage is the competent use of fundamental skills uniquely applied with quality of touch and using the 12 modifiers that adapt the massage application (Box 10.1).

QUALITY OF TOUCH

SECTION OBJECTIVES

Chapter objective covered in this section:

1. Evaluate and adapt massage manipulations based on 12 criteria.

Using the information presented in this section, the learner will be able to perform the following:

- Adapt massage methods based on 12 criteria, or modifiers, according to qualities of touch.
- Effectively establish and adjust the physical contact with the client.

Gertrude Beard (2007), a highly respected educator in massage therapy who emphasized massage as an integral part of physical therapy, described the components of massage as follows: "The factors that must be considered as components in the application of massage techniques are the direction of the movement, the amount of pressure, the rate and rhythm of the movements, the medium used, the frequency and duration of the treatment, and the position of the patient and of the physical massage therapist."

The ELAP terminology expanded on Beard's concepts of quality of touch, resulting in 12 ways to modify a massage application.

Variations in Touch: The 12 Modifiers

- Pressure
- Point of application (location and broadness of contact)
- Magnitude (intensity)
- Direction
- Drag
- Speed
- Pacing
- Rhythm
- Sequencing and transitioning
- Frequency
- Duration
- Intention for outcome

Pressure can be light, moderate, heavy/firm/deep, or variable. **Depth of pressure** is extremely important. Most soft tissue areas of the body consist of three to five layers of tissue, including the skin; the superficial fascia; the deep fascia; the superficial, middle, and deep layers of muscle; and the various fascial sheaths and connective tissue structures. Pressure must be delivered through each successive layer, displacing the tissue to reach the deeper layers without causing tissue damage or client discomfort. The heavier the pressure, the broader the base of contact with the surface of the body. More pressure is required to address thick dense tissue compared to thin delicate tissue. Pressure is typically a force that pushes tissues and delivers compressive stress to the tissue (Fig. 10.1). A 1–7 level pressure scale was presented in Chapter 8 related to biomechanics and tissue layers of the body. Tracy Walton, a researcher, writer, award-winning

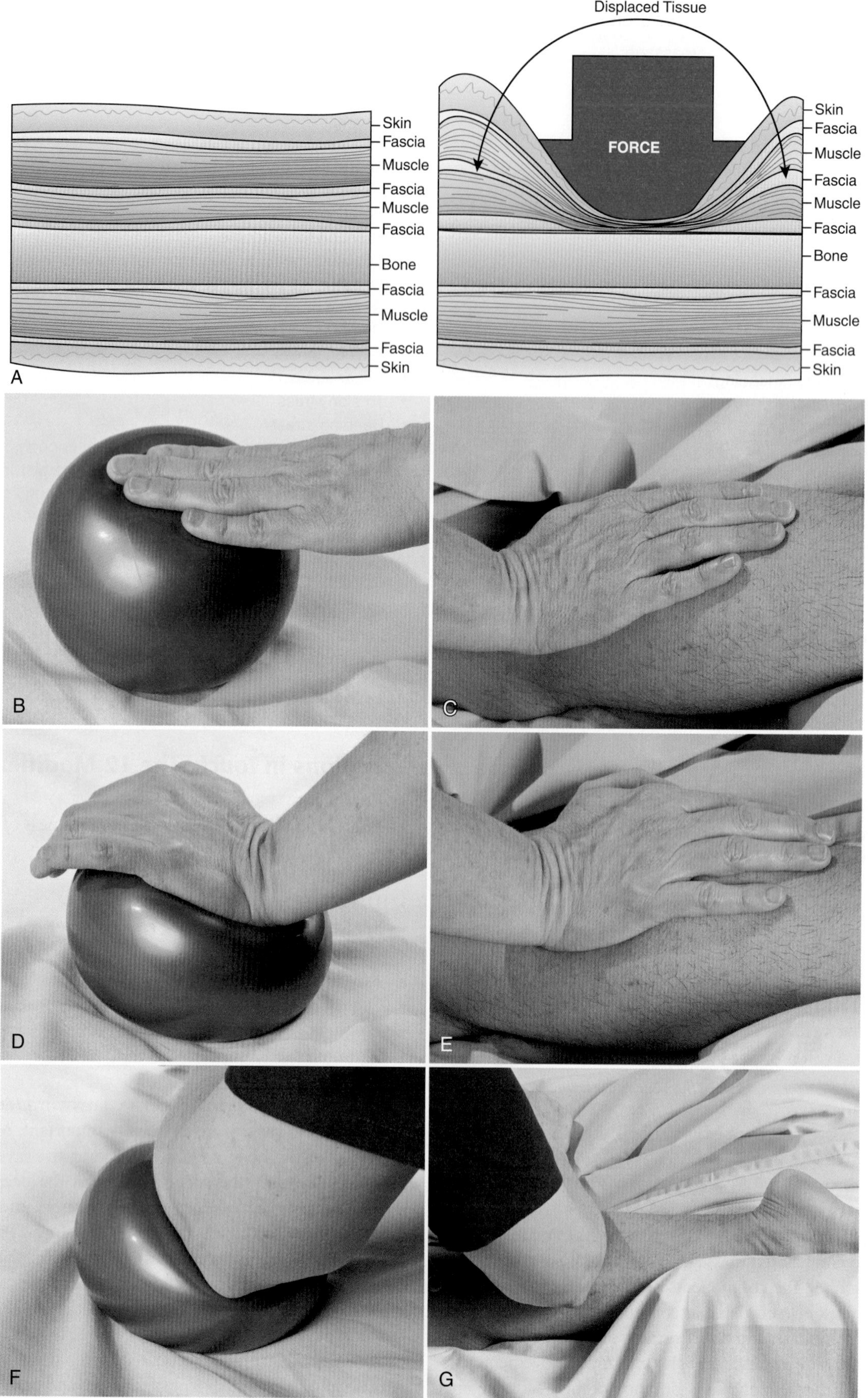

FIG. 10.1 A, Massage applications systematically generate force through each tissue layer. This figure provides a graphic representation of the application of force. It begins with a light, superficial application and progresses with increased pressure to the deepest layer. The varying degrees of pressure are light **(B, C),** medium **(D, E),** and heavy/firm/deep **(F, G).**

educator, and specialist in massage therapy and cancer care developed a 1–5 pressure scale. On the Walton pressure scale a level 1 would be the amount of pressure used to apply lotion to the skin and then increase gradually through levels 2–5. Clients may respond to pressure described as soft/light, medium/moderate, firm/hard, and heavy/deep to evaluate their experience of pressure . These descriptors can be adapted to a 1–10 scale with light being 1–2, medium 3–5, firm 6–8, and heavy 9–10.

Point of application refers to the location and broadness of contact. For example, massage applied to the face must be adapted and applied differently than massage on the thigh. The anatomy is different; the size of the area is different.

Magnitude is the intensity of the application. Magnitude includes elements such as how long and how strong or concentrated a massage application is. For example, a lot of pressure in a small area for a long time is going to feel more intense and therefore have more magnitude than light pressure in the same area for a short time.

Direction means that the massage may proceed from the center of the body outward (centrifugal) or from the extremities inward to the center of the body (centripetal). It can proceed from proximal to distal attachments of the muscle (or vice versa), following the muscle fibers, transverse to the tissue fibers, or in circular motions.

Drag is the amount of pull (stretch) on the tissue (tensile stress) and can result in tissue tautness (pulled or drawn tight; not slack). In this context, the term *drag* refers to the effort required to overcome resistance. Dry skin has a high resistance to slip. Lubricant is used during massage to increase slip and thus reduce drag. When a tensile stress application is used during assessment or to bring about a physiological change during the massage application, the amount of drag on the tissue increases or decreases in relation to the degree of slipperiness of the skin.

Speed of application can be fast, slow, or variable.

Pacing is the process of regulating or changing the timing, intensity, or rate of movement. Pacing is the means by which the massage therapist adapts to match the client's ease of movement, breathing rate, and mood when beginning the session and then leads the client toward indicated outcomes by altering the speed and rhythm of the massage application.

Rhythm refers to the regularity of application. A method that is applied at regular intervals is considered even, or rhythmic. A method that is disjointed, or irregular, is considered uneven, or nonrhythmic.

Sequencing and transitioning is a two-part modifier. *Sequencing* refers both to the sequence of methods (the order in which methods are applied to a particular body area) and to the overall sequence of the massage (the order in which body areas are massaged). *Transitioning* involves smooth, enjoyable movement from one type of method to another type, or the efficient progression of skills, such as the change from undraping a body area to placing the therapist's hands on the client's body.

Frequency is the rate at which the method repeats itself within a given time frame. In general, each method is repeated about three times before the therapist moves or switches to a different approach.

Duration is the length of time the method is applied or the technique remains in one location.

Intention for outcome is the therapist's focus on the client and their goals with a clear concept of outcome; this is related to the four main goals of massage.

Through these modifications, simple massage methods are adapted to produce the client's desired outcomes. Modifiers are used to alter massage application when a contraindication or caution for massage exists. For example, when a person is fatigued, the duration of application often is shortened; if a client has a fragile bone structure, the pressure is altered. As you strive to perfect your practice of massage application, remember that the quality of touch is more important than the method.

Establishing and Adjusting Physical Contact

The massage professional contacts the client's body in a secure, confident way. An unsure touch is difficult to interpret and unsettling to the client. Make sure your hands are warm and then tell the client you are about to touch them. Your touch should be steady, not abrupt.

After touch contact has been made with the client and the massage has begun, the intention of the contact should not be broken. This means that the massage therapist remains focused on the client for the entire session. Maintaining contact does not mean that the therapist never removes their hands from the client. Draping effectively, having the client change position, or applying lubricant to a different area is nearly impossible without removing your hands from the client's body. When removing your hands, simply establish verbal contact by telling the client you will be removing your hands for a moment, shifting the draping, or altering position. Before reestablishing touch, tell the client you will be touching their body and where so that the person does not startle. Once the client becomes familiar with the sequence of the massage, it is not as important to verbally cue the client. Mindfulness facilitates this process of remaining focused on the client.

Positioning the Client

The four types of client positioning are prone, supine, side-lying, and seated. All four are commonly used in combination during a massage. Making sure the client is comfortable is important when positioning and supports can be used for this purpose (see Chapter 9). The client may appreciate a positional shift during the massage to maintain general comfort. Let clients know before the massage begins that they should tell you if they are uncomfortable in any way and that you will adjust. If the client does not say anything during the session, check in about every 15 minutes to make sure they remain comfortable. Avoid keeping the client in the prone position for extended periods, and place a pillow, folded towel, or other support under the client at the abdomen and just above the pubic bone to support a neutral spine position and limit hyperextension of the lumbar spine (this is especially important related to low back disfunction). Side-lying position best supports adaptions for client comfort.

Positioning of the client also supports ergonomics and body mechanics (Chapter 8). Each position has advantages and disadvantages for massage application. Having the client change position during the massage session allows for the most effective access to each body area. Ergonomics recommendations support working at the sides of the table and limiting work from the ends of the table at the head and feet. This issue applies primarily to long gliding application from the head to the low back or from the feet to the upper thigh, which mostly occurs when the client is positioned prone. Massage of the feet when positioned at the end of the table is appropriate especially when the client is side lying, which also supports working from the side of the table. Massage of the upper shoulders, neck, head, and face is typically performed from the head of the table and is ergonomically sound if long gliding is avoided.

TYPES OF MECHANICAL FORCE AND MASSAGE MANIPULATIONS

SECTION OBJECTIVES

Chapter objective covered in this section:

2. Use massage manipulations to apply mechanical force to the soft tissue.

Using the information presented in this section, the learner will be able to perform the following:

- Demonstrate and explain the push or pull of a mechanical force to create the five kinds of load stresses that affect body tissues.
- Perform 9 basic massage manipulations and techniques.
- Combine the 9 basic massage manipulations and techniques adapted appropriately by the 12 modifiers into a basic full-body massage.

Massage must be simple. Many endeavor to introduce improvements into the science of massage but fail to gain adherents to their preventive methods. It would be well to advise these witty inventors of the new submethods to keep their improvements to themselves.

Albert Baumgartner, *Massage in Athletics,* **1947**

Soft Tissue Deformation Methods

The following terminology describes the ways forces are applied during massage based on the Entry Level Analysis Project (also see Chapter 4). These approaches can also be called soft tissue mobilization.

Each of these methods has the potential to load tissue and create a variety of mechanical stresses, such as compression, tension, shear, torsion, and bending stress (Archer et al., 2013).

- Static methods
- Compression methods
- Gliding methods
- Torsion/twisting methods
- Shearing methods
- Elongation methods
- Oscillating methods
- Percussive methods
- Movement methods

Force may be perceived as mechanical or as field forces (e.g., gravity and magnetism). Actions that involve pushing or pulling are examples of mechanical/physical force; these are the types of forces presented in this text. Mechanical forces can act on the body in a variety of ways by loading tissues and thus creating tissue stress. The different types of load stress and the ways they are applied therapeutically are important aspects of massage.

The five kinds of tissue loading that occur from force application are compression, tension, bending, shear, and torsion. Not all tissue is affected the same way by each type of force loading. We will look at each of the five types of tissue stress, the different ways each type can cause tissue injuries, and the ways each type produces important therapeutic benefits when applied by a skilled massage therapist.

Compression

Compressive stress occurs when two structures are pressed together. Compressive stress is an essential component of massage application because the magnitude and depth of pressure is primarily determined when applied mechanical force pushes and presses down into the tissues. This kind of application may be sudden and strong, as with a direct blow (percussion), or it may be slow and gradual, as with gliding. The magnitude and duration used during loading by pushing and pressing are important in determining the outcome of tissue loads and response to compression stress (Fig. 10.2).

Some tissues are resilient to compressive stress, and others are more susceptible. Nerve tissue is an interesting example. Nerve tissue can withstand a moderately strong compressive stress if the force does not last long (e.g., a sudden blow to the back of your elbow that hits your "funny bone"). However, even slight force applied for a long time, as occurs with carpal tunnel syndrome, can cause severe nerve damage. The therapist must take this into account when determining the duration of a massage application that involves compression over

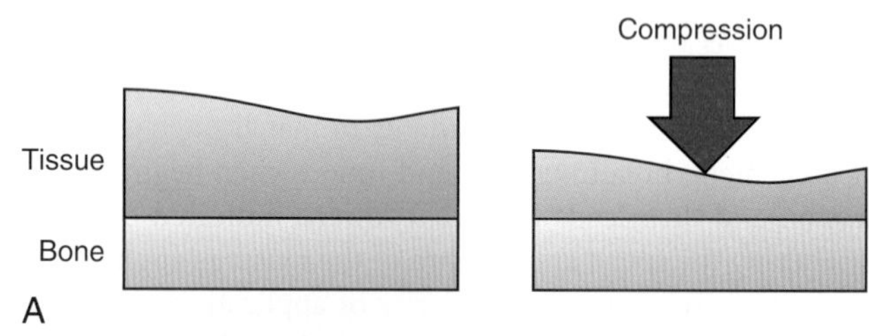

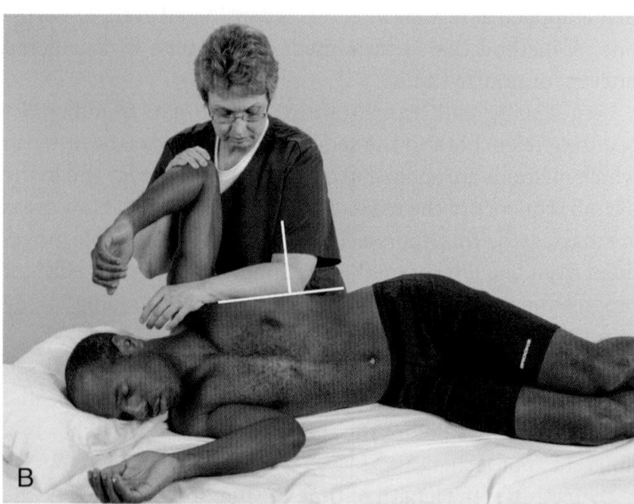

FIG. 10.2 Illustration **(A),** and example **(B),** of compression.

nerves. Compression should not be maintained on a specific area for extended periods during massage. Generally, a compression need not be sustained for longer than 15 to 30 seconds to achieve results.

Ligaments and tendons are sturdy and resistant to strong compressive loads. Muscle tissue, on the other hand, with its extensive vascular structure, is not as resistant to compressive stress. Excess compression can rupture or tear muscle tissue, causing bruising and connective tissue damage. This is a concern when pressure is applied to deeper layers of tissue. To prevent tissue damage, the therapist must distribute the pushing/pressing force application over a broad contact area on the body; the more force used, the broader the base of contact with the tissue.

Compression stress is used therapeutically to affect local circulation, sensory and autonomic nerve stimulation, neurochemicals, and connective tissue pliability.

Tension

Tension stress occurs when two ends of a structure are pulled in opposite directions. Certain tissues, such as bone, are highly resistant to tension stress. An extreme amount of pulling force is required to break or damage a bone by pulling its two ends apart. Soft tissues, on the other hand, are very susceptible to tension stress injuries. In fact, tension stress injuries are the most common soft tissue injuries. Such injuries include muscle strains, ligament sprains, tendinitis, fascial pulling or tearing, and nerve traction injuries (i.e., sudden stretching of nerves, such as occurs in whiplash).

Tension stress during massage occurs with applications that drag, glide, lengthen, and stretch tissue to elongate connective tissues and lengthen short muscles (Fig. 10.3). A tension stress created by pulling is not the same as what someone might describe as muscle tension. This tense sensation in muscle is created by excess muscular contraction, which results from an increase in nerve firing or an increase in tissue density caused by fluid accumulation and connective tissue changes. However, muscle tissues that are long as a result of being pulled apart are affected by tension stress.

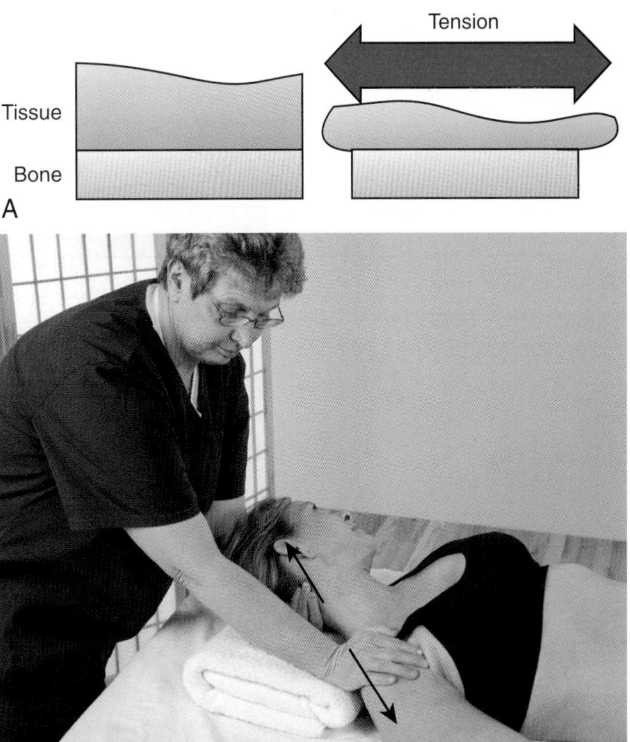

FIG. 10.3 Illustration **(A),** and example **(B),** of tension.

Bending

Bending stress is a combination of compression and tension stress. One side of a structure is exposed to compressive stress as the other side is exposed to tension stress. Bending stress occurs during many massage applications. The force application can be either a push or a pull. Think of pushing into a balloon and causing an indentation. At the same time, the other side of the tissue will expand out and experience tension stress. Bending stress can also be created by pulling. For example, if an elastic band is anchored down and you reach your fingers around and pull one side toward you, where your fingers are holding will be under compressive stress and the other side under tension stress (Fig. 10.4).

Bending stress rarely damages soft tissues; however, it is a common cause of bone fractures. Bending stress is effective in increasing connective tissue pliability and affecting proprioceptors in the tendons and belly of muscles (Fig. 10.5).

Shear

Shear stress is created when the mechanical force application causes tissues to slide against other tissues. Shear stress

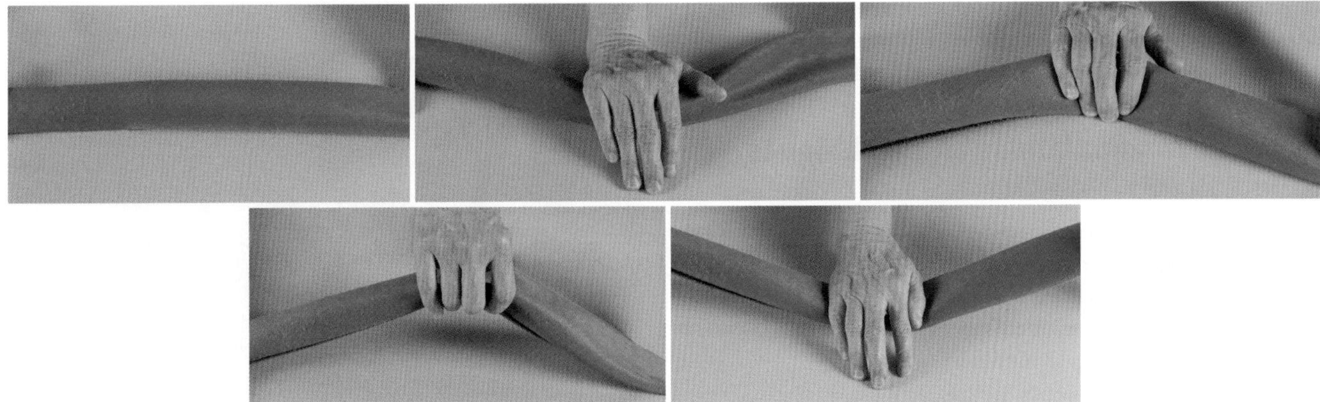

FIG. 10.4 Various applications that illustrate bending stress and how it affects tissues.

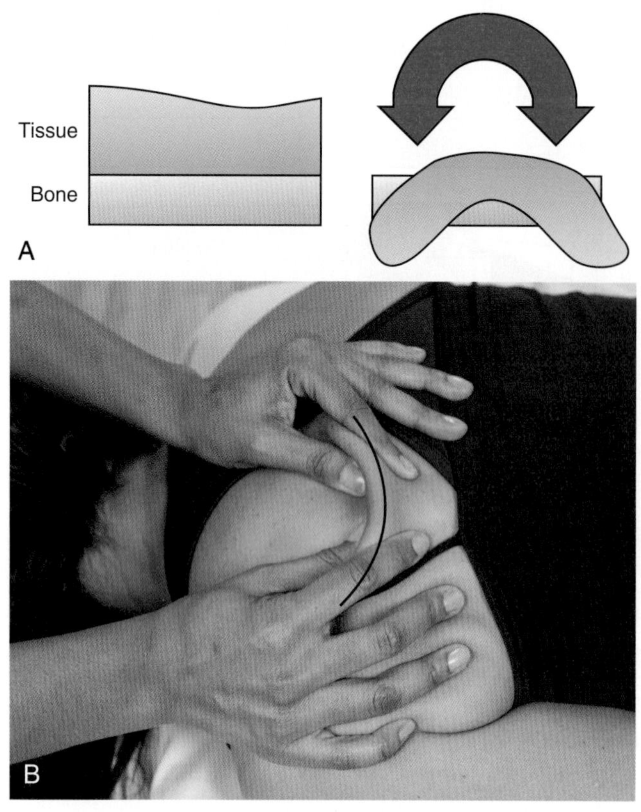

FIG. 10.5 Illustration (A), and example (B), of bending.

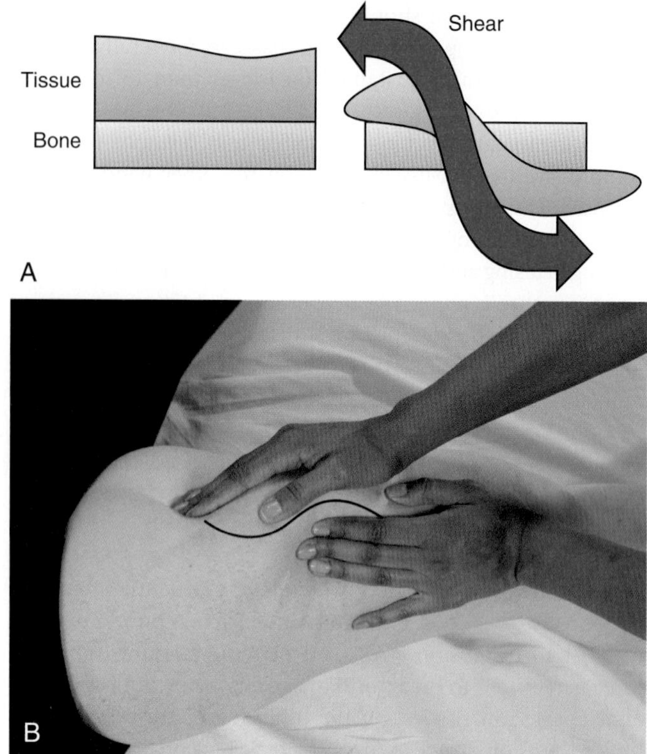

FIG. 10.6 Illustration (A), and example (B), of shear.

is created by a push/pull force application. Significant friction often is created between the structures that slide against each other. The massage method of friction uses shear stress to generate physiological change by increasing connective tissue pliability and creating therapeutic inflammation. However, excess friction may produce an inflammatory irritation that causes many soft tissue problems (Fig. 10.6).

Torsion

Torsion stress is best understood as pushing and pulling forces that load tissues so the tissues twist. Application of torsion stress to a single soft tissue structure is not very common and is rarely the cause of significant tissue injury. Torsion stress applied to a group of structures (e.g., a joint) is much more likely to be the cause of significant injury. For example, when the foot is on the floor and the individual turns the body, the knee as a whole is exposed to significant torsion stress (Fig. 10.7). Massage methods that use kneading introduce torsion stress and target connective tissue changes and fluid movement.

Massage Manipulations and Techniques (Mode of Application)

The methods of massage described in the following sections use push, press, pull, and twist to load tissue, resulting in one or a combination of the five types of mechanical stresses with the intent to achieve a therapeutic benefit (Fig. 10.8). This process is influenced by the 12 modifiers:

- Pressure
- Point of application (location and broadness of contact)
- Magnitude (intensity)
- Direction
- Drag
- Speed
- Pacing

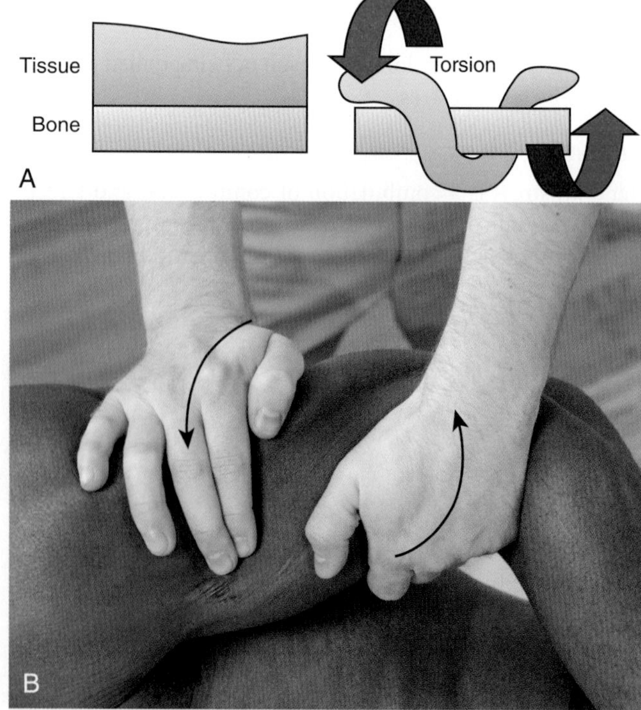

FIG. 10.7 Illustration (A), and example (B), of torsion.

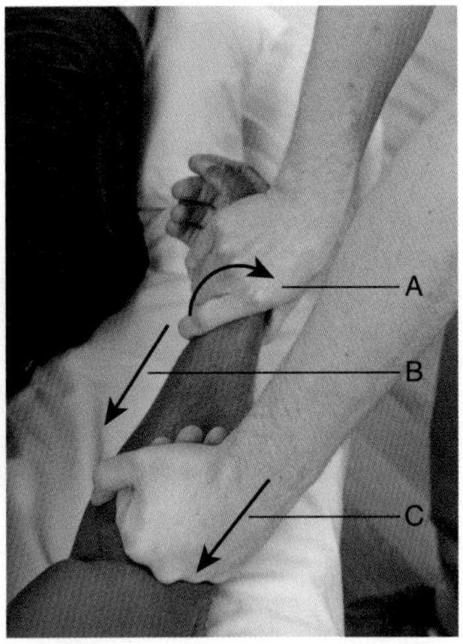

FIG. 10.8 Example of combined loading: Torsion loading **(A),** + Tension loading **(B),** + Compression loading **(C)**.

- Rhythm
- Sequencing and transitioning
- Frequency
- Duration
- Intention for outcome

Appropriate use of mechanical force is necessary. If insufficient magnitude or the wrong type of mechanical load stress is used, the application will not be effective; conversely, excessive or inappropriate use of force can damage tissues.

The variety of massage and bodywork modalities can be clarified by describing what is done during the application—that is, the type of force and load stress created, the mode of application, and the intended result.

EXAMPLE

The modality called *deep tissue massage* is not a unique form of massage, but rather appears to be an adaption of a push or pull (force) with enough magnitude (intensity) to load (change the shape of) the "deeper" (point of application) tissues with an intention of therapeutic adaptation (primarily through the nervous system) by the body.

Those studying this textbook should be able to modify the massage application from surface to deep, fast to slow, and long to short, as appropriate, based on the client's individual needs. The intention and outcome of the massage application appropriately influences nervous system function, mechanotransduction (Box 10.2), tissue layer sliding, musculoskeletal function, and fluid movement. Connective tissue pliability in both acute and chronic conditions influences the viscosity of loose connective tissue within fascia. Called *densification,* this alteration in ground matrix pliability appears to be reversible using massage methods. A much more difficult outcome is modifying fascial fibrosis that occurs from trauma, surgery, diabetes, and aging, all of which alter the fibrous layers of connective tissue.

MENTORING TIP

It is unclear how various massage manipulations and techniques specifically affect the physiology to provide massage benefits. Research has provided clues, and we can make educated guesses, but we do not know the exact mechanisms for how massage helps us feel and do better. For each massage method in this chapter, there is a description, theories of effect, and instruction in how to apply the methods. The theories of effect are biologically plausible and justifiable based on what we do know about massage. The instructions about application are consistent with historical data and reflect current recommendations by experts. It is difficult to reach a consensus because there are so many different opinions and ideas about massage. Learn from this textbook, your instructors, your classmates, and yourself. There is no absolute right or wrong way to give a massage, as long as no harm is done and safety is a priority for both you and the client.

The following massage manipulations, which are considered *modes* (ways or manners in which something is done) of application, are used to apply mechanical force during massage in an appropriate way to achieve the determined outcome for the massage without causing tissue damage. Review Chapter 8 for application recommendations related to ergonomics and body mechanics. Specifically, see Chapter 8 for pressure levels and drag intensity.

Box 10.2 What Is Mechanotransduction?

The term *mechanotransduction* describes physical forces that are converted into intracellular biochemical responses that influence cell behavior and differentiation. Mechanical forces influence the growth and shape of every tissue and organ. Pulling forces generated by cells through the cytoskeleton and external pulling through movement of the body influence many biological processes, such as tissue regeneration, healing, and differentiation. Found in the cytoskeleton of nearly all cells, actin forms dynamic microfilaments that provide structure and sustain forces. A cell's ability to assemble and disassemble actin allows it to rapidly move or change shape in response to the environment. Actin is fundamental to how cells accomplish most of their functions and processes. This research gives us a whole new way of thinking about how a cell can do things, such as rearrange its cytoskeleton in response to external forces.

The external forces affecting a cell could arise from mechanical actions such as blood flow, trauma to the body, or the loading of bones and other tissue as organisms move around. The force intensity needs to be sufficient to change the shape of the target tissue and sustained long enough to be effective. At the same time, the applied force must not damage tissue. So what is intense enough and long enough? There is no simple answer because tissue type and adaptive changes in the tissues will make a difference. Mechanotransduction is just starting to be recognized as a possible mechanism of benefit of massage therapy (Ingber, 2008; Kolahi and Mofrad, 2010).

From Ingber DE: Tensegrity-based mechanosensing from macro to micro, *Prog Biophys Mol Biol* 97:163, 2008; Kolahi KS, Mofrad MRK: Mechanotransduction: a major regulator of homeostasis and development, *WIREs Syst Biol Med* 2:625, 2010 (doi: 10.1002/wsbm.79).

Static Methods: Resting Position (Holding)

Description

The act of placing your hands on another person seems so simple, yet this initial contact must be made with respect and a client-centered focus, with the intention of meeting the client's goals.

Theories of Effect

With the resting position (holding, static), we enter the client's personal boundary space, as defined by sensitivity to changes in air movement and heat picked up by the sensory receptors in the skin. The root hair plexus is one of the most sensitive receptors to the movement of air. Activation of the heat sensors indicates that something is close enough to cause physical harm. Because of these sensors, the fight-or-flight responses of the sympathetic autonomic nervous system often are activated with the initial contact. The instinctive survival and protective mechanisms designed to protect human beings from hand-to-hand combat dictate that the physiological safety zone generally is an arm's length. If another person is at this distance, the sensory mechanisms of sympathetic arousal are less sensitive than if the person is close enough to touch. For this reason, the first approach to touch by the massage professional is very important. Holding provides time for the client to become acclimated to the proximity of another human being. It gives the client time to evaluate, on a subconscious level, whether this touch is safe. This first application of touch sets the stage for the first 15 to 30 minutes of the massage because it takes that long for the sympathetic arousal fight-or-flight response, which causes the release of adrenaline into the blood, to reverse itself. Holding also allows stillness when intermixed with the other movements of massage. The body needs time to process all the sensory information it receives during massage. Stopping the motions and simply resting the hands on the body provides this moment of stillness.

Applying Holding

An open, soft, relaxed, warm, dry hand is best for the application of holding (Fig. 10.9). This signals to the physiological survival mechanism that no weapon is nearby nor is there any intent to strike. A cool, clammy hand suggests sympathetic activation in the therapist. Subconscious survival mechanisms in the client can recognize this and will respond to perceived danger by tensing for protection.

Practice extending an open, relaxed hand. Rub your hands together to warm them, and then towel-dry them to remove any perspiration before touching the client. In most circumstances a slow, steady approach by the therapist, with deliberate hesitation at the arm's length boundary, accompanied by a verbal announcement that you will begin touching, is the best way to prevent excessive sympathetic arousal. Most of the time, the massage therapist seeks to activate the restorative parasympathetic state for the client. Yet even when the massage is designed to stimulate sympathetic activation, the first touch should be slow, gradual, and deliberate, using pressure level 1 or 2 (see Chapter 8).

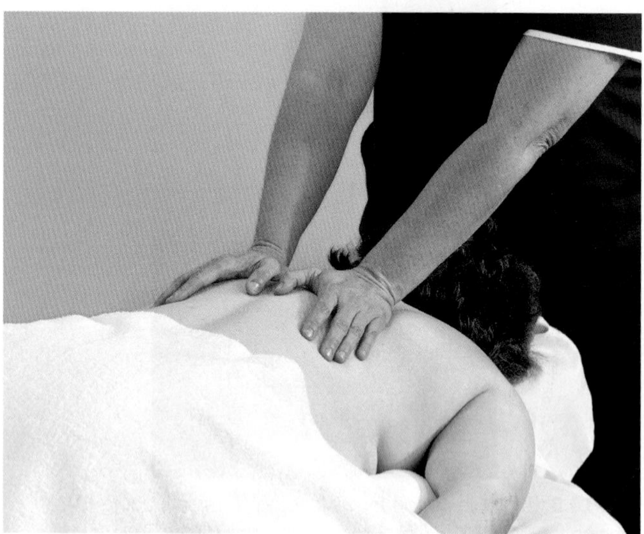

FIG. 10.9 Open, relaxed hands in the holding position.

Apply the holding technique slowly and gradually, in a confident, secure manner. As part of the survival mechanism, the body innately responds to a hesitant touch by withdrawing. Holding is an excellent way to call attention to an area through stimulation of the cutaneous (skin) sensory receptors. Simple, sustained touch over an area of imbalance often is enough stimulation to cause a reflexive response. This technique also adds body heat from the massage therapist's hand to an area of the client's body. In addition, it is an excellent way to reestablish contact with the client if the flow of the massage is interrupted or if physical contact is broken. Mastering the application of the holding technique makes flowing into the other methods easy (Proficiency Exercise 10.1).

PROFICIENCY EXERCISE **10.1**

1. Purposeful touch may be simple, but it is not easy. Diligent practice is required. If you enjoy animals, practice your approach with them. They do not hide responses as people do. Practice using holding to touch a dog, cat, or other animal while the animal is asleep and see if you can do it without waking the animal.
2. Babies and young children also are good for practice. Practice the holding techniques with a baby or child. Acceptance of the touch is indicated if the child does not startle or move away.

Compression

Description

Compression is used to apply pressure by pressing/pushing into tissue. Compression also can modulate the depth of pressure penetration into different tissue layers, from the skin surface sequentially through to the deep layers next to bones. Compression directs pressure downward into the tissues (Fig. 10.10), and varying depths of pressure add bending and compressive stress. Compression can be used alone or in combination with other methods. Even and consistent pressure delivery achieved with compression is the first aspect of

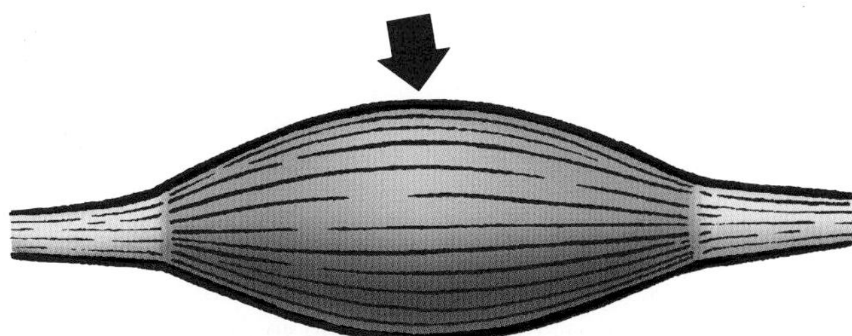

FIG. 10.10 The focus of compression is a vertical, downward pressure.

most other methods. Think compression first, then glide or knead. Compression targets and identifies tissue depth, dictating which layer is affected by gliding or kneading.

Much of the effect of compression results from pressing tissue against the underlying bone. This causes it to spread and be squeezed from two sides, similar to flattening out a tortilla or a ball of clay or pressing pizza dough into a pan. This is called *tissue displacement*. Compression is particularly suited for use when a lubricant is undesirable. This manipulation can be done over the clothing or without lubricant. Compression can replace gliding if gliding methods cannot or should not be used, such as in areas of excessive body hair, areas where a person is ticklish, and areas where the skin is sensitive to lubricant. Compression bypasses the tickle response by activating deep touch receptors. Specific, pinpoint compression is called *direct pressure, ischemic compression*, or *inhibitory pressure*.

Theories of Effect

Pressing tissue against the underlying hard bone spreads the tissue mechanically, enhancing the softening effect on the connective tissue component of the muscle. Tissues are affected by mechanotransduction. Compression applied to the belly of a muscle spreads the spindle cells, causing the muscle to sense that it is stretching. To protect the muscle from overstretching, the spindle cells signal the muscle to contract. The press-lift application stimulates the muscle and nerve tissues. The combination of these two effects makes compression a good method for stimulating muscles and the nervous system. Because of this stimulation, compression is a little less desirable for a relaxation or soothing massage. If the client wants to be alert and energized, a stimulating massage using compression can be done.

A muscle must contract or at least have the nerve "fire" (as occurs in a contraction) before it can relax. This is due to the threshold stimulation pattern of the nerve and its effects on muscle tone. Nerves build up the energy needed to stimulate the nerve impulse. The automatic response of muscle fibers to contraction is a period of relaxation called the *refractory period*. Sometimes the signals are enough to get everything ready to fire, but they are not strong enough to actually cause the contraction of the muscle fibers or discharge of the nerve. If stimulation of the nerves can be increased just enough to prompt the nerve to discharge, the muscle contracts and can reset to a normal resting length. Applying compression to the belly of the muscle, and the resultant effect on the spindle cells, seems to elicit this response. Any sustained, repetitive use of

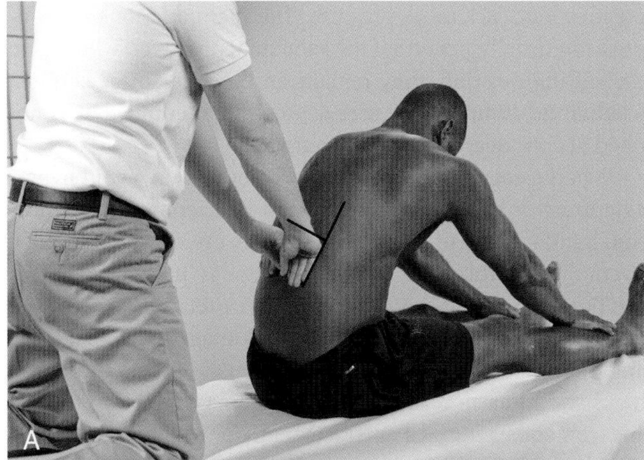

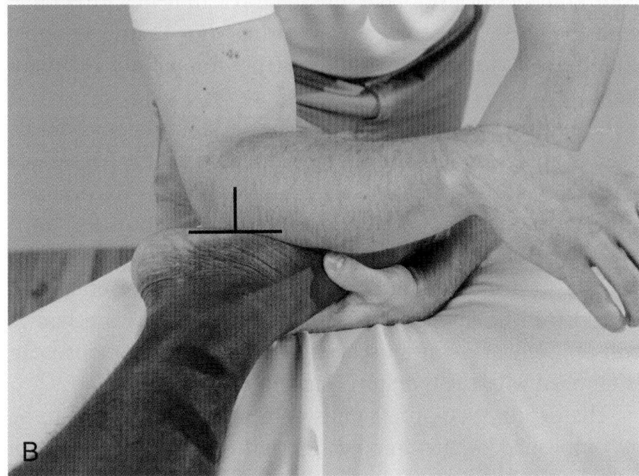

FIG. 10.11 Two examples of compression.

a stimulation method that causes muscle fibers to maintain a contraction or to contract repeatedly eventually fatigues the muscle fibers. Compression used in this manner initiates a relaxation response in muscles.

Compression can be justified as a method for enhancing local circulation. The hypothesis is that the pressure against the capillary beds changes the pressure inside the vessels and encourages fluid exchange. Compression appropriately applied to arteries allows back pressure to build, and release of the compression encourages increased arterial flow.

Applying Compression

Compression can be applied with stabilized fingers, the palm and heel of the hand, the fist, the knuckles, the forearm, and, in some systems, the leg and heel of the foot (Fig. 10.11). Limit using the thumb to apply compression. The joint structure of the thumb is susceptible to injury due to compressive loading. Compression is applied perpendicular to the tissue (i.e., 90 degrees). Usually it is applied against the contours (hills) of the body that are oriented at around 45 degrees. Compression is applied at a 90-degree angle against the tissue and adds depth of pressure to take the slack out of the tissue (the barrier) to produce bind (a sense of resistance). Then the angle changes to push or pull at a 45-degree angle without slipping to produce a drag (tension stress) that affects connective tissue. The superficial application of compression resembles the resting position but uses more pressure. The manipulations of compression usually penetrate the subcutaneous layer, whereas in the resting position, they remain on the skin surface. When used alone compression uses a press-lift method that is applied at a 90-degree angle to the tissue.

When using your palm to apply compression, avoid hyperextending or hyperflexing your wrist by keeping the application hand in front of rather than directly under your shoulder. Even though the compressive pressure is perpendicular to the tissue, the position of the forearm in relation to the wrist is about 120 to 130 degrees. Application against a 45-degree angle of the body plus the 45-degree angle of the therapist's hand and forearm results in the 90-degree contact on the tissue (remember from Chapter 8 to lean uphill). If you are using your knuckles or fist, make sure the forearm is in a direct line with the wrist. Remember, avoid using your thumb to apply compression, because the thumb structures cannot maintain stability.

The tip and the radioulnar side of the elbow should not be used to apply compression, because the ulnar nerve passes just under the skin and damage can result from extensive compression on the nerve. Use the forearm near the elbow for compression. The massage professional's arm and hand must be relaxed, or neck and shoulder tension develops. Leverage and weight transfer applied through appropriate body mechanics will do the work, not muscle strength. Compression also can be applied with the therapist's leg and foot.

The depth of compression is determined by what is to be accomplished, where compression is to be applied, and how broad or specific the contact is with the client's body. Heavy compression presses tissue against the underlying bone. Because of the diagonal pattern of the muscles, the massage therapist should stay perpendicular to the bone, with actual compression somewhere between a 60- and 90-degree angle to the body. Beyond those angles, the stroke may slip and turn into a glide (Proficiency Exercise 10.2).

PROFICIENCY EXERCISE 10.2

1. Inflate a series of balloons with different internal pressures. Fill some with water and others with gelatin and use these to represent the density and pliability of different tissue types. Balloons are great for practicing the angle and pressure of the manipulation. The best angle allows compression into the balloon without it slipping out from under you.
2. Use pieces of foam of various densities and place them over objects of different sizes and shapes. Determine how much pressure it takes to feel each object. Pay attention to the difference between the low-density foam and the high-density foam.
3. Design a complete massage using only compression. Pay close attention to ways in which you can use compression techniques to access the client's body successfully. Adjust depth of pressure, speed, rhythm, frequency, and duration, and observe the different physiological effects. Have a client lie on a mat, and experiment with using your leg and foot to apply compression.

Gliding/Stroking

Description

The historical term for gliding is **effleurage**. The term *effleurage* originates from the French verb meaning "to skim" and "to touch lightly on." A *stroke* is a single uninterrupted movement over the surface. The most superficial applications of **gliding** do this, but the full spectrum is determined by pressure, drag, speed, direction, rhythm, and so forth, making this one of the most versatile massage manipulations. The most common loads introduced by gliding are tension stress, bending stress, and compression stress.

After application of the initial touch, gliding often is next in the sequence, especially if a lubricant is used. As previously described, compression modulates the pressure level of gliding. The long, broad movements of this method are excellent for spreading the lubricant on the skin surface. The ease of application makes this an effective manipulation to use repetitively while gradually increasing the depth of pressure. This is one of the preferred manipulations to warm or prepare the tissue for more specific bodywork. Because of the horizontal nature of the manipulation, the flow pattern of the massage can progress smoothly from one body area to another. Gliding also is a good method to use to evaluate tissue texture, hot and cold areas, or areas that seem "stuck" (i.e., areas of binding). When gliding is performed as an assessment method, the pressure moves the application from surface to deep through distinct tissue layers, and the direction is variable. The frequency of the application relates to how many different directions and how many layers of tissue are being targeted. Typically each area is covered three or four times. When gliding is used as an intervention, the most common adaptation is to focus, shorten, and slow the application.

Theories of Effect

Slow superficial strokes (pressure level 2 or 3) are soothing, whereas fast superficial strokes (pressure level 1 or 2) are stimulating. If heavier pressure (levels 3–5) is applied at a slower rate, the effect is more due to tissue deformation and stimulates parasympathetic dominance (see Chapter 8). Moderate to heavy pressure that exerts sufficient drag on the tissue affects the connective tissue and the proprioceptors in the muscle (i.e., spindle cells and Golgi tendon organs). Heavy pressure produces a distinctive compressive force on the soft tissue, pressing it against the bone. Gliding is the preferred method for abdominal massage and can be justified as a massage method to facilitate local circulation (Proficiency Exercise 10.3).

Gliding applications that use moderate pressure from the fingers and toes toward the heart, are justifiable for stimulation of blood flow, particularly as it affects venous return and lymphatic flow. Light to moderate pressure with short, repetitive gliding that follows the patterns for the lymph vessels is the basis for manual lymphatic drainage (see Chapter 12).

Applying Gliding

The distinguishing characteristic of gliding methods is their horizontal application in relation to the tissue fibers, which generates a tension stress (Fig. 10.12). Gliding also can be applied across fibers to create a bending stress. The intensity and result of the mechanical force application are influenced

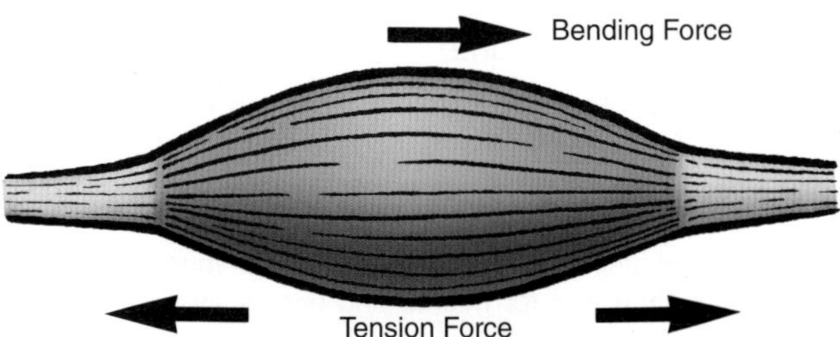

FIG. 10.12 The focus of gliding is horizontal applications.

PROFICIENCY EXERCISE 10.3

Do five massages, and experiment with the following suggestions, plus any other application of gliding you can create.

1. Use finger stroking of the face, first following the direction of the muscle fiber and then moving across the muscle fibers. Have a chart of the facial muscles available.
2. Use the forearm on the back, first following the muscle fiber directions from proximal to distal attachment and then moving across the muscle fiber direction. Keep a muscle chart nearby.
3. Use the palm or the pads of the fingers to lightly stroke the dermatome pattern from the spine to the fingers and toes. This method is sometimes called *nerve stroking.* Have a chart of dermatome distribution available.
4. Use the palm to glide from the toes and fingers toward the heart along the main pathways of the superficial veins. Use an anatomy chart as needed.
5. Grasp the fingers and toes, and "milk" the tissue with gliding.
6. Use the forearm to glide on the quadriceps, hamstrings, and abductors of the thigh. Use a muscle chart to follow the fiber direction. Then glide across the fibers.
7. Grasp the foot at the toes with both hands, and glide to the ankle.
8. Use the knuckles to glide on the bottom of the foot from the toes to the base of the heel.
9. Use the hand to glide in a specific pattern to gently separate the muscles in the hamstring and quadriceps groups.
10. Design an entire massage with only gliding approaches using variations of depth, drag, direction, speed, rhythm, frequency, and duration.

by drag and depth of pressure and the other modifiers. For example, when gliding is used to influence superficial fascia, significant drag occurs on the tissue. During a palliative (relaxation) massage approach, lubricant typically is used to reduce the drag. Compression is used to determine the layer of tissue affected by the tension or bending stress created by the gliding manipulation.

All gliding techniques begin with compression (excluding very light skin applications). Compress down into the target tissue first and then begin the glide. During gliding, light pressure remains on the skin, and moderate pressure extends through the subcutaneous layer to reach muscle tissue; however, it is not so heavy as to compress the tissue against the underlying bony structure.

The *excursion* (i.e., the distance across which the method is applied) is usually a few inches to no more than a foot. Other-

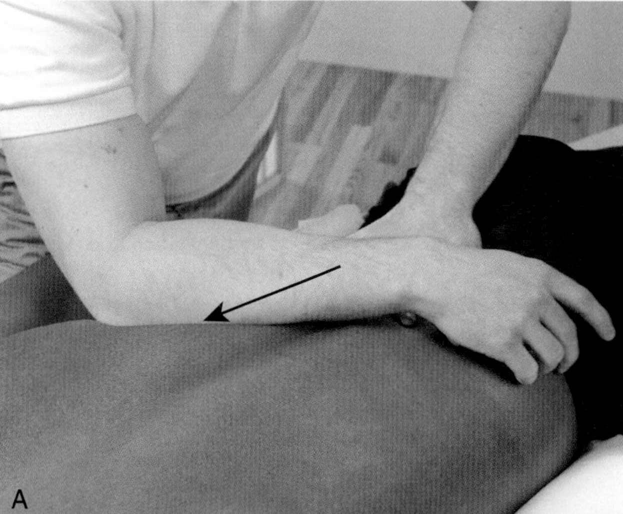

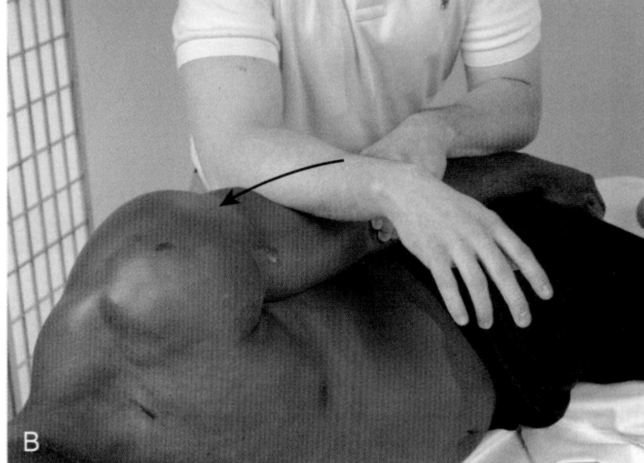

FIG. 10.13 Two examples of gliding.

wise, body mechanics are strained due to excessive reaching. Gliding against a slope (up-hill) allows for the most efficient use of body mechanics during pressure delivery. Increasing pressure adds a compressive force and drag to the application. Light stroking is done with the fingertips or palm. Small body areas, such as the fingers, can be grasped and surrounded (squeezed). The surface contact increases with full hand and forearm application (Fig. 10.13).

Kneading

Description

The historical term for **kneading** is **pétrissage**, which comes from the French verb *petrir,* meaning "to knead." In kneading, the soft tissue is lifted, rolled, twisted, and squeezed (Fig. 10.14).

Just as gliding is focused horizontally on the body, kneading is focused vertically with a lifting action and involves twisting. The main purpose of this manipulation is to lift tissue, applying bend, shear, and torsion stress to challenge the tissue to adapt toward normal function.

Skin/Superficial Fascia Rolling

Skin/superficial fascia rolling (Fig. 10.15) is a variation of the lifting technique. Firm kneading attempts to lift the muscular component away from the bone; skin/superficial fascia rolling,

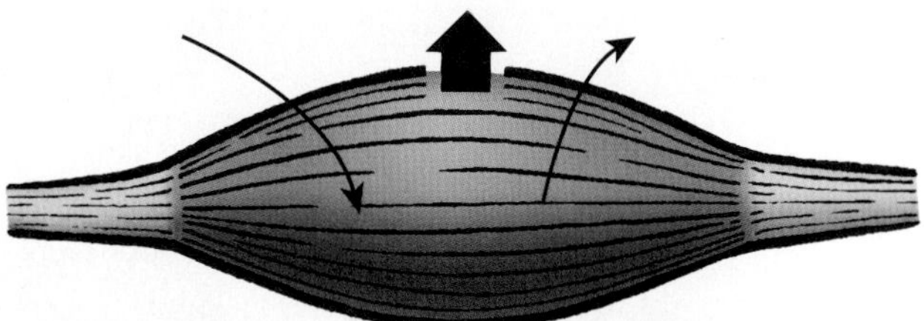

FIG. 10.14 The focus of kneading is vertical lifting and twisting.

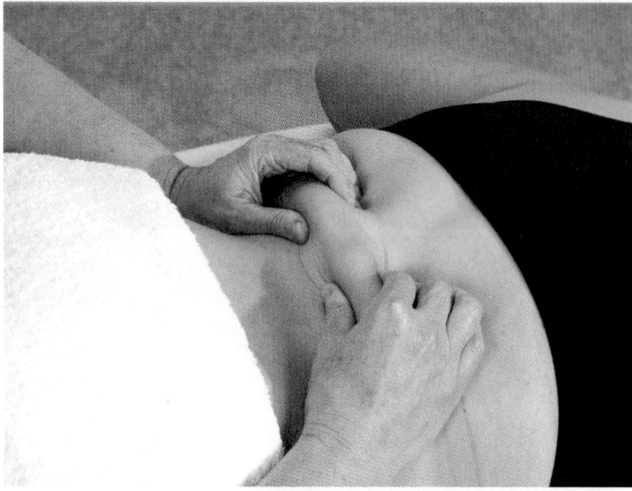

FIG. 10.15 Skin/superficial fascia rolling.

however, only lifts the skin and superficial fascia from the underlying deep fascia and muscle layer. It has a warming and softening effect on the superficial fascia, causing stimulation of the superficial nerves, and is an excellent assessment method. Areas of stiff skin/superficial fascia (bind) often suggest underlying problems. Skin/superficial fascia rolling is one of the few massage methods that can safely be used directly over the spine. Only the superficial tissue is accessed, and the direction of pull on the tissue is up and away from the underlying bones; therefore no risk of injury is posed to the spine, unlike with methods that involve any type of downward pressure.

Theories of Effect

Kneading is good for reducing muscle tone related to the nervous system and tissue stiffness (Box 10.3).

The lifting, rolling, and squeezing action affects the spindle cell proprioceptors in the muscle belly. As the belly of the muscle is squeezed, the spindle cells also are squeezed, and it is thought that muscle tension decreases. The tendons, when lifted, are stretched, which increases tension in both the tendons and the Golgi tendon receptors. The result of this sensory input is thought to be a reflexive relaxation of the muscle to protect it from harm, restoring a more normal resting length of the muscle.

Kneading hypothetically softens the superficial fascia, making it less dense and more pliable. This type of connective tissue, located under the skin, is similar to gelatin. It is made up of a glycol (sugar) protein that binds with water. If gelatin is mixed with water and allowed to sit, it becomes thick and solidifies, resulting in reduced pliability and increased density. If the gelatin is pressed into smaller pieces and stirred, it softens.

Box 10.3 What Is Tone?

Resting muscle tone provides structural and functional support to skeletal muscle and associated myofascial structures (tendons, fascia). Tone involves two elements: the nervous system and stiffness related to connective tissues and fluid. Muscle tone and stiffness are considered fundamental to muscle function and for maintaining energy efficient muscle contractions

Muscle tone is primarily the nervous system regulation of the resting tension in a skeletal muscle. It occurs because there are always a few motor units contracting in a resting muscle. Muscle tone is a physiologically complex network of neural circuits in the brain, spinal cord, and muscle spindle.

Stiffness is related to the viscoelastic component of surrounding connective tissues, osmotic pressure from the fluid in the cells, blood and lymph vessels, and interstitial spaces in the tissue

This is similar to the effect of kneading on connective tissue ground substance with the bend, shear, and tension stress exerted on the tissue. The difference in feeling in the muscles before and after kneading can be compared with the difference between the stiffness of a brand-new pair of shoes or jeans and the comfort of an old pair of jeans or a broken-in pair of shoes.

The fascia also forms a major part of each muscle. Kneading appears to have the mechanical effect of softening and creating space around the muscle fibers, making the tendons more pliable. The tension on the tendon as it is pulled during kneading deforms the connective tissue and mechanically warms it in a manner similar to that by which a piece of metal bent back and forth becomes warm. Instead of metal fibers, collagen fibers are bent and warmed. When something is warm, its molecules are moving faster and are farther apart. The space, which is created at the molecular level, translates into a softer, more pliable structure.

Kneading methods can be justified for supporting local circulation because they squeeze the capillary beds in the tissues and support fluid exchange.

Kneading may incorporate a wringing or twisting component (torsion) after the tissue has been lifted. Changes in magnitude by modulating depth of pressure and drag determine whether the client perceives the manipulation as superficial or deep. By the nature of the manipulation, the pressure and pull peak when the tissue is lifted to its maximum and are less at the beginning and end of the manipulation.

Sometimes the tissue will not lift. This may be a result of excessive edema (swollen tissue), a heavy fat layer, scarring that extends into the deeper body layers, or thickened areas of connective tissue, especially over aponeuroses (flat sheets of superficial connective tissue). If these conditions are present, kneading or skin/superficial fascia rolling applications are uncomfortable for the client. Shifting to gliding and compression may soften the tissue enough that kneading can be used more effectively later in the session.

Excessive body hair may hamper the use of kneading or skin/superficial fascia rolling. The massage therapist must be careful not to pull the client's hair when using these massage manipulations.

Applying Kneading/Skin Rolling

Kneading must be rhythmic to feel correct. The speed of the technique is limited. The speed and frequency of the application are determined by how much tissue can be lifted and how long it takes to roll, twist, and squeeze the tissue through the hand. Lifting the tissue quickly or squeezing it too fast is uncomfortable for the client. After the tissues have been lifted, the full hand is used to squeeze the tissue as it rolls out of the hand while the other hand prepares to lift additional tissue and repeat the process (Fig. 10.16). Because skin and the underlying muscles cannot be lifted without first pressing into them, compression is a component of kneading and is done first. Kneading is a rhythmic combination of pushing and pulling to twist tissue. Although the concept is difficult to explain, it is much like kneading bread dough; the consistency of the material determines how it is to be kneaded.

Think of kneading as three distinct movements—push, pin, pull. Push tissue forward with one hand. Pin the tissue in place with the same hand. Use the other hand to grasp around the tissue and then pull. Proper body mechanics are always necessary. The push hand dictates the therapist's stance and is applied exactly how gliding is. The opposite or "pull" hand creates counterpressure and increases lift. The push/pull together create torsion stress.

Kneading begins with one hand (the push hand) applying palmar compression on a 45-degree angle to move the tissue forward. The opposing hand (the pull hand) is placed so the tissue is pushed toward it. As the tissue bunches into the hand, the fingers, used as a unit with the palm, close over the mound of tissue. The tissue then is lifted, rolled, and squeezed through the hand as the therapist leans backward. Enough lubricant is needed so the tissues naturally pull free from the grasping hands. The massage therapist again rocks forward and the movements are repeated to create a rhythmic pattern of kneading. Except in delicate areas, such as the face, the fingers and thumbs should not be used to lift the tissue because of a tendency to pinch and cause the client discomfort.

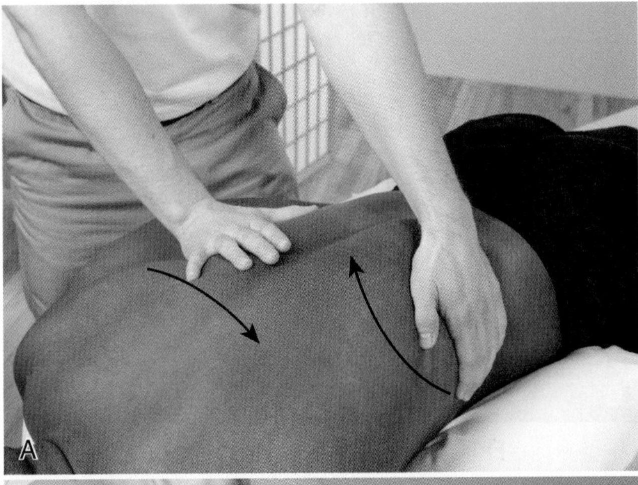

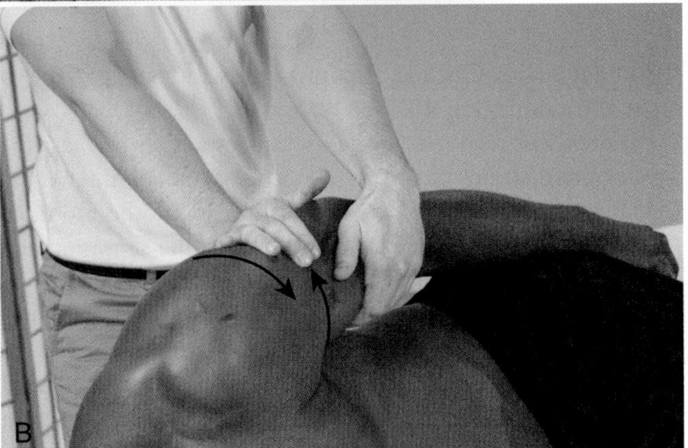

FIG. 10.16 Two examples of kneading.

To get a feel for the method, practice with some clay. The goal is to use as large a part of the palmar surface as possible. Press your fingers together, using them as a single unit pressed against the thenar eminence (the pad at the base of the thumb). Do not use the thumb itself. As pressure is applied, the tissue (or clay) is squeezed. It should feel as though the palm is pushing the tissue *into* the fingers. The fingers simply help gather the tissue. Once the tissue is gathered between palm and fingers, pull until you feel the end of the elastic give; this is where a sense of resistance (bind) is felt. This type of kneading works on both the skin and the tendons. One hand at a time can be used to lift, squeeze, and twist the tissue. Kneading becomes continuous when a hand-over-hand rhythm is established. Two hands also can be used against each other on larger areas, such as the hamstring muscle.

In skin/superficial fascia rolling, the entire hand is used to lift the tissue. The thumbs then are used to feed the skin to the fingers in a rolling motion.

Note: Although kneading is effective for softening and relaxing tissue, it is energy consuming for the massage therapist. As mentioned earlier, the fingers should be used as a unit with the thenar eminence of the thumb. The massage therapist should take care not to use this manipulation excessively. A better practice is to use kneading intermittently with gliding and compression, which do not require such labor-intensive use of the hands. Constant attention must be paid to body mechanics (Proficiency Exercise 10.4).

PROFICIENCY EXERCISE **10.4**

1. Knead a variety of sizes of bread dough. Small pieces can be used to practice the delicate applications used on the face and anterior neck; larger pieces can mimic big muscles, such as the gluteals. Bread dough is good for practice because it is resilient (like body tissue) and will not allow you to knead too fast.
2. Knead a partially inflated balloon. If it slips out of your grasp, you just pinched your "client." Using a balloon develops the use of the palm in place of the fingers.
3. For learning purposes only, practice kneading each area of the body. Because of the repetitive use of the hand for kneading, practice on a different body area each day over a week's time. Make sure to practice different depths of pressure, drag, direction, speed, rhythm, frequency, and duration of application. Notice that some parts of the body are more easily kneaded.

Shear Stress Methods/Friction

Description

Friction causes the force between two surfaces moving across one another. Friction is the mechanism of generating forces causing shear stresses. When a shear stress is applied to an object, the force tries to cut or slice through. The push/pull force application to create shear stress is typically applied transverse to the fiber direction. Friction is best applied to areas of high concentrations of connective tissue, such as the musculotendinous junction. Friction also can be combined with compression, a combination that adds a small stretch component. The movement created by friction does not slide on the skin surface.

One method of friction, formalized by James Cyriax, consists of small, focused movements performed on a local area. This method uses transverse friction massage without the application of lubricant (Cyriax, 1938).

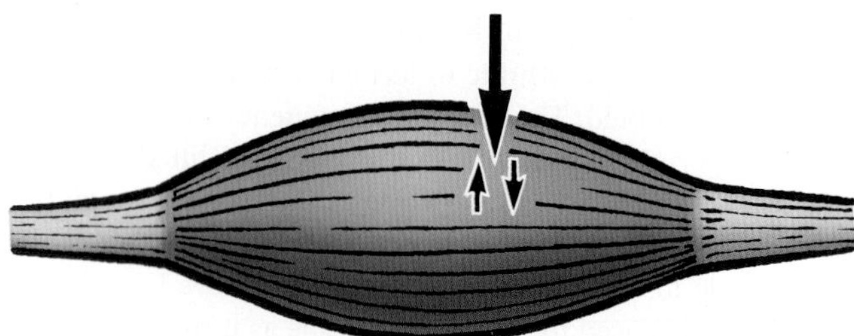

FIG. 10.17 The focus of friction is a vertical, downward pressure applied with a back-and-forth movement to underlying tissues.

Theories of Effect

The Cyriax type of friction initiates therapeutic inflammation. The chemicals released during inflammation result in activation of tissue repair mechanisms, with reorganization of the connective tissue. The Cyriax application also reduces pain through the mechanisms of counterirritation and hyperstimulation analgesia. Microtrauma predisposes the musculotendinous junction to inflammatory problems and connective tissue changes. This type of work can be coupled with other proper rehabilitation techniques to aid injury healing.

Friction manipulation may affect connective tissue, especially over tendons, ligaments, and scars, by creating therapeutic inflammation, which could trigger tissue remodeling. The area being frictioned may be tender to the touch for 48 hours after use of the technique. The sensation should be similar to a mild postexercise soreness but only in the local area. Because the focus of friction is the controlled application of a small inflammatory response, heat and redness are caused by the release of inflammatory chemicals. Also, increased circulation results in a small amount of puffiness. The area should not bruise. This method is not used over an acute injury or fresh scars. Modified use of friction, after the scar has stabilized or the acute phase has passed, may promote a more normal healing process.

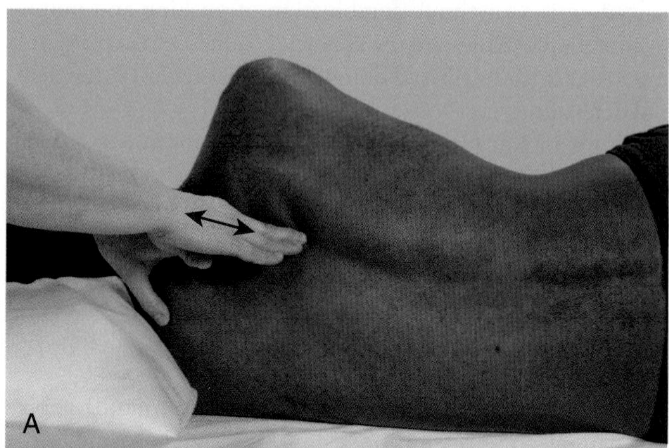

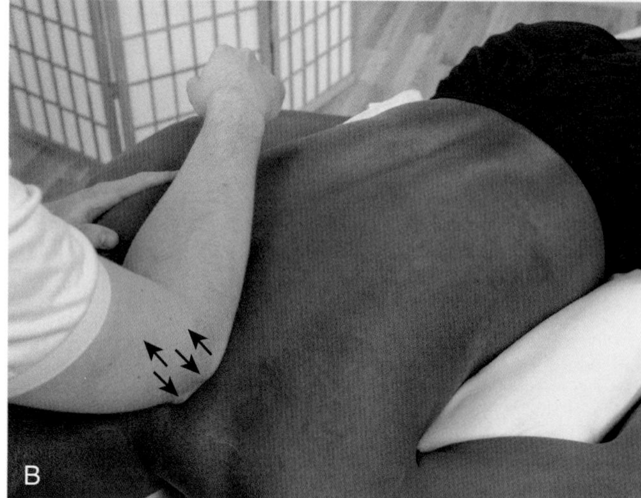

FIG. 10.18 Two examples of friction.

Applying Friction

When friction is used, the main focus is to move tissue under the skin. The skin moves with the fingers (Fig. 10.17). No lubricant is applied because the fingers or other part of the body used to apply friction (e.g., the forearm) must not slide. Friction burns may occur on the client if the fingers are allowed to slide back and forth over the client's skin or if friction is used excessively. Friction of this type generally is performed for 30 seconds to 5 minutes. The area to be frictioned should be placed in a soft or slack position. The movement is produced by beginning with a specific and moderate to heavy compression using the fingers, palm, or flat part of the forearm near the elbow. After the pressure required to contact the tissue has been reached, the upper tissue is moved back and forth over the under tissue. Transverse or cross-fiber friction moves the upper tissue perpendicular to the grain or fiber direction of the under tissue. Circular friction moves the upper tissue in circular motions (Fig. 10.18).

As the tissue responds to the friction, gradually increase the pressure and stretch the area. The feeling may be intense for the client; if it is painful, the application should be modified to a tolerable level so that the client reports the sensation as a "good hurt." It is recommended to use enough pressure so the client feels the specific area is being affected but does not complain of pain. Friction should be continued until the sensation diminishes. Gradually increase the pressure until the client again feels the specific area. Begin friction again and repeat the sequence for up to 5 minutes. (This method is discussed in greater detail in Chapter 12.)

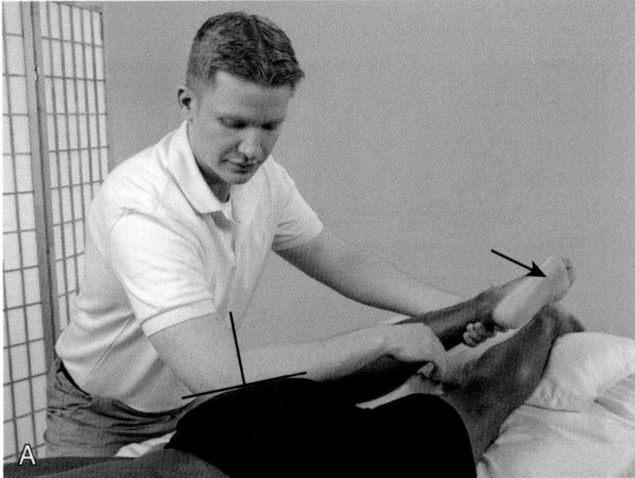

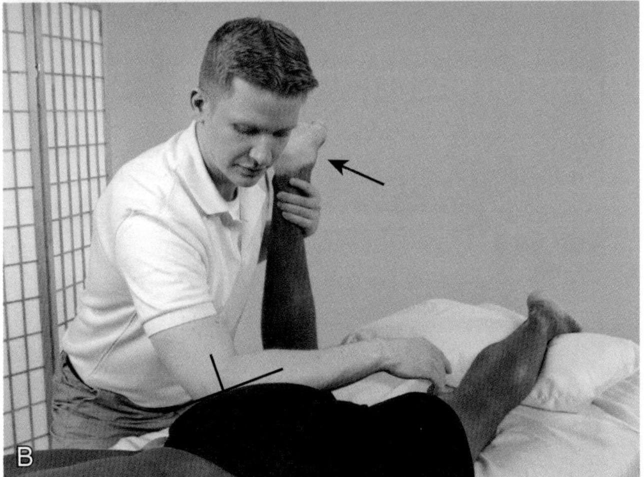

FIG. 10.19 Compression + Movement = Friction.

A modified application of friction that is used to keep high-concentration areas of connective tissue soft and pliable and to support normal tissue layer sliding is appropriate for general massage application. The modified application is essentially the same as transverse friction in that the focus is transverse to the muscle fiber direction and moves the tissue beneath the skin; however, the duration and specificity are reduced. The direction can be transverse or circular, pinpointed or more generalized, but the tissue under the skin is still affected.

Another effective way to produce friction is a combination of compression and passive joint movement, with the bone under the compression used to perform the friction (Fig. 10.19). The process begins with compression as just described, but instead of moving the tissue back and forth or in a circle, the massage therapist moves the client's body under the compression. This automatically adds the slack and elongation positions for the friction methods. The result is the same. This method is much easier for the massage professional to perform and also may be more comfortable for the client. The movement of the joint provides a distraction from the specific application of the pressure and generalizes the sensation. Broad general methods can be used with a higher degree of intensity than a pinpointed specific focus.

Elongation

Description

Elongation methods use mechanical/physical force to pull or push soft tissue in order to lengthen shortened areas. Elongation methods are typically called *stretching* and *traction.* Stretching is a natural and instinctive activity. Stretching is more related to soft tissues. Traction is the application of pulling force to stretch soft tissue and increase space in the joint (Box 10.4). Elongation methods do not have to be aggressive to be effective. Research has indicated that a slight pull on the tissue is optimal for benefit.

Longitudinal stretching pulls or pushes tissue in the direction of the fiber configuration. *Cross-directional stretching* pulls or pushes the tissue against the fiber direction (Figs. 10.20 and 10.21).

The two approaches accomplish the same thing, but longitudinal stretching is often done in conjunction with movement at the joint and gliding manipulations applied with drag in the direction of the force. If longitudinal stretching is not advisable, is ineffective in situations of joint hypermobility, or if the area cannot be effectively stretched longitudinally, cross-directional stretching is a better choice. Cross-directional stretching focuses on the tissue itself and does not depend on joint movement. Tissues tolerate the stretching sensation better when muscle energy methods are used before the actual elongation. These methods are described in the massage techniques section of this chapter.

Theories of Effect

Stretching is the deliberate lengthening of muscle/fascia units by changing the consistency and configuration of the connective tissue matrix to increase flexibility and joint range of motion. There also seems to be an increase in stiffness induced by stretch and subsequent rest. Tissues show decreases in fluid content immediately after stretching, allowing for more mobility in the tissue. When sufficient resting time is allowed, matrix hydration returns to higher than initial levels, increasing stiffness. These results seem contrary to the increase in flexibility that remains over a period of time after stretching. It is plausible that tissue sliding may have been restored when the hydration of the tissue was altered. Loose connective tissue responds to light tissue stretch. Hyaluronan, which lubricates between tissues layers so sliding occurs, may be distributed more effectively. There is likely influence on mechanoreceptors, neurological signaling, interstitial osmotic pressure, and blood flow modulation.

Studies about the benefits of stretching are mixed. Some show that stretching helps flexibility but that the stretching must be done daily over a period of weeks and regularly maintained. Random or occasional stretching does not support functional flexibility. Thus, because massage is not used daily, incorporating stretching into massage sessions may be of little value. Other studies show that stretching before or after exercise has little if any benefit and does not reduce muscle soreness after exercise. Regardless, the intent of elongation methods such as stretching is to make tissues longer. Do not aggressively stretch tissues around a joint. Proceed gently over multiple sessions to increase tissue length. Apply stretching only to identified areas of hypomobility. Overstretching creates hypermobility. Hypermobility

Box 10.4 How Much Elongation?

Paul Standley, PhD (University of Arizona, College of Medicine), researched the effects of the magnitude of elongation on bioengineered tendons. The tendons were "wounded," and the healing process was observed in relation to different versions of applied tension stress, using 3%, 6%, 9%, or 12% of stretch/elongation of the tissues, for 1, 2, 3, 4, or 5 minutes. The optimal result in terms of wound closure was achieved with 6% of load for 3 minutes.

How does this information translate into effective application of elongation methods during massage? According to the study, brief (1 minute), light (3%) tension stress had no effect on wound healing, and strong (12%), long (5 minutes) tension stress aggravated and interfered with wound healing. During general massage, we are not dealing with wound healing specifically. However, we can identify from this study a therapeutic range of benefit: 6% elongation of the tissue for 3 minutes. Any more applied strain to the tissue for a longer period seems to interfere with tissue health.

Elongation of 6% is not much. Let's explore how to find about 6% stretch. Refer to the figures as you perform the following activity.

- Elongation begins at tissue bind. Find a rubber band (or a balloon) and measure the length before stretching it; that measurement would be the start point (Figure 1).
- Let's say the rubber band is 2 inches long at the first point of bind. When it is stretched out as far as it will go, it elongates to 6 inches (Figure 2); that would be considered 100% stretch.
- If you reduce the pull so that the rubber band is stretched only 3 inches from the start point, that would be 50% elongation (Figure 3).
- Reduce the pull again so that the increase in length is only 2 inches; that would be 25% elongation (Figure 4).
- Reduce the pull again so that the rubber band is ¾ inch longer than the start point; that is about 12% elongation, which is still too much (Figure 5).
- Reduce the pull so that the rubber band lengthens only about ¼ to ½ inch from the original point of bind at 2 inches; that is approximately 6% elongation (Figure 6).

When you elongate tissue, you need to find where it first binds and then just move into the motion barrier. You can practice feeling the sensation of bind or motion barrier with two pieces of paper towel joined together at the perforations.

- As you begin to separate the two paper towels and the perforations become taut, that is bind/barrier (Figure 7).
- If you continue to pull apart, you will see the spaces between the perforations. This amount of elongation is about 6% (Figure 8).

Now compare Figures 1 and 7. This is the start point of tissue bind for elongation. Figures 6 and 8 represent the amount of pull on the tissues needed for benefit. Figures 2 is too much force application and can result in tissue damage. Even Figures 3, 4, and 5 add too much pulling force into the tissue. Effective elongation occurs when tissue is moved into bind or the first subtle natural stop point, and then just a little more force is applied into the tissue.

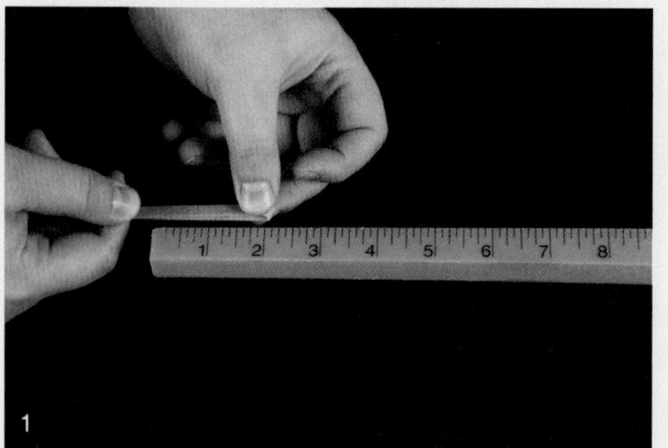

1

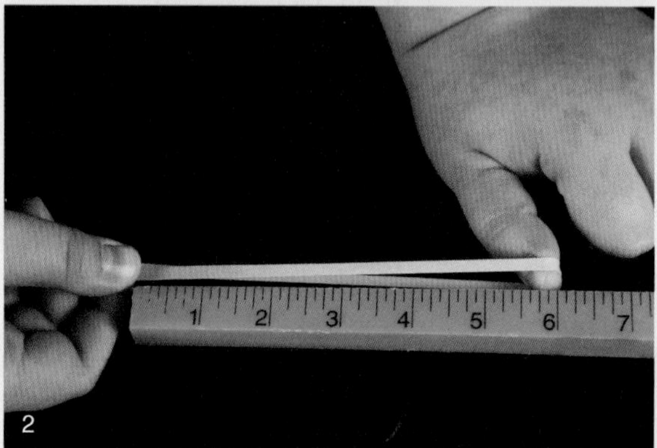

2

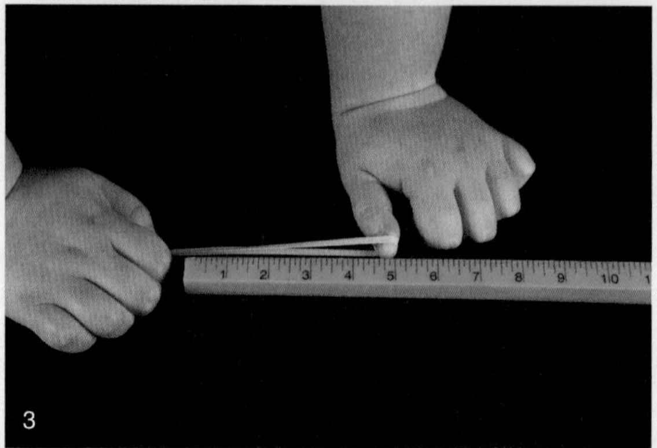

3

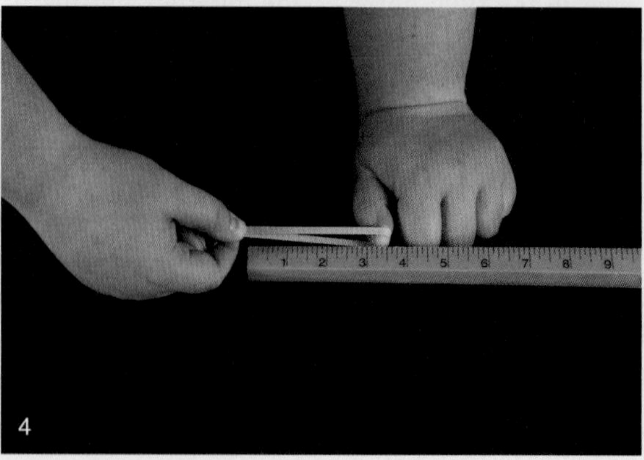

4

Box 10.4 How Much Elongation?—cont'd

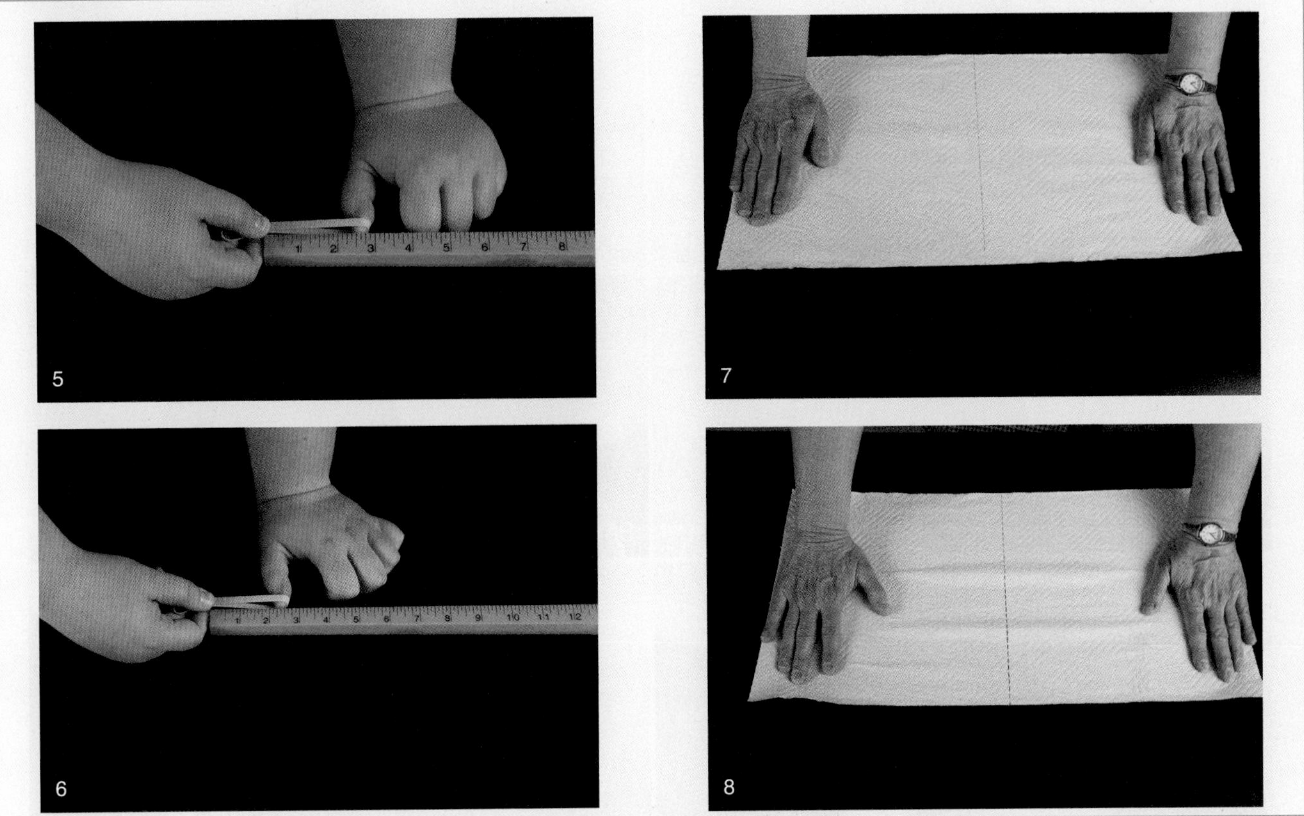

From Standley PR, Cao TV, Hicks MR, et al: Dosed myofascial release in three-dimensional bioengineered tendons: effects on human fibroblast hyperplasia, hypertrophy, and cytokine secretion, *J Manipulative Physiol Ther* 36:513, 2013.

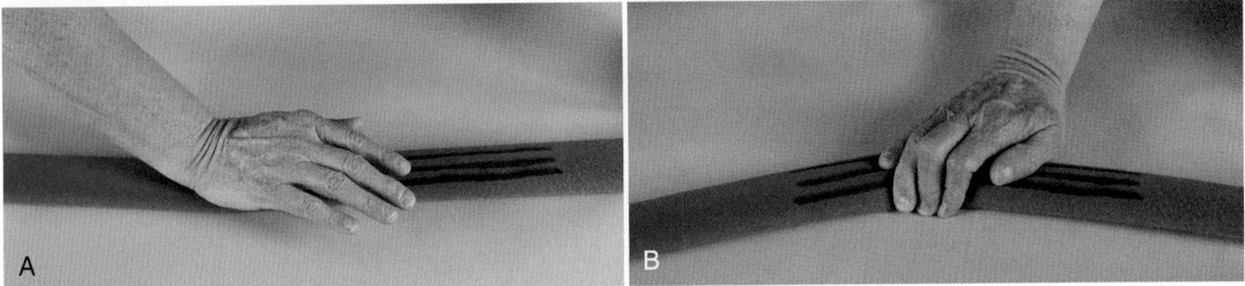

FIG. 10.20 A, Longitudinal stretching pulls or pushes tissue in the direction of the fiber configuration. **B,** Cross-directional stretching pulls or pushes the tissue against the fiber direction.

is a common cause of soft tissue discomfort because stability is provided by the soft tissues instead of the joint structure. Stretching should not be painful. Stretching should not strain the joints or move beyond functional ranges of motion. Forcing tissues into an elongated state can cause injury. Study and practice the elongation concepts described in Box 10.4.

Applying Elongation Methods

The following procedure is used for longitudinal stretching:

1. Position the target soft tissue in ease, which is the direction opposite the motion barrier/bind.
2. Choose a method to prepare the target soft tissue to stretch (e.g., gliding, compression, kneading).
3. After the target soft tissue has been prepared, elongate the soft tissue to its physiological or pathological barrier or to wherever protective contraction is engaged; this is the point of bind. Back off slightly to prevent protective spasm. Stay in line with the soft tissue fibers. Stretch tissue gently as the client exhales at about one-quarter to one half-inch increments.

The following two approaches are used for the actual stretch phase:

1. Hold the position just off the physiological or pathological barrier for at least 10 seconds to allow for the neurological reset of protective stretch receptors.
2. Take up slack by further lengthening the soft tissue for up to 20 seconds to create longitudinal pull (tension stress) on the tissue. Hold the soft tissue stretch up to 3 minutes to allow for changes in the connective tissue component of the target tissue.

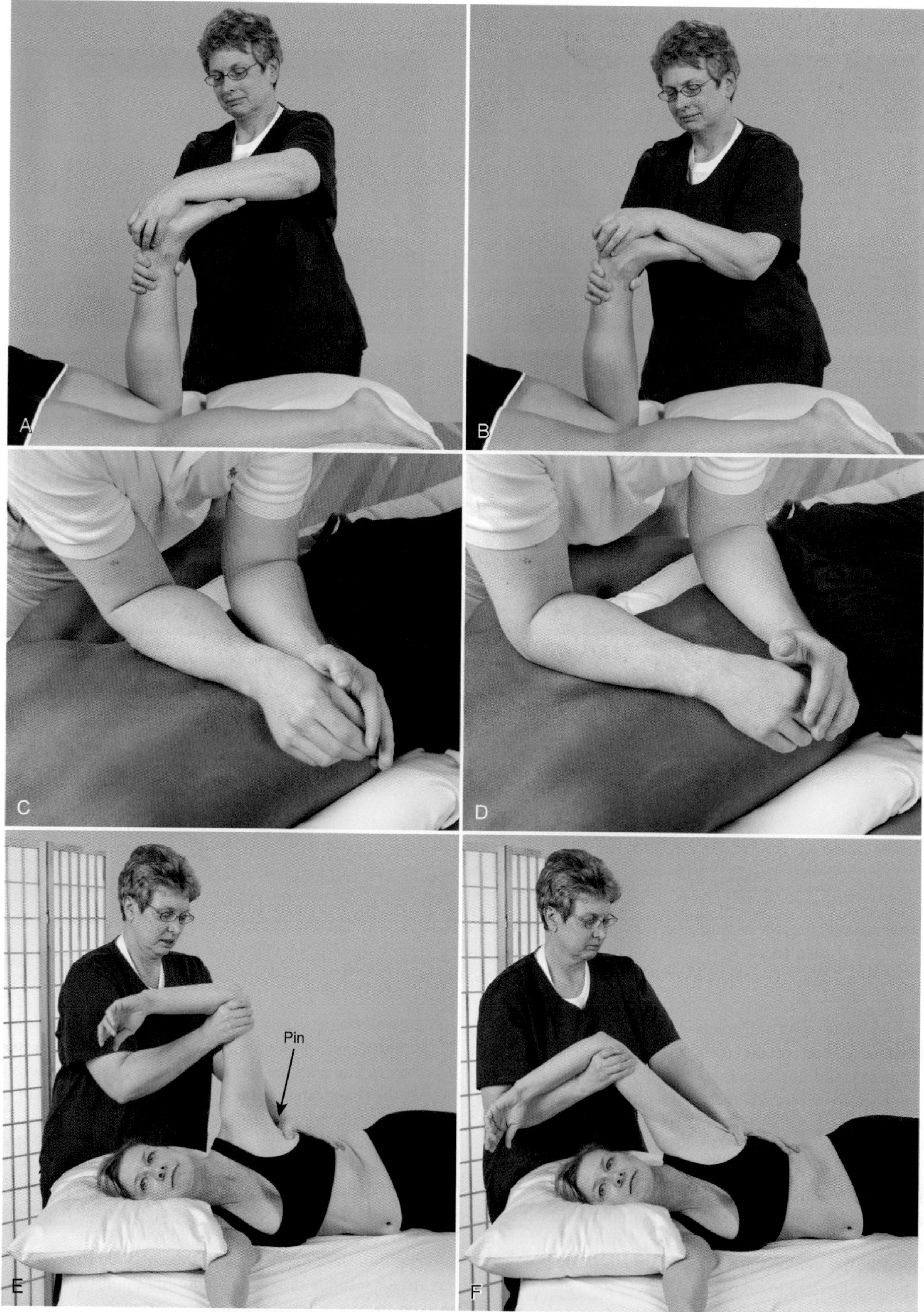

FIG. 10.21 Beginning **A,** and end **B,** of passive longitudinal stretch. Beginning **C,** and end **D,** of direct tissue stretch. **E, F** Pin and stretch.

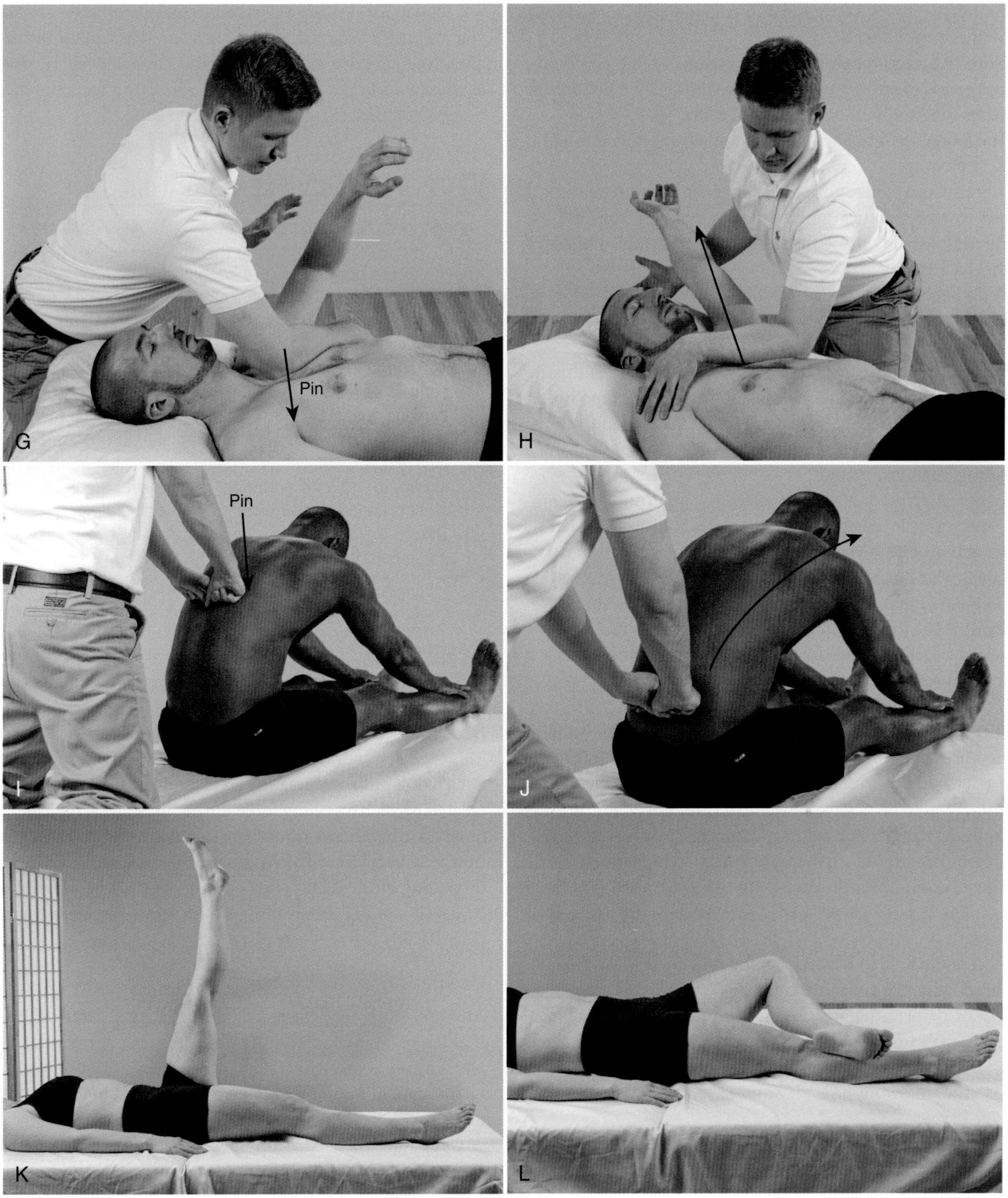

FIG. 10.21, cont'd Active release: pin. **G,** and client moves to stretch. **H,** Active release: pin **I,** and client moves to stretch **J. K, L,** Examples of active self-stretching.

Alternate Procedures for Longitudinal Stretching

If only a small section of soft tissue needs to be elongated, if the soft tissue does not lend itself to stretching with joint movement, or if the joints are so flexible that not enough pull is put on the soft tissues to achieve an effective tension stress to the tissues, the following alternate procedure for longitudinal stretching should be used:

1. Locate the short soft tissue to be stretched.
2. Place the hands, fingers, or forearms in the belly of the soft tissue or directly over the area to be stretched.
3. Contact the soft tissue with sufficient pressure to reset the neuromuscular mechanism.
4. Separate the fingers, hands, or forearms (tension stress) or lift the tissue with effort sufficient to stretch the soft tissue (bending or torsion stress). Take up all slack in the tissue, and then increase the intensity slightly and wait for the

connective tissue component to respond (this may take as long as 3 minutes).

Note: All requirements for preparation of the soft tissue and direction of stretch are the same as those described for the previous longitudinal stretching procedure.

The following procedure is used for active assisted longitudinal stretching:

1. Identify and isolate the short soft tissue, making sure it is not working against gravity in this position. Remind the client to exhale during the stretching (elongation) phase of this technique.
2. Lengthen the soft tissue to its physiological or pathological barrier, move slightly beyond this point, and stretch gently for 1 to 2 seconds.
3. Return the soft tissue to its starting position. Repeat this action in a rhythmic, pulse like fashion for 5 to 20 repetitions.
4. The client can benefit from contracting the antagonist muscle groups while the target soft tissue is elongated using a slow gentle movement.

Other effective methods involve the application of compression into the short binding tissue to hold it, followed by either active or passive movement:

1. Locate the area to be stretched, and passively move the distal joint so that the target tissue is soft (at ease). The movement of the joint is typically toward the target tissue.
2. Apply compression into the short tissue and hold it in a fixed position.
3. The client moves the adjacent joints and lengthens the tissue (sometimes called *active release*), or the massage therapist uses the other hand to move the tissue or joint into a stretched position (sometimes called *pin and stretch*). In either active or passive movement, the movement is away from the short tissue held with compression.

Cross-directional tissue stretching uses a push, pull, and twist component, introducing torsion, shear, and bend stress. The procedure for cross-directional stretching is as follows:

1. Access the area to be stretched by moving against the fiber direction using compression.
2. Lift or deform the area slightly and hold for 30 to 60 seconds, up to no longer than 3 minutes, until the area gets warm or seems to soften.

Use the following procedure for skin and superficial connective tissue:

1. Locate the area of restriction.
2. Lift and pull (like taffy), first moving into the restriction and then pulling and twisting out of it, keeping a constant tension on the tissue. Take up slack until the area warms and softens.

Deep Fascial Planes

Accessing deep fascial planes requires an understanding of the deep structures involved (Chapter 12 expands on this information). It is important to realize that the human body is made up of interconnecting parts; consequently, all stretching affects deep connective tissue structures. The body cannot be divided into separate layers; the only difference is the access point. A house may have three or four doors, each of which will let you inside. Where you enter may be different, but once you are inside, you are able to have an effect on all the areas. Therefore effective elongation of the more superficial tissues, as presented in this chapter, also indirectly affects the deeper tissue structures (Proficiency Exercise 10.5).

PROFICIENCY EXERCISE 10.5

Knead extra flour into bread dough so that the consistency is quite firm. Practice stretching the dough. Feel for the give of the dough as opposed to the dough breaking.

1. Design a lengthening and stretching sequence for yourself that accesses the major muscle groups and connective tissue areas. Pay attention to the difference in the feel of neuromuscular lengthening, with its quick release, and connective tissue stretching, with its softer, slower give.
2. Working with a partner, see how many massage manipulations and techniques you can combine and perform at one time (e.g., joint movement combined with compression, gliding combined with a stretch, percussion combined with a stretch, kneading combined with muscle energy methods).
3. Design a massage incorporating at least two massage or movement techniques for every body area.

Traction

Traction means pulling on part of the body to separate two or more parts. Traction is also used to keep a group of muscles (e.g., the neck muscles) stretched to reduce muscle spasms. This type of traction is usually accomplished with some sort of device that pulls the area for an extended time. Tension stress created by such a pulling force during massage is typically sustained for much less time than traction using a device. Traction is typically performed during massage at the limb joints by pulling at the distal ends of joints and at the cervical area by gently pulling the head in a direction away from the neck (Fig. 10.22).

Oscillation

Attempts to clarify massage terminology cluster vibration, shaking, and rocking under the umbrella term *oscillation*. **Oscillation** is any effect that varies in a back-and-forth, or reciprocating, manner. The term *vibration* sometimes is used more narrowly to mean a mechanical oscillation.

Very simply, oscillation involves action in the form of springs and swings. In terms of springs, it is logical to include massage methods that bounce off the tissue (later called *percussion*), just as beating a drum creates oscillation. The concept of swings can be related to any massage method that moves the body. Vibration is an action of moving back and forth rapidly; shaking is moving back and forth but is much bigger than vibration; and rocking is a rhythmic, swinging motion.

Vibration

Description

Vibration is powerful if it can be done long enough and at an intensity sufficient to produce reflexive physiological effects. Often a mechanical device is used to create vibration.

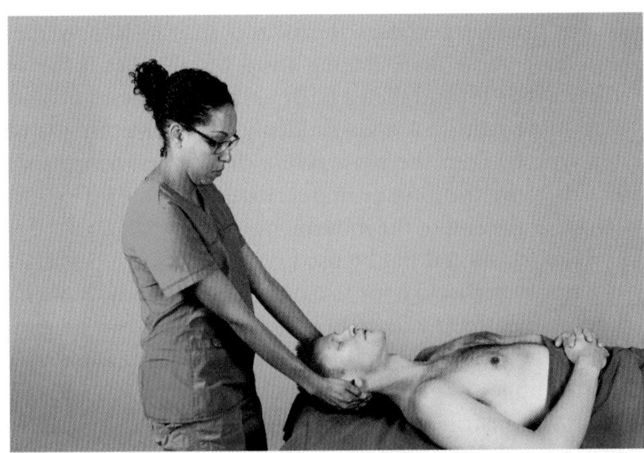
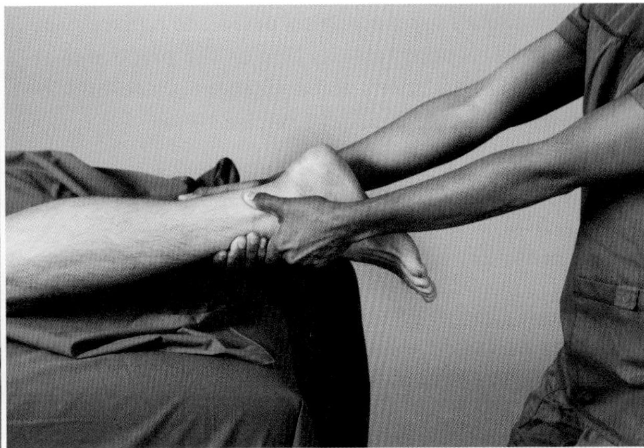

FIG. 10.22 Traction.

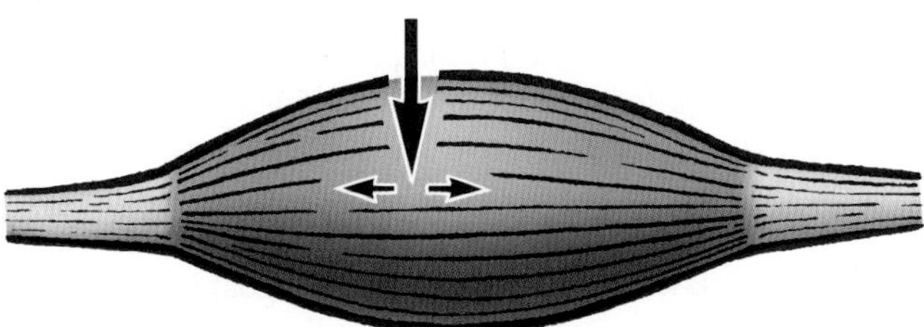

FIG. 10.23 The focus of vibration is downward and back and forth in a fast, oscillating manner.

Vibration also can be used to break up the monotony of the massage. If the same methods are used repeatedly, the body adapts and does not respond as well to the sensation or stimulation.

Theories of Effect

Manual vibration may facilitate neuromuscular function by applying the technique at the muscle tendons for up to 30 seconds. When this is complete, the antagonist muscle pattern relaxes through neurological reciprocal inhibition. Because vibration seems to "wake up" nerves, it is a good method for stimulating nerve activity. The nerves of the muscles around a joint also innervate the joint itself. Clients often interpret muscle pain as joint pain and vice versa. Used specifically and purposefully, vibration may shift the muscle-joint pain perception.

Applying Vibration

All vibration begins with compression. After the depth of pressure has been achieved, the hand needs to tremble and transmit the action to the surrounding tissues (Figs. 10.23 and 10.24).

To start with coarse vibration, place one hand on the client and compress lightly. Begin moving the hand back and forth using only the forearm muscles and limiting the motion to about 2 inches of space. Gradually quicken the back-and-forth movement, checking to make sure your upper arm stays relaxed. Next, make the back-and-forth movement smaller until the hand does not move at all on the tissue but is trembling at a high intensity. This is vibration.

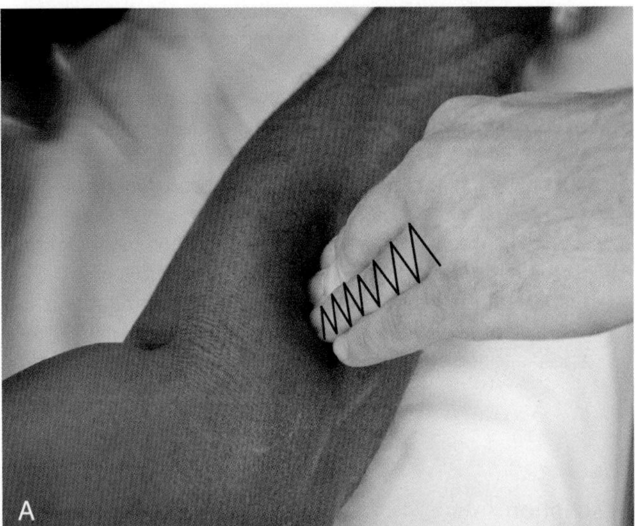

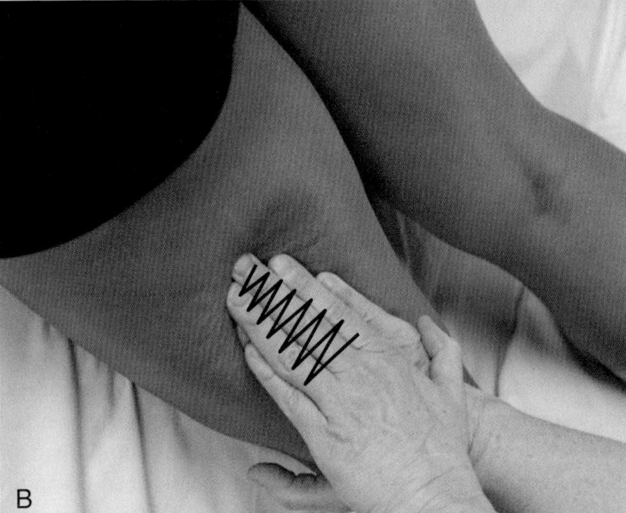

FIG. 10.24 Two examples of vibration.

Because considerable energy is needed to perform this manipulation, it should be used sparingly and only for short periods. A forearm gliding method should be used after vibration because the gliding action essentially massages and relaxes the therapist's arm, protecting it from repetitive use problems.

Some professionals use mechanical devices to replace manual vibration. This is acceptable as long as the practice is allowed by licensing regulations, the equipment is safe, and the client approves its use (Proficiency Exercise 10.6).

PROFICIENCY EXERCISE 10.6

The first two exercises to teach vibration were developed by a professional magician who is also a massage therapist and instructor. Many sleight-of-hand movements required for his illusions use the same movements as vibration. Perfecting these two balloon exercises will enhance your vibration skills.

1. Get a clear, 5-inch balloon. Put a penny inside it, and then inflate and tie the balloon. Grasp the tied end of the balloon, cupping it in the palm of your hand. Using wrist action only, circle the balloon until the penny begins to roll inside. Once you can do this, make the wrist circles smaller and smaller while continuing to roll the penny in the balloon. Eventually the action will be the movement required for vibration.
2. Use the same balloon and put the fattest part in the palm of your hand. Place your other hand on top of the balloon. Using just the bottom hand, use a coarse vibration to get the penny to jump and dance in the balloon. Once you can do this, make the movements smaller and smaller until you can make the penny dance with fine vibration movements.
3. Combine all the methods presented so far into a massage. Incorporate vibration at each tendon, paying attention to the results as the muscles contract or tense slightly in response to the stimulation.

Shaking

Description

Shaking is effective for relaxing muscle groups or an entire limb. Shaking sometimes is classified as a form of vibration; however, the application is different, because vibration begins with compression and shaking begins with lifting. Shaking warms and prepares the body for deeper bodywork and addresses the joints in a nonspecific manner. It is effective when the muscles seem extremely tight.

Theories of Effect

Shaking manipulations confuse the positional proprioceptors because the sensory input is too disorganized for the brain's integrating systems to interpret; muscle relaxation is the natural response in such situations. Shaking has a neurological effect, but a small mechanical influence also may be exerted on the connective tissue because of the lift-and-pull component of the method. Because shaking moves the superficial fascia on the deep fascia, there should be movement of interstitial fluid into lymph capillaries.

Applying Shaking

Shaking begins with a lift-and-pull technique. Either a muscle group or a limb is grasped, lifted, and shaken. To begin to understand shaking, think of a dog shaking water from its coat, a person shaking out a rug or blanket, a dog or cat tugging on a toy, or a horse swishing its tail.

For massage purposes, the focus of shaking is more specific and less intense than shaking a rug, but the idea is the same. It involves a lift and then a fairly abrupt downward or side-to-side movement that ends suddenly, as if something is being thrown off. Even the most subtle shaking movements deliberately move the joint or muscle tissue with the intention of a "snap" at the end of the movement.

Shaking should not be used on the skin or superficial fascia, nor is it effective for use on the entire body. Rather, it is best applied to any large muscle groups that can be grasped and to the synovial joints of the limbs. Good areas for shaking are the upper trapezius and shoulder area, biceps and triceps groups, hamstrings, quadriceps, gastrocnemius, and, in some instances, the abdominals and the pectoralis muscles close to the axilla. The joints of the shoulders, hips, and extremities also respond well to shaking.

The larger the muscle or joint, the more intense the method. If the movements are performed with all the slack out of the tissue, the focal point of the shaking is small and the technique is extremely effective. The more purposeful the approach, the smaller the focus of the shaking. The therapist should always stay within the limits of both joint range of motion and the elastic give of the tissue. The goal is to see how small the shaking action can be and still achieve the desired physiological effect. To accomplish this, first lift the tissue or limb, grasp it, and then lean back gently until the tissue becomes taut. Begin the shaking movement from this position (Fig. 10.25).

Rocking

Description

Rocking is a soothing, rhythmic method used to calm people. During rocking, nothing is abrupt; the methods have an even ebb and flow. All movement is flowing, like a wind chime in a gentle breeze or a porch swing on a hot summer night. Rocking is one of the most effective relaxation techniques the massage therapist can use.

Theories of Effect

Rocking has both neurological and chemical effects. Many parasympathetic responses are elicited by the rocking of the body during gliding, kneading, and compression. Rocking also works through the vestibular system of the inner ear and feeds sensory input directly into the cerebellum. Other reflex mechanisms probably are also affected. For rocking to be most effective, the client's body must move so that the fluid in the semicircular canals of the inner ear is affected, initiating parasympathetic mechanisms. Caution is needed if the client has any sort of inner ear vestibular dysfunctions where whole body rocking may cause dizziness and balance issues.

Applying Rocking

Rocking is rhythmic and should be applied with a deliberate, full-body movement. Rocking involves the up-and-down and side-to-side movement of shaking, but no flick or throw-off snap occurs at the end of the movement. The action moves the body as far as it will go, then allows it to return to the original position (Fig. 10.26).

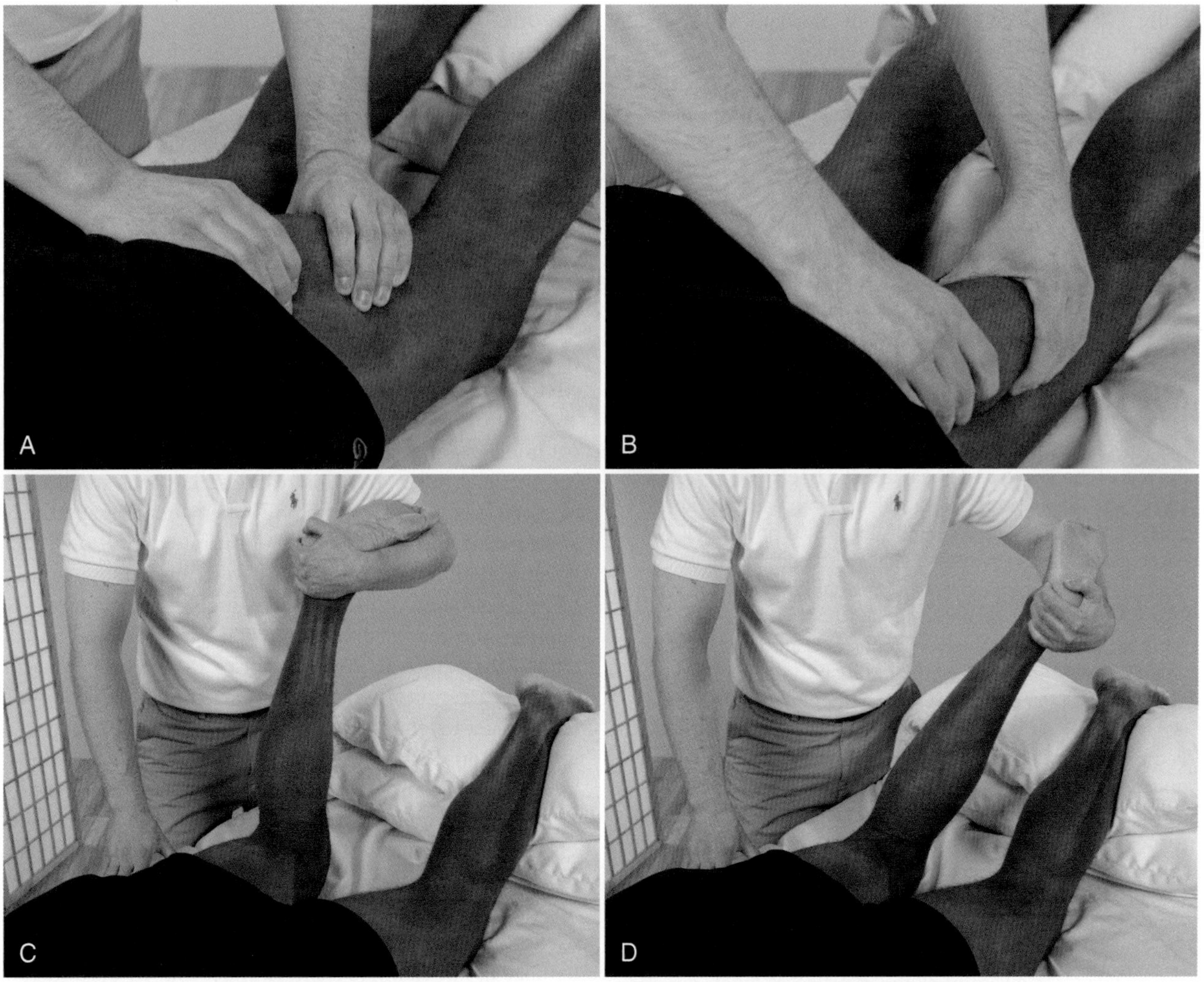

FIG. 10.25 Examples of shaking. **A, B,** Shaking tissue. **C, D,** Shaking a limb.

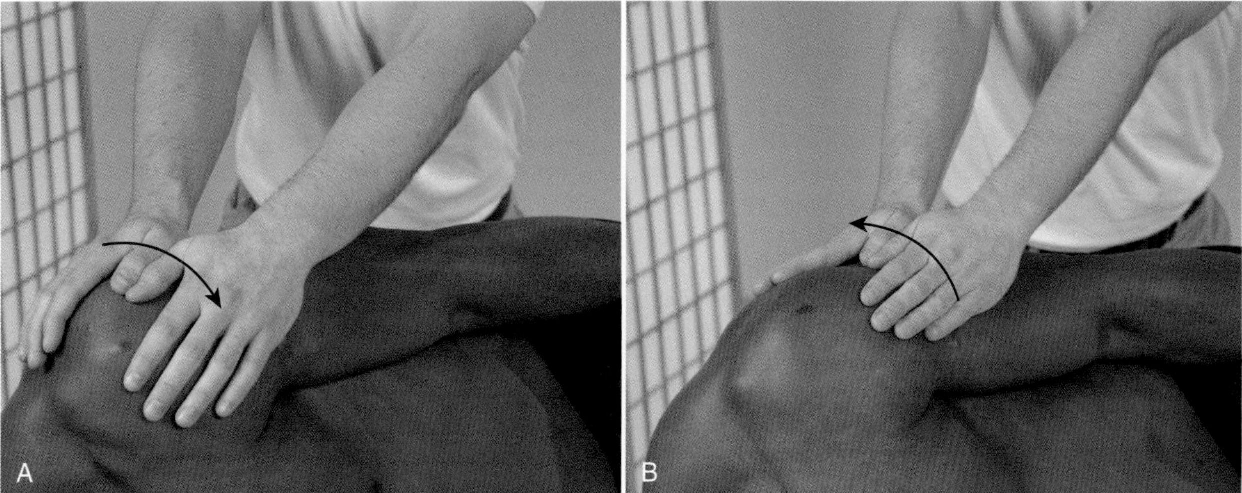

FIG. 10.26 Example of rocking.

After two or three rocks, the therapist can sense the client's rhythm. This attunement to the client's rhythm is a powerful point of interface for determining the pacing of the application. The massage therapist works within the rhythm to maintain and amplify it by attempting to gently extend the limits of movement or by slowing the rhythm. The client seems to relax more easily when a subtle rocking movement, matching his or her innate rhythm pattern, is incorporated as part of the generalized massage approach, along with such applications as gliding, kneading, compression, and joint movement, especially passive movements. The body mechanics described in this text tend to produce a rocking motion.

With a tense, anxious client who initially may resist rocking, begin the process with slightly bigger and more abrupt shaking manipulations. As the muscles begin to relax, switch to rocking methods (Proficiency Exercise 10.7).

PROFICIENCY EXERCISE 10.7

1. Lay a sheet on your massage table or other flat surface. Lift one end, and practice shaking the sheet to achieve a wave-like motion from one end of the sheet to the other. Practice directing the ripple to various locations on the table.
2. While sitting in a playground swing, using your legs to pump yourself. This exercise gives the full-body effect of the shake. Pay close attention to the feeling as you reach the top of the swing and begin to head back.
3. Using your own body for practice, systematically shake each joint, lying down to do the legs. See how small you can make the movement and still feel the effects. Grab the muscles of your arm and leg. Lift and shake the tissue, paying attention to the sensations.
4. Sit in an old-fashioned rocking chair and let the chair rock you. See what happens when you rock the chair. Vary the speed to go faster and slower than the chair's movement. Put the chair on different surfaces, such as carpet, hard floor, sand, and grass. Again, let the chair rock you and notice the difference. Remember, each person has an individual rhythm that needs to be identified, supported, and respected.
5. Play various types of relaxing music. Pick up the sway of the music and rock with it. Repeat the exercise with different beats of music.
6. Design an entire massage using a combination of shaking and rocking. Be aware of all the qualities of touch during the application.

Percussion

Description

Percussion (tapotement) moves up and down on the tissue. The term *tapotement* comes from the French verb *tapoter,* which means "to rap, smack, drum, or pat." In percussion techniques, the hands or parts of the hand administer springy blows to the body at a fast rate. The blows are directed downward, creating rhythmic compression of the tissue (Fig. 10.27).

Percussion is characterized as light or heavy. In light percussion, the compressive force of the blows penetrates only to the superficial tissue of the skin and subcutaneous layers; in heavy percussion, the force penetrates deeper into the muscles, tendons, and visceral (organ) structures, such as the pleura in the chest cavity.

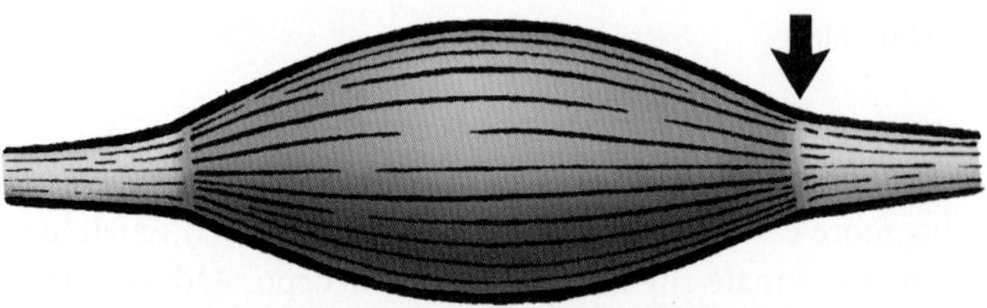

FIG. 10.27 The focus of percussion (tapotement) is a vertical, abrupt downward snapping.

Theories of Effect

Percussion is a stimulating application that operates through the response of the nerves. Because of its intense stimulating effect on the nervous system, it initiates or enhances sympathetic activity of the autonomic nervous system. However, percussion also can have mechanical results, which involve loosening and moving mucus in the chest. People with cystic fibrosis are treated with percussion, but massage therapy of this type is beyond the beginning skill levels of the massage therapist.

The most noticeable effect of percussion results from the response of the tendon reflexes. A quick blow to the tendon stretches it. In response, protective muscle contraction occurs. To obtain the best result, stretch the tendon first. The most common example of this reflex mechanism is the knee-jerk (or patellar) reflex, but this response happens in all tendons to some degree. This is helpful when the massage therapist is preparing the muscles for elongation applications, such as when a client indicates that the hamstrings are tight and need to be lengthened. With the client supine, the hip flexed to 90 degrees, and the knee flexed to 90 degrees, percussion on the stretched quadriceps tendon causes the quadriceps to contract. As a result, the hamstrings are inhibited, which makes them easier to lengthen to a more normal resting length.

When applied to the joints, percussion affects the joint kinesthetic receptors responsible for determining the position and movement of the body. The quick blows confuse the system, similar to the effect of joint-focused rocking and shaking, but the body muscles are stimulated rather than inhibited. This method is useful for stimulating weak muscles. The force used must move the joint but should not be strong enough to damage it. For example a single finger may be used to administer percussion over the carpal joints, whereas the fist may be used over the sacroiliac joint.

Percussion is effective when used at motor points that usually are located in the same area as the traditional acupuncture points, which in turn are located at neurovascular bundles. The repetitive stimulation causes the nerve to fire repeatedly, stimulating the nerve.

Percussion focused primarily on the skin affects the superficial blood vessels of the skin, initially causing them to contract. Heavy percussion or prolonged lighter application dilates the vessels by causing the release of histamine, a vasodilator.

Applying Percussion

Two hands usually are used alternately to do percussion. One or two fingers can be used to tap a motor point located at the center of the muscle mass where the motor nerve enters the muscle (this sometimes is called *neurotapping*). The forearm muscles contract and relax in rapid succession to move the elbow joint into flexion and then allow it to release quickly. This action travels down to the relaxed wrist, extending it; the wrist then moves back and forth to provide the action of the percussion. Percussion is a controlled flailing of the arms as the wrists snap back and forth. Remember that the wrist must stay relaxed. Beginning students usually want to use the wrists to provide the snap action. This is especially tempting when using small movements of the fingers; however, it will damage the wrist.

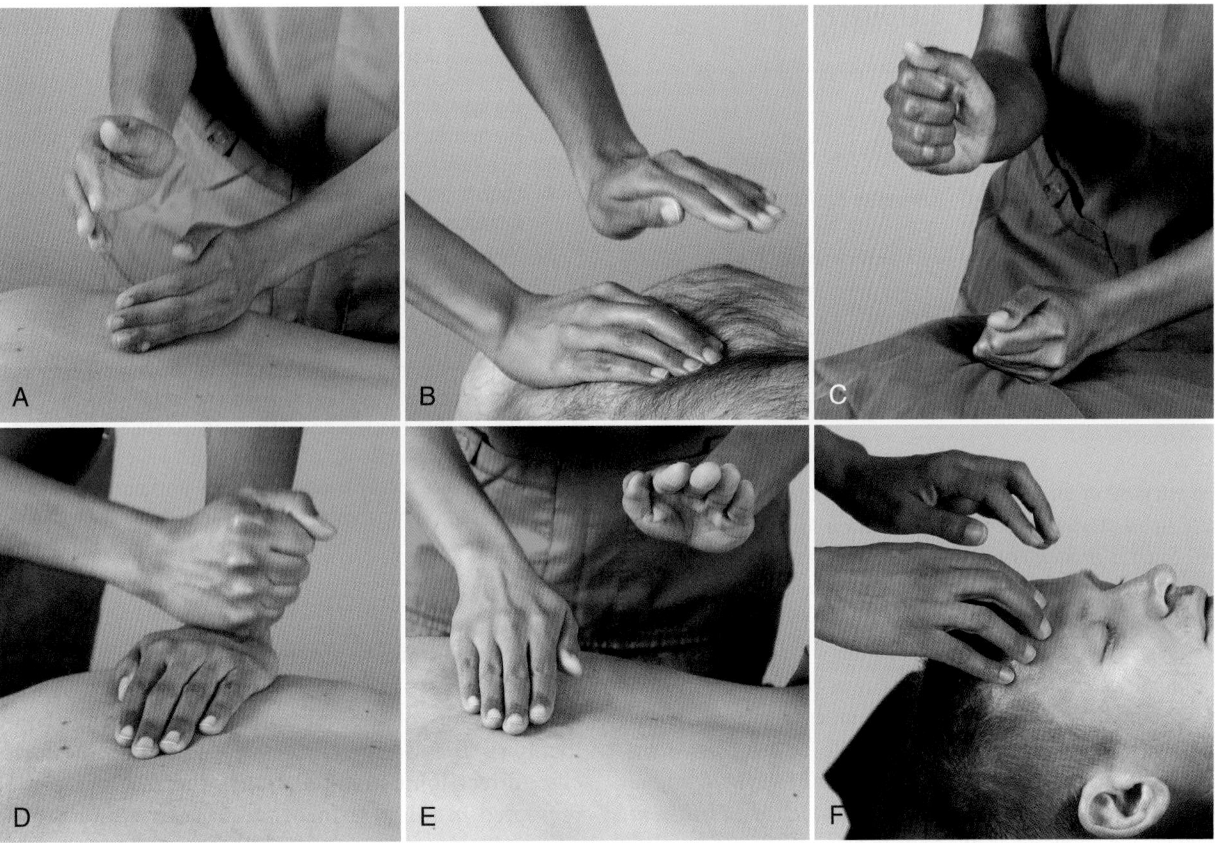

FIG. 10.28 Examples of percussion. A, Hacking. **B,** Cupping. **C,** Fist beating. **D,** Beating over the palm. **E,** Slapping. **F,** Finger tapping.

Heavy percussion should not be done in the kidney area, directly over joints, or anywhere pain or discomfort is present. The following are methods of percussion (Fig. 10.28):

1. *Hacking.* Hacking is applied with both wrists relaxed and the fingers spread, with only the little finger or the ulnar side of the hand striking the skin surface. The other fingers hit each other with a springy touch. Point hacking can be done by using the fingertips in the same way. Hacking is done with the whole hand on the larger soft tissue areas, such as the upper back and shoulders. Point hacking is used on smaller areas, such as the individual tendons of the toes, or over motor points.
2. *Cupping.* To perform cupping, the fingers and thumbs are positioned as if making a cup. The hands are turned over, and the same action used in hacking is performed. When done on the anterior and posterior thorax, cupping is good for stimulating the respiratory system and for loosening mucus. If the client exhales and makes a monotone noise during cupping, enough intensity is used so that the tone begins to break up, changing from "AAAAAAAAAAAAH-HHHHH" to "AH AH AH AH AH AH."
3. *Beating* and *pounding.* These moves can be performed with a soft fist with the knuckles down or with the fist held vertically and the action performed with the ulnar side of the palm. This technique is used over large muscles, such as the buttocks and upper leg muscles.
4. *Slapping (splatting).* For this technique, the whole palm of a flattened hand contacts the body. This is a good method for causing the release of histamine, thereby increasing vasodilation and its effects on the skin. It also is a good method to use on the bottoms of the feet. The broad contact of the whole hand disperses the force laterally instead of downward, and the effects remain in the superficial tissue. Kellogg (2010) called this movement *splatting.*
5. *Tapping.* For this technique, the palmar surface of the fingers alternately taps the body area with light to medium pressure. This is a good method to use around the joints, on the tendons, on the face and head, and along the spine (Proficiency Exercise 10.8).

PROFICIENCY EXERCISE **10.8**

1. Play a drum or watch a drummer. Pay attention to the action of the arms and wrists and the grasp of the drumsticks. Notice that the drummer holds the drumsticks loosely.
2. Get a paddleball or yo-yo and see what actions it takes to make these toys work. Play with a rattle or tambourine.
3. Use the foam from the compression exercises and practice the different methods and intensity of percussion (light to heavy, slow to fast).
4. While shaking your hands quickly, use hacking to strike the foam or a practice client. Without stopping, change hand positions so that all the methods are used.
5. Design a stimulating massage with various applications of percussion. Notice which qualities of touch are most reflected with these methods.

MASSAGE TECHNIQUES USING JOINT MOVEMENT

SECTION OBJECTIVES

Chapter objective covered in this section:

3. Incorporate movement of the joints as an aspect of massage application.

Using the information presented in this section, the learner will be able to perform the following:

- Use movement in a purposeful way to create a specific physiological response.
- Explain the proprioceptive mechanisms and their importance in the physiological effects of massage techniques.
- Move the synovial joints through the client's physiological range of motion using both active and passive joint movement.

The purpose of an active movement is to convey to and concentrate upon a selected point, the nutrition and energies of the system. Such a movement may accomplish a twofold purpose, that of supplying a part and of relieving another part more or less distant.

The mode of effecting this purpose is as follows: the person to receive the application is placed in an easy, unconstrained position, sitting, lying, half lying, kneeling, or in a convenient position that will suitably adjust all parts of the body to the purpose. The body is fixed either by the hands of an assistant or by means of an apparatus so as to prevent as much as possible any motion of all parts of the body, except the acting part. The patient is in some cases directed to move the free part in a particular direction, the effort to do so is resisted by the operator, with a force proportionate to the exertion made very nicely graduated to the particular condition of the part and of the system at large. The resistance is not uniform, but varies according to the varying action of muscles, as perceived by the operator. In other cases the operator acts while the patient resists. The action is the same, but in one case the patient's acting muscles are shortened and in the other lengthened. The operation is a wrestle, in which a very limited portion of the organism is engaged. The motion must be much slower than the natural movement of the part engaged, which strongly fixes the attention and concentrates the will. The act is repeated two or three times with all the care and precision the operator can command, being cautious not to induce fatigue.

George H. Taylor, *An Illustrated Sketch of the Movement Cure*, 1866

The use of movement as described in the next section follows Taylor's guidelines and recommendations, which were his interpretations of Ling's gymnastics, or active movements (Box 10.5). The principles of massage today are built on the principles described in the historical literature. The names may be different and the physiological explanations more precise, but the methods are similar.

The efficient use of movement techniques reduces the need for repetitive massage manipulations. If these techniques are used well, the neuromuscular mechanism can be activated and influenced quickly, with less physical effort by the massage professional.

Box 10.5 Taylor's Principles for the Application of Movement and Techniques

1. Be specific.
2. Be mindful of patterns of "too much" and "not enough."
3. Position the client purposefully.
4. Stabilize the body so that only the focused target area is affected.
5. You may move the area (client passive) or may cooperate in the effort with the client (client active).
6. Make sure the force and exertion are gradual and vary with the demand.
7. Remember that the purpose is to lengthen shortened tissue and stimulate weakened muscles.
8. You enable the lengthening or stimulation process by assisting the client.
9. Make sure the application is slow and purposeful.
10. Repeat the movement two or three times but not to fatigue.

It is important to distinguish between the soft tissue manipulations of the massage professional and the joint manipulations of the chiropractor, osteopath, or physical therapist. The massage professional does not perform specific, direct joint manipulations. The massage techniques presented in this text incorporate passive and active joint movement, in addition to lengthening and stretching methods, within the comfortable limits of the joint. These methods may indirectly affect the range of motion of a joint through changes in the soft tissue. The particular focus of the massage professional is the soft tissue, not the osseous structure of the joint.

Often a combination of soft tissue work and specific joint manipulation is required to achieve the functional goals of the client. In these instances the massage therapist, with appropriate training, becomes part of the multidisciplinary team under the supervision of the health care professional. This team approach provides the skills and expertise of multiple professionals to best serve the client.

Joint Movement and Range of Motion

Description

Range of motion (ROM) is the angle through which a joint moves from the anatomical position to the ends of its motion in a particular direction. It is measured in degrees. Each joint has a normal range of motion. Assessment methods that move a joint can determine whether a joint is able to move within a normal range of motion. If the joint moves less than the normal range or more than the normal range, a problem may exist.

The range or amount of movement at a joint is determined by a number of factors: (1) the shape of the bones that form the joint, (2) the tautness or laxity of the ligament and capsule structure of the joint, (3) the length of the soft tissue structure that supports and moves the joint, and (4) whether the joint moves independently of other joints (open chain) or is linked to other joints in a combined movement (closed chain).

To understand joint movement, you must first understand the structure and function of joints. A simplified review is presented here; anatomy and physiology resources can further clarify and describe individual joints and are valuable learning aids.

How Joints Work

Joints allow us to move. Joint position and velocity (movement) receptors inform the central nervous system where and how the body is positioned in gravity and how fast it is moving. These sensory data are the major determining factors for muscle tone patterns.

Joint movement techniques focus on the *synovial,* or freely movable, joints in the body (see Chapter 4). To a lesser extent, the joints of the vertebral column, hand, and foot also are considered, as are other joints, such as the facet joints of the ribs, the sacroiliac joint, and the sternoclavicular joint. These joints are not directly influenced by muscles, but rather move through indirect muscle action.

We can control some joint movements voluntarily; we can move our limbs through various motions, such as flexion, extension, abduction, adduction, and rotation. These are referred to as *physiological movements,* or osteokinematic movements. For normal physiological movement, other types of movements (*accessory movements,* or arthrokinematic movements) must occur as a result of the inherent laxity, or joint play, that exists in each joint. This laxity allows the ends of the bones to slide, roll, or spin smoothly on each other inside the joint capsule. These essential movements occur during movement of the joint and are not under voluntary control.

Comparing a Joint to a Door Hinge

A door provides a good example of joint motion. The hinge holds the door both to the casing and away from the casing. For the door to open and close efficiently *(osteokinematic movement),* the space between the door and the door casing must be maintained and the fit must be correct. If the fit of the door in the door casing is incorrect or if the space is not maintained, the door will not open and close correctly. In the body, ligaments act as the hinges.

The door hinge must be oiled. In the joint, the synovial membrane secretes synovial fluid, produced on demand by joint movement. If a joint does not move or is not moved, it will lock up like a rusty door hinge, and movement will be restricted or lost.

If you look closely at a door hinge, you will notice the space around the pin in the hinge. If you move the hinge back and forth (not swing the door), the hinge-and-pin mechanism moves a little *(arthrokinematic movement).* This little movement can be likened to joint play. If the ligaments and connective tissue that make up the joint capsule are not firm enough to maintain joint space, joint play is lost. Joint play is also lost if the capsule is too tight. Muscles around a joint can shorten, pulling the bone ends together and affecting joint play.

If the ligaments and joint capsule are not pliable, flexibility is lost. If the ligaments and joint capsule do not support the joint, the fit is disrupted. Muscle contraction may pull the joint out of alignment. Muscle groups that flex and adduct the joints are about 30% stronger and have more mass than the extensors and abductors. If the body uses muscle contraction to stabilize a joint, the uneven pull between flexors and extensors and adductors and abductors disturbs the fit of the bones at the joint.

Limitations on the Ability to Move a Joint

Joints have various degrees of range of motion. Anatomical, physiological, and pathological barriers to motion exist. A barrier is a point of resistance and can feel hard, such as when bone contacts bone, or more leathery and binding, such as when soft tissue is short.

Anatomical barriers are determined by the shape and fit of the bones at the joint. The anatomical barrier is seldom reached because the possibility of injury is greatest in this position. Instead, the body protects the joint by establishing physiological barriers. Physiological barriers are the result of the limits in range of motion imposed by protective nerve and sensory function to support optimum function. The sensation at the barrier is soft and pliable. An adaptation in a physiological barrier that causes the protective function to limit instead of support optimum functioning is called a pathological barrier. Pathological barriers often are manifested as stiffness, pain, or a "catch."

When massage therapists use joint movement techniques, they must remain within the physiological barriers. If a pathological barrier exists that limits motion and this motion limit is not resourceful compensation, then techniques are used to gently and slowly encourage the joint structures to increase the limits of the range of motion to the physiological barrier.

Joint End-Feel

When a normal joint is taken to its physiological limit, usually still a bit more movement is possible, a sort of springiness in the joint. This type of joint end-feel is called a *soft end-feel.* When a joint movement is restricted or soft tissue is shortened by a pathological barrier, resulting in reduction of the range of motion, movement is always limited in some direction. As the limit is reached and exceeded, comfortable movement is no longer possible. In the case of abnormal restriction, the limit does not have any spring, as is found at a physiological barrier. Rather, similar to a jammed door or drawer, the joint is fixed at the barrier, and any attempt to take it farther causes discomfort and has a "binding" or leathery feel. A distinct jamming rather than springy sensation is called a *hard end-feel.*

Joint Movement as Assessment

Joint movement is a primary assessment process to determine range of motion of a joint. Normal joint movements often are indicated by the degree of movement available, with the anatomical, or neutral, position labeled 0 degrees. The "normal" range of motion for each joint should be identified for each individual. Box 10.6 presents some examples of normal range of motion for common joints addressed during massage. For additional study, consult a comprehensive anatomy and physiology book for the degrees of movement for joints.

Remember that each person is unique, and many factors influence the available range of motion. Just because a joint does

Box 10.6 Normal Range of Motion for Major Joints

Available range of motion is measured from the neutral anatomical position (0). If 0 appears first, the movement begins in the anatomical position. If numbers appear first, the movement begins out of the anatomical position and returns to the neutral (0) position.

Normal Values (in degrees)

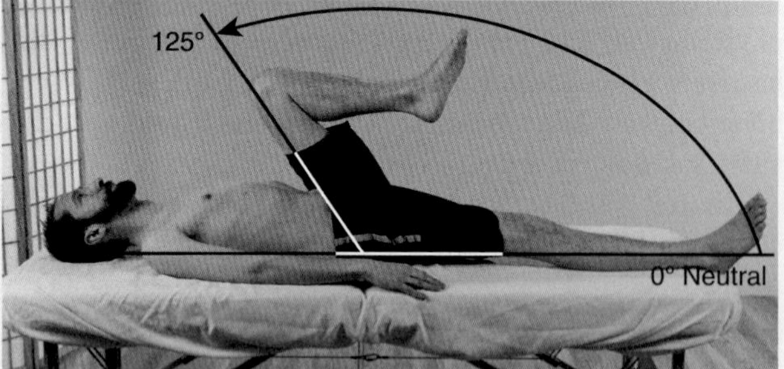

Hip flexion (0 to 125 degrees).

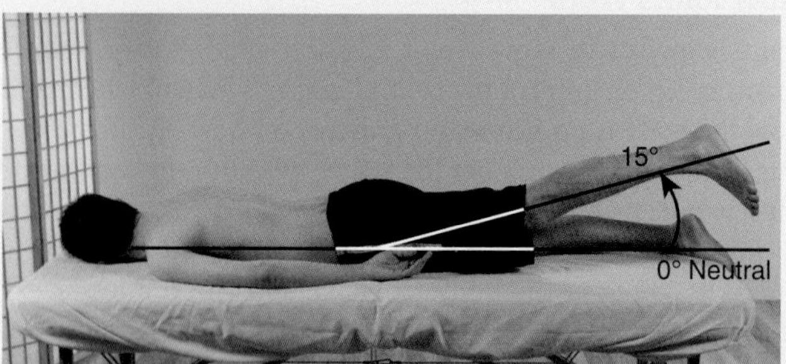

Hip hyperextension (0 to 15 degrees).

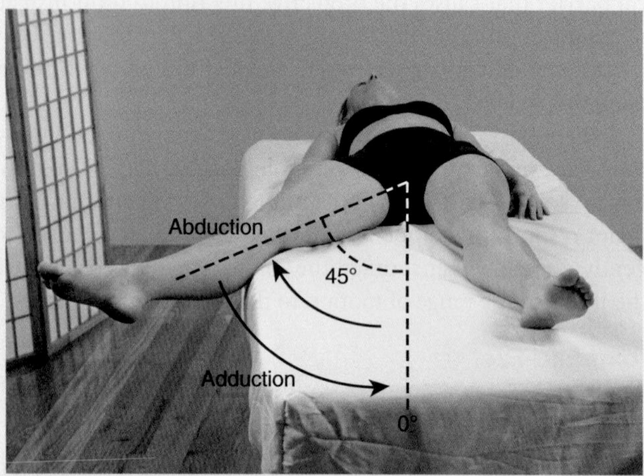

Hip abduction (0 to 45 degrees) and hip adduction (45 to 0 degrees).

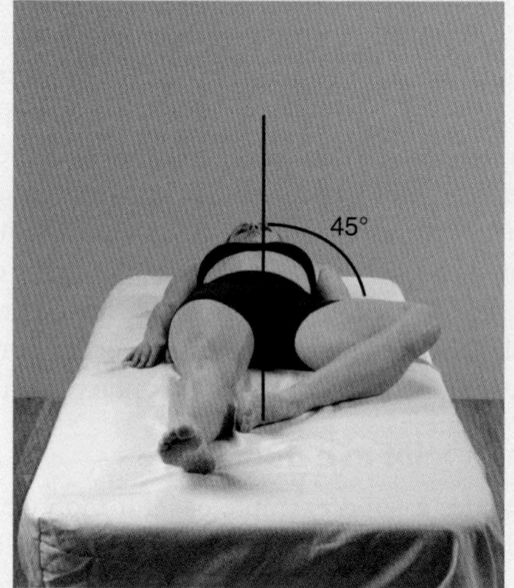

Hip lateral (extended rotator 0 to 45 degrees).

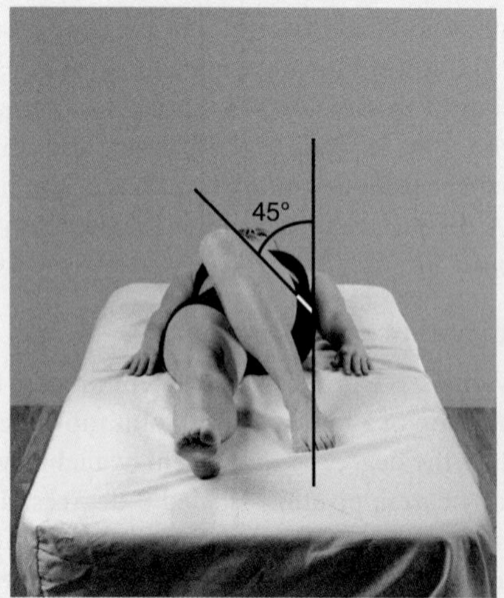

Hip medial (internal) rotation 0 to 45 degrees.

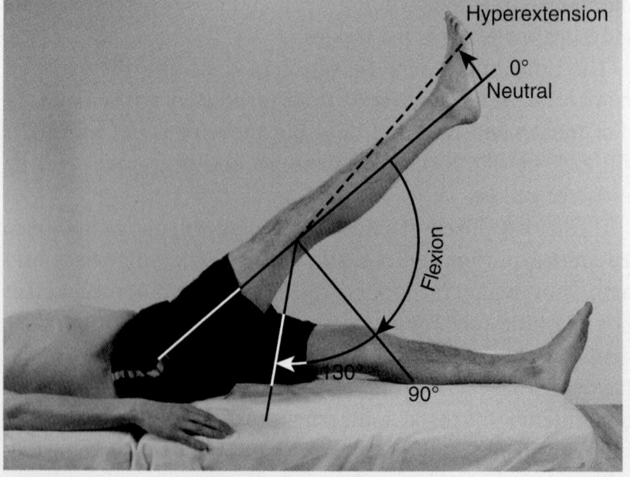

Knee flexion (0 to 130 degrees) and knee extension (120 to 0 degrees).

Box 10.6 Normal Range of Motion for Major Joints—cont'd

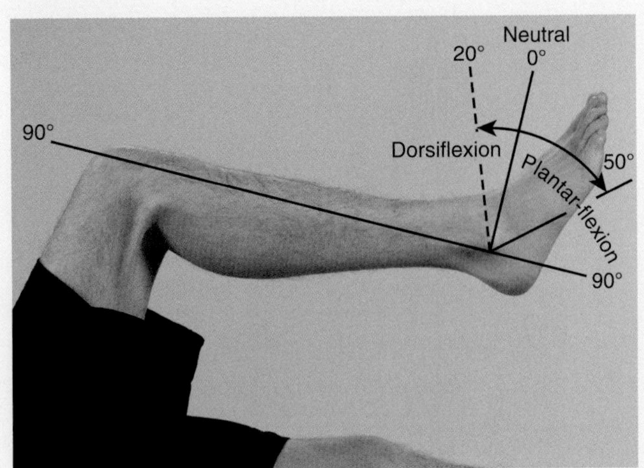

Ankle plantar flexion (0 to 50 degrees) and ankle dorsiflexion (0 to 20 degrees).

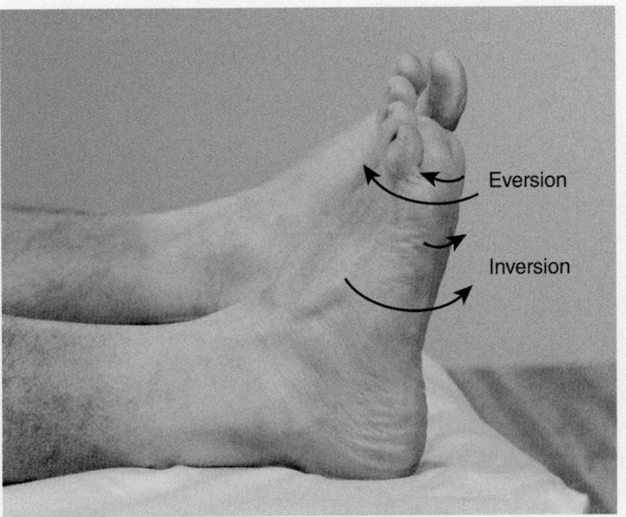

Foot inversion (0 to 35 degrees) and foot eversion (0 to 25 degrees).

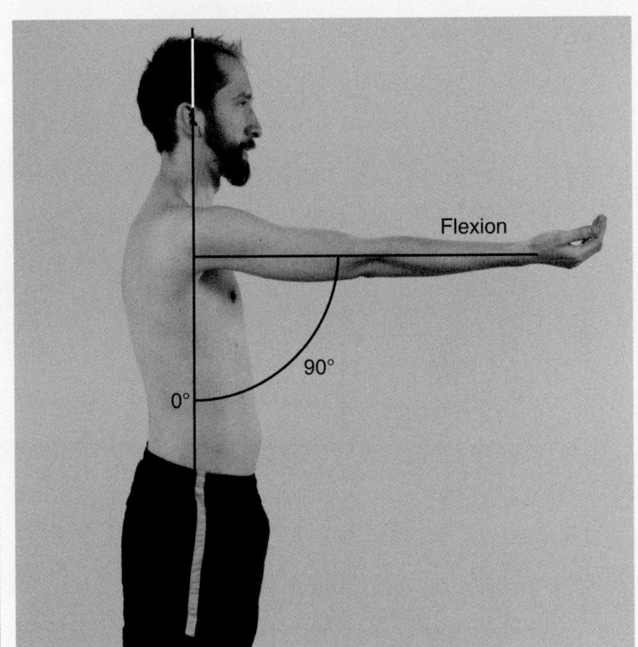

Shoulder flexion (0 to 90 degrees) and shoulder extension (90 to 0 degrees).

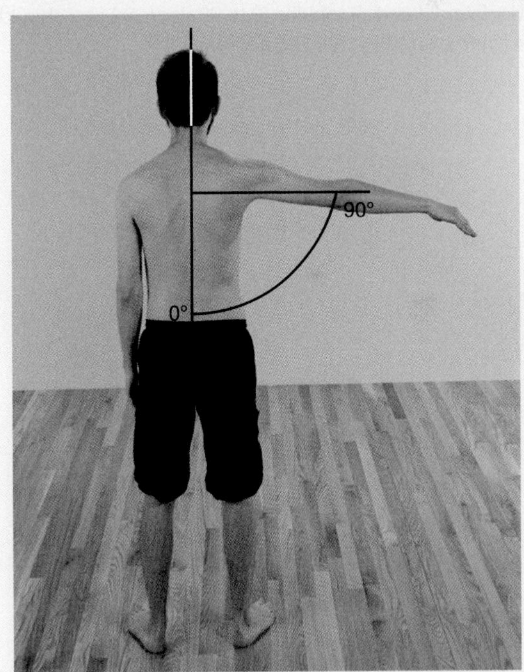

Shoulder abduction (0 to 90 degrees) and shoulder adduction (90 to 0 degrees).

Continued

Box 10.6 Normal Range of Motion for Major Joints—cont'd

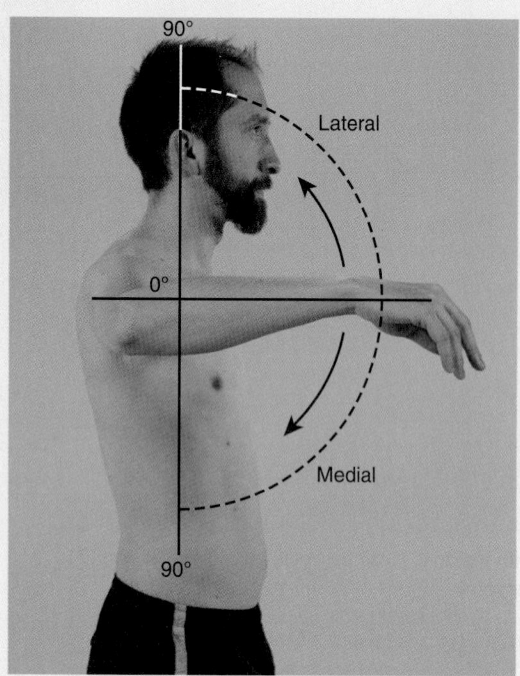

Shoulder lateral (medial) rotation (0 to 90 degrees) and shoulder medial (internal) rotation (0 to 90 degrees).

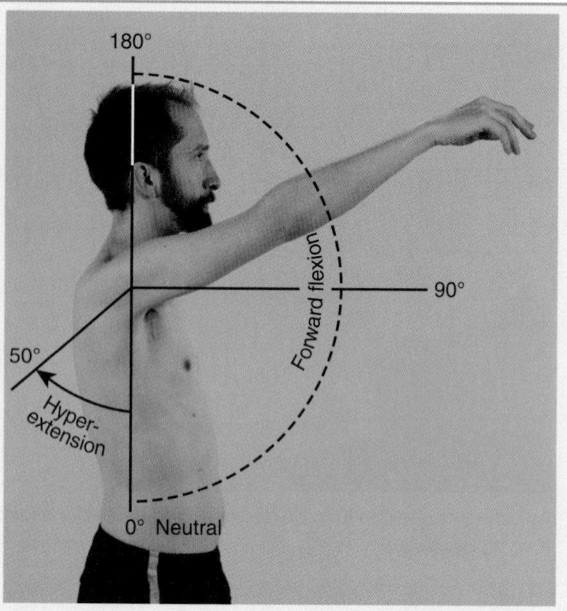

Combined shoulder and scapular movement forward flexion (0 to 180 degrees); extension (180 to 0 degrees).

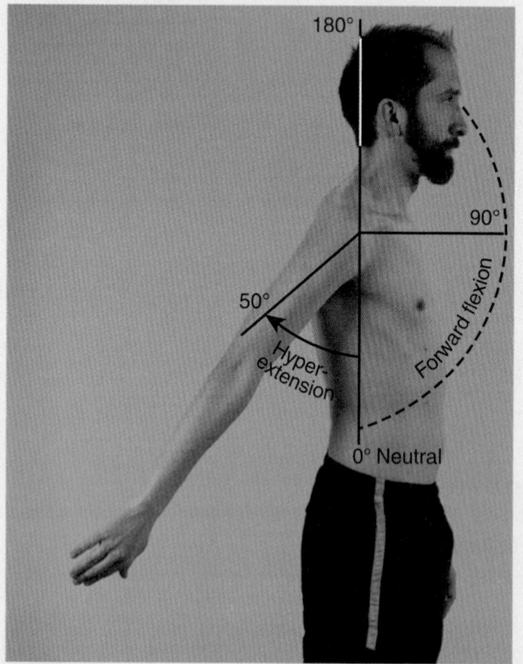

Combined shoulder and scapular movement hyperextension (0 to 50 degrees).

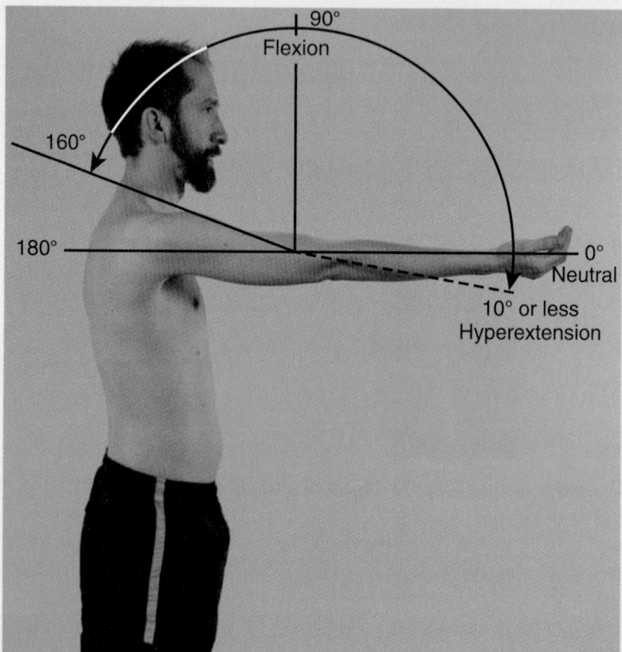

Elbow flexion (0 to 160 degrees); elbow extension (160 to 0 degrees); elbow hyperextension (0 to 10 degrees).

Box 10.6 Normal Range of Motion for Major Joints—cont'd

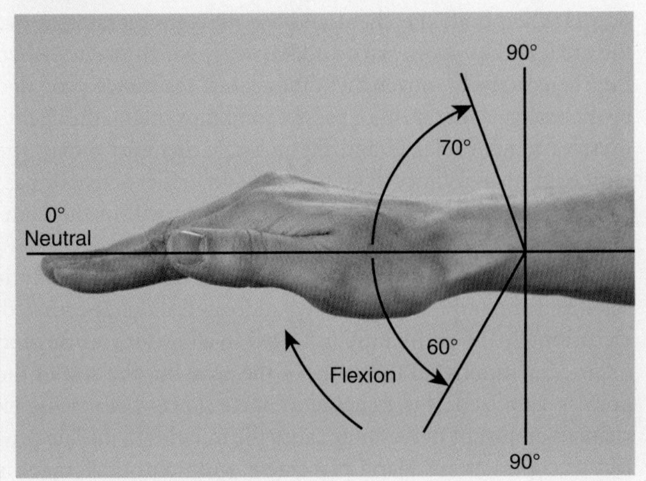

Wrist flexion (0 to 60 degrees); wrist extension (0 to 70 degrees).

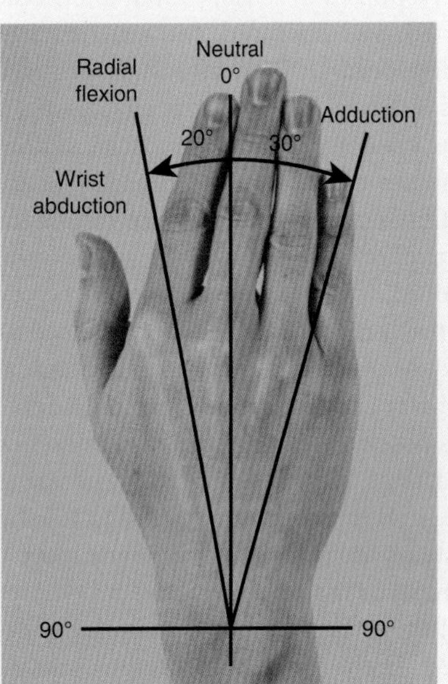

Wrist abduction (0 to 20 degrees); wrist adduction (0 to 30 degrees).

not have the textbook range of motion does not mean that what is displayed is abnormal. Abnormality is indicated by nonoptimal function. This can be either a limit (hypomobility) or an exaggeration (hypermobility) in the "textbook normal" range of motion. Study Box 10.6 carefully. When working with clients, use it as a guide for moving each joint through its full range of motion, as both a general massage application and a major assessment process. Always remember to move slowly and stay within the client's comfort limits. (A video of a joint movement sequence is presented on the Evolve website.)

Relationship of Joint Movement to Elongation Methods

Joint movement is the way we position an area for elongation. Joint movement is how we position an area to apply muscle energy techniques (discussed later) that will elongate short tissues. For this reason, the massage professional should concentrate on developing the ability to use joint movement efficiently and effectively.

Physiological Influences

Theories of Effects for Joint Movement Methods

Joint movement is effective because it provides a means of controlled stimulation to the joint mechanoreceptors. Movement initiates muscle tension readjustment through the reflex center of the spinal cord and lower brain centers. As positions change, the supported movement gives the nervous system an entirely different set of signals to process. The joint sensory receptors can learn not to be so hypersensitive. As a result, the protective spasm and movement restriction may lessen.

Joint movement also encourages lubrication of the joint and contributes an important addition to the lymphatic and venous circulations. Much of the pumping action that moves these fluids in the vessels results from compression against the lymph and blood vessels during joint movement and muscle contraction. The tendons, ligaments, and joint capsule are warmed from the movement. This mechanical effect helps keep these tissues pliable. The passive and active joint movement and muscle energy techniques presented in this chapter work with the neuromuscular reflex system to lengthen short tissues. In contrast, stretching has both a neurological and a mechanical aspect. Joint movement should be regularly incorporated into the massage session. Precise and aggressive stretching should only be cautiously used as an intervention.

A working knowledge of the proprioceptive interaction between the prime mover (muscle shortening) and the antagonist (muscle elongating), in addition to body-wide reflex patterns, is necessary to understand and implement massage techniques based on movement. With this knowledge, the massage therapist can choose methods that encourage a reset to a more normal or neutral muscular function state, which allows the optimum range of functioning. The neuromuscular mechanism (nerve muscle fascia unit) adjusts based on the information it receives. If the information is clear and accurate, the muscle structures operate as designed; if the information is unclear, incorrect, or inconsistent, imbalances can occur.

For example, if a client spends the day talking on the phone by holding the phone with the shoulder, the lateral neck flexors and shoulder elevators are held short (tight, concentric action), whereas the other side of the neck is held long (taut, eccentric action). An adaptation takes place, and painful resistance occurs when the neck muscles are used differently from the new reset position. This type of interaction is responsible for some types of muscle discomfort or reduced functioning.

Muscle system imbalances result because the body adapts to a different muscle spindle set point and a new muscle resting length (usually shortened). As altered function perpetuates, the central nervous system may become less precise in interpretation and response to signaling from sensory receptors. Motor responses to sensory input often become exaggerated, distorted, and confused. Movement becomes labored, and stiffening occurs. The stiffness is primarily related to changes in soft tissue–related connective tissue, especially fascia. Nervous system regulation of fascial stiffness (densification) contributes to stability and mobility of soft tissue. Imbalance of this regulatory mechanism results in increased or decreased myofascial tonus coupled with diminished neuromuscular coordination. Interpretation in the central nervous system can result in pain behavior and reduced function. Massage techniques can provide clearer neurological information so that the body can restore optimum function or as close to optimum as possible. Massage can also influence the stiffness of the fascia. This allows the body's homeostatic mechanism to restore neutral muscle positions and to redefine the central nervous system's internal perceptual body map.

All the massage manipulations described previously affect proprioception reflexively but usually have a general, nonspecific effect. In the sections that follow, you will learn ways to deliver accurate, specific information to the neuromuscular system that supports normal functioning. The difference is similar to providing a general announcement to a group of people (massage manipulations) and calling out individuals' names and delivering a message (movement techniques).

Caution in Working With Joints

Joint-specific work, including any type of high-velocity thrust manipulation, is beyond the scope of practice of the massage professional. Because of the interplay among the joint proprioceptors, muscle tone, fascial tone, innervation of the joint, and surrounding muscles by the same nerve pattern, any damage to a joint can cause long-term problems. Working within the physiological ranges of motion for the particular client is within the scope of practice of the massage professional. Specific corrective and rehabilitative procedures for pathological range of motion related to hypermobility, hypomobility, changes in joint end-feel, and painful or stiff movement are best applied in a supervised medical care setting as part of a multidisciplinary team or as part of a comprehensive care plan with oversite.

Application of Joint Movement Techniques

Types of Joint Movement Methods

NOTE: Range of motion (ROM) is the measurement of the distance and direction a joint can move. Joint movement is performed to assess the range of motion of a joint. Range of motion is an assessment finding, not a method. Joint movement is an action and therefore can be a method. However, confusion exists related to terminology. The terms *active range of motion* (AROM), *passive range of motion* (PROM), *active assisted range of motion* (AAROM), and *active resisted range of motion* (ARROM) may be used instead of joint movement terms used in this text.

Joint movement involves moving the jointed areas within the client's physiological limits of range of motion. The two types of joint movement are **active joint movement** and **passive joint movement**. In active joint movement, the client moves the joint by active contraction of muscle groups. The two variations of active joint movement are **active assisted movement**, which occurs when both the client and the massage therapist move the area, and **active resistive movement**, which occurs when the client actively moves the joint against resistance provided by the massage therapist. In passive joint movement, the client's muscles remain relaxed and the massage therapist moves the joint with no assistance from the client. Whether active or passive, joint movements are always performed within the comfortable limits of the client's range of motion.

When using joint movement methods, the client's body is stabilized and only the joint being addressed should be moved. Occasionally the entire limb is moved to allow for coordinated interaction among all the joints of the area, but the rest of the body is stabilized. It is essential to move slowly, because quick changes or abrupt moves may cause the muscles to initiate protective contractions. Hand placement with joint movement is important. Make sure the area is not squeezed, pinched, or restricted in its movement pattern. One hand should be placed close to the joint to act as a stabilizer and allow evaluation. The other hand is placed at the distal end of the bone; this is the hand that actually provides the movement. The stabilizing hand must remain in contact with the client and must be placed near the affected joint. As an alternative method of positioning the stabilizing hand, the jointed area can be moved without stabilization while the massage therapist observes where the client's body moves most in response to the range of motion action. The stabilizing hand then is placed at this point.

Active Joint Movement

In active joint movement, the client moves the area without any interaction by the massage therapist. This is a good assessment method and should be used before and after any type of soft tissue work because it provides information about the limits of range of motion and the improvement after the work is complete. Active joint movement is also great to teach as a self-help tool. As mentioned previously, the two variations of active joint movement are active assisted methods and active resistive methods.

Active Assisted Joint Movement. In active assisted joint movement, the client moves the joint through the range of motion and the massage therapist helps or assists the movement. This approach is useful in cases of weakness or pain with movement. The action remains within the comfortable limits of movement for the client. The focus is to create movement within the joint capsule, encourage synovial fluid lubricant, warm and soften connective tissue, and support muscle function.

Active Resistive Joint Movement. In active resistive joint movement, the massage therapist firmly grasps and holds the end of the bone just distal to the affected joint. The massage therapist leans back slightly to place a slight traction on the limb to take up the slack in the tissue. The therapist then instructs the client to push slowly against a stabilizing hand or arm while the therapist moves the joint through its entire range of motion. A tap or light push against the limb to begin the movement works well to focus the client's attention.

Another method is to stabilize the entire circumference of the limb and instruct the client to pull gently or move the area. The massage therapist's job is to maintain a gentle traction to prevent slack in the tissue, keep the movement slow, and give the client something to push or pull against, discharging the nervous system so that the area can relax.

The counterforce applied by the massage therapist does not exceed the pushing or pulling action of the client, but rather matches it and then allows movement.

Passive Joint Movement

If a client is paralyzed or extremely ill, only passive joint movement may be possible. Some clients do not wish to participate in active joint movement and prefer to take a passive role during the massage. Client participation is not necessary. When performing passive joint movement, the massage therapist should feel for the soft or hard end-feel of the joint range of motion. This is an important evaluation for determining the state of the joint and associated tissues.

Proper use of body mechanics is essential when performing passive joint movement that may require lifting action by the massage practitioner. The massage practitioner should not perform passive joint movement if they feel as if the activity and effort could cause them injury. Avoid working cross-body. Usually, the hand closest to the joint is the stabilizing hand. The actual movement comes from the massage therapist's whole body, not from the shoulder, elbow, or wrist. The movements are rhythmic, smooth, slow, and controlled. Before joint movement begins, the moving hand lifts the area, and the therapist leans back to produce the slight traction necessary to put a small stretch on the joint capsule. If this is not done, the technique is much less effective. When tractioning has been mastered and the joint is moved simultaneously, the size of the movement becomes smaller and the effectiveness increases. It is neither necessary nor desirable to have the client's limbs flailing about in the air (Fig. 10.29).

Because of the protective system of the joints it takes time to prepare the body for passive joint movement. Shaking, rocking, and the active joint movement sequence previously described work well for this purpose. To perform passive joint movement methods, instruct the client to relax the area by letting it lie heavy in your hands. Slowly and rhythmically move the joint through a comfortable range of motion for the jointed area. Repeat the action three or more times, increasing the limits of the range of motion as the muscles relax (Proficiency Exercise 10.9).

PROFICIENCY EXERCISE 10.9

1. Using Box 10.6 for reference, move each of your joints, using a variety of speeds, one at a time, through the normal range of motion. Notice the difference when you move slowly.
2. Pretend that a piece of plastic wrap is a joint. Hold one end tightly in your "stabilizing" hand. Now move the plastic wrap around, but do not stretch it or put drag on the "tissue." Use your "moving hand" to traction the plastic wrap. Pull on it as far as it will go without stretching the tissue. Pretend to assess range of motion from this point and feel the difference. Last, pull the plastic wrap just a little more. Feel the pliability and do the joint movement from this position. Feel for the difference in effect.
3. Design and perform a massage incorporating joint movement. As always, remain aware of the variation in depth of pressure, drag, direction, speed, rhythm, frequency, and duration.

PROFICIENCY EXERCISE 10.10

1. Design a progressive relaxation sequence for yourself using the concept of antagonist contract and then relax.
2. Design a lengthening sequence for yourself using pulsed muscle contraction.
3. Experiment with positional release concepts to relax sore spots on your body.
4. Design a complete massage incorporating all the muscle energy methods presented.
5. Repeat the massage sequence in the General Massage Protocol at the end of the chapter from step 5 using the "making it simple" pattern. Compare the results.

Suggested Sequence for Joint Movement Methods

When incorporating joint movement into the massage, follow these basic suggestions:

- If possible, perform active joint movement first. Assess range of motion by having the client move the area without participation by the therapist.
- Have the client move the area against a stabilizing force supplied by the therapist to increase the intensity of the signals from the contracting muscles.
- Incorporate any or all of the previously discussed massage methods.
- After the tissue is warm and the nervous system calmed, perform passive joint movement.
- During a massage session, strive to move every joint approximately three times. The first movement is to assess whether the range of motion is appropriate, hypermobile, or hypomobile. If the joint is hypomobile, take up any slack in the tissues and gently encourage an increase in the range of motion. If the area is hypermobile, do not increase the mobility. Only move the joint within the physiological range.
- Joint movement should be incorporated into every massage, when possible (Proficiency Exercise 10.10).

MUSCLE ENERGY TECHNIQUES

SECTION OBJECTIVES

Chapter objectives covered in this section:

4. Incorporate muscle energy techniques into the massage application.
5. Incorporate elongation methods into the massage application when appropriate.

Using the information presented in this section, the learner will be able to perform the following:

- Identify the types of muscle energy techniques.

Muscle energy techniques are used to increase tolerance to stretch sensation in some elongation methods. Methods that involve client muscle contraction against practitioners' counterforce have different names based on the discipline. These methods are known as *muscle energy technique* (MET), a term used by osteopathic physicians and in the massage community largely due to the influence of Dr. Leon Chaitow; *autogenic inhibition* (AI), the term used by chiropractors; and *proprioceptive neuromuscular facilitation* (PNF), the term used by physical therapists (Newey et al., 2018) (Box 10.7).

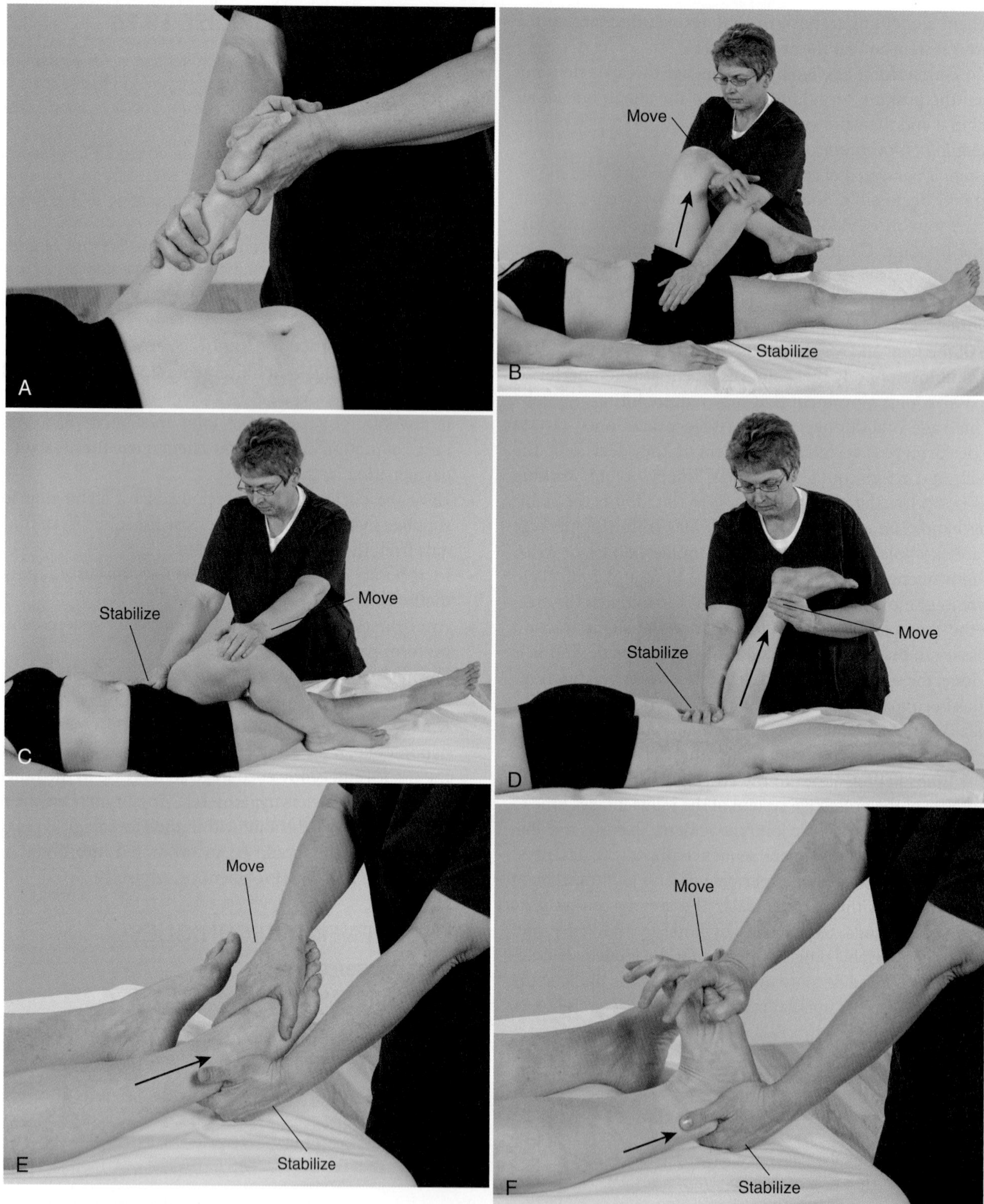

FIG. 10.29 Examples of joint movement. A, Wrist joint. The stabilizing hand holds below the wrist while the moving hand produces a slight traction and moves the joint through circumduction. (*Circumduction* is a circular movement of a jointed area.) **B,** Hip joint. The stabilizing hand holds above the anterosuperior iliac spine while the moving hand and arm produce a slight traction and move the joint through circumduction. **C,** Hip joint (alternate position). The stabilizing hand holds at the hip while the moving hand moves the hip through internal and external rotation. No traction is produced in this position. **D,** Knee. The stabilizing hand holds above the knee while the moving hand produces a slight traction and moves the joint through flexion and extension. **E, F,** Ankle. The stabilizing hand holds above the ankle. The moving hand produces a slight traction and moves the joint through circumduction.

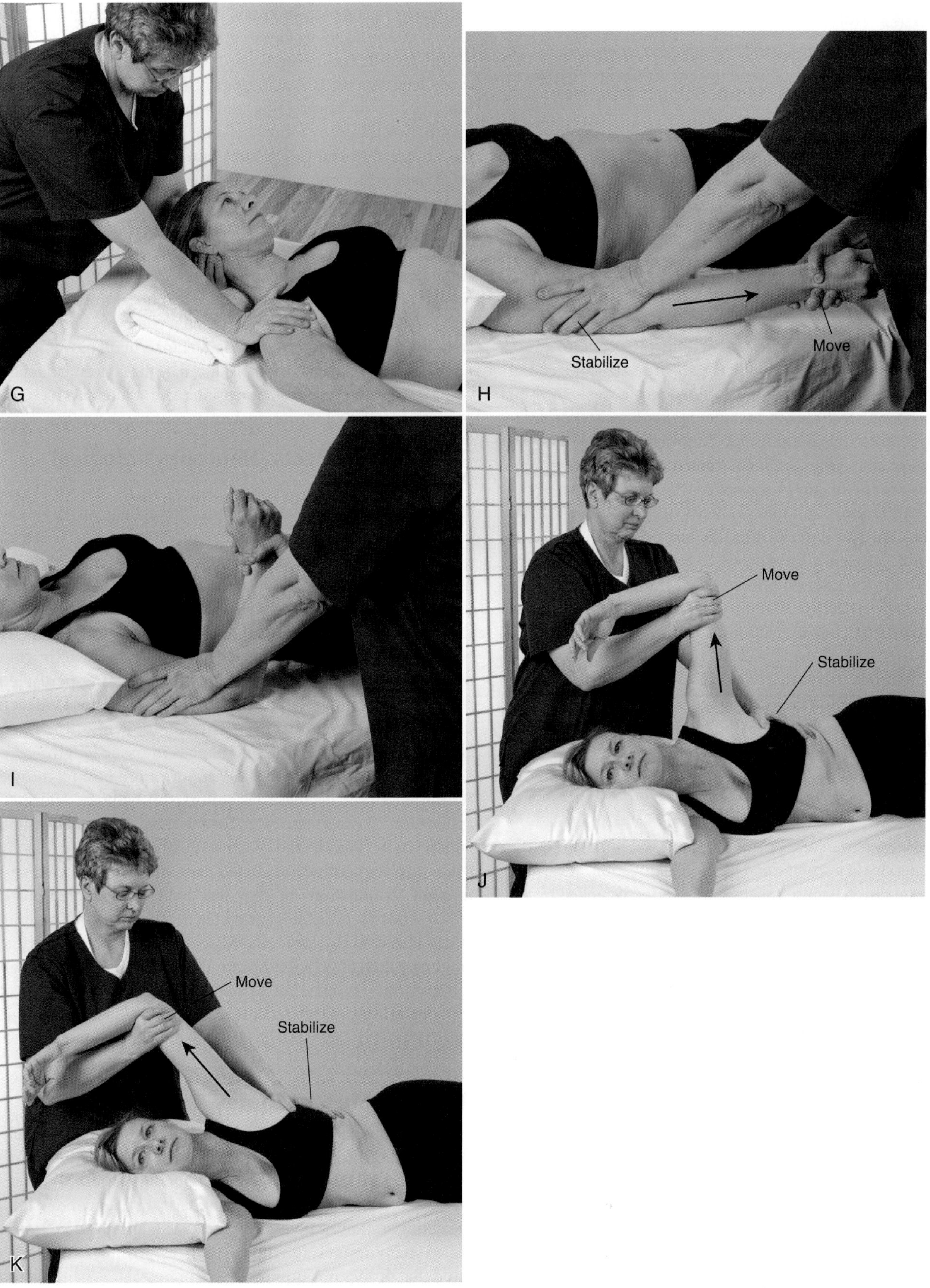

FIG. 10.29, Cont'd G, Neck. The stabilizing hand holds at the occipital base and produces slight traction while the moving hand moves the shoulder toward the feet. **H, I,** Elbow joint. The stabilizing hand holds above the elbow while the moving hand produces a slight traction and moves the joint through flexion and extension. Supination and pronation can also be achieved. **J, K,** Shoulder joint. One hand stabilizes at the shoulder joint. The other hand produces a slight traction to the shoulder joint and moves the shoulder through circumduction range of motion.

Box 10.7 Pioneers in Muscle Energy Techniques

Dr. T.J. Ruddy: Developed resistive induction technique.
Dr. Fred K. Mitchell: The father of muscle energy techniques. He built on Dr. Ruddy's method, turning it into a whole-body approach (Greenman, 2010).
Dr. Karel Lewit: Described the importance of methods that use post-isometric relaxation (Lewit, 1998).
Dr. Leon Chaitow: Synthesized the methods of Ruddy, Mitchell, and Lewit.
Margaret Knott and Dorothy Voss: Wrote the first book on proprioceptive neuromuscular facilitation techniques, which grew out of physical therapy approaches during the 1950s (Knott and Voss, 1985).

Muscle energy techniques fall within the scope of practice of therapeutic massage when they are used for general body normalization. Other names for approaches based on muscle energy techniques include *manual resistance techniques, contract-relax–antagonist contract (CRAC),* and *active isolated stretching.* The main differences among common methods are the origin of the approach, the intensity of the muscle contraction, and the specificity of the approach. Massage techniques as described in this text are incorporated as nonspecific aspects of a general massage. However, adaptive methods for intervention are used if massage outcomes are based on condition management or therapeutic change (see Chapter 6). Just as friction is an adaptive intervention method used only if changes in the tissue are desired, muscle energy methods are used as intervention approaches to address shortened muscles and associated soft tissues and support optimum muscle, soft tissue, or joint function (Burns and Wells, 2006; Chaitow and Fritz, 2023).

Description

Muscle energy techniques involve a voluntary contraction of the client's muscles in a specific and controlled direction, at varying levels of intensity, against a specific counterforce applied by the massage therapist. Muscle energy procedures have a variety of applications and are considered active techniques in which the client contributes the corrective force. The amount of effort may vary from a small muscle twitch to the maximum muscle contraction. The duration may be a fraction of a second to several seconds. All contractions begin and end slowly, gradually building to the desired intensity. No jerking is done in the movement.

The focus of muscle energy techniques is to stimulate the nervous system to allow a more normal muscle resting length. The **direction of ease** is the way the body allows for postural changes and muscle shortening or weakening compensation patterns, depending on its balance in gravity. Although compensation patterns may be inefficient, the patterns developed serve a purpose and need to be respected. It may seem logical to locate a shortened muscle structure (including fascia) or a rotated movement pattern and use direct methods to reverse the pattern. However, this may not be the best approach. Protective sensory receptors prevent any forced stretch out of a compensation pattern. Instead, the pattern of compensation is respected, and the body position is exaggerated and coaxed into a more efficient position by moving the body out of a position causing discomfort and into the direction it wants to go, thereby taking proprioception into a state of safety, which may allow it to stop signaling for protective spasm.

The term **lengthening** is used to describe this process, because lengthening is a neurological response that allows the muscles to stop contracting and return to a normal resting length. **Stretching** is more correctly defined as a mechanical force applied to elongate tissue. However, the terms are used interchangeably, which can be confusing.

Muscle energy techniques focus on specific muscle groups that form functional units. For example, a functional unit would be the medial compartment of the thigh that adducts the thigh. Another example is the functional unit of hip extension. It is almost impossible to isolate a specific anatomical muscle as seen in the textbooks. Muscles are packaged together within fascia to work together. It is more logical to think in terms of movement at joints, such as wrist extension produced by the concentric action of the wrist extensors, or shoulder internal rotation produced by concentric action of the internal rotators of the shoulder.

Theories of Effects: Neurophysiological Principles

Two neurophysiological principles have been used to explain the effect of muscle energy techniques as a result of physiological laws, not of mechanical force, as in stretching. These principles are **postisometric relaxation (PIR) and reciprocal inhibition (RI)**. However, research indicates that the physiological mechanism for benefit may not be directly related to PIR or RI. Rather, any type of muscle activation seems to increase tolerance to stretch by altering perceived pain and stretching sensation. In addition, some evidence indicates that the connective tissue component of the muscle is influenced, allowing for changes in tissue length.

Muscle energy techniques to support more normal muscle resting length and decrease discomfort is an evidence-informed application (Payla et al., 2018; Saadat et al., 2018; Shinde and Jagtap, 2018; Wendt and Waszak 2020). Pain reduction by MET involves centrally mediated pain inhibitory mechanisms through stimulation of low-threshold mechanoreceptors, which leads to possible gating effects. There may also be an effect related to rhythmic muscular contraction on interstitial and tissue fluid flow (Rayudu and Alagingi, 2018). Even though the scientific rationale for benefit is changing, the process of applying muscle energy techniques remains basically the same; these techniques are described in the following sections.

Applying Muscle Energy Techniques

Muscle groups should be positioned so that the proximal muscle attachment (origin) and the distal attachment (insertion) are either close together or in a lengthening phase with the attachments separated. Study muscle charts until you understand the configuration of the muscle structures and practice isolating as many muscle functional units as possible, keeping in mind that proper positioning is very important. When practicing, make sure the muscles can be isolated whether the client is supine, prone, or in a side-lying or seated position (Fig. 10.30).

Counterpressure is the force applied to an area that is designed to match the effort or force exactly or partially. The person providing the resistance (the massage therapist) can apply this holding force with one or both hands, or it can be applied against an immovable object or against gravity where appropriate. The response to the method is specific to a certain muscle or muscle group, referred to as the target muscle (or muscles).

Types of Muscle Contractions

The massage therapist uses three types of muscle contraction to activate muscle energy techniques: *isometric contraction*, *isotonic contraction*, and *multiple isotonic contractions*.

In an isometric contraction, the distance between the proximal and distal attachments (origin and insertion) of the target muscle is maintained at a constant length. A fixed tension develops in the target muscle as the client contracts the muscle against an equal counterforce applied by the massage therapist; this prevents shortening of the muscle. In this contraction, the effort of the muscle or group of muscles is exactly matched by a counterpressure so that no movement occurs, only effort.

In an isotonic contraction, the effort of the target muscle or muscles is not quite matched by the counterpressure, which allows a degree of resisted movement. With a concentric isotonic contraction, the massage therapist applies a counterforce but allows the client to move the proximal and distal attachments of the target muscle together against the pressure. In an eccentric isotonic contraction (more accurately described as an eccentric isotonic action because the term *contraction* specifically describes a shortening, and eccentric action results in lengthening), the massage therapist applies a counterforce but allows the client to move the jointed area so that the proximal and distal attachments of the target muscle separate as the muscle lengthens against the pressure.

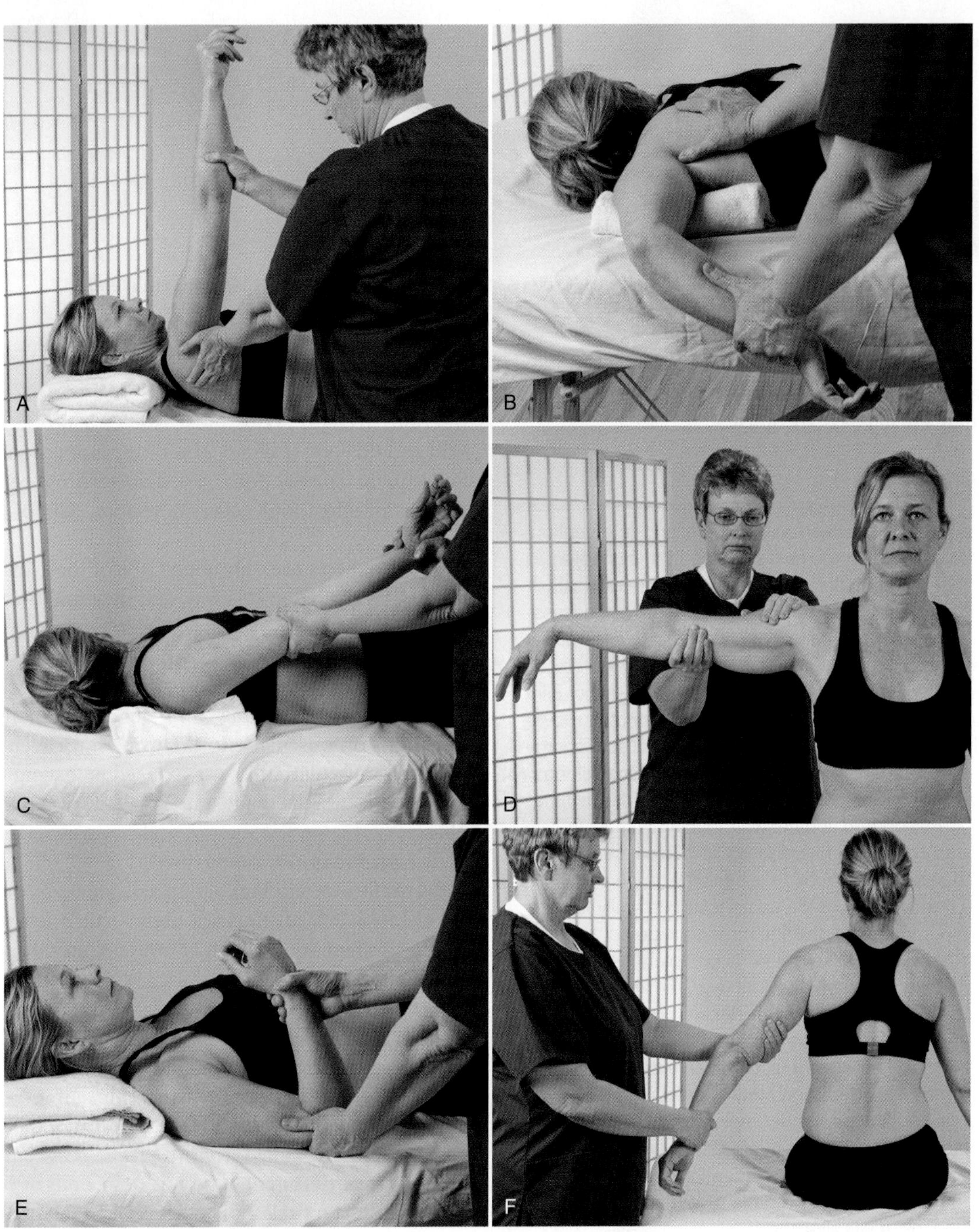

FIG. 10.30 Positions for muscle isolation. A, Serratus anterior. **B,** Subscapularis. **C,** Latissimus dorsi. **D,** Deltoid. **E,** Biceps and brachialis. **F,** Triceps.

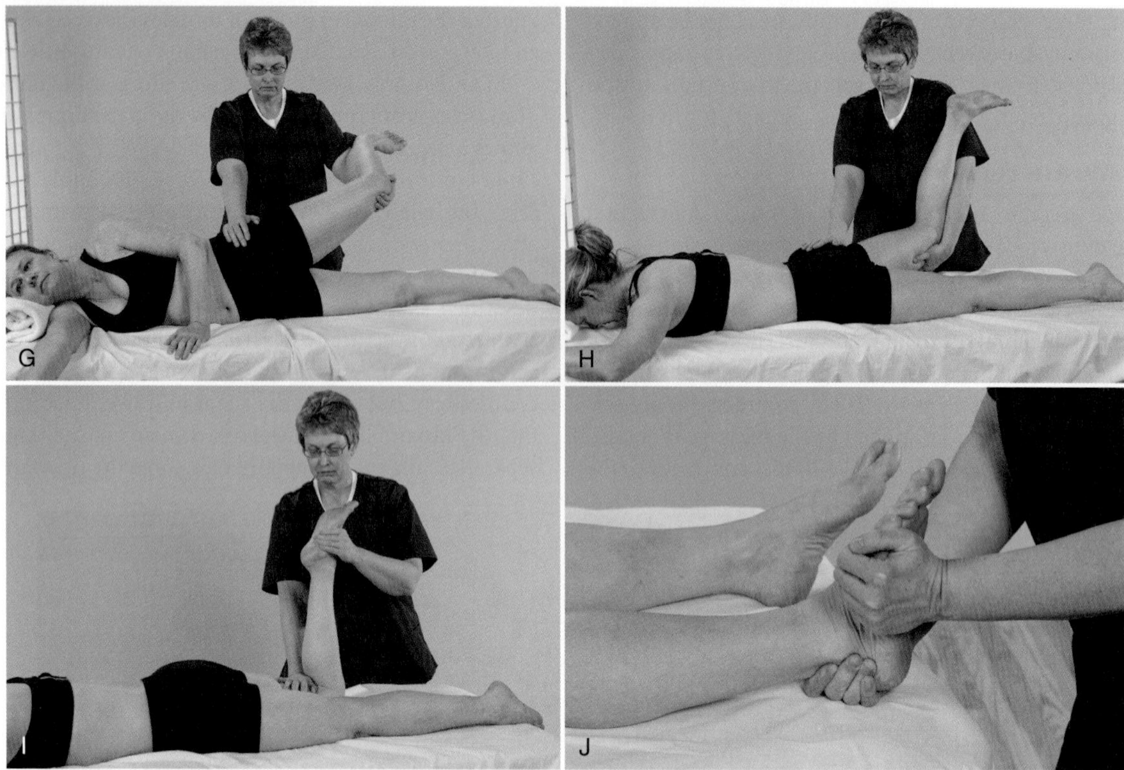

FIG. 10.30, Cont'd G, Gluteus medius. **H,** Gluteus maximus and hamstrings. **I,** Gastrocnemius and soleus. **J,** Fibularis.

Multiple isotonic contractions require the client to move the joint through a full range of motion against partial resistance applied by the massage therapist.

MENTORING TIP

There is a difference between assessment and intervention. Assessment is covered in the next chapter. In this chapter, as you learn about methods and modes of massage application, it may be difficult to recognize the difference between assessment and intervention, especially when we begin to learn about muscle energy techniques. Muscle energy techniques are an intervention. The method is used after assessment—either joint movement or tissue palpation—when there is restricted movement and the reason is shortened tissue. Then muscle energy techniques that support lengthening and stretching (elongation) are used as the intervention to change the tissue function toward normal. Stated another way, joint movement (active or passive) is used during massage on all jointed areas in the limbs on both sides of the body to assess the range of motion of the joints. If movement of the same joint bilaterally is similar and within normal range, the finding is considered "normal" and the joint movement assessment is complete. However, if movement differs and one of the joints (e.g., the knee) has less range of motion, the therapist must decide whether it is appropriate to introduce an intervention to assist the movement to be more normal. There are multiple intervention strategies. The area could be kneaded, or a slow glide could be used to elongate the tissue. Maybe the decision would be to use longitudinal stretching. If stretching is the choice, muscle energy methods are used as part of the intervention process to make the stretching more effective. Be patient with yourself. By the end of the textbook, it will all make much more sense.

Strength of Contraction

Muscle energy techniques do not use the client's full contraction strength. With most isometric work, the contraction should start at about 25% of the strength of the muscle. Subsequent contractions can involve progressively greater degrees of effort, but never more than 50% of the available strength.

Many experts use only about 10% of the available strength in muscles treated in this way, and they find that they can increase effectiveness by using longer periods of contraction. Pulsed contractions (a rapid series of repetitions) using minimal strength also are effective.

Coordinated breathing can be used to enhance particular directions of muscular effort. During muscle energy applications, all muscular effort is enhanced by having the client inhale as the effort is made and exhale during the lengthening phase.

Eye positions also can be used (Fig. 10.31). Looking down activates flexors and looking up activates extensors; when the client looks left, all muscles used to turn left are activated; when the client looks right, all muscles used to turn right are activated.

Agonist Contract

In muscle function terminology, the functional muscle unit that produces the movement by shortening and pulling is called the *agonist.* Muscle energy techniques using agonist contraction are called *contract/relax (CR)* and *hold/relax (HR).* In the brief latent period of 10 seconds or so after such a contraction, a muscle can be lengthened farther than it could before the contraction because of an increased tolerance to

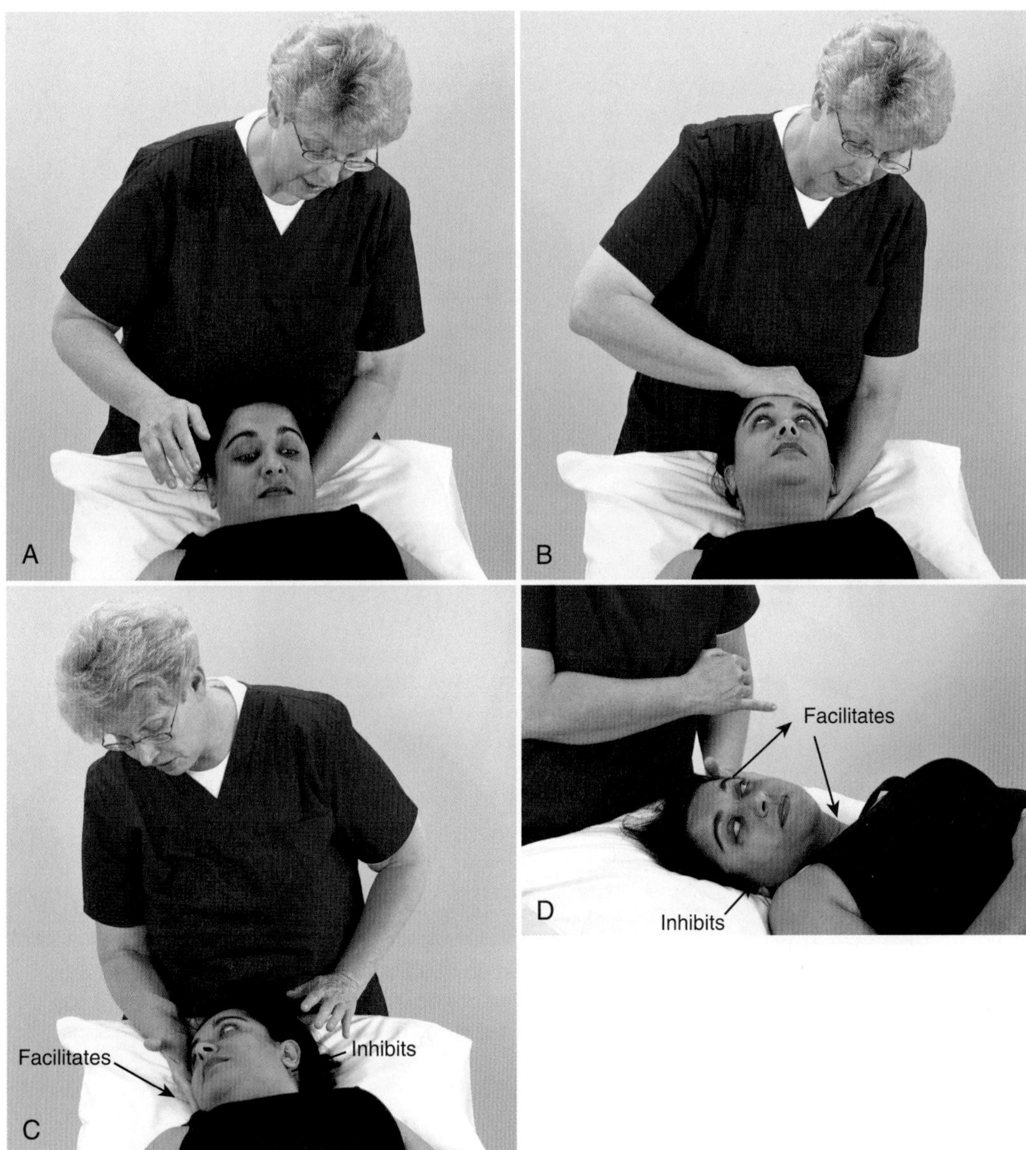

FIG. 10.31 Eye positions. A, Eyes down facilitates flexors. **B,** Eyes up facilitates extension and inhibits flexors. **C,** Eyes to the right facilitates muscles that move to the right and inhibits opposing muscles. **D,** Eyes to the left inhibits previously facilitated muscle and facilitates those previously inhibited.

the stretch sensation. After the contraction, the target muscle can be lengthened passively to its comfort barrier. The comfort barrier is the first point of resistance before the client perceives any discomfort at either the physiological or pathological barrier. The concept of bind discussed earlier in the chapter can be used interchangeably with the term *comfort barrier*. This may occur before the client's end range of motion is reached. The contraction of the target muscles involves minimal effort lasting 7 to 10 seconds. Repetitions continue until no further gain is noted or normal range of motion is achieved. The procedure for agonist contract methods is as follows (Fig. 10.32):

1. Lengthen the target muscle (agonist) to the comfort barrier (first indication of bind). Then back off slightly.
2. Tense the target muscle for 7 to 10 seconds.
3. Stop the contraction and lengthen the target muscle.
4. Repeat steps 1 through 3 until no results are achieved or the normal full resting length is obtained.

Antagonist Contract

Antagonist contract methods were thought to activate reciprocal inhibition in the opposing short muscles. RI takes place when a muscle contracts, causing its antagonist to function eccentrically (lengthen) to allow for more normal movement. Although this response is no longer considered the mechanism of action, using the antagonist of the target muscle is a MET variation. Such contractions usually begin in the midrange rather than near the barrier of resistance and last 7 to 10 seconds. The procedure for antagonist contract is as follows (Fig. 10.33):

1. Isolate the target muscles by putting them in passive contraction (the massage therapist moves the proximal and distal attachments of the muscles together using joint positioning).

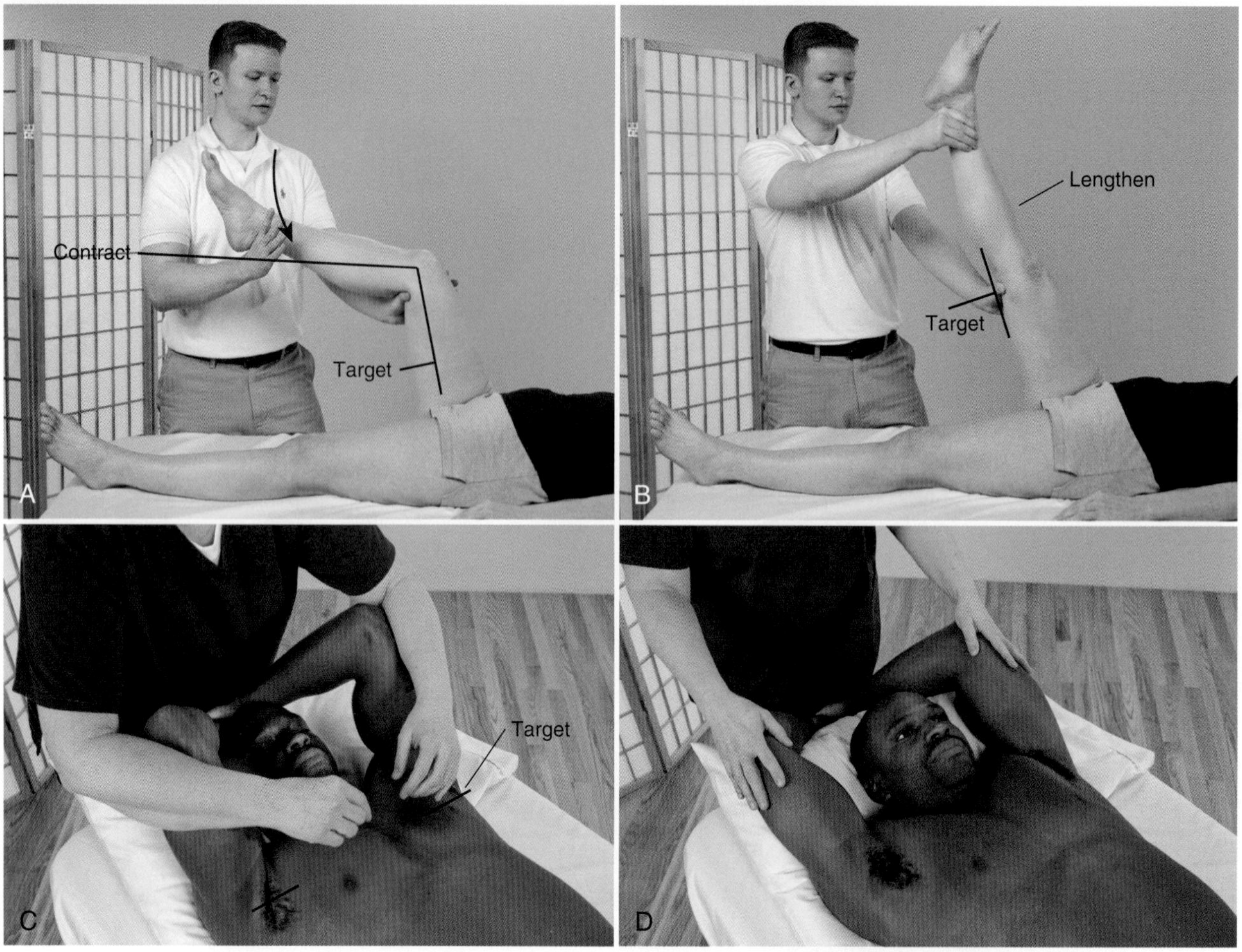

FIG. 10.32 Muscle energy techniques using agonist contract. A, Isolate target muscles (hamstrings and gastrocnemius), and have client contract by pushing calf down. **B,** Lengthen the target muscle. **C,** Isolate target muscles (latissimus dorsi and pectoralis major) and have client contract by pushing arms down toward chest. **D,** Relax and lengthen.

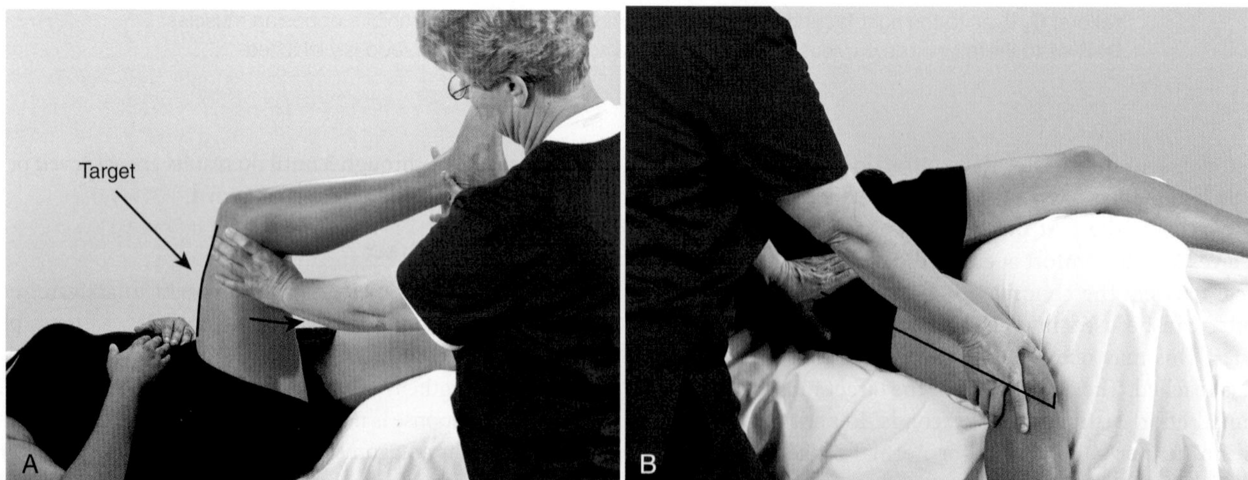

FIG. 10.33 Muscle energy technique using antagonist contraction. A, Antagonist contraction (hamstrings)—target quadriceps. **B,** Lengthen quadriceps.

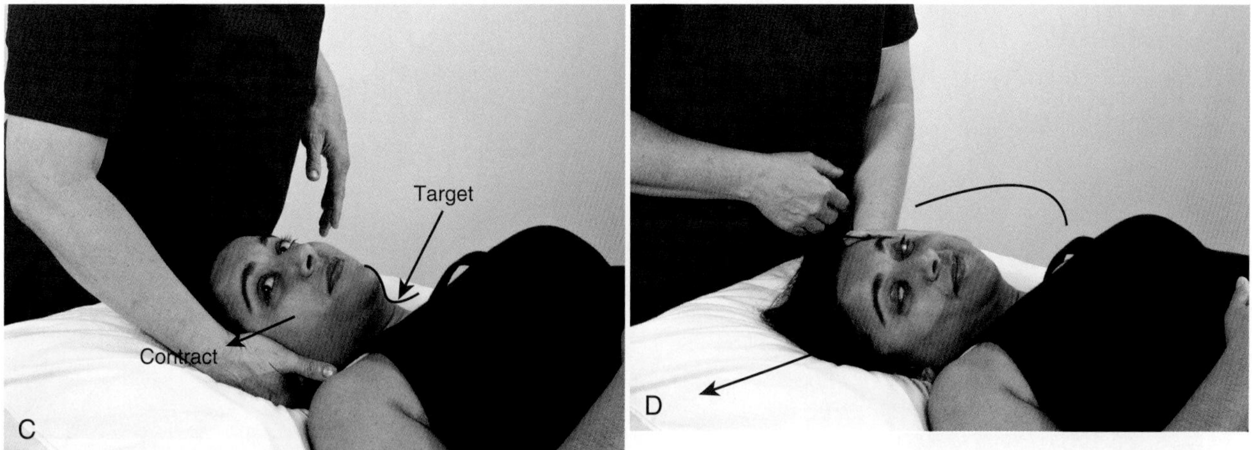

FIG. 10.33, Cont'd C, Identify antagonist muscles (lateral neck flexors) and contract antagonist. **D,** Lengthen target muscles.

2. Contract the antagonist muscle group (the muscle in extension).
3. Stop the contraction and slowly bring the target muscle into a lengthened state, stopping at resistance.
4. Place the target muscle slightly into passive contraction again.
5. Repeat steps 2 through 4 until no results are achieved or the normal full resting length is obtained.

Combined Methods: Agonist Contract–Relax–Antagonist Contract–Lengthen

The combined MET method (often called *CRAC,* or contract and relax and antagonist contract) can be used to enhance the lengthening effects. The procedure for CRAC is as follows (Fig. 10.34):

1. Position the target muscles as in agonist contract procedures.
2. Lengthen the target muscle to the barrier. Then back off slightly.
3. Contract the target muscle for 7 to 10 seconds, and then relax.
4. Contract the antagonist.
5. Stop the contraction of the antagonist.
6. Lengthen the target muscle to a more normal resting length.

Pulsed Muscle Energy Procedures

Pulsed muscle energy procedures involve engaging the comfort barrier and using small, resisted contractions (usually 20 in 10 seconds). The procedure for pulsed muscle energy is as follows (Fig. 10.35):

1. Isolate the target muscle by putting it into a passive contraction.
2. Apply counterpressure for the contraction.
3. Instruct the client to contract the target muscle rapidly in small movements for about 20 repetitions. Go to step 4 or use this variation: Maintain the position but switch the counterpressure location to the opposite side and have the client contract the antagonist muscles for 20 repetitions.
4. Slowly lengthen the target muscle.
5. Repeat steps 2 to 4 until the normal full resting length is obtained.

NOTE: All contracting and resisting efforts should start and finish gently.

Direct Applications

In some circumstances the client does not want to participate actively in the massage or cannot. The principles of muscle energy techniques can still be used through direct manipulation of the muscle tissue. Pushing muscle fibers together in the direction of the fibers in the belly of a muscle may reduce tone. Pushing muscle fibers together in the belly of the muscle is a way to relieve a muscle cramp. This is sometimes called **approximation**.

Separating the muscle fibers in the belly of the muscle in the direction of the fibers is thought to strengthen the muscle. Manipulation of the muscle or at the ends of the muscle where it joins the tendons is also an option. To inhibit the muscle, separate the tendon attachments of the target muscle. To strengthen the muscle, push the tendon attachments together. The pressure levels used to elicit the response must be sufficient to contact the muscle fibers. Pressure that is too light does not access the proprioceptors, and excessive pressure negates the response by activating protective reflexes. Moderate pressure, which allows the muscle itself to be palpated, is most effective.

Direct Manipulation to Initiate the Relaxation and Lengthening Response

The procedure is as follows (Fig. 10.36):

1. Place the target muscle in comfortable passive extension.
2. Press the tissues together on the target muscle.
3. Pull the tissues apart on the antagonist muscle.
4. Lengthen the target muscle.

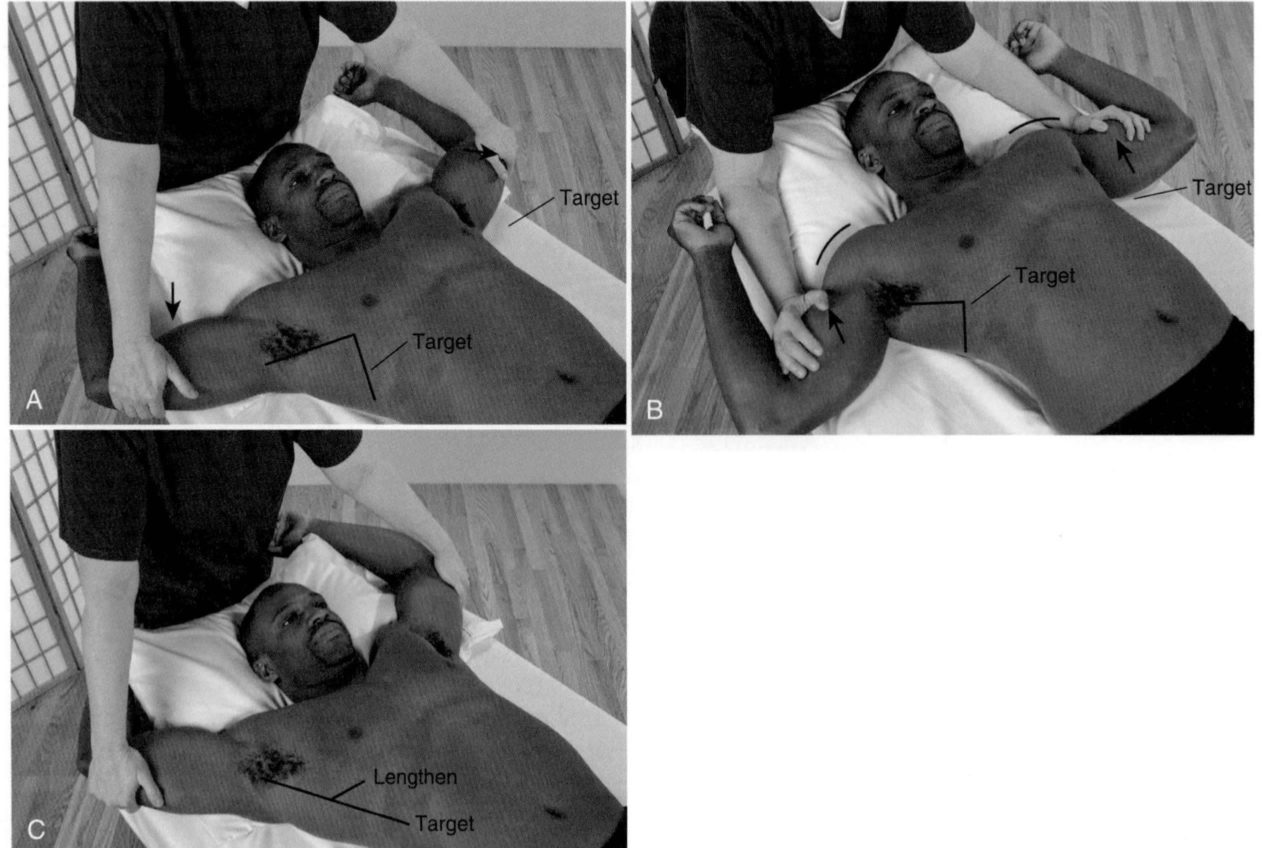

FIG. 10.34 A, Example of agonist contract–relax–antagonist contract (CRAC). Contract target muscles and then relax. **B,** Contract antagonist muscles. **C,** Relax and lengthen target muscles.

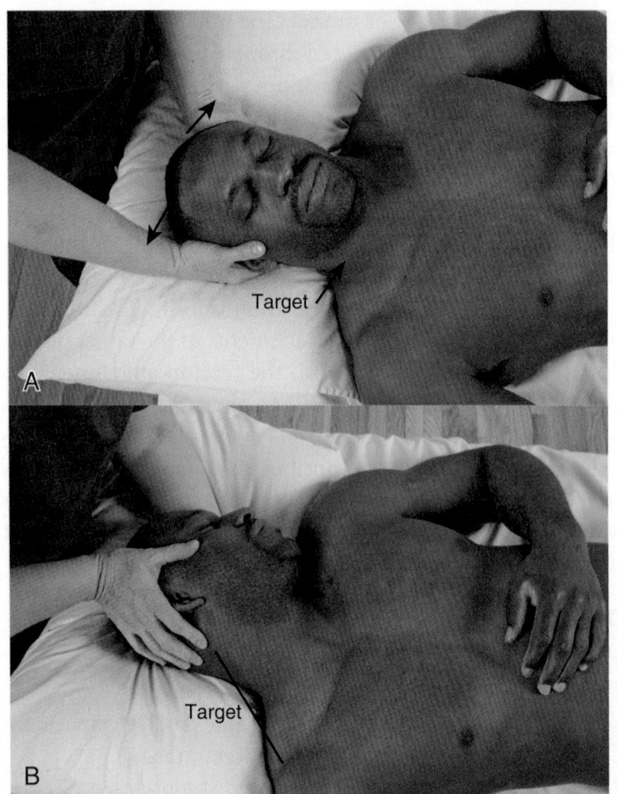

FIG. 10.35 Pulsed muscle energy. A, Target muscle at upper trapezius. Hold area firmly and have client move back and forth. **B,** Lengthen target muscle.

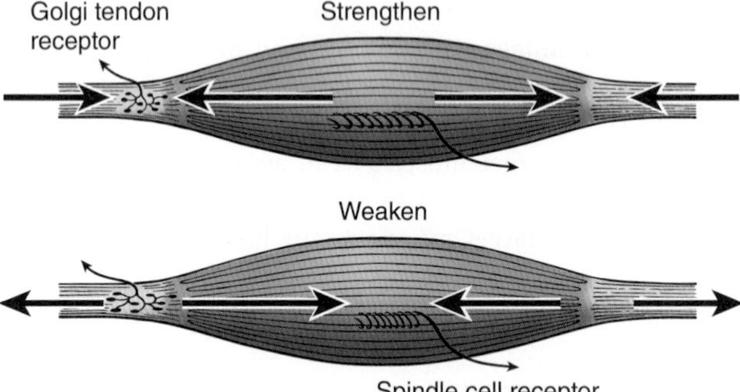

FIG. 10.36 Proprioceptive manipulation of muscles. Modified from Chaitow L: *Modern neuromuscular techniques,* Edinburgh, 1996, Churchill Livingstone.

5. Repeat steps 2 through 4 until no results are achieved or the normal full resting length is obtained.

Direct Manipulation of the Golgi Tendon Organs to Initiate the Lengthening Response

The procedure is as follows (Fig. 10.37):

1. Place the target muscle in comfortable passive extension.
2. Pull apart the tendon attachments of the target muscle.
3. Push the tendon attachments together on the antagonist muscle.
4. Lengthen the target muscle.
5. Repeat steps 2 through 4 until no results are achieved or normal full resting length is obtained.

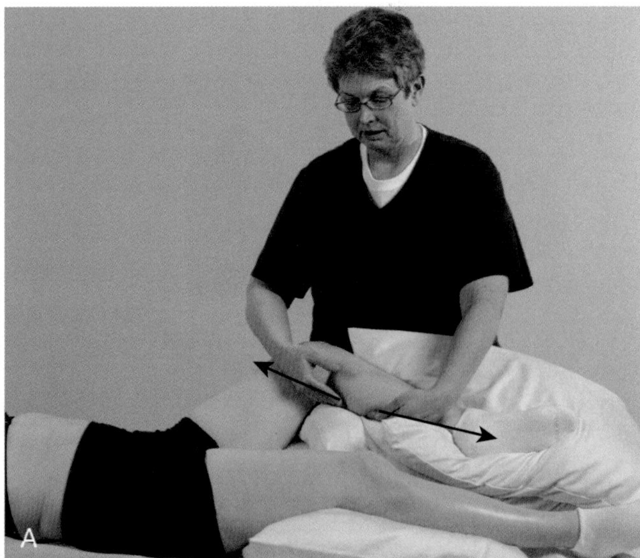

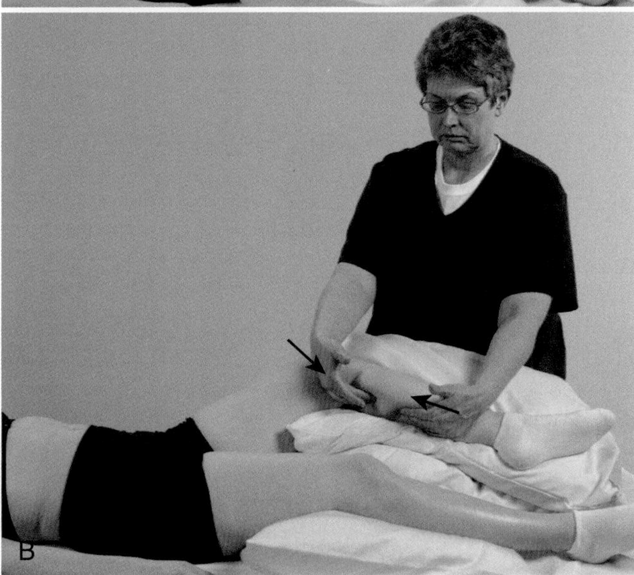

FIG. 10.37 Direct manipulation of proprioceptive muscle. **A,** Strengthen. **B,** Weaken.

Positional Release and Strain/Counterstrain

Strain/counterstrain, a technique formalized by Dr. Lawrence Jones, involves the use of tender points to guide the positioning of the body into a space where the muscle tension can release on its own. Positional release is a more generic term used to describe these methods.

According to Dr. Chaitow (2013, 2015), during a positional release technique (PRT), a muscle's spindles are influenced by methods that take them into an ease state and that theoretically allow them an opportunity to reset and reduce hypertonicity. Strain/counterstrain and other positional release methods use the slow, controlled return of distressed tissues to the position of strain as a means of offering the spindles a chance to reset and thus normalize function. This is particularly effective if the spindles have inappropriately held an area in protective splinting, such as occurs around a sprain or strain to hold the injured area to avoid tissue damage.

Repositioning of the body into the original strain, often the position of a prior injury, allows proprioceptors to reset and stop firing protective signals. By moving the body into the direction of ease (i.e., the way the body wants to go and out of the position that causes the pain), the proprioception is taken into a state of safety. Remaining in this state for a time allows the neuromuscular mechanism to reset itself. The massage therapist then gently and slowly repositions the area into neutral.

Positional release techniques gently allow the body to reposition and restore balance. Positional release methods are used on painful areas, especially recent strains, before, after, or instead of muscle energy methods. The tender points are often located in the antagonist of the tight muscle because of the diagonal balancing process the body uses to maintain an upright posture in gravity. These methods are highly effective ways of dealing with tender areas regardless of the pathological condition. Sometimes the reason the point is tender to the touch cannot be determined. However, if tenderness is present, a protective muscle spasm surrounds it. Positional release is an excellent way to release these small areas of muscle spasm without causing additional pain.

The positioning used during positional release is a full-body process. Remember, an injury or loss of balance is a full-body experience. For this reason, areas distant to the tender point must be considered during the positioning process. For example, the position of the feet likely will have an effect on a tender point in the neck.

The procedure for positional release is as follows (Fig. 10.38):

1. Locate the tender point.
2. Gently initiate the pain response with direct pressure. Remember, the sensation of pain is a guide.
3. Slowly position the body until the pain subsides.
4. Wait at least 30 seconds or longer until the client feels the release, lightly monitoring the tender point.
5. Slowly lengthen the muscle.
6. Repeat steps 1 through 5 until no results are achieved or the normal full resting length is obtained.

Integrated Approach

Muscle energy techniques can be used together or in sequence to enhance their effects. Recall that muscle tension in one area of the body often indicates imbalance and compensation patterns in other areas of the body. Tension patterns can be self-perpetuating. Often, using an integrated approach introduces the type of information the nervous system needs to self-correct. The procedure outlined here relies on the body's innate knowledge of what is out of balance and how to restore a more normal functioning pattern.

The following procedure is an integrated approach. Use the position from either option A, steps 1 and 2, or option B, steps 1 and 2, as the starting point for the rest of the process, which begins at step 3. (A) Identify the area of pain or postural distortion. (B) Identify the position of release or increased postural distortion. (C) Instruct the client to move out of the distortion pattern while providing resistance. (D) Lengthen.

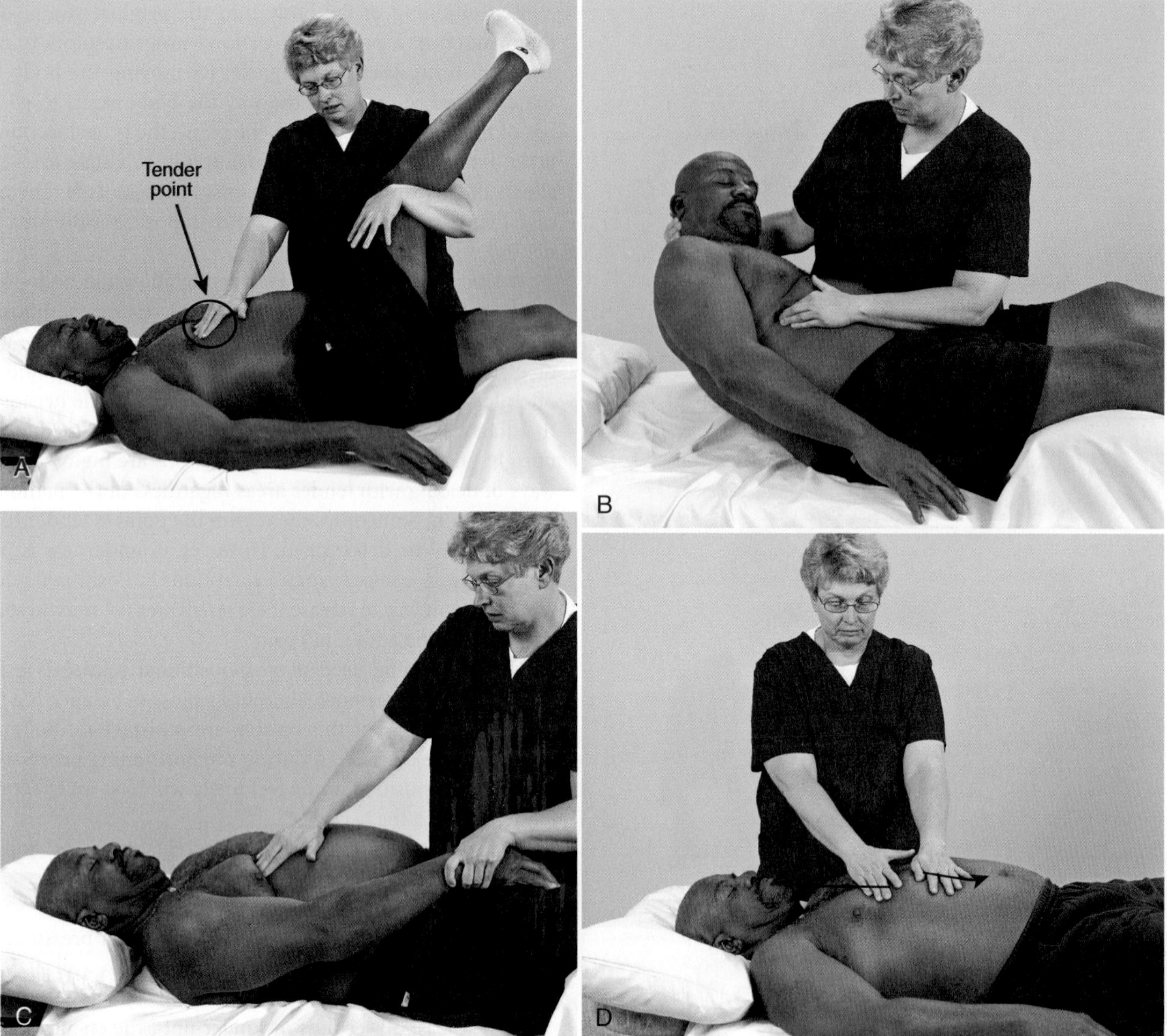

FIG. 10.38 Generalized positional release. A, Identify tender points in **B** and **C,** and begin to move the client into pain-relieving positions. **D,** Direct lengthening of tender area.

Option A

1. Identify the most obvious of the postural distortion symptoms.
2. Exaggerate the pattern by increasing the distortion, moving the body into ease. This position becomes the pattern of isolation of various muscles that will be addressed in the next part of the procedure (e.g., if the left shoulder is elevated and rotated forward, exaggerate and increase the elevation and rotation pattern). Continue with step 3.

Option B

1. Identify a painful point.
2. Use positional release to move the body into ease until the point is substantially less tender to pressure. The position of ease found becomes the pattern of isolation of various muscles that will be addressed in the next part of the procedure. Continue with step 3.

After choosing from option A or option B, continue the procedure as follows:

3. Stabilize the client in as many different directions as possible.
4. Instruct the client to move out of the pattern. Be as vague as possible and do not guide the client because it is important for the client to identify the resistance pattern.
5. Provide resistance for the client to push or pull against.
6. Modify the resistance angle as necessary to achieve the most solid resistance pattern for the client.
7. Spend a few moments noticing when the client's breathing changes; then, while still providing modified resistance, allow the client to move through the pattern slowly.
8. When the client has achieved as much extension on their own, recognize that they have achieved the lengthening pattern.
9. Gently increase the lengthening. If additional elongation in this position is desired, connective tissue stretching can be achieved.
10. Pay attention to the body areas that become involved in addition to the one addressed. This is your guide to the next position.

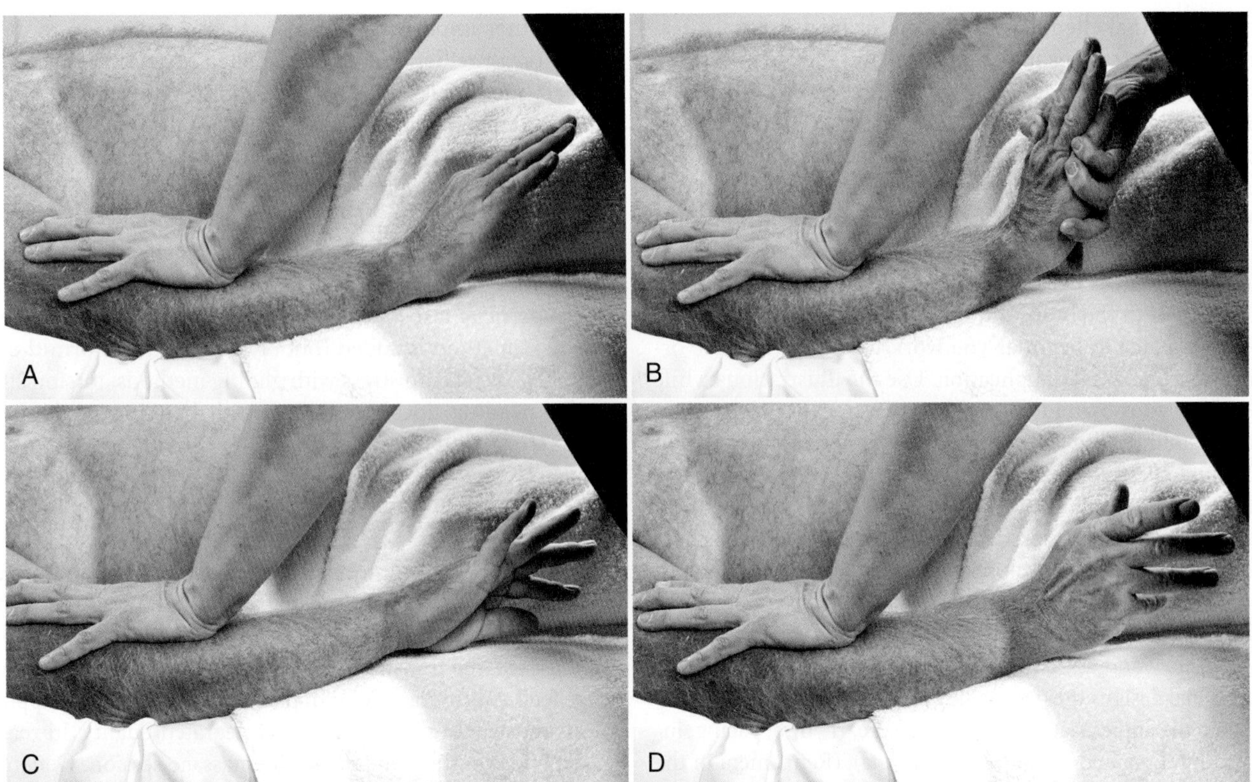

FIG. 10.39 Making it simple. A, Identify short tissue. **B,** Increase passive shortening of tissue. **C, D,** Move distal joints in circle.

Making It Simple

The various muscle energy techniques can be simplified. The act of contracting the muscles appears to be involved in a movement pattern to facilitate lengthening of the short muscles. Movement patterns occur at each jointed area and involve groups of muscles all neurologically linked: prime mover, agonist and synergist, and antagonist (eccentric control function). The eye position also influences the neurological signaling to the muscles.

The following is a combined simplified approach (Fig. 10.39):

1. Assess movement patterns with passive and active joint movement and identify short tissue (the target).
2. Position short tissue in the increased passively shortened position and hold it in that position.
3. Stabilize in all directions at the distal end of the area (e.g., for the elbow, stabilize just above the wrist; for the hip, just above the knee; and for the ankle, at the toes).
4. Instruct the client to push and pull back and forth for hinge joints (fingers/toes, elbows, knees) or move the area in a circle (wrist, ankle, shoulder/hip, neck, spine) while at the same time moving the eyes in a circle. The movement should be rhythmic and of moderate strength. This back and forth or circular movement against applied resistance activates all muscles in the movement pattern.
5. Slowly lengthen the target area (short tissue) to the bind (resistance barrier) and hold for a few seconds.
6. Repeat steps 3 to 5 two or three more times.
7. Massage the target tissue, primarily using gliding, compression, and kneading, both with and against the muscle fiber direction; this manually stimulates receptors, connective tissue, and fluid. Then shake or rock the area and lengthen again.

This sequence basically uses all the muscle energy methods described (see Proficiency Exercise 10.10).

SEQUENCE AND TRANSITIONING: THE BASIC FULL-BODY MASSAGE

SECTION OBJECTIVES

Chapter objective covered in this section:

6. Perform a full-body massage using the methods and techniques presented in the chapter.

Using the information presented in this section, the learner will be able to perform the following:

- Understand how to deal with difficult or unusual situations regarding body hair, skin problems, and avoidance of tickling.
- Make thoughtful decisions about the application of massage methods by body region.
- Adapt massage application based on the needs of individual clients.
- Design and perform a basic full-body massage.

The preceding section presented movement methods of massage. The next step is learning how to combine the methods into a focused massage session. A massage can be given in many ways. The choices massage therapists make each time they give a massage need to come from an understanding of the principles and practice of therapeutic massage. Each massage is different because the client is different each time, even if that client has been seen for many massage sessions. The illustrations in the protocol and the video clips on the Evolve website included with this text show body placement. Any methods and techniques can be used in any combination in a particular body area. Some learners will find these simple guidelines helpful, whereas others will find it easier to develop a structure themselves. For learning purposes, beginning with the suggestions provided and then modifying them as needed is a good way to start. Remember, the examples in the book and the clips on the Evolve website are only a place to begin as you work to understand the organization of massage application. Use the illustrations while generating your own ideas, and be open to experimentation, creation, and modification of massage applications based on individual clients according to body shape, style of massage, and equipment available.

The focus of the session depends on the outcomes the client is seeking. To understand those outcomes, the massage therapist must be able to take a general history and do a basic assessment of the client (see Chapter 4). Based on the information gathered in the history and assessment process, the therapeutic massage professional designs the best massage for that particular client by choosing the appropriate methods, pressure, rhythm, pacing, intensity, duration, and amenities (e.g., music). (Refinement of the assessment process and the criteria for decision making are addressed in Chapter 11 and in the case studies in Chapter 16).

When doing a massage, the massage therapist uses a variety of methods in a manner that allows easy transition from one method to another as a particular part of the body is addressed. Once you have learned the technical aspects of performing methods, it is time to learn to perfect the massage sequence—that is, to combine the methods in a logical way to address specific body areas and eventually to generate specific outcomes, such as relaxation, stress management, pain management, and functional mobility support. Also remember the four main approaches to care: palliative/pleasure, restorative, condition management, and therapeutic change. Outcomes and approaches to care are the foundation of a treatment/care plan and the platform for what is being called *outcome-based massage, custom massage,* or *therapeutic massage.*

General sequencing principles guide the massage application. These principles describe the direction and progression of manipulations:

General → Specific → General
Superficial → Deep → Superficial

General to specific to general and *superficial to deep to superficial* refer to the ways in which methods are applied to an area of the body. The first application of a method is done generally and superficially; this is followed by applications that are more specific and deeper. The methods then return to more general and superficial techniques before the therapist moves to another area.

This sequencing has many effects. It accustoms the client to the touch, and it allows the therapist to palpate through layers of tissue in a systematic manner for assessment or intervention for therapeutic change.

Another important concept is that compression to determine pressure depth is always applied first. After that, a secondary method is added, such as gliding or kneading. A good rule to remember is "Down first, then out or around." Compression (down) is used to determine the tissue layer being targeted. For example, holding methods typically are at skin level, so light pressure is applied. The superficial fascia is below the skin; therefore the compression generates pressure to move your hand, forearm, or foot through the skin and into the superficial fascia. Once the tissue layer has been reached, the next method is added (out or around), to deform the tissue; such as tension stress with gliding methods, torsion stress with kneading, local stretching with bending methods, or shear stress with frictioning.

Transitions

Massage application moves from one area of the body to another and from one method to another. The way the shift is made is called a *transition.* Because of the relaxation outcome of massage, the transitions need to be smooth so that the massage feels continuous. A myth persists that all massage applications must have this continuous integrated quality. In reality, it depends on the outcome of the massage session. Generally, massage application should include the relaxation/pleasure goal, and integrated transitions are important. However, there are exceptions, especially when the outcome is primarily related to functional movement. Transition methods primarily involve gliding and rocking. The major difference between gliding as a massage application for assessment and intervention and gliding as a transition method is the magnitude of pressure, direction, duration, and frequency. When gliding is performed as an assessment method, the pressure moves from surface to deep through distinct tissue layers with the direction variable. The frequency of the application relates to how many directions and how many layers of tissue are being targeted. Typically, each area is covered three or four times.

As mentioned previously, the excursion usually is in inches to no more than a foot, or the body mechanics are strained. Because of the depth of pressure, massage application needs to be applied against a slope (hill) to support weight transfer to create the mechanical force.

When gliding is used as an intervention, the most common adaptation is to focus, shorten, and slow the application. When gliding is used as a transition, however, the pressure is light and focused primarily on the skin and superficial fascia. The drag is minimal. The intention is not to specifically assess tissue or alter tissue. The intention is to get from one part of the body to another in a pleasurable, connected way. The stroke length can be longer, the frequency of application is limited to one or two times, and the method is rhythmic and of short duration. The speed is moderate to slow. The application can follow the contours of the body because pressure is not a primary quality of transition.

The transition application is performed with the forearm or with open, relaxed hands. The hands can be used during transition application because pressure levels are light to moderate, there is little drag, and no specific sustained pressure is necessary. Avoid any type of light fingertip stroking to prevent tickling or activation of "goosebumps," which increases sympathetic autonomic nervous system activity. Goosebumps occur when small muscles in the hair follicles contract. These contractions make the hairs stand up and increase sensory awareness.

Rocking is an effective and underused transition method. Slow, rhythmic rocking creates sensations that help calm the body's alert system. Rocking can be applied on the skin or over the drape. The application is rhythmic and slow and efficiently allows movement from one body area to another. Rocking is easy to apply, does not strain the therapist's body, and naturally supports the relaxation response. When employing rocking to transition from one area or method to another, use broad contact with forearms or relaxed open hands, and rock from your feet through your whole body, transferring the movement to the client's body.

Basic Full-Body Massage

The basic full-body massage is a common approach. The session lasts 45 to 60 minutes. The full-body general massage affects sensory nerve receptors, contacts multiple layers and types of tissues, and moves the major joints of the body. The general protocol is found at the end of the chapter and also in the video clips on the Evolve website.

The purpose of the full-body general massage is twofold:

- To assess the soft tissues and joint function
- To support normal function and well-being

The body is massaged primarily using gliding, compression, oscillation, and movement of the joints, along with limited use of kneading, shaking, and general friction methods. The other manipulations and techniques are chosen as needed as an intervention to address specific problem areas.

Regardless of the type of massage approach, the first and perhaps most important massage technique is holding, or the first touch. The next massage manipulations are used for general, broad applications and to transition between methods during the massage session. The methods most commonly used for general broad applications are gliding, compression, rhythmic rocking and shaking, and joint movement (Box 10.8).

The full-body general massage has a sense of wholeness, with a beginning point and an ending point. The massage should have a general sense of continuity. It needs to flow, to feel connected, like one continuous experience made up of all the applications of the massage methods chosen to achieve the individual client's outcomes.

The general sequence of contact is holding, compression, gliding, kneading, oscillation (rocking, shaking), and movement (usually passive joint movement). Remember, compression is used to determine the depth of pressure for gliding and kneading.

Each body area is addressed. Each method usually is applied three or four times (frequency), becoming slower and deeper with each application. The rhythm, duration, and direction vary, depending on the goal of the massage. The therapist then can move (transition) to a different body area and repeat the sequence (Box 10.9). It is important to learn to use the basic sequence as assessment for tissues and joints. In the next chapter you will learn about the specifics of assessment.

Box 10.8 When to Use Which Massage Method

The following methods are effective when used in the situations listed.

Gliding

- A lubricant will be used.
- A large surface area must be covered efficiently.
- Changes (transitions) are made between manipulations and techniques.
- The therapist moves/transitions from one area to another.
- The client prefers a soothing massage with generalized body responses.

Compression

- A lubricant will not be used.
- The client is hairy or ticklish.
- The client prefers a more stimulating massage.

Rhythmic Rocking and Shaking

- A lubricant will not be used.
- Excessive rubbing or pressing on the skin or underlying tissue is not desirable.
- The client wants a soothing massage with generalized body responses.

Joint Movement

- A lubricant will not be used.
- The client is hairy or ticklish.
- Excessive rubbing or pressing on the skin or underlying tissue is not desirable.
- The client wants a general increase in mobility.

Blending these four methods to provide the general base of the massage is beneficial. The other massage techniques create a unique massage.

MENTORING TIP

For now, while you are perfecting your skill in the basic massage application, consider assessment as a conversation with the body. Every aspect of the massage is asking this question: "How is this tissue functioning, and how are these joints moving?" If the body responds with "All good here," then transition to the next segment of the body and begin again. If the body's response is "Not functioning the best," then decisions must be made about the appropriateness of introducing an intervention.

General Massage Suggestions

Body Hair

Excessive body hair requires an alteration in the massage procedure. Gliding and kneading methods can pull the hair. A lubricant may feel uncomfortable. Compression and oscillation (vibration, rocking, and shaking), coupled with lengthening and stretching procedures, can be an effective alternative.

Box 10.9 Sequence of a Basic Massage

Five initial methods are used on each part of the body:

- Holding
- Compression
- Gliding
- Kneading
- Rocking

Three methods are used on areas of the body that allow the application:

- Joint movement/passive and active
- Shaking
- Percussion, type depending on the body area

Three methods are more specific for intervention:

- Focused compression/inhibitory pressure
- Elongation/stretching
- Shearing methods/friction

Once mastered, these methods become the foundation for palpation and movement assessment and intervention. Each method, whether used alone or in combination with other therapeutic intervention methods, can be adapted using the 12 modifiers.

Basic Sequence

The following basic sequence is performed on each body area.

1. *Holding:* Make contact using holding, then transition to compression.
2. *Compression:* Cover the area three times, with each application becoming slower and deeper. Use a broad base of the whole hand, double hand, forearm, or leg. To replace kneading, compress tissue away from bone and have the client move the joint below (distal to) the pressure. Move the joint back and forth or in small circles. Combine compression with rocking and then transition to gliding.
3. *Gliding:* Use four applications to cover the area. The first is light and superficial and can be done with the full, relaxed hand. The second is slower and deeper and moves the skin; it is applied with the forearm unless the area being massaged is too small (e.g., the fingers). Then use the hands. The third application is progressively slower and deeper to access muscle layers. Use forearms. The fourth application is superficial again and can be done with the full relaxed hand. Transition to kneading.
4. *Kneading:* Cover the area three times, with each application becoming slower and lifting more tissue. Make sure to use a broad base and do not pinch. Identify areas where compression plus movement is better than kneading. Transition to oscillation methods.
5. *Oscillation* or *percussion:* Apply the appropriate method to the area for about 30 to 60 seconds. Transition to joint movement.
6. *Joint movement:* Move each joint through a comfortable range of motion and introduce elongation (stretching and traction) if indicated.
7. Repeat gliding or introduce rocking as a transition method. Begin again on next body area.

Appropriate sanitation, draping, and body mechanics are used consistently.

The following is an example of body sequence using four positions.

Client lies on stomach (prone).

- Use bolster under ankles (possibly also under abdomen)
- Right side back from top of gluteus to top of shoulder blade
- Left side back from top of gluteus to top of shoulder blade
- Left and right side glutes

Turn client on left side.

- Use bolster as needed
- Right arm
- Right forearm
- Hand
- Left arm
- Left forearm
- Hand
- Right upper shoulder
- Right side of the neck
- Right side of the head

Move to legs.

- Left inner thigh
- Left calf
- Left foot
- Right outer thigh
- Right calf
- Right foot

Turn client on right side.

- Use bolster as needed
- Left arm
- Left forearm
- Hand
- Right arm
- Right forearm
- Hand
- Left upper shoulder
- Left side of the neck
- Left side of the head

Move to legs.

- Right inner thigh
- Right calf
- Right foot
- Left outer thigh
- Left calf
- Left foot

Turn client on back (supine).

- Use bolster under knees and head
- Left thigh
- Right thigh
- Abdomen
- Left chest
- Right chest

Wash or sanitize hands.

- Face
- Have client move to a seated position (you may have to assist some clients).
- Bilateral upper shoulders

Also see the General Massage Protocol at the end of the chapter and video clips on the Evolve site for examples and variations.

Skin Problems

Massage procedures must be altered for people with rashes, acne, psoriasis, and other skin problems. The integrity of healthy skin prevents the transmission of pathogens. Massage usually can be provided by placing a clean, white bath towel or triple-folded sheet over the affected area and using compression methods over the fabric. Be careful to avoid contact with any body fluids.

Working over a clean towel or sheet can be helpful for clients who have sensitive skin and find the movement of massage irritating. Any method that does not glide on the skin can be used over a towel, a sheet, or loose, nonrestrictive clothing. Using a towel to lift tissue, especially the tissue of the abdomen, is helpful for gaining an effective grip and is more comfortable.

Avoiding Tickling

Tickling usually can be avoided by using a broad contact point, reducing the speed and increasing the pressure of the method. Also, because tickling oneself is difficult, the problem often can be solved by placing the client's hand on the area you want to massage and massaging with it. Tickling frequently can be avoided by working over a towel or sheet.

Considerations and Suggestions for Massage Applications by Body Region

Head and Face Massage

Because of the extensive motor/sensory sensitivity of the face, massage can stimulate considerable nervous system activity, which may be beneficial for relaxation and pain control. Also, the facial muscles create the expressions that reflect our moods and emotions. Changes in expression are processed in the emotional centers of the brain. Careful massage of the face may gently interact with the way the client feels emotionally.

Key Points

- Always ask before massaging the head and face to confirm if the client does not want their hair or makeup disrupted.
- Use lubricants carefully, keeping in mind the sensitivity of the facial skin. Avoid using lubricant on the face if possible.
- Remember that the delicate nature of the facial skin and muscles requires a confident yet moderate approach.
- Always clean your hands before massaging the face. Pathogens can easily be spread through the mucous membranes of the eyes, nose, and mouth. Avoid direct contact with these areas.

Neck Massage

The neck is a crowded, complex area. It can be affected by responses to stress and by chest and shoulder breathing, which can cause the neck muscles to become rigid and hypertonic. Effective massage of the neck is necessary to provide for relaxed breathing and to reduce the perception of stress.

Careful study of the anatomy of the neck shows that the direct soft tissue influence extends from the forehead to the second and third ribs, the middle thoracic vertebrae, and the middle of the humerus. Because the neck area balances the head against gravity, postural distortion anywhere in the body is reflected in the neck. Massage to this area, in conjunction with an entire body approach, is most beneficial.

The brachial nerve plexus exits from the neck. It is helpful to think of most arm, wrist, and hand problems as beginning at the neck. Problems result either from direct dysfunction of the neck or from difficulties in the arm and hand, which often indirectly cause a neck problem. Nerves, blood, and lymph vessels permeate the area.

Key Points

- Although the neck can be massaged effectively with the client lying supine or prone, side-lying is also an effective position for massage of the neck. The head is stabilized against the table, and the neck area is opened up for easy access.
- Always provide lengthening and stretching for the neck from the shoulder with the head held still. Injury may result if the neck is lengthened or stretched by moving the head.
- Avoid excessive extension of the head where it joins the cervical vertebrae. Lying with the head back in this position on a hard surface can cause tearing in the neck's arteries. This position can also cause vertebrobasilar insufficiency (VBI), or vertebral basilar ischemia, which is a temporary set of symptoms caused by decreased blood flow in the posterior circulation of the brain.
- Avoid moderate to heavy pressure into the anterior triangle of the neck (the general area between the sternocleidomastoid muscle and the trachea). Such pressure can damage blood vessels and nerves in this area. Other than very light pressure the anterior triangle of the neck is avoided.
- When massaging the neck, use broad, generalized methods of massage applied with the forearm or the whole hand; this feels less invasive to the client than when you use the fingers and thumbs.

Shoulder Massage

The shoulder complex (scapula, clavicle, humerus, and associated muscles, fascia, ligaments, and tendons) floats on the trunk. It is constructed with a loose fit at the shoulder (glenohumeral) joint to provide for a wide range of motion. Soft tissue (muscles, tendons, ligaments, and fascia) connects the shoulder to the trunk, with multidirectional forces coming from the back, chest, and neck. Nerves, blood, and lymph vessels permeate the area. The therapist should consider all these tissues and areas when massaging the shoulder.

The joint design reflects the fact that flexor muscles (which narrow a joint angle) and adductor muscles (which pull toward the midline of the body) exert more pull and are stronger than the extensors (which increase the joint angle) and abductors (which pull away from the midline). Joint alignment may be compromised by an imbalance in the tone pattern of these muscles. The therapist should keep this in mind when working with the shoulder.

The brachial nerve plexus, which supplies the arm, may be affected by soft tissue dysfunction in the shoulder area. This is an important consideration for clients who have arm pain and discomfort, often resulting from repetitive use injury. Massaging the shoulder may reduce muscle tension and soften connective tissue in the area, which may alleviate discomfort in the shoulder and arm.

Key Points

- Although the shoulders can be massaged with the client lying supine or prone, side-lying is an effective position for massage, range of motion, and lengthening and stretching of the shoulder.
- The shoulder is stabilized at the iliac crest and sacrum by the latissimus dorsi muscle and the lumbar dorsal fascia. With any shoulder massage, the therapist should consider massage of the low back area.

Arm and Forearm Massage

The nerves of the brachial nerve plexus run the entire length of the upper limb. Nerve impingement from soft tissue at the neck, shoulder, and elsewhere in the entire length of the arm and forearm needs to be considered if pain is radiating into the area. Blood and lymph vessels permeate the area.

When massaging the arm and forearm, it is useful to remember that the fingers actually begin at the elbow, and the shoulder mechanism extends to the elbow. The elbow joint area is more complex than a hinge joint because of the pronation (palm down)/supination (palm up) action at the elbow. Flexion, extension, pronation, and supination movement patterns need to be considered when massaging the arm.

Key Points

- Positioning and stabilization of the upper limb for massage can be aided by massaging the arm and forearm in all the basic positions: supine, prone, and side-lying. Each offers advantages.
- Massage only the areas of the limb that are easily accessible in each position. Return to the arm or forearm as the client changes position.
- Massage the area using the forearm stabilized against the massage table in the prone or supine position or against the body in the side-lying position.

Wrist and Hand Massage

The wrist and hand have an intricate, complex joint and soft tissue structure. Thorough attention to massage of these structures and range of motion of the wrist and hand requires time and a focus on detail. Because of the extensive motor/sensory sensitivity of the hand, massage can provide intense neurological stimulation. The hand is an effective area for massage to initiate relaxation and pain control.

Massage of the hand can be a time of increased connection between the client and the massage therapist. This is a result of the hand-in-hand position. The sense of intimacy created by the act of holding hands may shift the therapeutic focus from the client to the massage therapist. Extra care is suggested to prevent transference/countertransference and professional boundary issues without disturbing the closeness created at this time.

Slow circumduction (moving in a circle) of the wrists, both passive and active against resistance, accesses the joint movement patterns of the wrist. The carpal and metacarpal (palm) joints of the hand can be addressed with a scissoring action. The phalangeal (finger) joints are hinge joints that respond well to active movement against resistance and **passive joint movement**.

Key Points

- Because the hand usually is in a flexed position, opening and spreading the tissue of the palm is beneficial.
- Using compression to provide a pumping action on the palm stimulates the lymphatic plexus in the palm, which in turn encourages lymphatic flow. This can be helpful for clients whose hands swell.

Chest Massage (Anterior Thorax)

The pectoralis muscles and associated connective tissue are involved in arm and shoulder movement. This large soft tissue area often is shortened, not only affecting shoulder and arm action, but also causing breathing difficulties. Effective massage, lengthening, and stretching are beneficial when this tissue is short and dense.

The intercostal muscles (those between the ribs) are important in respiratory function. Slow, deliberate work between the ribs with the client in the side-lying position can be valuable for restoring mobility and breathing function.

Key Points

- On females, the breast area can pose difficulties in accessing the chest. The side-lying position is effective for massage of the chest area, because the breast tissue falls toward the table, allowing access to the side of the chest and the axilla. Using the client's hand as a "buffer" between the therapist's hand and the client (e.g., as when avoiding tickling) can be helpful when working around the clavicles and ribs.
- Broad compressive applications to the rib area in the side-lying position are effective in providing general joint movement to the ribs.
- Avoid the breast tissue and nipple area. No reason exists to massage this area during general massage, and the tissue often is sensitive to touch and can be easily irritated.
- Be extra attentive to changes in the tissue in the chest area. Without any alarm reaction, refer clients to their physician if you notice any lumps or tissue changes.

Abdominal Massage

Many times the abdomen is given only superficial attention during massage; avoid this tendency. This is an important area that deserves effective massage application. Abdominal muscles maintain a taut fascial girdle surrounding the entire thorax and influence lumbar and core stability via connection to the deep fascia laterally and posteriorly. Lifting methods applied to this connective tissue can be beneficial. During supine position, using a towel to lift the abdominal tissue provides grip and protects against pinching.

Be careful of pressure down into the abdomen. Always move slowly, allowing the tissue to soften under the touch. If you feel a pulse or throbbing, immediately reduce the pressure.

Not all researchers agree that massage has a substantial effect on peristalsis or even that mechanical emptying of the colon is possible. Nonetheless, with abdominal massage, it seems prudent to approach the area as though massage does have an effect. Theoretically, to support peristalsis and mechanical emptying of the colon, all massage manipulations are directed in a clockwise fashion. To prevent any chance of impaction of fecal material, the manipulations begin in the lower left quadrant at the sigmoid colon. The methods progressively contact the large intestine and eventually end up encompassing the entire colon area. The abdomen often is ticklish; this is a protective mechanism. Follow the instructions given earlier to avoid tickling.

Key Points

- The abdomen can be massaged with the client in the supine or side-lying position. Side-lying on the left is the most effective position. During abdominal massage, the knees usually are bent about 90 degrees to the trunk to tilt the pelvis and allow for more relaxed abdominal tissue.
- Because the abdomen contains no bony structure against which to apply pressure, much abdominal work is done with lateral pressure. The tissue is pushed against pressure from the massage therapist's opposing hand or with kneading that lifts the tissue.

Abdominal Sequence

Standing on the left side of the body when the client is in supine position allows for best use of therapist body mechanics (Fig. 10.40). Large intestine elimination patterns are also facilitated with the client lying on their left side.

The direction of flow for emptying the large intestine and colon is as follows:

1. Massage down the left side of the descending colon, using short strokes directed to the sigmoid colon.
2. Massage across the transverse colon to the left side, using short strokes directed to the sigmoid colon.
3. Massage up the ascending colon on the right side of the body, using short strokes directed to the sigmoid colon.
4. End at the right ileocecal valve, located in the lower right quadrant of the abdomen.
5. Massage the entire flow pattern, using long, light to moderate strokes, from the ileocecal valve to the sigmoid colon. Repeat the sequence.

Back Massage

The back often is the starting place for the massage because for many clients, the back does not feel as vulnerable an area as the abdomen. Even if shortening of the anterior tissues is causing the client's backache, beginning massage on the back directly addresses the client's experience of discomfort. Nerve roots are located all along the spine. Massage close to but not on the spine is beneficial. The low back, including the deep fascial connections and the relationship to the quadratus lumborum muscle, is easily massaged with the client in the side-lying position with the arm raised over the head to lift the rib cage away from the iliac crest. Firm, even pressure with the forearm often feels best to the client. Gentle movement to provide for rotation of the spinal column is most effectively done in the side-lying position.

Key Points

- Avoid spending excessive time on massage of the back. Often the reason for back pain or stiffness is shortening and weakness of muscles in the chest and abdomen. The resulting change in posture is responsible for the back tension.
- The back is effectively massaged in the prone, side-lying, and seated positions.
- Use of the forearm is effective for back massage. The lumbar dorsal fascia area responds well to **skin rolling** (tissue lifting) and connective tissue stretching methods. Pressure directly over the spine is not appropriate. However, skin rolling techniques that lift the skin over the spine are effective.

Hip Region Massage

The lumbar and sacral plexuses both innervate the gluteal and hip region. The client may be more confident if the words *gluteal* or *glutes* are not used; that the area is called the *hip region.* Nerve distribution patterns include the entire lower body, and the largest nerve is the sciatic nerve. When using heavy pressure to address the soft tissue, avoid sustained deep pressure on the nerve tracts.

The sacroiliac joints are large joints that are not directly moved by muscular action. Joint movements are indirectly achieved through movement of the leg through an active and passive joint movement sequence.

The coxal articulations (hip joints) are massive joints with an extensive ligament structure. The joint provides considerable range of motion, second only to the shoulder joint. When doing joint movement methods, include as many variations of flexion, extension, abduction, adduction, and internal and external rotation as possible to involve all the soft tissue elements.

Key Points

- Massage of the hip region is most effective when the client is in the side-lying or prone position. Stretching/elongation methods are most easily done in the side-lying or supine position. This area is heavily muscled and reinforced with extensive deep fascia, ligament, and tendon structures. The bones and joints in this area are large compared with those in other body areas. Increased pressure and duration may be required to address these tissues.
- Methods need to work slowly into the tissue. Avoid working with the hands, and make extensive use of the forearm, knee, or foot; these are less intimate, which may be an important consideration when working with the hip region.

Thigh and Leg Massage

The lumbosacral plexus nerves supply the lower limb, with the sciatic nerve running the entire length of the thigh and leg. Impingement can occur anywhere along the nerve

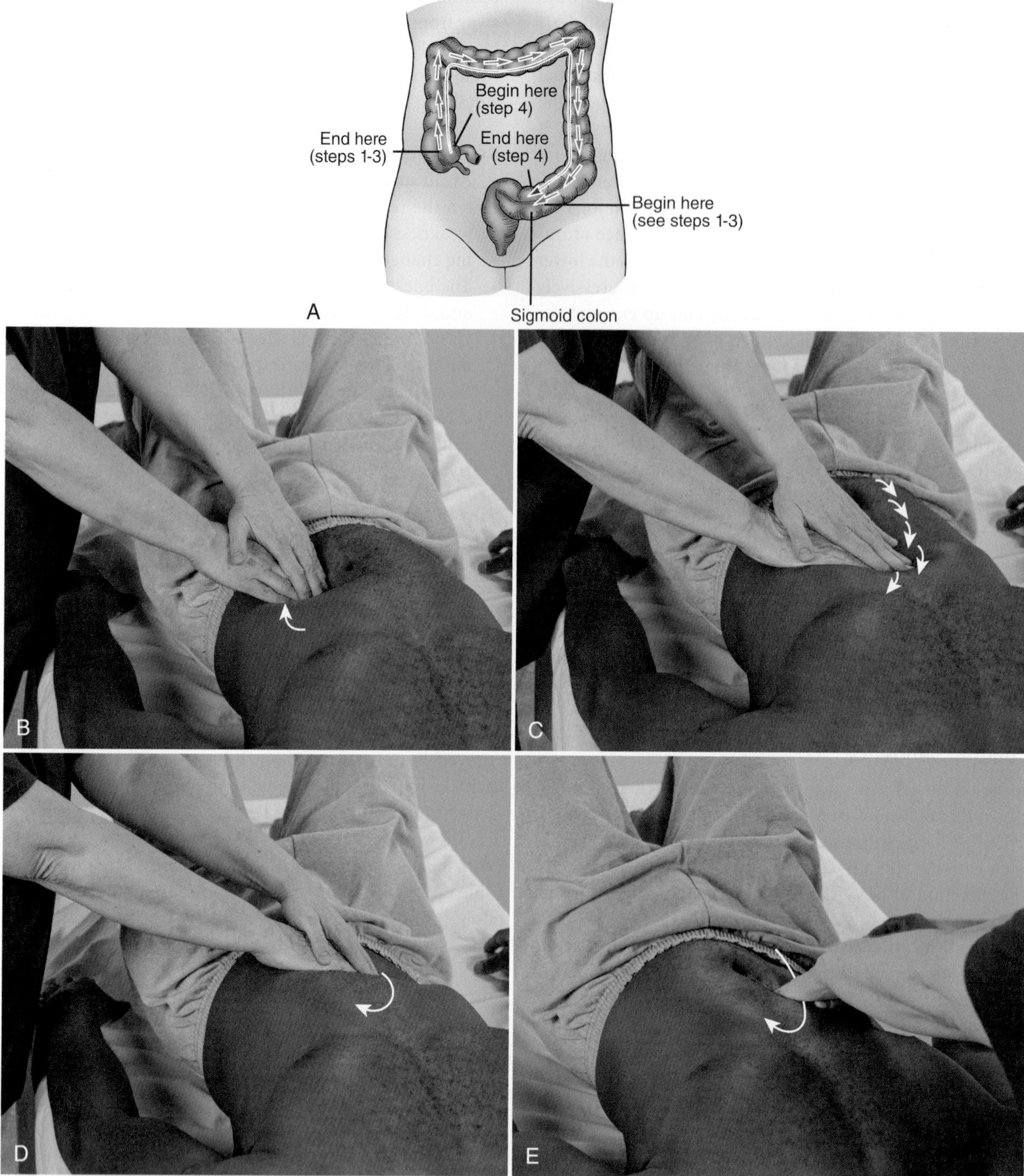

FIG. 10.40 A, Colon (arrows indicate the flow pattern). All massage manipulations are directed in a clockwise fashion. The manipulations begin in the lower left quadrant (on the right side as you view the illustration **[A]**) at the sigmoid colon. The methods progressively contact all of the large intestine and eventually cover the entire colon area. **B,** Abdominal sequence. The direction of flow for emptying of the large intestine and colon. Massage down the left side of the descending colon using short strokes directed toward the sigmoid colon. **C,** Massage across the transverse colon to the left side using short strokes directed toward the sigmoid colon. **D,** Massage up the ascending colon on the right side of the body using short strokes directed toward the sigmoid colon. End at the right-side ileocecal valve, which is located in the lower right quadrant of the abdomen. **E,** Massage the entire flow pattern of the abdominal sequence, using long, light to moderate strokes, from the ileocecal valve to the sigmoid colon. Then repeat the sequence.

pathways. The distribution of leg pain can indicate the nerve portion affected. When located, the entire nerve tract needs to be searched above and below the impingement site for soft tissue restriction to provide soft tissue normalization around the nerves. Light stroking along the nerve tracts is soothing.

The knee is a complex joint influenced by muscles from above and below the joint. Knee instability often is compensated for by increased muscle tone in the leg muscles and thickening and shortening of the iliotibial tract (a large connective tissue structure on the outside of the thigh). This is resourceful compensation, and the protective nature of the muscle and connective tissue tension must be considered. The gluteus maximus and tensor fascia lata muscle exert a pull at the iliotibial crest. Address these muscle/fascia structures to reduce tension on the iliotibial tract and knee. If the client has a hypermobile knee, you can use the proper methods to reduce excessive muscle tone and connective tissue shortening, but you should not try to remove the splinting action entirely. To do so may result in increased knee pain.

Key Points

- Supine, prone, and side-lying are all effective positions for massage of the thigh and leg and are best used in combination to access all parts of the lower limb easily. For the most efficient use of time in the general massage session, make sure each area of the thigh and leg is massaged only once. For instance, if you massage the back of the thigh or leg in the prone position, it is not necessary to repeat the back of the area again in the supine position unless a specific reason exists for doing so.
- The side-lying position offers the easiest access to the medial and lateral aspects of the thigh and leg. The supine position provides access to all aspects of the lower limb, whereas the prone position is the most limited.
- The soft tissue mass of the lower limb lends itself to massage with the forearm, leg, and foot. Kneading often is uncomfortable on the leg because of body hair and the tight adherence of the skin and superficial fascia to the underlying tissue. Gliding and compression in multiple directions combined with shaking are effective methods to use instead.
- Varicose veins most often occur in the leg, particularly in the saphenous veins. Thromboembolism and thrombophlebitis are serious conditions involving a blood clot in a vein. If the clot moves, it can lodge in the heart, lung, kidney, or brain, with serious consequences. Symptoms of deep vein thrombophlebitis in the lower limb are aching and cramping that can be mistaken for muscle pain. Massage of any type is contraindicated, and immediate referral is indicated for thromboembolism and thrombophlebitis. Diagnosis is beyond the scope of practice for therapeutic massage; therefore massage therapists should remain cautious of any leg pain and refer the client to the appropriate health care professional.
- Isolated joint movement of the hip requires stabilizing at the pelvis. Stabilizing pressure in this area can be uncomfortable. A small pillow or folded towel can be used over the stabilizing point to ensure comfort.

Ankle and Foot Massage

The ankle and foot mechanism is a complex structure. It has many joints, muscles and extensive fascia, and nerves that provide stability and neurological position information during walking and standing. An extensive connective tissue network provides stability. Any disruption of normal ankle and foot action often results in a compensatory pattern through the entire musculoskeletal system.

Massage of the foot is one of the best ways to provide a high degree of nervous system input for relaxation and pain control. Many beneficial effects are obtained with foot massage because of the stimulation of parasympathetic activity, which results in the relaxation or quieting response.

The sole of the foot contains a vast lymphatic plexus that acts as a pump to move lymphatic fluid in the foot and legs. Compression used in a rhythmic pumping action during massage would logically be effective in stimulating the lymphatic system.

The tibial nerve, off the sciatic nerve, branches into the medial and lateral plantar nerve, which in turn branches to provide extensive nerve distribution in the foot. Sciatic nerve impingement can be felt into the foot. Nerve pain in the foot can indicate impingement anywhere along the nerve tract from the lumbosacral plexus to the foot. Nerve pain in the foot needs to be addressed with massage of the entire lower limb, and the therapist should notice which areas of restriction refer pain to the foot.

Key Points

- For a client who is nervous or in pain, the feet often are a safe place to begin a massage.
- Because of the number of joints in the ankle and foot, careful and deliberate joint movement work is beneficial in this area. Slow circumduction (circular movements), both passive and active against resistance, accesses the ankle movement patterns. The tarsal and metatarsal (main foot) joints can be accessed with a scissoring or bending movement of the foot. Phalangeal (toe) joints are hinge joints that benefit from both active joint movement against resistance and passive joint movement.

Designing a Massage

The following series of photographs provides one example of how a massage can be designed. Examples of massage applications are provided, incorporating the various methods and techniques described in this chapter. It is assumed that the learner would perform the approaches on both sides of the body where appropriate. Variations also are shown, providing options for massage of a particular area. This series of photographs is complemented by the video demonstration provided on the Evolve website. By studying these examples, you should be able to modify and adapt applications to make each massage unique (Proficiency Exercise 10.11).

PROFICIENCY EXERCISE 10.11

Design a 1-hour massage sequence on paper using a variety of methods and techniques from this chapter. Trade papers with another learner and perform the other person's massage sequence on them. When you are finished, list what you learned from the experience and share the list with your partner in this exercise. Have your partner critique his or her massage design.

The series of photographs is organized as an example of a full-body massage in three positions: prone, side-lying, and supine. Draping is shown, but not in such a way as to obstruct the view of the application. The demonstration client is male. Female clients require comprehensive anterior thorax/breast draping. Ideally, the massage is applied using all of the best positioning. Most areas of the body can be massaged in the three positions; however, some positions related to body areas support optimum body mechanics, and circumstances may require that variations be used. The demonstration begins on the back in the prone position. To begin in the supine position on the head and face reverse the protocol.

GENERAL MASSAGE PROTOCOL

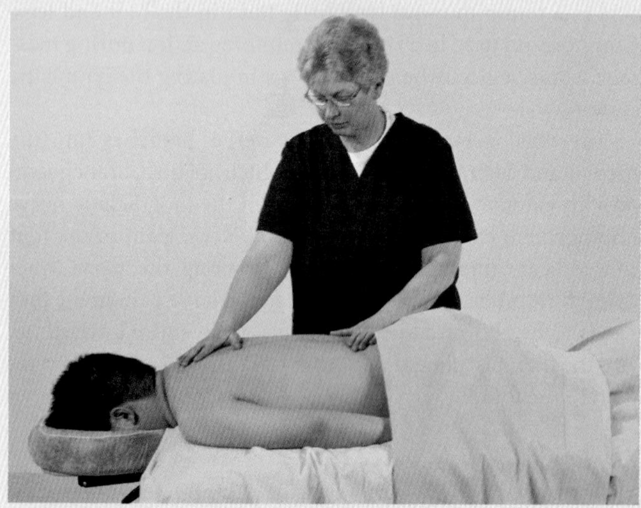

1. Calmly and with compassion approach the client, with intention focused on massage outcomes. Focus. Then apply a holding.

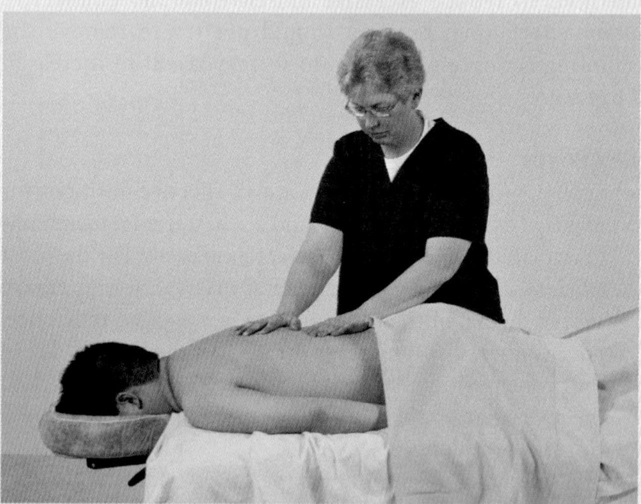

2. Palpation. Wet/dry skin drag, ease/bind, hot/cold, rough/smooth.

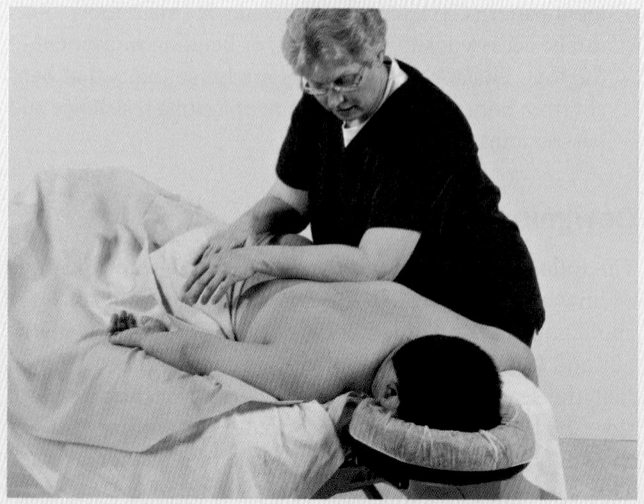

3. Glide on back. Vary speed, drag, and depth of pressure.

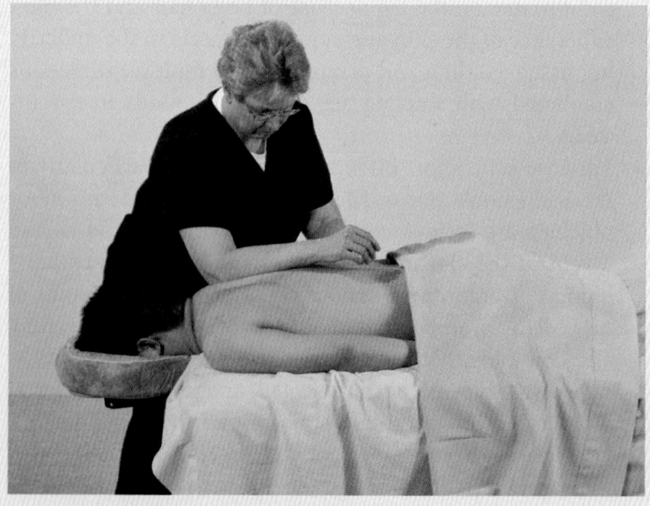

4. Shift position. Glide/compress.

GENERAL MASSAGE PROTOCOL—cont'd

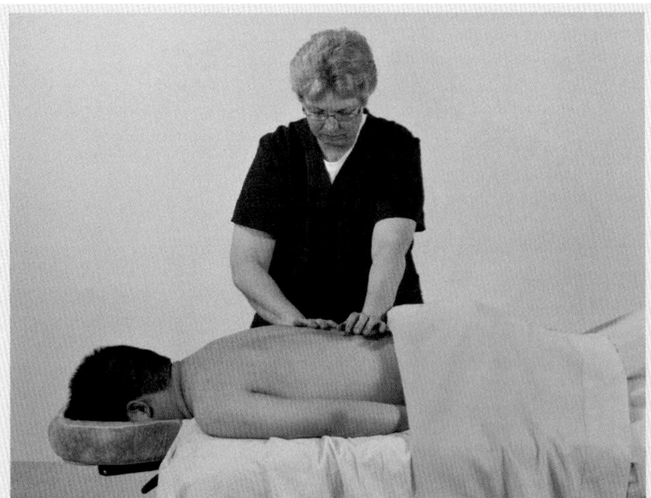

5. Knead.

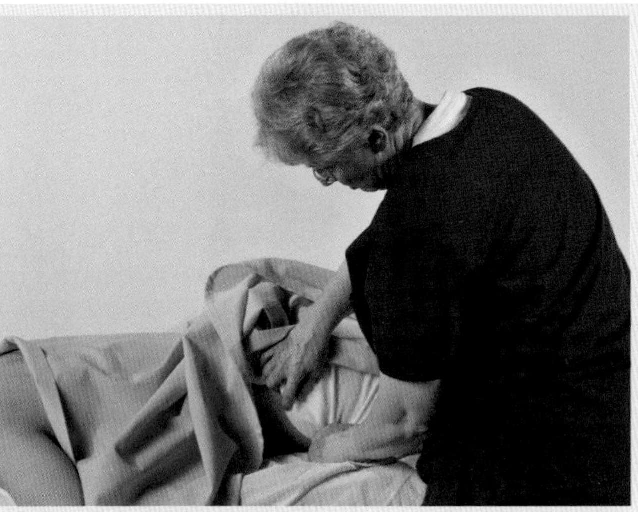

6. Move underwear with permission, have client move the garment, or work over the drape.

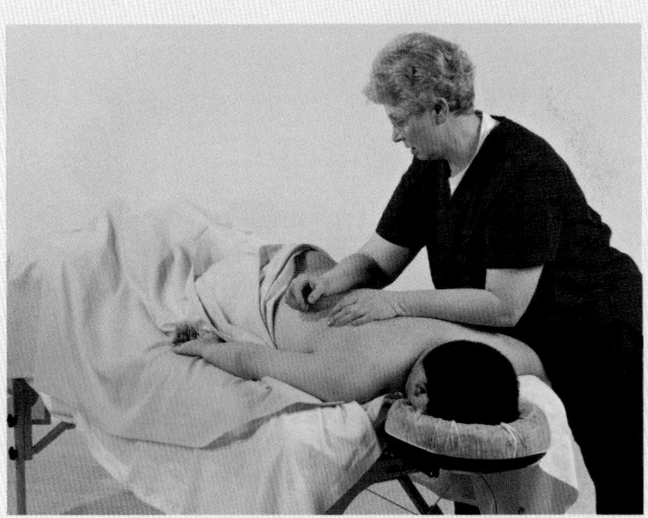

7. Glide the lumbar and hip region.

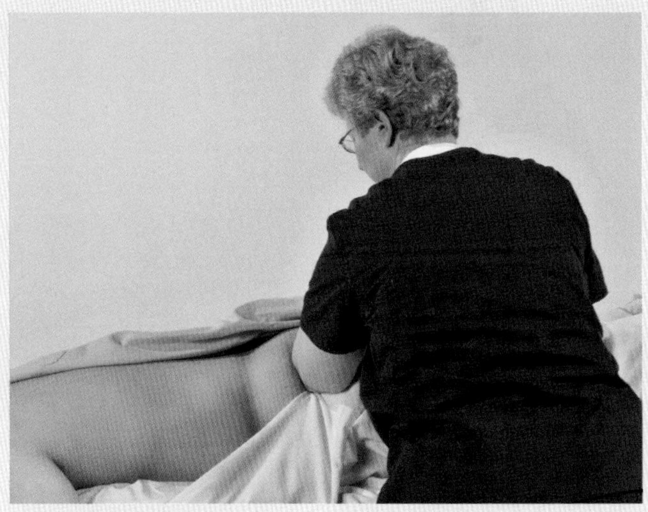

8. Compression to hip area.

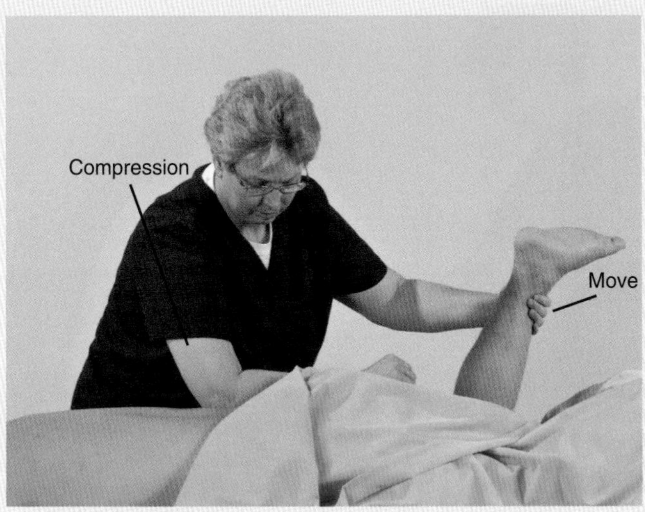

9. Combined loading. Compression and movement.

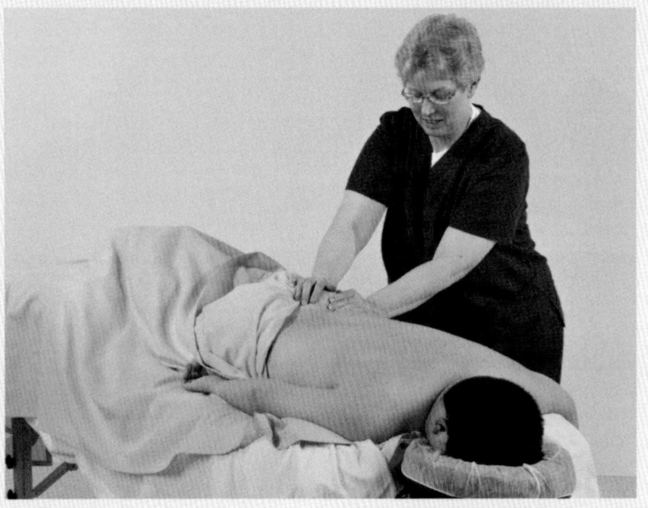

10. Knead.

Continued

GENERAL MASSAGE PROTOCOL—cont'd

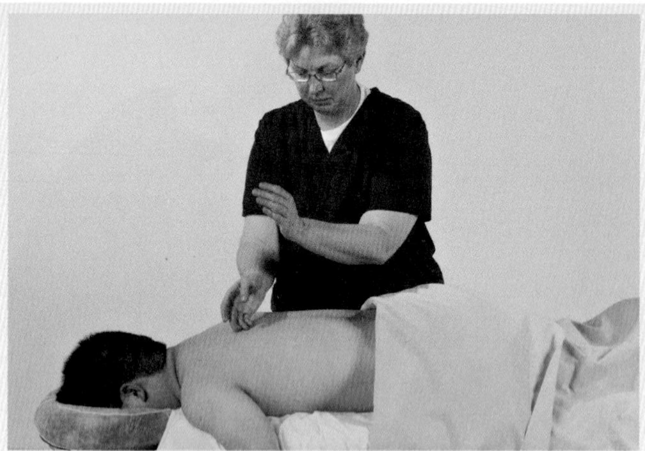

11. Percussion. Repeat opposite side (steps 2–11).

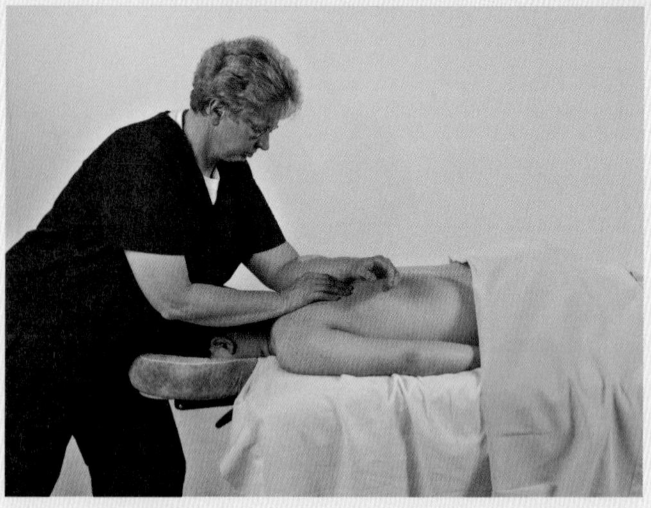

12. Shift position. Compression/glide upper back/shoulder.

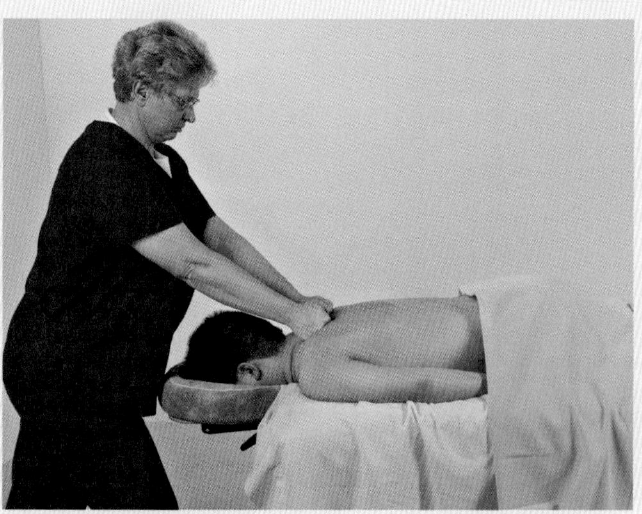

13. Compression.

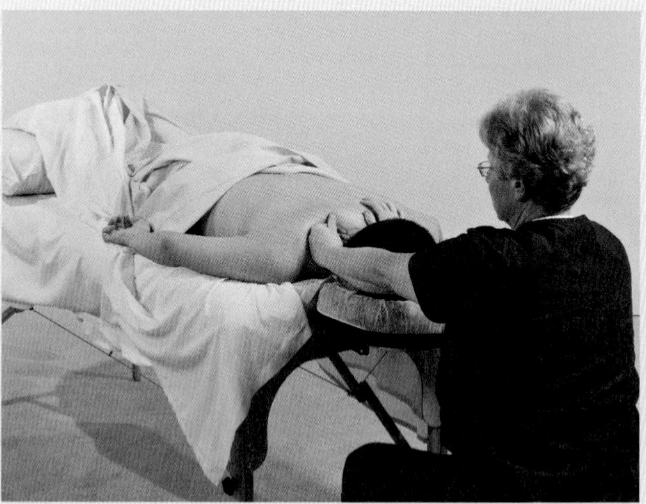

14. Compression with therapist kneeling or seated.

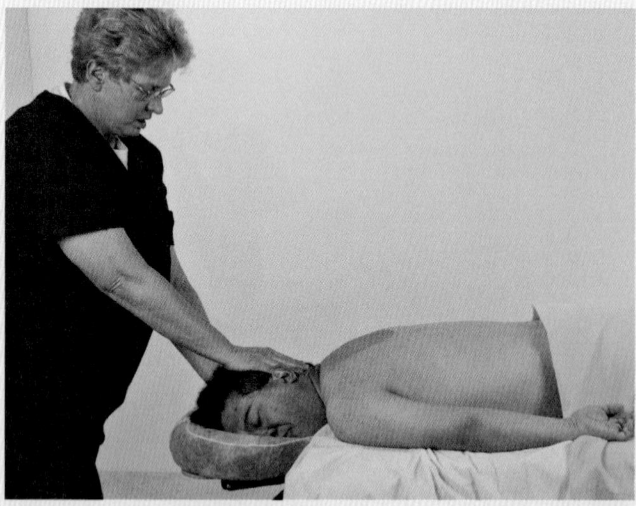

15. Turn head, massage scalp.

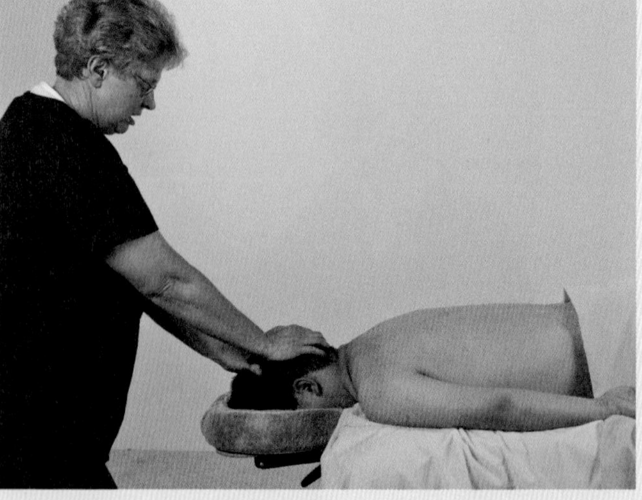

16. Reposition head. Compress muscles of the head.

GENERAL MASSAGE PROTOCOL—cont'd

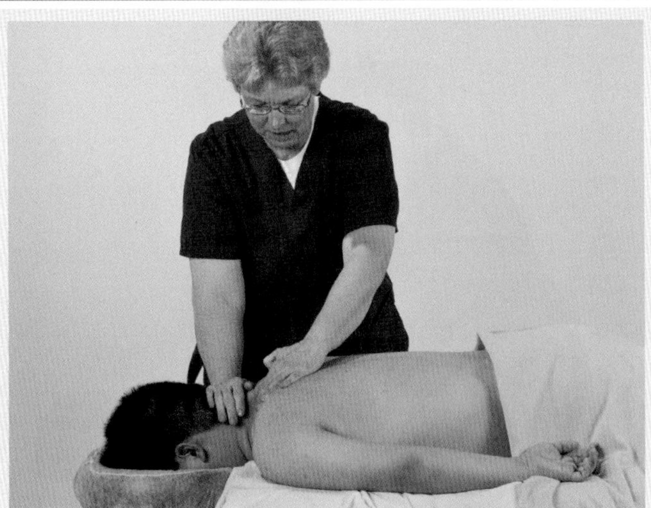

17. Knead neck.

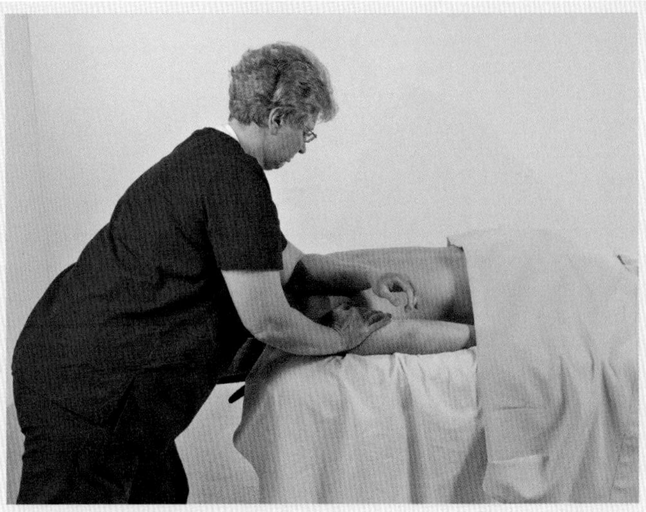

18. Compression/glide on shoulder.

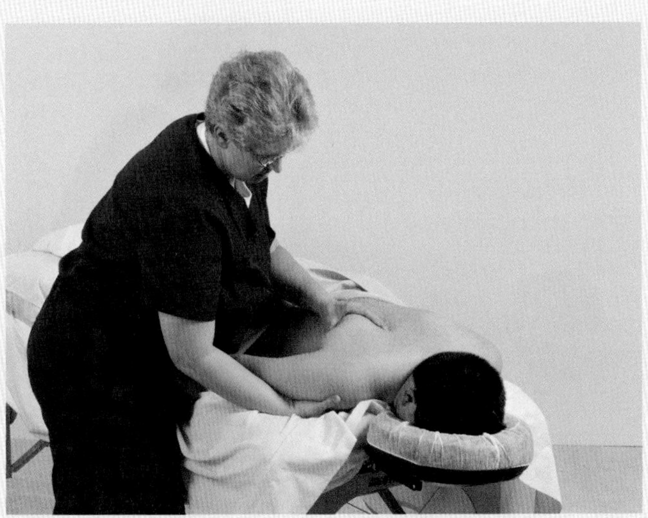

19. Oscillation. Shaking and move scapula.

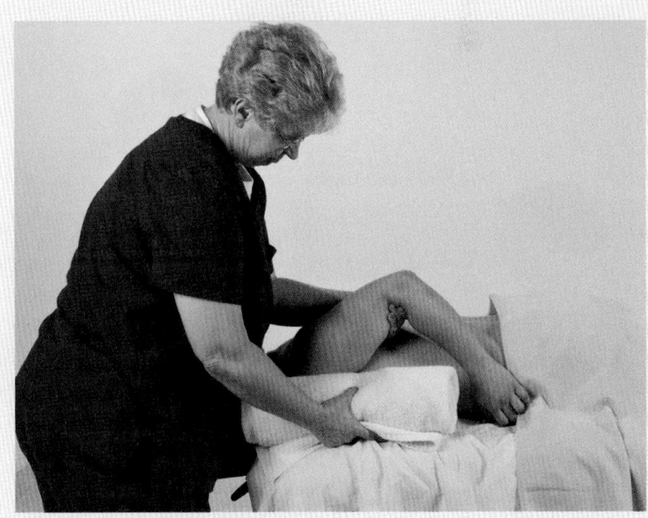

20. Bolster shoulder.

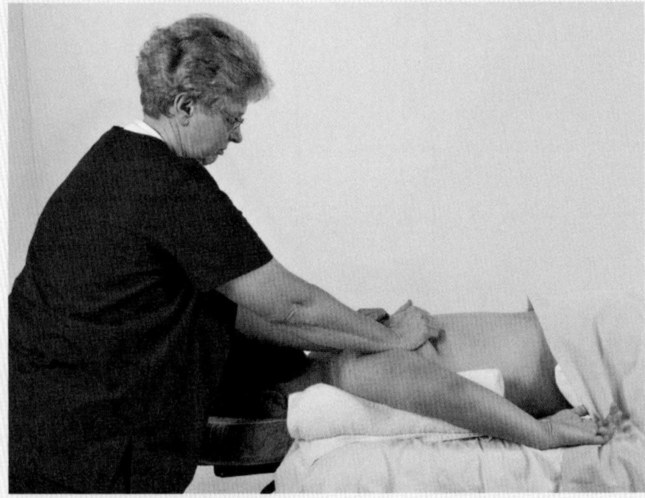

21. Knead and glide around scapula.

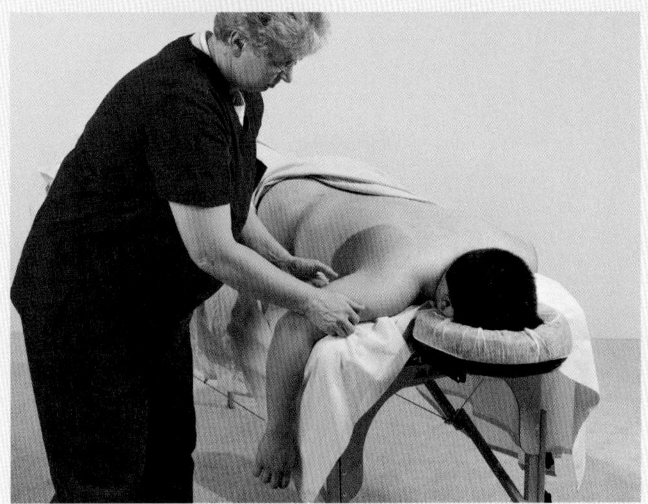

22. Position arm, rock and shake, then assess.

Continued

GENERAL MASSAGE PROTOCOL—cont'd

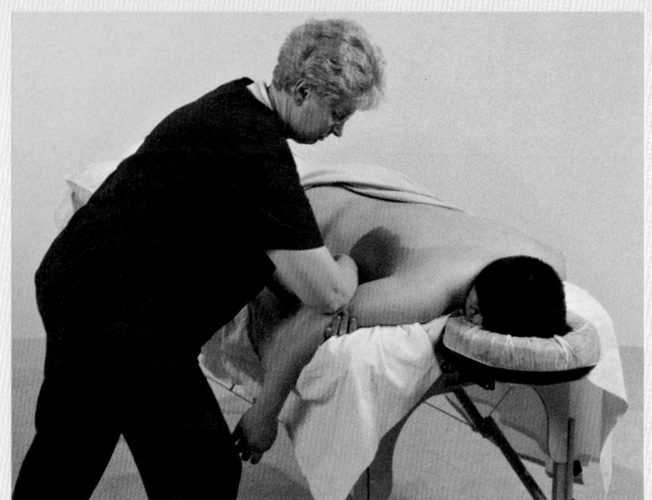

23. Glide arm using forearm.

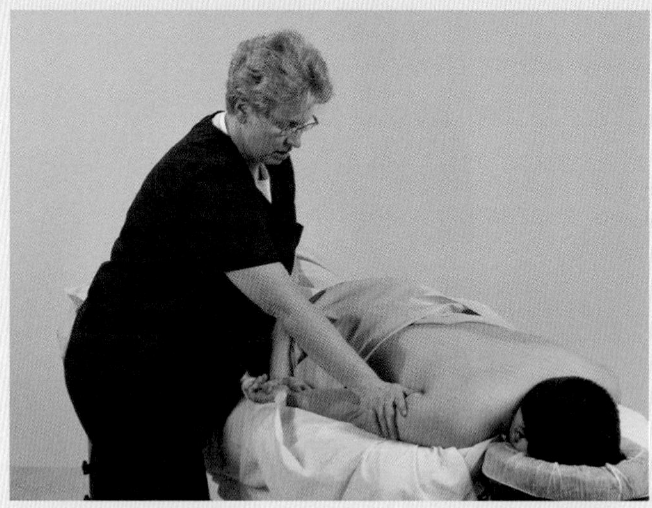

24. Glide using palm.

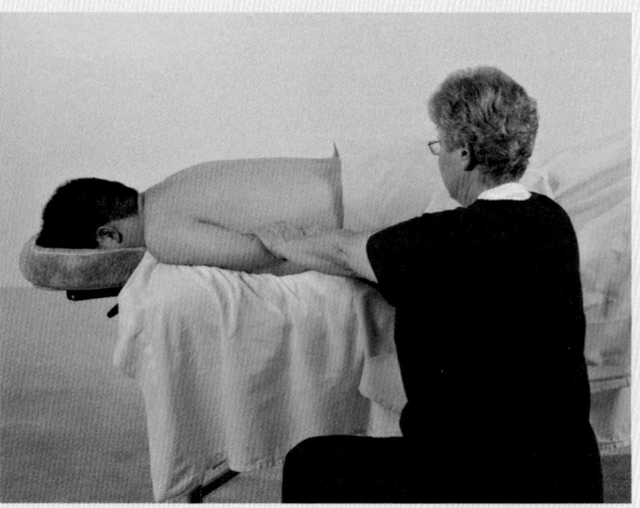

25. Knead arm and forearm. Massage therapist kneeling or seated.

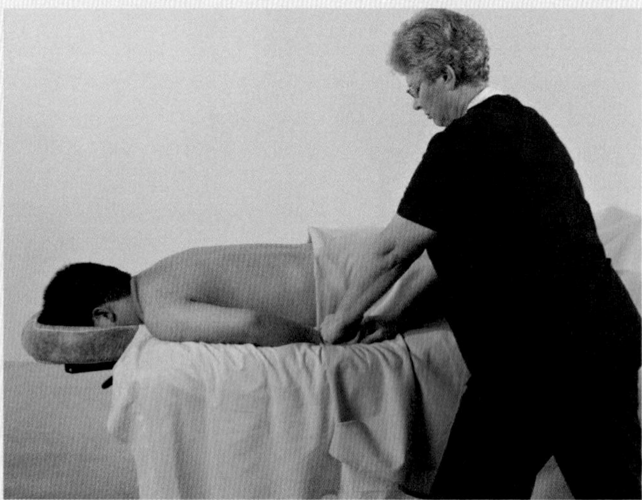

26. Compress forearm and hand. Repeat on opposite side (steps 18–26).

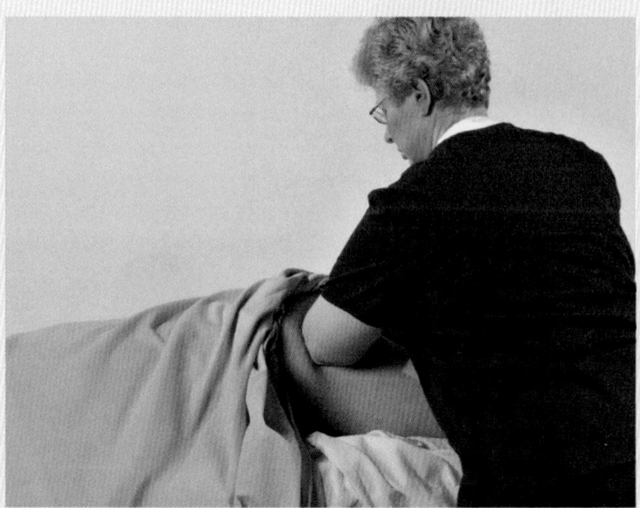

27. Move to hip and thigh. Compression/glide with forearm.

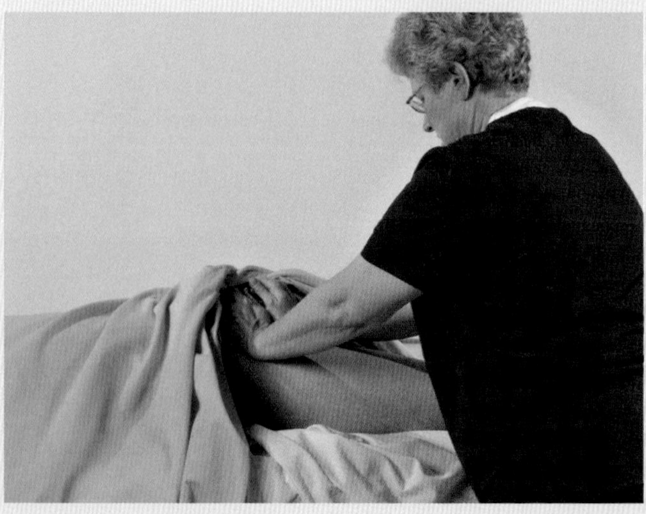

28. Palm compression.

GENERAL MASSAGE PROTOCOL—cont'd

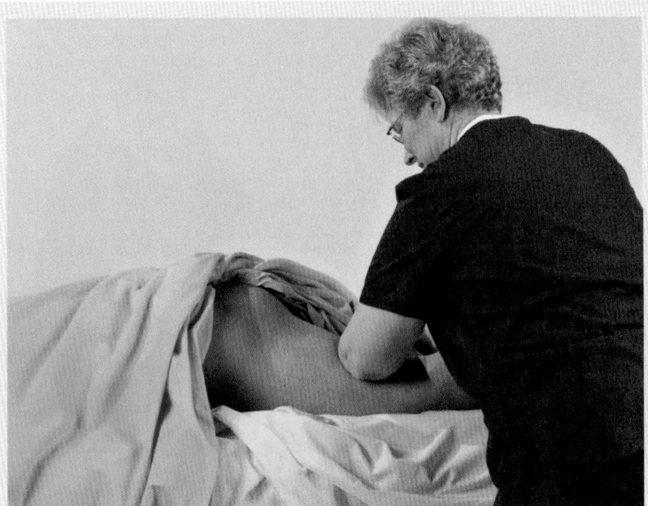

29. Repeat gliding, slower and deeper.

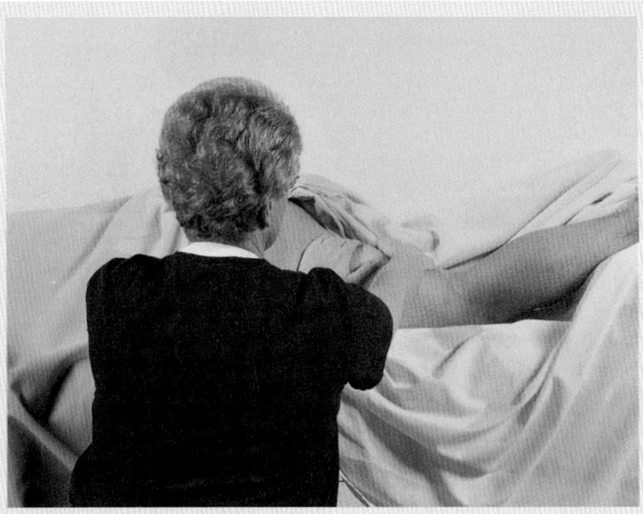

30. Knead posterior thigh while kneeling or seated.

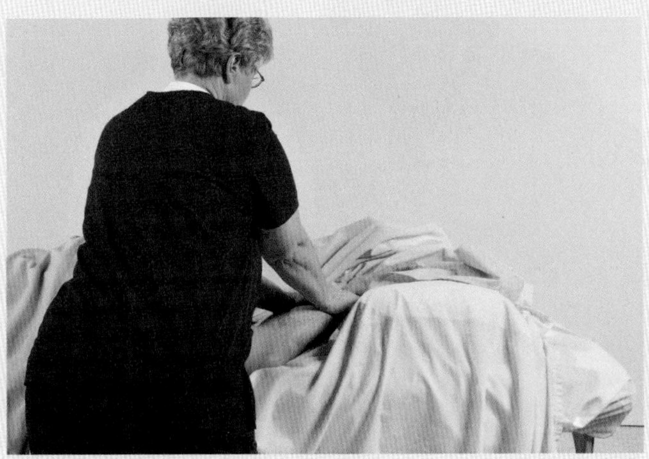

31. Glide on calf.

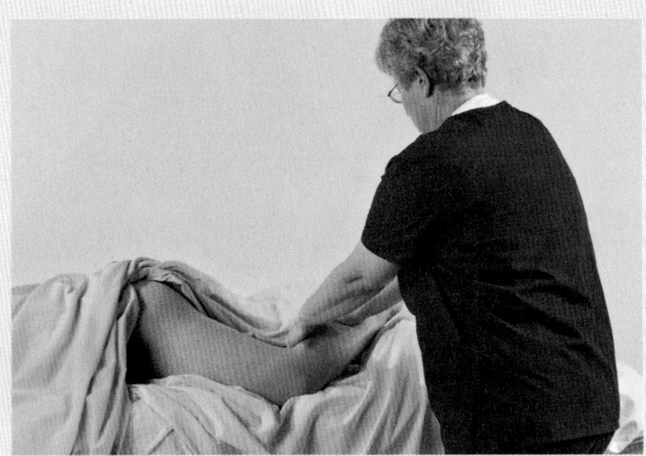

32. Reposition leg and knead calf.

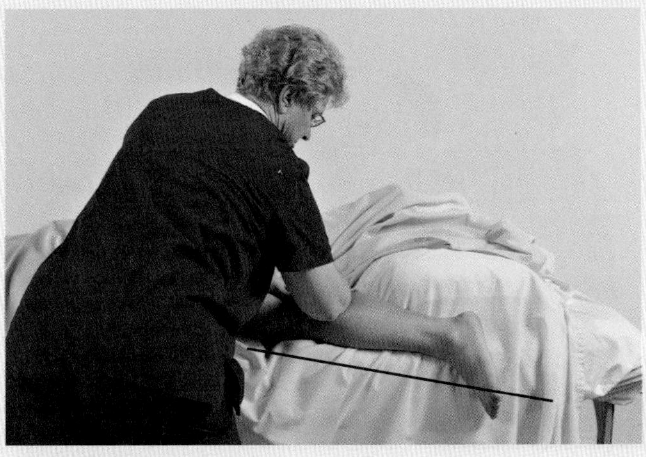

33. Reposition leg, straighten knee, compress, glide, and knead.

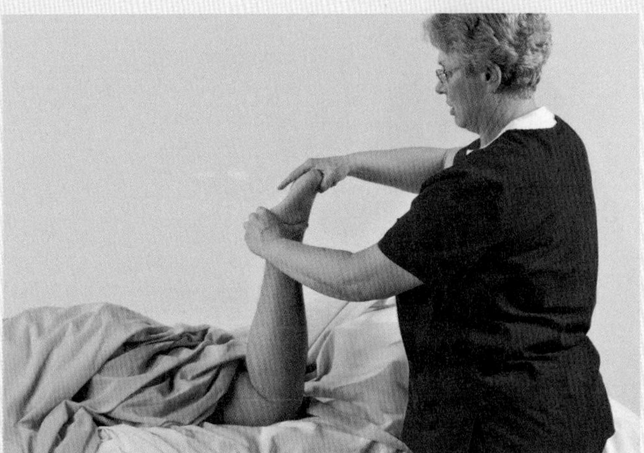

34. Joint movement of knee, ankle, foot.

Continued

GENERAL MASSAGE PROTOCOL—cont'd

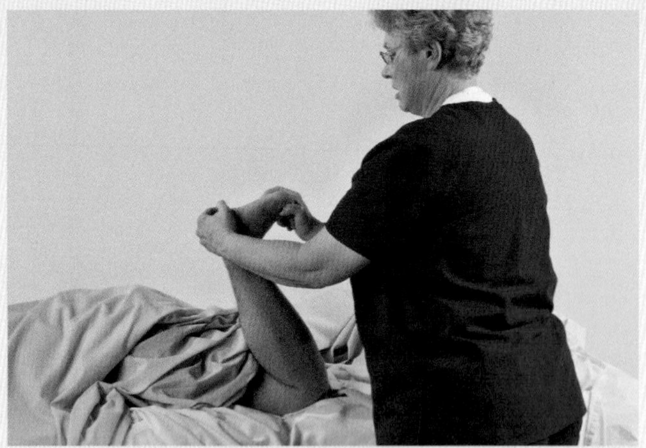

35. Elongate and move. Position leg for foot massage.

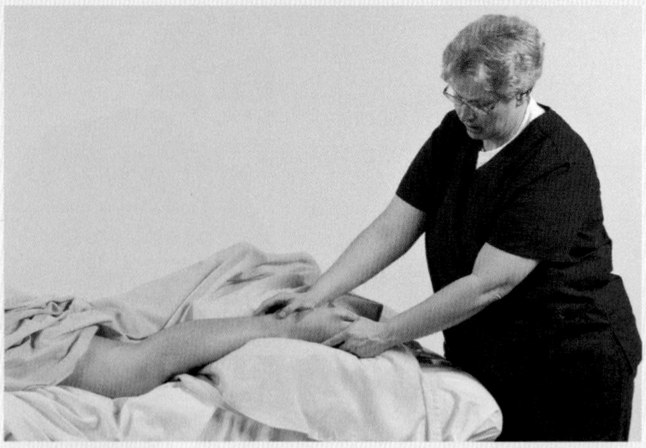

36. Compression of lateral foot using palm. Reposition leg.

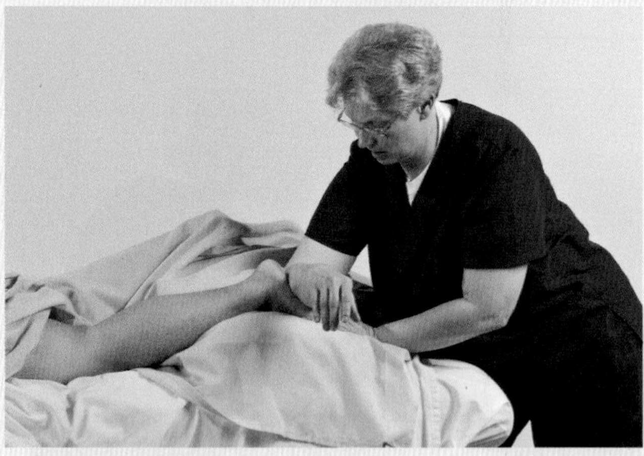

37. Compression of sole of foot using forearm. Repeat steps 27–37 on opposite side.

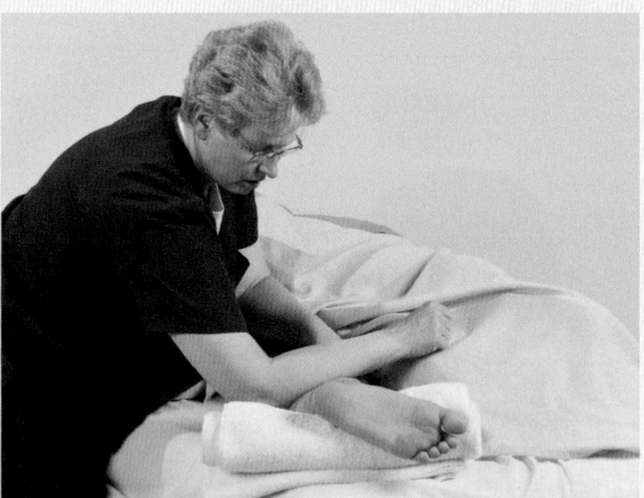

38. Reposition client side-lying with glide/compression of calf and foot.

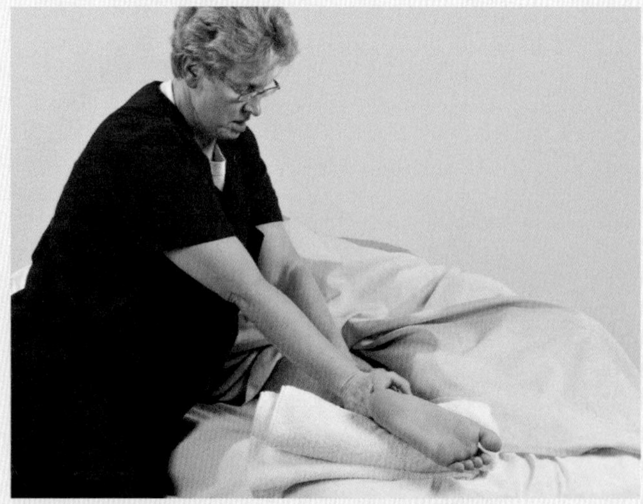

39. Compression/glide of ankle and heel, medial side.

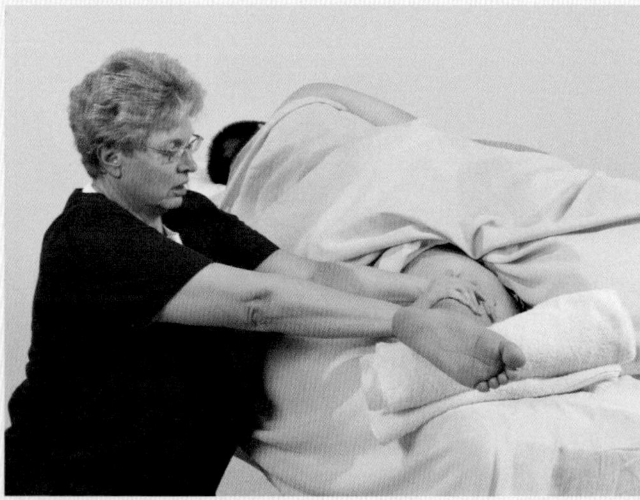

40. Knead calf.

GENERAL MASSAGE PROTOCOL—cont'd

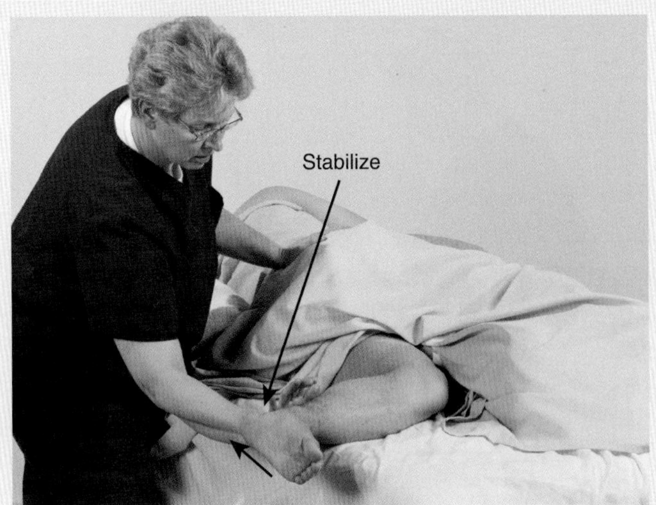

41. Muscle energy techniques using antagonist contraction.

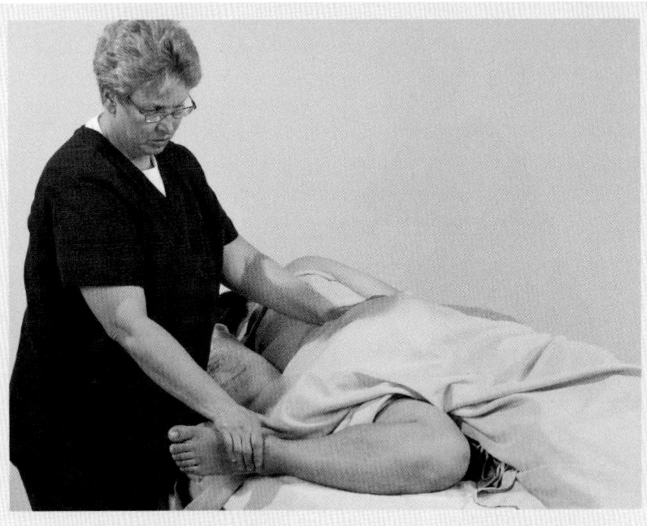

42. Lengthen anterior thigh.

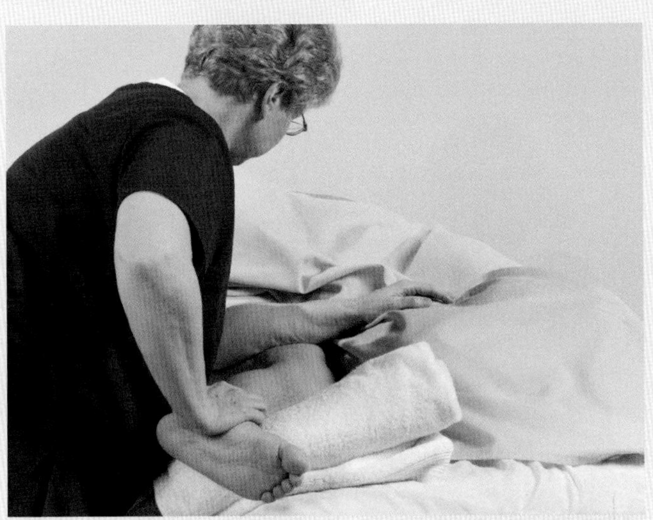

43. Glide of the inner (medial) thigh.

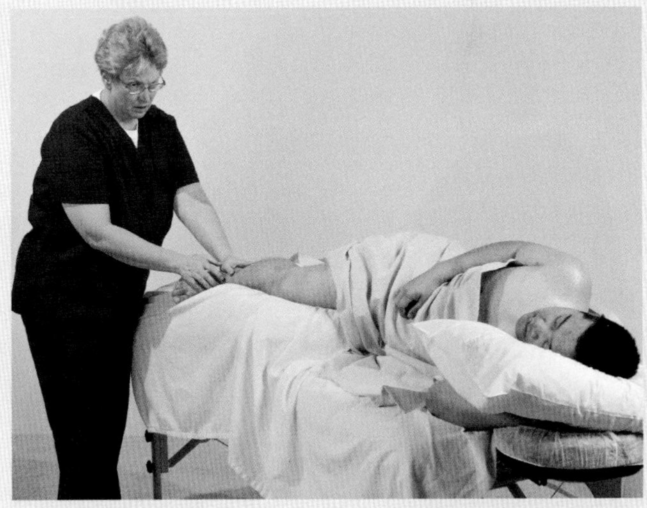

44. Client remains side-lying. Switch to opposite leg.

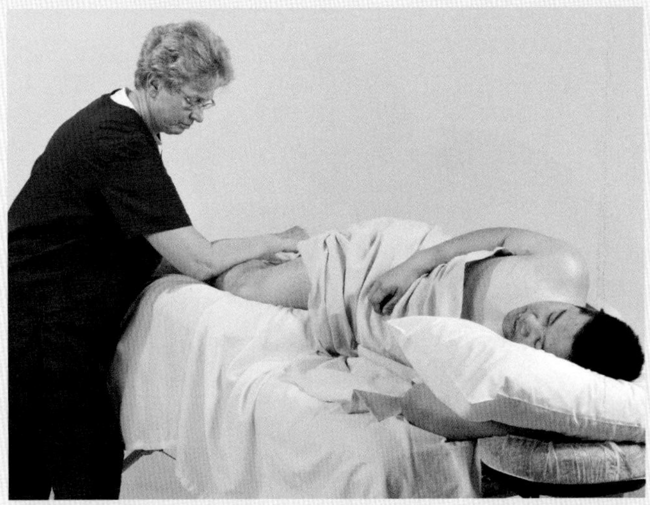

45. Compression/glide on calf, lateral side.

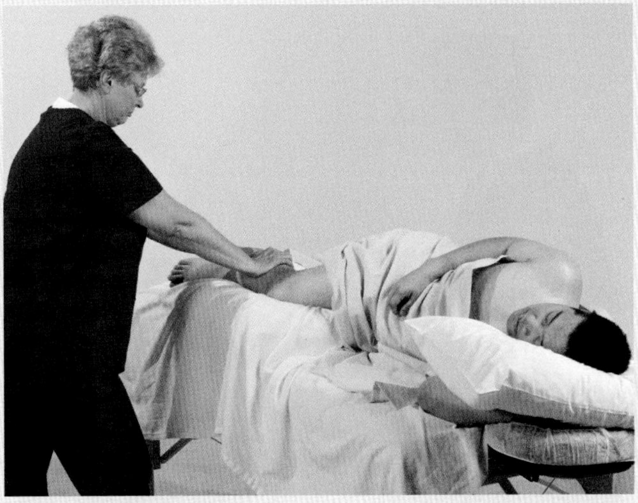

46. Knead calf.

Continued

GENERAL MASSAGE PROTOCOL—cont'd

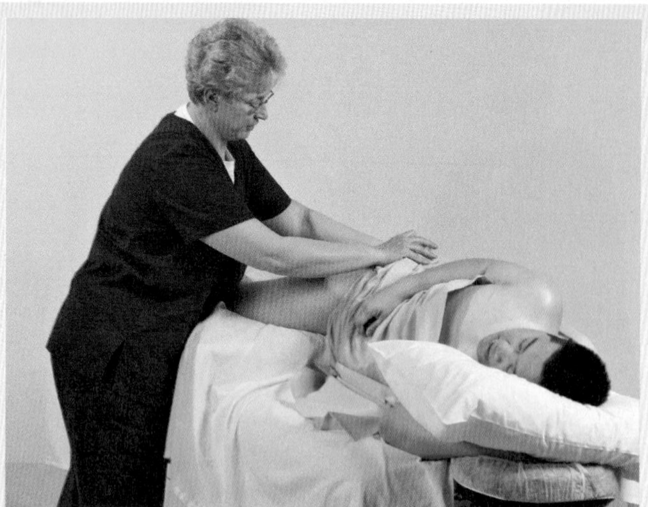

47. Move drape to provide access to thigh and hip.

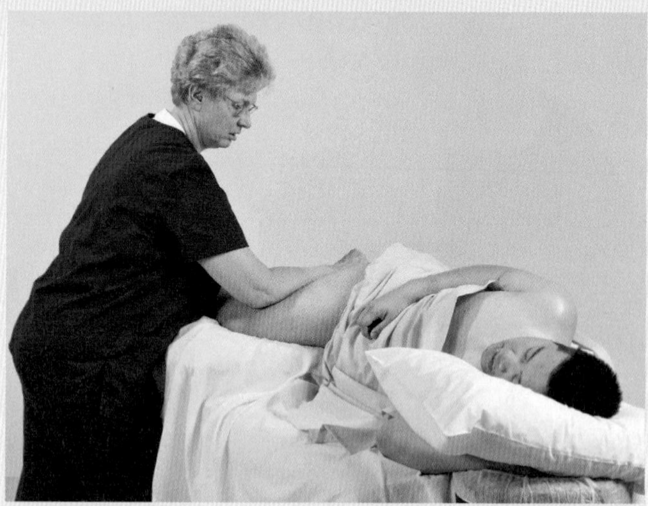

48. Glide, lateral thigh. Caution: Do not compress tissue into underlying bone.

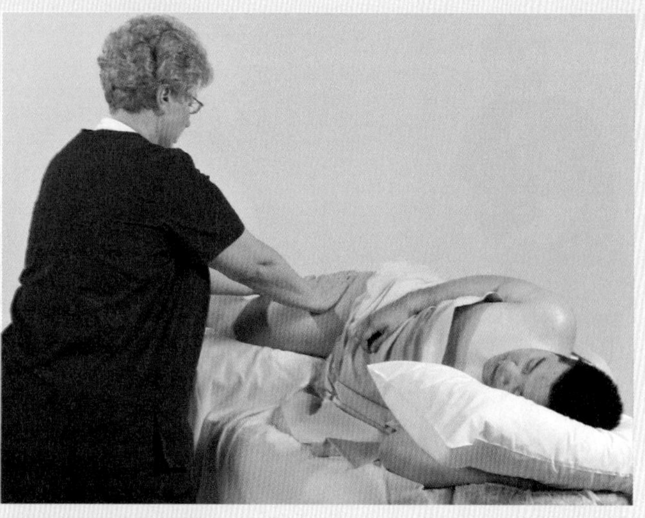

49. Knead lateral thigh.

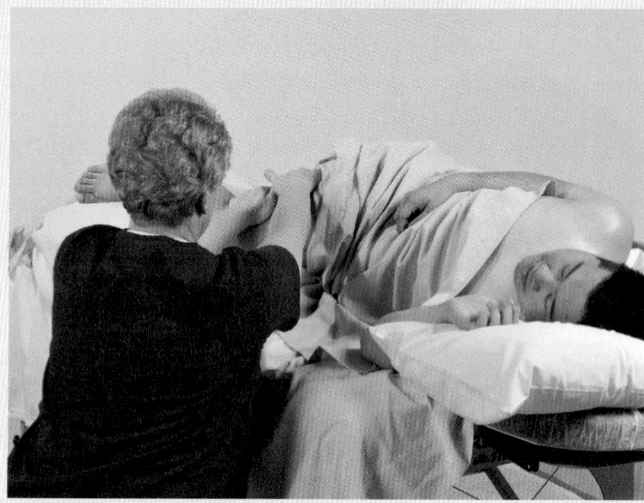

50. Knead while kneeling or seated.

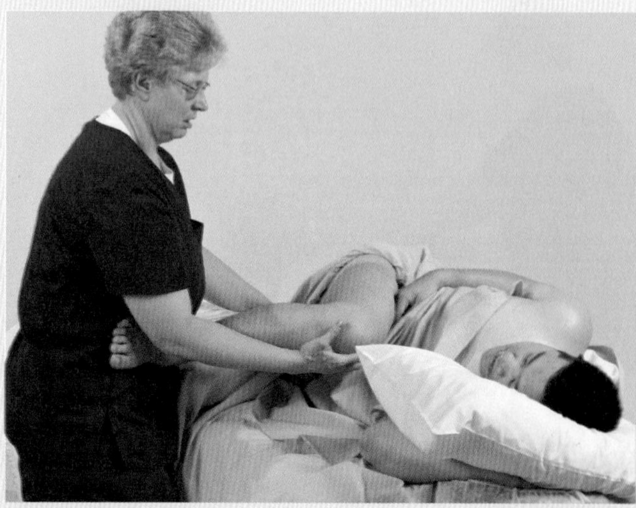

51. Joint movement.

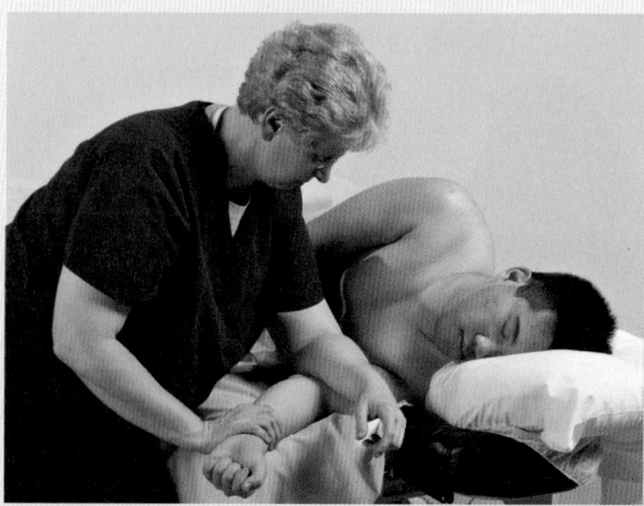

52. Arm. Compression/glide using forearm.

GENERAL MASSAGE PROTOCOL—cont'd

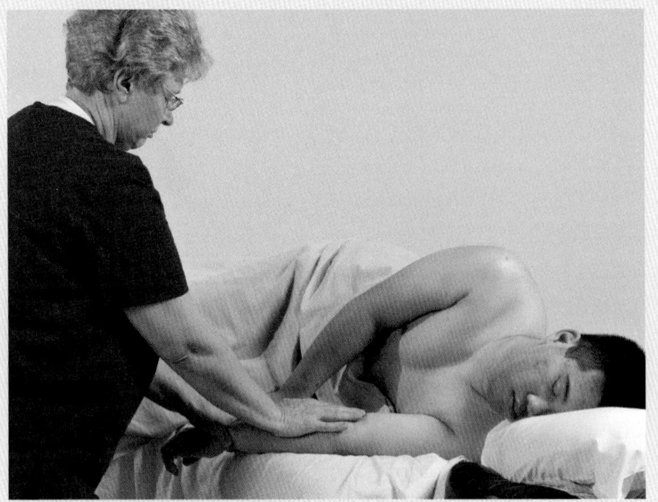

53. Glide using palm.

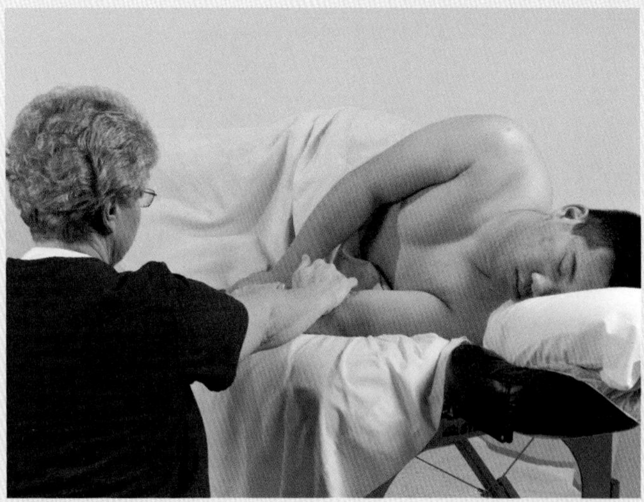

54. Knead while kneeling or seated.

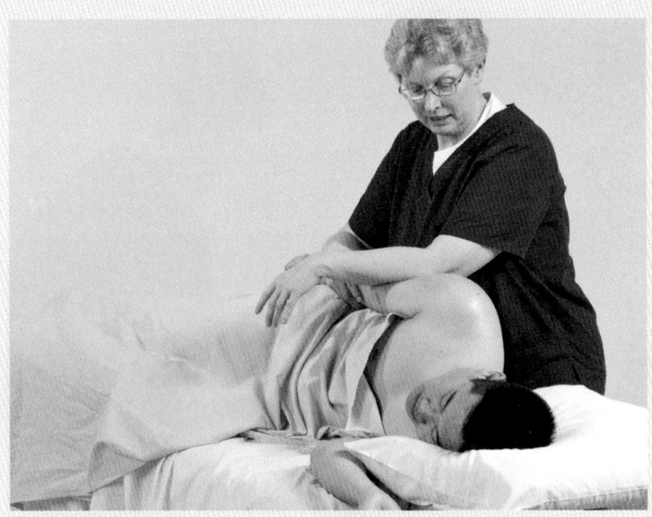

55. Move to opposite arm. Compression/glide.

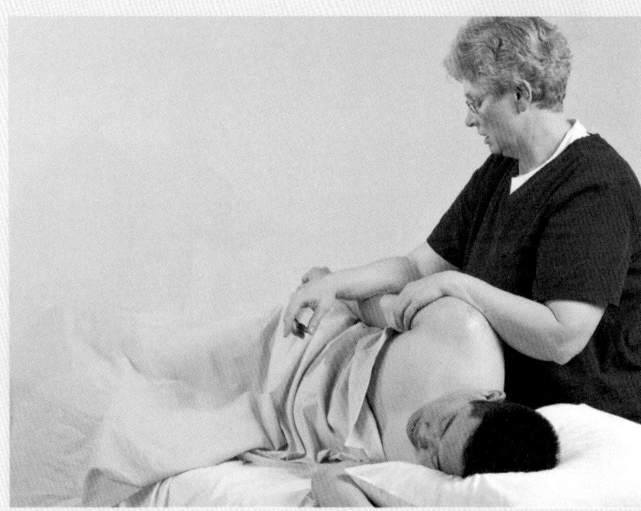

56. Change position to access forearm. Compression/glide using forearm.

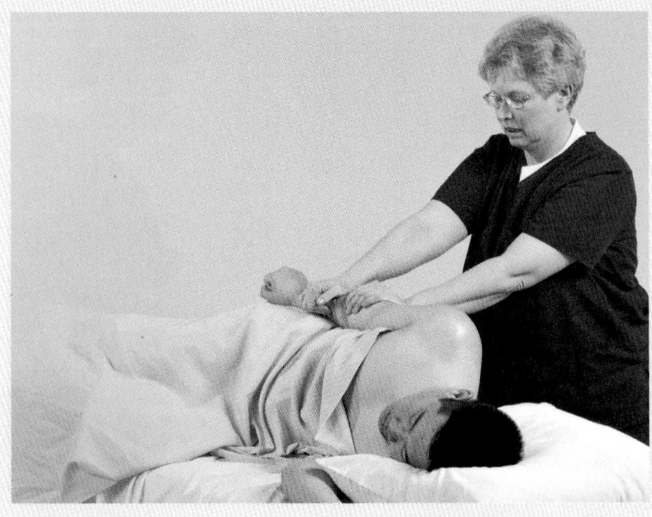

57. Knead arm.

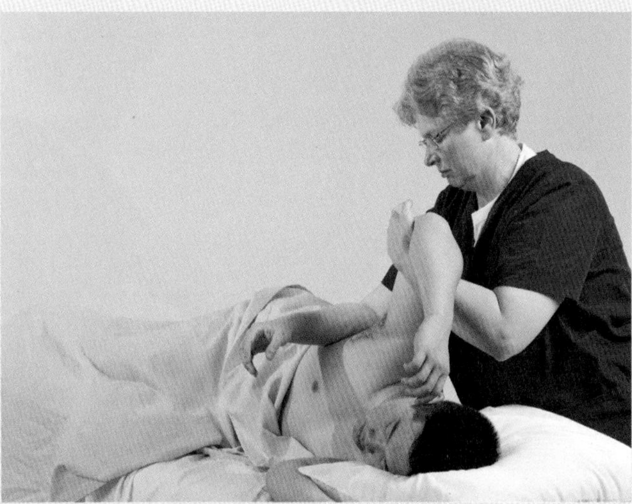

58. Joint movement and compression combined with glide.

Continued

GENERAL MASSAGE PROTOCOL—cont'd

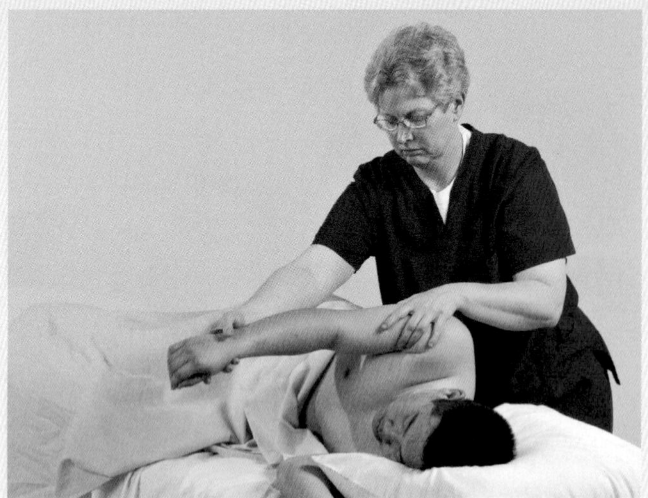

59. Joint movement and position arm.

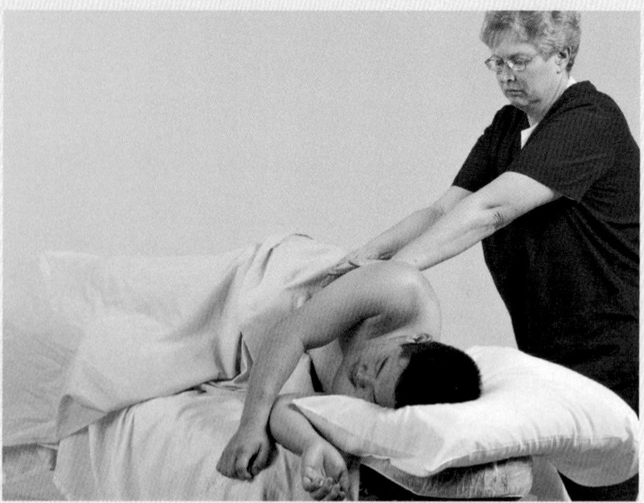

60. Knead lateral chest and back.

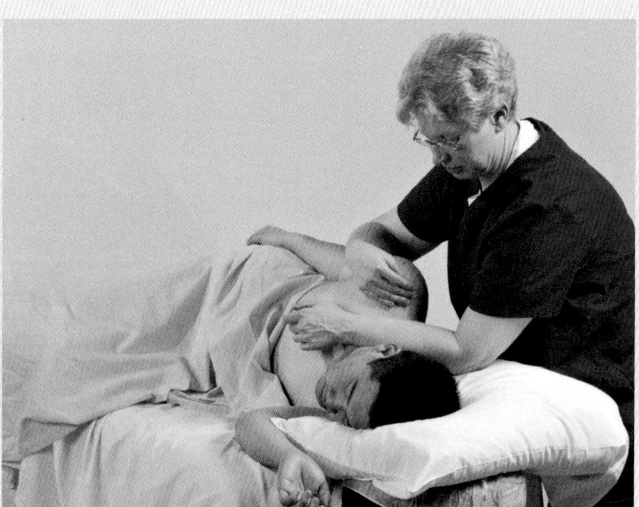

61. Compression of neck: Stay behind the sternocleidomastoid muscle.

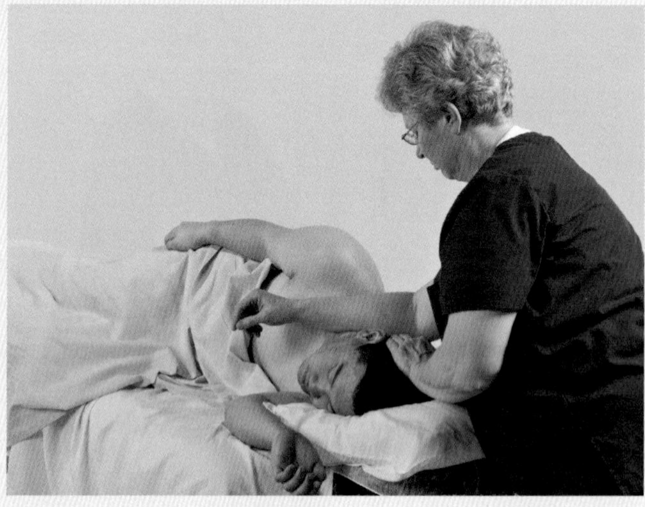

62. Compression of shoulder.

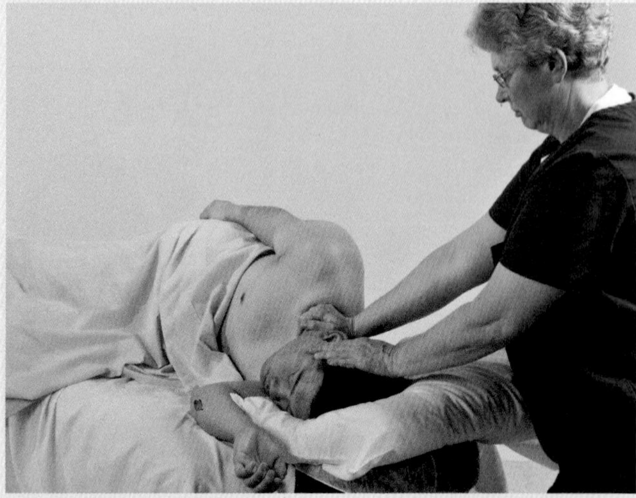

63. Knead neck.

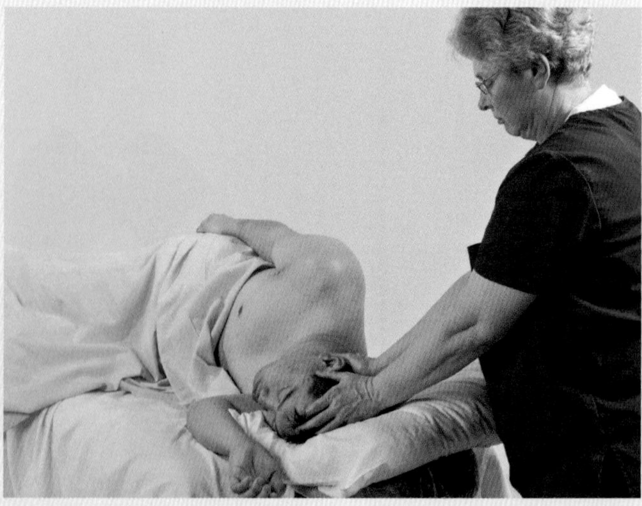

64. Massage the head. Repeat steps 38–64 on opposite side.

GENERAL MASSAGE PROTOCOL—cont'd

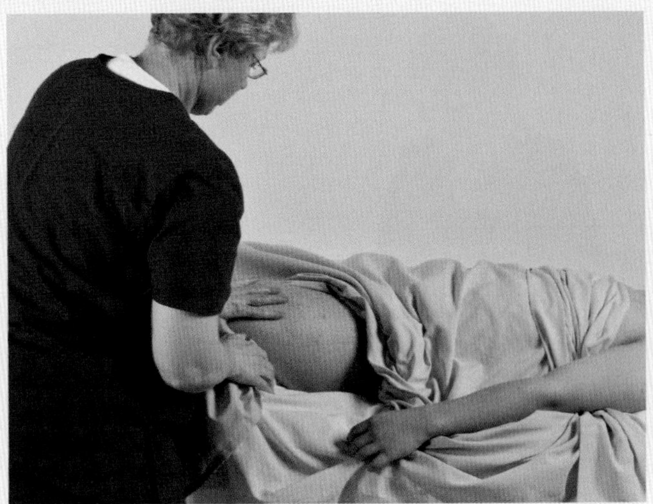

65. Turn client supine, begin with leg. Assess and palpate.

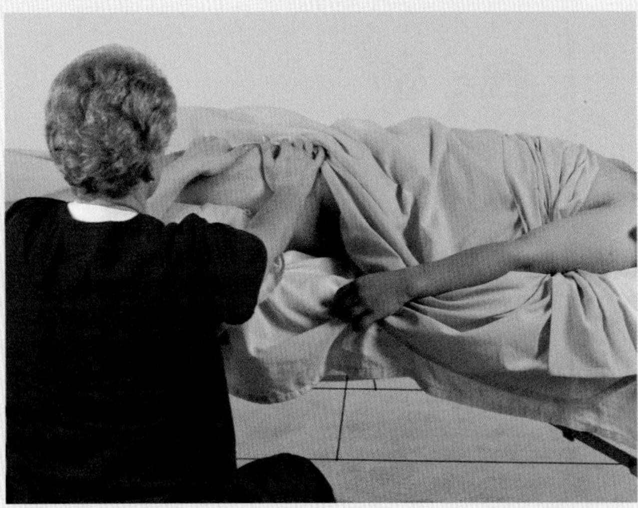

66. Knead anterior thigh. Massage therapist kneeling or seated.

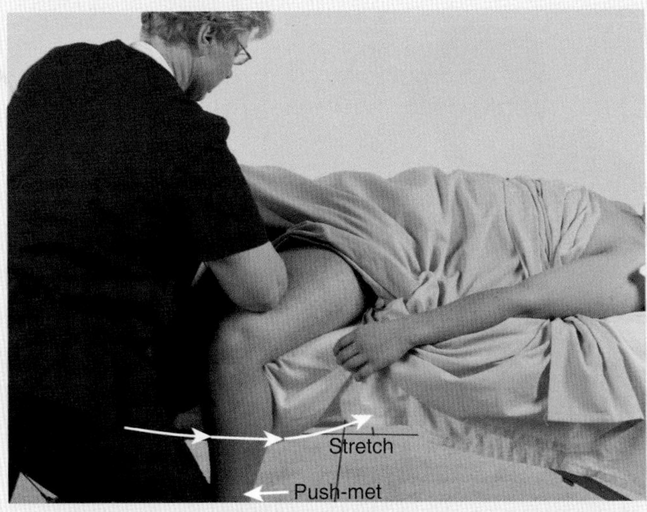

67. Position leg. Glide anterior thigh combined with muscle energy technique and lengthen and stretch using the therapist's leg as the point where the client pushes as well as for stretch.

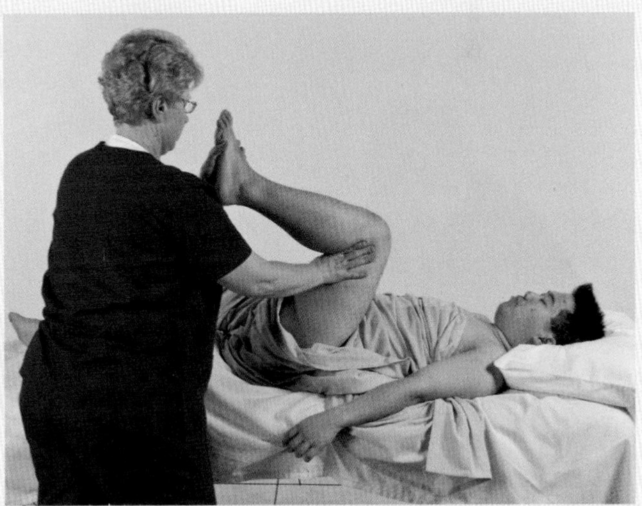

68. Joint movement of hip/assessment.

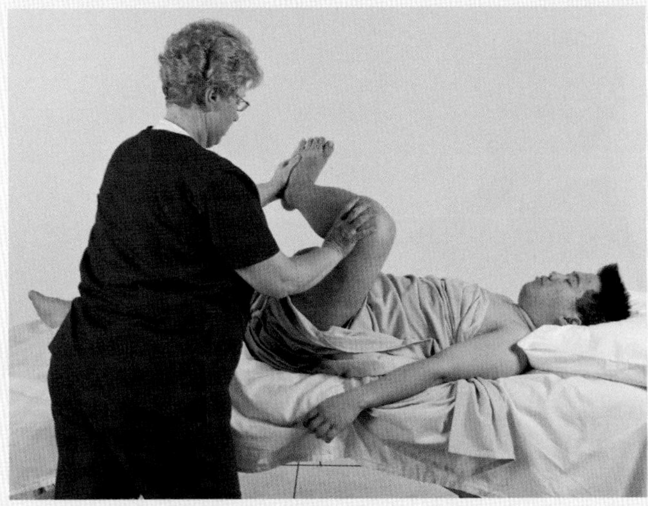

69. Joint movement/assessment, muscle energy techniques.

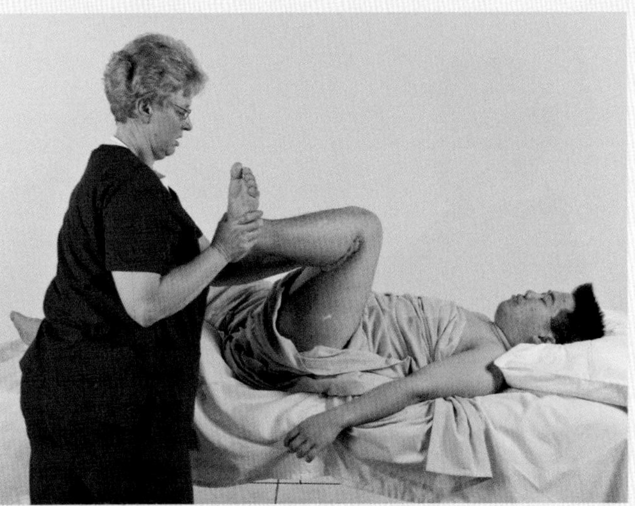

70. Joint movement/muscle energy techniques, lengthen.

Continued

GENERAL MASSAGE PROTOCOL—cont'd

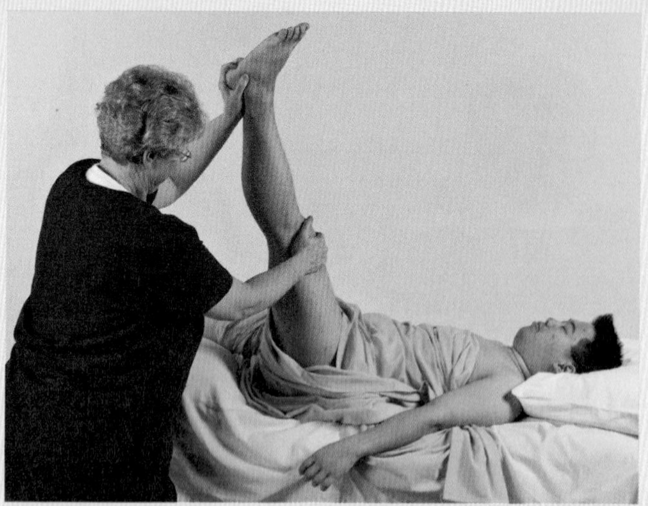

71. Assessment/joint movement, lengthen (hip and knee).

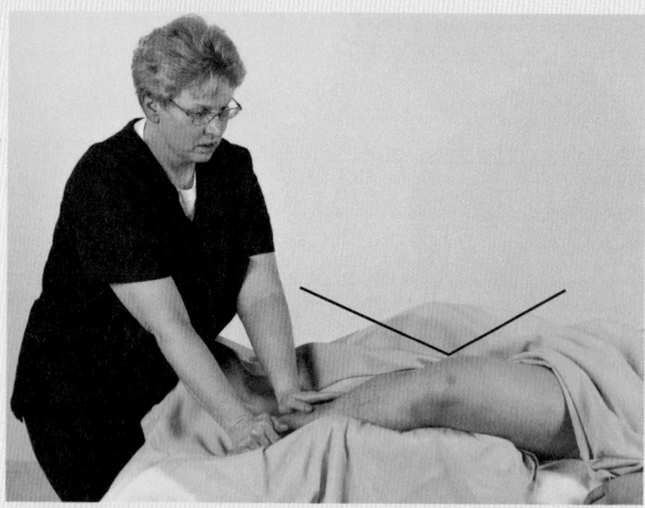

72. Position leg to massage foot, medial leg.

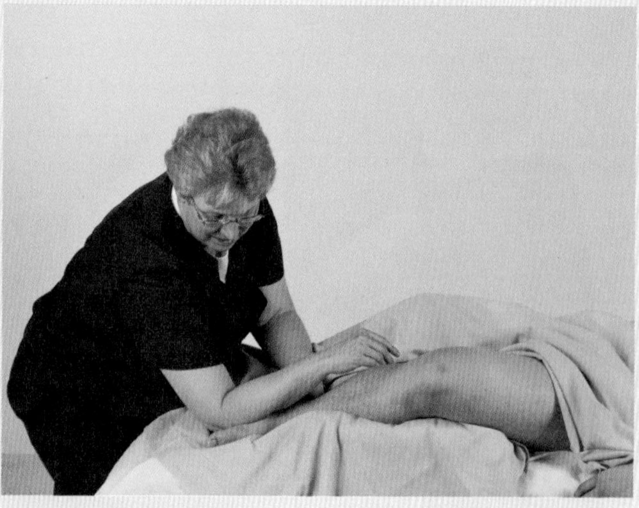

73. Compression of foot.

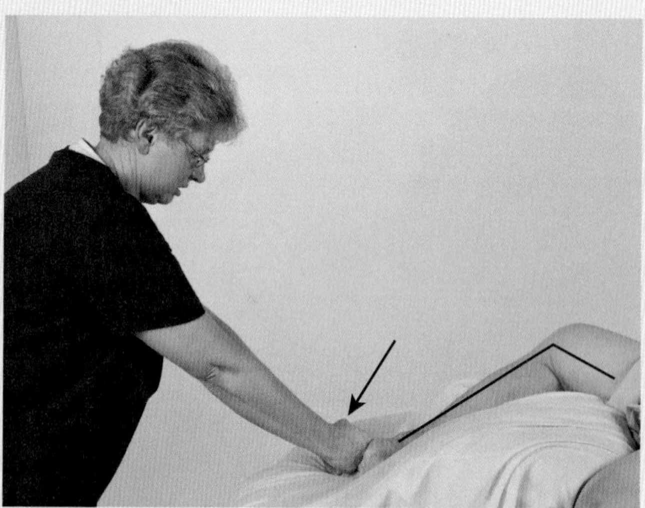

74. Compression of foot. Note leg position.

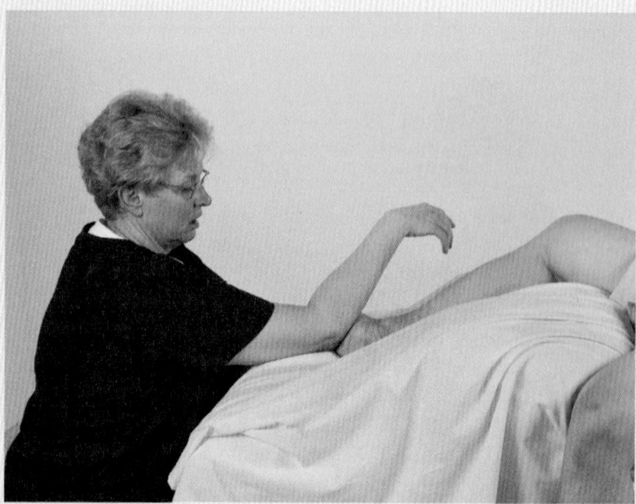

75. Compression of foot while therapist kneels or is seated.

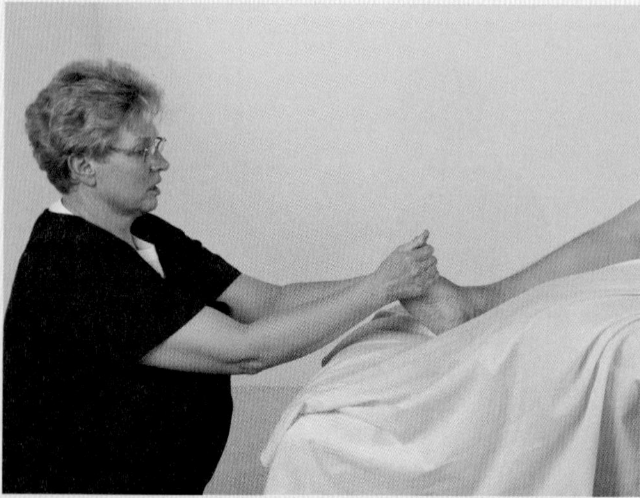

76. Elongate tissue between toes. Repeat steps 65–76 on opposite side.

GENERAL MASSAGE PROTOCOL—cont'd

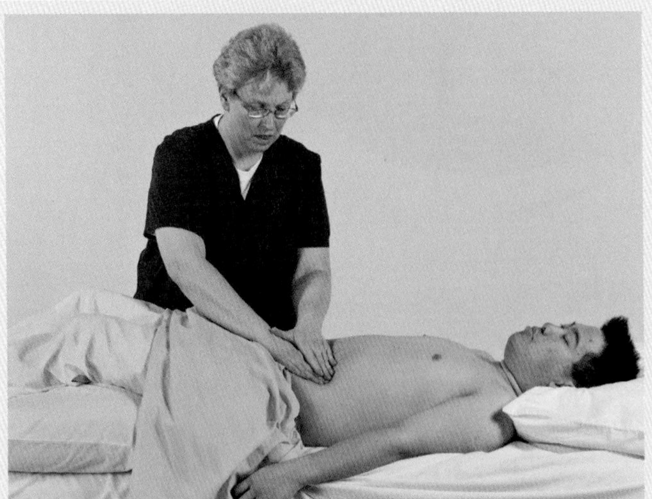

77. Massage abdomen.

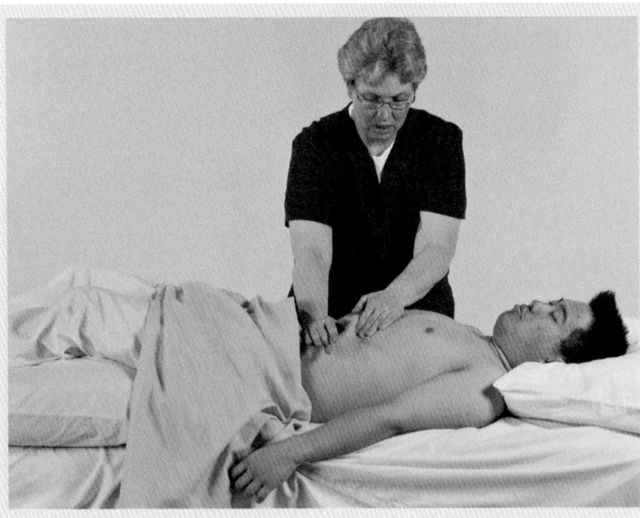

78. Knead abdomen.

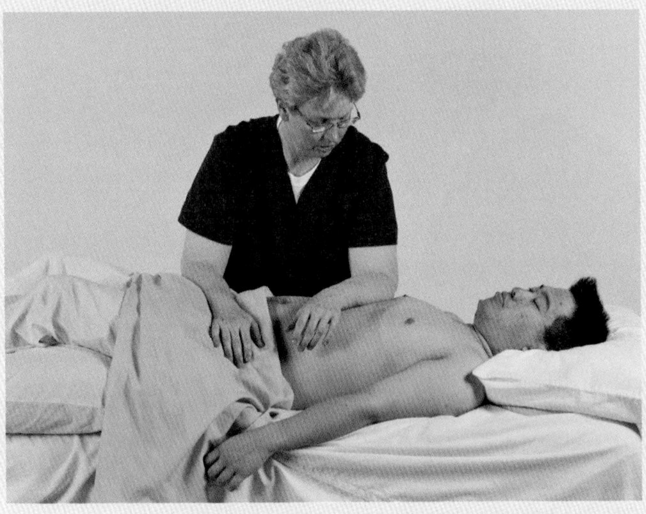

79. Compression/glide on chest. Drape appropriately for females.

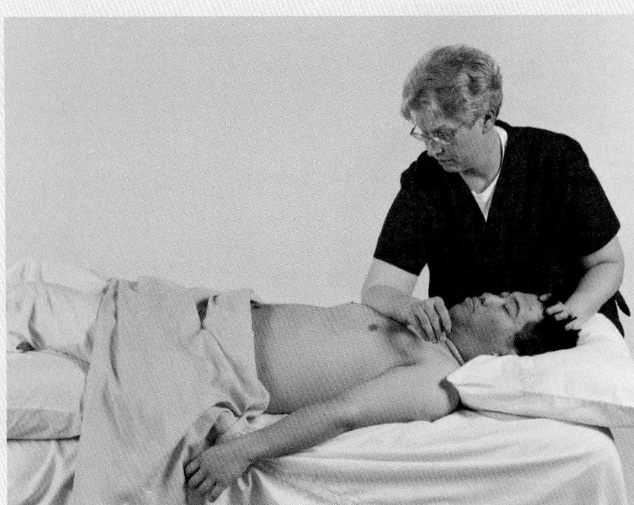

80. Change position and massage anterior thorax.

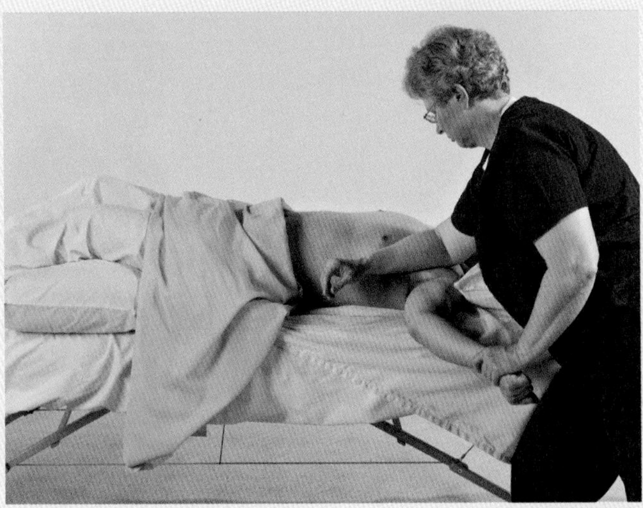

81. Move arm. Compression/glide on pectoralis muscle and associated fascia.

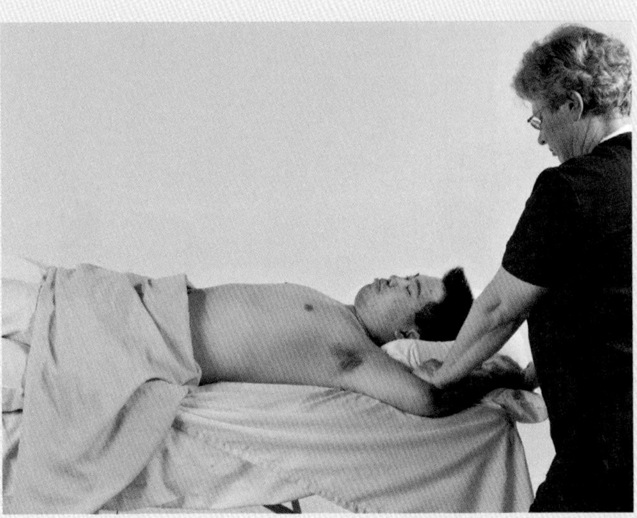

82. Position arm. Compression and kneading.

Continued

GENERAL MASSAGE PROTOCOL—cont'd

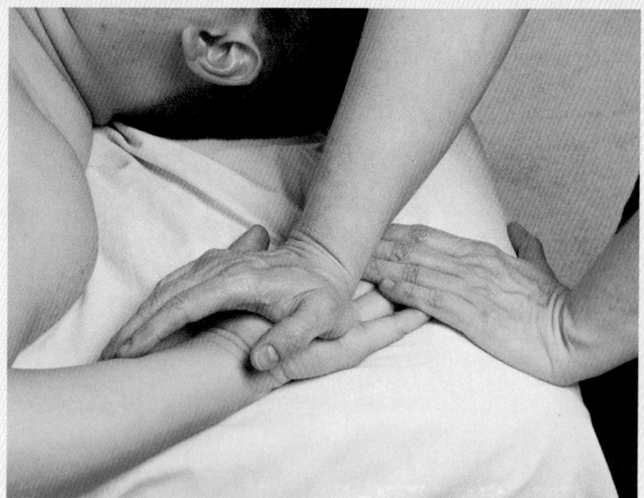

83. Compression of hand.

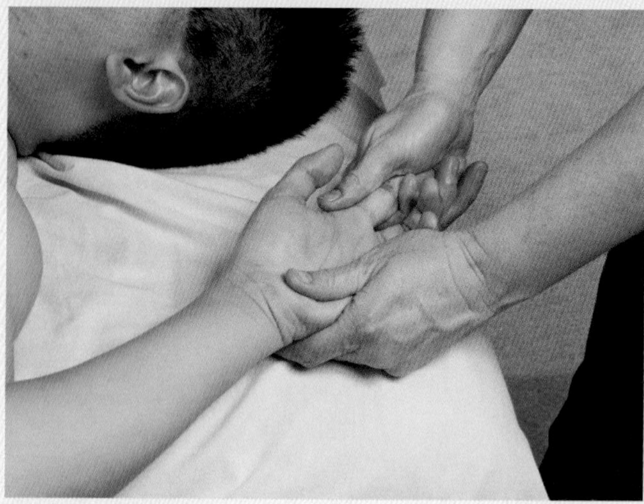

84. Massage fingers.

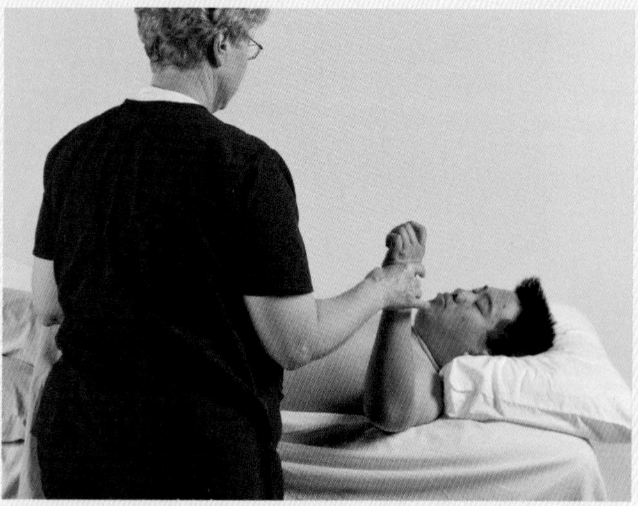

85. Joint movement of shoulder and elbow.

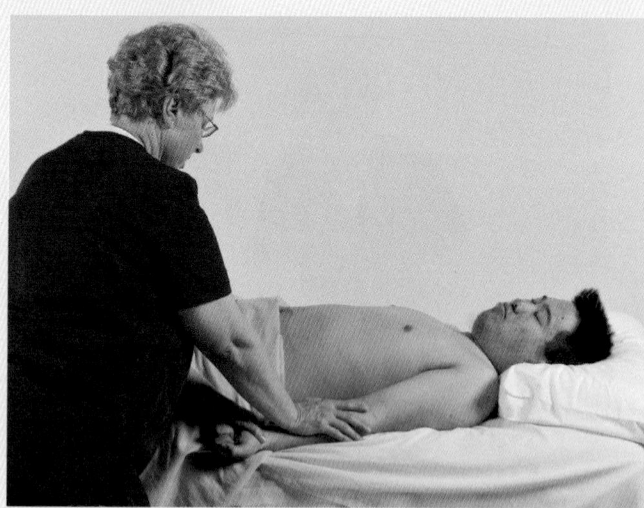

86. Position arm. Compress/glide forearm and arm.

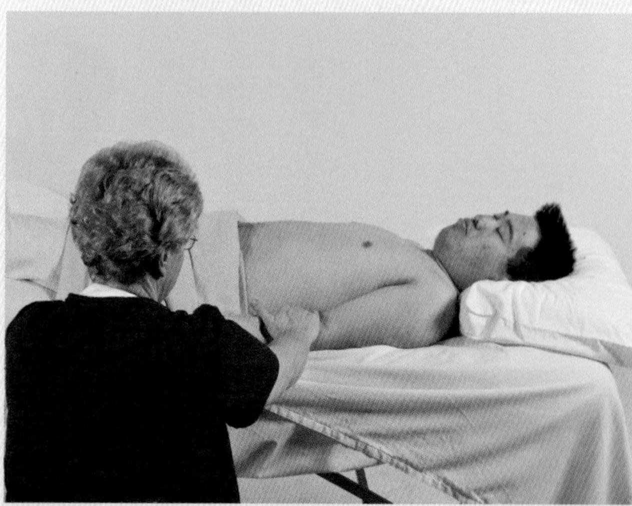

87. Kneading of forearm and arm, therapist kneeling or seated. Repeat steps 79–87 on opposite side.

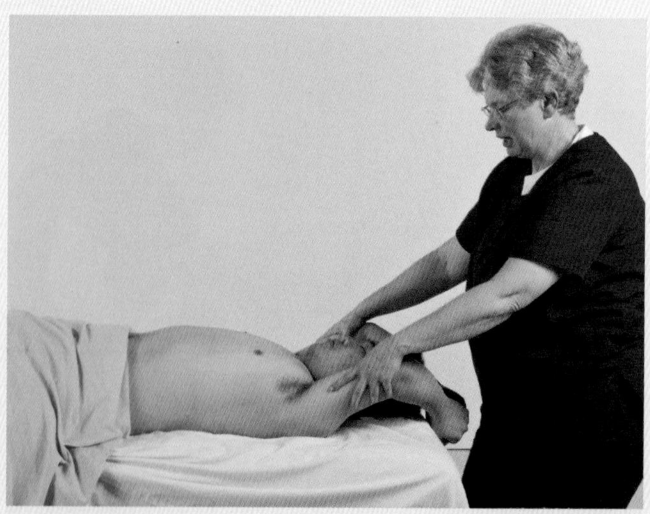

88. Bring arms up. Joint movement and muscle energy techniques.

GENERAL MASSAGE PROTOCOL—cont'd

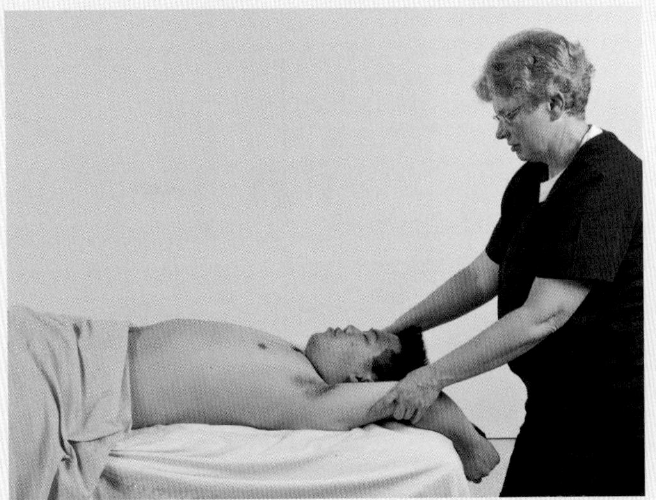

89. Lengthen.

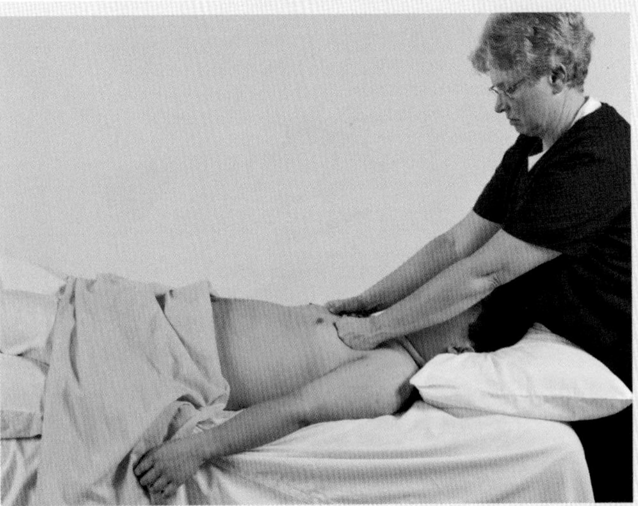

90. Compression of upper anterior thorax.

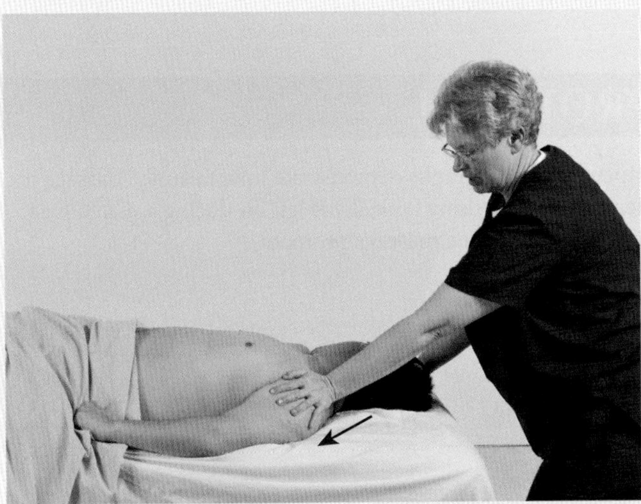

91. Joint movement of neck. Force is applied at shoulder for lengthening. Repeat step 91 on opposite side.

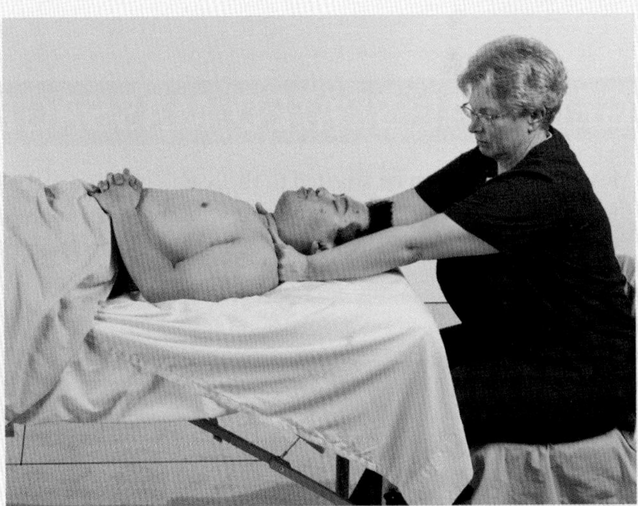

92. Compression of shoulder and neck massage, therapist seated.

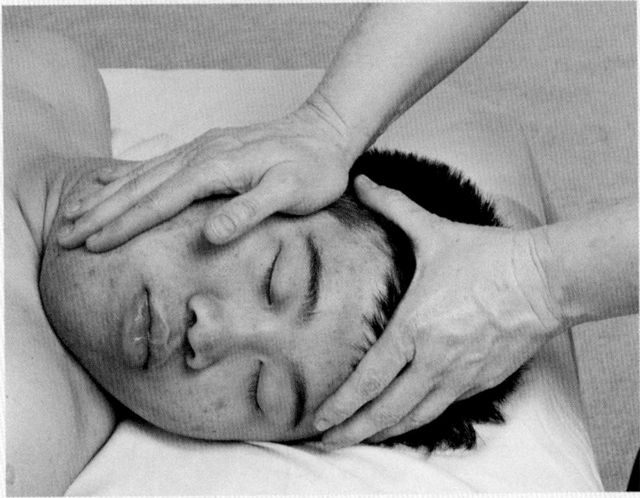

93. Compression/glide muscles of mastication. Repeat step 93 on opposite side.

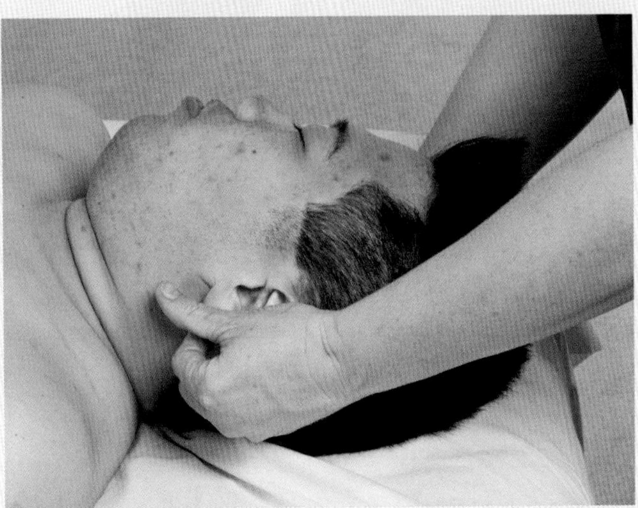

94. Ears.

Continued

GENERAL MASSAGE PROTOCOL—cont'd

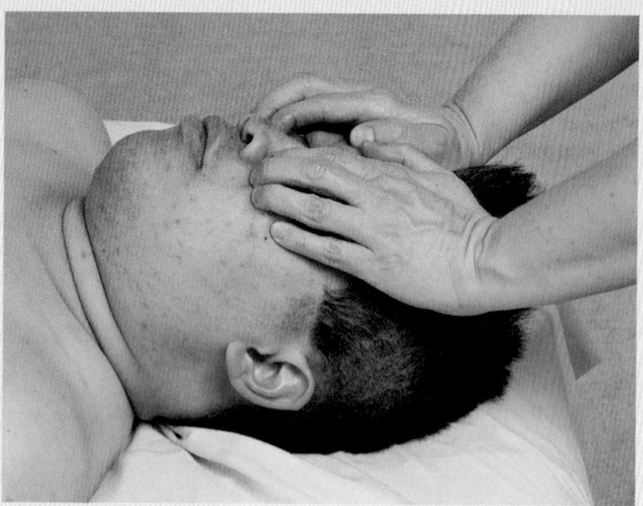

95. Face/compression.

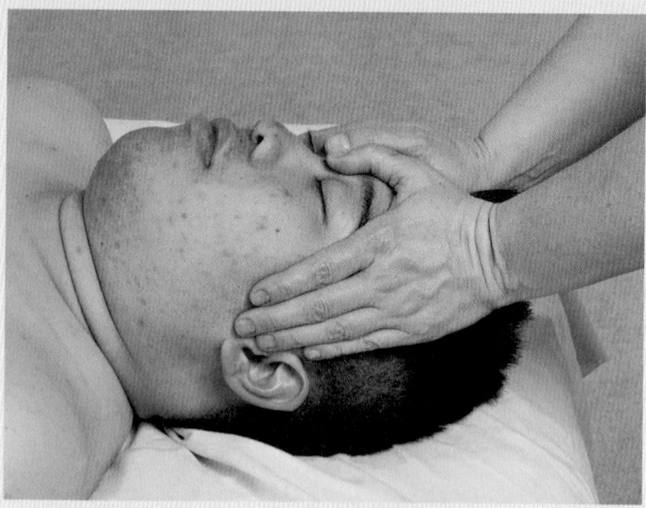

96. Finish. Note: If you want to begin with the client supine, start here and work backward through the figures.

GENERAL SEATED MASSAGE PROTOCOL

Massage methods can be adapted to the seated position. The accompanying photographs demonstrate how to apply massage to the various body regions using primarily compression and movement because clothing typically is left on during a seated massage (see the Evolve website for a complete video demonstration of the general seated massage protocol).

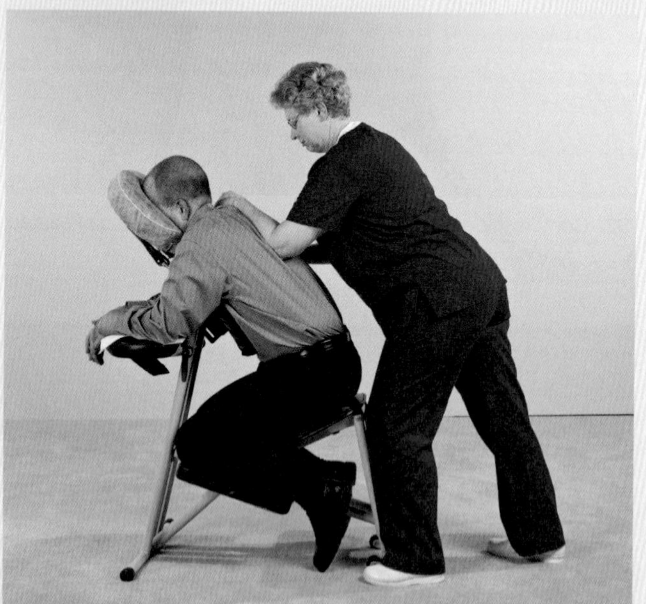

1. Forearm compression, standing.

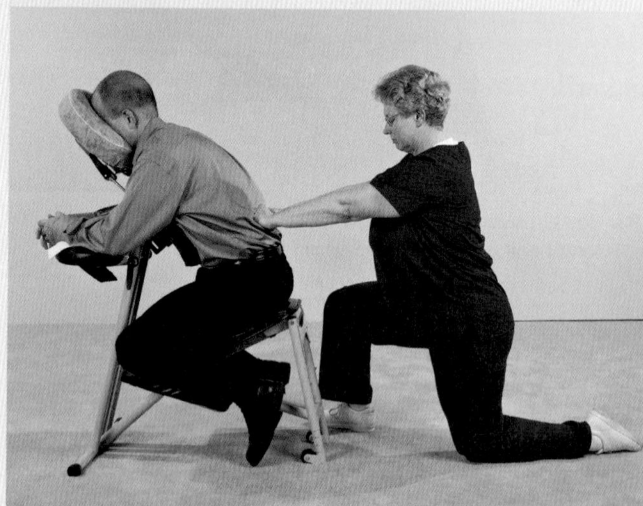

2. Fist compression, kneeling.

GENERAL SEATED MASSAGE PROTOCOL—cont'd

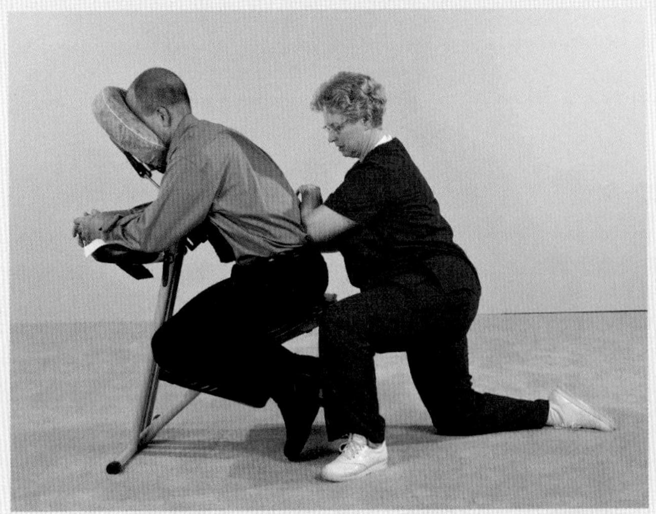

3. Forearm position, kneeling.

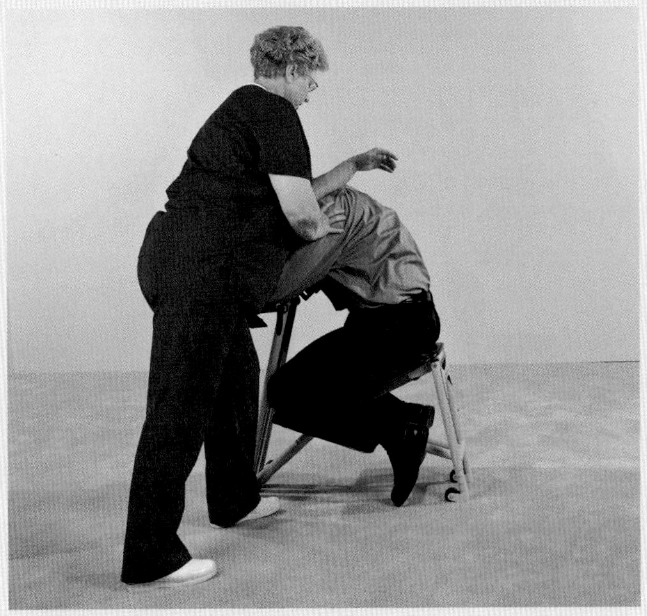

4. Forearm compression, shoulder.

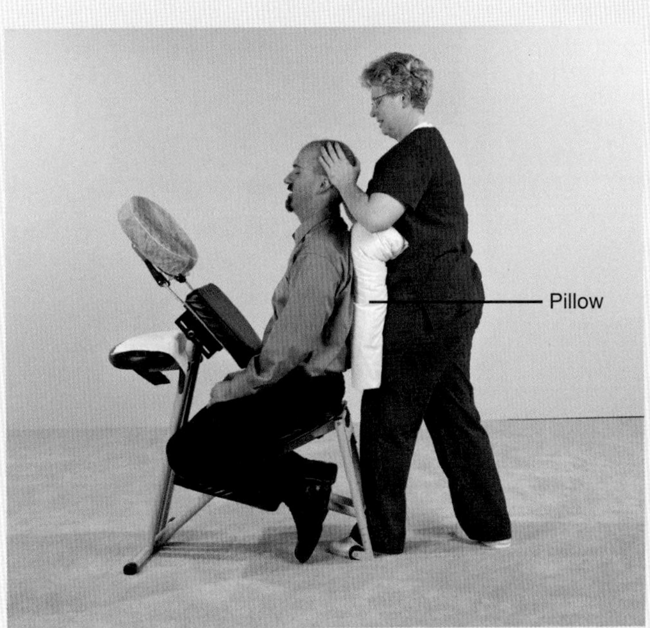

5. Position client against pillow.

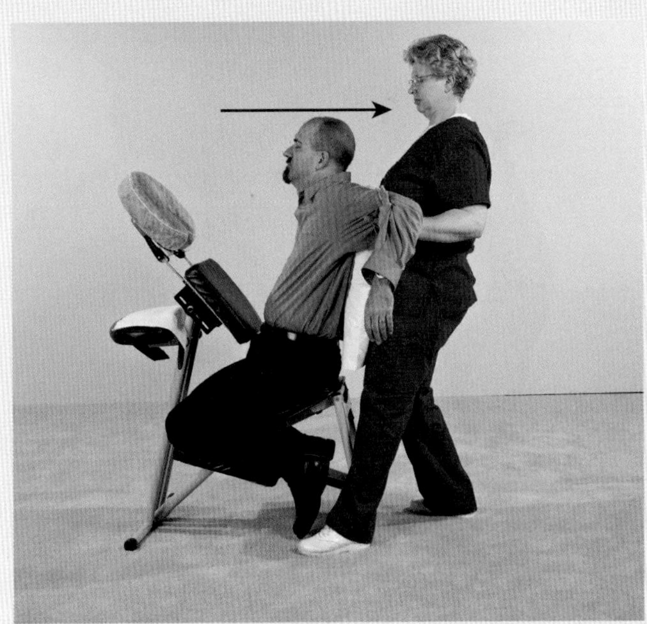

6. Lengthen, lean back.

Continued

GENERAL SEATED MASSAGE PROTOCOL—cont'd

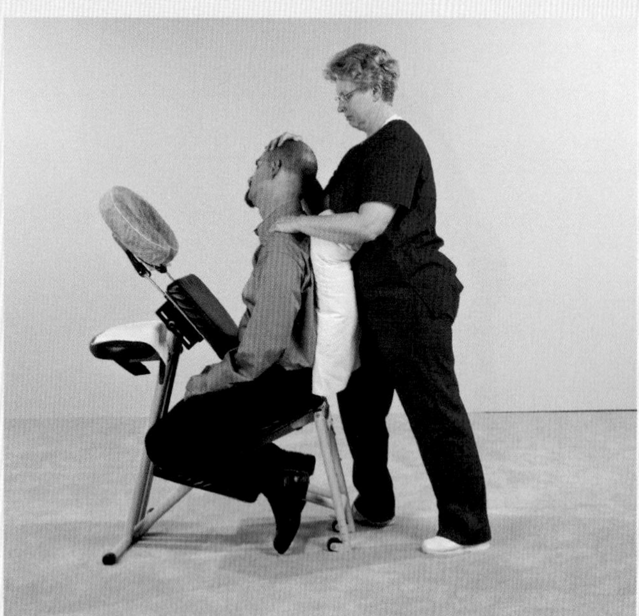

7. Movement of the neck.

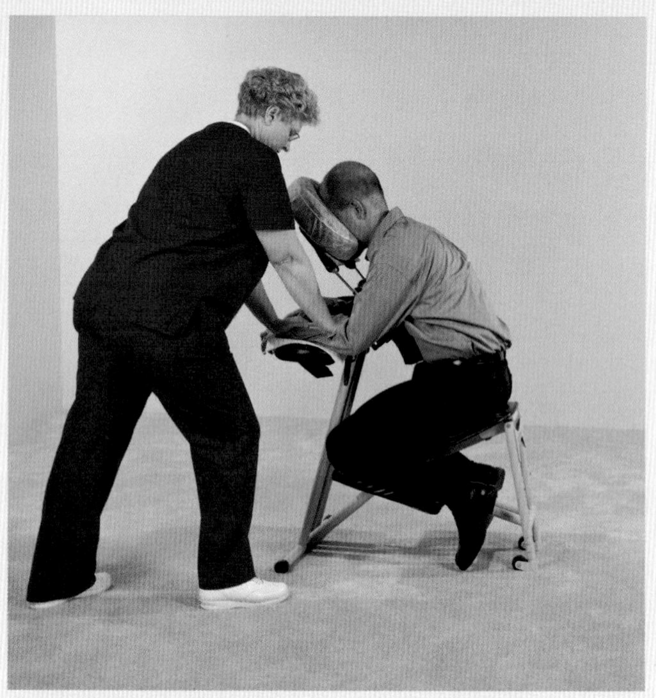

8. Palm compression, forearm.

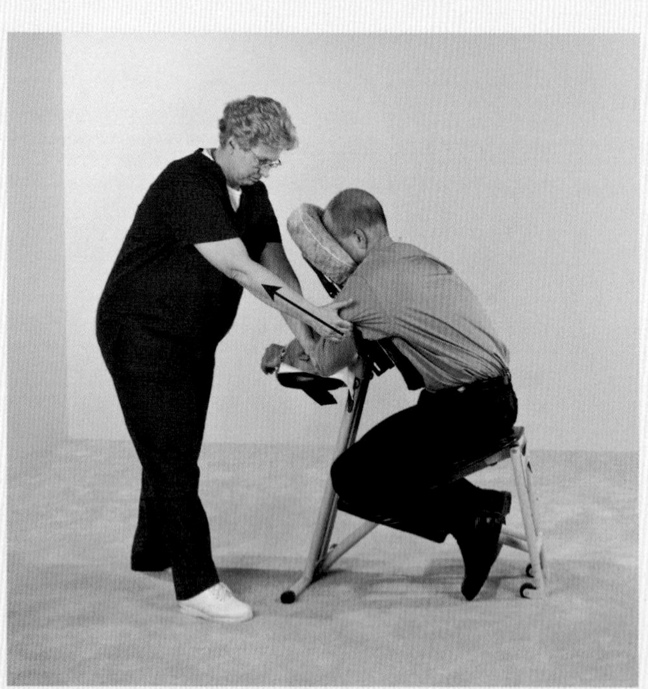

9. Pull back to massage upper arm.

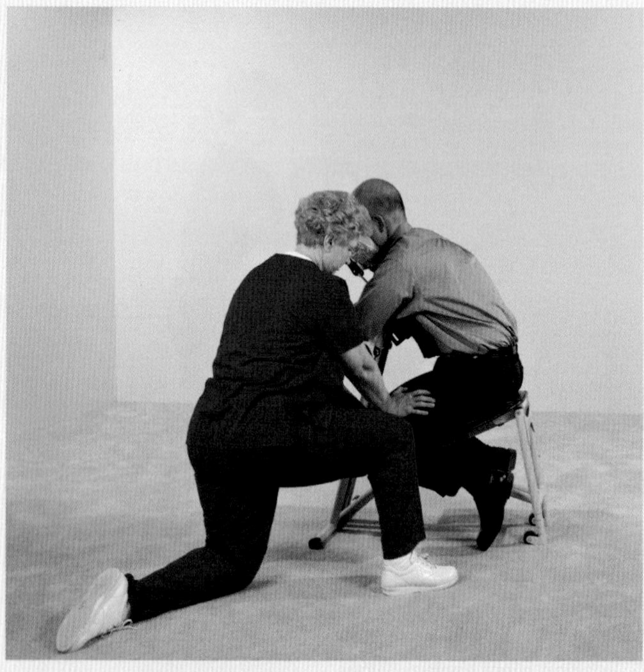

10. Kneel to compress thigh.

GENERAL SEATED MASSAGE PROTOCOL—cont'd

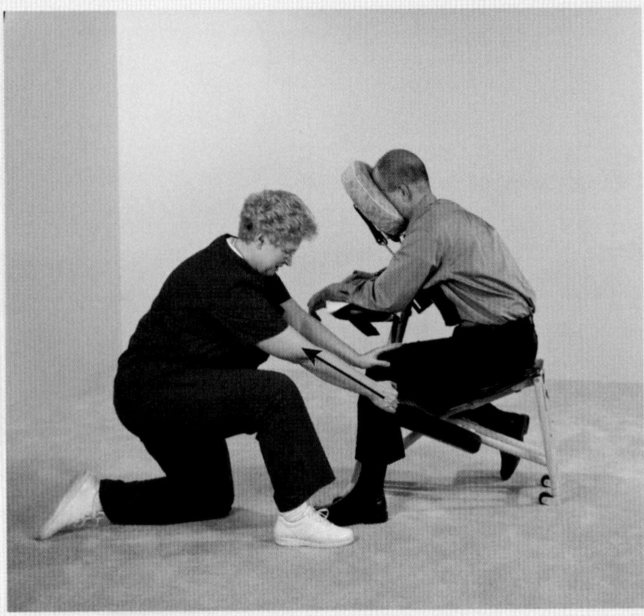

11. Pull and lean back to massage calf.

MAT MASSAGE PROTOCOL

The following series of photographs provides an example of massage application using a mat. An entire sequence is not provided, but the photographs show positioning, bolstering, sequencing, and body mechanics, along with examples of gliding, kneading, and compression, the three basic components of general massage. It is impossible to show all the massage variations, but the examples given should provide enough structure to allow you to begin to perfect techniques for massage on a mat (see the Evolve website for a complete demonstration of the mat massage protocol).

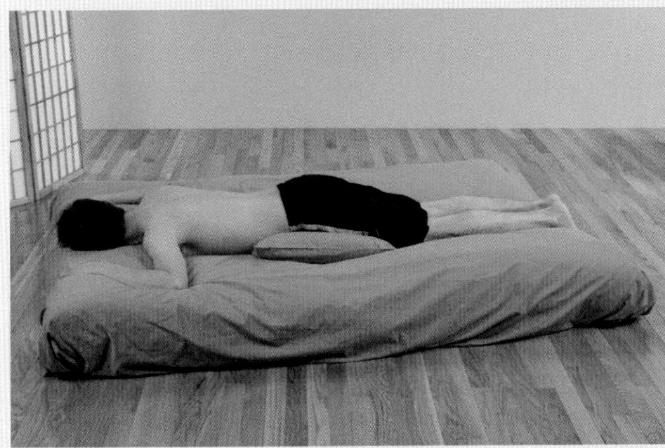

1. Client positioned prone on mat.

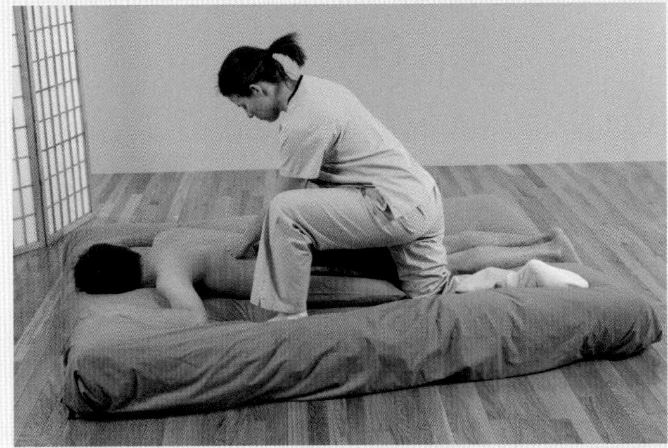

2. Kneeling body mechanics.

Continued

MAT MASSAGE PROTOCOL—cont'd

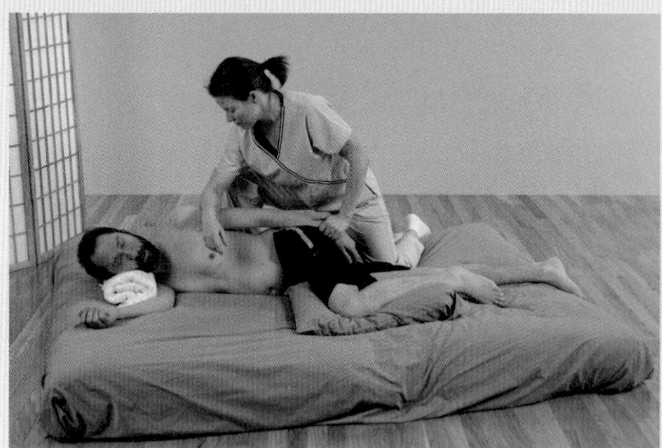

3. Side-lying using forearm compression/glide.

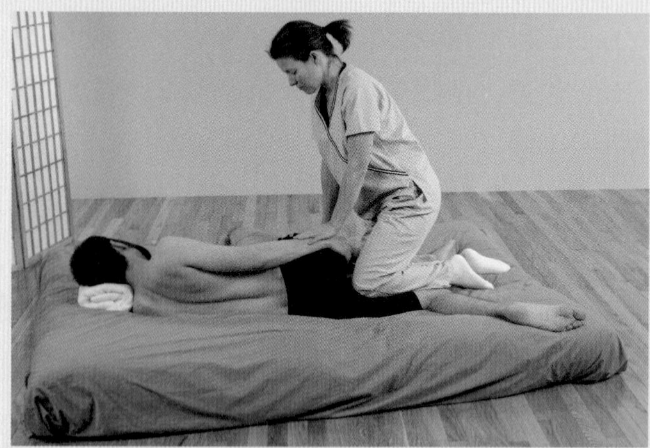

4. Using leg to apply compression.

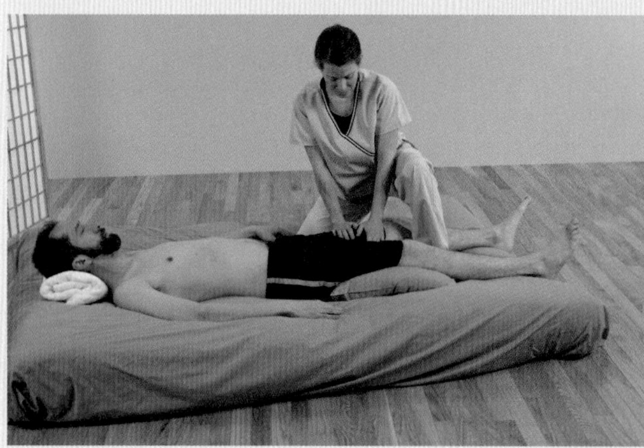

5. Working on legs in supine position.

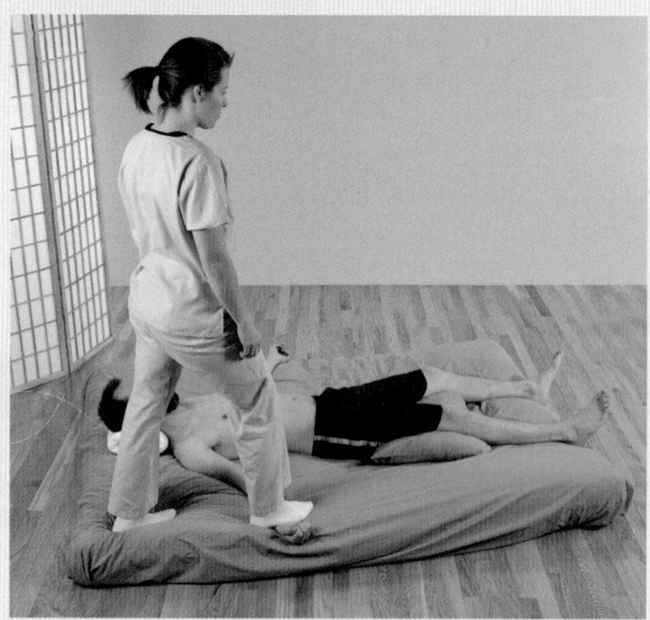

6. Using foot to perform massage.

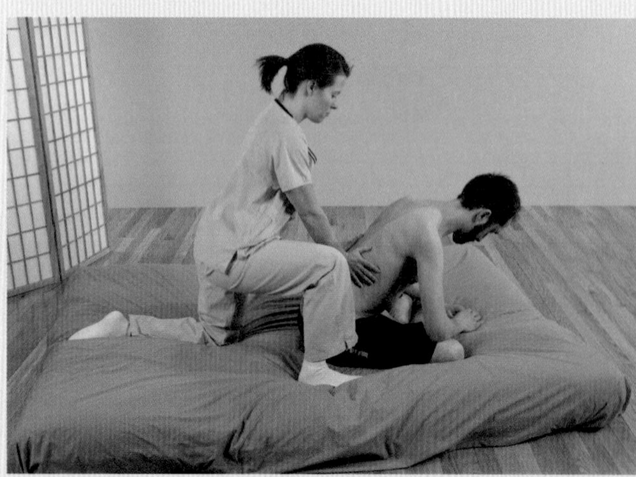

7. Back massage, client seated.

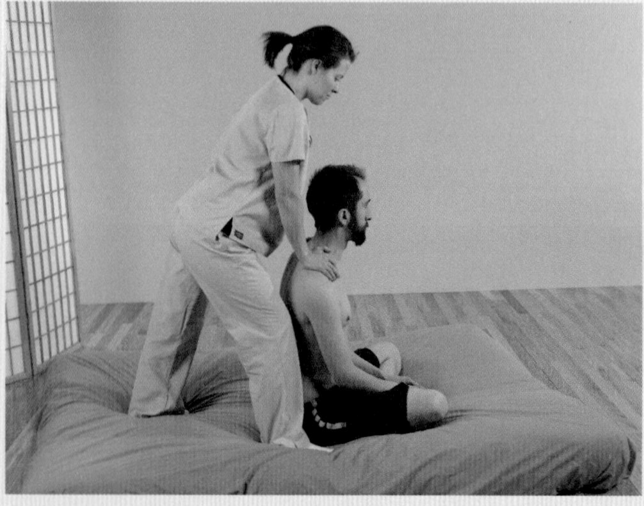

8. Shoulder and neck compression.

Foot in the Door

Offering to provide a massage to the person interviewing you for a job is an excellent way to showcase your skills. Once you have your foot in the door, be prepared to provide a massage to potential employers. Make sure you have a uniform, massage table, and supplies conveniently available (i.e., in your car). If you consistently provide quality massage to clients, they will refer their friends and acquaintances to you. Referral from a satisfied client is the best career builder there is. Incidentally, a foot massage is a great "massage sample."

SUMMARY

Now that you have all the individual skills to give a great massage, your job is to practice using them in combination. It is common to be clumsy with massage applications at first. Skills evolve with experience and practice. Few people, if any, do something perfectly on their first attempt. Expertise is a never-ending process of learning, modification, and change. If you work with a client-centered focus, allow the client's needs to direct the massage, and do not try to force a particular response, the client should experience beneficial results.

Massage manipulations and techniques can be combined to produce an infinite number of therapeutic massage applications. Give yourself permission to practice and improvise. As you practice, ask the client for feedback on how a particular application of a technique or massage manipulation feels and what its effects are. Always be open to innovation, and do not be afraid to experiment with new techniques.

LEARN MORE ON THE WEB

Science.gov searches more than 60 databases and 2200 selected websites from 15 federal agencies, offering 200 million pages of authoritative US government science information, including research and development results. Search terms: massage, mechanical forces.

Evolve

Visit the Evolve website: http://evolve.elsevier.com/Fritz/fundamentals/.

Evolve content designed for massage therapy licensing exam review and comprehension of content beyond the textbook. Evolve content includes:

- Content Updates
- Science and Pathology Animations
- Body Spectrum Coloring Book
- MBLEx exam review multiple choice questions

FOR EACH CHAPTER FIND:

- Answers and rationales for the end-of-chapter multiple-choice questions
- Electronic workbook and answer key
- Chapter multiple choice question quiz
- Quick content review in question form and answers
- Technique videos when applicable
- Learn more on the Web

REFERENCES

Archer P, Chandler C, Garbowski R, et al. *The core: Entry-Level Analysis Project report. Coalition of National Massage Therapy Organizations (Alliance for Massage Therapy Education, American Massage Therapy Association, Associated Bodywork & Massage Professionals, Commission on Massage Therapy Accreditation, Federation of State Massage Therapy Boards, Massage Therapy Foundation, and National Certification Board for Therapeutic Massage & Bodywork)*; 2013. Available at Elapmassage.org.

Baumgartner AJ. *Massage in Athletics*. Minneapolis: Brugess Publishing; 1947.

Beard G. *A History of Massage Technique*. 5th ed. St Louis: Saunders; 2007.

Beyer L, Vinzelberg S, Loudovici-Krug D. Evidence (-based medicine) in manual medicine/manual therapy—a summary review. *Manuelle Medizin*. 2022:1–20.

Brian D, Patrick LS van Dun, Eric J, Sandy F, Paul M, Norman K, Franklin G, Kendi H, David L, Giacomo C, Leah F, William RR, Cameron M, Vaclav K, Crystal M, Bernie L, Paul S. Profession-based manual therapy nomenclature: exploring history, limitations, and opportunities. *J Man Manip Ther.* 2023. doi:10.1080/10669817.2023.2288495.

Burns DK, Wells MR. Gross range of motion in the cervical spine: the effects of osteopathic muscle energy technique in asymptomatic subjects. *J Am Osteopath Assoc.* 2006;106:137.

Chaitow L. *Muscle Energy Techniques*. 4th ed. Edinburgh: Churchill Livingstone; 2013.

Chaitow L. *Positional Release Techniques with on-line videos E-Book*. Elsevier Health Sciences; 2015.

Chaitow S, Sandy F, eds. Chaitow's muscle energy techniques E-Book. *Elsevier Health Sciences*; 2023.

Cyriax E. Some misconceptions concerning mechano-therapy. *Br J Physical Med.* 1938.

Rayudu GM, Alagingi NK. Efficacy of mulligan technique versus muscle energy technique on functional ability in subjects with adhesive capsulitis. *Int J Recent Sci Res.* 2018;9(4):25638–25641. http://dx.doi.org/10.24327/ijrsr.2018.0904.1898.

Greenman PE. *Principles of Manual Medicine*. 4th ed. Baltimore: Lippincott Williams & Wilkins; 2010.

Ingber, DE. Tensegrity-based mechanosensing from macro to micro. *Prog Biophys Mol Biol.* 2008;97(2–3):163–179.

Kellogg JH. *The Art of Massage: A Practical Manual for the Nurse, the Learner and the Therapist*. Kila, Mont: Kessinger Publishing; 2010.

Knott M, Voss D. *Proprioceptive Neuromuscular Facilitation: Patterns and Techniques*. 3rd ed. Baltimore: Lippincott Williams & Wilkins; 1985.

Kolahi KS, Mohammad RKM. Mechanotransduction: a major regulator of homeostasis and development. *Wiley Interdisciplinary Reviews: Systems Biology and Medicine.* 2010;2(6):625–639.

Lewit K. *Manipulative Therapy in Rehabilitation of the Locomotor System*. 3rd ed. Oxford: Butterworth-Heinemann; 1998.

Newey OMS, Son DO, Rita M, Hensel DO. *Defining Muscle Energy: A Multidisciplinary Approach*; 2018.

Payla M, Gill M, Singal SK, Shah N. A comparison of the immediate and lasting effects between passive stretch and muscle energy technique on hamstring muscle extensibility. *Indian J Physiother Occup Ther.* 2018;12(1).

Saadat Z, Hemmati L, Pirouzi S, Ataollahi M, Ali-mohammadi F. Effects of integrated neuromuscular inhibition technique on pain threshold and pain intensity in patients with upper trapezius trigger points. *J Bodyw Mov Ther.* 2018.

Shinde M, Jagtap V. Effect of muscle energy technique and mulligan mobilization in sacroiliac joint dysfunction. *Global J Res Analysis.* 2018;7(3).

Taylor GH. *An Illustrated Sketch of the Movement Cure: Its Principal Methods and Effects*. New York: The Institute; 1866.

UK National Guideline Centre. "Evidence review for manual therapy for chronic primary pain." (2021).

Wendt M, Waszak M. Evaluation of the combination of muscle energy technique and trigger point therapy in asymptomatic individuals with a latent trigger point. *International Journal of Environmental Research and Public Health.* 2020;17(22):8430.

MULTIPLE-CHOICE QUESTIONS FOR DISCUSSION AND REVIEW

The answers, with rationales, can be found on the Evolve site. Use these questions to stimulate discussion and dialogue. Each question offers the opportunity to review terminology, practice critical thinking skills, and improve multiple choice test taking skills. Answers and rationales are on the Evolve site. It is just as important to know why the wrong answers are wrong as it is to know why the correct answer is correct.

1. A massage practitioner uses massage methods in a brisk and specific way. Which of the following client goals is best served by this approach?
   a. Decreased alertness
   b. Increased parasympathetic response
   c. Decreased sensory awareness
   d. Increased alertness
2. A massage client is unhappy with the massage. The main complaint is a feeling of choppiness and lack of continuity. Which of the following qualities of touch does the massage therapist need to improve?
   a. Depth of pressure
   b. Drag
   c. Rhythm
   d. Direction
3. Which of the following methods is most beneficial for abdominal massage to mechanically encourage fecal movement in the large intestine?
   a. Gliding
   b. Resting/holding
   c. Percussion
   d. Compression
4. A client requests that percussion be used at the end of the massage to stimulate the nervous system. Which is the best choice for the face?
   a. Hacking
   b. Cupping
   c. Tapping
   d. Slapping
5. Which of the following methods would be best for assessing the physiological and pathological motion barrier?
   a. Passive joint movement
   b. Active resistive movement
   c. Post-isometric relaxation
   d. Concentric isotonic contraction
6. Which component is essential for effective application of joint movement?
   a. Stabilization to isolate the movement to the targeted joint
   b. Percussion to stimulate the joint kinesthetic receptors
   c. High-velocity manipulative movement
   d. Cross-directional tissue stretching to cause traction on the joint capsule
7. A client's muscles cramp when the massage professional attempts to use agonist contract to lengthen a shortened group of muscles. Which of the following methods would be a better choice to lengthen the muscle group?
   a. Skin rolling
   b. Active resistive joint movement
   c. Antagonist contract
   d. Stretching
8. When the outcome for the massage is to support parasympathetic dominance, which combination of methods would be the best choice?
   a. Gliding, rocking, and passive joint movement
   b. Compression, shaking, and friction
   c. Active joint movement, elongation, and rocking
   d. Tapotement, compression, and vibration
9. A client is requesting extensive massage to the neck and upper shoulders. Which is the most efficient client position to massage these areas?
   a. Prone
   b. Supine
   c. Seated
   d. Side-lying
10. Which method is beneficial to use on the hands and feet to stimulate lymphatic movement?
    a. Superficial gliding
    b. Skin rolling
    c. Vibration
    d. Pumping compression
11. A client complains of a stiff and stuck feeling in the lumbar area. Assessment indicates that the fascia in that area is thick and with reduced sliding. Which method would best restore pliability to this tissue?
    a. Skin rolling
    b. Shaking
    c. Resting position
    d. Vibration
12. A client has a lot of body hair on the back. During the first massage, lubricant was used. At the return visit the client requests that lubricant not be used where there are large amounts of hair. Which method could be used?
    a. Gliding
    b. Kneading
    c. Compression
    d. Petrissage
13. A client has an outcome goal for the massage of increased circulation and range of motion for the knee. Which of the following is the best approach?
    a. Restorative
    b. Condition management
    c. Therapeutic change
    d. Palliative
14. A client complains of restricted range of motion in the shoulder. The primary outcome for the massage is to increase shoulder mobility. Which method would be the best choice?
    a. Friction
    b. Muscle energy
    c. Hydrotherapy
    d. Resting position
15. A client has been receiving massage weekly for 2 months. The main goal for the massage is increased mobility in the lumbar and hip region. The client has experienced

stiffness and reduced ability since a fall off a bike 2 years ago. General massage and muscle energy methods with lengthening have produced mild improvement. Which of the following mechanical tissue based methods has the potential to improve results?
   a. Lymphatic drainage
   b. Stretching
   c. Contract/relax
   d. Strain-counterstrain
16. A client asks that most of the massage time be focused on the back. The client continues to complain that the massage is not effective in reducing back pain. What explanation can be given to the client?
   a. The soft tissue of the back often is symptomatic because of extensive pulling and shortening of the tissues in the anterior thorax; massage of the chest may help.
   b. Massage to the back limits blood flow, so the soft tissues remain in contracture.
   c. Massage on the extremities would be better to reduce the pain in this area because the effect is more concentrated.
   d. The connective tissues of the back respond best to percussion methods and using a more generalized approach would provide relief.
17. A client is complaining about pain and stiffness in the neck but is particularly sensitive to pressure used in the neck area and responds by flinching and stiffening whenever the neck is massaged. The current approach is primarily to use kneading with the client in the prone position. What is the best alternative?
   a. Change position to supine and use gliding.
   b. Use side-lying position and broad-based compression.
   c. Combine passive range of motion, muscle energy, and friction with the client seated.
   d. Have the client sit, and then use firm kneading.
18. A client arrives late for a massage appointment. The remaining time is 30 minutes. The goal for the session is general relaxation. Which combination of body regions should you focus on to achieve the desired outcomes in the allotted time?
   a. Back, gluteals, and hips
   b. Face, hands, and feet
   c. Hands, arms, and back
   d. Face, neck, and shoulders
19. A client requests heavy/deep pressure during the massage but no sensations of sharpness or pain. Which of the following modifiers is the focus of this application?
   a. Duration
   b. Pacing
   c. Point of application
   d. Rhythm
20. A client is describing a massage received while on vacation. The session was provided on a mat using the feet. An oil was used. Which was most likely the method applied?
   a. Gliding methods
   b. Torsion twisting methods
   c. Movement methods
   d. Shearing methods

Exercise

Using the foregoing questions as examples, write at least three more questions, one of each type: factual recall and comprehension, application and concept identification, and clinical reasoning and synthesis. Take care to develop plausible wrong answers and be sure that the correct answer is clearly correct. Then write a rationale for each question. The more questions you write, the better you will understand the material.

CHAPTER 11

Assessment Procedures for Developing a Care/Treatment Plan

http://evolve.elsevier.com/Fritz/fundamentals/

CHAPTER OBJECTIVES

After completing this chapter, the student will be able to perform the following:

1. Conduct an effective client interview.
2. Explain subjective and objective instruments and implement them into the assessment process.
3. Identify and address during massage elements relating to function and dysfunction of posture.
4. Explain the process of walking and identify and address gait dysfunction.
5. Integrate joint movement into the massage for assessment purposes.
6. Define and use simple orthopedic tests during the assessment process.
7. Use massage application as palpation assessment.
8. Adapt joint movement methods to perform muscle testing assessment.
9. Interpret and categorize assessment information.
10. Use clinical reasoning skills to apply assessment data to treatment plan development for the four main outcome goals related to massage therapy.

CHAPTER OUTLINE

KEY TERMS

4-Element Movement System Model	Orthopedic tests
Assessment	Palpation
End-feel	Phasic muscles
Functional movement	Postural muscles
Kinesiology	Rapport
Neurological muscle testing	Resourceful compensation
	Strength testing

Every intervention must be preceded by assessment and followed by post-assessment to evaluate effectiveness.

As you begin your education in massage therapy, it is important that you understand the value of the sequence and general flow of the massage application. Modeling precise massage routines is a valuable learning exercise; however, after you grasp the concepts, the routine must evolve to meet the unique needs of the individual client. Massage practitioners who have the ability to modify and alter the application of therapeutic massage are better able to serve their clients. People do not fit neatly into a routine sequence of massage techniques. To achieve the best results, the learner must use the concepts derived from performing the routines to design an application based on physiological outcomes, rather than trying to make the client fit the routine.

Instead of providing the structure of a precise, step-by-step routine, this chapter teaches you to perform an assessment to evaluate current function and ways to determine short- and long-term outcome goals for the client. Because most of the physiological changes and benefits of massage result from the most basic technical skills, expertise comes from the decisions made in applying those skills. The practitioner's ability to make those decisions depends on the ability to gather the client's history data, perform assessment and analysis, and interpret the information collected during assessment. Then, with the information gathered and the client outcomes determined, the massage methods and variations (pressure, drag, frequency, direction, speed, rhythm, etc.) are identified to develop an individualized treatment plan.

The assessment process can be as basic as ruling out contraindications for a one-time session in a day spa, cruise ship or resort, or as comprehensive as determining a client's needs for therapeutic massage provided as a medical care component, as part of a rehabilitation or pain management program, or in the development of coping strategies for addressing the physical effects of anxiety disorder. The care/treatment plan also can be simple (e.g., providing a 1-hour vacation from daily stress) or complex (e.g., using massage to aid the management of asthma, depression, stroke rehabilitation, side effects caused by chemotherapy, and sports training protocols).

This chapter also presents the assessment skills a massage therapist needs to adapt massage application to meet the four main outcome goals in the wellness massage setting and to function effectively with supervision in a medical care setting, providing massage as part of a comprehensive treatment plan. The massage professional should be able to participate in this process by providing reliable information to be considered in the development of the treatment plan. The ability to reason clinically at this level supports the effectiveness of all massage interactions, be they for relaxation and restorative outcomes or for the management of complex health conditions.

To understand the results of the massage session, the learner must separate assessment information obtained before, during, and after the massage from methods of intervention. To support the learning process, this chapter is divided into two distinct areas:

- Assessment procedures
- Interpretation of assessment information with general suggestions for massage intervention

Always begin each massage session with this question: "What information do I need to develop a safe, effective massage therapy treatment plan for this client?"

Assessment and intervention are different. Assessment takes the form of a uniform protocol. For massage therapy, the general massage should be considered assessment. As the massage is performed, palpation assessment occurs. As the joints are moved during the massage, joint range of motion is assessed. The same moves are used on both sides of the body and compared with what is considered a normal response.

EXAMPLE

Superficial fascia should slide similarly in similar locations. During the general (assessment) massage, the superficial fascia is moved in an area such as on the upper shoulder. Both sides when compared are similar. Then as the massage continues and is focused on the anterior thigh, the superficial fascia moves more on the left than the right. Inspection of the area indicates a scar on the right thigh—a logical reason for the difference in the tissue mobility. Then the decision needs to be made about whether the decrease in superficial fascia movement is helpful (resourceful compensation) or is interfering with effective movement or causing uncomfortable sensation. More focused assessment might occur to determine whether changing the tissue function is desirable and possible. Finally, the decision is made to do an intervention to produce change. The intervention is to hold the stiff, stuck tissue still while the client moves the knee back and forth.

Most of the time available is for massage assessment *not* intervention. The actual intervention type is usually quite simple. For example: slow down, increase drag, and increase repetitions; or pull the tissue up and move the adjacent joint; or apply pressure on the area and move the client so that the sensation decreases and hold there for 15 seconds. The intelligence about where to work is much more important than the specific method to use.

MENTORING TIP

The full body general massage is your primary palpation and movement assessment. As you perform the massage, you have a little conversation with each tissue layer you touch and each joint that you move. The conversation goes something like this: "Hello, skin, how are you doing? Anything you would like help with? All feels fine, so let's communicate with the superficial fascia. Hello, fascia. Do you slip and slide like designed? No, a little more stuck right here? I wonder why? Let's investigate more. Hello, shoulder adductor muscles and deep fascia. Is everyone comfortable? You all have enough room? Is the shoulder joint stable? No! Well that hypermobile joint is making soft tissue shorten to keep the bones in the right alignment. I understand why this spot might be tender when I touch it. Let's do some more investigation, and maybe I can figure out something to help so you don't have to work so hard. Hello, shoulder joint. I am going to move you around and see if the range of motion is functional. Pectoralis major muscle and fascia have some tender points, and that can happen when the joint is troubled. Wow, shoulder, I can tell you are not happy. I could try some METs (muscle energy techniques) and connective tissue focus to bring down the muscle tone and increase the pliability of the dense fascia." And the conversation continues.

Yes, you can go through the steps of giving a massage and not pay attention, functioning as a massage technician. If you want to function as a massage therapist, you use the massage methods to ask assessment questions so you can provide appropriate intervention when needed.

ASSESSMENT

SECTION OBJECTIVES

Chapter objective covered in this section:

1. Conduct an effective client interview.

Using the information presented in this section, the student will be able to perform the following:

- Explain the importance of assessment.
- Identify resourceful compensation.
- Define *rapport* and establish rapport with a client.
- Interview a client effectively.
- Use effective listening skills.
- Use a sample script for the assessment interview process.

Assessment is a learned skill. The ability to incorporate this skill into massage sessions enhances the quality of treatment given by the massage professional. **Assessment** is the collection and interpretation of information provided by the client, the client's consent advocates (parent or guardian), and the referring medical professionals, in addition to information gathered by the massage practitioner. In a growing number of clinical medical care settings, the massage professional's assessment is considered in the treatment plan developed by the multidisciplinary health care team. Therefore, being able to perform standard assessment and charting procedures is crucial. Chapter 4 introduced these concepts; this chapter refines and integrates them. Although the massage professional observes, interprets, and makes decisions based on information gathered during assessment procedures, it is important to remember that the massage professional is not equipped to diagnose any specific medical condition or to treat one except under the direct supervision of a licensed medical professional.

Components of the Assessment

For the massage practitioner, the information gathered during a pre-massage assessment has four purposes:

- To determine whether the client should be referred to a medical professional
- To discover any cautions that would modify the massage application
- To obtain input from the client that is used to help develop the massage care/treatment plan
- To design the best massage for the client, specifically the types of methods used and the mechanical loads generated by those methods, in addition to the proper application of depth of pressure, drag, direction, speed, rhythm, frequency, and duration of each method, to achieve the desired physiological outcome (Fig. 11.1)

Assessment is related to outcome goals. The outcome for relaxation/well-being will require a much different assessment process than the outcome for functional mobility (Box 11.1).

In reality, the assessment and the application of massage techniques are almost the same thing. Often massage manipulations and techniques are first used during a massage to evaluate the tissue, then they are altered slightly in intensity to support tissue-appropriate change, and finally they are used to reassess for tissue changes. Therefore, massage professionals must keep the following in mind:

- Assessment does not change a condition; rather, it is an attempt to understand it.
- Interventions are intended to change the abnormal findings revealed by the assessment.

Compensation Patterns

Compensation patterns are the result of the body's adjustment to some sort of dysfunction. Years of clinical experience have

FOCUS ON PROFESSIONALISM

Scope of practice defined by licensing laws relates to entry level practice. The purpose of licensing is to protect the public from harm. This is an important concept when considering assessment procedures and interventions to achieve client outcomes for the massage session. A necessary aspect of assessment, as part of massage therapy practice, is to identify WHAT NOT TO DO, WHEN TO REFER, AND HOW TO CONSULT WITH OTHER HEALTH AND MEDICAL PROFESSIONALS. This is especially important for those newly licensed and just beginning their professional journey as a massage therapist.

Massage therapy is a spectrum of care beginning at entry level. Experience and ongoing professional development expand assessment and intervention within the scope of practice, allowing massage therapists to work with clients having more complex issues as part of multidisciplinary teams. More detailed assessment is needed to make clinical decisions. The massage therapist may perform the assessments or need to interpret assessment information provided by other professionals to contribute to an integrated care plan.

Almost all massage therapy scope of practice language includes "The purpose of massage is to enhance and benefit the general health and well-being, establishing and maintaining good physical condition of the client"; while medical practice scope of practice statements contain language such as "diagnose and treat, injury and acute and chronic disease, the alleviation of impairments, functional limitations, or disabilities." The concepts of enhance, benefit, maintain, general health, wellbeing are quite different from diagnose, treat, alleviate, injury, disease.

This distinction is important when performing assessment procedures and determining appropriate massage therapy–based intervention.

It can be confusing for clients to understand the limits of scope of practice and intention for care from the massage therapists because the data collection process of assessment is similar among health professionals. The expectation of "find and fix" by both the massage therapist and clients can lead to ethical issues. The entry level massage therapist is generally clear about massage therapy limits of practice. However, with experience, education, and professional development the distinctions can begin to blur.

This is an entry level textbook that is preparing the learner for a professional journey and a massage therapy practice that evolves beyond entry level. Assessment is essential for critical thinking and critical thinking is essential for professional development.

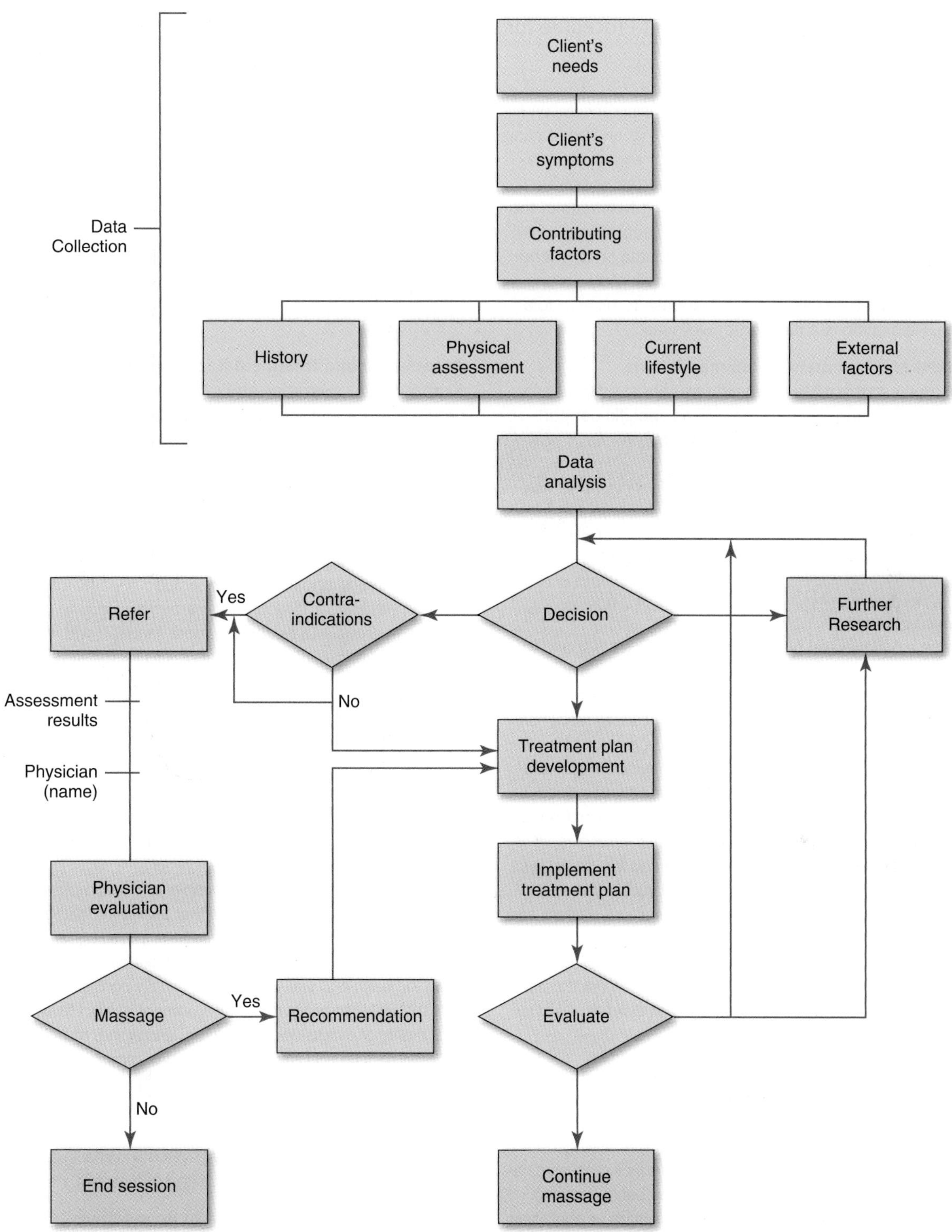

FIG. 11.1 Algorithm for the development of a care/treatment plan.

taught many therapists that most symptoms are compensatory patterns. Some problems are recent, and some developed in early life and compounded over time. Compensatory patterns often are complex, but the client's body frequently can show us the way if we listen to the story it tells. The importance of compensation must be considered in an assessment.

Resourceful Compensation

Assessment identifies what is functioning normally, what is abnormal, and whether the abnormal condition is problematic (maladaptive), requiring attention, or is a resourceful and successful adaptive compensation.

Patterns of **resourceful compensation** develop when the body has been required to adapt to some sort of trauma or repetitive use pattern. Permanent resourceful adaptive changes, although not as efficient as optimal functioning, are the best patterns the body can develop in response to an irreversible change in the system. Resourceful compensation must be supported, not eliminated. Determining whether the changes in the body are helpful or harmful can be difficult.

Box 11.1 Recommended Assessment Procedure for Each of the Four Outcome Goals

Relaxation

Massage outcome: Relaxation well-being

Relaxation: General all-over feeling of well-being; mental and physical relief after effort; tranquil, soothing, and comforting

The goal of relaxation is the foundation for almost all massage therapy interventions. Relaxation is a normal, general, and physiologically inclusive process involving functions of the parasympathetic autonomic nervous system supporting recovery from daily life activities. A relaxation outcome is not pathology based; therefore, specific massage-related interventions are minimal, and the results occur in response to pleasurable sensation. Relaxation is a function of wellness.

Assessment and Treatment Recommendations

Client history is gathered to determine positional adaptations, contraindications, and cautions, as well as specific comfort needs, such as the use of a blanket and components of how each client expects to feel when relaxed.

During general nonspecific moderate pressure massage, use palpation, rocking, shaking, and rhythmic joint movement to assess for general tension holding, and if areas are found, simply slow down the method and maintain the application for 15 to 30 seconds.

Stress Management

Stress is the emotional and physical way in which we respond to demands to respond and adapt. Stress is a physiological response that enables people to cope with strain and anxiety. Stress management includes strategies to support a normal stress response and prevent, control, or reverse stress-related pathology. Many people use massage to manage stress-related symptoms including irritability, inability to concentrate, fatigue, and trouble sleeping. As stress increases, pathology can occur, resulting in anxiety and depression. The physical symptoms of stress include rapid heart rate, muscle tension including headache and low back pain, digestive upset, and many other symptoms related to changes in breathing and the regulation of the autonomic nervous system and endocrine system. Many addictive behaviors are linked to a stressful lifestyle, such as overeating, smoking, drinking, and drug abuse. Constant stress can increase blood pressure and the risk for stroke and contributes to many diseases such as heart disease, diabetes, and multiple autoimmune conditions.

Assessment and Treatment Recommendations

Include procedures from relaxation/well-being outcome and add the following:

Client history to determine the manifestation of stress symptoms and behaviors, current interventions including medications being used and effectiveness, sleep behaviors, and target areas that are responding to stress such as shoulders and back.

Physical assessment: Breathing and postural assessment.

Palpation: During general nonspecific moderate pressure massage, use palpation, rocking, shaking, and rhythmic joint movement to assess for general tension holding, especially involving breathing and in indicated tension target areas. Also palpate for changes in superficial fascia, especially densification. If dysfunctional areas are found related to the stress symptom areas found, slow down the assessment method and maintain application for 15 to 30 seconds. Increase drag and elongate and twist superficial fascia where densification is identified. Use shaking and active and passive joint movement with muscle energy methods to reduce stiffness and tension in the limbs related to the fight-or-flight response.

Pain Management

Pain is a complex topic. Pain theories are evolving to help us better understand different types of pain sensations. Two basic types of pain are acute pain and chronic/persistent pain. Acute pain is a natural outcome of tissue damage, warning us that we have been harmed. Chronic pain is persistent pain without tissue damage and is a serious health care problem. Strategies to manage pain such as medication can lead to even more problems related to side effects and abuse.

Assessment and Treatment Recommendations

Incorporate all relaxation and stress management goal assessment and intervention procedures in addition to the following:

Add increased history assessment to include pain history, pain scales, pain drawings of location and type of pain, treatments being used, and functional physical capacity (what can the client do and not do); expand palpation to full range of 12-level palpation assessment.

Intervention guidelines: Focus on stress management massage application and include specific intervention methods for targeted pain areas by slowing down over the areas and becoming more focused with applications. Use various force applications to increase pliability of dense soft tissue and muscle energy methods, especially positional release, to slightly elongate areas of short tissue. Carefully use cross-fiber friction in one or two areas of fibrotic tissue. Do not overfocus on painful tissue areas. Sensations of "good hurt" can be incorporated in target areas if pressure reproduces the familiar pain sensation.

Functional Mobility

Functional mobility means that people can accomplish the movements desired to live in a manner that allows for taking care of daily life activities, pursuing occupational pursuits, and being able to physically move to support play and exercise, thereby contributing to health and well-being. We typically connect quality of life with the ability to move in our environment easily. However, due to a variety of events, including injury and aging, movement can become difficult and limiting. The most common concerns are stiffness and pain. Developing and maintaining control of posture and movement is often attributed primarily to the muscle system, but evidence has suggested that the intricate relationship between the nervous, muscular, and fascial systems is vital in developing and maintaining control of posture and movement.

Assessment and Treatment Recommendations

Incorporate all relaxation/well-being, stress management, and pain management goal assessment and intervention procedures in addition to the following:

Gait assessment, joint range of motion, orthopedic tests if appropriate, specific sequence for joint assessment, full range of palpation at all 12 levels, and targeted muscle testing including gait and muscle activation sequences. Focus on kinetic chain relationships.

Intervention: The massage foundation should be the stress management massage used as the assessment platform, and corrections should be applied as needed with no more than 10 minutes of specific intervention in a 50-minute massage session.

The main reason for physical change in the body is adaptive demand. Recall that anatomy is form and physiology is function. Form and function influence each other. If a person breaks a bone, the healing process changes the shape of the bone to some extent; the bone typically becomes thicker at the point of the healed fracture. This can be both a help and a hindrance to the body. For example, the healed bone may be strong, but the changes in the bone's shape caused by the thickening process may result in impingement on another tissue or interference with range of motion.

This situation often arises when the clavicle is broken. It usually heals well, but because of the clavicle's proximity to the ribs, the change in shape might cause pinching or rubbing of structures between the clavicle and the ribs, resulting in nerve impingement, inflammation, and pain. Massage cannot change the shape of bone. However, it can be used to maintain as much tissue pliability as possible, which may reduce symptoms.

Another example of resourceful compensation is swelling and muscle tension around a joint sprain. The increased stiffness of the area prevents movement during the early stages of healing, almost in the same way that a cast does. This type of compensation should not be altered. However, if these tissue changes persist into the later stages of healing, they will interfere with a return to normal function. Massage may be used to reduce unproductive tissue changes and support a full return to function.

In massage, a general guideline for detecting resourceful compensation is that the body resists the changes introduced by massage. This resistance to change may occur as follows:

- During massage, the client stiffens or flinches away from the application. This also may be caused by inappropriate application of a method. However, if the application style is altered and the tissues continue to resist change, a beneficial reason likely exists for the adaptation in the body. Do not force tissue changes. Massage the area in general and manage symptoms.
- Immediately after the massage, the client indicates that they feel good. Then 24 to 48 hours after the massage, the client is sore and symptoms have increased, indicating the massage has caused tissue damage or destabilized a resourceful compensation pattern.

During assessment procedures, if you are unable to identify a logical reason for the tissue and movement changes, the best course is to use general methods in the area and to avoid aggressive specific intervention procedures during the massage. A referral for diagnosis may be indicated. When resourceful compensation is present, therapeutic massage methods are used to support the altered pattern and prevent any greater increase in distortion than is necessary to support the body change (compensation).

Some compensatory patterns develop to accommodate short-term conditions that do not require permanent adaptation. Having a leg in a cast and walking on crutches for a time is a classic example. The body catching itself during an "almost" fall is another classic setup pattern. Unfortunately, the body often habituates these patterns and maintains them well beyond their usefulness. Over time, the body begins to show symptoms of pain, stiffness, inefficient function, or combined symptoms.

A simple means of differentiating resourceful from unresourceful compensation is as follows:

1. If the client reports improvement immediately after the massage and at least 50% of the improvement remains 24 to 48 hours later, the compensation pattern likely is reversible. The outcome for massage application is therapeutic change (see Chapter 6).
2. If the client reports improvement immediately after massage, but 24 to 48 hours later the symptoms return at the same or greater intensity, the compensation pattern likely is resourceful and cannot be reversed at this time. Massage application becomes condition management.
3. If the client has no significant reduction in symptoms immediately after massage (adaptive capacity is exhausted), only palliative care is appropriate.

Dysfunction as a Solution

No education on assessment is complete without a discussion of whether the pattern discovered is a problem or a solution. The previous section defined resourceful compensation as the best that can be expected under the circumstances. The concept of dysfunction as a solution is similar to the patterns of resourceful compensation. If all the information gathered during assessment can be viewed as an attempt at a solution, this broadens the practitioner's perspective in the decision making required for effective massage care plans. As discussed in Chapter 6, it is important to consider the client's whole situation in determining whether a condition is a dysfunction or a solution. This is client centered focusing on whole person care and reflects a biopsychosocial approach. Consider these examples:

- A workaholic client has continual tension headaches. When the client has a headache, they tend to slow their pace and work fewer hours. Is the headache a problem or a solution?
- A massage therapist who regularly provides massage sessions for 25 clients a week develops a low back condition that prevents them from working with more than 10 clients a week. Management of the low back condition requires the massage professional to receive regular massages, exercise regularly, and manage stress. The massage therapist is able to reduce their workload, which opens time for teaching and community service. Is the low back dysfunction a problem or a solution?

Understanding the bigger picture when analyzing assessment information adds an important dimension to the development of essential and appropriate massage care plans. View each pattern as a solution and realize that current problems are past solutions that no longer provide benefit. Solutions are to be supported. Problems must be understood and possible solutions offered. Massage effectively provides both for the body.

Establishing Rapport

The client is the most significant resource involved in the assessment process. A massage professional needs four primary skills for gathering information from a client:

- The ability to establish rapport
- Keen observation

- Successful interviewing methods
- Active listening

Rapport is the development of a relationship based on mutual trust and harmony. It is the massage professional's responsibility to establish a sense of rapport with clients. The massage practitioner needs to show a genuine interest in the person that goes beyond the problems and goals the person presents.

Rapport is enhanced if the massage professional uses words, a tone of voice, and body language similar to those of the client. The process of rapport involves neurons in the brain, called *mirror neurons*, which coordinate the process of looking and acting like the person with whom we are communicating. This process is an instinctual survival mechanism. If the body language and tone of voice are similar (like a dance), the client and massage therapist connect. If the mirroring is not established for some reason, the people communicating will feel odd and may avoid contact. This is an overlooked issue in client retention. Unless the client feels rapport, they will not be able to relax during the massage and likely will avoid further contact.

Some massage practitioners may have difficulty mirroring their mannerisms or tone of voice to their potential clients, which may result in difficulty establishing rapport. Social conditioning or some sort of physical issue may be the cause of this disconnect. For example, a person who has suffered a closed head injury may not be able to modulate eye contact or body language. If the reason for the disconnect is not evident, the potential client will not understand why they feel uncomfortable.

Medication also can interfere with rapport mechanisms, as do almost all substances if abused. Massage professionals who have a physical condition that makes mirroring difficult for them should briefly explain the situation to clients and coworkers. Massage professionals who find that they have clients with whom they are out of sync benefit from learning more effective rapport skills. This may require taking communication classes or seeking help to understand the nature of their own behavior and that of the client.

How to Observe

Attention to detail and the client's needs provide a sensitive, well-trained massage therapist with essential information. Clients notice the difference between a massage professional who takes the time to honor the client's space and adjust to it and one who tries to make the client fit into a routine method of massage application. During the initial conversation, it is important to pay close attention to the client visually. If the practitioner has a visual impairment, information gathered from the interview and physical assessment replaces visual assessment. An effective therapist uses all the senses—hearing, sight, smell, touch, and intuition—in the assessment of the client.

At the beginning of each session, the massage therapist should get a sense of the client's general presence. What is the *vitality* of the client based on their strength, activity, and energy for living? How well does the client move and breathe? Does the client's presence suggest sympathetic or parasympathetic dominance? Sympathetic dominance is the display of restlessness, anxiety, fear, anger, agitation, elation, or exuberance. Parasympathetic dominance is indicated by a generally relaxed appearance, contentment, slowness, or, in the extreme, depression. Because therapeutic massage can either stimulate or inhibit the neuroendocrine function, this needs to be considered in the massage design.

If a client is active and exuberant (sympathetic dominance), the initial massage approach and the massage practitioner's energy level need to match the client's energy level. If the focus of the session is to calm the client, the therapist begins to slow down as the massage progresses to provide a calming effect.

If the client is fatigued and slow moving (parasympathetic dominance), the therapist should proceed slowly in the initial pace of the massage. During the session, the energy and activity level of the massage practitioner and the methods used can be increased as the client's energy increases, so long as the client has sufficient adaptive capacity. In general, excessive sympathetic activation would be balanced by a relaxing, full-body rhythmic massage with a general nonspecific approach. Excessive parasympathetic activation would be balanced by a stimulating massage with a specific focus. If the client seems "out of sorts," operating more as a collection of parts than the sum of the parts, the focused, coordinated presence of the professional providing a harmonized, rhythmic approach to the massage is beneficial.

Gestures

People tend to be consistent with their gestures and word phrases within their internal body language system. However, body language is as individual as the person. Particular gestures or styles of body language cannot be generalized to mean one specific thing. The professional is responsible for learning what a gesture means for a particular individual.

Because of nervous system patterns and the basic universal body language connected with survival emotions such as fear, anger, distress, and happiness, some body language is fairly consistent from person to person. However, the massage practitioner cannot assume that a certain gesture means the same thing with every person. Time and careful observation are required to decipher an individual's body language code. This is done by watching for repetitive body language and connecting the particular gesture or posture to the client's mood and state and the content of the conversation. Eventually the client repeats the body language patterns often enough that the individual pattern is evident.

The skilled massage practitioner pays attention to where and how a client indicates a problem on the body. These gestures often reveal whether a client has a muscle, joint, or visceral problem. It also is important for the therapist to observe the client's body language and nonverbal responses while discussing various topics. Everything the person does is important. Everyone's behavior has a pattern, and all the bits of information combine to reveal that pattern (Proficiency Exercise 11.1).

The following are common gestures and indications:

- If the client points to a specific area, this suggests hyperactivity of a trigger point or a motor point or possibly a joint problem. The meaning depends on the area indicated.
- If the client points to a specific area but the hand then swipes in a certain direction, a trigger point or nerve entrapment problem may be the issue.

PROFICIENCY EXERCISE 11.1

1. Watch people in a public place. Is the general presence of each person you observe sympathetic or parasympathetic in nature?
2. Ask 10 people to explain a physical ache or pain to you. Watch their gestures carefully. What similarities do you notice in their explanations?
3. Walk into your own treatment space or that of a fellow learner. Look at it the way a client would see it. Are the sheets wrinkle free; the lotion dispensed from a closed, single-use container; the counters clean; the doorknobs free of a greasy feeling; and the lighting adequate but not glaring? Also, do you see a therapist who is calm and welcoming, not nervous, rushed, or unengaged?

- Grabbing, pulling, or holding and moving an area as if to stretch it often indicates muscle or fascial shortening or binding.
- If movement is needed to show the area of tightness, the area may need elongation combined with muscle energy work to prepare for stretching and for resetting of neuromuscular patterns.
- If the client moves into a position and then acts as if stuck, the area may need connective tissue focus.
- Drawing lines on the body may indicate nerve entrapment in the fascial planes or grooves.

Interviewing and Listening: Subjective Aspect of Assessment

Communication skills first were presented in Chapter 2. These skills are used during interviewing sessions and throughout client–practitioner interactions.

The point of the interview is to help the client communicate their health history and to reveal the goal for the massage. During an interview information is only gathered, not interpreted—resist the urge to try to understand what all the information means. Interpretation comes after all the information has been gathered, which may take several sessions. Any massage provided at this initial stage is a form of assessment. Although the client experiences generalized benefits from the assessment-focused massage, only when sufficient information has been gathered can the client's expected outcomes be specifically addressed using an intervention.

When you speak to a client, it is important to use words the client can understand. Although professionalism is important, medical terminology need not be used if it will confuse the client. If the client uses a word that is unclear, the therapist should ask what the person means. Asking for clarification enhances knowledge and understanding of the information obtained from the client. Do not use slang or jargon when speaking in the professional setting to either co-workers or clients.

Certain specific information must be obtained from the client. The massage professional can easily forget to ask the important questions. A client information form provides a framework for obtaining necessary and essential information during the interview.

Open-ended questions encourage conversation. Questions that can be answered with only one word should be avoided. The question "Have you ever had a professional massage?" requires the client to answer only yes or no. A better question would be, "What is your experience with therapeutic massage?" This question requires the client to give more detail when answering.

When listening, the massage therapist must do nothing but listen. You cannot listen while thinking about what is going to be said or while writing or interpreting information. An active listener nods or shows other signs of interest to encourage the person to continue speaking.

Many people need time to sort out their thoughts and feelings and develop their statements. The conversation should proceed slowly, and the client should never be rushed. Some people rehearse what they say internally before speaking. They speak with pauses between statements, and you must wait for the client to complete thoughts before speaking. If interrupted, clients often forget what they were going to say. Other clients talk quite a bit. They may need to sort through their information by saying it aloud. Practitioners who give the person their full attention and observe what makes the client most comfortable find it easier to resist the urge to treat everyone in the same manner.

When the client provides information, the massage practitioner should restate what the client has said. The client then has the opportunity to correct any information and is reassured that the therapist was listening and understands what has been said. It is amazing how often information is misinterpreted (Proficiency Exercise 11.2). In addition, a competent professional is careful about having preconceived ideas and keeps an open mind while the assessment is in progress (Box 11.2).

The documentation form used for this aspect of assessment is the Health History Intake Form (see Chapter 4).

PROFICIENCY EXERCISE 11.2

1. With a partner, practice asking three open-ended questions that you might use during an interview.
2. Hold conversations with 10 people. Practice restating information you are given in response to a question you had asked.
3. Practice using and modifying the script example provided in Box 11.2.

PHYSICAL ASSESSMENT: OBJECTIVE ASPECT OF ASSESSMENT

SECTION OBJECTIVES

Chapter objective covered in this section:

2. Explain subjective and objective instruments and implement them into the assessment process.

Using the information presented in this section, the student will be able to perform the following:

- Define biomechanics and kinesiology.
- Use standardized documentation instruments to measure and record assessment findings.

After the subjective assessment has been completed, the massage therapist may choose to do a physical assessment before be-

Box 11.2 Sample Script for the Assessment Interview

1. Greet the client. Smile, introduce yourself.

   Example:
   - Hi. My name is ______, and I will be your massage therapist.
2. Initiate conversation. Ask how the client would like to be addressed: First name, Last name. Ask for pronouns the client uses: She/Her/Hers, He/Him/His, They/Them/Their

   You have completed the personal data in the intake form.

   Example:
   - Names are important. Can you confirm how you would like to be addressed?
3. Explain the assessment process and the forms used. Include information on confidentiality.

   Example:
   - Because this is your first massage session, we will be doing an information-gathering process.
   - Together we will gather information about your health history relevant to massage so that I will be able to plan the safest and most beneficial massage for you.
   - I will use two forms. One is a history form, on which I will record the information you give me. The other is a physical assessment form, on which I will record the results of various physical assessment procedures. Examples of these procedures include a postural symmetry assessment, in which I will compare the left and right and front and back of your body for evenness; muscle assessments to identify how the muscles are functioning; and joint assessments for stability and ease of movement.
   - I will analyze this information, and we will discuss it to determine whether there may be any reason for you to be evaluated by another health professional (referral) and also to determine the goals for the massage outcome. Finally, we will agree on a massage care plan.
   - This process is always more extensive for the first visit.
   - When you return for future massage sessions, we will recap what was done in the previous session and update the records for anything new.
   - At least once a year, we will again do a comprehensive reassessment and review of the outcomes of previous massage sessions.
   - I want to assure you that all the information gathered will be maintained in a secure system to protect your privacy.
   - You may have a copy of your records at any time.
   - If I ask a question and you do not wish to answer, feel free to tell me.
   - At all times, if you are uncomfortable with any conversation, questions, or massage assessment or method, please tell me right away.
   - Please feel free at any time to ask questions or give me feedback, and please do not be concerned about hurting my feelings. I depend on you to make sure that what I am doing during the assessment and massage is safe and beneficial.
   - Do you have any questions or comments?
4. Give the client time to respond.
5. Begin the health history.

   Example:
   - Let's start with your reasons for wanting a massage.
   - What results do you want from the massage? For example, is your goal better sleep, reduced neck stiffness, decreased knee discomfort, more energy, a mini vacation from everyday life?
   - Another way to think about your goals for massage would be to tell me how you want to feel or what you want to be able to do more easily after the massage.
6. Give the client the history form.

   Example:
   - I am going to use the history form to help me ask questions so that I stay on track and do not forget something.
   - Would you like to fill out this form first and then we can discuss it, or would you prefer that I ask the questions and fill in the responses you give?
7. Follow the sequence on the form to gather the information. Any areas indicating some sort of past illness, injury, experience with massage, and so forth should be explored in more detail.

   Example:
   - You indicated that you are taking some vitamins and herbs. Would you please tell me what you are taking and the reason for it? Sometimes I have to alter the massage because of an unwanted effect that massage could cause.
   - For example, if you are taking fish oil and aspirin, both of which are anticoagulants and can thin the blood, I would want to make sure that the pressure and the type of application do not cause any bruising.
   - On the basis of the information you provided on the history form, am I correct that you have a family history of cardiac disease?
   - Have you been monitored by your physician for these types of conditions?
   - What is your current health status with regard to cardiovascular disease?
8. After completing the history form, summarize the information.

   Example:
   - Let's see if I understand all this data.
   - Your primary reasons for receiving massage are to relieve shoulder stiffness to see whether that reduces the frequency of tension headaches, and you would like relaxation, as well as support for well-being. Correct?
   - These are all reasonable goals and within my scope of practice.
   - Because your doctor suggested massage for the headaches, we know they are aware of your condition and has made a diagnosis.
   - If you want, I can forward them the summaries of the results of the massage sessions.
   - You will need to sign a release of information form for me to be able to do this.
   - It may be enough for you to keep them updated.
   - You indicated that you will take over-the-counter pain medication for the tension headache, so please tell me before each massage session if you have taken any medication, when you took it, and what you took so I can alter the massage application if necessary.
   - I will also observe the condition of your skin because you indicated that you work out in the sun and you have had some areas of possible skin cancer treated.
   - When I do massage, I see parts of your body that you usually do not, such as your back or your neck.
   - If I find any areas that look as if the doctor should see them, I will let you know, and then please follow up with your physician. Okay?

Continued

Box 11.2 Sample Script for the Assessment Interview—cont'd

- Is there anything you would like to add, or do you have any questions?

9. Respectfully wait for a moment, and then move to the physical assessment process.

   Example:
   - Now we will begin the physical assessment.
   - Actually, the entire time I am giving you a massage, I am performing assessment.
   - When I move your tissues by gliding and kneading, for example, I am performing palpation assessment.
   - It is kind of like listening to your tissues with my hand or forearm.
   - Your skin, fascia, muscles, and joints give me information, such as hot, cold, wet, dry, rough, smooth, stiff, short, long, and so forth.
   - I will also move your joints during the massage to assess for range of motion.
   - Sometimes I might ask you to maintain a position I place you in or to push or pull against me.
   - These are all forms of muscle testing assessment.
   - I will ask for feedback, for example, "Is this painful?" or "Does this feel stiff to you?"
   - Even if I don't ask the question and you have those types of sensations, tell me, okay?
   - If the way your tissues feel or your joints move seems to be somewhat less than optimal, I may do a more specific assessment.
   - When I do these assessments, I am checking to see whether there might be something I need to be particularly cautious about or whether I think I should refer you to your doctor.
   - For example, if I think your leg feels swollen, I might press into it to identify whether the swelling is pitting edema or simple edema.
   - I may ask a couple of questions to see whether the situation has a logical explanation, for example, "Have you been sitting a long time?"
   - If the condition does not appear to have a logical explanation, I may suggest that you see your physician.
   - Before the massage I will do postural and walking assessments and some simple assessments to check for efficient breathing function.
   - I may do some specific assessment procedures based on something you tell me.
   - For example, if you tell me your low back is aching, I might have you bend forward, sideways, and backward.
   - After the massage we will redo some of the assessments to see whether any change has occurred, either for better or for worse.
   - This is called post-assessment, and the information collected helps me plan the next massage session.
   - I also will explain things during the massage.
   - These assessment procedures will be performed in a relaxing way so that you are also relaxed at the end of the massage.
   - Do you have any questions or comments?

10. Hand the client the physical assessment form and explain it briefly.

    Example:
    - This is the form I will use so that I stay organized.
    - I will show you how to do the things I ask you to do.
    - For example, if I want you to move your shoulder a certain way, I will demonstrate first.
    - If anything I ask you to do is uncomfortable or painful, stop doing it and tell me.
    - If any of the assessments reproduce the symptoms you are experiencing, such as re-create headache pain, tell me right away.
    - I really appreciate your participation, so let's get started.

11. Use the physical assessment form to perform the assessments. Do as many as possible as part of the massage. All of the passive and active joint movement assessments and palpation assessments can be incorporated into the massage session. Summarize your findings.

    Example:
    - Because your physician indicates that the discomfort in your knee is likely osteoarthrosis, I performed various assessments to help me determine the safest and most beneficial approach to massage. Because there is joint pathology, massage will be best targeted to managing symptoms and supporting movement.
    - There appears to be some fascia binding in the area of the surgical scar that could be contributing to the stiffness in your shoulder. Massage should be able to soften that up somewhat. We will reevaluate in five or six sessions to see whether the connective tissue methods have been beneficial.
    - Your left ankle moves beyond the normal range of motion. This is called hypermobility, and often the joint is unstable. You told me you sprained it a couple of times, and that could be the cause. You also said that it does not bother you, so unless you ask or I think it may be contributing to some other situation, such as knee pain, I will include the area in the general massage application but not specifically target it for intervention.

12. In writing up the history and the physical assessment, follow these rules:
    - Record all pertinent data
    - Avoid extraneous data
    - Use common terms
    - Avoid abbreviations
    - Be objective
    - Use diagrams when indicated

ginning the massage. For a single-session general massage, the physical assessment usually is limited to having the client show the massage therapist any movements that feel restricted or may be causing discomfort. It is important to ask the client to point out any bruises, varicose veins, or areas of inflammation so that they can be avoided or the methods used over them can be altered. The massage practitioner should ask, "Are there any areas you feel I should avoid?" Be sure the information is indicated on the client information form/health history or the SOAP/session form, and then take care to avoid those areas.

The assessment for basic therapeutic massage, including the development of a care/treatment plan and agreed-on outcomes over a series of massage sessions, includes a general evaluation of the client's posture, gait (walking pattern), and biomechanical function. To understand posture and gait function, we must learn a bit about biomechanics and kinesiology.

Table 11.1 Applied Force Stress and Resulting Injuries

Force Stress	Injury
Tension	Soft tissue stretching: tears, strains
Compression	Contusions, direct blows
Bending	Ligament tears, fractures
Shearing (forces occur perpendicular to tissue fibers)	Ligament tears, blisters, abrasions
Rotational/torsion (combined tension and shearing forces)	Ligament tears, spiral fractures

Biomechanics and Kinesiology

Biomechanics is the science of the action of forces, internal or external, on the living body. *Kinetics* is a branch of the study of biomechanics that describes the effect of forces on the body. The topic of kinetics is introduced here as it applies to the musculoskeletal system.

A force can be considered a push or a pull that can produce, stop, or modify movement. Force application is what a massage professional does when giving a massage. In Chapter 10, each massage method was explained in terms of the force applied and the expected outcome as the tissues responded to the force. These same forces and the stress applied to the tissue also can cause injury (Table 11.1). When we perform various assessments, these forces are applied to identify whether the area is injured.

Kinesiology is the science of the study of movement and the active and passive structures involved, including bones, joints, muscle tissues, and all associated connective tissues. The following are elements of kinesiology:

- *Stability* is required to provide a steady base for functioning. Stability concerns usually focus on the proximal musculature in the trunk, shoulders, and hips, which allow for movement of the extremities. Stability is required before balance can exist.
- *Balance* is the ability to execute complex patterns of movement with the right timing and sequence. Balance is essential to motor function, as is the ability to maintain the center of gravity over the available base of support.
- *Coordination* is the efficient execution of a movement. Coordination usually involves motor learning and practice.
- *Endurance* (lasting power) is based on efficiency and stamina.

The components of biomechanics and kinesiology appear throughout this chapter each time a specific type of assessment is presented.

Outcome Documentation Instruments

Because health care intervention is based on evidence of benefit, the massage therapist must be able to show that beneficial changes occur in the client's status as a result of massage. Both the value and quality of evidence-based interventions can be assessed using standardized assessment tools, or instruments.

Two important aspects of the development of a care/treatment plan and effective documentation (charting) are pre-assessment and post-assessment. When the pre-assessment and post-assessment data are compared, the benefits of massage can be identified, as can parts of the care/treatment plan that may need to be adjusted in future massage sessions. To assess outcomes accurately, massage therapists must use the same instruments for follow-up evaluations that they used for the baseline (beginning) evaluation.

Instruments for evaluating outcomes can be divided into two categories: those that use subjective measurements, which focus on data provided by the client, and those that use objective measurements, which focus on data provide by the practitioner's assessment.

Subjective Measurements

Pain Evaluation

The evaluation of pain classically has been a subjective measurement. Pain assessment tools help people describe their pain experience. Three examples of assessment instruments that focus on subjective outcomes are as follows:

- Pain scales (measure the intensity of pain)
- Pain drawing (measures the location and quality of pain)
- McGill Pain Questionnaire (MPQ; measures the sensory and cognitive experience of pain)

Pain scales are commonly used to describe the intensity of the pain or how much pain the person feels. Types of pain scales include the numerical rating scale, the visual analog scale, the categorical scale, and the pain faces scale:

- On the numerical rating scale, individuals are asked to identify how much pain they are having by choosing a number from 0 (*no pain*) to 10 (*the worst pain imaginable*).
- The visual analog scale is a straight line on which the left end represents no pain and the right end represents the worst pain. Individuals are asked to mark the line at the point they think represents their level of pain.
- The categorical pain scale has four categories: none, mild, moderate, and severe. Individuals are asked to select the category that best describes their pain.
- The Defense and Veterans Pain Rating Scale, DVPRS, was created in 2010 to increase the understanding of pain intensity levels specifically among military personnel and veterans experiencing acute or chronic pain (Fig. 11.2).
- The pain faces scale uses six faces with different expressions on each face. Each face represents a person who feels happy because they have no pain or who feels sad because they have some or a lot of pain. Individuals are asked to choose the face that best shows how they are feeling. This rating scale can be used by people aged 3 years or older (Fig. 11.3).

Pain drawing involves providing documentation with generic human body forms representing the anterior, posterior, and lateral views of the body. Clients use colored pencils or pens to draw their symptoms on the body forms. It is possible to identify intensity and distribution of the pain or other symptoms based on the quality of the drawing. Those areas that are heavily marked indicate intense pain. Large or small symptom distribution can be determined by when and what shape the client has drawn. Colors such as orange and red can be used to indicate intense pain. See the physical assessment

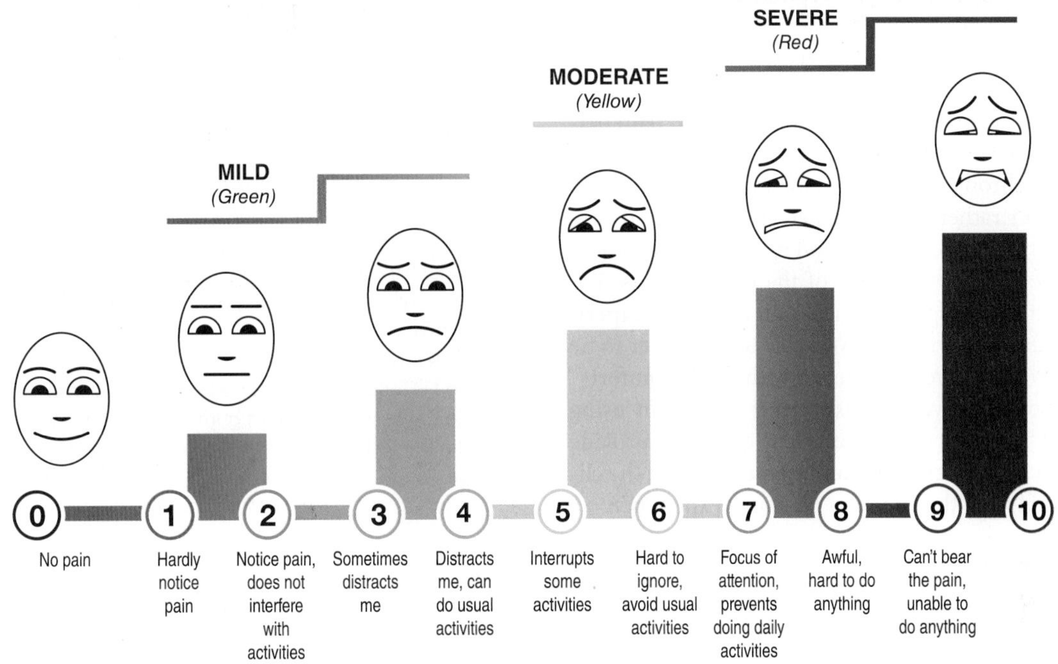

FIG. 11.2 Defense and veterans pain rating scale. (From Polomano RC, Galloway KT, Kent ML, et al. Psychometric testing of the Defense and Veterans Pain Rating Scale [DVPRS]: A new pain scale for military population. *Pain Medicine*, 2016;17(8):1505–1519. https://doi.org/10.1093/pm/pnw105.)

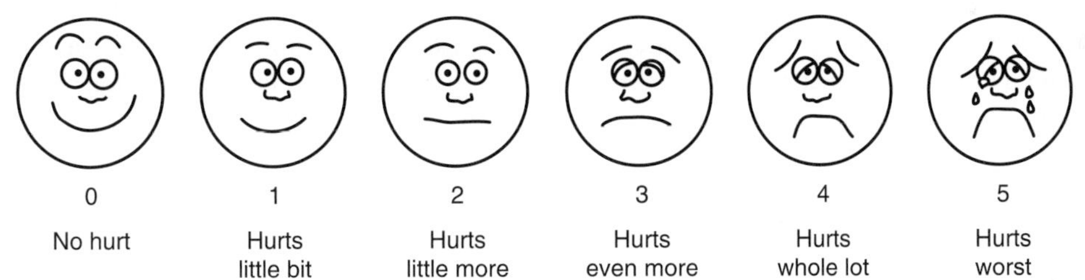

FIG. 11.3 Categorical/numerical pain scale. (Modified from Whaley L, Wong D. *Nursing care of infants and children*, ed 3, St. Louis, 1987, Mosby.)

form in Chapter 4 for an example of figures that can be used for pain drawing.

On the McGill Pain Questionnaire, individuals use sensory, affective, and evaluative word descriptors to specify their subjective pain experience. The three primary measures are (1) the pain rating index, which is based on two types of numerical values that can be assigned to each word descriptor; (2) the number of words chosen; and (3) the present pain intensity, which is rated on a 1-to-5 intensity scale (Melzack, 1983).

The short form of the McGill Pain Questionnaire (SF-MPQ) has 11 questions related to the sensory dimension of the pain experience and 4 related to the affective dimension (Melzack, 1987). Each descriptor is ranked on a 4-point intensity scale (0 = none, 1 = mild, 2 = moderate, 3 = severe). The pain-rating index of the standard MPQ is included, as is a visual analog scale. You may encounter these types of pain measurement documents in various work environments, especially medical settings. Search the internet for access to the various forms available.

Questioning the Use of Scales

Pain scales are effective assessments for acute pain. These same pain scale assessments may not reflect accurate information when assessing chronic pain. There is a trend to avoid overemphasizing the concept of pain, especially when working with clients with chronic conditions. The relationship between pain and the injury state of the tissues becomes less predictable as the acute phase blends into a more chronic pain pattern. The relationship between pain ratings and nociceptor activation is variable. Psychosocial factors are important in most chronic pain states, and many individuals have a distorted understanding of pain, which drives much of their discomfort. There is a need for pain neuroscience education (PNE) to help individuals better understand how pain perception can alter and the difference between acute pain related to actual tissue damage and a chronic nonproductive pain sensation more related to fear and neurobiological sensitivity. When pain scales are used to evaluate chronic pain, the fear state and increased pain perception is reinforced.

For assessing chronic pain, it may be more productive to focus on function rather that pain perception. Instead of a pain scale, an activity of daily living and functional movement assessment may be more reflective of the client's status. For example, instead of asking how much pain a client is experiencing, ask about an activity: "Are you able to bend over to tie your shoes?" "What are you able to do without discomfort?" "Describe the sensation you are experiencing without using the word *pain*." These types of assessment questions provide usable insight to how the chronic condition is affecting the client without reinforcing the attention on a pain experience.

Box 11.3 Standardized Palpation of Tenderness

The American College of Rheumatology has developed a quantifiable method of assessing tissue tenderness (Wolfe et al., 1990). The examiner observes the response to palpatory stimulus by noting pain behaviors, such as facial grimacing and signs of withdrawal. By comparing the painful sites to uninvolved body areas, the examiner can determine whether the response is due to increased physiological activity; this same assessment process can be used to detect a change in pain perception at the same pressure. Instruments for gauging pressure, called algometers, can further objectify the assessment.

A baseline of 4 kg of pressure is used (enough to blanch the tip of a thumbnail pressed on a table), and results are rated as follows:

Grade 0—No tenderness
Grade I—Tenderness with no physical or verbal response
Grade II—Tenderness with grimacing, flinching, or both
Grade III—Tenderness with withdrawal (positive jump sign)
Grade IV—Withdrawal from non-noxious stimuli

Objective Measurements

Physical Evaluation

Physical assessment procedures typically are classified as objective. The main considerations are body balance, efficient function, and basic symmetry. These assessment procedures cover the isolated function of muscles or joints (or both), range of motion, strength, and endurance. These functions are measured and compared with what is considered normal function, and the differences (deviations from the norm) are recorded.

Symmetry

People are not perfectly symmetrical, but the right and left halves of the body should be similar in shape, range of motion, and ability to function. For example, the ear, shoulder, hip, and ankle should be in a vertical line. The greater the discrepancy in symmetry, the greater the potential for soft tissue and joint dysfunction.

Functional Capacity

Whole body movement capabilities also can be measured. Functional assessment considers posture, gait, and range of motion. Disruption of the gait (walking) reflexes creates the potential for many problems. Common gait problems include a functional short leg caused by soft tissue shortening, short neck and shoulder muscles, aching feet, and fatigue.

Examples of functional capacity tests include lifting, carrying, walking, sitting, standing, balancing, and hand function. These types of assessment procedures are especially helpful for measuring qualitative goals, such as improvement in performing activities of daily living and occupation-related rehabilitation. Functional capacity tests measure functions such as joint mobility and muscle strength and endurance, cervical rotation mobility, hip range of motion, and trunk extensor endurance. Such tests may include the following:

- Walking 1 mile
- Climbing two flights of stairs (16 steps)
- Squatting
- Kneeling
- Sitting for prolonged periods with the knees bent in one position
- Running a short distance (100 yards, the length of a football field)
- Standing on one foot
- Walking a short distance (1 block)
- Reaching above the head

Assessment data can be quantified in a number of ways, such as by using the Standardized Palpation of Tenderness and the Muscle Testing Assessment. A number of questionnaires also can help identify the client's perception of their own well-being, distress, or activity intolerance. These include the Oswestry Low Back Pain Disability Questionnaire, Roland-Morris Questionnaire, and Functional Assessment Screening Questionnaire (FASQ). Conduct an internet search for access to the questionnaires (Box 11.3).

Muscle Testing Assessment

Various instruments have been developed to measure muscle and joint function (Fig. 11.4). Box 11.4 presents an example of an efficient assessment procedure.

POSTURE ASSESSMENT: STANDING POSITION

SECTION OBJECTIVES

Chapter objective covered in this section:

3. Identify and address during massage elements relating to function and dysfunction of posture.

Using the information presented in this section, the student will be able to perform the following:

- Complete a basic postural assessment.

Functional posture is considered to be a state of musculoskeletal balance involving minimal body stress or strain. Modern life

Muscle Strength Grading Scale (Oxford Scale)
Medical Research Council [MRC] grading scale

Grade	Value	Muscle Strength
5	Normal	Complete range of motion (ROM) against gravity with full resistance
4	Good	Complete ROM against gravity with some resistance: Full range of motion with decreased strength Sometimes this category is subdivided further into $4^{-}/5$, 4/5, and $4^{+}/5$
3	Fair	Complete ROM against gravity with no resistance; active ROM
2	Poor	Complete ROM with some assistance and gravity eliminated
1	Trace	Evidence of slight muscular contraction, no joint motion evident
0	Zero	No evidence of muscle contraction NT: Not testable

FIG. 11.4 Muscle strength grading scale (Oxford scale). (From Medical Research Council: *Aids to the examination of the peripheral nervous system*, London, 1976, Her Majesty's Stationary Office.)

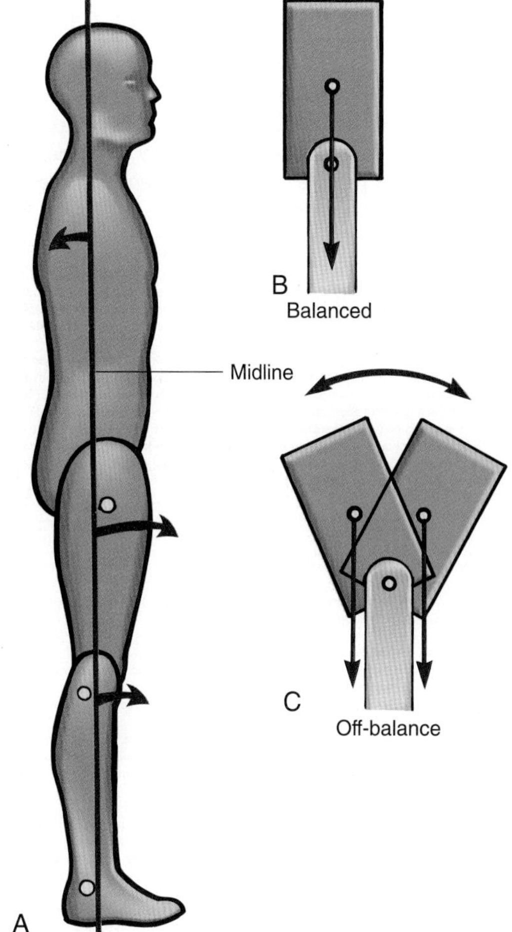

FIG. 11.5 A, In a normal, relaxed stance, the leg and trunk tend to rotate slightly off the midline of the body but maintain a counterbalance force. Balance is achieved in **B,** but not in **C.** Any time the trunk moves off this midline balance point, the body must compensate.

and the rise in a sedentary lifestyle have had a negative effect on most human motor behavior (Kiruthika et al., 2018; Gouveia et al., 2021; Solanki and Mehta 2022). Common postural distortions are lumbar lordosis, thoracic kyphosis, forward head, rounded shoulder, and pronated foot. Primarily, on talking about good–bad posture, there is no gold standard definition for it. Second, there is no single correct posture. Apart from common postural perceptions, there is no sound evidence that there is one ideal posture or that preventing "incorrect postures" will eliminate back pain (Kripa and Kaur 2021).

When assessing posture, the massage practitioner must take care to note the complete postural pattern, head to toe. Every action has a reaction, and the reaction can be compensation. Most compensatory patterns (reactions) occur in response to external forces imposed on the body. The body makes countless compensatory changes daily. This is normal, and if other pathological conditions are not present, they seldom become problematic. However, if the client has had an injury, maintains a certain position for a prolonged period, or overuses a body area, the body may not be able to return to a normal dynamic balance efficiently. The balance of the body against the force of gravity is the fundamental determining factor in a person's posture, or upright position. Even subtle shifts in posture demand a whole body compensatory pattern (Fig. 11.5 and Box 11.5).

The cervical, thoracic, lumbar, and sacral curves (Fig. 11.6) develop because of the body's need to maintain an upright position against gravity. In adults, the cervical vertebrae, when viewed laterally, form a symmetrical anterior convex curve. The thoracic vertebrae curve posteriorly, and the lumbar vertebrae reverse and curve in the anterior direction, with a posterior curve of the sacrum. The sharp angulation above C1, the atlas, which allows the head to maintain a level, horizontal plane, also has been considered a curve. Changes in the normal spinal curves result in scoliosis, lordosis, and kyphosis.

Mechanical Balance

A mechanically balanced, weight-bearing joint is in the gravitational line of the mass it supports and is located exactly through the axis of rotation. The axis of rotation is the center around which something rotates. Placement of the feet influences the stability of the standing position by providing a base of support. The most common position is one leg in front of the other, with mild external rotation of the forward leg. People commonly have a functionally long and short leg. When a person is standing, the long leg often is the front one. When the person is seated with the legs crossed, the long leg often is on top.

The standing posture requires various segments of the body to cooperate mechanically as a whole. Passive tension of ligaments, fascia, and the connective tissue elements of the

Box 11.4 Efficient Intake, Assessment, Care/Treatment Plan, and SOAP/Session Note Documentation Process

The content of this box leads you through the process and documentation forms for the four basic massage outcomes: relaxation, stress management, pain management, and functional mobility outcomes.

All outcomes require informed consent and client intake, a health history form, and a SOAP note form.

INFORMED CONSENT

I, (client's name) ________________, have received a copy of the policies for Massage Works operated by Sue and John Grey. I have read Massage Works' policies, and I understand them. The massage procedures, information about massage in general, general benefits of massage, contraindications to massage, and possible alternatives have been explained to me. The qualifications of the massage professional and reporting measures for misconduct have been disclosed to me.

I understand that the massage I receive is for the purpose of stress reduction and relief from muscular tension, spasm, or pain and to increase circulation. If I experience any pain or discomfort, I will immediately inform the massage practitioner so that the pressure or methods can be adjusted to my comfort level. I understand that massage professionals do not diagnose illness or disease or perform any spinal manipulations, nor do they prescribe any medical treatments, and nothing said or done during the session should be construed as such. I acknowledge that massage is not a substitute for medical examination or diagnosis and that I should see a health care provider for those services. Because massage should not be performed under certain circumstances, I agree to keep the massage practitioner updated as to any changes in my health profile, and I release the massage professional from any liability if I fail to do so.

Client's signature ________________ Date ________

Therapist's signature ________________ Date ________

Consent to Treat a Minor

By my signature I authorize (therapist's name) to provide therapeutic massage to my child or dependent.

Signature of Parent or Guardian ________________ Date ________

For clients who will have several sessions, the next step is completion of the needs assessment and initial care or treatment plan (presented in detail in Chapter 4).

Modified Informed Consent Form for Single Session

For clients who will be seen only once (e.g., the professional is working on a cruise ship, doing sports massage at an event, or doing promotional chair massage at a health fair), the following modification in informed consent can be made.

I, (client's name) ________________, have received a copy of the policies for (name of business) ________________, operated by (owner) ________________. I have read the rules and policies, and I understand them. The general benefits of massage and contraindications to massage have been explained to me. I have disclosed to the therapist any condition I have that would contraindicate massa[...] tions, I understand that no specific needs assessment has been performed. The qual[...] reporting measures for misconduct have been disclosed to me.

I understand that the massage I receive is for the purpose of stress reduction an[...] pain and to increase circulation. If I experience any pain or discomfort, I will immed[...] that the pressure or methods can be adjusted to my comfort level. I understand tha[...] illness or disease or perform any spinal manipulations, nor do they prescribe any[...] massage is not a substitute for medical examination or diagnosis and that I sho[...] services.

I understand that a single massage session or massage used on a random basis is[...] massage approach using standard massage methods and does not include any m[...] function specifically.

Client's signature ________________

Therapist's signature ________________

Consent to Treat a Minor

By my signature I authorize (therapist's name) to provide massage work to my child[...]

Signature of Parent or Guardian ________________

CLIENT INTAKE AND HEALTH HISTORY FORM

Name: ________________ Date: ________

Address: ________________ City: ________ State: ________ Zip: ________

Phone: (day) ________ (eve) ________ Date of Birth: ________

Occupation: ________________ Employer: ________________

Referred by: ________________ Physician: ________________

Previous experience with massage:

____

Primary reason for appointment / areas of pain or tension:

____

Emergency contact—name and number: ________________

Please mark (X) for all conditions that apply now. Put a (P) for past conditions, an (F) for family history of illness.

Pain Scale: minor-1 2 3 4 5 6 7 8 9 severe-10

____ headaches, migraines	____ chronic pain	____ fatigue
____ vision problems, contact lenses	____ muscle or joint pain	____ tension, stress
____ hearing problems, deafness	____ muscle, bone injuries	____ depression
____ injuries to face or head	____ numbness or tingling	____ sleep difficulties
____ sinus problems	____ sprains, strains	____ allergies, sensitivities
____ dental bridges, braces	____ arthritis, tendinitis	____ rashes, athlete's foot
____ jaw pain, TMJ problems	____ cancer, tumors	____ infectious diseases
____ asthma or lung conditions	____ spinal column disorders	____ blood clots
____ constipation, diarrhea	____ diabetes	____ varicose veins
____ hernia	____ pregnancy	____ high/low blood pressure
____ birth control, IUD	____ heart, circulatory problems	
____ abdominal or digestive problems	____ other medical conditions not listed	

Explain any areas noted above:

____

Current medications, including aspirin, ibuprofen, herbs, supplements, etc.:

____

Surgeries: ________________

Accidents: ________________

Please list all forms and frequency of stress reduction activities, hobbies, exercise, or sports participation:

____

Client completes Intake Health History Form.

Continued

Box 11.4 Efficient Intake, Assessment, Care/Treatment Plan, and SOAP/Session Note Documentation Process—cont'd

Care/Treatment Plan-General Relaxation/Well-Being

Goal for massage: Relaxation/well-being, general classical nonspecific massage, moderate nonpainful pressure, 50 minutes in duration. Positioning prone and supine or left/right side.

Client signature ______________________

Date ______________

Massage therapist ______________________

Date ______________

Complete Soap or Similar Charting Method Each Session

Outcome Goal: Relaxation___

S

O

A

P

NOTES:

End Process for Relaxation Outcome

Goals for massage: stress relief, pain relief, or mobility

Postural Assessment

For outcomes goals related to stress, pain, or mobility, continue with more comprehensive assessment beginning with postural assessment. View the client from three standing positions: front, back, and side. Note any areas of asymmetry on the figure. Assess for upper and lower crossed syndrome.

MASSAGE ASSESSMENT/PHYSICAL OBSERVATION/PALPATION AND GAIT PRE POST

Client Name: ______________________ Date: ______________

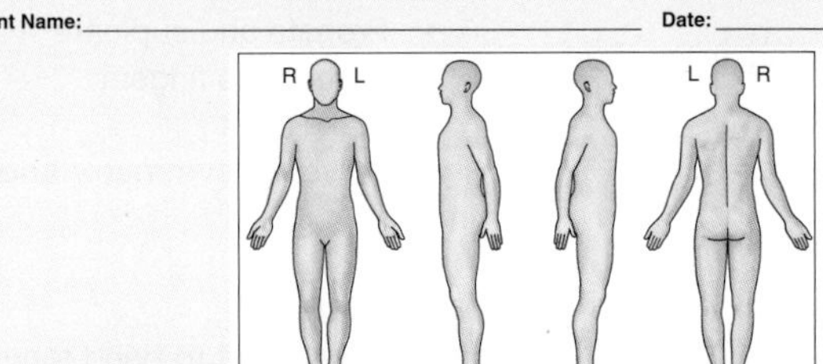

OBSERVATION & PALPATION

ALIGNMENT	RIBS	SCAPULA
Chin in line with nose, sternal notch, navel	Even	Even
Other:	Springy	Move freely
HEAD	Other:	Other:
Tilted (L)	**ABDOMEN**	**CLAVICLES**
Tilted (R)	Firm and pliable	Level
Rotated (L)	Hard areas	Other:
Rotated (R)	Other:	**ARMS**
EYES	**WAIST**	Hang evenly (internal) (external)
Level	Level	(L) rotated □ medial □ lateral
Equally set in socket	Other:	(R) rotated □ medial □ lateral
Other:	**SPINE CURVES**	**ELBOWS**
EARS	Normal	Even
Level	Other:	Other:
Other:	**GLUTEAL MUSCLE MASS**	**WRISTS**
SHOULDERS	Even	Even
Level	Other:	Other:
(R) high / (L) low	**ILIAC CREST**	**FINGERTIPS**
(L) high / (R) low	Level	Even
(L) rounded forward	Other:	Other:
(R) rounded forward	**KNEES**	**PATELLA**
Muscle development even	Even/symmetrical	(L) □ movable □ rigid
Other:	Other:	(R) □ movable □ rigid

ANKLES	TRUNK	LEGS
Even	Remains vertical	Swing freely at hip
Other:	Other:	Other:
FEET	**SHOULDERS**	**KNEES**
Mobile	Remain level	Flex and extend freely through stance and swing phase
Other:	Rotate during walking	Other:
ARCHES	Other:	**FEET**
Even	**ARMS**	Heel strikes first at start of stance
Other:	Motion is opposite leg swing	Plantar flexed at push-off
TOES	Motion is even (L) and (R)	Foot clears floor during swing phase
Straight	Other:	Other:
Other:	(L) swings freely	**STEP**
SKIN	(R) swings freely	Length is even
Moves freely and resilient	Other:	Timing is even
Pulls/restricted	**HIPS**	Other:
Puffy/baggy	Remain level	**OVERALL**
Other:	Other:	Rhythmic
HEAD	Rotate during walking	Other:
Remains steady/eyes forward	Other:	
Other:		

Box 11.4 Efficient Intake, Assessment, Care/Treatment Plan, and SOAP/Session Note Documentation Process—cont'd

Continue with expanded assessment for stress management, pain management, and functional mobility outcomes.

Functional Capacity Assessment

Ask the client if they have any issues with the following:

- Rolling over in bed
- Getting in or out of chair
- Getting up and down on the floor
- Getting in or out of car
- Climbing stairs
- Bending, twisting, or turning
- Squatting or kneeling
- Pushing, pulling, lifting, or reaching with arm(s)
- Throwing
- Gripping objects
- Breathing
- Sleeping

Explain any areas indicated.

Adaptive Capacity Assessment

Functioning effectively __________ Functioning with effort __________

Functioning with fatigue and pain______________ Function limited______________

Explain any areas indicated:

Postural Assessment

View the client from three standing positions: front, back, and side. Note any areas of asymmetry on the figure. Assess for upper and lower crossed syndrome.

Physical Assessment

Back

Instruct the client to bend forward, keeping the knees straight. Observe for the following:

- Scoliosis
- Kyphosis
- Asymmetry

Instruct the client to side-bend by sliding the hand down the side of the leg; compare the two sides. Instruct the client to twist the torso left and right; compare the two sides. Observe for symmetry and range of motion. Explain your findings.

Cervical Spine Range of Motion

Instruct the client to do the following:

- Look at ceiling (extension)
- Look at floor (flexion)
- Look over each shoulder (rotation)
- Bend the ear to each shoulder (abduction/lateral flexion)

Observe for symmetry and range of motion. Explain your findings.

Shoulder Range of Motion

Instruct the client to do the following:

- Scratch the back with each hand from over the shoulder (external rotation and abduction)
- Scratch the back with each hand from under the shoulder (internal rotation and adduction)

Observe for symmetry and range of motion. Explain your findings.

Upper Extremity Range of Motion

Instruct the client to do the following:

- Flex and extend the elbows
- Pronate and supinate
- Spread the fingers
- Make a fist

Observe for symmetry and range of motion. Explain your findings.

Lower Extremity

Instruct the client to bend forward at the hip joints to touch the toes.

- Observe for hamstring shortening at the hip and the knee.

Instruct client to sit on chair and stand.

- Observe for hip flexion and extension, knee flexion and extension, and overall leg strength.

Instruct the client to do the following:

- Rise up on toes; observe for calf strength
- Rise up on heels; observe for leg strength

Instruct the client to perform the one leg standing balance test:

- Have the client stand first on one foot and then on the other; compare the two sides, and observe for balance and coordination

Instruct the client to perform the squat test: Have the client raise the arms over the head and then squat by pretending to sit down in a chair; observe for symmetry and reduced or excessive movement; core strength; hip, knee, and ankle flexion; hip adduction; shoulder abduction; and latissimus shortening. Record your findings on the figure.

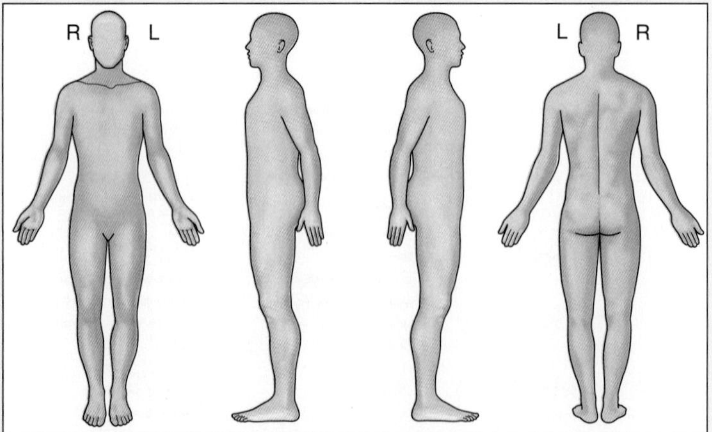

Explain your findings.

Indications for more specific assessment/findings:

Breathing	Muscle testing	Firing patterns
Pain	Specific joint movement	
Gait		

Continued

Box 11.4 Efficient Intake, Assessment, Care/Treatment Plan, and SOAP/Session Note Documentation Process—cont'd

Palpation Assessment

Completed during massage. Indicate your findings on the figure.

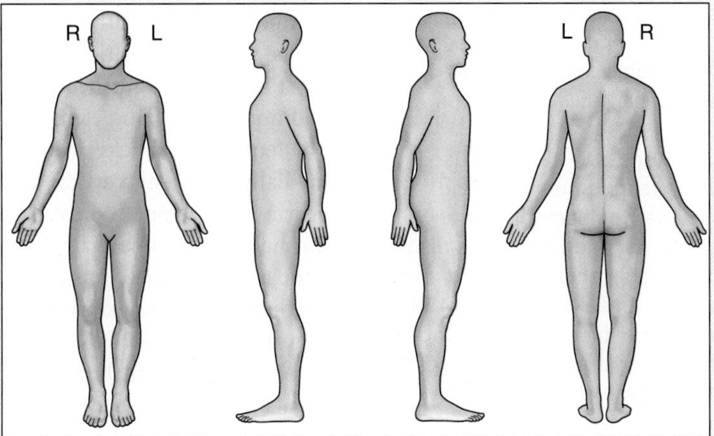

Impressions and Critical Thinking Summary of Assessment Findings

Care/treatment plan: Multiple sessions for outcome goals of stress management, pain management, or functional mobility

CARE/TREATMENT PLAN

Client Name:____________________

Choose One: ☐ Original plan ☐ Reassessment date__________

Short-term client goals:
Quantitative:
Qualitative:

Long-term client goals:
Quantitative:
Qualitative:

Therapist objectives:

1) Frequency, 2) length, and 3) duration of visits:
1) ______ 2) ______ 3) ______

Progress measurements to be used: (Ex.— pain scale, range of motion, increased ability to perform function)

Dates of reassessment:

Categories of massage methods to be used: (Ex.— general constitutional, stress reduction, circulatory, lymphatic, neuromuscular, connective tissue, neurochemical, etc.)

Additional notes:

Client Signature:____________________ Date:________

Therapist Signature:____________________ Date:________

Outcome Goals: Relaxation__ Stress Management__ Pain Management__ Functional Mobility__

S
O
A
P
Notes:

Note: Forms and figures are examples only. See Chapter 4 for actual forms.

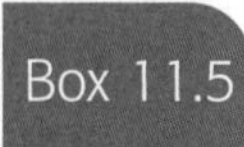

Box 11.5 Habitual Factors Leading to Posture Distortion

Three major factors influence posture: heredity, disease, and habit. These factors must be considered in the evaluation of posture. The easiest factor to adjust is habit.

- Occupational habits (e.g., a shoulder raised from talking on the phone) and recreational habits (e.g., a forward-shoulder position in a bike rider) can have an effect on posture.
- Clothing and shoes can affect the way a person uses the body. Tight collars or ties restrict breathing and contribute to neck and shoulder problems. Restrictive belts, control-top undergarments, and tight pants also limit breathing and affect the neck, shoulders, and mid-back. Shoes with high heels or those that do not fit the feet comfortably interfere with postural muscles. Shoes with worn soles imprint the old postural pattern, and the client's body assumes the dysfunctional pattern if she puts them back on after the massage. To maintain postural changes, the client must change to shoes that do not have a worn sole.
- Sleep positions can contribute to a wide range of problems such as neck strain when sleeping on one's stomach or sleeping on one's side, which can affect the shoulders.
- Furniture that does not support the back or that is too high or too low perpetuates muscular dysfunction.

By normalizing the soft tissue and teaching balancing exercises, the massage therapist can play a beneficial role in helping clients overcome habitual postural distortion.

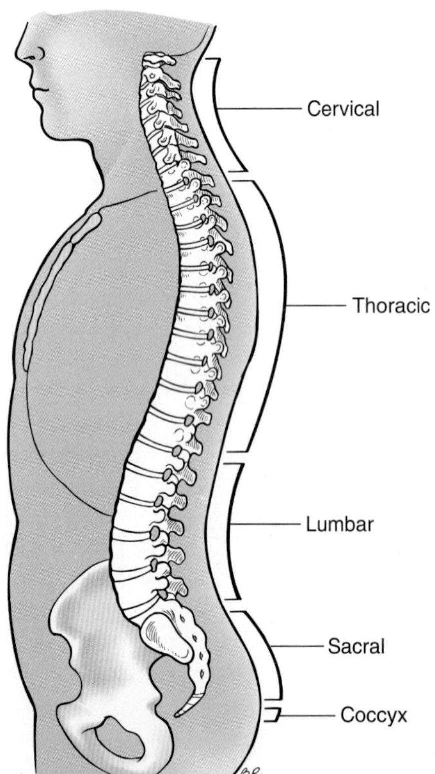

FIG. 11.6 Normal spinal curves.

muscles supports the skeleton. Muscle activity plays a small but important role. Postural muscles maintain small amounts of contraction that stabilize the body upright in gravity by continually repositioning the body weight over the mechanical balance point.

In relaxed symmetrical standing, both the hip and the knee joints assume a position of full extension to provide for the most efficient weight-bearing position. The knee joint has an additional stabilizing element in its screw-home mechanism. The femur rides backward on the medial condyle and rotates medially about its vertical axis to lock the joint for weight bearing; this happens only in the final phase of extension. The normal screw-home extension pattern of the knee is not hyperextension, which puts a strain on the knee. The hamstrings are the major muscles that resist the force of gravity at the knee (Smith et al., 1996; Norkin and Levangie, 2005).

At the ankle joint, bones and ligaments do little to limit motion. Passive tension of the two-joint gastrocnemius muscle (i.e., the muscle crosses two joints) becomes a key factor. This stabilizing force is diminished if high-heeled shoes are worn. The heel of the shoe puts the gastrocnemius on a slack. If these heels are worn constantly, the muscle and the Achilles tendon shorten.

During prolonged standing, the average person shifts position frequently. The two basic positions used are the symmetrical stance, with the weight distributed equally on both feet, and the asymmetrical stance, in which nearly all the weight rests on one foot (Fig. 11.7). The asymmetrical stance is the most common, with the weight shifted back and forth between the two feet. This allows for rest periods and shifting of the gravitational forces. Body sway is limited by the intermittent action of appropriate antigravitational postural muscles.

Asymmetry usually results when short muscles (increased tone), shortened connective tissue, or both pull the body out of alignment. Direct trauma pushes joints out of alignment. Weak stabilizing mechanisms, such as overstretched ligaments or inhibited antagonist muscles, contribute to the problem. A chiropractor, an osteopath, or another trained medical professional skilled in skeletal manipulation is needed for these conditions. Often a multidisciplinary approach to client care is required.

Postural Assessment: Procedure for the Standing Position

1. To assess posture in the standing position, have the client use the symmetrical stance.
2. The feet are about shoulder width apart, and the eyes are closed.
3. With the eyes closed, most of the client's postural patterns are exaggerated, because the client is unable to orient the body visually.
4. Often the client tips the head or rotates it slightly to feel balanced; this indicates muscular imbalance and internal postural imbalance information relayed by positional receptors.

Box 11.6 presents a list of indicators of lack of symmetry. The physical assessment form in Chapter 4 is a helpful tool for performing the physical assessment.

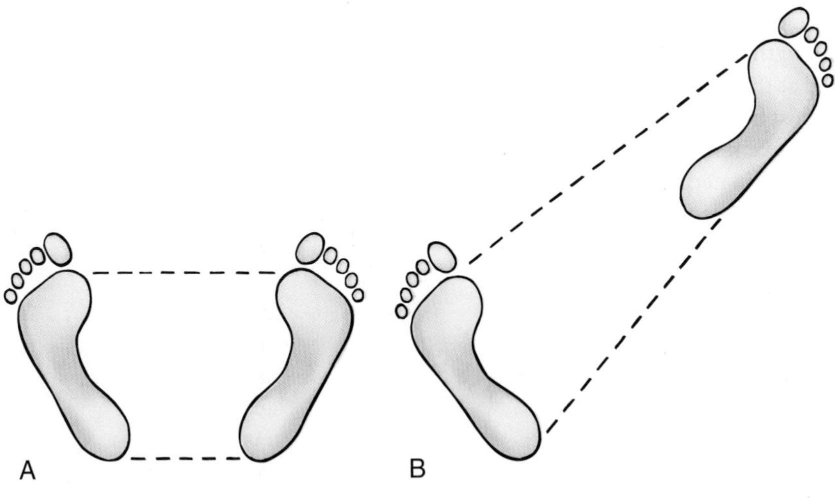

FIG. 11.7 A, Symmetrical stance. **B,** Asymmetrical stance. The asymmetrical stance, with the weight shifted from foot to foot, is the most efficient standing position.

Box 11.6 Landmarks That Help Identify Lack of Symmetry

The following landmarks can be used to compare the symmetry of the body in various aspects. Be sure to observe the client from the back, the front, and the left and right sides:

- The middle of the chin should sit directly under the tip of the nose. Check the chin alignment with the sternal notch. These two landmarks should be in a direct line.
- The shoulders and clavicles should be level with each other. The shoulders should not roll forward or backward or be rotated with one forward and one backward.
- The arms should hang freely and at the same rotation out of the glenohumeral (shoulder) joint.
- The elbows, wrists, and fingertips should be in the same plane.
- The skin of the thorax (chest and back) should be even and should not look as if it pulls or is puffy.
- The navel, located on the same line as the nose, chin, and sternal notch, should not look pulled.
- The ribs should be even and springy.
- The abdomen should be firm but relaxed and slightly rounded.
- The curves at the waist should be even on both sides.
- The spine should be in a direct line from the base of the skull and on the same plane as the line connecting the nose and the navel. The curves of the spine should not be exaggerated.
- The scapulae should appear even and should move freely. You should be able to draw an imaginary straight line between the tips of the scapulae.
- The gluteal muscle mass should be even.
- The tops of the iliac crests should be even.
- The greater trochanter, knees, and ankles should be level.
- The circumferences of the thigh and calf should be similar on the left and right sides.
- The legs should rotate out of the acetabulum (hip joint) evenly in a slight external rotation.
- The knees should be locked in the standing position but should not be hyperextended. The patellae (kneecaps) should be level and pointed slightly laterally.
- A line dropped from the nose should fall through the sternum and the navel and should be spaced evenly between.

Intervention Guidelines

Misalignment of body areas can be caused by muscles that pull or that do not stabilize, by connective tissue shortening or laxity, or, more likely, by a combination of these factors. The best course is to follow the lead provided by the client's body. When performing massage, the practitioner should honor what the body is doing. This can be done by creating an exaggeration of the asymmetrical pattern found and then slowly encouraging the body to shift to a more symmetrical pattern. The integrated muscle energy approach explained in Chapter 10 is effective in these situations. Working with superficial fascia dysfunction often requires slow, sustained elongation (15–30 seconds) that puts sufficient mechanical force into the tissue, in addition to specific application of friction (shear stress) massage techniques. Connective tissue approaches normalize the twists and pulls of shortened connective tissue (see Chapter 12).

GAIT ASSESSMENT

SECTION OBJECTIVES

Chapter objective covered in this section:

4. Explain the process of walking and identify and address gait dysfunction.

Using the information presented in this section, the student will be able to perform the following:

- Complete a basic gait assessment.

Factors Affecting Gait

Gait is the way we walk. Two major abilities are essential to walking: equilibrium and locomotion. *Equilibrium* is the ability to assume an upright posture and maintain balance. *Locomotion* is the ability to initiate and maintain rhythmic stepping. Many other contributing factors also are involved in the process of walking.

The musculoskeletal system must provide intact bones, well-functioning joints, and adequate muscle strength. Normal muscle tone, which is important, is controlled at the subcortical level of the nervous system. Muscle tone must be high enough to resist gravity but low enough to allow movement. Reciprocal innervation of muscles allows for the coordinated action of agonists and antagonists that is necessary for skilled movements.

Vision also is vital to normal walking, particularly when other sensory input is reduced. Vision gives information about the movement of the head and body relative to the surroundings and is important for the automatic balance responses to changes in surface conditions. People with visual impairments are likely to have gait alterations.

Other sensory systems that are important in this process are the vestibular, auditory, and sensory motor systems.

Abnormal Gait

Abnormal gait or gait abnormality occurs when the body systems that control the way a person walks do not function in the usual way. Causes of walking/gait disorders can range from arthritis to a neurological condition to something as simple as ill-fitting footwear. Observation during assessment may identify abnormal gait such as:

- Walking with head and neck bent forward
- Dragging or shuffling feet
- Irregular, jerky movements
- Smaller steps and walking slowly or stiffly
- Waddling

Some walking abnormalities have been given names:

- Propulsive gait – a stooped, stiff posture with the head and neck bent forward
- Parkinsonian gait – stooped posture, with the head and neck bent forward; difficulty initiating steps and walking with slow, small steps
- Scissors gait – legs flexed slightly at the hips and knees like crouching, with the knees and thighs hitting or crossing in a scissors-like movement
- Spastic gait – a stiff, foot-dragging walk caused by a long muscle contraction on one side
- Steppage gait – foot drop where the foot hangs with the toes pointing down, causing the toes to scrape the ground while walking, requiring someone to lift the leg higher than normal when walking
- Ataxic, or broad-based, gait – feet wide apart with irregular, jerky, and weaving or slapping when trying to walk
- Hemiplegic gait – affects one side of the body with dragging the affected leg
- Diplegic gait – characterized by bent hips and knees with the ankles internally rotated, resulting in a swinging gait on both sides of the body
- Myopathic gait – waddling from side to side when walking due to weakness in the pelvic region

Procedure for Gait Assessment

Understanding the basic body movements of walking can help the massage practitioner recognize dysfunctional and inefficient gait patterns. It is important to observe the client from the front, the back, and both sides. The process of gait assessment proceeds in the following way:

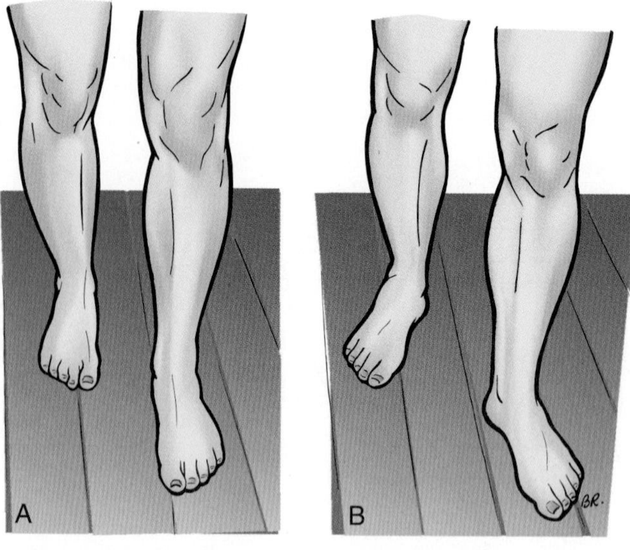

FIG. 11.8 Proper **(A)** and improper **(B)** foot position in walking.

1. Watch the client walk, noting the heel-to-toe foot placement. The toes should point forward with slight external rotation with each step (Fig. 11.8).
2. Observe the upper body. It should be relaxed and fairly symmetrical. The head should face forward with the eyes level with the horizontal plane. A natural arm swing should occur opposite the leg swing. The arm swing begins at the shoulder joint. On each step, the left arm moves forward as the right leg moves forward and vice versa. This pattern provides balance. The rhythm and pace of the arm and leg swing should be similar. Increasing the walking speed should increase the speed of the arm swing. The length of the stride determines the arc of the arm swing (Fig. 11.9).
3. Observe the client walking and note the person's general appearance. The optimal walking pattern is as follows:
   a. The head and trunk are vertical, with the eyes easily maintaining forward position and level with the horizontal plane; the shoulders are level and perpendicular to the vertical line.
   b. The arms swing freely opposite the leg swing, allowing the shoulder girdle to rotate opposite the pelvic girdle.
   c. The step length and timing are even.
   d. The body oscillates vertically with each step.
   e. The entire body moves rhythmically with each step.
   f. At the heel strike, the foot is approximately at a right angle to the leg.
   g. The knee is extended, not locked, in slight flexion.
   h. The body weight is shifted forward into the stance phase.
   i. At push-off, the foot is strongly plantar flexed, with defined hyperextension of the metatarsophalangeal joints of the toes.
   j. During the leg swing, the foot easily clears the floor with good alignment, and the rhythm of movement remains unchanged.
   k. The heel contacts the floor first.
   l. The weight then rolls to the outside of the arch.

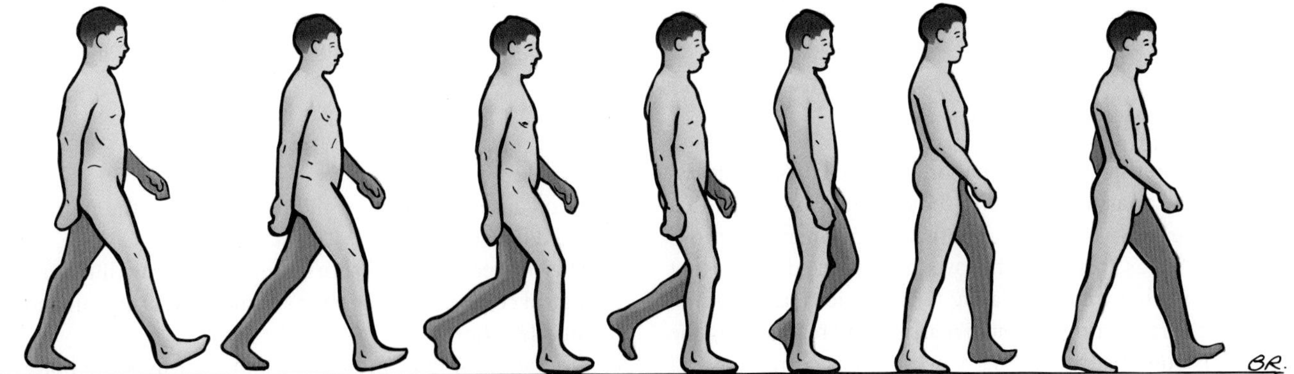

FIG. 11.9 Efficient gait position.

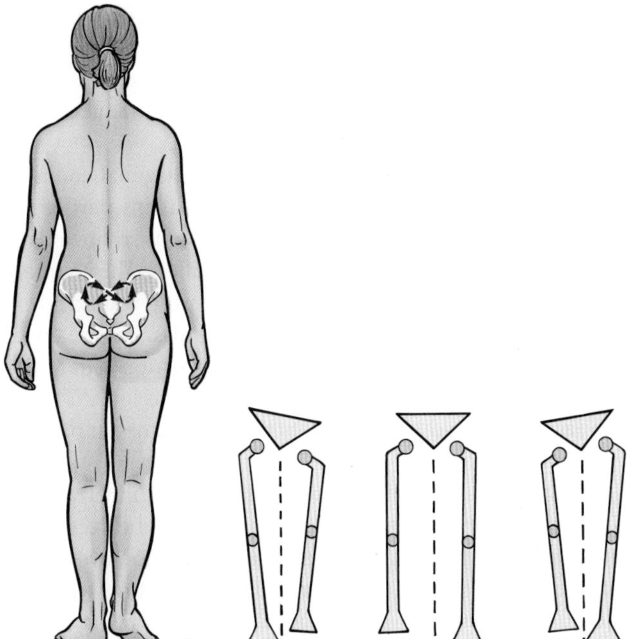

FIG. 11.10 Mechanism of the slight rocking movement of the sacroiliac joint.

m. The arch flattens slightly in response to the weight load.
n. The weight then is shifted to the ball of the foot in preparation for the spring-off from the toes and the shifting of the weight to the other foot.

During walking, the pelvis moves slightly in a side-lying, figure-eight pattern. The movements that make up this sequence are transverse, medial, and lateral rotation. The stability and mobility of the sacroiliac (SI) joints play important roles in this alternating side, figure-eight movement. If these joints are not functioning properly, the entire gait is disrupted. The SI joint is one of the few joints in the body that is not directly affected by muscles that cross the joint. It is a large joint, and the bony contact between the sacrum and the ilium is broad. The rocking of this joint often is disrupted (Fig. 11.10).

The hips rotate in a slightly oval pattern, beginning with a medial rotation during the leg swing and heel strike, followed by a lateral rotation through the push-off.

The knees move in a flexion and extension pattern opposite each other. The extension phase never reaches enough extension to initiate the normal knee-lock pattern that is used in standing.

The ankles rotate in an arc around the heel at heel strike and around a center in the forefoot at push-off.

Maximum dorsiflexion at the end of the stance phase and maximum plantar flexion at the end of push-off are necessary.

Muscle Group Interaction of Gait Patterns

It also is important to consider the pattern of muscle interactions that occurs with walking. Remember that gait has a certain pattern for efficient movement. For example, if the left leg moves forward for the heel strike, the right arm also moves forward. This results in activation of the flexors of both the arm and leg and inhibition of the extensors. One muscle out of sequence with the others can set up increased muscle tone (too strong) or inhibited (unable to hold) muscle imbalances. Whenever a muscle contracts with too much force, it overpowers the antagonist group, resulting in inhibited muscle function. The imbalances can occur anywhere in the pattern.

Practical Application

It is helpful to break apart the gait cycle and look at the relationship of the arms and legs (see Fig. 11.9). You can use your own body to learn how the muscles of the shoulders and arms and hips and legs work in sequence. Begin to take a step and then stop and notice the position of the body. Notice what part of the body is moving forward and what is behind the body. Now continue the step and freeze. Observe again. Continue this process until you complete an entire gait cycle.

Careful study of this interaction is important for work with individuals such as athletes or dancers. An understanding of this interaction also is helpful in working with people who have various forms of spastic paralysis and spastic muscle conditions. For example, a child with a head injury that causes flexor spasms in the right arm may be helped temporarily by a reduction in the spasm pattern through activation of left leg extensor patterns, especially if the child has more coordination in that area. All other possible interactions follow suit.

Common Findings from Gait Assessment

Any disruption of the gait demands that the body compensate by shifting movement patterns and posture. Observing areas of the body that do not move efficiently during walking is a good means of detecting dysfunctional areas.

Intervention Guidelines

When interpreting the information gathered from gait assessment, the massage therapist should focus on areas that do not move easily when the client walks and areas that move too much. Areas that do not move are restricted; areas that move too much are compensating for inefficient function. By releasing the restrictions through massage and reeducating the reflexes through neuromuscular work, such as correcting gait reflexes and exercise, the practitioner can help the client improve the gait pattern.

The techniques used are similar to those for postural corrections. The shortened and restricted areas are addressed with massage, and then the neuromuscular mechanism is reset with muscle energy technique and soft tissue/muscle tissue lengthening. During visual and palpation assessment, shortened and restricted areas form concavities or metaphorical caves. Accompanying the adaptation of short tissues, long taut tissues form into convexities or metaphorical hills. This simplification can quickly provide assessment information and guide massage intervention plans (i.e., massage and lengthen the short tissues in the caves and exercise the long taut tissues on the hills).

The client should be taught slow lengthening and stretching procedures for the short areas (caves). After stimulating the muscles in weakened areas, the practitioner can teach the client strengthening exercises for the long areas (hills). The therapist must make sure to incorporate the adaptation methods into a complete, full-body massage rather than doing spot work on isolated parts of the body to support adaptation and integration. Suggestions could be made to the client to evaluate factors that may contribute to identified dysfunctions, such as posture, footwear, chairs, tables, beds, clothing, shoes, workstations, physical tasks (e.g., shoveling), and repetitive exercise patterns.

Proper functioning of the SI joint is a key factor in walking patterns. Because SI joint movement has no direct muscular component, it is difficult to use any kind of muscle energy lengthening when working with this joint. The joint is embedded deep in supporting ligaments. To keep the surrounding ligaments pliable, direct and specific connective tissue techniques are indicated unless the joint is hypermobile. If that is the case, external bracing combined with rehabilitative movement may be indicated. Sometimes the ligaments restabilize the area. Stabilization of the jointed area should be interspersed with massage to ensure that the ligaments remain pliable and do not adhere to each other. This process takes time.

The diagnosis of specific joint problems and fitting for external bracing are outside the scope of practice for therapeutic massage, and the client must be referred to the appropriate professional. Recall that all dysfunctional patterns are whole body phenomena. Working only on the symptomatic area is ineffective and offers limited relief. Therapeutic massage with a whole-body focus is extremely valuable for dealing with gait dysfunction (Proficiency Exercise 11.3). Gait assessment prior to the general massage compared with a post-massage assessment often indicates more efficient walking patterns even when no specific interventions are used.

Key Points

- Pain causes the body to tighten and alters the normal relaxed flow of walking.
- Muscle weakness and shortening interfere with the neurological control of the agonist (prime mover) and antagonist muscle action.
- Limitation of joint movement and joint hypermobility result in protective muscle contraction. If the situation becomes chronic, shortening of both muscle groups (agonist and antagonist) and muscle weakness result.
- Changes in the soft tissue, including all superficial fascia, the connective tissue elements of the tendons, ligaments, and fascial sheaths, restrict the normal action of muscles and joints. Connective tissue usually displays reduced sliding and becomes less pliable.
- Amputation disrupts the body's normal diagonal counterbalance function. Obviously, amputation of any part of the leg disturbs the walking pattern; what is not so obvious is that amputation of any part of the arm affects the counterbalance movement of the arm swing during walking. The rest of the body must compensate for the loss. Loss of any of the toes greatly affects the postural information sent to the brain from the feet. These details may be overlooked when in fact they could be major contributing factors in posture and gait problems.
- Soft tissue dysfunction can exist without joint involvement.
- Any change in the tissue around a joint has a direct effect on the joint function. Changes in joint function eventually cause problems with the joint. Any dysfunction with the joint immediately involves the surrounding muscles and other soft tissue.

ASSESSMENT OF JOINT RANGE OF MOTION

SECTION OBJECTIVES

Chapter objective covered in this section:

5. Integrate joint movement into the massage for assessment purposes.

Using the information presented in this section, the student will be able to perform the following:

- Complete a range-of-motion assessment.

Recall from Chapter 10 that active and passive joint movement can assess the range of motion of a joint. Active joint movement is performed when the client moves the joint through the planes of motion that are normal for that joint. Any pain, crepitus, or limitation that manifests during the action is reported. This assessment identifies how the client is willing or able to move their body.

Passive joint movement to assess range of motion is performed when the massage therapist moves the joint passively through the planes of motion that are normal for the joint. The assessment identifies limitation (hypomobility) or excess

PROFICIENCY EXERCISE 11.3

Protocol for Gait Muscle Testing

The body has many gait-related kinetic chain patterns. The coordination between the upper and lower limbs allows for normal arm swing in relation to leg movements. The figures illustrate these patterns and how to assess for function. If assessment identifies altered function intervention may be indication.

Intervention

Use massage methods to inhibit muscles that assess as too strong by remaining in concentric contraction patterns when they should inhibit. Appropriate methods are slow compression, kneading, gliding, and shaking. Strengthen muscles that inhibit when they should hold strong. Appropriate methods are percussion and rhythmic contraction of inhibited muscles. Then retest the pattern; it should be normal.

This procedure is demonstrated in detail on the EVOLVE website video clips for this chapter.

To perform this assessment, you must understand two important definitions:

- Control group: For this particular purpose, the control group is the group of muscles that initiates the reflex response.
- Test group: Also in this case, the test group is the muscle group that responds to the stimulus from the control group.

Activate the control group first by having the client hold against resistance applied by the practitioner. Maintain the activation of the control group while accessing the response from the text group by applying resistance. The test group should remain strong or inhibit depending on the part of the gait being assessed.

For testing of the arm flexors and extensors, the humerus should be stabilized superior to the elbow joint, and the femur should be stabilized above the knee.

A–D are contralateral (opposite arm and leg) assessments

E–H are unilateral (same side arm and leg) assessments.

A

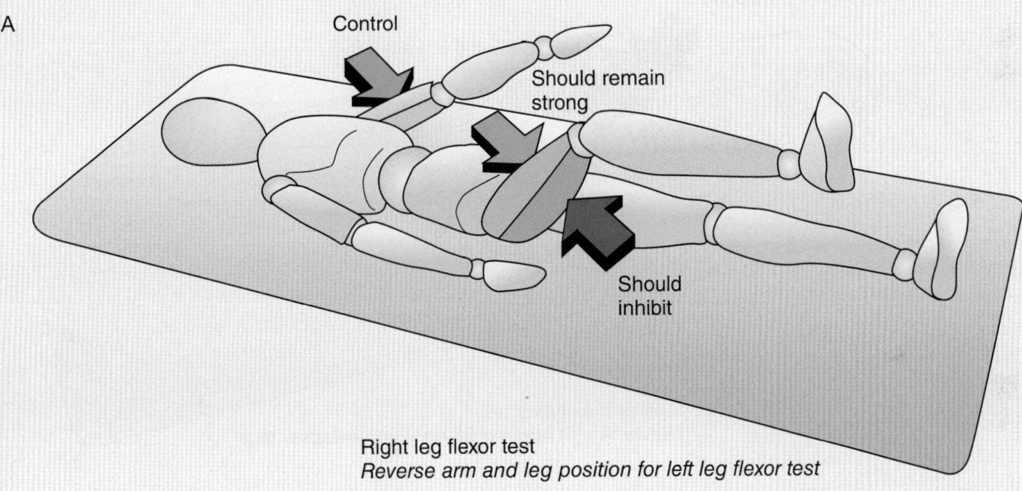

Right leg flexor test
Reverse arm and leg position for left leg flexor test

B

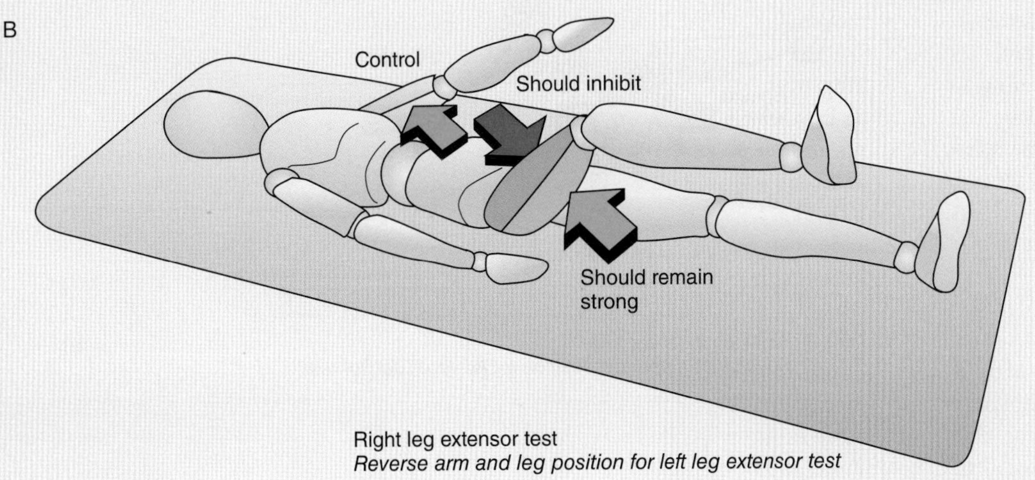

Right leg extensor test
Reverse arm and leg position for left leg extensor test

PROFICIENCY EXERCISE 11.3—cont'd

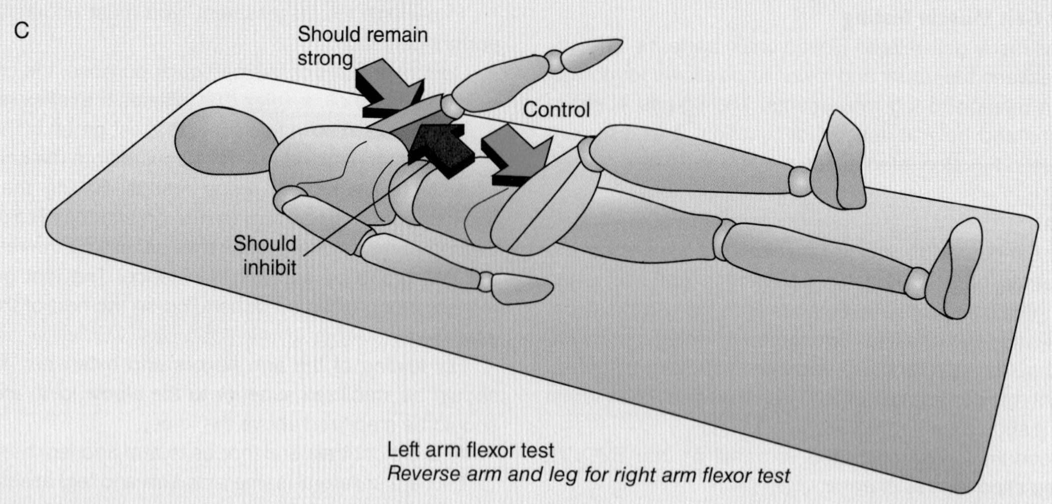

Left arm flexor test
Reverse arm and leg for right arm flexor test

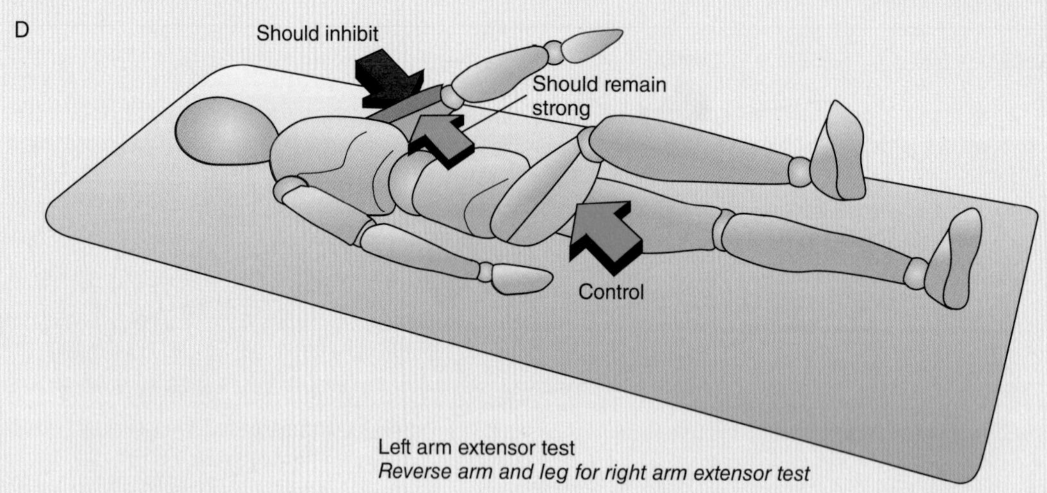

Left arm extensor test
Reverse arm and leg for right arm extensor test

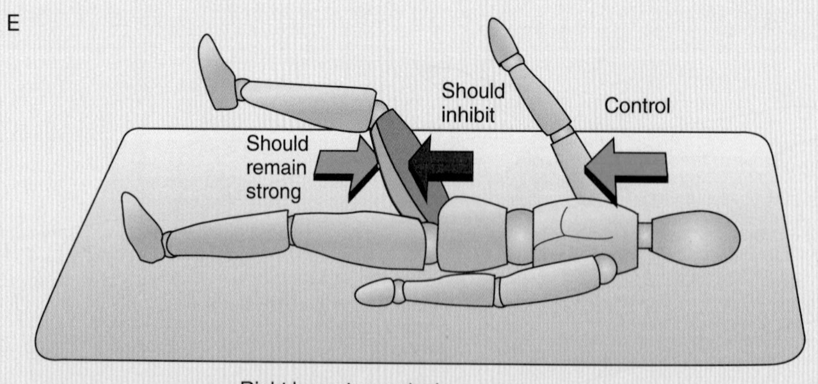

Right leg extensor test
Reverse arm and leg position for left leg extensor test

Continued

PROFICIENCY EXERCISE 11.3—cont'd

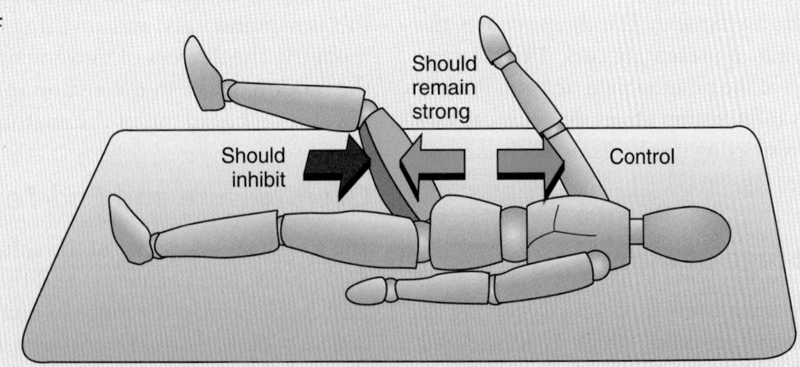

Right leg flexor test
Reverse arm and leg position for left leg flexor test

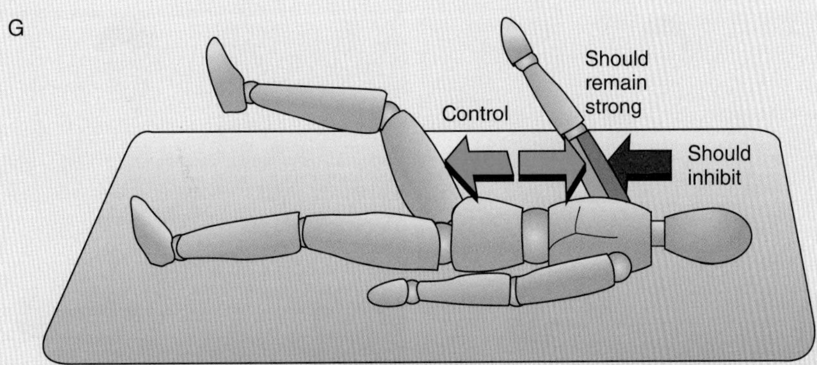

Right arm extensor test
Reverse arm and leg position for left arm extensor test

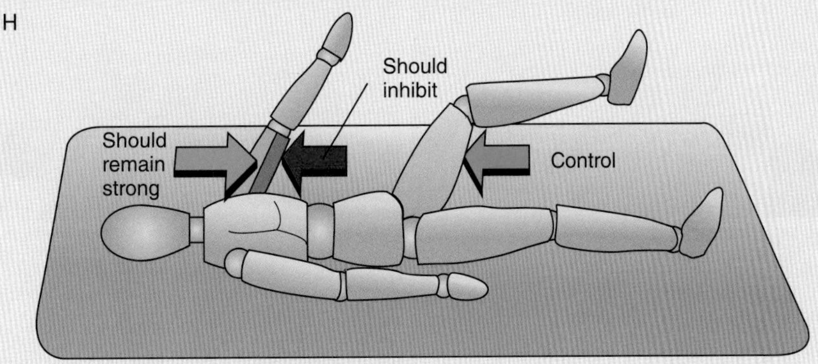

Left arm flexor test
Reverse arm and leg position for right arm flexor test

movement (hypermobility) of the joint. Passive movement is performed carefully and gently to allow the client to fully relax the muscles during the assessment. The client reports the point at which pain or bind, if present, occurs. The massage therapist stops the motion at the point of pain or bind. Passive joint movement provides information about the joint capsule and ligaments and other restricting mechanisms, such as muscles and connective tissue (Fig. 11.11).

Measuring Joint Range of Motion

Joint range of motion is measured in degrees, starting at the neutral line of anatomic position, which is considered 0. Movement of a joint in the sagittal, frontal, or transverse plane is described as the number of degrees of flexion, extension, adduction, abduction, and internal and external rotation (Fig. 11.12). For example, the elbow has approximately 150 degrees of flexion at the end range. Anything less than this is hypomobility, and anything more is considered hypermobility. The degrees of movement are recorded as 0 to X° if the motion began in the anatomic position and as X° to 0 if the motion began out of the anatomic position.

Overpressure and End-Feel

The length and elasticity of the soft tissues (i.e., muscles, tendons, fascia, and ligaments) and the arrangement of the joint surfaces determine the range of motion of the joint and therefore the joint's normal end-feel (see Chapter 10). In using overpressure, the massage therapist gradually applies just a bit more pressure when the end of the available passive range of joint motion has been reached. The sensation transmitted to

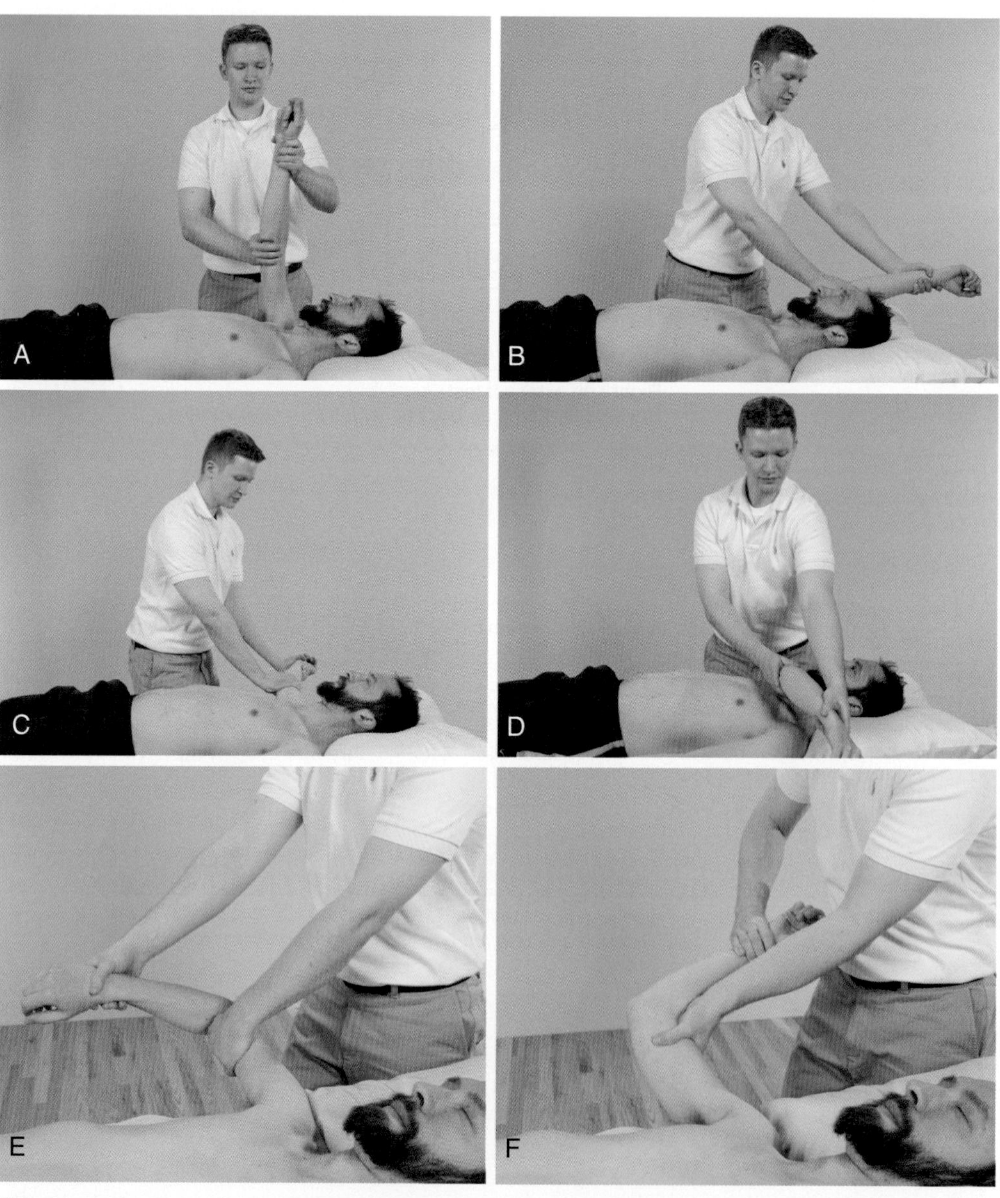

FIG. 11.11 Assessment of shoulder using passive joint motion. A, Flexion glenohumeral joint only. **B,** Full flexion shoulder complex including glenohumeral joint and scapular movement. **C,** Horizontal abduction. **D,** Horizontal adduction. **E,** Internal/medial rotation. **F,** External/lateral rotation.

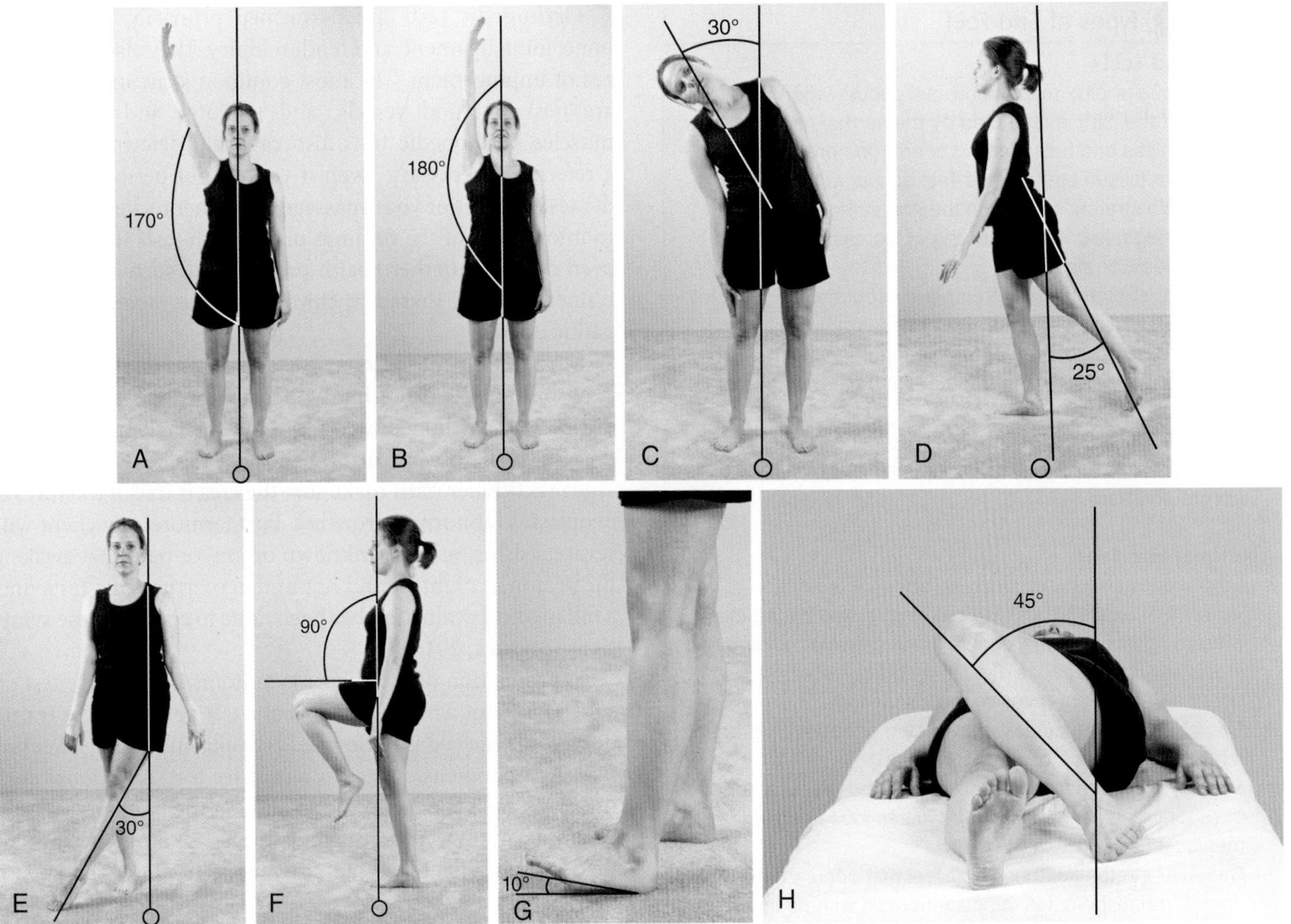

FIG. 11.12 Examples of visual assessment of active joint movements and degrees of range of motion. A, 170 degrees, shoulder abduction. **B,** 180 degrees. **C,** 30 degrees, lateral trunk flexion. **D,** 25 degrees, leg extension. **E,** 30 degrees, hip adductor. **F,** 90 degrees, hip flexion. **G,** 10 degrees, dorsiflexion. **H,** 40 to 45 degrees, internal hip rotation.

the therapist's hands by the tissue resistance at the end of the available range is the end-feel of a joint (Box 11.7).

Assessment of Range of Motion

Active and passive joint movement can identify limits or excess of movement. Joint movement determines the joint position. In the *closed packed position*, the articular surfaces of the bones within most joints are closest together and the shapes of the bones best fit together. This position is the most stable position for a joint and usually in or near the very end range of a motion. In this position, most ligaments and parts of the capsule are pulled taut, providing an element of natural stability to the joint. For many joints in the lower extremity, the closed packed position is essential to normal function. At the knee, for example, the closed packed position, which is full extension, provides stability to the knee in the standing position through the combined effect of maximum joint congruity and stretched/taut ligaments. All positions other than a joint's closed packed position are referred to as the joint's *loose packed positions*. In these positions, the ligaments and capsule are relatively slackened, allowing increased mobility. A joint in the loose packed position, especially midrange, is most mobile but least stable.

Intervention Guidelines

Effusion is a buildup of excess fluid inside the joint capsule. This condition looks and feels like a water balloon. Effusion is an indication of joint injury or other pathology inside the joint capsule. If effusion is identified, the client should be referred to the physician. Massage can be performed but avoid the area.

Simple edema from an increase in fluid in the tissue spaces around a joint is managed with lymphatic drainage (see Chapter 12). If any unexplained edema develops, the client should be referred for diagnosis. In general, if a joint range is reduced (hypomobile), massage should target the short soft tissues to increase length and pliability, which would allow for more joint range of motion. Muscle energy methods and elongation methods can also be used to improve joint movement. Do not stretch a joint area beyond the typical physiological barriers. Never stretch beyond functional normal joint range. Never force an increase in range of motion; instead, allow it to occur as a natural outcome of effective massage application to the soft tissues of the body. Range of motion should improve as the client's tissues normalize with general massage. Do not stretch tissues around joints that are hypermobile. Although functional flexibility is desirable, being too flexible is a major cause of dysfunction and pain (Bettini et al., 2018; Eccles et al.,

Box 11.7 Types of End-Feel

Normal End-Feel

- Soft tissue approximation end-feel occurs when the full range of the joint is restricted by the normal muscle bulk; it is painless and has a feeling of soft compression.
- Muscular (tissue stretch) end-feel occurs at the extremes of muscle stretch, such as in the hamstrings during a straight leg raise; it has a feeling of increasing tension, springiness, or elasticity.
- Capsular stretch (leathery) end-feel occurs when the joint capsule is stretched at the end of its normal range, such as with external rotation of the glenohumeral joint; it is painless and has the sensation of stretching a piece of leather.
- Bony (hard) end-feel occurs when bone contacts bone at the end of normal range, as in extension of the elbow; it is abrupt and hard.

Abnormal End-Feel

- Empty end-feel occurs when no physical restriction to movement exists except the pain expressed by the client.
- Muscle spasm end-feel occurs when passive movement stops abruptly because of pain; a springy rebound may occur as a result of reflexive muscle spasm.
- Boggy end-feel occurs when effusion or edema is present; it has a mushy, soft quality.
- Springy block (internal derangement) end-feel is a springy or rebounding sensation and indicates loose cartilage or meniscal tissue within the joint.
- Capsular stretch (leathery) end-feel that occurs before normal range indicates capsular fibrosis with no inflammation.
- Bony (hard) end-feel that occurs before normal range indicates bony changes or degenerative joint disease or malunion of a joint after a fracture.

2018; Nicholson et al. 2022). When working with clients who are hypermobile, focus on the soft tissue between the joints and avoid active stretching using joint movement.

If an empty capsular or hard end-feel is identified, the joint is damaged. Referral is needed for acute conditions. Joint movement limited by muscle contraction may indicate an underlying problem with joint laxity or injury, and caution is indicated before muscle guarding is reduced. Proceed slowly until a balance is achieved between increased range of motion and maintaining joint stability. If joint stability is reduced, the client usually experiences pain in the joint for a day or two after the massage; also, increased stiffness in the area may be noted as stability is restored.

BASIC ORTHOPEDIC TESTS

SECTION OBJECTIVES

Chapter objective covered in this section:

6. Define and use simple orthopedic tests during the assessment process.

Using the information presented in this section, the student will be able to perform the following:

- Perform basic orthopedic tests to assess for the need for referral.

Orthopedic tests are performed primarily to assess for bone, joint, ligament, and tendon injury. They also identify areas of impingement. The most common structures impinged are nerves, blood vessels, and tendons, and occasionally muscles. Orthopedic tests also can help determine whether a referral is necessary. Even if you do not perform orthopedic tests as part of your massage assessment, clients are likely to inform you of the findings of any such tests that may have been done by another health professional, such as an athletic trainer, physical therapist, chiropractor, or medical or osteopathic doctor.

Most orthopedic tests assess areas to evaluate pain, joint play, and muscle extensibility. Because of the strain involved during some orthopedic tests, care must be taken to avoid further injury. Before any orthopedic tests can be done, the massage practitioner must make sure the area is free of fractures or neoplasms (abnormal growths). Furthermore, any client with severe spasms, pain of unknown origin, or pain that awakens the person at night should not undergo orthopedic tests until a full medical evaluation has been done to address these symptoms (Manske, 2016).

Reproduction of the client's symptoms is a positive test result. Any client who does not want a test performed or is cautious while the test is performed is displaying an *apprehension sign.* An apprehension sign is a positive test. Additional positive signs are a change in the stability of the joint and changes in pulses. Many types of orthopedic tests can be performed. Box 11.8 presents those that are most relevant to therapeutic massage practice.

Sequence for Joint Assessment

Learning any new process, such as joint assessment, is easier when there is a procedure to follow, such as this example of a sequence of questions to ask when assessing joint function.

History

1. Have you been injured? If yes, how and when did the injury happen?
2. Do you have any pain, impaired mobility, or stiffness? If yes, where is it located? Can you show me?
3. Do your joints feel and move evenly on both sides of your body? If no, please explain. Can you show me?
4. If an injury or symptoms such as stiffness are present, continue with the following questions.
   a. Does it hurt all the time or only when you bump or press on it or when you move?
   b. Did you hear or feel a "pop" or "snap"?
   c. Have you had a similar injury? If yes, please explain.

Observation

1. Is there any obvious deformity that suggests a fracture or dislocation?
2. Is the area swollen, including edema and effusion?
3. Is there any discoloration?
4. Compare injured and uninjured areas and identify changes.

Note: When performing the following assessments, remember that pain is the indication of a pathological condi-

Box 11.8 Orthopedic Assessment Tests

This box briefly describes a few common orthopedic tests.

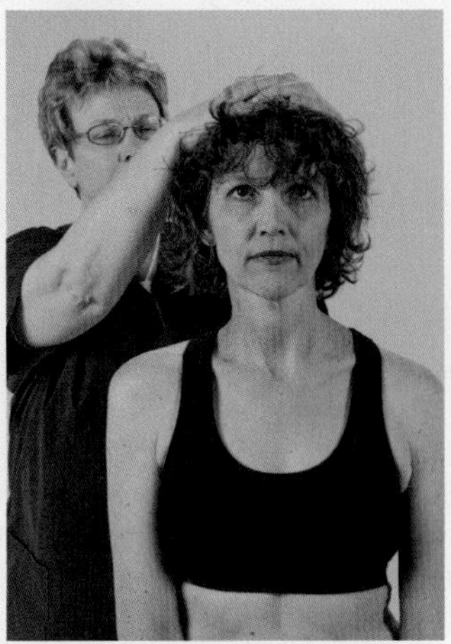

Axial Compression Test

- The client is either sitting or lying, and you press down on the top of the client's head, causing narrowing of the neural foramen and pressure on the facet joints, or muscle spasm.
- A positive test causes increased pain and indicates that there is some type of pressure on a nerve. *Refer client.*

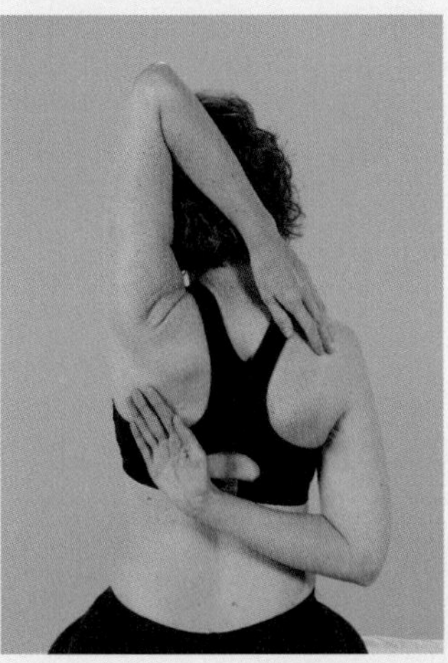

Apley's Scratch Test

- The client is seated or standing. Ask the client reach over the head with one hand to scratch their back while keeping the other hand behind the back.
- Or tell the client to touch the opposite scapula to test range of motion of the shoulder.
- Reaching over the head allows you to assess abduction and external rotation.
- Reaching behind the back allows you to assess adduction and internal rotation.
- Compare both sides for symmetry.
- If the client experiences pain or limited range of motion, there may be a rotator cuff tear or shoulder impingement (there may also be a potential for adhesive capsulitis or glenohumeral osteoarthritis). *Refer client.*

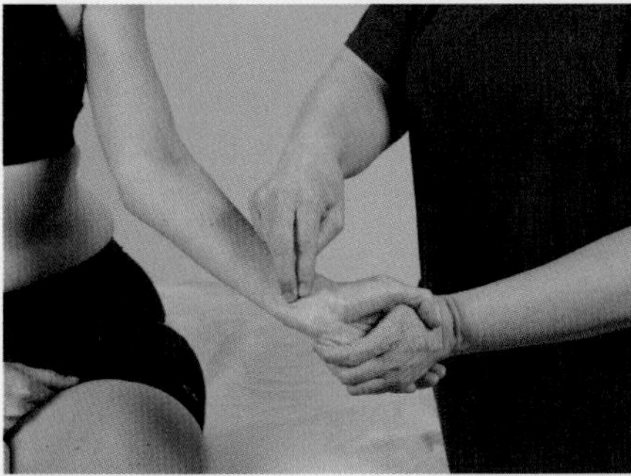

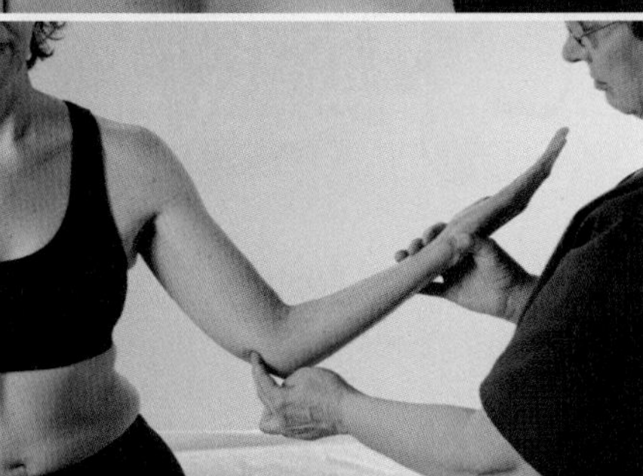

Tinel's Test

- Assesses for ulnar nerve irritability.
- Assessment is performed at elbow and wrist.
- Place elbow flexion and wrist in extension.
- Tap at the cubital or carpal tunnel.
- A positive test produces paresthesia (numbing) or tingling along the distal course of the ulnar, indicating irritability or impingement of the ulnar nerve. *Refer client.*

Box 11.8 Orthopedic Assessment Tests—cont'd

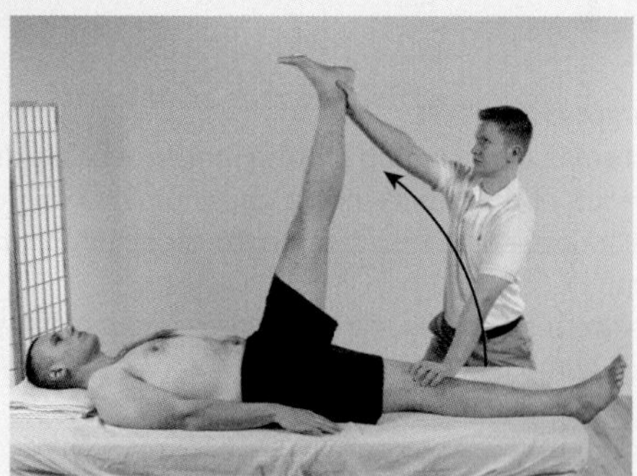

Straight Leg Raising Test

- With the knee extended and the client supine, the hip is flexed (with the leg straight).
- A positive test results in pain in the sciatic nerve pathway down the leg and suggests a disk herniation. *Refer client.*

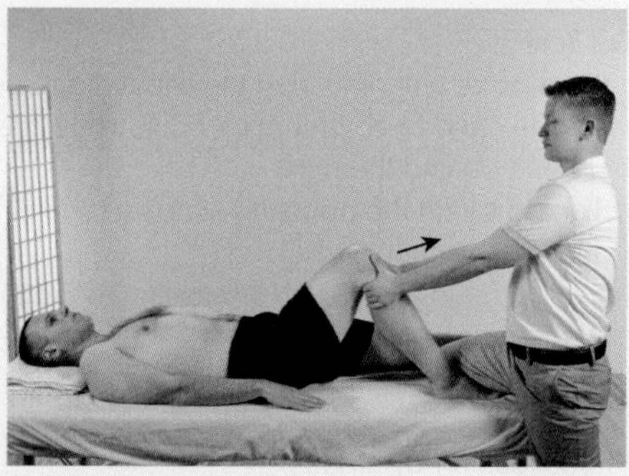

Anterior Drawer Test

- The client reclines with the knee flexed to 90 degrees.
- Grasp the proximal tibia and pull forward.
- If the tibia displaces anteriorly, the anterior cruciate ligament may be injured. *Refer client.*

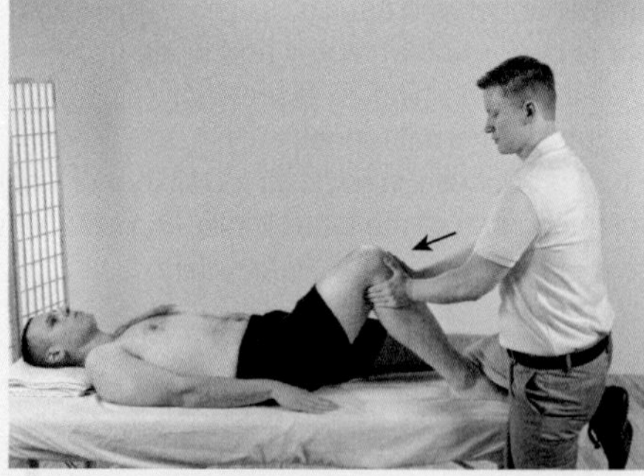

Posterior Drawer Test

- With the knee flexed approximately 90 degrees, push the proximal tibia posteriorly.
- Excessive movement indicates a tear of the posterior cruciate ligament. *Refer client.*

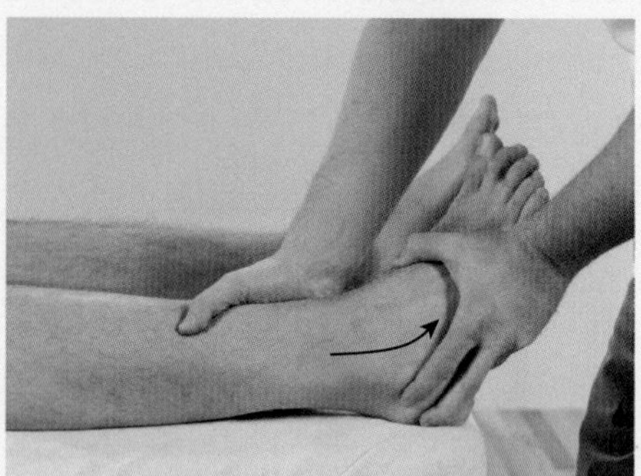

Talar Tilt Test

- The distal tibia is stabilized while the other hand "tilts" the talus to test the integrity of the lateral ligament complex.
- A positive sign would indicate injury such as a sprain. *Refer client.*

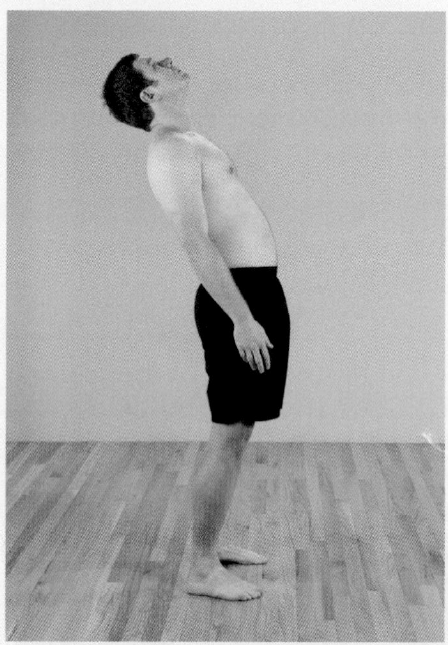

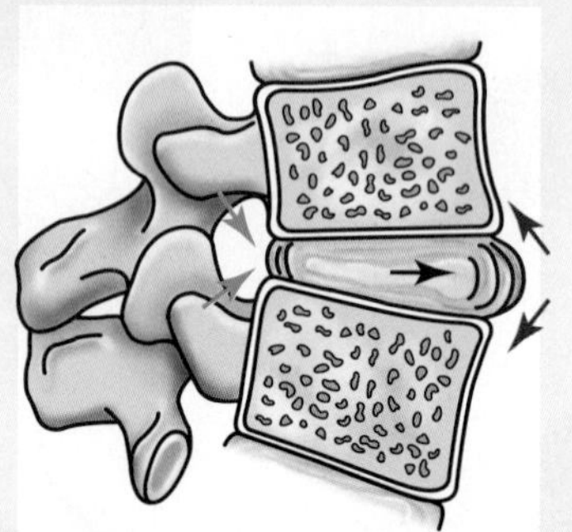

Trunk extension—an anterior herniation in which the gel-like nucleus has pushed forward.

Continued

Box 11.8 Orthopedic Assessment Tests—cont'd

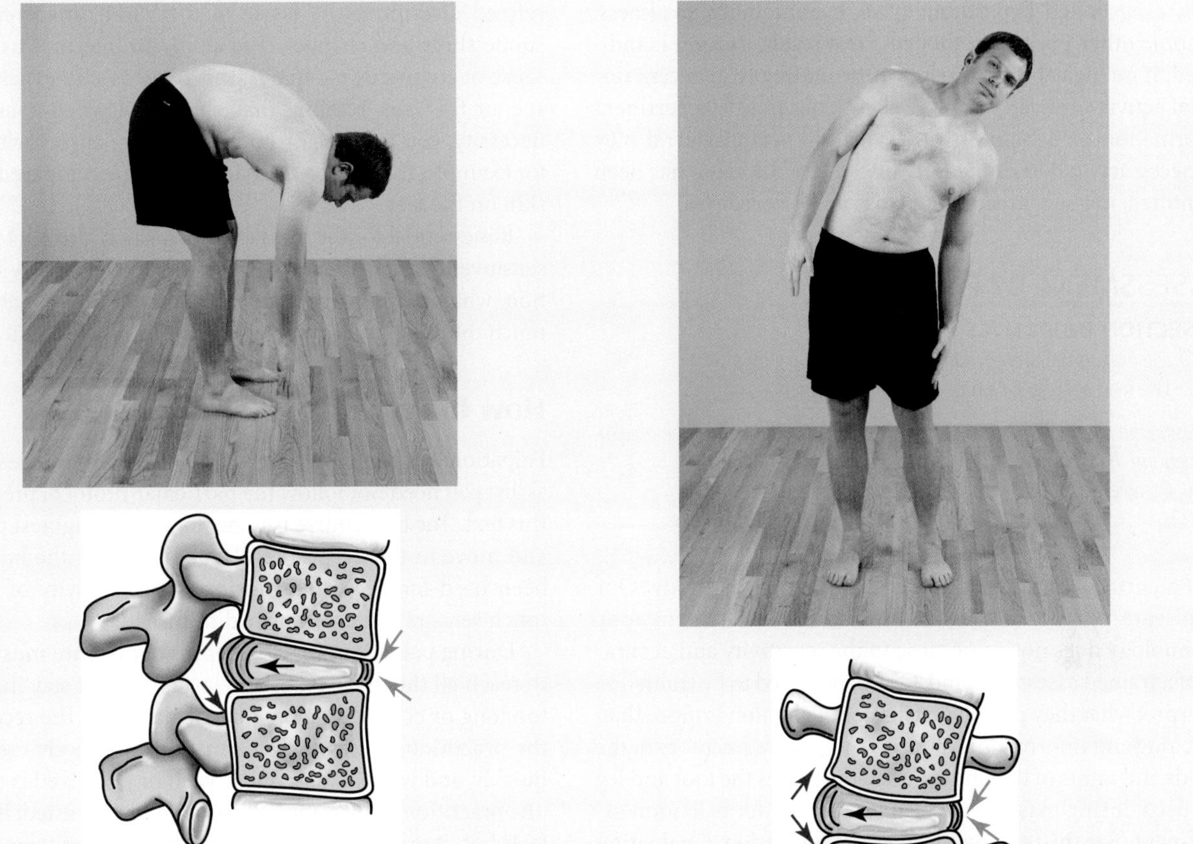

Trunk flexion—a posterior herniation in which the gel-like nucleus has pushed backward.

Trunk lateral flexion—a lateral herniation in which the gel-like nucleus has pushed to the side.

tion—do not cause an increase in pain; only locate the source of the pain.

Palpation

1. Perform palpation on the uninvolved side first. The uninvolved area is "normal."
2. Palpate all bony landmarks.
3. Briskly tap the bone and ask the client if they felt an increased pain sensation. If so, this may indicate a stress fracture. Avoid the area during the massage and refer the client.
4. Palpate all ligament and tendon attachments.
5. Palpate all muscles that act on the area.
6. Palpate for edema and effusion.

Range of Motion

1. Perform active joint movement assessments to evaluate for changes in range of motion.
2. Perform a passive joint movement assessment and compare the range of motion to that seen with active movement assessment.

Manual Muscle Testing

1. Perform testing on the normal side.
2. Perform testing on the affected area. Do not cause additional pain or strain the injured area.

Specific Orthopedic Tests

1. Carefully perform appropriate orthopedic tests.

Intervention Guidelines

If the practitioner notes no pain, stiffness, mobility issues, or other concerns during the assessment, the joint can be considered normal. General massage for the jointed area is indicated to support normal function.

If the practitioner notes pain with movement or on palpation, discoloration, indications of inflammation, unusual stiffness, exaggerated hypermobility or hypomobility, weakness, or some other positive orthopedic test result, caution is indicated. If no logical cause exists for the finding (e.g., recent unusual activity or a fall) or if the client does not have pertinent information or is being treated by a physician, referral may be necessary to determine the cause. Once the cause has been identified, massage treatment plans can be developed.

ASSESSMENT BY PALPATION

SECTION OBJECTIVES

Chapter objective covered in this section:

7. Use massage application as palpation assessment.

Using the information presented in this section, the student will be able to perform the following:

- Complete a 12-level palpation assessment.

Palpation is the use of touch to examine the body. Our hands are our most versatile and refined assessment tool. Technology does not come close to the sensitivity and accuracy of a trained assessing hand. Our hands need to be trained to interpret what they perceive accurately. Palpation is more than touching and information gathered by sensory receptors in the hands and joints of the upper limb. Sometimes the foot and leg are used during massage and can be effective for palpation assessment. For the therapeutic massage professional, palpation is an essential and continuous process, and the hands as well as other parts of the body used to perform massage become skilled with experience. *Massage is palpation assessment.*

With palpation assessment, the main considerations for basic massage are as follows:

- The ability to differentiate between types of tissue
- The ability to distinguish differences of tissue texture in the same tissue types
- The ability to palpate through the various tissue layers from superficial to deep

The tissues the massage therapist should be able to distinguish are the skin, superficial fascia, deep fascia and fascial sheaths, tendons, ligaments, blood vessels, muscle layers, and bone.

Palpation also includes assessment for hot and cold, and various body rhythms, including breathing patterns and pulses. During palpation of the skin, it is prudent to observe general skin condition and color.

Mechanisms of Palpation

Before learning actual palpation skills, it helps to understand the mechanism that makes palpation an effective assessment tool. The proprioceptors and mechanoreceptors of the shoulder, arm, and hand (or hip, leg, and foot) receive stimulation from the tissue being palpated. This is the reception phase. These impulses are transmitted through the peripheral and central nervous systems to the brain, where they are interpreted (DeStefano, 2011).

The somatosensory region of the brain that interprets this sensory information devotes a massive area to the hand. The refined discriminatory sense of the hand can perceive very subtle shifts and changes. The ability to interpret usually is a sense of comparison—that is, this tissue is softer than that tissue, or this feels rougher than that. Because comparison is a necessity, you must be careful to compare apples with apples; for example, the skin on the back cannot be compared with the skin on the feet.

It is essential for the massage therapist's entire self to become sensitive to subtle differences in the client's body. With palpation, what is going on must be felt and not thought about. Too much thinking shifts awareness away from kinesthetic input.

How to Palpate

Palpation can begin in many ways. After you have learned the skills, you need not follow the particular protocol presented in this text. The best course is to begin with the lightest palpation and move to the deepest levels, because after the hands have been used for deep compression, the sensitivity of the light touch sensors is momentarily diminished.

During palpation, varying depths of pressure must be used to reach all the tissue types and layers. Do not stay in one area too long or concentrate on a particular spot. The receptors in the practitioner's hands, forearms, or other body areas adapt quickly, and what is subsequently felt or perceived is then lost. The practitioner's first impression should be trusted; if the area feels hot, it probably is. The differences often are small.

For practice, put your thumb and first finger together. Close your eyes and move the finger on the thumb only enough so that you feel the movement. Open your eyes and notice that the observable difference is tiny. Palpation assessment occurs at this level of awareness.

Palpation assessment becomes part of the massage. In any massage, about 90% of the touching can be considered assessment as part of holding, gliding, kneading, compression, shaking and rocking, and joint movement. Palpation assessment contacts the tissue but does not override it or encourage it to change. This type of work generally relaxes or stimulates the client, depending on the type of strokes used and the rhythm, duration, and speed of application.

Near-Touch Palpation

The first application of palpation does not involve touching the body; rather, the intent is to detect hot and cold areas. This is best done just off the skin using the back of the hand, which is sensitive to heat. The general temperature of the area and any variations should be noted. It is important to move fairly quickly in a sweeping motion over the areas assessed because heat receptors adapt quickly.

Sensitive cutaneous (skin) sensory receptors also detect changes in air pressure and air movement. This is one reason we can feel someone come up behind us when we cannot see the person. The movement and change in the surrounding air pressure alert us; this is a protective survival mechanism. Being able to consciously detect subtle sensations is an invaluable assessment tool. It is important to realize where the information comes from and why it can be sensed, to dispel the notion that this is an extrasensory ability. We are subconsciously aware of all the sensory stimulation that we have receptor mechanisms to detect. With practice, we can become consciously aware of these more subtle sensory experiences. Sensitivity, or intuition, is the ability to work with this information on a conscious level.

Intervention Guidelines

Impaired circulation, fibrotic tissue, and inhibited muscle activity often develop in underactive and cool areas. Hot areas may be caused by inflammation, muscle spasm, or increased surface circulation. When the focus of intervention is to cool the hot areas, a method such as application of ice can be used (see the section on hydrotherapy in Chapter 12). A hot area can also be cooled by reducing the muscle spasms and encouraging more efficient blood flow in the surrounding areas.

Cold areas often are areas of diminished blood flow, dense connective tissue formation, or muscle flaccidity. Heat can be applied to cold areas. Stimulation massage techniques increase muscle activity, heating up the area. Connective tissue approaches soften connective tissue, help restore space around the capillaries, and release histamine, a vasodilator, to increase circulation. These approaches can warm a cold area (Fig. 11.13).

Palpation of the Skin

The second application of palpation is light surface stroking of the skin. First, determine whether the skin is dry or damp. Damp areas feel a little sticky, which causes fingers to drag. This light stroking also causes the root hair plexus that senses light touch to respond. It is important to notice whether a particular area gets more goose bumps (i.e., the pilomotor reflex) than other areas. This is a good time to observe for color, especially blue or yellow coloration. In addition, the practitioner should note and keep track of all moles and surface skin growths. It is important to recognize potential skin cancer and refer clients to physicians when suspicious areas are identified. Pay attention to the quality and texture of the hair and observe the shape and condition of the nails.

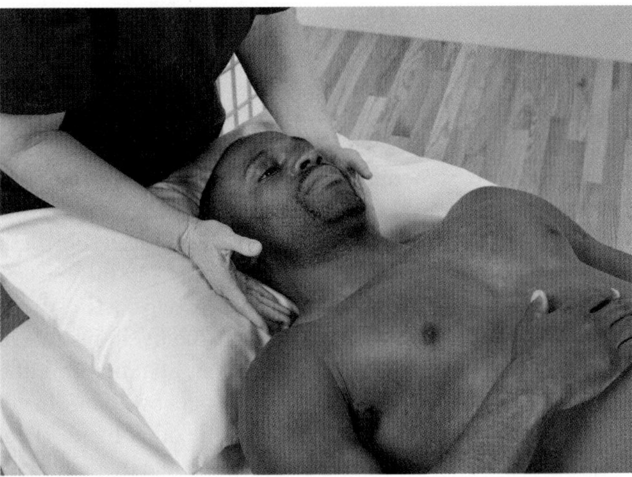

FIG. 11.13 Near-touch palpation to determine hot-cold temperature differences.

In palpation, the massage practitioner uses gentle, small stretching of the skin in all directions and compares the elasticity of these areas (Fig. 11.14). The skin also can be palpated for surface texture. Roughness or smoothness can be felt by applying light pressure to the skin surface.

Intervention Guidelines

Skin should be contained, hydrated, resilient, elastic, even, and have rich coloring. If the skin does not spring back into its original position after a slight pinch, this may be a sign of dehydration (Fig. 11.15). The skin should have no blue, yellow, or red tinges. Blue coloration suggests lack of oxygen; yellow indicates liver problems, such as jaundice; and redness suggests fever, alcohol intake, trauma, or inflammation. Color changes are most noticeable in the lips, around the eyes, and under the nails. Skin pigmentation can influence assessment. Individuals with dark skin may not have the same signs as those with lighter skin.

- Pallor is the result of inadequate circulating blood or hemoglobin and subsequent reduction in tissue oxygenation. In clients with dark skin, pallor may be observed as the absence of underlying red tones and the skin may appear ashen gray or yellowish brown. Pallor is most evident in areas with the least pigmentation such the front surface of the eye and the inner surface of the eyelids, nail beds, palms of the hand, and soles of the feet.
- Cyanosis (a bluish tinge) is most evident in the nail beds and lips. In clients with darker skin, cyanosis may present as gray or whitish (not bluish) skin around the mouth, and

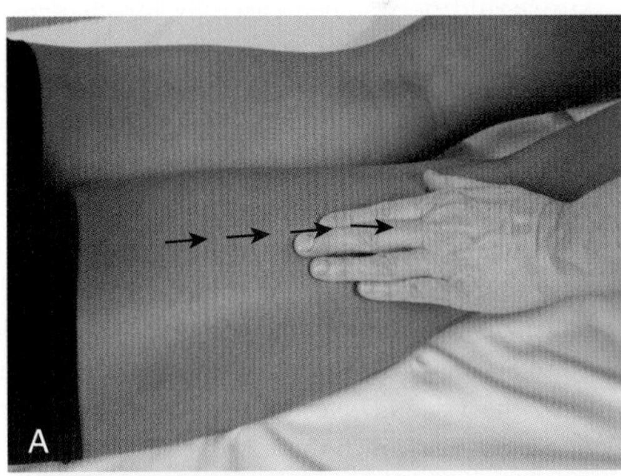

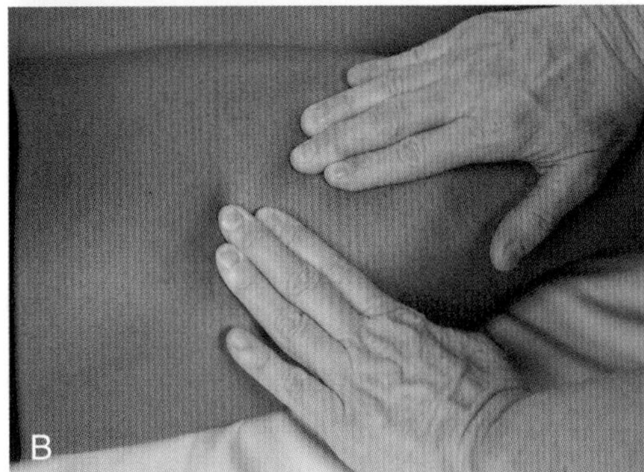

FIG. 11.14 A, Skin drag assesses for hot/cold, wet/dry, rough/smooth. **B,** Skin stretch palpation assesses for local areas of ease and bind.

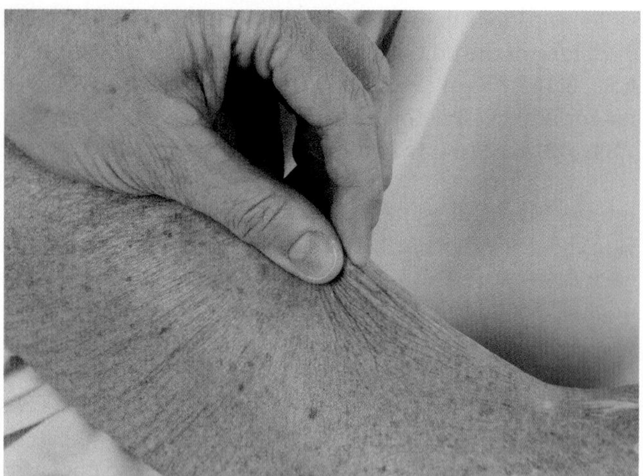

FIG. 11.15 Dehydration test.

the eyes may appear gray or bluish. In clients with yellowish skin, cyanosis may present as grayish-greenish skin tone.

- Jaundice (a yellowish tinge) may first be evident in the sclera of the eyes and then in the mucous membranes and the skin.
- For clients with darker skin, inflammation appears to be more gray or violet in color rather than red.

Bruises must be noted and avoided during massage except for simple lymphatic drainage (see Chapter 12). A client whose body shows any hot redness or red streaking should be referred to a physician immediately. This is especially important with the lower leg because of the possibility of deep vein thrombosis (blood clot).

The skin should be watched carefully for changes in any moles or lumps. As massage professionals, we often spend more time touching and observing a person's skin than anyone else, including the person. If we keep a keen eye for changes and refer clients to physicians early, many skin problems can be treated before they become serious.

Depending on the area, the skin may be thick or thin. The skin of the face is thinner than the skin of the lower back. The skin in each particular area, however, should be similar. The skin loses its resilience and elasticity over areas of dysfunction. It is important to know the visceral referred pain areas on the skin. If changes occur in the skin in these areas, the client should be referred to a physician.

The superficial skin is a blood reservoir. At any particular time, it can hold 10% of the available blood in the body. The connective tissue must be pliable to allow the capillary system to expand to hold the blood. Histamine, which is released from mast cells found in the connective tissue of the superficial fascial layer, dilates the blood vessels. Histamine is also responsible for the client's reported sense of "warming and itching" in an area that has been massaged.

Damp areas on the skin are indications that the nervous system has been activated in that area. This small amount of perspiration is part of a sympathetic activation called a *facilitated segment.* Surface stroking with enough pressure to drag over the skin will identify these slightly damp areas because there is a tiny sensation of stickiness. In addition, repeated stroking over the sticky area elicits a red response over the area of a hyperactive muscle. Deeper palpation of the area usually elicits a tender response. The small erector pili muscles attached to each hair also are under the control of the sympathetic autonomic nervous system. Light fingertip stroking produces goose bumps over areas of nerve hyperactivity. All of these responses can indicate potential activity, such as tender points in the layers of muscle under the indicated area.

Hair and Nails

The hair and nails are part of the integumentary system and can reflect health conditions. The hair should be resilient and secure; hair loss should not be excessive when the scalp is massaged.

The nails should be smooth. Vertical ridges can indicate nutritional difficulties, and horizontal ridges can be signs of stress caused by changes in circulation that affect nail growth. Clubbed nails may indicate circulation problems. The skin around the nails should be soft and free of hangnails.

During times of stress, the epithelial tissues are affected first. Hangnails; split skin around the lips and nails; mouth sores; hair loss; dry, scaly skin; and excessively oily skin are all signs of prolonged stress, medication side effects, or other pathological conditions. Only a physician can diagnose the cause of the condition (refer to the contraindications in Appendix A for more information).

Palpation of the Superficial Connective Tissue

The third application of palpation is the superficial connective tissue, also called superficial fascia, which separates and connects the skin and muscle tissue. The skin is tightly bound to the superficial fascia. During movement, the skin and superficial fascia need to glide over the sheet-like deep fascia covering the muscles. There is a thin layer of a slippery substance called hyaluronic acid or hyaluronan between the superficial fascia and deep fascia to allow for this sliding.

This layer of tissue is found by using compression until the fibers of the underlying muscle are felt. The pressure should then be lightened so that the muscle cannot be felt, but if the hand is moved, the skin and superficial fascia also move. In some body areas, such as the back of the hands, the superficial fascia is thin; in other areas, such as on the back, the tissue is thicker. The tissue should feel resilient and springy, as if you were touching gelatin.

The superficial fascia holds fluid and fat. If surface edema is present, it is in the superficial fascia layer. This water-binding quality gives this area the feel of a water balloon, but it should not feel boggy or soggy or show pitting edema (i.e., the dent from the pressure stays in the skin). Fat is stored in the superficial fascia; the method known as skin rolling should really be called superficial fascia rolling. By lifting and rolling the tissue folds, the massage practitioner can compare binding and density (Fig. 11.16).

The sensation of bind comes from tissue being restrained from motion. To experience the sensation, hold one end of a rubber band or a piece of cloth, tissue, or paper with one hand; hold the other end of the material with the other hand. Then, keeping one hand still, slowly begin to pull the material with the other hand. When you feel a tiny tug on the hand that is still, you have reached bind.

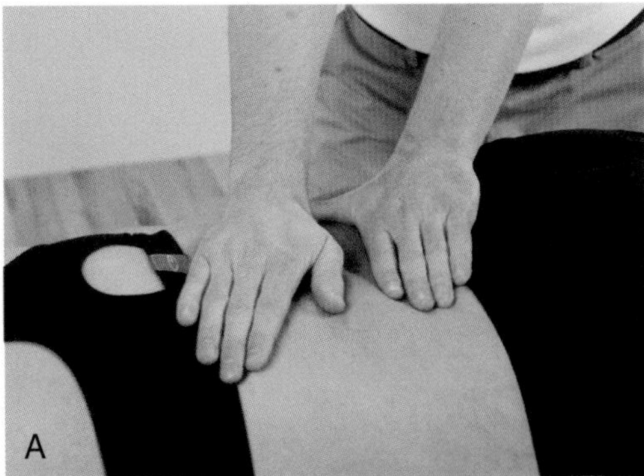

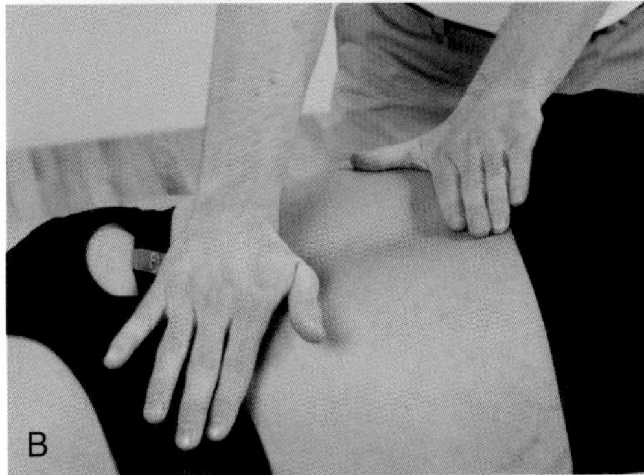

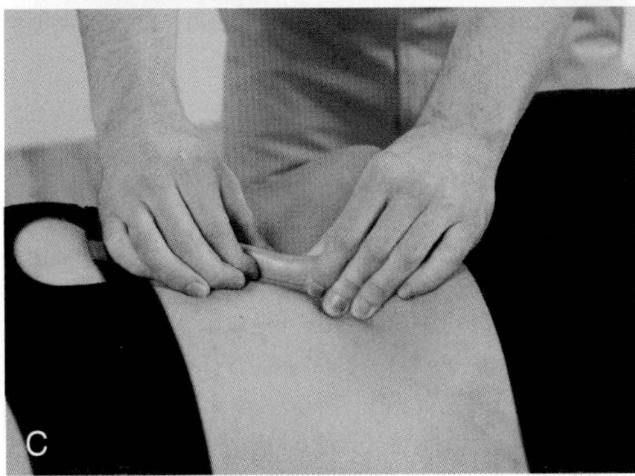

FIG. 11.16 Beginning **(A)** and end **(B)** for palpation assessment of superficial fascia for ease and bind mobility. **C,** Skin and superficial fascia rolling palpation assesses for ease, bind, mobility, and pliability in the superficial fascia.

The sensation of something dense can be understood as a thick consistency and firmness with a greater depth than typical. To experience the sensation of dense tissue, squeeze an orange or grapefruit and then a kiwi or strawberry; also try this with a couch or chair cushion compared with a bed pillow and a sponge compared with a cotton ball.

Methods of palpation that lift the skin and superficial fascia, such as kneading and skin rolling, provide much information. Depending on the area of the body and the concentration of underlying connective tissue, the superficial fascia should lift and roll easily.

The superficial fascia can become dense due to the fluid component of the tissue becoming less viscous and pliable. Dense tissue feels thick and stiff. The fascia can also become fibrotic where the fibers of the fascia become entangled and matted. This usually occurs because of an injury to the tissue and an extended inflammatory response. Fibrotic tissues feel hard, stuck, and knotty.

Intervention Guidelines

Supporting sliding and increasing the pliability of the superficial connective tissues is beneficial. This can be done by applying the assessment methods more slowly and deliberately, allowing for softening in the tissues. Slide is restored as the hyaluronan is able to spread evenly between the superficial and deep fascia.

Repetitive force loading of connective tissues, especially superficial fascia and the loose areolar (fluffy) fascia that occurs throughout the body, can help reduce densification and restore pliably. Lifting and twisting methods are effective.

Fibrotic tissue is more difficult to manage. Friction methods may be required to create a therapeutic inflammation process that will support tissue remodeling. It is important to mention that massage does not "break up" fibrosis.

Any areas that become redder than the surrounding tissue or that stay red or purple longer than other areas are suspect for connective tissue changes. Usually, lifting and elongation (bend, shear, and torsion stress) of the reddened tissue or use of the myofascial approaches presented in Chapter 12 normalizes these areas.

Palpation of Vessels and Lymph Nodes

The fourth application of palpation involves the circulatory vessels and lymph nodes. The more superficial blood vessels lie just above the muscle and in the superficial connective tissue. The vessels are distinct and feel like soft tubes. Pulses can be palpated, but the feel of the pulse is lost if the pressure is too intense. Feeling for pulses helps detect this layer of tissue.

In this same area are the more superficial lymph vessels and lymph nodes. Lymph nodes usually are located in joint areas and feel like small, soft gel caps. The compression of the joint action assists in lymphatic flow. A client with enlarged lymph nodes should be referred to a medical professional for diagnosis. Light, gentle palpation of lymph nodes and vessels is indicated in this circumstance (Fig. 11.17).

Vessels should feel firm but pliable and supported. If any areas of bulging, mushiness, or constriction are noted, the practitioner should refer the client to a physician.

The practitioner should compare the pulses by feeling for a strong, even, full pumping action on both sides of the body. If differences are perceived, the client should be referred to a physician. Sometimes the differences in the pulses can be attributed to soft tissue restriction of the artery or a more serious condition that can be diagnosed by the physician. To assess for capillary function of the circulatory system, press each nail in the fingers and toes firmly, but not painfully, until the nail bed blanches (whitens). Then release and observe how long it takes for the nail to return to normal color. Refill of capillaries in the nail beds should take approximately 3 to 5 seconds and should be equal in all fingers.

Intervention Guidelines

Enlarged lymph nodes may indicate local or systemic infection or more serious conditions. The client should be referred to a physician immediately if these are noted. Tissue should not be boggy and taut from water retention. It is important to refer the client to a physician if the person has unexplained and persistent

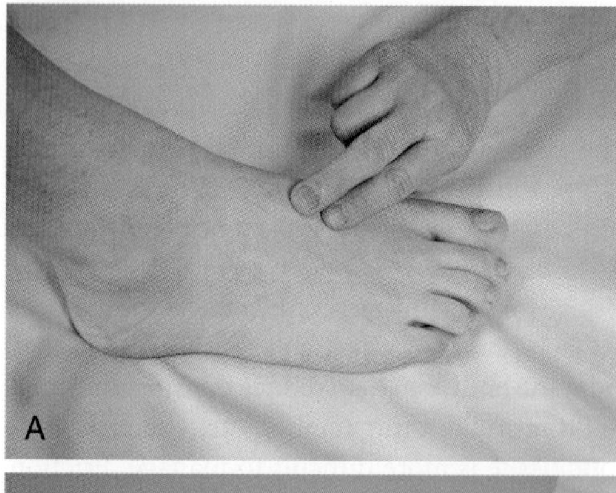

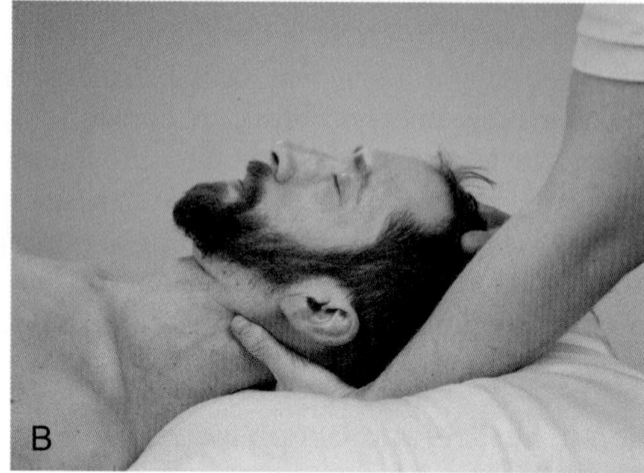

FIG. 11.17 A, Palpation assessment of vessels for circulation. **B,** Assessment of lymph nodes.

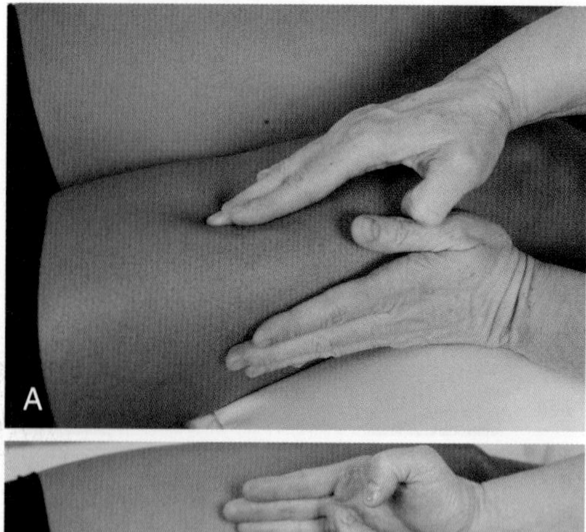

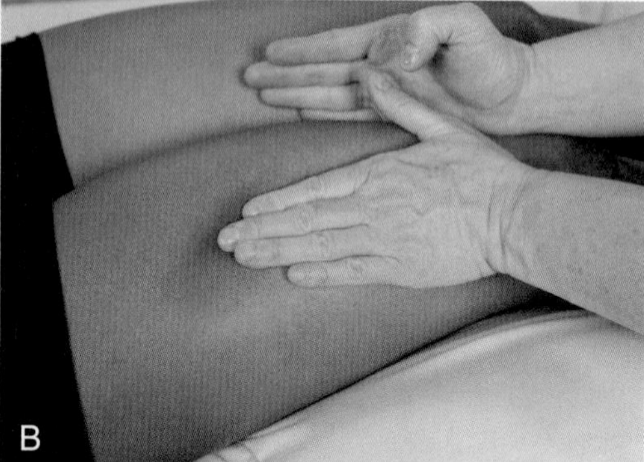

FIG. 11.18 Palpation of muscle and sliding assessment for mobility.

edema. General massage appears to support fluid movement, at least at a local level. (Specific applications that affect blood and lymph circulation are presented in Chapter 12.)

Palpation of Muscle Tissue

The fifth application of palpation is skeletal muscle. Muscle tissue has a distinct fiber direction that can be felt. This texture feels somewhat like corded fabric or fine rope. Muscle is made up of contractile fibers embedded in connective tissue. Individual muscles are wrapped and contained in layers of deep fascia. The area of the muscle that becomes the largest when the muscle is concentrically contracted is in the belly of the muscle. The tendons develop where the muscle fibers end and the connective tissue continues; this is called the *musculotendinous junction.* A good practice activity involves locating these areas for all surface muscles and as many underlying ones as possible. Almost all muscular dysfunctions, such as tender points or micro scarring from tiny muscle tears, occur at the musculotendinous junction or in the belly of the muscle.

Often three or more layers of muscle are present in an area. All of the layers in an area that function to create a joint movement are wrapped together into a function unit called a *compartment.* The layers of muscle in each compartment are separated by deep fascia, and each muscle layer should slide over the one beneath it (Fig. 11.18). It is important to carefully compress systematically through each layer until the bone is felt. Pressure used to reach and palpate the deeper layers of muscle must travel from the superficial layers down to the deeper layers. To accomplish this, the applied pressure must be even, broad based, and slow. The touch should not have a "poking" quality. Abrupt pressure should never be used because surface layers of muscle will tense up and guard, preventing access to deeper layers.

Muscle tends to push up against palpating pressure when concentrically contracting. Having the client slowly move the joint that the muscle moves can help the practitioner identify the location of muscles being assessed (Fig. 11.19).

Make sure to slide each layer of muscle back and forth over the underlying layer to detect any adherence between the muscle layers. The layers usually run cross-grain to each other. The best example is the abdominal muscle group. Even in the arm and leg, where all the muscles seem to run in the same direction, a diagonal crossing and spiraling of the muscle groups is evident. If a muscle layer becomes adherent to (stuck to) the one beneath it, movement is limited to the available movement of the tissue to which the muscle layer is attached. This limited sliding is not an adhesion, which is an abnormal connection of membranous surfaces due to inflammation or injury. Instead, the sliding and distribution of hyaluronan are affected.

Muscles can feel tense and ropy in both concentric (short) and eccentric (long) patterns. Therefore, think of muscle functioning as short/tight and long/taut.

Skeletal muscle is assessed for both texture and function. It should be firm and pliable. Soft, spongy muscle or hard, dense muscle indicates connective tissue and fluid dysfunction (muscle tone problems). Muscle atrophy results in a muscle that feels smaller than normal. Hypertrophy results in a muscle that feels larger than normal.

Intervention Guidelines

Application of the appropriate techniques can normalize the connective tissue component of the muscle, and circulation

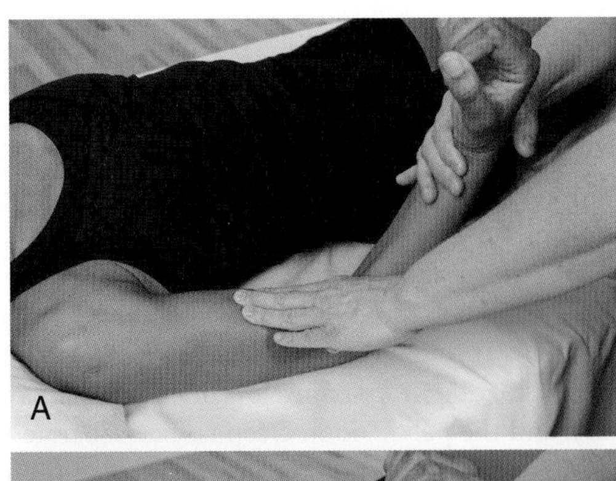

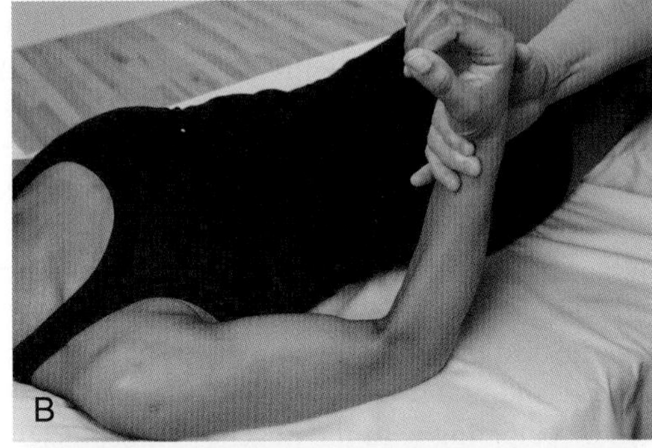

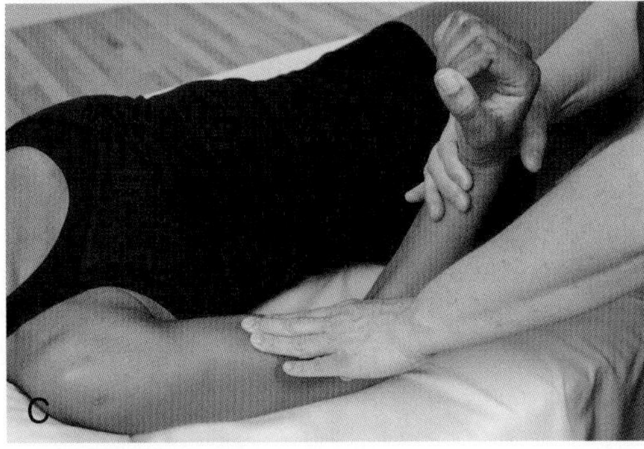

FIG. 11.19 Palpation of muscle. A, Contact the area. **B,** Have the client contract the muscles. **C,** Palpate the muscles as they contract.

methods can address fluid movement. Excessively strong or weak muscles can result from problems with neuromuscular control or imbalanced work or exercise demand. Weak muscles can be a result of wasting (atrophy) of the muscle fibers or neurological inhibition.

Tension/tightness can be felt in muscles that are either concentrically short or eccentrically long. Tension/tightness that manifests in short muscles that are concentrically contracted results in tissue that feels hard and bunched (caves). When muscles are tense/tight from being pulled into an extension pattern, they feel like long, taut bundles with some contraction and shortened muscle fiber groups (hills). Usually, flexors, adductors, and internal rotators become short, whereas extensors, abductors, and external rotators palpate tight but are really taut because they are long and have eccentric dysfunctional patterns.

Massage addresses the short concentrically contracted muscles (caves) to lengthen them, rather than the long muscles (hills), because massage methods usually result in longer tissues. Remember, massage is effective at making tissues longer and more pliable; it is not effective at making long tissues shorter. Therapeutic exercise is necessary to restore normal tone to the "long" muscles. Massage is applied to the long tissue areas, but the focus is on relieving discomfort by using massage as a form of counterirritation and hyperstimulation analgesia. The massage application does not include invasive intervention (e.g., frictioning or sustained inhibitory pressure), intense stretching, or pressure into the deep muscle layers.

Important target areas are the musculotendinous junction and the muscle belly, where the nerve usually enters the muscle. Motor points cause a muscle contraction with a small stimulus (somewhat like a pilot light for a gas stove). Disruption of sensory signals at the motor point causes many problems, including trigger points and referred pain (see Chapter 12), and restricted movement patterns caused by the increase in the physiological barrier and the development of pathological barriers. Typically, when these tissues are located in the short "cave" areas, compression is used to create inhibitory pressure at the muscle attachment or the muscle belly (or both) to reduce neurologically driven tone and restore normal resting length. These same methods are *not* used in the long, taut "hill" areas. These areas benefit from a more superficial general massage application coupled with exercise.

Skeletal muscle conditions depend on the person's heredity, activity level, and general health. Careful assessment of the entire pattern, use of clinical reasoning and critical thinking skills, and general full body massage addressing all tissue components are the best recommendations.

It is amazing what sorts itself out during a thorough generalized massage when the entire body is addressed. Do not discount the effectiveness of this type of massage when skeletal muscle imbalances are detected. Spot work on isolated areas is seldom effective. Neurological muscle imbalances interfere with the kinetic chain (linked reflex patterns), most notably the gait reflexes and the interaction between postural/stabilizing and phasic/moving muscles. The best intervention is a general full-body approach that is modified based on qualities of touch (e.g., depth, drag, and so on).

Palpation of Tendons

The sixth application of palpation is the tendons. Tendons have a higher concentration of collagen fibers and feel more pliable and less ribbed than muscle. Tendons feel like duct tape. Tendons attach muscles to bones. These attachments can be directly on the bone, but just as often tendons attach to ligaments, other tendons, and deep fascia for indirect attachment to the bone. The key point to remember is that these attachment areas are made up of several types of connective tissue. The difference in the connective tissue is the ratio of collagen, elastin, and water. Beneath many tendons is a fluid-filled bursa, or cushion, which assists the movement of the bone under the tendon. Bursae feel like small water balloons or bubbles.

Intervention Guidelines

Tendons should feel elastic and mobile. If a tendon has been torn (sprain), it may adhere to the underlying bone during the healing process. Some tendons, such as those of the fingers and toes, are enclosed in a sheath and must be able to glide

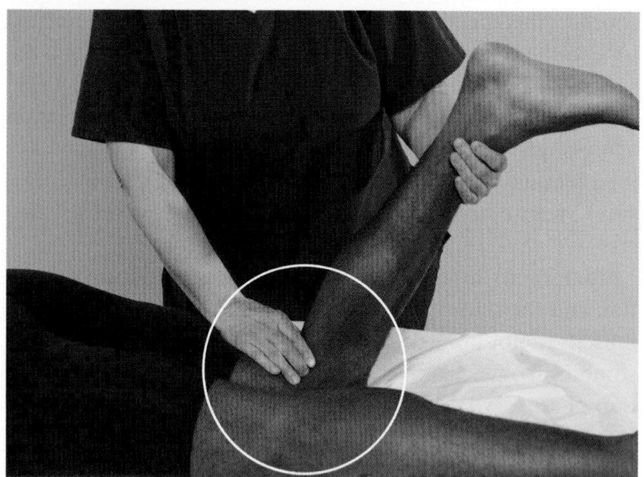

FIG. 11.20 Palpation of tendons assesses for stability, mobility, and pain.

within the sheath. If they cannot glide, inflammation occurs, and the result is tenosynovitis. Overuse also can cause inflammation. Inflammation signals tissue healing with the formation of connective tissue, which can interfere with movement and cause the tendons to adhere to surrounding tissue. Frictioning techniques may help these conditions. Usually, taut tendon structures normalize when the muscle's resting length is normalized (Fig. 11.20).

Palpation of the Deep Fasciae

The seventh application of palpation is the deep fasciae. The deep fasciae feel like sheets of plastic wrap and duct tape. Unlike the superficial fascia, which is thick and spongy, the deep fasciae are thin but very fibrous. Deep fasciae separate muscle structures into functional compartments and expand the connective tissue area of bone for muscular attachment. Some deep fasciae, such as the lumbodorsal fascia, the abdominal fascia, and the iliotibial band, run on the surface of the body and are thick, like a tarp. Other types of deep fasciae, such as the linea alba and the nuchal ligament, run perpendicular to the surface of the body and the bone, like a rope. Still others run horizontally through the body. The horizontal pattern occurs at joints, the diaphragm muscle (which is mostly connective tissue), and the pelvic floor. Deep fasciae separate muscle groups and provide a continuous, interconnected framework for the body that follows the principles of tensegrity. The shapes and sheets of deep fasciae are kept taut by the design of the cross-pattern and the action of muscles that lie between sheaths, such as the gluteus maximus, which lies between the iliotibial band and the lumbodorsal fascia.

The larger nerves and blood vessels lie in grooves created by the fascial separations. Careful comparison reveals that the location of the traditional acupuncture meridians corresponds to these nerve and blood vessel tracts. The fascial separations can be felt by palpating with the fingers. With sufficient pressure, the fingers tend to fall into these grooves, which can then be followed. These areas need to be resilient but distinct because they serve as both stabilizers and separators (Fig. 11.21). Deep fascial sheaths should be pliable, but because they are stabilizers, they may be more dense than tendons in some areas. Problems arise if the tissues that are separated or stabilized by these sheaths become stuck to the sheath.

Chronic health conditions almost always show dysfunction with the connective tissue. Any techniques discussed as connective tissue approaches are effective as long as the

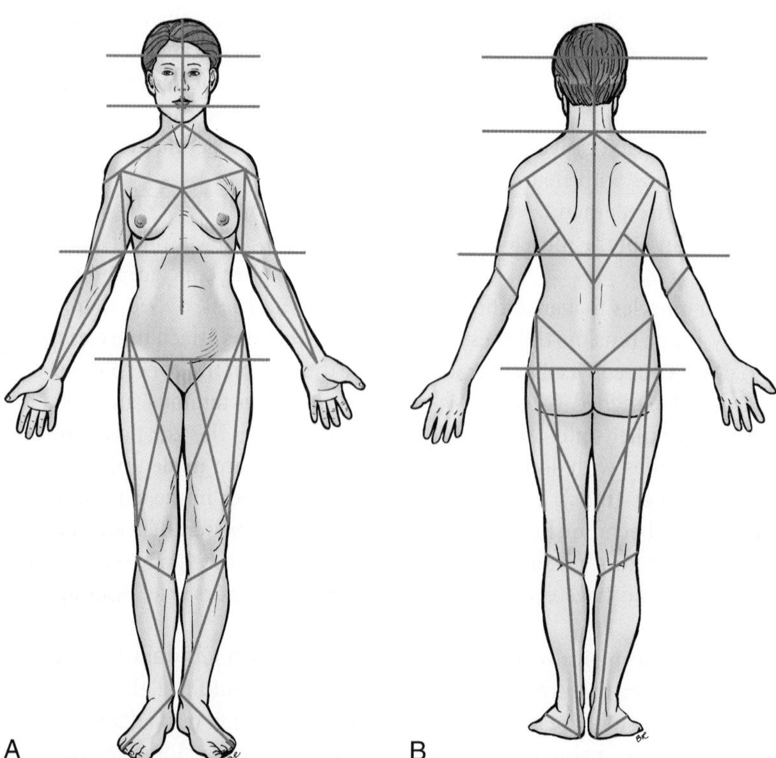

FIG. 11.21 Fascial sheaths. **A,** Anterior view. **B,** Posterior view.

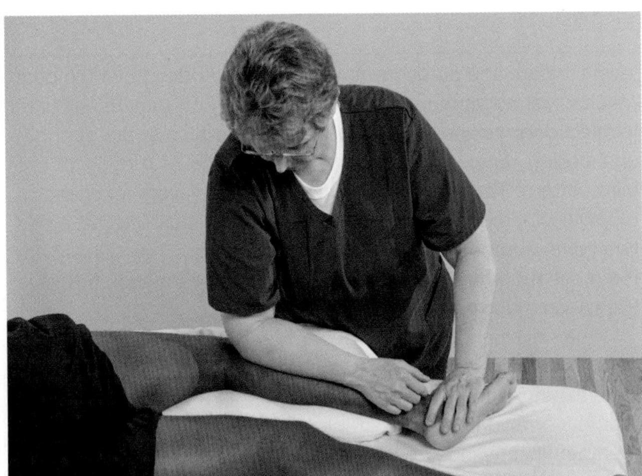

FIG. 11.22 Palpation of fascial sheaths assesses for bind and mobility. Here we see an example of the sheath between the lateral and posterior compartment of the leg.

practitioner proceeds slowly and follows the tissue pattern. The massage therapist should not override the tissue or force the tissue into a corrective pattern. The goal is to restore normal sliding.

Intervention Guidelines

Fascial separations between muscles create pathways for the nerves and blood vessels. When palpated, these pathways feel like grooves running between muscles. If these areas become narrow or restricted, blood vessels may be constricted and nerves impinged. A slow, specific, but careful stripping/gliding along these pathways can be beneficial. If the application is too aggressive, vessels and nerves can be damaged. As a general guide, the client should not grimace, flinch, or protectively tense up during the application. The nerves run in these fascial pathways, and the nerve trunks correlate with the traditional meridian system. Therefore, most meridian and acupressure work takes place along these fascial grooves.

Muscle layers and compartments are also separated by deep fascia, and because muscles must be able to slide over each other, the practitioner assesses for restrictive adherence between muscle layers. This situation often occurs in the legs. If assessment indicates that the muscles sheaths are stuck to each other, kneading and gliding can be used to slide one muscle layer over the other (Fig. 11.22).

Mechanical work, such as slow, sustained elongation, and methods that pull and drag on the tissue are used to support gliding of deep fascia. Working across the fiber direction rather than along the fiber orientation is especially beneficial. Because this work may feel uncomfortable, it should not be undertaken unless the client is willing to commit to regular appointments until the area has been normalized. This may take 6 months to 1 year. It is not possible to stretch deep fascia. Instead, the methods used either restore slide between tissue layers or soften the ground substance.

When deep fascia is compressed, twisted, or pulled, fluid is squeezed out of the fascial tissue. Eventually the fluid will be restored into the fascia, but for a short time (about 30 minutes) the deep fascia is more pliable. Once the water is reabsorbed, the deep fascia will again stiffen. During this short increase in pliability, the area is more mobile. This is only a short-term change, but it can be used to increase mobility in adjacent tissues. General massage methods that are applied slowly and that generate drag to introduce bend, shear, and torsion stress on tissues that are dense, stiff, and bind are indicated.

Palpation of Ligaments

The eighth application of palpation is the ligaments. Ligaments are found around joints. They are high in elastin and somewhat stretchy; they feel much like bungee cords, although some ligaments are flat. The ligaments hold joints together and maintain joint space in the synovial joints by keeping the joint apart. Ligaments should be flexible enough to allow the joint to move, yet stable enough to restrain movement for joint stability. It is important to be able to recognize a ligament and not mistake it for a tendon. With the joint in a neutral position, if the muscles are isometrically contracted, the tendon moves but the ligament does not.

Palpation of Joints

The ninth application of palpation is the joints (Box 11.9). Joints often feel like hinges. Careful palpation should reveal the space between the synovial joint ends. Most assessment, at the basic massage level, is done with active and passive joint movements. An added source of information is palpation of the joint while it is in motion. The sense should be that of a stable, supported, resilient, and unrestricted range of motion within a functional range.

With joint movements, it is important to assess for end-feel, as previously described. Simply, end-feel is the perception of the joint at the limit of its range of motion, and it feels either soft or hard. In most joints it should feel soft; this means that the body is unable to move more through muscular contraction, but a small additional force by the therapist produces some give. A hard end-feel is what the bony stabilization of the elbow feels like in extension. No more active movement is possible, and passive movement is restricted by bone.

It is important to assess for fluid changes around joints. Tissues around the joint can swell because of edema or excess fluid, which can build up inside the joint capsule. Edema typically occurs around the joint. Swelling caused by fluid inside the joint capsule is called *effusion.* A small amount of fluid exists in normal joints. This fluid acts as a lubricant for the bones moving against each other and maintains the space in the joint between the bones. Effusion can be a protective mechanism for arthritic joints, because a small amount of excess fluid keeps the bone ends apart. Excessive effusion can indicate serious injury or a pathological condition. Edema feels spongy, and pressure leaves an indentation. Effusion feels more like a water balloon.

Movement of the joints through comfortable ranges of motion can be used as an evaluation method. Comparison of the symmetry of range of motion (e.g., comparing the circumduction pattern of one arm against that of the other) is effective for detecting limitations of a particular movement.

Intervention Guidelines

Muscle energy methods supporting elongation to normal resting length, in addition to all massage manipulations,

Box 11.9 Joint Function

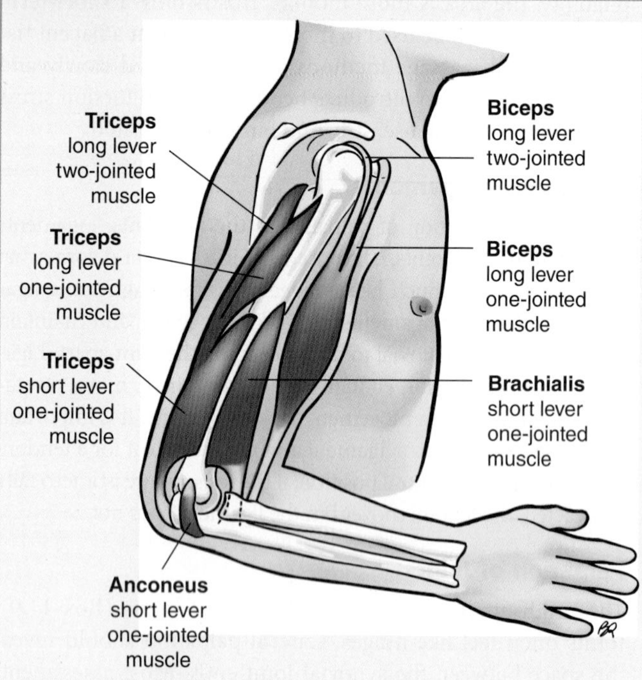

Joints consist of one-joint muscles or two-joint muscles functioning as either short or long levers.

For the most part, massage practitioners work with synovial (freely movable) joints. These joints are the focus of this text. The amount of joint movement depends on the bone structure, supportive elements of the ligaments, and arrangement of the muscles. Joints are designed to fit together in a specific way. For a joint to move, there must be a space between the bone ends. The bone ends must be smooth and lubricated to prevent friction. Also, the muscular elements must function properly, and the joint structure, including the cartilage, must be functional. Anything that interferes with these key elements interferes with joint function.

Balance is another key element in joint function. If the positional receptors in a joint relay information to the central nervous system indicating that damage to the joint may occur, motor activity (i.e., muscular action) is affected.

Joints are characterized as having one-joint muscles or two-joint muscles, depending on the basic configuration of the muscles around the joint. One-joint muscles are muscles that cross a single joint; they consist of short levers and long levers. Short levers initiate and stabilize movement. They often have the best mechanical advantage in joint movement, and they usually are located deep to the long levers. Long levers have the strength and pulling range to carry out the full range of motion of the joint pattern. They are superficial to the short levers and deep to the two-joint muscles. Two-joint muscles are muscles that cross two joints and coordinate movement patterns. They usually are the most superficial of the muscles. A noted exception to this is the psoas muscle.

When evaluating joint function, the massage professional is most concerned with pain-free, symmetrical range of motion. Determining whether pain on movement is a muscle or tendon problem or a ligament or joint problem can be difficult. Because therapeutic massage deals with nonspecific soft tissue dysfunction, treating joint dysfunction specifically is out of the scope of practice for massage professionals unless they are specifically supervised by a chiropractor, physician, physical therapist, athletic trainer etc.

It is important to be able to distinguish between the muscle and tendon components and the ligament and joint components in a restricted movement pattern. When in doubt, always refer suspected joint problems to a medical professional.

Muscle and tendon problems can be differentiated from ligament and joint problems in two ways:

- Pain on gentle traction usually indicates a soft tissue problem, such as a muscle or tendon condition; pain with gentle compression usually indicates a ligament or joint problem.
- If active range of motion produces pain and passive range of motion does not, the cause usually is a muscle or tendon problem. If both passive and active range of motion produce pain, the cause usually is a ligament or joint problem.

When massage practitioners work with joints, it is important that they distinguish between the *anatomical barrier* and the *physiological barrier.* The anatomical barrier is the bone contour and the soft tissue (especially the ligaments) that serve as the final limit to motion in a joint. Beyond this motion limit, tissue damage occurs. The physiological barrier is more of a nervous system protective barrier that prevents access to the anatomical barrier when damage to the joint could occur. A *pathological barrier exists* when the movement is limited by some sort of injury, dysfunction, or inappropriate compensation pattern. The massage therapist must stay within the limits of the physiological barrier to avoid possible hyper-movement of a joint. Therapeutic massage may increase the range of motion of a jointed area by resetting the confines of the pathological barrier.

can be used to support symmetrical range-of-motion functions. All these tissues and structures are supported by general massage applications, which result in fluid movement shifts, increased soft tissue pliability, maintenance of normal fascial sliding, and balance of neuromuscular patterns.

Massage can positively affect the normal limits of the physiological barrier. When joints are traumatized, the surrounding tissue becomes "scared," almost as if saying, "This joint will never get in that position again." When this happens, all the proprioceptive mechanisms reset to limit the range of motion, setting up a pathological barrier. Massage and appropriate muscle lengthening, combined with muscle energy techniques and self-help, can have a beneficial effect on ligaments, joint function, and bone health. Ligaments are relatively slow to regenerate, and sustained improvement takes time.

Massage to the soft tissue around joints can increase tissue pliability; however, the most common soft tissue dysfunction around joints is laxity, not shortening. Lax (loose) joint structures should not be massaged directly; instead, the muscles around the joint should be the main target. Joint laxity, with the resulting instability, is a common factor in the chronic pain pattern. Intervention will require stability training and strengthening exercises.

Palpation of Bones

The tenth application of palpation is the bones. Those who have developed their palpation skills find a firm but detectable pliability to bone. Bones feel like young sapling tree trunks and branches. For the massage practitioner, it is important to be able to palpate the bony landmarks that indicate the tendinous attachment points for the muscles and to trace the bone's shape (Fig. 11.23).

Palpation of Abdominal Viscera

The eleventh application of palpation is the viscera, which are the internal organs of the body. The abdomen contains much of the viscera. It is important for the massage professional to be able to locate the organs in the abdominal cavity and to know their positioning.

The massage therapist should be able to palpate the distinct firmness of the liver and the large intestine. Although deep massage to the abdomen is not suggested for those trained in basic massage, light to moderate stroking of the abdomen is beneficial for the large intestine. The massage therapist should be able to locate and palpate this organ. Refer the client to a physician if any hard, rigid, stiff, or tense areas are noted in the abdomen. Close attention must be paid to the visceral referred pain areas (see Chapter 6). If tissue changes are noted, the practitioner must refer the client to a physician.

Intervention Guidelines

It is important to include the abdominal area in the general massage session. The soft tissue in this area is part of core stability. The fascial girdle in this area includes the following:

- The lumbar dorsa fascia
- The abdominal fascia
- The raphes where the fascia layers join in the front along the linea alba, on the sides between the iliac crest and rib, and the ligament structures along the spinous processes of the vertebral column.

The raphes can be considered fascial hubs or connecting points that are major areas to address because these areas are where many structures converge.

The skin/superficial fascia often is taut in areas of visceral referred pain. As a result of cutaneous and visceral reflexes, benefit may be obtained by stretching the skin in these areas. There is some indication that normalizing the pliability of the skin/superficial fascia over these areas has a positive effect on the functioning of the organ. If nothing else, circulation may be increased and peristalsis (intestinal movement) may be stimulated.

In accordance with the recommendations for colon massage (see Chapter 10), repetitive stroking in the proper directions may stimulate smooth muscle contraction and can improve elimination problems and excessive intestinal gas. A professional practitioner is prepared for the results and will inquire as to whether the client wants to visit the restroom (Fig. 11.24).

Palpation of Body Rhythms

The twelfth application of palpation is the body rhythms, which are felt as tiny, swaying undulations and pulsations. Body rhythms are designed to operate in a coordinated, balanced, and synchronized manner. In the body, the rhythms all entrain (synchronize). When palpating body rhythms, the practitioner should get a sense of this harmony. Although the trained hand can pick out some of the individual rhythms, just as one can hear individual notes in a song, it is the whole connected effect that is important. When a person feels "off" or "out of sync," they often are speaking of disruption in the entrainment process of their body rhythms.

The three basic rhythms assessed are the respiration, blood circulation, and lymph circulation. Some bodywork systems also concentrate on proposed craniosacral rhythms. Subtle energetic rhythms may be present in the body but currently cannot be substantiated using available technology. The three basic rhythms supported by the most scientific understanding are described as follows:

- *Respiration.* The breath is easy to feel. It should be even and should follow good principles of inhalation and exhalation (see Chapter 15). Palpation of the breath is done by placing the hands over the ribs and allowing the body to go through

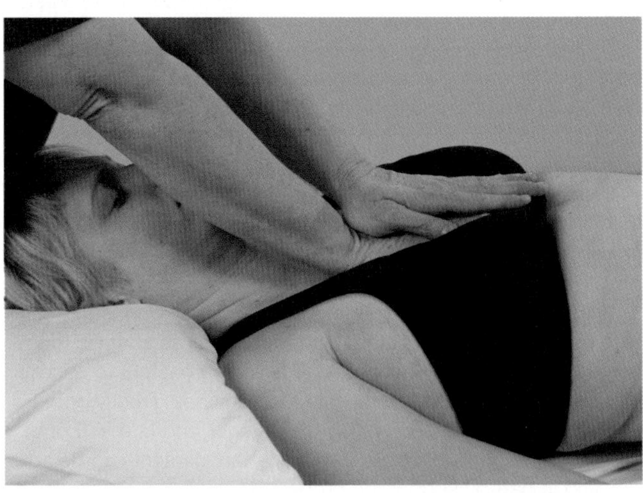

FIG. 11.23 Palpation of bone (e.g., the sternum).

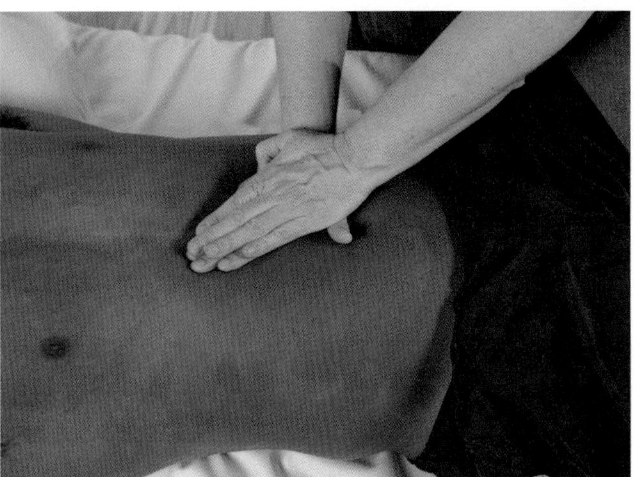

FIG. 11.24 Palpation of viscera assesses for pliability, mobility, and pain.

three or more cycles as the practitioner evaluates the evenness and fullness of the breath. Relaxed breathing should result in a slight rounding of the upper abdomen and lateral movement of the lower ribs during inhalation. Movement in the shoulders or upper chest indicates potential difficulties with the breathing mechanism.

- *Blood circulation.* The rhythmic beating of the heart moves the blood in the body. The movement of the blood is felt at the major pulse points. The pulses should be balanced on both sides of the body. Basic palpation of the movement of the blood is done by placing the fingertips over pulse points on both sides of the body and comparing for evenness. The vascular refill rate is another means of assessing the efficiency and rhythm of the circulation. To assess this rate, press the nail beds until they blanch (push blood out), and then let go and count the seconds until color returns. The nail bed color should return within a few seconds.
- *Lymph circulation.* Lymph vessels have an undulating, peristalsis type of rhythm. The movement is subtle and wavelike. The sensation is full body and not limited to vessels, as with the blood circulation.

Intervention Guidelines

The body rhythms are assessed before and after the massage. An improvement in rate and evenness should be noticed after the massage. The massage practitioner must remain focused on the natural rhythm of the client. Supported by rocking methods, a rhythmic approach to the massage, and the appropriate use of music, the body can reestablish synchronized rhythmic function.

Breathing

Improved breathing function helps the entire body. Recall from Chapter 5 that the muscular mechanism for inhalation and exhalation depends on unrestricted movement of the musculoskeletal components of the thorax. The muscles of respiration include the scalenes, intercostals, anterior serratus, diaphragm, abdominals, and pelvic floor muscles. If a breathing pattern disorder (see Chapter 5) is a factor and the person is prone to anxiety, massage intervention can help normalize the upper body and support the breathing mechanism.

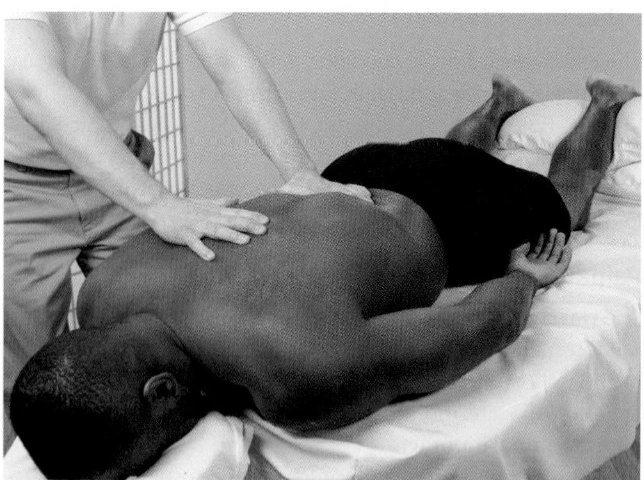

FIG. 11.25 Palpation assessment of breathing and body rhythm.

Because of the whole body interplay between muscle groups in all actions, tight lower leg and foot muscles often are found to interfere with breathing. By contracting the lower legs and feet and taking a deep breath, a person can discover that breathing is a whole body function (Fig. 11.25). Disruption of function in any of these muscle groups inhibits full and easy breathing. (For additional information on breathing, see Chapter 15.)

General massage and stress reduction methods seem to help breathing the most. The client can be taught slow tissue lengthening methods and the breathing retraining pattern found in Chapter 15. The client also can be advised to avoid wearing restrictive clothing (Box 11.10).

Box 11.10 Relationship Between Functional Movement and Breathing Function

Normal breathing, also known as diaphragmatic breathing, involves integrated motion of the upper rib cage, lower rib cage, and abdomen and the main breathing muscle, the diaphragm. The diaphragm is the main muscle of the respiratory pump. It attaches onto the lower six ribs, the xiphoid process of the sternum, and the lumbar vertebral column (L1–3). Abnormal breathing, known as thoracic or upper chest breathing, involves using axillary respiratory muscles that attach on the ribs and are involved in upper rib cage and shoulder motion. Breathing pattern disorder (BPD) can be defined as *inappropriate breathing that is persistent enough to cause symptoms with no apparent organic cause.* These symptoms are usually related to increased sympathetic autonomic nervous system activity and related endocrine function. Breathing pattern disorder can have an effect on respiratory chemistry, specifically a decrease in the level of carbon dioxide (CO_2) in the bloodstream. This causes the pH of the blood to increase, and a state of respiratory alkalosis occurs, causing many symptoms such as anxiety, dizziness, chronic cough, numbness and tingling (especially in hands, feet, and face), or changes in heart rate and blood pressure. A thoracic/upper chest–dominant breathing pattern can lead to hypertonicity of the accessory muscles of breathing, explaining the occurrence of shoulder and neck pain and headache.

Individuals with poor posture, scapular movement dysfunction, low back pain, neck pain, temporomandibular joint pain, and headache often have faulty breathing mechanics. The diaphragm performs both postural and breathing functions. Disruption in one function of the diaphragm will affect the other. Diaphragmatic function is essential for stabilization of the trunk by increasing intra-abdominal pressure, which stiffens the lumbar spine. There can be altered motor control strategies and respiratory dysfunction in subjects with sacroiliac joint pain.

Massage therapy that targets normal thoracic function can help reverse breathing pattern disorder as well as address functional movement dysfunction. A general approach is to assess and address all fascia and muscle that attaches directly or indirectly on the ribs, especially on the anterior and lateral thorax. The outcome goals of stress and pain management can be addressed in part by supporting proper breathing.

PROFICIENCY EXERCISE 11.4

1. Palpate several objects with different textures. Then palpate the same objects through a sheet, a towel, a blanket, and foam. See how many you can identify.
2. Have people walk up to you while you are blindfolded. Pay attention to when you sense the person's presence.
3. Feel for heat radiating off various objects. How far away can you get from the object before you cannot feel the heat?
4. Feel appliances or machinery as the motor runs. Pay attention to the vibrations. How far away can you get and still feel the vibrations?
5. Put a dime in a phone book under two pages. Locate the dime. Keep increasing the number of pages over the dime until you cannot feel it.
6. Get two magnets and play with them. Feel for the "force field."
7. Palpate or observe all of the following on five clients:
   - Heat and cold
   - Air pressure and current shifts
   - Damp or dry skin
   - Goose bumps
   - Color
   - Hair
   - Nails
   - Skin texture
   - Skin roughness or smoothness
   - Superficial connective tissue and superficial fascia
   - Blood vessels
   - Pulses
   - Lymph nodes
   - Direction of skeletal muscle fiber
   - Musculotendinous junction
   - Motor points
   - Muscle layers
   - Tendons
   - Fascial sheaths
   - Ligaments
   - Bursae
   - Joints
   - Joint space
   - Joint movement
   - Joint movement end-feel
   - Bone
   - Bony landmarks
   - Bone shape
   - Viscera
   - Breathing

Proficiency Exercise 11.4 provides a palpation exercise. Follow Fig. 11.26 for the palpation of arterial pulses.

ASSESSMENT PROCEDURES FOR MUSCLE TESTING

Traditional anatomy involves learning about individual muscles in the body as they have been dissected and named by anatomists. However, the most current research indicates that this is an artificial way of understanding the body. No such structure as an individual muscle actually exists. Instead, the body functions in movement patterns, and all of the elements involved in the movement are connected. The contractile structures that we call *muscles* are concentrated within connective tissue networks that also hold nerves and blood vessels. The *tendons*, as we call them, are not separate but consist of this same material, although with fewer contractile fibers; as they approach the jointed areas, they become part of the material that makes up the ligaments, joint capsule, and bone. As these structures cross over the joints, they again begin to increase in contractile fibers and start to look like muscles.

If the body were dissected in a way to identify function, these long chains would appear. The connective tissue sheaths bundle up functional units such as the structures that flex the knee or stabilize the back. These units collectively would be called by the function performed, such as elbow flexors or cervical extensors. Even this level of separation is not quite correct. The functional relationships of the muscles surrounding a jointed area cannot be separated. For example, knee flexion occurs when what we call the hamstring muscles shorten. However, all of the structures that act on the knee are active and communicating during this specific movement. One segment is shortening, another is controlling the speed and direction of the movement, and yet another is providing stability, and so forth. If the massage practitioner understands the interconnectedness of the body, the muscle testing assessment makes more sense.

TYPES OF MUSCLE TESTING

SECTION OBJECTIVES

Chapter objective covered in this section:

8. Adapt joint movement methods to perform muscle testing assessment.

Using the information presented in this section, the student will be able to perform the following:

- Complete a basic muscle testing assessment.

Muscle testing procedures are used for different purposes. The purpose of strength testing is to discover whether the muscle responds with sufficient strength to perform the required body functions. The purpose of **neurological muscle testing** is to discover whether the neurological interaction of the muscles is working smoothly.

Strength Testing

In general, the purpose of **strength testing** is to determine whether the muscle or muscle groups are able to respond with adequate force to a demand without excessive recruitment of other muscles and whether the muscle strength patterns are similar on both sides of the body. Strength testing determines a muscle's force of concentric contraction.

Procedure for Strength Testing

1. The preferred method is to isolate the muscle or muscle group by positioning the joint that the muscle acts on in the middle of the available range of motion.
2. The muscle or muscle group being tested should be isolated as specifically as possible.
3. The client holds or maintains the contracted position of the muscle isolation while the therapist slowly and evenly applies a counterpressure to pull or press the muscle out of its isolated position.

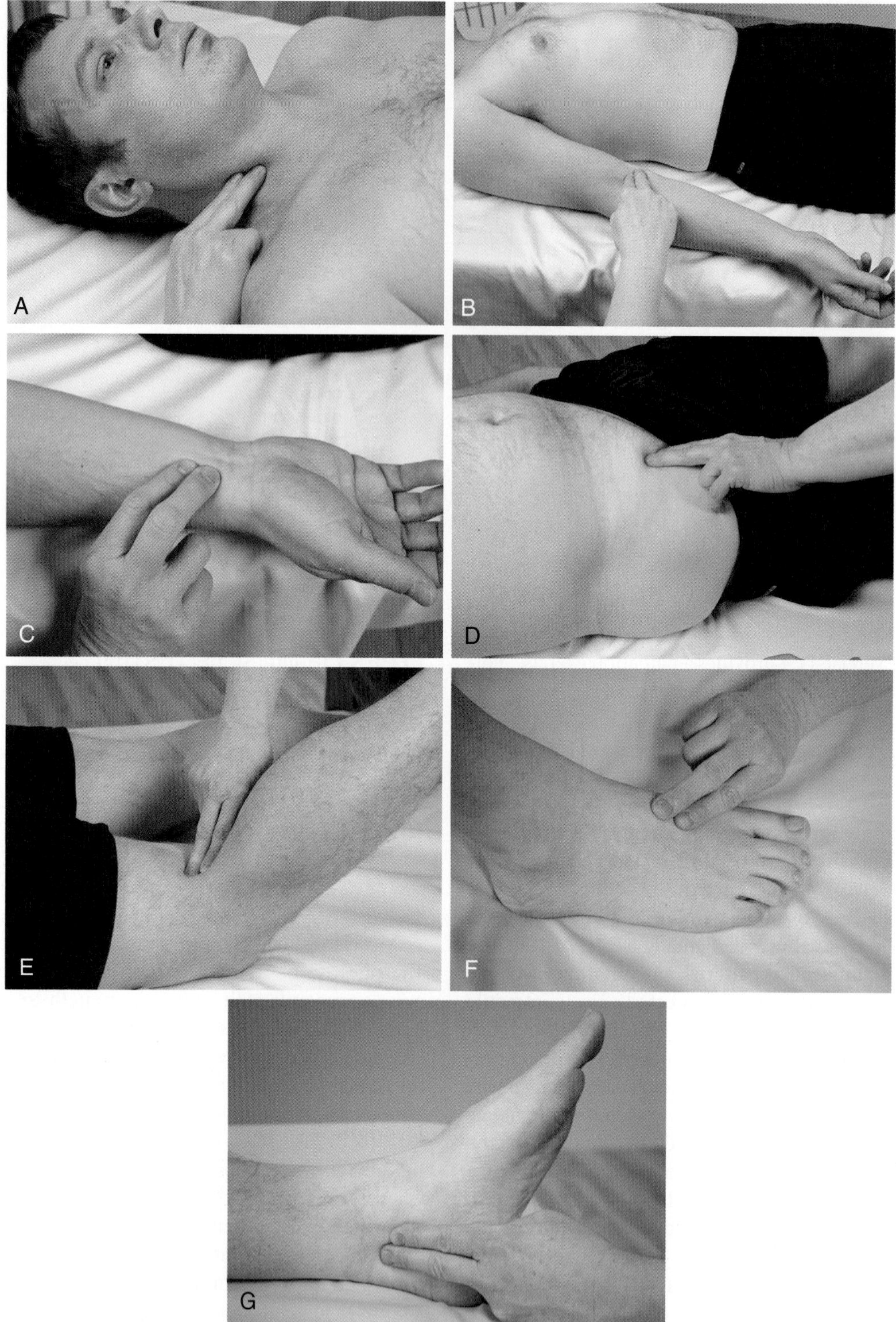

FIG. 11.26 Palpation of the arterial pulses. A, Carotid pulse. **B,** Brachial pulse. **C,** Radial pulse. **D,** Femoral pulse. **E,** Popliteal pulse. **F,** Dorsalis pulse. **G,** Posterior tibial pulse.

4. The massage therapist must use sufficient force to recruit a full response by the muscles being tested but not enough to recruit other muscles in the body.

If strength testing is done this way, there is little chance the therapist will injure the client. As with palpation, the muscle test must be compared with a similar area, usually the same muscle group on the opposite side.

Various assessment scales are used to describe the findings from strength testing. The most common is a numerical scale. Grades for a manual muscle test are recorded as numerical scores ranging from 1, which represents no activity, to 5, which represents a "normal" or best possible response to the test or as great a response as can be evaluated by a manual muscle test. The grades are as follows:

5—Normal strength
4—Movement against gravity and resistance
3—Movement against gravity (resistance eliminated)
2—Movement with gravity eliminated
1—Only a flicker of movement

Because this text is based on tests of motions rather than tests of individual muscles, the grade represents the performance of all muscles in that motion.

Procedures for Muscle Testing

Muscle strength is assessed by making the muscles hold against an imposed force. The term *resistance* is used to describe a force that acts in opposition to a contracting muscle. Manual resistance should always be applied in the direction of the "line of pull" of the participating muscle or muscles. Resistance is applied at a 90-degree angle to the primary axis of the body part tested.

1. To ensure correct positioning and stabilization for the test, place the muscle group to be tested in the test position rather than have the client actively move it there.
2. Stabilize the rest of the body so that only the joint targeted for assessment will move in response to the muscle contraction.
3. Apply resistance near the distal end of the segment to which the muscle attaches.
4. Make sure the application of manual resistance to a part is never sudden or uneven (jerky). Apply resistance slowly and gradually, allowing it to build to the maximum tolerable intensity.

A tested muscle or muscle group may be unable to hold against applied force for many reasons, including atrophy, joint dysfunction, and neurological inhibition (Fig. 11.27).

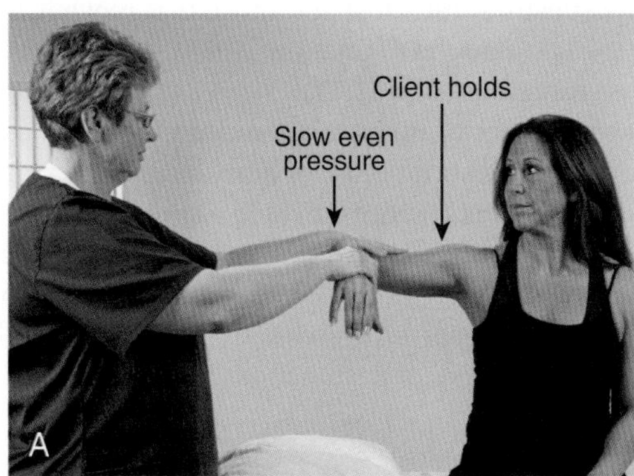

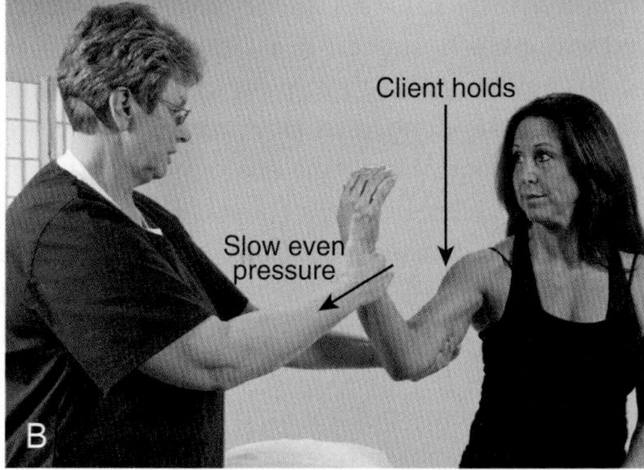

FIG. 11.27 A, Muscle test for medial deltoid. **B,** Muscle test for biceps.

Assessing the Coordination of the Agonist–Antagonist Interaction

Another muscle testing method used for assessment is to compare a muscle group's strength with its antagonist muscle group pattern. The body is designed so that the flexor, internal rotator, and adductor muscles are about 25% to 30% larger and therefore stronger than the extensor, external rotator, and abductor muscles. It also is designed so that flexors and adductors usually work against gravity to move a joint. The main purposes of extensors and abductors are to restrain and control the flexor and adductor movement and to return the joint to a neutral position. Less strength is required because gravity is assisting the function.

Strength testing should reveal a difference in the pattern between the flexors, internal rotators, and adductors, and the extensors, external rotators, and abductors in an agonist/antagonist pattern. These groups should not be equally strong (i.e., able to hold against the same applied force). Flexors, internal rotators, and adductors should show more muscle strength than extensors, external rotators, and abductors.

Neurological Muscle Testing

Neurological muscle testing focuses more on the patterns of muscle communication. A small force is used for testing, because only the nervous system is assessed. An efficient pattern is one in which the muscles contract evenly, without jerking and without a lot of synergistic (helper muscle) activity. The same isolation of muscle groups is used as in strength testing. The client holds the contraction, and the massage therapist provides moderately light pressure against the muscle. Different neurological interactions can be assessed, including muscle group interactions, muscle activation sequences and firing patterns, and postural (stabilizer) and phasic (mover) muscle interactions.

As always, the goal is to locate the muscle interaction pattern—not only for the muscle directly tested but also for all other muscles linked through functional units and gait and postural reflexes. In tests of neuromuscular activity, it is important that the massage practitioner notice what the rest of the body does when the isolated muscle group is tested. For example, if testing of the neck flexor muscles causes the left leg to roll in, a pattern of interaction has shown itself. These patterns may be natural, such as the gait reflexes, but they often are a mixed-up set of signals that cause the body to respond inappropriately. Inefficient patterns cause some muscles to contract with more force than is necessary. After contraction, muscles may not be able to resume a normal resting length; they may remain short and thus maintain tension patterns. Whenever a pattern of overly short muscles exists, a pattern of inhibited and weak muscles also is present. When the prime mover for a particular function does not respond appropriately, the synergist attempts to compensate, altering optimal movement. Synergistic dominance is a common form of neuromuscular dysfunction. These imbalances use energy and contribute to fatigue and pain.

Muscle Group Interactions

Remember that most joints in the body are moved by muscles that cross a single joint or muscles that cross two joints. Muscles are tested in groups because isolating a single muscle is almost impossible; the brain does not process movement of individual muscles. It is more important to work with muscles in patterns of flexion and extension, adduction and abduction, internal and external rotation, or elevation and depression than to be concerned with the function of individual muscles. The movement pattern of each synovial joint is based on the flexion and extension principle. To move in gravity, each joint must be stabilized by some sort of diagonal pattern that functions as a counterbalance. Therefore, the entire body is involved in all movement patterns.

Muscle Synergies: Muscle Activation Sequences/Muscle Firing Patterns

Movement requires groups of muscles working together in sequence to produce coordinated movements and is called muscle synergy. The most basic **functional movements** produced by skeletal muscles are standing and walking, and synergistic coordination occurs to efficiently accomplish tasks such as reaching, grasping, lifting, and running. Each muscle synergy pattern consists of co-activation of multiple muscles in an efficient sequence. Depending on the movement outcome, these patterns shift. These patterns also provide a more generalizable assessment of motor function in neuromotor deficits that may guide more targeted rehabilitation interventions. Synergistic muscle patterns are important in all types of functional movement demands. However, just how the nervous system integrates the concurrent control of locomotion and balance function remains elusive. Neural circuits for locomotion have been identified in the mammalian spinal cord and can endogenously produce rhythmic motor patterns to muscles. Reflex patterns also regulate the order in which muscles contract to produce movement. The pattern of contraction typically involves the following sequence: (1) agonist supported by synergists, (2) fixators and co-contraction of antagonist, and (3) neutralizers. Support muscles in other body areas also act to integrate the movement body wide. This pattern is general, and exceptions occur, but the pattern provides a framework for understanding muscle interaction (Tresch and Jarc, 2009; Bizzi and Cheung, 2013; Dischiavi et al., 2018; Kamel et al., 2021). In clinical practice these muscle synergies of motor function often are called muscle activation sequences or muscle firing patterns.

Muscles contract, or fire, in a neurological sequence to produce coordinated movement. If the optimal muscle activation sequence is disrupted and muscles fire out of sequence or do not contract when they should, labored movement and postural strain result. Firing patterns can be assessed by initiating a particular sequence of joint movements and palpating for muscle activity to determine which muscle is responding first, second, or third to the movement.

The central nervous system recruits the appropriate muscles in specific activation sequences to generate the appropriate muscle function of acceleration, deceleration, or stability. If these firing patterns are abnormal and the synergist becomes dominant, efficient movement is compromised and the joint position is strained. The general firing pattern is prime movers, then stabilizers, and then synergists. If the stabilizer must also move the area (acceleration) or control movement (deceleration), it typically becomes short. If the synergist fires before the prime mover, the movement is awkward and labored.

If one muscle is short and has increased tone, reciprocal inhibition typically occurs. Reciprocal inhibition exists when a short, tight muscle decreases nervous stimulation to its functional antagonist, causing it to reduce activity (i.e., inhibition). For example, a short psoas reduces the function of the gluteus maximus. The activation and force production of the prime mover (the gluteus maximus) decreases, leading to compensation and substitution by the synergists (hamstrings) and stabilizers (erector spinae), creating an altered firing pattern. The most common firing pattern dysfunction is synergistic dominance, in which a synergist compensates for a prime mover to produce the movement (Lee et al., 2018). For example, if a client has an inhibited gluteus medius, synergists (the tensor fasciae latae, abductor complex, and quadratus lumborum) become dominant to compensate for the weakness. This alters normal joint alignment, which further alters the normal length-tension relationships of the muscles around the joint. (The most commonly used assessment procedures and the intervention for altered firing patterns are presented in Proficiency Exercise 11.5.)

Postural (Stabilizer) and Phasic (Mover) Muscle Interactions

The two basic types of muscles are those that support the body in gravity (postural muscles) and those that move it through gravity (phasic muscles) (Chaitow, 1988). Muscles can perform both functions (Box 11.11).

These two types of muscles are made up of various kinds of muscle fibers. Postural muscles have a higher percentage of slow-twitch red fibers, which can hold a contraction for a long time before fatiguing. Phasic muscles have a higher percentage of fast-twitch white fibers, which contract quickly but tire easily. These two types of muscles are tested differently and develop different types of dysfunctions.

Postural Muscles

Postural (stabilizer) muscles are relatively slow to respond compared with **phasic (mover) muscles**. They do not produce bursts of strength if asked to respond quickly, and they may cramp. They are the deliberate, slow, steady muscles that require time to respond. Using the analogy of the tortoise and the hare, these muscles are the tortoise. Inefficient neurological patterns, muscle tension, reorganization of connective tissue with fibrotic changes, and trigger points are common in postural muscles (Chaitow, 1988).

If posture is not balanced, postural muscles must function more like ligaments and bones to provide stability. When this happens, an increase in tissue density, trigger points, and even fibrotic tissue can develop in the muscle to provide the

PROFICIENCY EXERCISE 11.5

Protocol for Assessing Common Muscle Activation Sequences and Muscle Firing Patterns

Trunk Flexion (Figures A1, A2)

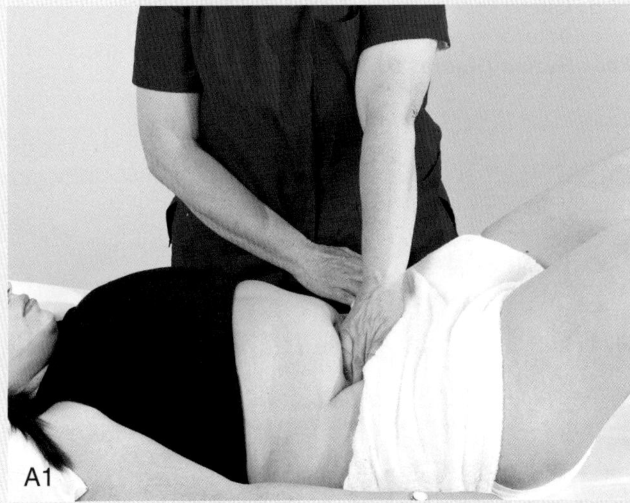
A1

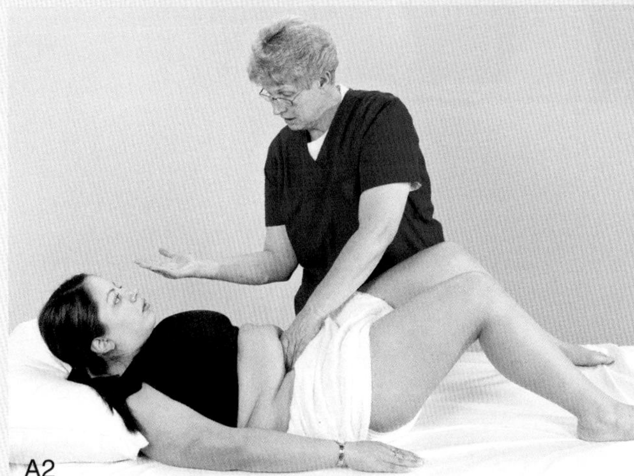
A2

Palpate either side of the rectus abdominis to assess contraction of the obliques and the transverse abdominis abdomen.

1. Normal firing pattern
   a. Transverse abdominis
   b. Abdominal obliques
   c. Rectus abdominis
2. Assessment
   a. Position the client supine with the knees and hips in approximately 90 degrees of flexion.
   b. Instruct the client to perform a normal curl up.
   c. Assess the abdominal muscles' ability to functionally stabilize the lumbar-pelvic-hip complex by having the client draw the abdominal muscle in (as when bringing the umbilicus toward the back), and then do a curl just lifting the scapula off the table while keeping both feet flat. An inability to maintain the drawing-in position or to activate the rectus abdominis during the assessment demonstrates an altered firing pattern of the abdominal stabilization mechanism.
3. Altered firing pattern
   a. Weak agonist—abdominal complex
   b. Overactive antagonist—erector spinae
   c. Overactive synergist—psoas, rectus abdominis
4. Symptoms
   a. Low back pain
   b. Buttock pain
   c. Hamstring shortening

Hip Extension (Figures B1, B2)

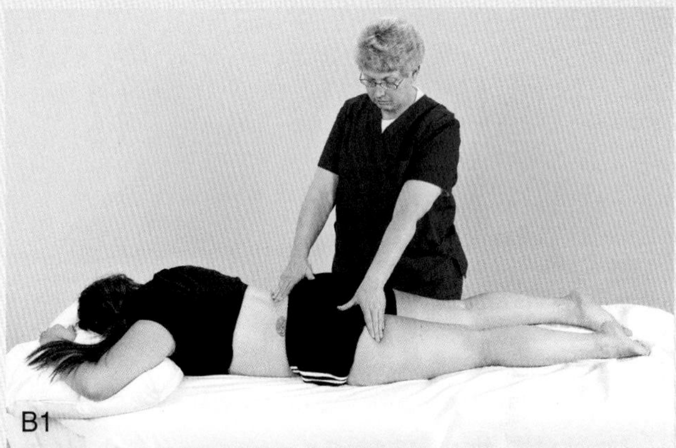
B1

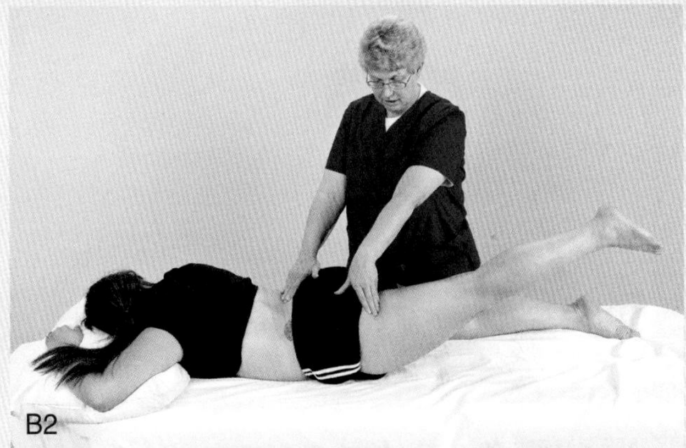
B2

1. Normal firing pattern
   a. Gluteus maximus
   b. Opposite erector spinae
   c. Same-side erector spinae and hamstring
   or
   a. Gluteus maximus
   b. Hamstring
   c. Opposite erector spinae
   d. Same-side erector spinae
2. Assessment
   a. Place the client in the prone position.
   b. Palpate the erector spinae with the fingers of one hand while palpating the muscle belly of the opposite gluteus maximus and hamstring with the little finger and thumb of the other hand.
   c. Instruct the client to raise the hip more than 15 degrees off the table.
3. Altered firing pattern
   a. Weak agonist—gluteus maximus
   b. Overactive antagonist—psoas

PROFICIENCY EXERCISE 11.5—cont'd

c. Overactive stabilizer—erector spinae
d. Overactive synergist—hamstring
4. Symptoms
   a. Low back pain
   b. Buttock pain
   c. Recurrent hamstring strains

Hip Abduction (Figures C1, C2)

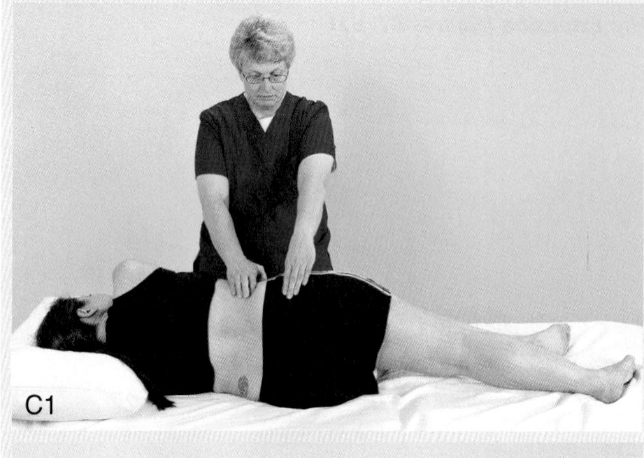

C1

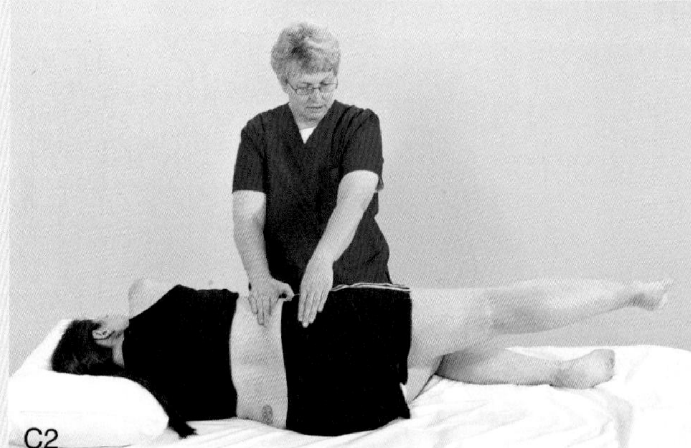

C2

1. Normal firing pattern
   a. Gluteus medius
   b. Tensor fasciae latae
   c. Quadratus lumborum
2. Assessment
   a. Place the client in the side-lying position.
   b. Stand next to the client and palpate the quadratus lumborum area with one hand and the tensor fasciae latae and gluteus medius with the other hand.
   c. Instruct the client to abduct the leg from the table.
3. Altered firing pattern
   a. Weak agonist—gluteus medius
   b. Overactive antagonist—adductors
   c. Overactive synergist—tensor fasciae latae
   d. Overactive stabilizer—quadratus lumborum
4. Symptoms
   a. Low back pain
   b. Sacroiliac joint pain
   c. Buttock pain
   d. Lateral knee pain
   e. Anterior knee pain

Knee Flexion (Figures D1, D2)

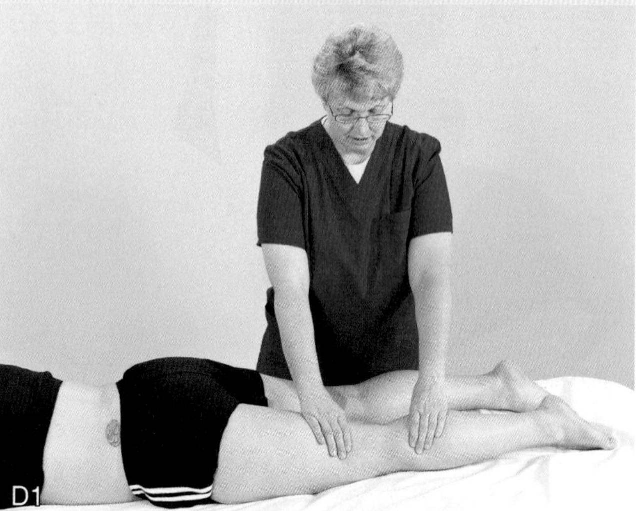

D1

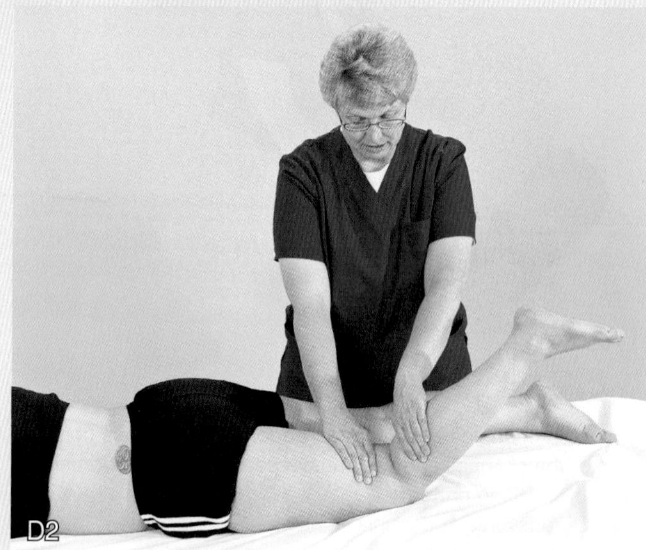

D2

1. Normal firing pattern
   a. Hamstrings
   b. Gastrocnemius
2. Assessment
   a. Place the client in the prone position.
   b. Place your fingers on the hamstring and the gastrocnemius.
   c. Instruct the client to flex the knee.
3. Altered firing pattern
   a. Weak agonist—hamstrings
   b. Overactive synergist—gastrocnemius
4. Symptoms
   a. Pain behind the knee
   b. Achilles tendinitis

Continued

PROFICIENCY EXERCISE 11.5—cont'd

Knee Extension (Figures E1, E2)

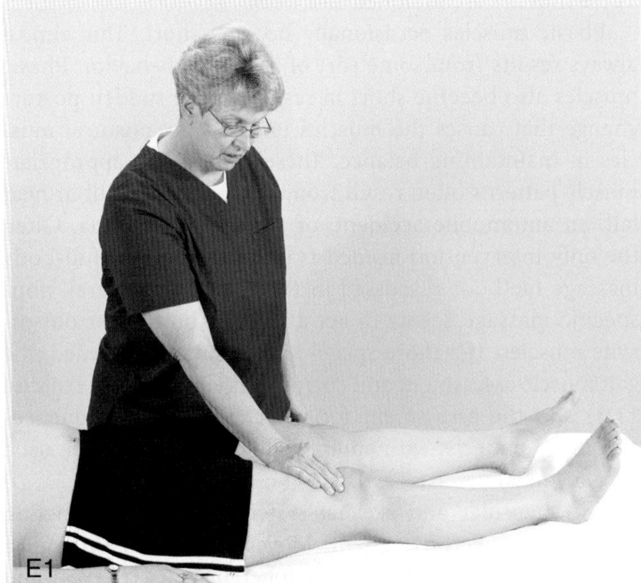
E1

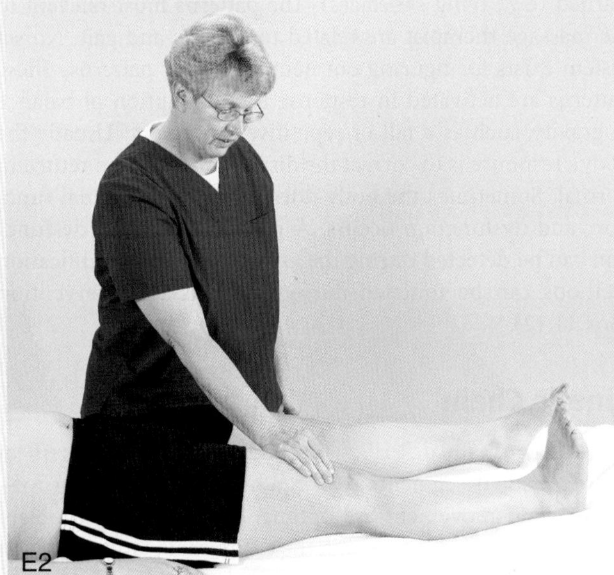
E2

1. Normal firing pattern
   a. Vastus medialis
   b. Vastus intermedius and vastus lateralis
   c. Rectus femoris
2. Assessment
   a. Place the client in the supine position with the leg flat.
   b. Instruct the client to pull the patella cranially (toward the head).
   c. Place your fingers on the vastus medialis oblique portion, vastus lateralis, and rectus femoris.
3. Altered firing pattern
   a. Weak agonist—vastus medius, primarily oblique portion
   b. Overactive synergist—vastus lateralis
4. Symptoms
   a. Knee pain under the patella
   b. Patellar tendinitis

Shoulder Abduction (Figures F1, F2)

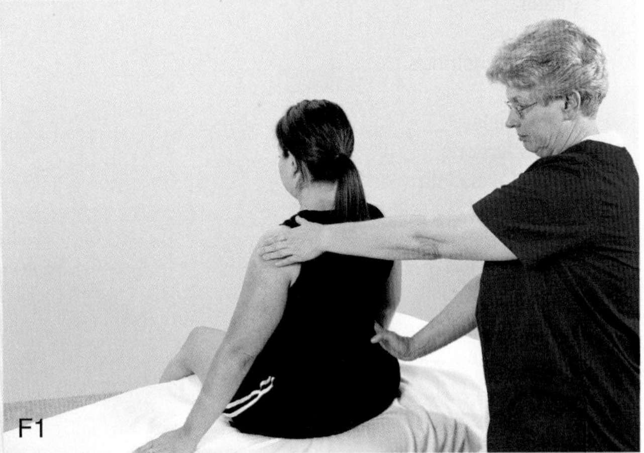
F1

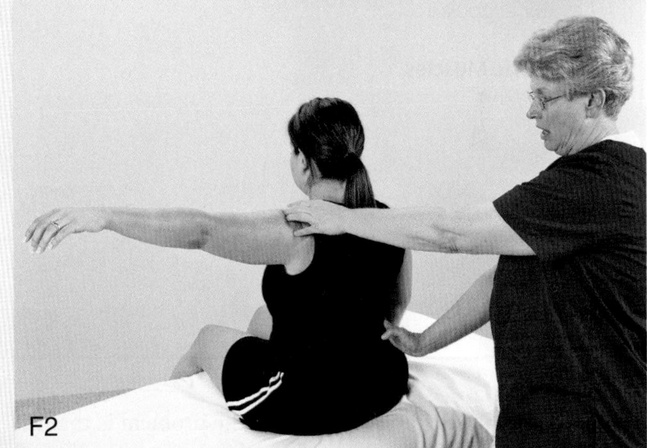
F2

1. Normal firing pattern
   a. Supraspinatus
   b. Deltoid
   c. Infraspinatus
   d. Middle and lower trapezius
   e. Contralateral lumbar area
2. Assessment
   a. Place the client in the seated position. Stand behind the client and put one hand on the client's shoulder and the other on the contralateral quadratus area.
   b. Instruct the client to abduct the shoulder to 90 degrees.
3. Altered firing pattern
   a. Weak agonist—levator scapulae
   b. Overactive agonist—upper trapezius
   c. Overactive stabilizer—ipsilateral quadratus lumborum
4. Symptoms
   a. Shoulder tension
   b. Headache at the base of the skull
   c. Upper chest breathing
   d. Low back pain

Intervention for Altered Firing Patterns

Use appropriate massage applications to inhibit the dominant muscle, and then strengthen the weak muscles.

Box 11.11 Major Postural and Phasic Muscles

Major Postural Muscles
- Gastrocnemius
- Soleus
- Adductors
- Medial hamstrings
- Psoas
- Abdominals
- Rectus femoris
- Tensor fascia lata
- Piriformis
- Quadratus lumborum
- Erector spinae group
- Pectorals
- Latissimus dorsi
- Neck extensors
- Trapezius
- Scalenes
- Sternocleidomastoid
- Levator scapulae

Major Phasic Muscles
- Neck flexors
- Deltoid
- Biceps
- Triceps
- Brachioradialis
- Quadriceps
- Hamstrings
- Gluteus maximus
- Anterior tibialis

ability to stabilize the body in gravity. The problem is that the connective tissue freezes the body in the dysfunctional position, because unlike muscle, which can actively contract and lengthen, connective tissue is more static.

Dr. Vladimir Janda, a neurologist of the Prague School of Manual Medicine and Rehabilitation, identified predictable compensatory postural patterns describing common postural changes. Postural muscles tend to shorten and have increased motor tone when under strain. This is an important consideration when massage practitioners attempt to assess which muscles are short, apt to develop trigger points and connective tissue changes, and require lengthening and stretching (see Chapter 12). Connective tissue shortening is dealt with mechanically through forms of stretch. Trigger points usually respond to muscle energy methods and inhibitory pressure. Short concentric contraction muscles are dealt with through muscle energy methods and lengthening procedures (see Chapter 10).

Phasic Muscles

Phasic (mover) muscles jump into action quickly and tire quickly. Musculotendinous junction problems are more common in phasic muscles. The four most common problems are microtearing of the muscle fibers at the tendon, inflamed tendons (tendinitis), adherence of muscles and tendons to underlying tissue, and bursitis.

Phasic muscles usually are inhibited (weaker) in response to postural muscle shortening. Sometimes the inhibited muscles also shorten as a form of compensation, which allows the weak muscle the same contraction power on the joint. It is important not to confuse this condition with hypertense muscles. These muscles are inhibited and weak.

Phasic muscles occasionally become short. This almost always results from some sort of repetitive behavior. Phasic muscles also become short in response to a sudden posture change that causes the muscles to assist the postural muscles in maintaining balance. These common, inappropriate muscle patterns often result from an unexpected fall or near fall, an automobile accident, or some other trauma. Often the only intervention needed is using the general full-body massage methods discussed in this text. This general, nonspecific massage seems to act as a reset button for out-of-sync muscles. If a more specific intervention is needed, the gait muscle assessment and corrections (Proficiency Exercise 11.3) and the assessment for muscle activation sequences and firing patterns with appropriate correction can be used (Proficiency Exercise 11.5).

The muscular and skeletal systems coordinate function through the nervous system. Movement occurs through a series of patterns that are both inherent (e.g., reflexes) and learned (e.g., tying shoelaces). The patterns most relevant to the massage therapist are related to posture and gait. No set system exists for figuring out neuromuscular patterns. These patterns are activated in response to a disruption of balance in gravity, such as a fall or repetitive movement. Usually the body's response is to correct the disruption and then return to normal. Sometimes the body does not resume normal function, and dysfunction occurs. A general pattern of dysfunction can be detected during the assessment, and modification methods can be initiated during the massage intervention (Box 11.12).

Kinetic Chain

The kinetic chain describes the body as a linked system of interdependent segments. When all segments function well, posture and movement are optimal. However, if a problem arises in any part of a segment, the entire chain is affected. Just as there is no such thing as an individual muscle, body segments do not exist in isolation. By understanding the relationship of the body segments to each other, we can maximize the effectiveness of massage application, because we understand the importance of whole body massage rather than isolated spot work.

Anatomically, the kinetic chain describes the interrelated groups of body segments, connecting joints, and muscles working together to perform movements and the portion of the spine to which they connect. The upper kinetic chain consists of the fingers, wrists, forearms, elbows, upper arms, shoulders, shoulder blades, and spinal column. The lower kinetic chain includes the toes, feet, ankles, lower legs, knees, upper legs, hips, pelvis, and spine. In both chains, each joint is independently capable of a variety of movements. The diagram in Fig. 11.28A shows the common areas of interrelated kinetic chain function. Follow the colored lines to locate the interconnections.

BOX 11.12 The 5 Primary Kinetic Chains

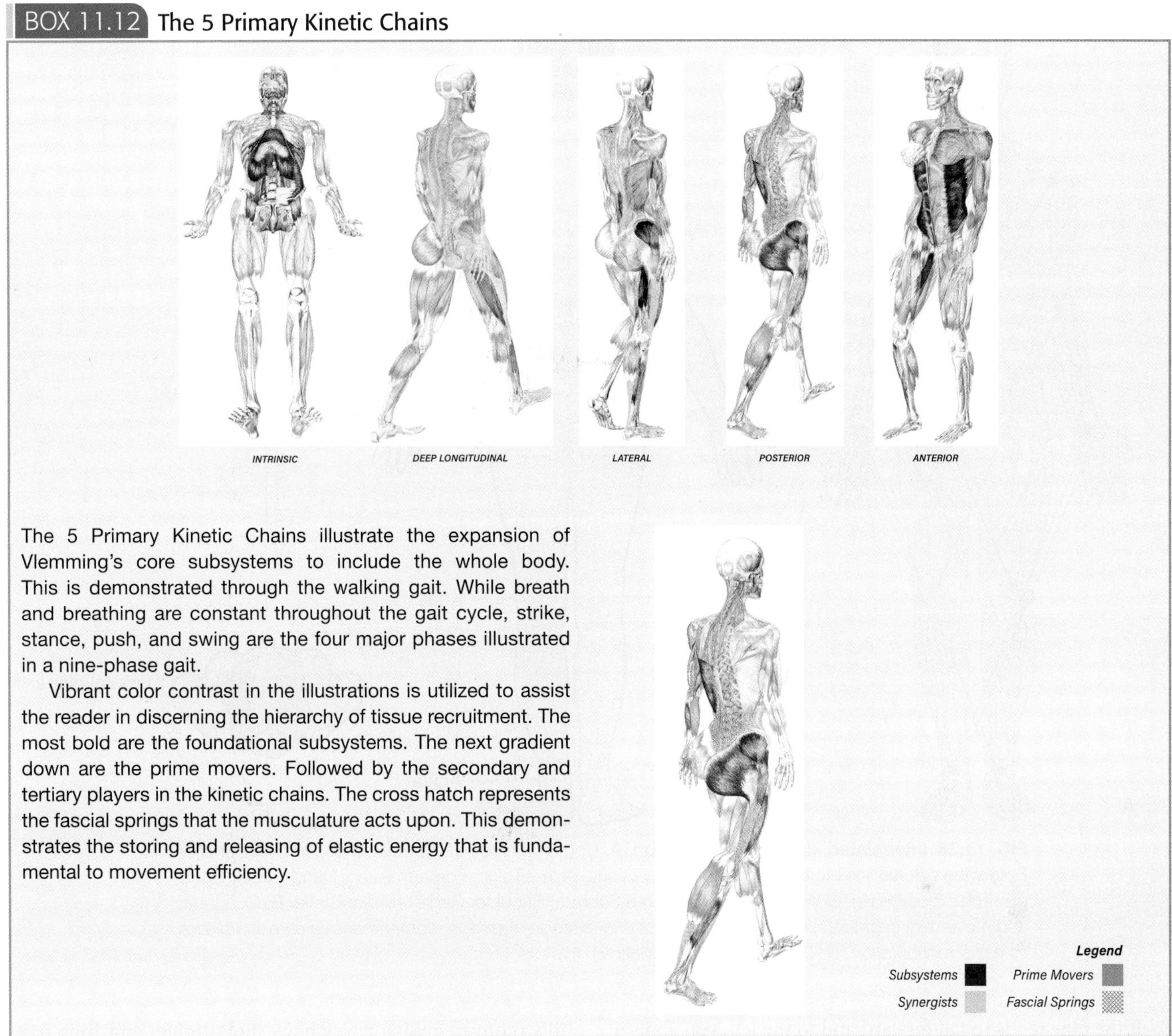

The 5 Primary Kinetic Chains illustrate the expansion of Vlemming's core subsystems to include the whole body. This is demonstrated through the walking gait. While breath and breathing are constant throughout the gait cycle, strike, stance, push, and swing are the four major phases illustrated in a nine-phase gait.

Vibrant color contrast in the illustrations is utilized to assist the reader in discerning the hierarchy of tissue recruitment. The most bold are the foundational subsystems. The next gradient down are the prime movers. Followed by the secondary and tertiary players in the kinetic chains. The cross hatch represents the fascial springs that the musculature acts upon. This demonstrates the storing and releasing of elastic energy that is fundamental to movement efficiency.

Kinetic Chain and Posture

The body is a circular form divided into four quadrants: a front, a back, a right side, and a left side. With divisions on the sagittal and frontal planes (Fig. 11.28B), the body must be balanced in three dimensions to withstand the forces of gravity and maintain normal function.

The body moves and is balanced in gravity in the following skeletal areas through the atlas: the C6 and C7 vertebrae; the T12 and L1 vertebrae (the thoracolumbar junction); the L4, L5, and S1 vertebrae (the sacrolumbar junction); and at the hips, knees, and ankles (see Fig. 11.28), with stabilization at the shoulder. If a postural distortion exists in any of the four quadrants or within one of the jointed areas (e.g., the tissue between the atlas and the axis or the hip and the knee), the entire balance mechanism must be adjusted to maintain upright posture and keep the eyes horizontal. This occurs as a pinball-like effect that jumps front to back and side to side in the soft tissue between the movement lines at the joints.

For example, if one segment, such as the area between L1 and L4–5 and S1 (lumbar, low back area) is altered (e.g., tipped or rotated), the segments above and below must tip or twist in the opposite direction to provide counterbalance and maintain the eye position and center of gravity. As expected, the next segments up and down also adjust, and the eventual result is distortion from head to toe.

The following demonstration can help you gain an understanding of postural balance:

1. Get a pole of some type (a broom handle without the broom portion will work).
2. Tie a string around the pole.
3. Try to balance the pole on its end with the string.
4. Note that in trying to counter the fall pattern of the pole, you work opposite that fall pattern.

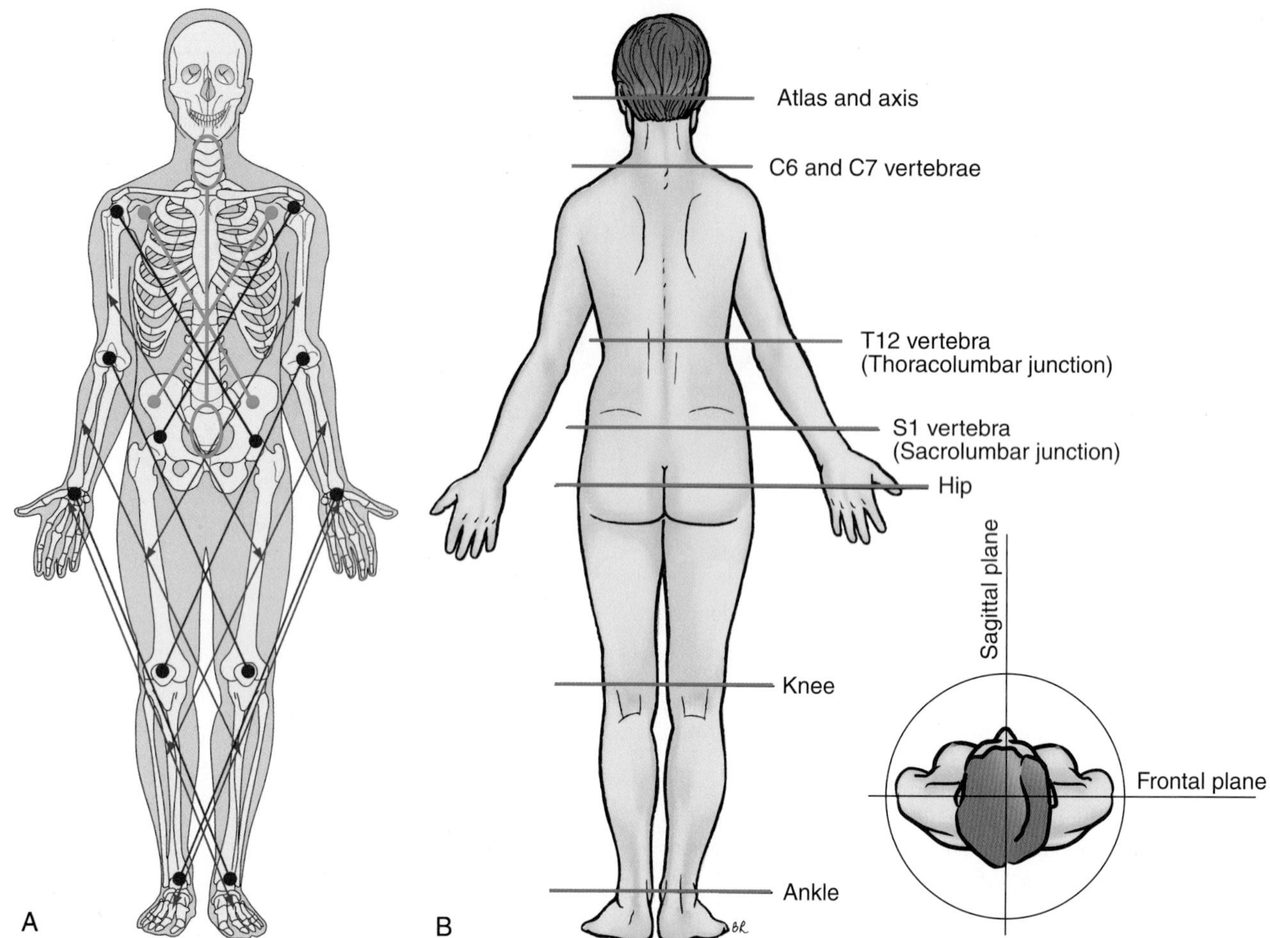

FIG. 11.28 Interrelated kinetic chain function. A, Common areas of interrelated kinetic chain function. Follow the colored lines to locate the interconnections. Arm—Thigh; Forearm—Leg; Hand—Foot; Shoulder—Hip; Elbow—Knee; Wrist—Ankle; Cervical—Sacrum; Shoulder Girdle—Pelvic Girdle. **B**, Quadrants and movement segments. (From Fritz S: *Sports and exercise massage: comprehensive care in athletics, fitness & rehabilitation*, ed 2, St. Louis, 2013, Mosby.)

5. If the pole tends to fall forward and to the left, you apply a counterforce back and to the right.

This concept can be explained in another way. The body is made up of many different poles stacked on top of one another. The poles stack at each of the jointed areas previously mentioned. Muscles and other soft tissue between the joints form movement segments that must be three-dimensionally balanced in all four quadrants to support the pole in that area. Each area must be balanced. If one pole area tips a bit to the right, the body compensates by tipping the adjacent pole areas (above, below, or both) to the left. If a pole area is tipped forward, adjacent poles are tipped back. A chain reaction occurs, such that when compensating poles tip back, their adjacent areas must counterbalance the action by tipping forward. As explained previously, this is how the body-wide compensation pattern is set up.

Whether the pole areas sit nicely on top of each other with evenly distributed muscle and other soft tissue action or whether they are tipped in various positions and counterbalanced by compensatory muscle and fascial actions, the body remains balanced in gravity. However, the "tippy pole" pattern is much more inefficient than the balanced pole pattern (Fig. 11.29). Tippy poles create caves (concave areas) and hills (convex areas); caves have short tissue, and hills have long tissue. Because massage affects short tissue most and supports elongation and relaxation, most massage intervention occurs in the concave areas; tissues that are long need to be exercised.

Interventions focus on normalizing the balance process by lengthening short, tight areas and strengthening muscles in corresponding long, taut, weak areas, allowing the poles to straighten out. If a pole is permanently tippy, such as with scoliosis or kyphosis, intervention plans attempt to support the appropriate compensation patterns and prevent them from increasing beyond what is necessary for postural balance.

Kinetic Chain and Movement

Movement can occur either in a closed kinetic chain or open kinetic chain.

A closed kinetic chain occurs when the most distal aspects of the extremity are fixed to the earth or another solid object. This fixed position alters the movement of the joints and surrounding musculature up the chain. Closed-chain movements promote joint stabilization and have the potential to recruit more muscles and their associated joints.

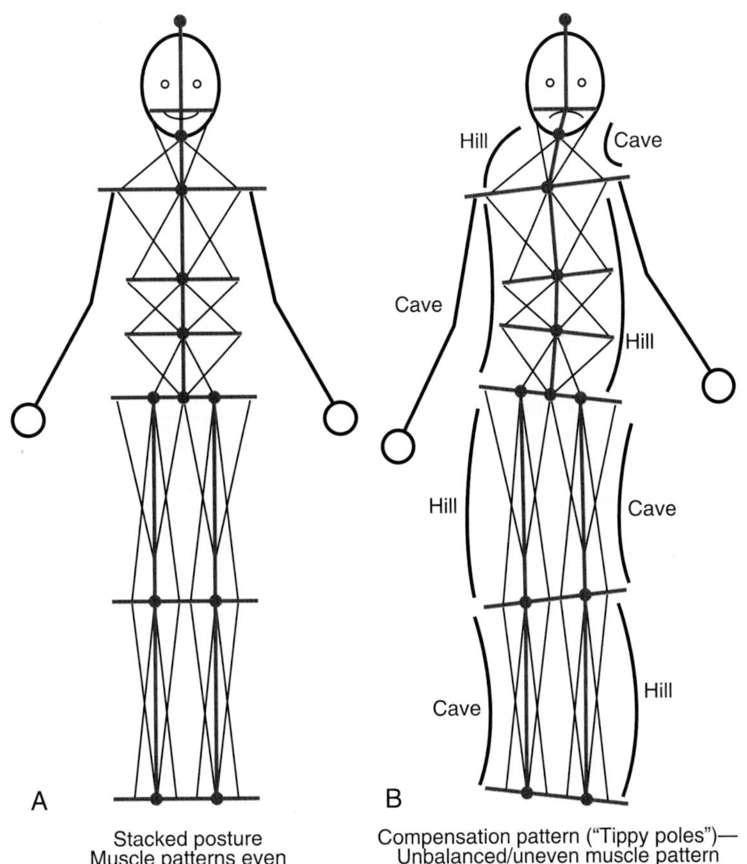

FIG. 11.29 Stacked pole **A,** versus tippy pole **B,** postural influences on the body.

An open kinetic chain refers to the distal end of an extremity not being fixed to an object, thus allowing free movement in space. Open-chain movements tend to recruit the musculature associated with only a single working joint.

For example, if you move an arm (or a leg) and your hand (or foot) also is free to move, an open kinetic chain exists. Waving your hand is an open kinetic chain movement. However, if your arm (or leg) is fixed against a surface, such as the floor or a desk, and you push, this is a closed kinetic chain movement. Closed kinetic chain movements provide simultaneous movements of the interconnected segments. As in our example, if you place your hands against a wall and push, the joints of the wrist, elbow, and shoulder all work together. Problems arise when the joints are not mobile enough to function independently during open kinetic chain movements or when they cannot remain stable in closed kinetic chain movements. Intervention involves increasing soft tissue pliability in a joint with limited mobility and supporting exercise for a joint that is unstable.

Each jointed area has an ideal movement activation sequence (firing pattern). The movement is a product of the entire mechanism, including bones; joints; ligaments; capsular components; tendons; muscle shapes and fiber types; interlinked fascial networks; nerve distribution; myotactic units (muscles that work together) of prime movers, antagonists, synergists, and fixators; neurological kinetic chain interactions; the body-wide influence of reflexes, including the positional and righting reflexes of vision and the inner ear; circulatory distribution; general systemic balance; and nutritional influences. Assessment of a movement pattern as normal indicates that all parts are functioning in a well-orchestrated manner. When a dysfunction is identified, the causal factors may arise from any one or a combination of these elements. Often a multidisciplinary diagnosis is necessary to identify clearly the interconnected nature of the pathological condition.

Intervention Guidelines

Muscle dysfunction, discovered through muscle testing procedures, often indicates how the body is compensating for postural and movement imbalances. Muscle testing also can locate the main muscle problems. When the primary dysfunctional group of muscles is tested, the main compensatory patterns are activated, and other body-wide compensation patterns activate and exaggerate. The massage professional must become a detective, looking for clues to unwind the pattern. By concentrating on methods that restore symmetry of function, the practitioner can help the client's body to work out the details.

An example of a major muscle problem is short muscles with increased motor tone. If these muscles can be relaxed and lengthened, using elongation methods to support desirable connective tissue changes, the rest of the dysfunctional pattern often resolves.

If the extensors and abductors are stronger than the flexors and adductors, major postural imbalance and distortion result. Similarly, if the extensors and abductors are too weak to balance movement patterns, the body curls into itself, and nothing works properly. If gait and kinetic chain postural patterns are inefficient, more energy is required for movement, and fatigue and pain can result.

Shortened postural (stabilizer) muscles indicate the need for lengthening. This takes time and uses all the massage practitioner's technical skills. The fiber configuration of the muscle tissue (slow-twitch red fibers or fast-twitch white fibers) dictates that techniques must be sufficiently intense and must be applied long enough to allow the muscle to respond. Shortened and weak phasic (mover) muscles first must be lengthened. Eventually, strengthening techniques and exercises are needed.

If the hypertense phasic muscle pattern is caused by repetitive use, the muscles can be normalized with muscle energy techniques and then lengthened. Overworked muscles often increase in size (hypertrophy). The client must reduce the activity of that muscle group until balance is restored, which usually takes about 4 weeks. Muscle tissue that has undergone hypertrophy begins to return to normal if it is not used for the excessive activity during that time. Athletes often have this pattern and likely will resist complete inactivity. A reduced activity level and a more balanced exercise program, combined with flexibility training, can be beneficial for them. Refer these individuals to appropriate training and coaching professionals if indicated.

FOCUS ON PROFESSIONALISM 11.2

From the beginning of this textbook we have focused on four main outcome goals: relaxation, stress management, pain management, and functional mobility. Specific physical assessment for functional mobility is more complex than for the other goals because there are more assessments to perform. However, when clients have concerns with their ability to move easily, it is typically interpreted as pain and stress. Movement is not about parts. The parts (anatomy) of the body are important, but movement is about patterns of relationship. A client can have normal range of motion in the shoulder when assessed lying down, but if the same client stands up and combines shoulder motion with hip motion as they walk, you have a pattern of movement. A technician can be trained to perform a basic massage sequence quite easily in a short time. A professional massage therapist uses assessment data to inform the massage application for identifiable massage outcomes. This type of learning process is more in-depth and ongoing.

Inappropriate muscle activation sequences (firing patterns) can be addressed by inhibiting the muscles that are contracting out of sequence and stimulating the appropriate muscles to fire. Using compression at the attachment and in the muscle belly inhibits motor tone. Tapotement is a good technique for stimulating muscles. If the problem does not normalize easily, referral to an exercise professional may be indicated.

Recall that the range of motion of a joint is measured in degrees. A full circle is 360 degrees. A flat horizontal line is 180 degrees. Two perpendicular lines (as in the shape of a capital L) create a 90-degree angle. Various ranges of motion are possible. For example, when the range of motion of a joint allows 0 to 90 degrees of flexion, anything less is hypomobile and anything more is hypermobile. A great degree of variability exists among individuals as to the actual normal range of motion; the degrees provided are general guidelines. Range of motion is measured from the anatomic position. Whether the client is standing, supine, or side-lying, anatomic position is considered 0 degrees of motion.

PUTTING IT ALL TOGETHER: FUNCTIONAL BIOMECHANICAL ASSESSMENT

SECTION OBJECTIVES

Chapter objective covered in this section:

9. Interpret and categorize assessment information.

Using the information presented in this section, the student will be able to perform the following:

- Organize assessment information into categories of distortion and stages to develop a massage care/treatment plan.

Functional biomechanical assessment defines mobility based on active and passive movements of the body, through the use of palpation and observation to detect distortion in these movements.

The **4-Element Movement System Model** describes primary elements (motion, force, motor control, and energy) essential to the performance of all movements:

- Motion: ability of a joint or tissue to be moved passively.
- Force: ability of the contractile (i.e., muscles) and noncontractile structures (i.e., tendons) to produce movement and provide dynamic stability around joints during static and dynamic tasks.
- Motor control: ability to plan, execute and adapt goal-directed movements such that they are accurate, coordinated, and efficient.
- Energy: the ability to perform sustained or repeated movements and is dependent on the integrated functioning of the cardiovascular, pulmonary, and neuromuscular systems.

The 4-Element Model is a systematic observational assessment approach using five observation targets abbreviated as CASSS (control, amount, speed, symmetry, symptoms):

- Control: smoothness, coordination, and timing of movement
- Amount: amplitude (range, magnitude, or distance) of movement at each joint
- Speed is the length of time
- Symmetry: observed in bilateral tasks or comparing unilateral performance between limbs; speed is the length of time
- Symptoms: stiffness, pain, instability, or fatigue.

Potential impairments are identified to implement treatment strategies (Zarzycki et al., 2022).

Muscle testing and identification of the functional relationships of muscles also are performed.

Typical dysfunction includes the following:

- Local joint hypermobility or hypomobility
- Gait dysfunction
- Altered muscle synergies: firing patterns (activation sequences)
- Postural imbalance (tippy pole)

Any one or combination of these conditions can lead to changes in motor function and can be accompanied by temporary or chronic joint, muscular, and nervous system disorders.

Performing a Basic Functional Assessment

The assessment skills presented so far in this chapter are the tools used to perform a basic functional assessment of the client. Remember that each individual joint movement pattern is part of an interconnected aspect of the neurological coordination pattern of muscle movement (the kinetic chain) and of the tensegrity of the body's design. Both posture and movement dysfunctions identified in an individual joint pattern must be assessed and treated in broader terms of kinetic chain interactions, muscle length relationships, and the effects of stress and strain on the entire system and the person's ability to adapt and respond to intervention. When a movement pattern is evaluated, multiple types of information are obtained in one functional assessment.

When a jointed area moves into flexion and the joint angle is decreased, the prime mover and synergists concentrically contract, antagonists eccentrically function with controlled lengthening, and the fixators isometrically contract and stabilize. Body-wide stabilization patterns also come into play to assist in allowing the motion.

During assessment, resistance applied to load the prime mover groups and synergists is used to assess for neurological function of strength and, to a lesser degree, endurance as the contraction is held. At the same time, the antagonist pattern or the tissues that are lengthened when positioning for the functional assessment can be assessed for increased muscle or connective tissue shortening.

Dysfunction shows itself in limited range of motion by restricting the movement pattern. Therefore, when placing a jointed area into flexion, the examiner assesses the extensors for increased tone, which can cause shortening that would limit movement. When the jointed area moves into extension, the opposite becomes the case. The same is true for adduction and abduction, internal and external rotation, plantar and dorsal flexion, and so on.

Each movement pattern (e.g., flexion and extension of the elbow and knee, circumduction and rotation of the shoulder and hip, movement of the trunk and neck) is assessed by sequentially positioning each area in all available movement patterns and by testing for strength, range, and ease of movement.

Resistance (pressure against) applied to the muscles is focused at the end of the lever system. For example:

- When the function of the shoulder is assessed, resistance is focused at the distal end of the humerus, not at the wrist.
- Elbow function is assessed with resistance at the wrist, not the hand.
- When extension of the hip is assessed, resistance is applied at the end of the femur.
- When flexion of the knee is assessed, resistance is applied at the distal end of the tibia, not the foot.

Resistance is applied slowly, smoothly, and firmly at an appropriate intensity, as determined by the size of the muscle mass.

Stabilization is essential for accurate assessment of movement patterns. Only the area assessed is allowed to move. Movement in any other part of the body must be stabilized. The massage therapist usually applies a stabilizing force. As one hand applies resistance, the other provides the stabilization. Sometimes the client can provide the stabilization. Some methods use straps to provide stabilization.

The easiest way to identify the area to be stabilized is as follows:

1. Move the area to be assessed through the range of motion.
2. At the end of the range, some other part of the body begins to move; this is the area where stabilization is applied.
3. Return the body to a neutral position.
4. Provide the appropriate stabilization to the area identified and begin the assessment procedure.

During assessments, muscles should be able to hold against appropriate resistance without strain or pain from the pressure and without recruiting or using other muscles. Appropriate resistance is applied slowly and steadily and with just enough force to induce the muscles to respond to the stimulus. Large muscle groups require more force than small ones. The position should be easy to assume and comfortable to maintain for 10 to 30 seconds. Contraindications to this type of assessment include joint and disk dysfunction, acute pain, recent trauma, and inflammation.

Distortion Categories

Distortions in functioning are often measured and categorized in the following way:

- *First-degree distortion:* The person must use additional muscles from different parts of the body for usual and simple movements. As a result, movement becomes uneconomical and labored.
- *Second-degree distortion:* Moderately expressed shortening of postural muscles and inhibition and weakening of antagonist muscles. Moderately peculiar postures and movements of some parts of the body are present. Postural and movement distortion, such as altered firing patterns, begin to occur.
- *Third-degree distortion:* Clearly expressed shortening of postural muscles and weakening of antagonist muscles occur, and specific, nonoptimal movement develops. Significantly expressed peculiarity in postures and movement occurs. Increased postural and movement distortions result in defined changes in muscle and motor tone and related connective tissues.

It is important to determine which muscles are shortened and which are inhibited to choose the appropriate therapeutic intervention.

On the basis of the three levels of distorted function, the development of postural and movement pathological conditions is divided into three stages:

- Stage 1: *Functional tension.* In stage 1, the person tires more quickly than normal. This fatigue is accompanied by first- or second-degree limitation of mobility, painless local myodystonia (changes in the muscle length–tension relationship), postural imbalance in the first or second degree, and nonoptimal motor function of the first degree.

As a result: The person can do what they want but it takes more energy.

- Stage 2: *Functional stress.* Stage 2 is characterized by fatigue with moderate activity, discomfort, slight pain, and the appearance of singular or multiple degrees of limited mobility that is painless or that results in first-degree pain. It may be accompanied by local hypermobility or hypomobility. Functional stress is characterized by reflex vertebral-sensory dysfunction, fascial and connective tissue changes, and regional postural imbalance. It is also accompanied by distortion of motor function in the first or second degree and firing pattern alterations.

As a result: The person can still do most things but perhaps not as easily. The individual eventually begins to avoid certain activities and uses more energy to achieve reduced function.

- Stage 3: *Connective tissue changes in the musculoskeletal system.* The reasons for connective tissue changes are overloading, disturbances of tissue nutrition, microtrauma, microhemorrhage, unresolved edema, and other factors, both endogenous (inside the body) and exogenous (outside the body). Hereditary predisposition is also a consideration. In stage 3, changes in the spine and weight-bearing joints may appear, with areas of local hypermobility and instability of several vertebral motion segments, hypomobility, widespread painful muscle tension, fascial and other connective tissue changes in the muscles, regional postural imbalance in the second or third degree in many joints, and temporary nonoptimal motor function with second- or third-degree distortion. Visceral disturbances may be present. Individuals in stage 3 have significantly reduced function.

As a result: The person is no longer able to perform many common occupational and daily life activities. They avoid most activities, and when the person does participate, extreme fatigue occurs.

Distortion Management

Stage 1 (functional tension) often can be managed effectively by massage methods and by massage practitioners who are competent in the skills presented in this text. It is important that the client have all symptoms evaluated by the appropriate health care professional, because the early phases of many serious conditions present the same symptoms as those seen in stage 1 postural conditions. Working with stage 2 and stage 3 conditions (functional stress and connective tissue changes) usually requires more training and proper supervision within a multidisciplinary approach.

Assessment Results

The results of the assessment identify either appropriate function of each area or dysfunction, which is rated as first, second, or third degree. When all assessments have been completed, the overall result is described as normal or as stage 1, stage 2, or stage 3 dysfunction, as described previously. First-degree and stage 1 dysfunction usually can be managed by general massage application. (Remember to make sure the client has no underlying serious conditions.) Clients with stage 2 or stage 3 dysfunction should be referred to the appropriate health care professional, and cooperative multidisciplinary treatment plans should be developed (Fig. 11.30).

Intervention Guidelines

Guidelines for analyzing problems found through the functional biomechanical assessment include the following:

- If an area is hypomobile, consider increased muscle tone or shortening in the antagonist pattern as a possible cause.
- If an area is hypermobile, consider instability of the joint structure or muscle weakness in the fixation pattern or problems with antagonist/agonist co-contraction function as potential causes.
- If an area cannot hold against resistance, consider weakness from reciprocal inhibition of the muscles of the prime mover and synergist pattern and tension in the antagonist pattern as potential causes.
- If pain occurs on passive movement, consider joint capsule dysfunction and nerve entrapment syndromes as possible causes.
- If pain occurs on active movement, consider muscle firing patterns and fascial involvement as a possible cause.
- Always consider body-wide reflexive patterns, as discussed in the section on posture and gait and kinetic chain, as plausible causes.

The following guidelines also are important:

- The ability to easily resist the applied force should be the same or similar bilaterally.
- Opposite movement patterns should be easy to assume.
- Bilateral asymmetry, pain, weakness, inability to assume the isolation position or to move into the opposite position, fatigue, or a heavy sensation may indicate dysfunction.
- Intervention or referral depends on the severity of the condition (stage 1, 2, or 3) and whether the dysfunction is related to joint, neuromuscular, or myofascial problems.

A plan based on efficient biomechanical movement focuses on reestablishing or supporting effective movement patterns. Biomechanically efficient movement is smooth, bilaterally symmetrical, and coordinated, with an easy, effortless use of the body. Functional assessment measures the efficiency of coordinated movement. During assessment, noticeable variations need to be considered.

CLINICAL REASONING AND PROBLEM SOLVING

SECTION OBJECTIVES

Chapter objective covered in this section:

10. Use clinical reasoning skills to apply assessment data to treatment plan development for the four main outcome goals related to massage therapy.

Using the information presented in this section, the student will be able to perform the following:

- Use the clinical reasoning model as a decision-making tool in the development of massage care/treatment plans.

Once the assessment information has been gathered, it is time to connect all the pieces in an interpretation and analysis process to develop the best massage treatment plan for the individual client. The massage does not depend on a modality

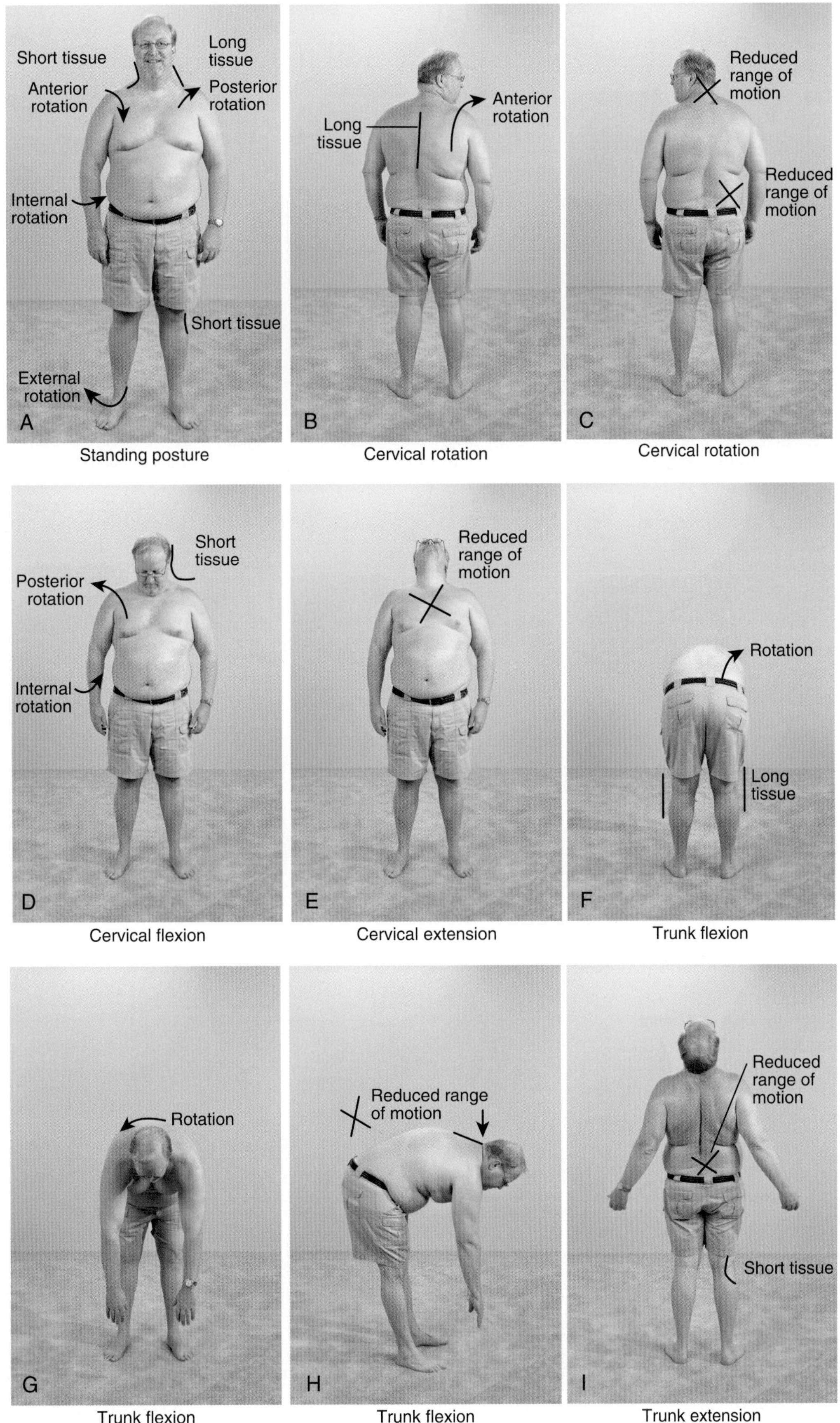

FIG. 11.30 Postural and functional movement assessment. Examples of dysfunction patterns.

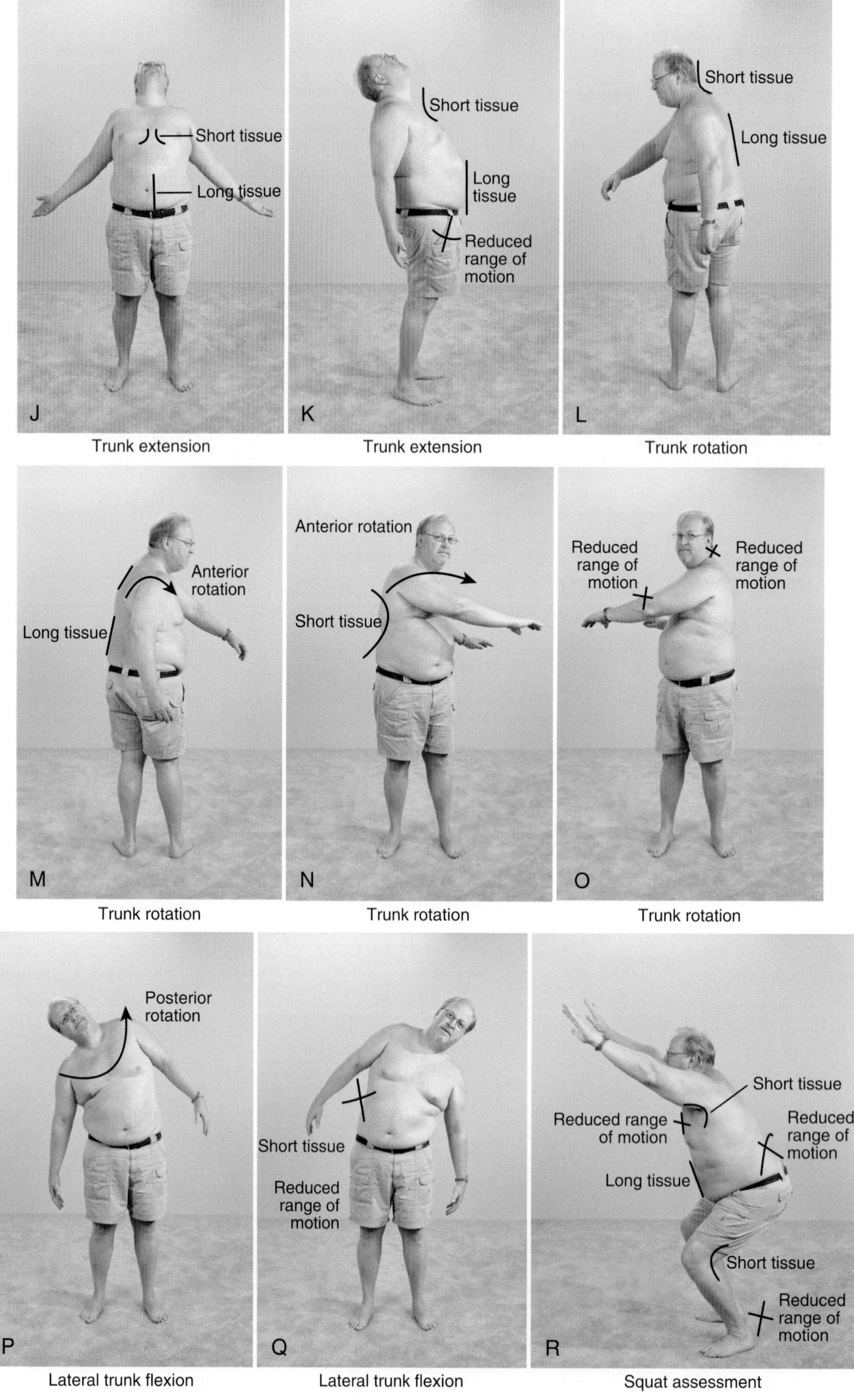

FIG. 11.30, cont'd

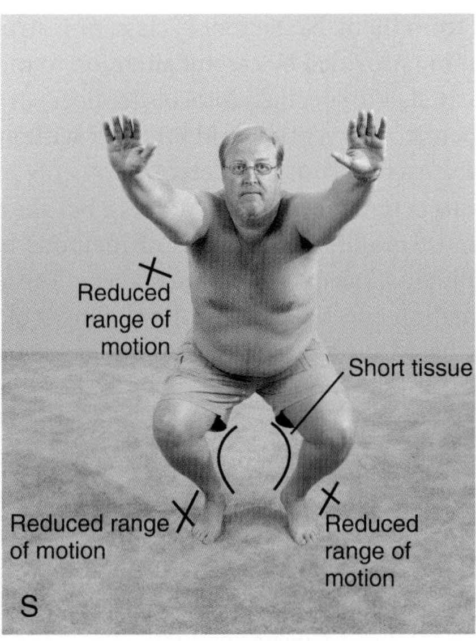

Squat assessment

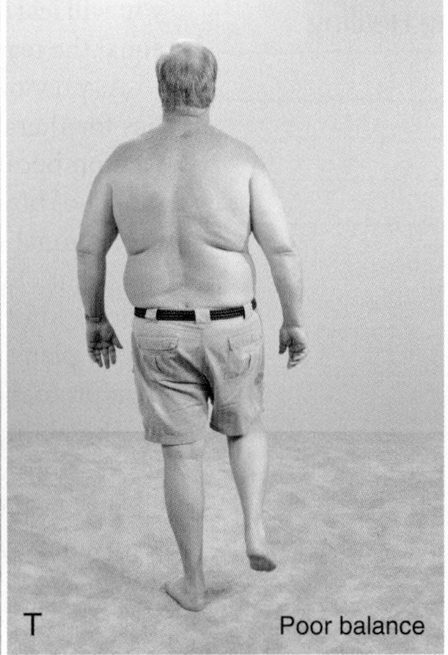

One-foot balance

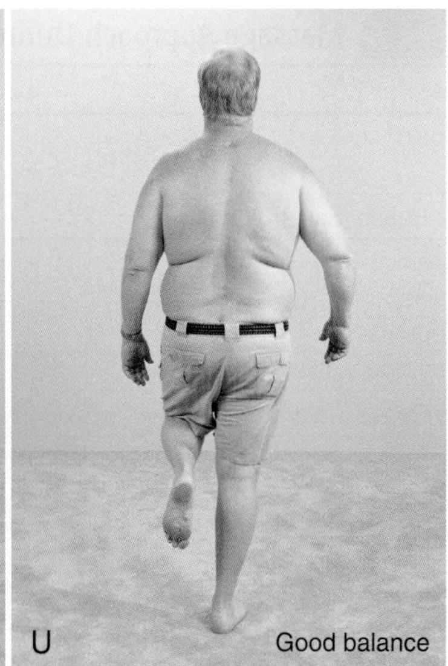

One-foot balance

FIG. 11.30, cont'd

Table 11.2 Stages of Tissue Healing and Appropriate Massage Interventions

	Stage 1 (Acute): Inflammatory Reaction	Stage 2 (Subacute): Repair and Healing	Stage 3 (Chronic): Maturation and Remodeling
Characteristics	Vascular changes Inflammatory exudate Clot formation Phagocytosis, neutralization of irritants Early fibroblastic activity	Growth of capillary beds into area Collagen formation Granulation tissue Fragile, easily injured tissue	Maturation and remodeling of scar Contracture of scar tissue Alignment of collagen along lines of stress forces (tensegrity)
Clinical signs	Inflammation Pain before tissue resistance	Decreased inflammation Pain during tissue resistance	Absence of inflammation Pain after tissue resistance
Massage intervention	(3–7 days after injury) *Main goal:* Protection Control and support effects of inflammation PRICE treatment (protection, rest, ice, compression, and elevation) Promote healing and prevent compensation patterns Passive movement midrange General massage and lymphatic drainage with caution Support for rest with full-body massage	(14–21 days after injury) *Main goal:* Controlled motion Promote development of mobile scar Cautious, controlled soft tissue mobilization of scar tissue along fiber direction toward injury Active and passive, open and closed-chain range of motion (midrange) Support for healing with full-body massage	(3–12 months after injury) *Main goal:* Return to function Increase strength and alignment of scar tissue Cross-fiber friction of scar tissue coupled with directional stroking along lines of tension away from injury Progressive stretching and active and resisted range of motion (full range) Support for rehabilitation activities with full-body massage

or protocol; rather, it is an individualized approach based on care/treatment plans. To provide an outcome-based massage, the practitioner must use clinical reasoning and critical thinking skills (Tables 11.2 and 11.3).

The main purpose of intervention is to help the body regain homeostasis, symmetry, ease of movement, and optimal function. Therefore, when observing gait or posture, the practitioner should note areas that seem pulled, twisted, low, or high. The massage therapist's job is to use massage methods to lengthen shortened areas, untwist twisted areas, raise low areas, lower high areas, soften hard areas, firm up soft areas, warm cold areas, and cool hot areas.

After rapport has been established, clients are comfortable and begin to trust the massage therapist. They will communicate a variety of information during the discussion or the massage session. The practitioner should listen for repeated phrases, such as "It's a real pain in the neck" or "I can hardly stand up to it." The massage therapist should not counsel or explain the ramifications of the information, only notice the pattern and keep general clinical notes.

Careful attention should be paid to the order of priority in which the client relays the information. If the headache is mentioned first, the knee ache second, and the tight elbow last, the areas should be dealt with in that order, if possible, in the

Table 11.3 Massage Approach During Healing

Acute Phase
Manage pain Support
Subacute Phase (Early)
Manage pain Support sleep Manage edema Manage compensation patterns
Subacute Phase (Later)
Manage pain Support sleep Manage edema Manage compensation patterns Support rehabilitative activity Support mobile scar development Support tissue regeneration process
Remodeling Phase
Support rehabilitation activity Encourage appropriate scar tissue development Manage adhesions Restore firing patterns, gait reflexes, and neuromuscular responses Eliminate reversible compensation patterns Manage irreversible compensation patterns Restore tissue pliability

From Fritz S: *Sports and exercise massage: comprehensive care in fitness, athletics, and rehabilitation*, St. Louis, 2013, Mosby.

massage flow. A client typically says "It's tight there" if a motor tone problem is the trouble. "Stiff" can apply either to a connective tissue problem or a fluid retention problem (muscle tone), and "stuck" often indicates a joint problem.

The importance of listening to understand is paramount. Many experienced professionals have learned that if we listen to our clients, they will tell us what is wrong and how to help them restore balance. The best way to do this is not to jump to conclusions, to pay attention, and to let the information unfold. Realize that each client is the expert about themselves. Clients are your teachers about themselves, and in teaching you, they often begin to understand themselves better. In every session, approach each client with fascination about what you will learn from them. No textbook, class, or instructor can equal the teaching provided by careful attention to the client.

As previously stated, specific protocols (recipes) or modalities for therapeutic intervention seldom work without modification because each person is different. Protocols provide a model of how to begin a therapeutic process, but the massage professional must modify applications of methods based on the client's individual needs and circumstances. The ability to process information effectively in the development of a therapeutic plan is based on a clinical reasoning approach rather than protocols.

The ability to apply what is learned comes from a clinical reasoning/problem-solving process. Effective work with clients becomes a continual learning process of performing a pre-massage assessment, determining intervention procedures, analyzing their effectiveness through post-massage assessment, and recognizing progress made from session to session. Even in the most basic sessions with a client, when the goals are pleasure and relaxation, decisions must be made about the best way to encourage the body to respond to meet the particular client's goals.

After a history has been completed and an assessment performed, the information gathered is analyzed and interpreted. The next step is to make decisions about what to do and how to develop the process into a coordinated, effective plan for achieving the client's goals. This information was first presented in Chapter 4; now we put it all together (Table 11.4).

As noted in Chapter 4, sessions with massage professionals are goal oriented. Goals describe desired outcomes. A primary reason for developing care/treatment plans is to set achievable goals and outline a general plan for reaching them. It is important to develop measurable, activity-based (functional) goals that are meaningful to the client. Goals must be *quantifiable* (measurable) and *qualifiable* (experiential—that is, related to what they can achieve for the client).

EXAMPLE

1. The goal for massage is to increase pliability in burn-related scar tissue to increase in range of motion of the shoulder from 80 degrees of abduction to 100 degrees of abduction. *(Quantifiable)*
2. The client will be able to reach above shoulder height. *(Qualifiable)*

Table 11.4 Assessment Procedures Related to Outcome Goals

Goal	Interview	Observe	Pain Evaluation	Postural Assessment	Functional Physical Capacity	Gait Assessment	Joint Range of Motion	Orthopedic Tests	Palpation	Muscle Testing
Relaxation/ well-being	x	x							x	
Stress management	x	x			x		x		x	x
Pain management	x	x	x	x	x		x	x	x	x
Functional mobility	x	x	x	x	x	x	x	x	x	x

The database developed in history taking and assessment procedures, combined with any health care treatment orders from other professionals, provides the foundation for clinical reasoning and decision making. Decisions are based on an analysis of the database information. The following five-part analysis process has been presented in many ways throughout this text:

1. Review the facts and information collected.

   Questions that can help with this process include the following:
   - What are the facts?
   - What is considered normal or balanced function?
   - What has happened? (Spell out events.)
   - What caused the imbalance? (Can it be identified?)
   - What was done or is being done?
   - What has worked or not worked?
2. Brainstorm the possibilities.

   Questions that can help with this process include the following:
   - What are the possibilities? (What could it all mean?)
   - What does my intuition suggest?
   - What are the possible patterns of dysfunction?
   - What are the possible contributing factors?
   - What are possible interventions?
   - What might work?
   - What are other ways to look at the situation?
3. Consider the logical outcome of each possibility.

   Questions that can help with this process include the following:
   - What is the logical progression of the symptom pattern, contributing factors, and current behaviors?
   - What is the logical cause and effect of each intervention identified during brainstorming?
   - What are the pros and cons of each intervention suggested? (Remember to look at both sides of the issue.)
   - What are the consequences of not acting?
   - What are the consequences of acting?
4. Consider how the people involved would be affected by each possibility.

   Questions that can help with this process include the following:
   - For each intervention considered, what is the impact on the people involved: client, practitioner, and other professionals working with the client?
   - How does each person involved feel about the possible interventions?
   - Is the practitioner within their scope of practice to work with such situations?
   - Does the practitioner feel qualified to work with such situations?
   - Does a feeling of cooperation and agreement exist among all parties involved?
5. Results of the process.

   Based on your analysis, answer the following questions:

1. Does the client need referral? If so, to which professionals?
2. What are the measurable function goals for the care/treatment plan?
3. What interventions would you choose to achieve those goals?
4. How would you use them to address the various imbalances?
5. What results do you expect?
6. How long do you think it will take to achieve the goals?

Creating the Care/Treatment Plan

The development of a care/treatment plan is based on the five-part analysis just described. After completing the analysis, the practitioner can decide what will be involved in the care/treatment plan. Methods are chosen to achieve the agreed-on goals for the session. The plan is not an exact protocol set in stone; rather, it is a guideline. The care/treatment plan may evolve over the first three or four sessions and may be altered if a change occurs in the therapeutic goals or the client's status.

Decision making becomes a part of each session. As the care/treatment plan unfolds with each successive session, an update on effects, progress, and setbacks is discussed with the client before the massage begins. An updated targeted assessment based on goals is performed, and clinical reasoning and problem solving are used to choose the most effective methods for achieving the best results for the current session. As the plan is implemented, it is recorded sequentially, session by session, in some form of charting or documentation process (e.g., SOAP notes; see Chapter 4).

The effectiveness or ineffectiveness of intervention procedures is analyzed and compared with the results of previous sessions. Review of the charting notes from previous sessions becomes the foundation for this analysis. The plan is refined, reevaluated, and adjusted as necessary as the sessions progress (See Chapter 16).

During the massage, assessment and intervention intermingle. Differentiating the two is difficult, except through careful observation. For the experienced massage therapist, assessment and intervention interact in the context of the massage session. An area of imbalance is discovered through various methods of palpation and passive and active range of motion. Assessment leads into intervention, often simply by gently increasing the intensity or duration of the original evaluation method and repeating the methods three or four times.

Reassessment

After the massage is complete, a reassessment must be done to determine what changes the body has made. This can be done efficiently by targeting a few major areas that were the core focus of the massage. The reassessment process helps the client integrate the body changes. The before-and-after awareness is also a reinforcing factor for the client regarding the benefits of massage.

The entire process of massage is an assessment, an intervention for adaptation, and then a reassessment to see whether the approach was beneficial. This takes practice. During the learning process, assessment and reassessment can feel choppy. The skilled massage therapist learns through practice to flow between the three steps of assessment, intervention/adaptation,

Box 11.13 Additional Mechanisms of Dysfunction

Additional powerful determinants of normal function are righting reflexes in the neck. These reflexes, when coordinated with the eyes, keep the body oriented perpendicular to a horizontal plane. Balance mechanisms of the inner ear also are a factor. Any inner ear difficulties or visual distortion affects neuromuscular interactions and postural balance patterns.

A common and often undiagnosed eye and ear problem is benign paroxysmal (or vestibular) positional vertigo, which occurs when otolith crystals in the inner ear become displaced and send erroneous positional information to the balance and muscle coordination centers in the lower brain. The eyes are linked through the righting reflex mechanism. Various muscle tension patterns can be linked to this and other, similar conditions. Referral to the appropriate health care professional is important for proper diagnosis.

and reassessment during the massage, providing a sense of continuity and fluidity to the session (Box 11.13).

Foot in the Door

If you want a successful career as a massage therapist, designing and adapting massage application to each individual is absolutely essential. If you want to get your foot in the door where health care insurance may pay for massage, you need to perfect your assessment skills and be able to justify the benefits of the massage treatment plan. You can get your foot in the door of health care practices such as chiropractors, hospitals, and clinics by demonstrating the ability to fine-tune massage application with assessment skills and treatment planning.

SUMMARY

Massage is a whole body discipline. Assessment skills are the basis for developing intuition; this is done by learning to pay closer attention and becoming more skilled in the interpretation of the assessment information. With practice and experience, these skills become almost second nature.

Trained massage professionals who consider themselves therapists modify methods to best address the client's needs. Massage therapists not only perform massage "routines," as does the massage technician, but they also adjust and adapt massage applications in an outcome-based approach. Massage methods are simple; however, when they are applied with the right intensity and in the right location, the body recognizes the stimulation and can respond resourcefully. This is the approach used by a competent massage therapist. This learning is continuous; the client never stops teaching the therapist.

The more reliable the assessment information, the more likely it is to be accurately interpreted. The more accurate the interpretation, the more specific the application of massage methods. Massage and bodywork techniques are relatively basic. Soft tissue can be pushed, pulled, shaken, stretched, and pounded, regardless of the bodywork system. Forces applied to accentuate change are tension, bend, shear, compression, and torsion. The only variables are the location of the application; the intensity, including drag, depth of pressure, and rhythm; the direction; the frequency; and the duration. The detective work and skills required to assist the client in figuring out each individual pattern prevent the massage therapist from becoming bored, which can occur if the same protocol is administered over and over.

The bottom line is the client knows their body best. The practitioner's job is to understand what the client says verbally, visually, through body language, and in the tissues and movement patterns. Each person's body language is unique. It takes time to learn it. Only through listening, observing, touching, and then using effective clinical reasoning skills can massage therapists begin to recognize the patterns, which ultimately allows them to find solutions for the individual.

The massage therapist should not hesitate to ask for help and should refer a client when the problem is beyond the professional skills determined by the scope of practice for massage therapy and the professional's individual training. By joining in the team approach with other health professionals, the massage practitioner can become an important part of the complex client treatment process.

Practice enables the massage professional's skills to grow. After completing 1000 massage sessions, the massage professional begins to own the information learned in school. After 5000 massage sessions, the massage professional has enough experience to begin to trust the process of massage. After 10,000 massages, the massage therapist mindfully intermingles assessment and intervention if needed into an elegant session.

Robert Fulghum (1991) tells a story about hiccups that epitomizes massage:

The reason most cures work, at some time on some people, is that hiccups usually last from between seven and 63 hicks before stopping of their own accord. Whatever you do to pass the time while the episode runs its course seems to qualify as a cure, so the more entertaining the cure is, the better. The hiccuper will be treated with great solicitation while in the throes of these mini convulsions, and the individual who has produced the winning cure will be looked upon with respect.

Applications of therapeutic massage certainly are "entertaining" for the body, and conditions often do improve with therapeutic massage. When a massage intervention allows more efficient functioning for a client, massage professionals should focus on educating the client about the body's responses so that the client begins to experience personal empowerment and recognizes the body's own healing potential.

Learn More on the Web

To learn more about assessment and biomechanics, visit the National Science Foundation, National Institutes of Health, and Neuromuscular Research Laboratory (NMRL), which is the applied research facility of the University of Pittsburgh's Department of Sports Medicine and Nutrition, within the School of Health and Rehabilitation Sciences. More suggestions and links are on the Evolve site.

Evolve

Visit the Evolve website: http://evolve.elsevier.com/Fritz/fundamentals/

Evolve content designed for massage therapy licensing exam review and comprehension of content beyond the textbook.

Evolve content includes:

- Content Updates
- Science and Pathology Animations
- Body Spectrum Coloring Book
- MBLEx exam review multiple choice questions

FOR EACH CHAPTER FIND:

- Answers and rationales for the end-of-chapter multiple-choice questions
- Electronic workbook and answer key
- Chapter multiple choice question quiz
- Quick content review in question form and answers
- Technique videos when applicable
- Learn more on the Web

REFERENCES

Bettini EA, Moore K, Wang Y, Hinds PS, Finkel JC. Association between pain sensitivity, central sensitization, and functional disability in adolescents with joint hypermobility. *J Pediatr Nurs*. 2018;42:34–38.

Bizzi E, Cheung VC. The neural origin of muscle synergies. *Front Comput Neurosci*. 2013;7:51.

Chaitow L. *Soft-Tissue Manipulation: A Practitioner's Guide to the Diagnosis and Treatment of Soft-Tissue Dysfunction and Reflex Activity*. 4th ed. Rochester, Vt: Inner Traditions/Bear & Co; 1988.

Chaitow L, Gilbert C, Bradley D. *Recognizing and Treating Breathing Dysfunction: A Multidisciplinary Approach*. 2nd ed. Edinburgh: Churchill Livingstone Elsevier; 2014.

DeStefano L. *Greenman's Principles of Manual Medicine*. 4th ed. Baltimore: Williams & Wilkins; 2011.

Dischiavi SL, Wright AA, Hegedus EJ, Bleakley CM. Biotensegrity and myofascial chains: A global approach to an integrated kinetic chain. *Med Hypotheses*. 2018;110:90–96.

Eccles JA, Scott HE, Davies KA, Bond R, Harrison NA. Joint hypermobility and its relevance to common mental illness in adolescents: A population-based longitudinal study. *J Psychosom Res*. 2018;109:100.

Fulghum R. *Uh-oh*. New York: Villard Books; 1991.

Gouveia JP, Forte P, Ribeiro J, Coelho E. Study of the Association between Postural Misalignments in School Students. *Symmetry*. 2021;13(10):1959.

Haas M, Cooperstein R, Peterson D. Disentangling manual muscle testing and applied kinesiology: critique and reinterpretation of a literature review. *Chiropr Osteopat*. 2007;15:11.

Hall S, Lewith G, Brien S, et al. A review of the literature in applied and specialized kinesiology. *Forsch Komplementmed*. 2008;15:40.

Kamel E, Abdelmajeed S, Khozamy H El, Hassan K. Trunk and hip muscles activation patterns in subjects with and without chronic low back pain: A systematic review. *Physiotherapy Quarterly*. 2021;29(2):79–88.

Kripa S, Kaur H. Identifying relations between posture and pain in lower back pain patients: a narrative review. *Bulletin of Faculty of Physical Therapy*. 2021;26(1):1–4.

Kiruthika S, Rekha K, Preethy G, Abraham M. Prevalence of postural dysfunction among female college students-a qualitative analysis. *Biol Med*. 2018;10(1):1–3.

Lee JH, Jeong HJ, Cynn HS, Kang TW. Metatarsophalangeal joint flexion affects dorsiflexor activity in subjects with a dominant extensor hallucis longus. *J Back Musculoskele Rehabil (Preprint)*. 2018:1–8.

Manske RC. *Fundamental Orthopedic Management for the Physical Therapist Assistant*. 4th ed. St Louis: Elsevier; 2016.

Melzack R. The McGill Pain Questionnaire. In: Melzack R, ed. *Pain Measurement and Assessment*. New York: Raven Press; 1983.

Melzack R. The short-form McGill pain questionnaire. *Pain*. 1987;30:191.

Nelson KE, Sergueef N, Glonek T. Recording the rate of the cranial rhythmic impulse. *J Am Osteopath Assoc*. 2006;106:337.

Nicholson LL, Simmonds J, Pacey V, De Wandele I, Rombaut L, Williams CM, Chan C. International Perspectives on Joint Hypermobility: A Synthesis of Current Science to Guide Clinical and Research Directions. *JCR: Journal of Clinical Rheumatology*. 2022;28(6):314–320.

Norkin CC, Levangie PK. *Joint Structure and Function: A Comprehensive Analysis*. 4th ed. Philadelphia: F.A. Davis; 2005.

Perrin RN. Lymphatic drainage of the neuraxis in chronic fatigue syndrome: a hypothetical model for the cranial rhythmic impulse. *J Am Osteopath Assoc*. 2007;107:218. Retrieved from: http://www.jaoa.org/cgi/content/full/107/6/218.

Smith LK, Weiss E, Lehmkuhl L. *Brunnstrom's Clinical Kinesiology (Brunnstrom's Clinical Kinesiology Series)*. 5th ed. Philadelphia: FA Davis; 1996.

Solanki R, Mehta M. Occupational health and postural discomfort faced by bankers due to computer usage. *Age*. 2022;20(30):16 (in years).

Tresch MC, Jarc A. The case for and against muscle synergies. *Curr Opin Neurobiol*. 2009;19(6):601–607.

Wolfe F, Smythe HA, Yunus MB, et al. The American college of rheumatology 1990 criteria for classification of fibromyalgia. Report of the multicenter criteria committee. *Arthritis Rheum*. 1990;33:160.

Zarzycki R, Malloy P, Eckenrode BJ, Fagan J, Malloy M, Mangione KK. Application of the 4-Element Movement System Model to sports physical therapy practice and education. *International Journal of Sports Physical Therapy*. 2022;17(1):18.

MULTIPLE-CHOICE QUESTIONS FOR DISCUSSION AND REVIEW

The answers, with rationales, can be found on the Evolve site. Use these questions to stimulate discussion and dialogue. You have to understand the meaning of the words in the question and possible answers. Each question provides you with the ability to review terminology, practice critical thinking skills, and improve multiple choice test taking skills. Answers and rationales are on the Evolve site. It is just as important to know why the wrong answers are wrong as why the correct answer is correct.

1. A massage practitioner identifies an area of restricted tissue and immediately uses skin rolling to increase connective tissue pliability. How did this interfere with assessment processes?
   a. The localized treatment did not prove effective.
   b. The pattern was changed before it was understood.
   c. The therapist did not chart the area before the massage.
   d. The method was not appropriate to the condition.
2. Which of the following is INCORRECT when using muscle strength testing?
   a. Isolate muscles and position at the mid-range of ROM.
   b. Use a force sufficient to recruit a full response of the tested muscles and the surrounding muscles.
   c. Use a slow and even counterpressure to pull or push the muscle out of the isolated position.
   d. Compare muscle tests bilaterally for symmetry.
3. During the interview process, a client continues to grab the tissue at the back of the neck and pull it. What is the most logical explanation for this gesture?
   a. Nerve entrapment
   b. Joint compression
   c. Trigger point
   d. Connective tissue shortening
4. A physician refers a client for massage for circulation enhancement to the limbs. The client complains of cold hands and feet. Assessment indicates decreased pliability of the tissues around the elbows and knees. Work-related

activities require repetitive movement in these areas. The massage professional presents three main approaches for the physician to consider:

1. General massage and rest
2. General massage with connective tissue stretching in the restricted areas
3. Compression focused specifically to the arteries to encourage circulation

After considering all three options, the physician eliminates option 1 as too time consuming. Option 2 seems viable, but the client does not respond well to methods that may be painful. Option 3 seems too limited an approach to the massage professional. The decision is to begin with option 3 and expand to connective tissue methods when the client is able to tolerate them. Which part of this process best reflects brainstorming possibilities?

a. Data collection
b. Analysis of outcomes based on pros and cons
c. Generating the options
d. Assessment for more facts

5. A client experienced an episode of severe low back pain 3 years ago. The diagnosis was a compressed disk at L4. The condition has stabilized and pain is experienced only occasionally. Assessment indicates shortened lumbar fascia, increased lateral flexion to the right, and a high shoulder on the right. The massage professional specifically addressed these areas and noted improvement following the massage. The next day the client called complaining that the low back was in spasm. What is the most logical reason for what happened?
   a. The phasic muscles were too weak to maintain posture.
   b. The gait shifted so that there was a more normal heel strike.
   c. Facilitated segments in the skeletal muscles went into spasm.
   d. Resourceful compensation patterns were disturbed.

6. When one is evaluating a treatment plan for successful client compliance, which of the following would provide the best information?
   a. Any referral information from the health care provider
   b. Completing a comprehensive physical assessment
   c. Generating multiple treatment options
   d. Indications of enthusiasm for the plan by the client and any support system

7. During walking and running, the upper and lower limbs function contralaterally for counterbalance. This being the case, if the shoulder flexion on the right is activated and the hip flexors on the left are assessed, what would be the most logical result?
   a. The muscles should be inhibited.
   b. The muscles should be facilitated.
   c. The muscles should be functioning eccentrically.
   d. The muscles should be fibrotic.

8. During assessment, the massage therapist identifies that the rectus abdominis is firing first during trunk flexion. What does this mean?
   a. This is a normal firing pattern for hip abduction.
   b. Trunk flexion firing pattern is normal.
   c. Trunk flexion firing pattern is synergistic dominant.
   d. The psoas is normal and hip extension is abnormal.

9. During postural assessment, the massage professional observes that the client's shoulder girdle is rotated to the left. Which of the following histories is most likely to be the cause?
   a. The client regularly reaches to the left when answering the phone.
   b. The client often wears boots when riding horses.
   c. The client does weight-bearing exercise with machines 3 times a week.
   d. The client wears tight clothing.

10. A regular client has a grade 2 left ankle sprain and is using a crutch to maintain balance when walking. During assessment of posture, the massage therapist notices an elevated right shoulder. What is happening to cause this?
   a. The client is closing an open kinetic chain pattern.
   b. The muscles of the right lower leg are inhibited.
   c. The symmetrical stance is enhanced.
   d. The body is displaying compensation patterns.

11. While observing a client walk, the massage professional notices that the pelvis does not move evenly. The client complains of focused pain in the right sacral area. Which of the following is most correct?
   a. Create a massage treatment plan describing specific treatment for sacroiliac dysfunction.
   b. May indicate the need for referral, with current massage focused on general nonspecific approaches.
   c. Design a massage to lengthen the left leg to balance the pelvic rotation.
   d. Immediately refer the client to a chiropractor for sacroiliac dysfunction.

12. A client is complaining of weakness and heaviness in the muscles that flex the left thigh. During muscle testing, the muscle group is found to be inhibited. Based on gait patterns, which of the following muscle groups also should be inhibited?
   a. Right arm flexors
   b. Left arm flexors
   c. Right thigh flexors
   d. Left thigh extensors

13. A client is experiencing spasms in the left thigh flexor muscles. An attempt to muscle test the area could result in a cramp. The massage professional remembers that activation of the gait reflexes can facilitate or inhibit muscle contraction. Which group of muscles would the massage professional have the client contract to inhibit the left thigh flexors?
   a. Left arm flexors
   b. Right arm flexors
   c. Left arm extensors
   d. Right thigh extensors

14. If the area between C7 and T12 is pulled forward, making the chest concave, with a right rotation pattern making the right shoulder more forward than the left, where are the shortened soft tissues?
  a. Anterior thorax on the right
  b. Right lumbar posterior
  c. Left thorax posterior
  d. Lower abdominal on the right

15. A client has increased internal rotation of the right shoulder. Which of the following is the best massage approach to reverse the condition?
  a. Frictioning and traction to the external rotators
  b. Muscle energy with lengthening of the internal rotators
  c. Compression and tapotement to the internal rotators
  d. Stretching of the flexors and extensors with lengthening to the external rotators

16. During range of motion assessment, if full extension of the shoulder has a hard end-feel, what would be a logical conclusion?
  a. The shoulder assesses as normal.
  b. The shoulder has a firing pattern dysfunction.
  c. The anatomic range of movement is dysfunctional.
  d. The shoulder has joint dysfunction.

17. A client has recurring hamstring strain and currently is experiencing low back pain. Which of the following is the most logical cause?
  a. Hip extension firing pattern dysfunction
  b. Soft end-feel of the hip joint
  c. Scapular fixation with external rotation
  d. Overpressure of the symphysis pubis

18. A massage professional positions the client's body to assess the strength of the hip flexors. Which is the correct position for the hand applying resistance?
  a. Near the hip
  b. At the ankle
  c. At the distal end of the femur
  d. On the tibia

19. A client is experiencing pain with any activity involving external/lateral rotation of the right shoulder. Range of motion is limited to 40 degrees. This condition has been coming on gradually. Muscle testing indicates weakness when resistance is applied to move the shoulder from external rotation to internal rotation. There is shortening in the muscles of internal rotation. Which of the following would be the most logical treatment plan?
  a. Muscle energy methods to support lengthening of the infraspinatus and methods to increase tone in the subscapularis
  b. Deep massage to the rhomboid muscles and stretching of the lumbar fascia
  c. Traction of the scapulothoracic junction
  d. Massage to reduce tension in the pectoralis major and latissimus dorsi with tapotement to stimulate tone in the infraspinatus and teres major

20. A client is lying supine, and observation indicates that the left leg is rotated internally. What should muscle testing reveal?
  a. Muscles that externally rotate the hip are short, and muscles that internally rotate the hip are inhibited.
  b. Muscles that externally rotate the hip are inhibited, and muscles that internally rotate the hip are overly strong.
  c. Gluteus medius should test weak.
  d. Adductor longus should test weak.

UNIT IV

Beyond the Basics

Complementary Bodywork Systems

CHAPTER 12

http://evolve.elsevier.com/Fritz/fundamentals/

CHAPTER OBJECTIVES

After completing this chapter, the student will be able to perform the following:

1. Describe the physiological mechanisms of complementary bodywork systems.
2. Explain and implement hydrotherapy as an adjunct to massage application.
3. Describe the use of stones and other tools used for thermotherapy.
4. Safely integrate aromatherapy into the massage process.
5. Describe the safe use of implements and kinesiology tape during a massage session.
6. Modify massage application to support beneficial blood and lymph movement in the body.
7. Modify massage application to target the connective tissues of the body.
8. Identify and effectively use massage to address trigger points.
9. Explain the fundamental concepts of Asian bodywork and incorporate the simple application of acupuncture and acupressure methods into massage therapy.
10. Compare shiatsu and Thai massage and incorporate mat methods into massage.
11. Explore the healing philosophy of Ayurveda.
12. Use the principles of polarity therapy as an energetic adjunct method.
13. Modify foot massage to incorporate the philosophy of reflexology.

CHAPTER OUTLINE

KEY TERMS

Acupressure	Lymphedema
Acupuncture	Meridians
Adjunct	Myofascial approaches
Aromatherapy	Neuromuscular therapy
Ayurveda	Polarity
Cryotherapy	PRICE first aid
Cultural appropriation	Reflexology
Essential oils	Shiatsu
Hydrotherapy	Systemic massage
Implement	Thai massage
Latent trigger point	Thermotherapy
Lipedema	Transverse frictioning
Lymphatic drainage	Trigger point

This chapter presents a brief overview of bodywork systems that can be incorporated into massage, suggestions for implementing the basic concepts and techniques that overlap well with massage therapy, and guidance for the development of an integrated system.

The chapter describes four classifications of bodywork:

- Therapeutic massage adaptation so specific it is often incorrectly classified as a system of bodywork outside of massage therapy
- Eastern- and Asian-based methods of bodywork from cultural traditions
- Adjunct approaches often included with massage
- Adjunct energy-based extremely light or no-touch methods

The many different systems of bodywork cluster into six categories:

- Stimulus/response reflex systems (e.g., hydrotherapy)
- Fluid movement systems (e.g., lymphatic drainage)
- Structural systems (e.g., Rolfing/structural integration and myofascial release)
- Neuromuscular methods (e.g., trigger point therapy)
- Eastern and Asian methods involving vital energy, chakras, meridians, and points
- Energetic systems (e.g., polarity)

Methods based on extreme specialization are often called soft tissue mobilization, manual therapy, or lymphatic drainage but use the same methods as massage adapted to target a specific tissue type or physiologic function or dysfunction. It is unfortunate that this separation has occurred. Therapeutic massage is soft tissue mobilization, manual therapy, and it can be adapted to affect body fluids or influence connective tissue. In this category the chapter describes fluid movement, connective tissue-targeted methods, and addressing trigger points.

Another layer of confusion involves aspects of Asian, Eastern, and other culturally based bodywork systems being incorporated into massage. This is called **cultural appropriation** which is the unacknowledged or inappropriate adoption of the customs, practices, ideas, etc. of one people or society by members of another and typically more dominant people or society: These healing systems are unique, complex practices that require extensive education and experience to truly embrace the philosophy and rich foundation of each system. It is questionable whether taking small segments out of the total system and adding these bits into massage is ethical. Yet this is currently the case in the massage profession. These pieces are often mixed into massage therapy as adjuncts. Adding to the confusion is that these culturally based healing systems typically have a component of massage-type application. To put it more directly, you cannot remove a part of a whole and expect the part will honor the whole. (Mentoring Tip).

Adjunct means an additional part added to something but not essentially a part of it, that is, something used in addition to the primary therapy but not part of the primary approach. In the massage community, the adjuncts commonly used are hydrotherapy, thermotherapy, aromatherapy, and implements and devices such as vacuum/suction cups (cupping) or mechanical percussion and vibration devices used to augment massage. Music can be used therapeutically as an adjunct method (Ilkkaya et al., 2014).

Another methodology often combined with massage is energy-based approaches. These methods do not have to include physical contact and often include a spiritual platform. Because physical contact is not made during an energy-based-type session, these approaches are not massage.

The chapter is organized to take advantage of similarities among bodywork systems. The first adjunct methods discussed are hydrotherapy, thermotherapy, and aromatherapy. Hydrotherapy and thermotherapy are excellent adjuncts to massage and can be included in the massage session by using hot and cold packs, stones, or footbaths in addition to the massage. Often aromatherapy is combined with hydrotherapy, such as in scented footbaths or steam inhalation during the massage. Essential oils typically are used as an additive to the massage lubricant.

MENTORING TIP

It is confusing. The easily classified adjuncts, such as hydrotherapy, which are common add-ons in the massage practice, require additional study for safe use. What is covered in this chapter primarily focuses on safety. If you are interested in the cultural healing systems, be respectful and realize that an introduction does not make you competent. The separation of connective tissue methods and fluid movement methods from massage is similar to separation of bits from culturally based systems. Adaptation of massage using the 12 modifiers targeted to a specific tissue should not be the foundation for a separate bodywork system; however, in the massage and bodywork realm this has occurred. Furthermore, tender/trigger points are a condition, not a method. Yes, all of this is confusing and unfortunate.

Various tools or implements are discussed next. Specific recommendations are provided for skin scraping methods and suction methods.

The next category of methods addresses the movement of fluids in the body. The lymphatic and circulatory systems are the main focus. Hydrotherapy, thermotherapy, and aromatherapy also influence fluid movement, or, in the case of aromatherapy, move through the body using blood as a means of transport.

The connective tissue, myofascial, and trigger point assessment and intervention methods are next. When combined, these approaches form the basic techniques of many fascia-based methods and neuromuscular therapy. Understand that just because something has a different name does not mean it is a different method. Usually the name of a method is a marketing strategy, especially if the name does not describe what anatomy, physiology, and pathology is being targeted by the approach. For example, this combination of approaches has been incorrectly called *deep tissue massage. Pressure* is a modifier used to adapt massage application. *Deep* as a descriptor is much too abstract and is a directional term. There are many layers of soft tissue in any given area, all superficial or deep to each other. The name *deep tissue massage* is inaccurate, confusing, and should be avoided.

Asian and Eastern bodywork systems are presented next. It is interesting that most trigger points (93%-97%) are in the same location as traditional Chinese acupuncture points. Another interesting fact is that acupuncture points and meridian locations are closely related to the enveloping deep fascia around muscle groups. Current thought is that trigger points and acupuncture points likely describe the same physiologic phenomena.

The Asian systems described are traditional Chinese medicine (TCM) and shiatsu (Japanese). Reflexology is actually based on TCM even though it has been westernized; therefore, it appears with this group. Also included in the Eastern system is Ayurveda from India and traditional Thai massage from Thailand, which has its roots in Ayurveda. The chakras are included in the Ayurvedic physiology. Dr. Randolf Stone combined these systems with principles of body energy flow into polarity therapy. A short segment on color therapy is included because the Asian and Eastern systems place importance on the value of color both in assessment and treatment.

The element that all these systems have in common with therapeutic massage is the application of touch in a structured way to introduce various forms of sensory and mechanical information to the body to effect positive physiologic change. The language of each system is different, and the theory bases vary. The methods of assessment for each approach are distinctive and generally unique to that approach. Do not become too concerned with, or overwhelmed by, the different terminologies that describe the same elements of anatomy and physiology in each bodywork method.

This text does not attempt to describe the various systems in depth; rather, it is devoted to the professional practice of therapeutic massage. Expertise in any of the systems requires specific study. Massage students have enough to learn about therapeutic massage; they should not be expected also to develop expertise in the other styles. Nor does it seem necessary to attempt to become proficient in multiple bodywork styles because the ultimate result of the application for all of them is essentially the same. In simple terms, pick one (maybe two) and learn it (them) well.

The information in this chapter is not sufficient training to enable the practitioner to understand and use these methods purposefully and intelligently for anything other than general enhancement of the skills already developed. However, with a commitment to further education, these methods can add efficiency, effectiveness, and enthusiasm for the benefits that therapeutic massage has to offer with regard to wellness, prevention, rehabilitation, and client-directed healing. It is important for massage practitioners to understand the basis of other methods so that they know when a client might be better served by referral to other practitioners.

As you practice the various methods presented, pay attention to areas in which you display a particular interest and talent; this can help direct you to specific avenues for continuing education.

COMPLEMENTARY BODYWORK SYSTEMS

SECTION OBJECTIVES

Chapter objective covered in this section:

1. Describe the physiological mechanisms of complementary bodywork systems.

Using the information presented in this section, the student will be able to perform the following:

- Identify similarities in bodywork methods.

In their book *Zen Shiatsu: How to Harmonize Yin and Yang for Better Health*, Masunaga and Ohashi (1977) describe the interface of various bodywork methods:

> *Some professional therapists insist that a great difference exists among the three (Amma [Chinese], Western massage, shiatsu [Japanese]) forms of treatment. I believe that a great difference cannot exist within a general field, in this case, manually applied stimulation to the human body. Of course, there are a variety of methods and schools, but basically they are similar. It is important to note that effectiveness of any treatment depends on both the practitioner and the method working together. So the effectiveness of any treatment can vary greatly from one practitioner to another. All three methods of manipulation aim at stabilizing the functioning of the human body, the difference being whether they stimulate blood circulation and nerve interactions directly or indirectly. The effectiveness of manipulative therapy has been proven by modern scientific experiments involving cutaneous stimulation. From this point of view, no difference exists among the basic three techniques, though they were developed from different principles. The purpose of manipulative therapy is to work with a person's natural healing force to correct any internal malfunctioning particular to that person.*

Many massage professionals continue their therapeutic massage learning through the comprehensive study of a single additional bodywork approach. Other practitioners study many different bodywork modalities, some in considerable depth and others more superficially. They then integrate the information into therapeutic massage, variations, concepts, and an expanded look at the body.

Basis of Bodywork

You can apply pressure, lift and pull tissue, rock the body, stroke the skin, move the joints, generate tissue repair by creating therapeutic inflammation, stimulate reflex responses, and provide the client with interpersonal and professional support, compassion, and acceptance. Regardless of the theoretical, historical, and cultural base, all the bodywork systems, including therapeutic massage, are built on this foundation.

Expertise in any bodywork system consists of quality assessment for the purpose of making effective decisions about the application of treatment to provide a service that benefits the client. Within these bodywork systems a unique form of assessment may exist. For example, traditional Chinese medicine includes assessment of the tongue for color, coating, and shape and of the pulse as it relates to various meridians. Information is gathered and analyzed, a plan is made and implemented, and results are evaluated.

Benefits derived from receiving these various methods range from pleasure and comfort to ongoing management of chronic conditions and stress, in addition to a therapeutic change process (Tick et al., 2018; Bayülgen and Gün, 2022).

Body, Mind, and Spirit

Bodywork—therapeutic massage as a complete system within the broader realm—serves the wholeness of the individual through a direct influence on the body and a respect for the mind and spirit. The concept of the body-mind-spirit connection found in many complementary systems of bodywork leads to the acceptance of the unity and integrity of the individual. Consideration must include various aspects of the person, although never separate from the whole. As discussed at the beginning of this textbook, the skin is not separate from the emotions, nor the emotions separate from the organs, nor the organs separate from the muscles. No part is separate from the spirit or the context of our influence on others, society, culture, and the larger expanse of the universe. These concepts are reflected in a whole person, client-centered approach within the biopsychosocial model of care.

In many bodywork traditions, this interconnectedness is also apparent. For example, the Ayurvedic medicine of India is similar to Asian medicine. These healing practices are similar to the Indigenous people around the globe. In Thailand, Tibet, Russia, and other parts of the world, the ancient traditions of medicine and folk health wisdom have a common difference with Western scientific thought: these systems identify body-mind-spirit lifestyle imbalance, a concept referred to in this text as dysfunction or "almost sick and not quite well." They introduce interventions to reverse this process before it cycles into body-mind-spirit disease. Western health care is beginning to embrace this concept of wholeness through prevention, and whole person care is now a consistent component of health care.

Therapeutic Massage, Relaxing Massage, Medical Massage, and All the Rest

Many names are attached to massage therapy, such as *wellness massage*, *sports massage*, *medical massage*, *prenatal massage*, *geriatric massage*, and so forth. This becomes confusing to students, massage therapists, and the public. For example, sports massage is massage that focuses on an athlete. Prenatal massage focuses on a person who is pregnant. Regardless of the population served (see Chapter 14), the most effective massage uses fundamental massage skills adapted to the client's unique circumstances (see Chapter 16). This type of massage is now called *outcome-based massage*, yet another name to confuse students, massage therapists, and the public.

The main purpose of this textbook is to train the massage professional to use massage methods intelligently, based on quality evidence (see Chapter 5), to promote health and well-being for anyone seeking massage. Massage is best used in the prevention of disease and the support of optimal health. Generally healthy people can benefit from the normalizing physiologic effects of hydrotherapy and massage adapted to address connective tissue, lymphatic and blood circulation, trigger points, and so forth. These targeted approaches can add another dimension to the effectiveness of the massage.

The current trend is toward expanding the role of the massage professional in the wellness center/spa industry. Typically, this setting reflects the integrated approach and offers clients many modalities in various combinations of service menus. For example, a hydrotherapy application, including the use of essential oils, mud and clay packs, and salt scrubs, may be combined with massage. (Specific information on spa applications is presented in Chapter 13.)

Sometimes the client may present the massage professional with minor problems that can be helped by the use of the techniques discussed in this chapter. These same methods can be used in various forms of medical care and rehabilitative procedures or with athletes. To use the methods in a more specific way, massage professionals require additional training, especially in pathophysiology, pharmacology, and medical treatment protocols, so that they can understand the integration of massage therapy into these approaches. Even when the massage practitioner deals with medical conditions and works in the medical care environment (see Chapter 13), the methods (i.e., massage manipulations and techniques as described in Chapter 10 or any of the methods described in this chapter) do not change. Some methods are more appropriate for certain conditions, and others are chosen for different outcomes. The difference is the condition of the person receiving the massage. Additional education focuses not only on learning new methods but also on learning how to choose and apply methods with clients who have various complex circumstances. It is also important to realize that different methods and approaches are beneficial but not as a stand-alone intervention or to replace massage therapy (Page, 2021).

Massage professionals who work with a client in the sports and fitness or medical setting need to increase their knowledge based on the function, dysfunction, or disease addressed. For example:

- Serving the athlete requires an understanding of training protocols, common stress patterns, and injury rehabilitation of that particular sport.
- Working with stroke rehabilitation requires increased knowledge of stroke etiology, rehabilitation, and the use of massage as part of the overall rehabilitation and management process.
- Working with clients who suffer from depression is enhanced by an understanding of the manifestations of depression, mental health interventions, and psychotropic pharmacology.

The massage professional should confer with the medical team when dealing with clients who are undergoing medical intervention (e.g., medications, physical therapy, psychotherapy, or chiropractic treatment). The massage should be integrated into the entire treatment protocol. Supervision by the medical team can help ensure that methods used for a client are monitored and evaluated for effectiveness and safety.

Before continuing with the specific content in this chapter, it is important to acknowledge that new discoveries are occurring that may change how we understand massage therapy and adjunct methods especially those that involve meridians and points (Gomes and Leão 2020; Dorsher and Helio da Silva 2022).

For example, the primo-vascular system (PVS) is distributed throughout the entire body and is composed of tiny primo-nodes (PN) storing many small cells and very small primo-vessels (PV) branching out from the nodes. The PVS integrates the features of the cardiovascular, nervous, immune, and hormonal system. Also called the *Hyaluronic Acid-rich Node and Duct System (HAR-NDS or NDS)* (Choi et al., 2019) this system has recently emerged as a third component of the circulatory system. The PVS is found in and on most organs, including the brain, and inside some lymph and blood vessels. The tiny vessels and nodes are difficult to see because they are semitransparent and very tiny, which may be the main reason it was not discovered until recently as the technology became available to identify the structures. There is fluid movement in the vessels, and it is speculated that this system has a role in regeneration. Another important finding is its potential relevance to cancer metastasis. Researchers are investigating if the PVS may be the physical location for the traditional acupuncture points and meridians. More research is needed (Kang et al., 2013; Soh et al., 2013; Lee et al., 2014, Shin et al., 2019; Stefanov 2022).

We now know that there is a lymphatic type clearing system in the brain (Absinta 2017, Kuo et al., 2018; Buccellato et al., 2022). A body wide structure called the *interstitium* has been identified influencing understanding of fascia and fluid movement. This newfound network drains into the lymphatic system and is the source of lymph, the fluid vital to the function of immune cells which generate inflammation (Benias et al., 2018; Cenaj et al., 2021). As massage professionals, we need to maintain ethical behavior and explain massage in an evidence-informed manner based on biologic plausibility. However, as more information becomes available, we need to be open to new understandings.

HYDROTHERAPY AND THERMOTHERAPY

SECTION OBJECTIVES

Chapter objective covered in this section:

2. Explain and implement hydrotherapy as an adjunct to massage application.

Using the information presented in this section, the student will be able to perform the following:

- Explain the general effects of hot and cold-water applications.
- Incorporate simple hydrotherapy methods into a massage session.
- Suggest easy, basic hydrotherapy self-help techniques for clients.

Hydrotherapy is a distinct form of treatment that combines well with massage. Water can be used in many ways, depending on the client's health needs and condition and the facilities available for therapy. Hydrotherapy is a component of the spa environment, sports treatment, and health care. **Thermotherapy** is the use of temperature for therapeutic purposes. Thermotherapy consists of application of heat or cold. Thermotherapy is often related to the use of heat. Cold therapy especially when using ice is called **cryotherapy**. Hydrotherapy and thermotherapy are often used together because water is an effective way provide temperature-based applications, Of all the adjunct methods hydrotherapy and thermotherapy are most aligned with massage therapy evidence-informed outcomes. The practical limitation of using water and temperature as part of a massage session is specialized equipment. However, many methods involve basic supplies such as hot and cold towels used as packs and compresses, smaller tubs for foot soaks and so forth. Hydrotherapy and thermotherapy can also be easily adapted for self-care and health messaging for clients.

History of Hydrotherapy

Water therapy is as old as the human race. One of the first recorded mentions of the use of water as medicine involves the temples of the Greek god of medicine, Aesculapius. At the temples, bathing and massage were part of the treatment of the sick. Hippocrates used water as a beverage for reducing fever and treating many diseases. He also stressed the value of using various types of baths, each with a different temperature, as a therapeutic tool to combat illness. Later, the ancient Roman physicians Galen and Celsus also recommended specific baths as an integral part of their remedies. Almost every warm-climate civilization has at some point in its history used baths for therapeutic purposes (Buchman, 1977; Chaitow, 2016).

These methods have powerful physiologic effects and have been used for centuries as part of the healing process. Before the development of antidepressant and stimulant medications, hot, warm, and cold applications were used to stimulate or sedate the autonomic nervous system. Cold shock was used instead of electric shock to treat depression. Warm baths of long duration were used to calm anxious individuals. For centuries, herb and mineral additives were used to enhance the effects of water treatments. *Balneotherapy* is the term used to describe the treatment of disease by bathing.

Hydrotherapy Uses and Indications

Based on available literature, hydrotherapy is used to improve immunity and for the management of pain. It produces different effects on various systems of the body depending on the temperature of water. The consistent findings were reductions in musculoskeletal pain, spasm, connective tissue distensibility, intramuscular temperature, nerve conduction velocity, reduction in inflammation and spasticity (except upon initial cold contact) (Mooventhan and Nivethitha, 2014; Archanah et al., 2018; Barker, 2018; Rafferty et al., 2018; Leutualy et al., 2022).

Water accounts for the largest percentage of our body weight. It is available in many forms, all of which have the potential to be therapeutically beneficial. Water can relax or stimulate, anesthetize, and reduce or increase circulation. It works naturally and is nonallergenic, tissue tolerant, inexpensive, and readily available.

Water's three forms (liquid, steam, and ice) allow it to be used at a variety of temperatures and in a variety of ways, such as full or partial baths, showers, compresses, packs, hot water bottles, frozen ice bandages, wrapped ice, and steam (Table 12.1).

The therapeutic properties of hydrotherapy are based on its mechanical or thermal effects (or both) and the body's reaction to hot and cold stimuli. Therapeutic effects also occur in response to the hydrostatic pressure exerted by the water when the body (or body part) is immersed in (surrounded by) water and in response to the sensation of the water against the skin. The peripheral nerves are stimulated by the temperature or pressure of the water, and impulses from the sensation on the skin are carried deeper into the body, stimulating the central nervous system, the autonomic nervous system, and, indirectly, all the other body systems (Sujatha et al., 2018; Joicy et al., 2021).

In general, heat quiets and soothes the body, slowing the activity of internal organs. Cold, in contrast, stimulates and invigorates, increasing internal activity. When the body is submerged in water, such as in a bath, a pool, or a whirlpool, the constant pull of gravity is reduced. Water also has a hydrostatic pressure effect; it has a massage-like effect, because water in motion stimulates touch receptors on the skin.

Rest and relaxation are potential benefits of hydrotherapy; it is useful for some anxious clients because it promotes general relaxation of the nervous system. Hydrotherapy usually is one component of an overall health and wellness program. It also can offer specific relief to people with a number of conditions, such as the following:

- Arthritis problems
- Back and neck pain
- Sports injuries
- Work-related injuries
- Cerebral palsy
- Orthopedic injuries

Table 12.1 Therapeutic Uses of Water

Use	Application
Analgesic (relieves pain)	Hot, warm, and cold applications
Anesthetic (reduces sensation)	Cold application
Antiedemic (reduces swelling)	Cold application
Antipyretic (reduces fever)	Cool to cold application
Antiseptic (kills pathogens)	Boiling water, high-pressure steam (not for use on the body)
Antispasmodic (reduces muscle spasms)	Hot, warm, and cold applications
Astringent (causes tissues to contract)	Cold application
Burn treatment (first-degree and mild second-degree burns only)	Cool application
Diaphoretic (produces sweating)	Hot application
Diuretic (increases urine formation)	Drinking water
Emetic (produces vomiting)	Drinking warm water
Expectorant (loosens mucus)	Hot and steam applications
Immunologic enhancement (increases white cell production)	Cold application
Laxative (promotes peristalsis of the bowel)	Drinking cold water or use of an enema
Sedative (reduces sympathetic arousal and encourages sleep)	Drinking warm water
Stimulant (increases sympathetic arousal)	Short hot and cold applications
Tonic (increases muscle tone)	Cold and alternating hot and cold applications

Modified from Nikola RJ: *Creatures of water: Hydrotherapy textbook,* Salt Lake City, 2005, Europa Therapeutic LLC.

Hydrotherapy has a scientific evidence-informed effect on various systems of the body, and it has essentially no side effects when used carefully (Mooventhan and Nivethitha, 2014; Krafft et al., 2022).

Key Points

Water is effective as a therapeutic agent for several reasons:

- It can store and transmit heat.
- It is a good conductor of heat.
- It is nontoxic.
- It can change states within a narrow, easily obtainable temperature range.
- In its solid form (ice), it is an effective cooling agent.
- It its liquid form (water), it may be applied using many pressures and temperatures, in addition to methods ranging from total immersion to local compression.
- In its gaseous form (steam), it may be used in vapor or steam baths or for inhalation treatments.

- The density of water is near that of the human body; therefore, it supports exercise for clients with joint disease, paralysis, or atrophy.
- The hydrostatic pressure exerted on the body surface during immersion increases urine output and venous and lymphatic flow from the periphery.

Effects of Hydrotherapy

Despite the commonly held conviction as to the efficacy of hydrotherapy in restoring a good psychophysical condition after physical exercise, positive reviews of athletes, and some published research, the actual efficacy of hydrotherapy still remains debatable (Slaga et al., 2018).

People are using hydrotherapy as self-care or care to support typical aspects of conventional care (Almassmoum et al., 2018).

The effects of water are primarily reflexive and focus on the autonomic nervous system. The addition of heat energy or the dissipation of heat energy from tissues can be classified as a mechanical effect. In general, cold stimulates sympathetic responses, and warmth activates parasympathetic responses. Short- and long-term applications of heat or cold differ in effect. For the most part, short cold applications stimulate and vasoconstrict and have a secondary effect of increased circulation as blood is channeled to the area to warm it. Long cold applications depress and reduce circulation. Short applications of heat vasodilate vessels and depress and deplete tone, while long heat applications result in a combined depressant and stimulant reaction (Lee and Yi Y, 2019).

Visceral Reflex

Cutaneous and Somatic Effects

Stimulation of certain nerve endings in organs results in both a muscle and a skin response in a reflex loop. Usually, the muscles spasm or increase in tension, and the skin becomes tauter. This reflex is responsible for visceral referred pain patterns (see Chapter 6). Theoretically the reflex is a loop; therefore stimulation of muscle and skin can reflexively affect the corresponding organ. In general, an organ is in a reflex pattern with the muscles and skin over it. Applications of hydrotherapy seem to have either sedative or stimulating effects on the specific organ.

Mechanical Effects

Different water pressures can exert a powerful mechanical effect on the nerve and blood supplies of the skin. Techniques that are used include a friction rub with a sponge or wet mitten and pressurized streams of hot and cold water directed at various parts of the body (Box 12.1 and Table 12.2).

Osmosis is a theoretic principle of hydrotherapy in which water moves across a permeable or semipermeable membrane from a mineral salt concentration that is low to a high concentration to equalize solution consistency. In theory, if the water used for hydrotherapy application is lower in salt content than body fluids, water moves from the outside of the body to the inside through the semipermeable superficial tissue of the skin and superficial fascia. If the salt content of the water external to the skin is higher, such as when mineral salt baths are used, water from the body moves into the external soak water. When this happens, surface edema might be reduced. Unfortunately, no research has either confirmed or discounted this effect.

Physiologic Effects

Hydrotherapy techniques with heat and cold are thought to produce physiologic effects that help improve circulation, stimulate the immune system, provide relief from pain, reduce stress, and tone the body. Water itself helps restore and rejuvenate the body.

The physiologic effects of hydrotherapy can be thermal and mechanical. Thermal effects are produced when the water temperature is higher or lower than the current body temperature. When the temperature difference is small, the effect is mild; when the temperature difference is large, the effect is strong. Mechanical effects occur from the pressure of the water on the body, such as occurs in showers or whirlpools, and hydrostatic pressure forces that occur in baths.

In hydrotherapy, heating and cooling effects occur when heat from the water is transferred to the body or vice versa.

Circulation Enhancement

Supporting circulation is an important aspect of promoting healing. Circulation can be effectively enhanced with hydrotherapy. Massage may also be effective for moving blood in the body. The combined effects of massage and hydrotherapy might increase the rate of blood flow, decrease the rate of blood, increase blood flow to an ischemic area (an area with too little blood), and decrease blood flow in a congested area (an area with too much blood) (Manjuladevi et al., 2018; Parker et al., 2018). To accomplish these changes in blood flow, three physiologic effects are necessary:

- The revulsive effect
- The derivative effect
- The collateral circulation effect

Revulsive Effect

The revulsive effect occurs when blood flow through an area increases. The most effective means of accomplishing this is to use alternating hot and cold applications. The revulsive effect depends on repeated application. A series of three hot/cold applications is typical. The cold application should last 20 to 30 seconds, which is long enough to produce vasoconstriction. The warm application typically lasts twice as long as the cold application.

The revulsive effect is most beneficial for conditions involving tissue congestion. For example, if the client is experiencing sinus congestion, alternating hot and cold compresses over the face can reduce sinus pressure.

Derivative Effect

The derivative effect is the opposite of the revulsive effect. Instead of encouraging blood flow to or through an area, the goal is to shift blood flow away from an area, thereby creating blood volume changes from one area of the body to another. An example of the derivative effect is application of heat to the feet to reduce congestion in the head. Vascular headaches, in

Box 12.1 Effects of Hydrotherapy Using Heat, Cold, and Ice Applications

Effects of Heat
Increases circulation
Increases metabolism
Increases inflammation
Increases respiration
Increases perspiration
Decreases pain
Decreases muscle spasm
Decreases tissue stiffness
Decreases white blood cell production

Applications of Heat Hydrotherapy
As a Sedative
Water is a very efficient, nontoxic, calming substance. It soothes the body and promotes sleep.

Techniques: Use hot and warm baths to quiet and relax the entire body. Salt baths, neutral showers, or damp sheet packs can be used to relax certain areas.

For Elimination
The skin is the largest organ of the body, and simple immersion in a long, hot bath or a session in a sauna or steam room can stimulate the excretion of toxins through the skin. Inducing perspiration is useful for treating acute diseases and many chronic health problems (Box 12.9).

Techniques: Use hot baths, Epsom salt or common salt baths, hot packs, dry blanket packs, and hot herbal drinks.

As an Antispasmodic
Water effectively reduces cramps and muscle spasm.

Techniques: Use hot compresses (depending on the problem), herbal teas, and abdominal compresses.

Effects of Cold and Ice
Cold
Increases stimulation
Increases muscle tone
Increases tissue stiffness
Increases white blood cell production
Increases red blood cell production
Decreases circulation (primary effect); increases circulation (secondary effect)
Decreases inflammation
Decreases pain
Decreases respiration
Decreases digestive processes

Ice
Increases tissue stiffness
Decreases circulation
Decreases metabolism
Decreases inflammation
Decreases pain
Decreases muscle spasm

Types of Applications
Ice packs
Ice immersion (ice water)
Ice massage
Cold whirlpool
Chemical cold packs
Cold gel packs (use with caution)

Contraindications to Use of Ice
Vasospastic disease (spasming of blood vessels)
Cold hypersensitivity; signs include the following:
Skin: Itching, sweating
Respiratory: Hoarseness, sneezing, chest pain
Gastrointestinal: Abdominal pain, diarrhea, vomiting
Eyes: Puffy eyelids
General: Headache, discomfort, uneasiness
Cardiac disorder
Compromised local circulation

Precautions for Use of Ice
Do not use frozen gel packs directly on the skin.
Do not use ice applications (cryotherapy) for longer than 30 minutes continuously.
Do not do exercises that cause pain after cold applications.
Do not use cryotherapy on individuals with certain rheumatoid conditions or those who are paralyzed or have untreated coronary artery disease.

Applications of Cold Hydrotherapy
Ice is a primary therapy for strains, sprains, contusions, hematomas, and fractures. It has a numbing, anesthetic effect and helps control internal hemorrhaging by reducing circulation to and metabolic processes within the area.

For restoring and increasing muscle strength and increasing the body's resistance to disease:

Cold water boosts vigor, adds energy and tone, and aids in digestion.

Techniques: Use cold water treading (standing or walking in cold water), whirlpool baths, cold sprays, alternate hot and cold contrast baths, showers and compresses, salt rubs, apple cider vinegar baths, and partial packs.

For Injuries
Application of an ice pack controls the flow of blood and reduces tissue swelling.

Technique: Use an ice bag in addition to compression and elevation.

As an Anesthetic
Water can dull the sense of pain or sensation.

Technique: Use ice to chill the tissue.

For Minor Burns
Water, particularly cold and ice water, has been rediscovered as a primary healing agent.

Technique: Use ice water immersion or saline water immersion.

To Reduce Fever
Water is nature's best cooling agent. Unlike medications, which usually only diminish internal heat, water both lowers temperature and removes heat by conduction.

Technique: Use ice bags at the base of the neck and on the forehead and feet; cold-water sponge baths; and drinking cold water.

which too much blood in the vessels causes pressure, also may respond to this type of intervention.

Cold or heat can be applied for lengthy periods (up to 30 minutes) and at varying temperature extremes, depending on the size of the treated area and desired effect.

Collateral Circulation Effect

In the body, superficial and deep tissues receive blood through the same arteries as they branch. These branches are called *collateral arteries.* The collateral circulation effect creates change in the deep, rather than superficial, collateral branches of the

Table 12.2 Classification of Water Temperatures Used for Treatment

	Temperature Range	Effect
Very cold	32–56°F	Painful
Cold	56–65°F	Uncomfortable
Cool	65–92°F	Goose bumps
Neutral	92–98°F	Normal skin temperature
Warm to hot	98–104°F	Comfortable
Very hot	104–110°F*	Reddened skin

*Temperatures higher than 110°F should not be used.

same artery. Application of heat to an area causes surface vessels to dilate, increasing blood flow to the superficial tissues while also reducing blood flow to the deep tissues. Application of cold has the opposite effect. Local application of hydrotherapy techniques (generally by compress or pack) is used to produce collateral circulatory changes in a specific area of the body.

Effects of Cold Applications

In the skin, cold receptors are more numerous than heat receptors. The temperature-regulating mechanism in the hypothalamus responds to signals by attempting to prevent cooling or overheating. The primary or direct effect of cold applications is depressant. A decrease in function can occur locally if cold is applied to an area of the body or systemically if the entire body is exposed to cold. When the application of cold lasts a long time and the temperature is significantly colder than body temperature, the effects require a more adaptive response from the body. Caution is required for those who do not have sufficient adaptive capacity to respond to cold.

Cold applications typically cause shivering, goose bumps, increased pulse and respiration, dilation of blood vessels, and increased muscle tone. These effects are referred to as a *tonic*, a stimulating reaction to cold. As the body responds to the cold application, the return to normal function results in the secondary, or indirect, effect of cold, called the *reaction*. The secondary effect, or reaction, occurs only when the body has the adaptive capacity to respond to the cold by warming the area by increasing blood flow. In general, the colder the application, the greater the reaction. Many hydrotherapy techniques are directed at producing the reaction to the cold application.

Effects of Hot Applications

Hot applications stimulate the body to eliminate heat and thereby prevent tissue damage. Heat applications have different effects, depending on the temperature, duration of application, and method used. Water temperatures between 98°F and 104°F (37–40°C) are generally considered "hot." A temperature above 104°F is considered very hot. Many people can tolerate hot air, such as in a sauna, for fairly long periods, even though temperatures in a sauna may reach as high as 200°F, well above an individual's tolerance for heat in water. Often, after exposure to heat, cold is applied, such as a cold shower.

Exposure to the high temperatures of hot tubs and saunas has become popular, but it can be dangerous. Prolonged use may weaken the individual or trigger dangerous changes in respiratory and cardiac function. In people who are pregnant, prolonged exposure to hot temperatures may harm the fetus.

Box 12.2 lists additional risks, cautions, and contraindications for heat and cold applications of hydrotherapy. Specific indications and contraindications are discussed with each particular application in the Hydrotherapy Treatments and Common Techniques section.

Box 12.2 Risks, Cautions, and Contraindications for Heat and Cold Hydrotherapy

Clients whose ability to sense temperature changes is impaired are at risk for burns, scalding, or frostbite because they are unable to determine whether or not tissue is being damaged.

Clients with diabetes should avoid hot applications to the feet or legs and full-body heating treatments, such as hot baths and body wraps.

Cold applications should not be used if the client has been diagnosed with Raynaud disease.

Elderly people and young children may not be able to adapt to prolonged exposure to heat and should avoid long, full-body hot treatments, such as whirlpools and saunas.

Long-duration exposure to hot treatments, such as immersion baths and hot saunas, are not recommended for individuals with multiple sclerosis, people who are pregnant, anyone with high or low blood pressure, or individuals with any type of heart condition.

Temperatures higher than 104°F should never be used because the body temperature increases quickly and cannot adapt.

Hydrotherapy Supplies

Hydrotherapy can be used as an adjunct to massage with the aid of a few basic supplies:

- Tubs, bowls, and other containers of various sizes to hold water
- Thermometer
- Large watering can
- Hot plate, large pot, slow cooker, or electric roaster to heat water
- Small refrigerator to cool water and make ice
- Cotton sheets
- Wool or acrylic blankets
- Flannel material or towels and washcloths
- Some sort of waterproof sheeting (e.g., tarp, vinyl, or plastic tablecloth)
- Plastic sheeting
- Classic hot water bottle
- Elastic bandages for wrapping around an area to hold a compress or pack in place
- Rice/seed-filled cloth bags
- Microwave oven

Optional Equipment

- Hydrocollator, which is a liquid heating device used to heat and store hot packs. These heating units are typically stainless steel and offer a constant supply of temperature-consistent packs.

- Hot towel steamers/warmers
- A paraffin bath machine, which contains a heat source and tank that holds paraffin wax. The machine melts the wax and maintains it in a liquid state. When you immerse your hand, foot, or other body part in the liquid paraffin, the wax coats the body part completely. The warm temperature from the wax is thought to penetrate the skin, muscles, and bones to provide a soothing effect that can help relieve the pain of arthritis, bursitis, joint inflammation, or muscular strains or spasms.
- Access to a tub and shower if immersion methods will be used

Note: The equipment required for techniques must be sanitized and maintained properly.

Hydrotherapy Treatments and Common Techniques

Hydrotherapy Baths

A *bath* is a full or partial immersion of the body into water. The water temperature and the duration of the bath depend on the desired outcome. Substances can be added to the water to produce specific results. Additives most commonly used are salts, essential oils, milk, oatmeal, and seaweed preparations. The water may be moving, as in a whirlpool, or still.

Hot Full Immersion Bath

- Water temperature range: 100°F to 104°F (38–40°C)
- Bath duration: Up to 20 minutes

Indications for a Hot Full Immersion Bath

- Muscular spasms
- Detoxification through sweating
- Relaxation and stress reduction

Note: Hot baths typically are followed by a brief cool treatment, such as a cool shower.

Caution: Prolonged hot immersion baths are contraindicated for the elderly, infants, young children, immunosuppressed individuals, pregnant individuals, and people with cardiac or kidney disease.

Neutral Full Immersion Bath

- Average temperature of the skin: 92°F to 95°F (33–35°C)
- Bath duration: 15 minutes to 4 hours

Note: If the bath lasts longer than 20 minutes, warm water must be added to maintain the temperature.

Indications for a Neutral Full Immersion Bath

- Supporting parasympathetic dominance (considered a sedative effect)
- Creating increased urinary output as a result of hydrostatic pressure of the water against the body
- Treating peripheral edema
- Reducing the surface temperature of the body (when the elevated temperature is the result of lack of the normal heat-producing stimulus of cool air on the skin)
- Anxiety and irritability
- Exhaustion from insomnia
- Chronic pain

Caution: Clients commonly feel chilled after a neutral bath, and care must be taken to keep them warm.

Variations of Full Immersion Baths

Whirlpool

A whirlpool is a tub with air jets that move the water to stimulate the tissues. Generally, the water temperature is hot. Whirlpools open pores and promote sweating. They also promote psychological and mechanical muscular relaxation.

Mud Bath

In a mud bath, a combination of volcanic ash or clay, peat moss, and natural spring water is used to exfoliate and nourish the skin.

Herbal Bath

For an herbal bath, herbs are added to the water, producing the combined therapeutic properties of the herbs and the water. Two preparation methods are used:

Method 1: One cup of herbs is added to 2 quarts of water and simmered for 15 minutes to create an infusion. The herbs then are strained from the infusion, and the liquid is added to the bathwater.

Method 2: A thin cloth or mesh bag is filled with about 1 cup of herbs. It is either placed in the bathwater or tied to the faucet so that the hot water runs through it as the tub fills.

Cold Foot Bath

The feet are placed in a tub filled calf deep with cold water. The client should stop soaking the feet when the water is no longer perceived as cold.

Indications for a Cold Foot Bath

- Varicose veins
- Edema
- Vascular headaches
- Low blood pressure
- Circulatory problems
- Ankle sprain, strain, or bruise
- Sweaty feet
- Aching feet

Caution: Cold foot baths are not used for clients who suffer from cold feet, very high blood pressure, diabetes, or peripheral vascular disease.

Rising Temperature or Warm Foot Bath

- *Rising temperature foot bath:* The feet are immersed in a foot bath filled with water at body temperature (Fig. 12.1*A*). Hot water is added gradually to produce a final temperature of 103°F to 104°F (39–40°C).
- *Warm foot bath:* The feet are immersed in a warm foot bath with the water at 100°F to 104°F (38–40°C). The foot bath should last 10 to 15 minutes and can be done daily.

Indications for a Rising Temperature or Warm Foot Bath

- Cold feet
- Onset of a common cold
- Preactivity/plantar fascia softening
- Relaxation

Caution: Do not use a rising temperature or warm foot bath if the client has varicose veins, lymphostasis, or edema.

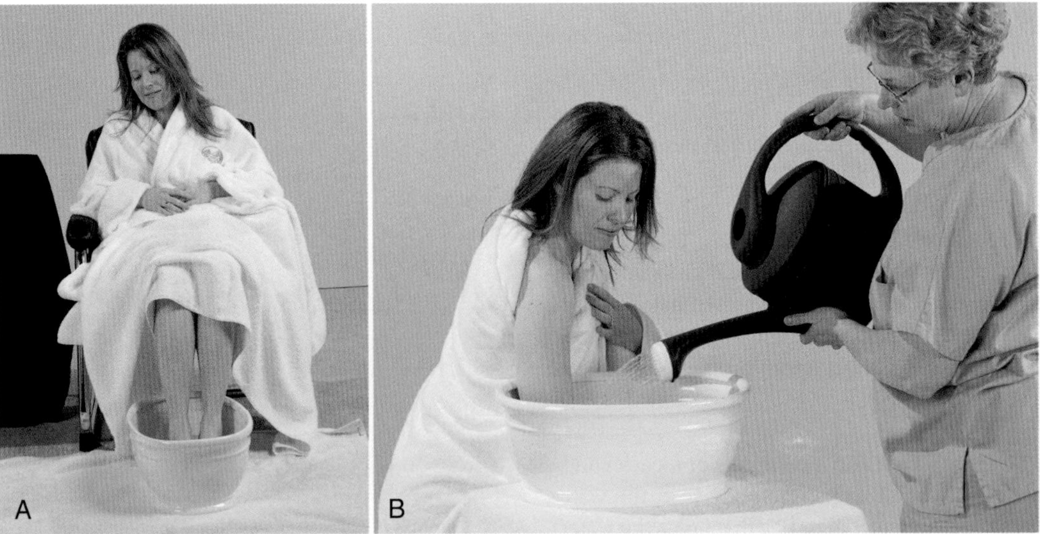

FIG. 12.1 A, Foot bath. **B,** Arm bath.

Cold Arm Bath

For a cold arm bath, a tub is filled with cold water until it reaches a depth several inches above the immersed elbow (Fig. 12.1*B*).

Indications for a Cold Arm Bath

- Headaches
- Shoulder, elbow, wrist, and hand pain

Caution: Do not use a cold arm bath if the client has heart or circulatory problems.

Rising Temperature and Warm Arm Bath

- *Rising temperature arm bath:* The arm is immersed in a tub filled with water at body temperature. Hot water is added gradually to produce a final temperature of 103°F to 104°F (39–40°C).
- *Warm arm bath:* The arm is immersed in a warm bath with the water at 100°F to 104°F (38–40°C). The arm bath should last 10 to 15 minutes and can be done daily.

Indications for a Rising Temperature or Warm Arm Bath

- Bronchitis
- Asthma
- Respiratory infection
- Circulatory conditions

Caution: Rising temperature or warm arm baths are not indicated in cases of acute inflammation.

Sitz Bath

An immersion bath of the pelvic region typically is performed using a specially constructed tub, but it also may be done in a regular bathtub. A sitz bath may be hot, neutral, cold, contrasting hot and cold, rising temperature, or warm. Before a sitz bath, the feet should be warmed with a warm foot bath.

Variations of Sitz Baths

Hot sitz bath: Water temperature generally is 105°F to 110°F (40–43°C); bath lasts 3 to 10 minutes. The primary effect is analgesic. Effects require a more adaptive response from the body.

Neutral sitz bath: Water temperature is 92°F to 95°F (33–35°C); bath lasts 15 minutes to 2 hours. To manage inflammation, the client must be kept warm during treatment.

Cold sitz bath: Water temperature is 55°F to 75°F (13–24°C); bath lasts 30 seconds to 5 minutes. Cold sitz baths are given to increase the tone of the smooth muscles of the uterus, bladder, and colon. Caution is required for those who do not have sufficient adaptive capacity to respond to cold. Cold temperatures range from 55°F to 65°F (13–18°C). Anything colder, such as ice, is considered very cold. Anything warmer is considered cool.

Contrast sitz baths: These baths usually are given in groups of three (i.e., three repetitions of hot to cold). Two separate tubs are needed. For the hot bath, the water temperature is 105°F to 110°F (40–44°C); for the cold bath, it is 55°F to 85°F (13–29°C). The client spends about 3 minutes in the hot bath and then 30 seconds in the cold bath. The water level in the hot tub is slightly higher than that in the cold tub. The client must be kept warm. A contrast sitz bath increases pelvic circulation and the tone of the smooth muscles in the area.

Indications for a Sitz Bath

- Uterine cramps
- Hemorrhoids or inflammation (cold sitz bath)
- Irritable bladder (warm or rising temperature sitz bath)

Note: All contrast hydrotherapy treatments finish with the cold application.

Caution: A warm or rising temperature sitz bath should not be used for hemorrhoids. Hot sitz baths are not indicated in cases of acute inflammation.

Saunas and Steam Baths

Saunas and steam baths have similar effects. A sauna is dry heat, and the heat acts to promote sweating and general relaxation. The moist air of a steam bath seems to have a greater effect on the respiratory system. The client should spend no more than 15 to 20 minutes at a time in a sauna and should wipe the face frequently with a cold cloth and drink cool water to prevent overheating. Infrared saunas may allow for longer duration.

Indications for Saunas and Steam Baths

- Increase blood flow
- Increase heart rate
- Support immune system
- Encourage secretions in the respiratory system and open the airways
- Support relaxation
- Reduce muscle aching from overexertion

CAUTION: Clients should not use a sauna if pregnant or unless supervised by a physician, if they have rheumatoid arthritis, acute infection, acute or chronic inflammation, vascular changes in the brain or heart, circulatory problems, or cancer.

Compresses and Packs

The difference between a bath and a compress or a pack can be understood in this way: with baths, the body is in the water; with a compress or pack (a material or bag that holds the water), water is layered on the body. The three basic types of compresses are hot, cold, and alternating hot and cold (Fig. 12.2).

Compresses and packs are applied using cloth or some other compress material, which is wrung out to the desired amount of moisture and then applied to any surface of the body. A single compress consists only of layers of the wet material. A double compress is a wet cloth completely covered by dry material (usually wool), which prevents cooling by evaporation or heat loss. With a cold double compress, the body warms the area, producing a secondary reaction to the cold. A water bottle filled with hot or cold water or ice also can be used.

Compresses are named according to the area of the body to which they are applied (e.g., a head compress or a knee compress).

Cold Compresses

For a cold compress, a cloth is immersed in cold water (sometimes ice water), wrung out, and then placed on the body. Substances often are added to the water, such as baking soda, Epsom salts, boric acid, herbs, or cider vinegar. A cold compress can remain on the body 1 to 5 minutes before losing its temperature, at which time a new cloth should be applied, thereby maintaining the cold effect. The optimal temperature for a cold compress depends on the problem, the desired outcome, and the client's adaptive capacity. In general, the colder the temperature, the less time is required.

A cold double compress is achieved by covering a cold compress with several layers of dry material, such as flannel, wool, or other heavy fabrics. These layers of dry material trap heat and prevent any heat loss by evaporation. The double compress remains on the area until it is warmed by the body. The primary effects of cold double compresses are to increase the local circulation and eliminate metabolic waste from the area.

A cold single compress has a primarily vasoconstrictive effect, both locally and distally. The temperature of the initial application depends on the client's adaptive capacity and the reason for use. In general, the colder the application, the stronger the secondary reaction to the cold.

CAUTION: Do not use a cold compress for pleurisy or acute asthma because these conditions may be seriously aggravated. Cold compresses should not be used for ill or weak individuals, who are unable to generate a secondary response to cold.

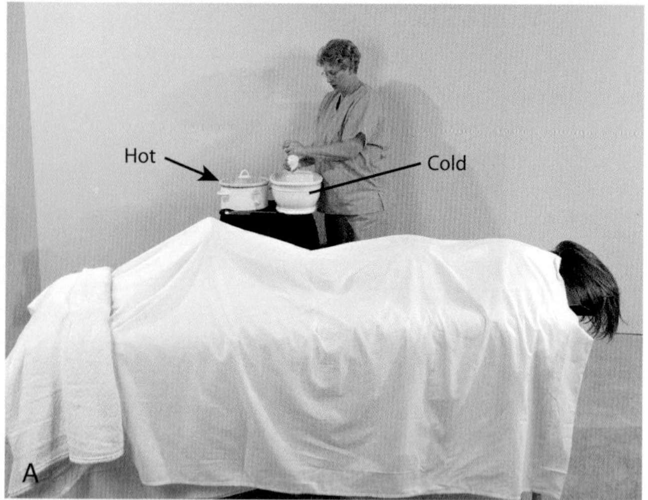

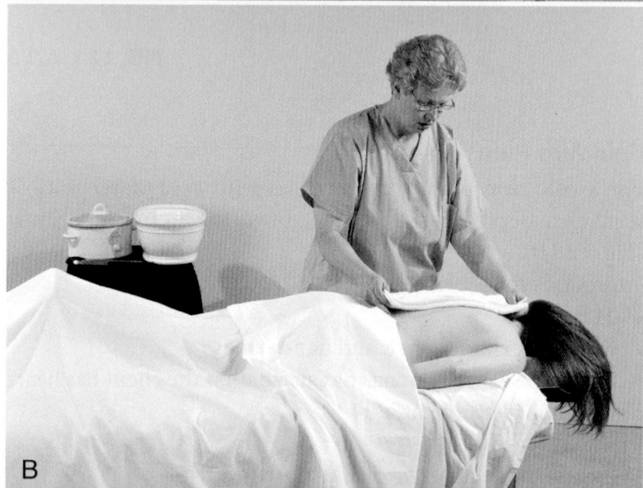

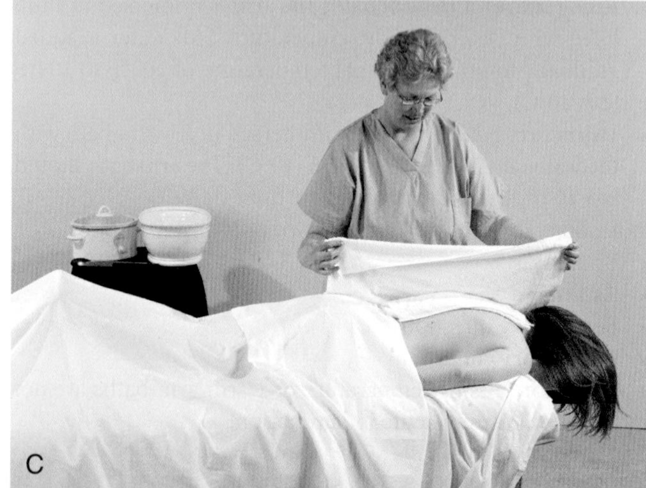

FIG. 12.2 Applying a compress. **A,** Wet the compress with hot or cold water and wring it out. **B,** Apply it to the area. **C,** Cover the compress with a towel.

Cold Packs

Crushed ice in a plastic bag is the most commonly used cold pack. It can be left in place for up to 20 minutes and then removed, or it may be applied repeatedly (i.e., left in place for 1 minute and then removed for 5 minutes). Reusable cold packs that contain gel can be used. A bag of frozen peas or corn makes an effective cold pack.

Indications for a Cold Compress or Pack

- Reduce edema after injury
- Inhibit inflammation
- Relieve pain caused by congestion
- Reduce body temperature (e.g., fever), especially when applied over a large area
- Upper respiratory infections
- Sore throat
- Swollen lymph nodes

CAUTION: When using ice packs, place a thin cloth between the pack and the skin to prevent frostbite.

Hot Compresses

A hot compress is a prolonged application of moist heat, generally to a local area of the body, which may create an analgesic effect, especially for pain caused by muscle spasm and intestinal or uterine cramping. Fairly hot compresses may be applied directly to the skin surface, with care taken to avoid burning the client.

A *fomentation* is a special type of hot compress that provides prolonged exposure at a higher temperature. Fomentations must be applied over a bath towel placed on the affected area, because the temperature of these compresses cannot be tolerated when applied directly to the skin.

Warm Packs

A warm pack can be created by soaking wrapping cloth in a hot infusion or decoction of herbs, wringing it out, and then applying it to the client's body. Alternatively, various sizes of bags can be filled with rice and then heated in a microwave oven. The typical heating time is 1 minute per pound, not to exceed 5 minutes. This type of pack stays warm longer than a water-based pack; therefore, it is important to monitor the client to prevent burns.

Indications for Hot Compresses or Packs

- Increase blood flow to the periphery
- Decrease internal congestion
- Tissue warming and relaxation
- Insomnia
- Nervous tension
- Mild muscular spasms
- Arthrosis
- Sluggish blood flow
- Headaches (muscle tension type)

NOTE: Extreme caution is required when electric heating pads are used. Burns are common because the device does not cool down as does a hot pack or hot water bottle.

CAUTION: Hot applications are contraindicated on the extremities of diabetic individuals. Special precautions must also be observed when treating the elderly, infants, and individuals with impaired neurologic function, edema, or decreased circulation. It is important to monitor the skin to make sure the client is not burned.

Wet Sheet Pack

Treatment with a wet sheet pack is one of the most useful hydrotherapy procedures. It requires 1 to 3 hours, depending on the client's condition (Fig. 12.3).

1. Place two wool or acrylic blankets lengthwise on the table with a small pillow at the head and a small bolster under the knees for comfort. The blankets must be large enough to cover the client.
2. Have the client take a warm shower or bath before applying the treatment. Soak a clean white cotton sheet in cold water and then wring it out as dry as possible. Open the sheet and place it lengthwise along the table with equal amounts draped over each side. The sheet should be slightly smaller than the blankets.
3. Have the client remove clothing (underwear can be left on) and lie down on the wet sheet. The shoulders should be 4 to 6 inches below the top of the sheet. Have the client raise both arms over the head. Wrap one side of the sheet around the client's body, tucking it in snugly on the opposite side. Below the hips, wrap the sheet around the leg on the same side.
4. Have the client lower the arms. Then bring the opposite side of the sheet over the body, covering both arms, and wrap the opposite leg.
5. Smooth the wet sheet over the body to ensure complete contact and tuck it in around the feet.
6. Quickly pull the blankets on the table over the client's body and tuck them in firmly, making sure there are no drafts around the client's neck or feet.
7. Additional blankets may be placed over the client, and a stocking cap can be pulled over the head to increase the heating effect.
8. Supervise the client closely. If the person feels claustrophobic or anxious, first remove the sheet from the feet. If this is unsuccessful, the procedure may need to be stopped. If the client complains of chilliness, add blankets, place a hot water bottle on the feet, or provide warm drinks.

A wet sheet pack proceeds through four stages: tonic (cooling), neutral, heating, and eliminative. Depending on the desired effect, the therapist may prolong any specific stage.

- *Tonic stage:* This stage lasts 2 to 15 minutes and is finished when the client no longer perceives the sheet as cold. The tonic stage creates an intense thermic reaction. The duration of this stage depends completely on the amount of water left in the sheet. For a shorter duration (used for those who are ill or fragile), the sheet should be wrung out as completely as possible. If the client is relatively healthy, more moisture can be left in the sheet to prolong this stage.
- *Neutral stage:* The neutral stage begins when the client is no longer cold. It may last 15 minutes to 1 hour, depending on the client's adaptive capacity. During this phase, the client experiences a sense of calm similar to that experienced during a neutral bath. Very often the client falls asleep during this stage.
- *Heating stage:* Heat from the client accumulates beneath the blankets, and light perspiration eventually begins to appear on the forehead; the interval between the sense of feeling warm and the appearance of perspiration is the heating stage. This stage may last 15 minutes to 1 hour.
- *Eliminative stage.* In the eliminative stage, the client begins to perspire.

The entire procedure can take up to 3 hours. If an individual cannot remain confined (e.g., needs to use the restroom frequently), do not use this technique.

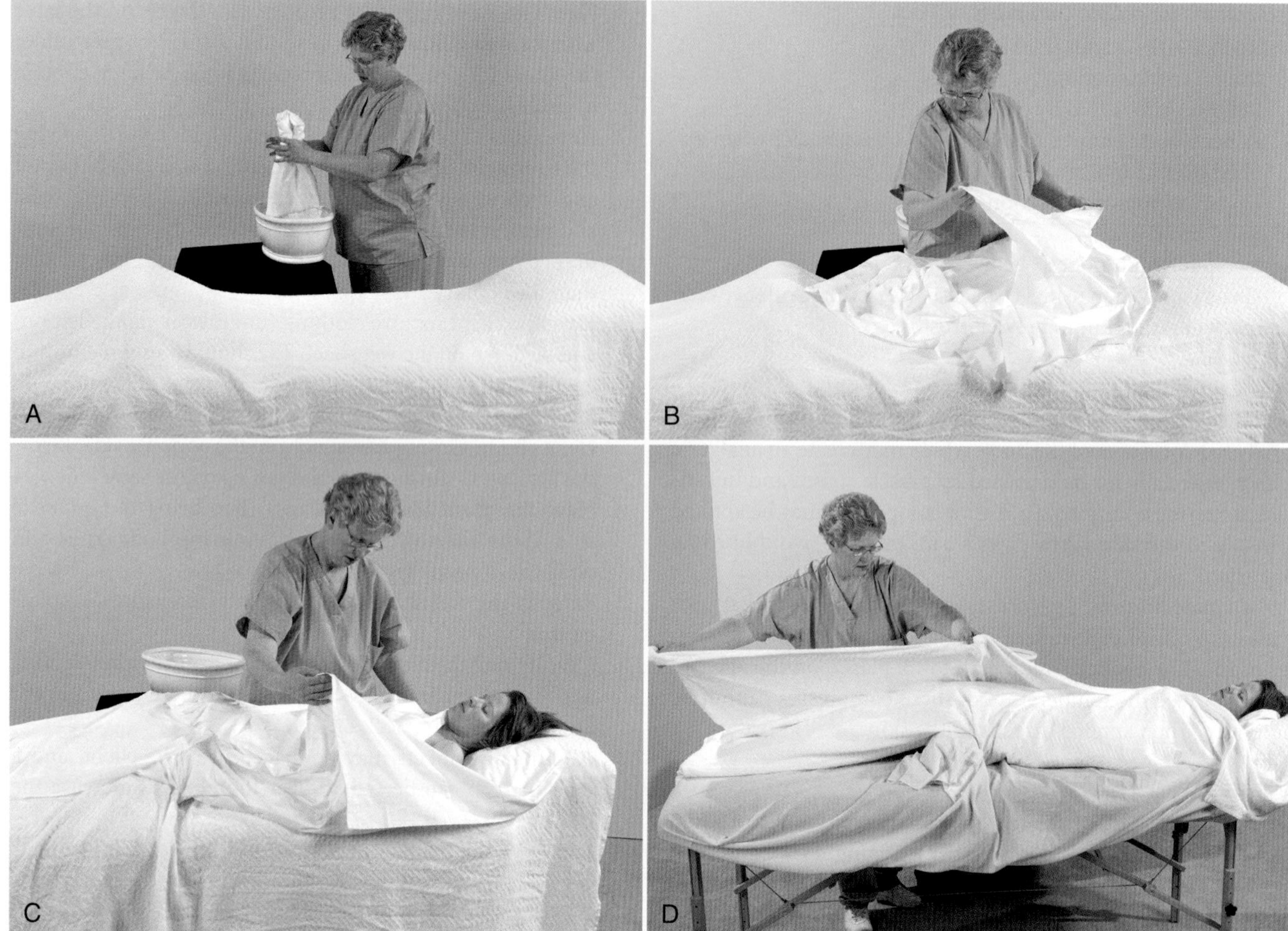

FIG. 12.3 Using a wet sheet pack. **A,** Place two blankets on the table. Wet a sheet and wring it out. **B,** Place the wet sheet over the top blanket. **C,** Have the client lie down on the wet sheet and then wrap the sheet around the person. **D,** Wrap the surface blanket around the client and then finally wrap the second blanket for warmth.

Integrating Hydrotherapy Into Therapeutic Massage

It is likely that hydrotherapy and thermotherapy will be integrated into a variety of nonpharmacology pain management strategies based on effectiveness and low risk. It may be that the pain reduction experienced by ice application provides the most benefit. Between ice applications, rub the body part briskly with the hand. When heat is ineffective for muscle spasms, use ice. Often a sciatica attack that does not respond to moist heat responds to one or two frozen packs.

A wrapped ice bag is the most common application, but an ice bath or ice massage is also effective. To prevent frostbite, place a layer of fabric between the ice and the skin. Apply ice periodically, not continuously. Ice application continues through four sensations (over a 10- to 15-minute period): appreciation of cold (pain), warming, ache or throbbing, and skin anesthesia (numbness).

The effects of alternating hot and cold include constriction and dilation of vessels and decreased congestion. Techniques include hot and cold compresses, ice bags, warm or hot baths, hot packs, whirlpool baths, and alternating hot and warm or hot and cold showers (Proficiency Exercise 12.1).

PROFICIENCY EXERCISE 12.1

Gather some of the recommended supplies for hydrotherapy (e.g., bowls, towels, and a watering can). Experiment with hot and cold applications that you feel are convenient to offer as part of the massage process, such as a warm foot bath and a cool eye compress.

Clients can be taught the basic techniques of hydrotherapy as self-help measures. Although many massage therapy facilities do not have access to hydrotherapy equipment, simple hot and cold compresses or packs can be used. A warm foot bath is easy to incorporate into a massage and serves the dual purpose of relaxing the client and freshening "stale" feet before the massage. A bag of frozen peas makes a great cold pack because it can mold to almost any area. Hot water bottles or seed bags warmed in a microwave oven are safer to use than electric heating pads because they naturally cool down before they can cause a burn. It is efficient to have a hot towel warmer in the area with both dry and damp wet towels. Water frozen in a paper cup (Fig. 12.4) makes an effective massage tool (freeze with a stick in it for even better results), especially when the practitioner uses ice as a counterstimulant to assist in lengthening and stretching procedures.

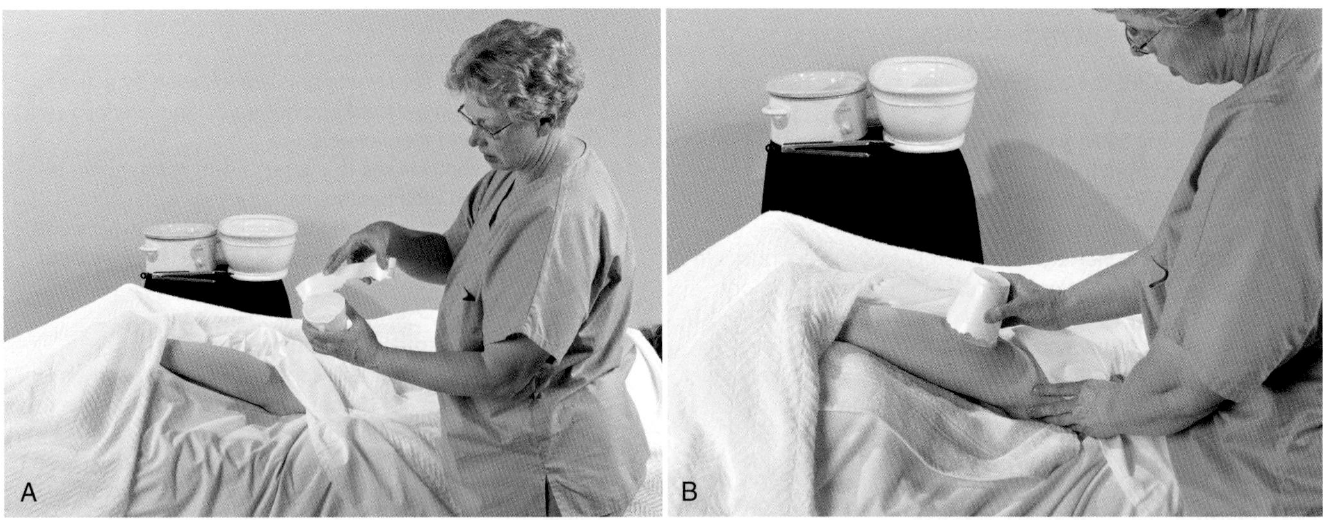

FIG. 12.4 Ice massage. A, To use the ice pop, peel away the edge of the cup or freeze the ice with a stick inserted and peel away the cup. **B,** Apply ice massage to a local area. Catch dripping water with a towel.

Drinking water also should be available for both the client and the therapist. Meticulous attention to sanitation is necessary when water applications are used (Boxes 12.3 and 12.4).

HOT AND COLD STONES

SECTION OBJECTIVES

Chapter objective covered in this section:

3. Describe the use of stones and other tools used for thermotherapy.

Using the information presented in this section, the student will be able to perform the following:

- Describe the physiological effects of thermotherapy (the use of stones) as an aspect of massage.
- Use hot and cold stones safely.

The use of stones is an ancient healing art that has been rediscovered, particularly in the spa setting. Its modern form came in the early 1990s, when massage therapist Mary Hannigan of Tucson trademarked her particular style and called it LaStone Therapy. Since then, it has quickly become a popular treatment in the spa industry in North America, and it has taken many forms. Most spas offer their own versions.

Stone therapy is a type of *thermotherapy* and *implement assistant massage.* It uses deep penetrating heat from smooth, heated stones and alternating cold from chilled stones. There is nothing magical about stones. The simple fact is that stones have an innate ability to hold heat well. As shown in the hydrotherapy section, the physiologic benefits of applying alternating temperatures to the body have long been scientifically investigated and validated. The weight of the stones also has value for providing a sustained compressive force against the tissue while the stone is in place. The stone can also be used as a tool to augment massage application.

Types of Stones Commonly Used for Massage

Basalt stones are commonly used. Basalt is an igneous rock (explained later in the chapter) and holds heat well, but many other types of stones work fine. The size, weight, and shape of the stone are more important than the type of stone. When the stones are wet or oiled, they change color, becoming darker and acquiring a satin-like appearance.

River rock is commonly used for stone thermal applications in massage. River rocks have smooth rounded edges from movement in riverbeds and streambeds. It is also important that the river rock used have some flat surfaces. Quality is determined by the type of parent rock (e.g., sandstone, granite, basalt) and the distance the rock has traveled in the river. Some stones are smoother than others, and color varies; not all river rock is smooth and black. A stone's ability to hold heat depends on the amount of ore in the stone. Ore can appear in the rock as tints of green, gray, rust, blue, and other colors. Black stones do not necessarily hold heat better than lighter colored ones.

Another rock commonly used for stone massage is nephrite (jade). Nephrite is composed of calcium, magnesium, and iron silicate. Nephrite is unique and versatile because it can hold heat just as well as it can hold cold.

Manufactured ceramic "stones" are also available on the market which can be heated in a microwave.

Healing Properties of Minerals

The properties of the crystalline structures of minerals have led to a belief in the healing qualities of various stones. The rarer the stone, the greater its value, and therefore the more healing properties or mystical qualities that are attributed to the mineral.

Gemstones and crystals exhibit rather unusual electrical properties. Four types of electrical phenomena have been described for gemstones:

- *Frictional electrical charges.* Certain gemstones develop an electrical charge when rubbed by a particular material. Thales recognized this quality in amber around 600 BC; in fact, the Greek word for amber is *electron.* In essence, the outer layers of electrons are exchanged between the two materials, and the charge generated depends on the

Box 12.3 Rules of Hydrotherapy

See Table 12.2 for the classification of water temperatures for treatments.

Hydrotherapy has a powerful effect on the body. The following rules, taken from the Ontario, Canada, curriculum guidelines for massage therapy, should be followed when hydrotherapy is used in the massage setting.

1. Always take a thorough case history to check for possible contraindications. Contraindications include circulatory and kidney problems and skin conditions.
2. Always adapt the method to the individual, not vice versa. The time, temperatures, and other variables used in procedures should be considered guidelines, not absolutes.
3. Have the client go to the bathroom before treatment begins.
4. Stay with the client during treatment or have some way for the client to contact you, such as by using a bell.
5. Explain the complete treatment to the client beforehand so they know what to expect and what is expected.
6. Make sure the room is draft free, clean, and quiet. All equipment should be sanitary and in good working condition. Each client should have clean towels and sheets.
7. Keep the client from becoming chilled during or after the treatment.
8. For cold-water treatments, the water should be as cold as possible, within the client's tolerance. A difference of 10°F from the client's body temperature (hydrotherapy application) is the minimum needed to produce stimulation and change in the circulation.
9. For warm-water treatments, the water should be as warm as necessary, within the client's tolerance. A temperature that is too hot can be debilitating.
10. More is not better. Using greater extremes of temperature or longer durations is not always more effective. The aim is to achieve a positive change, and too much can overtax, damage, or set back the condition.
11. Ask pertinent questions during the treatment, including questions about comfort level and thirst, but keep talking to a minimum to allow the client to relax.
12. Check the client's respiratory rate and pulse before, during, and after treatments as required, especially with prolonged hot treatments. The pulse should stay fairly even.
13. Watch for discomfort or negative reactions or both to the treatment.
14. Stop the treatment if a negative reaction occurs.
15. Generally, short cold treatments are followed by active exercise. Prolonged cold and hot treatments are followed by bed rest and then exercise.
16. Apply cold compresses to the head with hot treatments and prolonged cold treatments.
17. Never give a cold treatment to a cold body. Always warm the body first. The easiest method for this is a warm foot bath.

Water Applications for Health Purposes

1. *Local heat:* Apply heat to a specific area of the body, such as a joint or the chest, throat, shoulders, or spine. Use a hot, moist compress or a hot water bottle.
2. *Local cold:* Apply cold to a specific area of the body. Use a cold compress, ice bag, ice pack, ice hat, or frozen bandage.
3. *Sponging:* Use alcohol, water, or witch hazel applied with a sponge to wash the body.
4. *Tonic friction:* Combining water sponging and washing with some form of friction, either from the hand or a rough washcloth, produces a tonic effect in the body. Use cold friction massage or a cold sponge rub.
5. *Baths:* Baths involve immersion of the body in cold, hot, or tepid water. Use foot, sitz, full, mineral, or herb baths. Any part of the body may be partly bathed, as in an arm, eye, or finger bath. A whirlpool is a bath in which the water is moving under pressure.
6. *Compresses and packs:* Compresses and packs are folded cotton, flannel, or gauze soaked in water or liquid medications or herbs. A pack covers a larger area than a compress.
7. *Showers:* Several kinds of water streams can be directed against the body. Alternate streams can also be directed against the body, or large amounts of water can be poured from a height.
8. *Shampoo:* Using soap and water together on one or all parts of the body creates a shampoo. Use shampoo to cleanse the hair after a sauna or steam room session.
9. *Steam:* A vaporizer can cleanse the upper respiratory system, and a steam room or sauna increases body perspiration and releases many stored toxins. Cold steam, as from a humidifier, moistens dry rooms in winter and is important in preventing colds and sinus headaches.
10. *Sauna (dry heat):* A sauna is an intense but tolerably heated room. A tepid or cold shower should be taken after a sauna treatment.

materials. For instance, glass develops a positive charge when rubbed with silk and a negative charge when rubbed with flannel. Diamond, tourmaline, and topaz can be electrically charged by friction.

- *Pyroelectricity.* Pyroelectricity is electrical forces induced by heat. Tourmaline and quartz exhibit this effect, which is the reason they attract dust in a display case if they are located near a heat source, such as a light bulb. This effect was first recognized in tourmaline by Theophrastus in 315 BC and was fully researched during the 18th century. The German name for tourmaline originally was *aschentrekker*, which means "ash drawer," a reference to the gem's tendency to attract dust when charged. The color of the tourmaline seems to make a difference; black is the least chargeable, and red is the most chargeable.
- *Piezoelectrical charges.* Piezoelectrical charges are created by mechanical compression of a material; that is, the electrical charge is generated by squeezing, pulling, or compressing the material. Quartz and tourmaline show this property. Even more important is the reverse effect; that is, when an electrical current is passed through the material, it thickens or lengthens. This is the process by which quartz is used to regulate a clock. An electric current causes the quartz to oscillate (vibrate) at a consistent rate. The same principle was used in submarine detection as early as 1918 and in radio broadcasting frequency control in 1922. An

Box 12.4 ICE/RICE/PRICE/POLICE/MEAT/MCE/MICE/CRIME

ICE/RICE/PRICE/POLICE/MEAT/MCE/MICE/CRIME are all acronyms for methods to manage acute soft tissue injury such as a sprain or strain. The process began with ICE and has since evolved, altering methods and letters to the acronyms:

I—Ice. Ice therapy, or cryotherapy, is the application of cold typically with and ice pack applied to the injured area.
Ice lowers skin and tissue temperature which decreases nociceptive signally and can lead to a reduction in pain sensation. There is some controversy over the use of ice since it can reduce the productive acute inflammatory response. However, ice is a much better pain management strategy than pain medication. When applying ice to a local area do not apply it direct to skin to prevent frost bite. Ice application should not exceed 20 minutes.

C—Compression. Compression after an injury helps in the prevention of further swelling and a bit of immobilization. Compression to a local area is usually applied using an elastic bandage wrap. The bandage should not be so tight that it causes discomfort or interferes with blood flow.

E—Elevation. Elevating the injured area results in a decrease in hydrostatic pressure which in turn, reduces the accumulation of interstitial fluid and manages edema.
Next R and P were added:

R—Rest. The intention of rest is to support the healing process. Not excessive rest but taking it easy for 24 hours may be prudent.

P—Protection. Protection prevents further injury and involves some type of immobilization such as the compression bandage, reduced weight bearing, or demand such as crutches or a sling.

The result is PRICE. However, over time, best practices indicated that PRICE needed updating, and POLICE came into being. The R was removed, and the O and the L were added:

OL—Optimal Loading. Optimal Loading uses movement, weight bearing, and resistance to stimulate the healing process of bone, tendon, ligament, and muscle. The intensity of the loading increases as the healing progresses. The right amount of activity can help manage swelling.

Then the use of ice/cryotherapy was thought to interfere with the productive inflammatory response in the acute phase of healing, so MEAT immerged.

MEAT—The acronym stands for Movement, Exercise, Analgesics, Therapy.
The MEAT protocol has elements of Optimal Loading by recommending movement, exercise, and therapy (physical therapy in particular). The use of analgesics is to reduce pain enough to support movement, exercise, and therapy. Analgesic medication is usually also antiinflammatory which will certainly interfere with the normal healing process; ice therefore remains best for pain management.

And the variations continue:

MCE—Move safely, Compression, Elevation
Ice is again part of the protocol...maybe.

MICE—Motion, Ice, Compression, Elevation

CRIME—Compression, Rest, Ice, Motion and Elevation.

intriguing and still unanswered question remains as to whether piezoelectric forces in certain of the earth's minerals may be what animals sense, either in their systems or on the ground, to "predict" earthquakes by exhibiting strange behavior. Strong changes in atmospheric pressure may cause this effect. Piezoelectrical forces are known to exist in the bones, cartilage, and tendons of vertebrates.

- *Electrical conduction.* Some gemstones also conduct electricity.

Gliding Tool

The smoothness and shape of stones allow some to be used for gliding techniques (see the section on implement-assisted massage later in this chapter). A little oil applied to the stone allows a smooth gliding movement as the muscle is warmed; this is similar to "ironing" a muscle. However, some body mechanics concerns for the practitioner arise with regard to gripping the stone. When the massage therapist holds the stone, the muscles in the forearm are activated, which has the potential to cause damage; therefore, the stone should be held with a light grip. The use of stones for actual massage should be limited.

Pressure Point Tool

Stones of a certain shape can be used for compression. For example, reflexology or trigger point treatments can be provided with stones. Client safety is always a concern when implements are used, and caution is necessary.

Compression Tool

The weight of the stones provides physical and mental comfort and enhances compression applications. As the stones cool, they can remain on the body while massage is applied to other areas. Care must be taken to ensure that stones are not overly hot because they can cause burns.

Thermotherapy Tool

Because of their ability to hold heat and cold, stones make excellent thermotherapy tools. Warm stones transfer heat to the client's muscles and produce relaxation. When frozen or chilled, stones can be used in all cases in which ice would be appropriate. Alternating hot and cold is a well-practiced method of increasing circulation. Stones provide a uniform element for applying temperature without the drawback of drips, as may occur with ice bags.

Note: Stones used as massage tools must be polished smooth so that they do not catch or pull the client's body hair or scrape the skin.

Proper Body Mechanics While Using Stones

Some applications of stone massage include holding the stone in the hand and using it to apply gliding or compression on a trigger point or acupuncture point. However, body mechanics concerns arise. Gripping the stone while using it to apply pressure strains the practitioner's forearm muscles. The hand must remain relaxed during the massage application or the muscles in the forearms are strained. Even if the stone is not gripped but rather slid around the body, just using the palm of the hand tends to activate the forearm muscles.

Another safety concern when using stones, or any object, to apply compression is that the massage practitioner's hand is not in direct contact with the client's body, monitoring feedback and pressure depth. Therefore injury might occur.

Justifying the Use of Stones with Massage

Massage therapists should avoid using gimmicks, fads, and buzzwords, because this compromises the practitioner's professionalism and the validity of the treatment. Some may question the justification of stones used in the massage setting. However, the unique properties of stones support their use as an adjunct therapy.

If you are going to use stones during massage, you should do some research about them. *Petrology* is the study of the classification and mineral and chemical composition of rocks (the term *petrology* is derived from the word *petroleum*). The terms *stones* and *rocks* can be used interchangeably.

Body parts that can be treated with stones include the following:

- Forehead
- Area between the toes
- Thigh and back of the calf
- Arm (elbow joint, forearm)
- Sternum, stomach
- Back
- Shoulder
- Neck
- Lumbar area
- Gluteals
- Scapulae

Stones typically are placed on areas of the body with concentrated neurovascular activity including joints, nerve plexuses, acupuncture points, meridians, and chakras.

Simply allowing the room temperature stones to rest on the body is beneficial. The therapeutic quality of the stone, coupled with the sustained compressive force from the weight of the stone, as well as speculative energetic influences from crystal structure and color, may be sufficient to achieve a therapeutic effect. Static placement avoids the potential for repetitive strain injuries caused by using the stones to apply the massage, and because the stone is room temperature the client is protected from burns.

Selecting Stones

Make the stone selection process unique by searching for your own or, for convenience, purchase a set from a distributor. To select stones, you can go to a quarry, the beach, a landscaper, or your garden. Many distributors sell crystals. You can find smooth or tumbled stones in many places. Make it a fun practice to search for stones that intrigue you and begin your collection.

Stones used therapeutically have to have a weight and shape that are conducive to body placement. The stones must be fairly flat so that they do not roll around on the body, and they should be fairly smooth so that they do not cause injury. Typically, a flat, oval shape lies on the body without rolling off. River rock often has these shapes. Different sizes of stones can be used on different areas. For example, a stone for the forehead would be flat, rectangular, approximately 2 inches by 3 inches, and 0.5-inch thick. A stone used for placement on the sacrum could be flat, triangular, and about the size of your hand.

Keep in mind that stones used during massage must be able to withstand constant immersion in hot or cold water and must be sanitized by washing the stones, the heater, and other equipment in hot soapy water and then soaking them in a sanitizing agent (e.g., 10% bleach solution) after each use.

Procedure for Using Stones During Massage (Fig. 12.5)

SAFETY FIRST

Never put a hot stone directly on the skin and leave it in place on the skin. Only stones that are being constantly moved by the practitioner should directly touch the skin.

1. Before the client arrives, sanitize and then cool the stones to between 100°F and 104°F (38–40°C) for hot and warm application. Cool in ice water or refrigerate for cold applications. Stones should be warmed in a specific device designed for hot stones. A cooking thermometer is effective to ensure a beneficial and safe temperature.
2. Use a gliding manipulation with the heated stone and keep the hot stone moving at all times to prevent burns. When the stone loses heat, replace it with another. Observe precautions for body mechanics.
3. Preferably, use the warm stone to heat your hands. Then use your warm hands for massage and place the stone as described in the next step.
4. Place warm stones on top of a sheet or towel at specific points on the body, especially where neurovascular bundles occur, such as on either side of the spine or in the palms of the hand. Instruct the client to speak up if the stones are too warm or the pressure is too intense.
5. If the client has inflammation or a muscle injury, use cold stones in those areas.
6. Cover the area with a towel and then place the stones on the towel rather than directly on the skin; this is the safest and most sanitary method. With direct application to the skin, the most serious concern is burning the client if the stone is too hot for the individual's skin and/or if it is left on too long. Always use warm, not hot, stones and place stones over a towel.
7. Apply the stones with an intentional, centered approach.
8. Placement of stones can be combined with general massage. Also, it might be fun to have a selection of stones to give clients for self-help methods. However, make sure the client understands the importance of safe temperature.
9. If the therapeutic benefit of stone application depends on temperature and weight, cloth bags filled with rice or other grains can be used as an alternative. A pair of socks makes a great bag for this purpose. Fill one sock with the grain (the most inexpensive rice you can buy works fine) and tie the end tightly with string. Then slip the other sock over

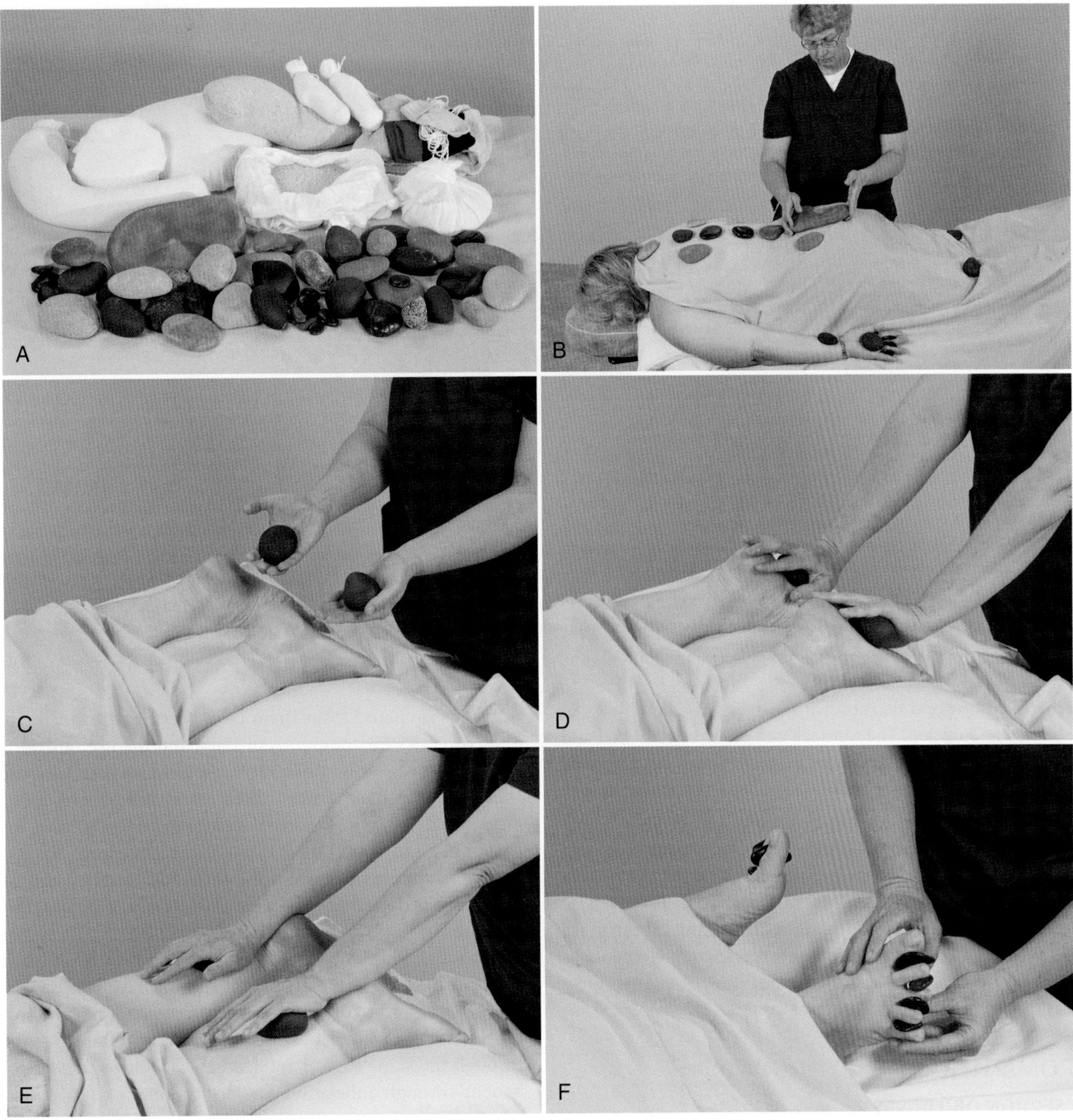

FIG. 12.5 Stone massage and the use of rice bags, which can be used for hot and cold applications. A, Examples of stones and rice bags. **B,** Application of stones on the posterior of the body. Hot stones must be placed over a sheet or towel; cold stones can be placed on the skin. **C–E,** Examples of using stones to perform massage. **F,** Example of placing stones between the toes.

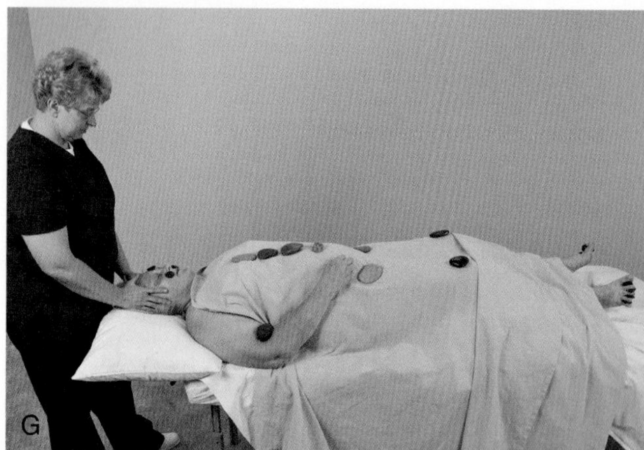

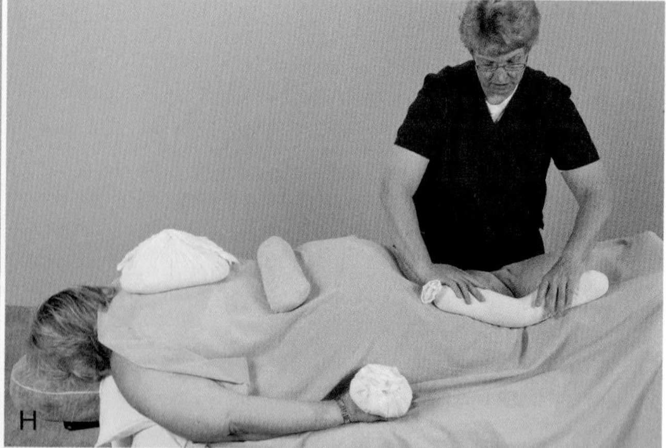

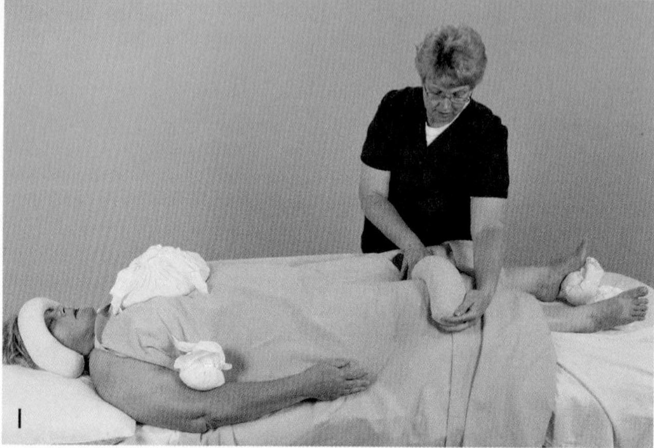

FIG. 12.5, cont'd G, Application of stones on the anterior of the body. Hot stones must be placed over a sheet or towel; cold stones can be placed on the skin. **H–I,** Examples of using rice bags for compression and thermotherapy.

the filled one and tie it off with a string in a bow that can be tied and untied. The top sock can easily be removed and laundered. Various sizes and shapes of bags can be made using different sizes of socks.

Different colors of socks can be used to add a color element to the process. These bags—rice, socks, and string—cost less than $5 to make. Sock bags can be heated in the microwave or cooled in the freezer. They can also be molded to the area where they are placed, and they tend to stay put. These grain bags provide all the same proposed therapeutic elements as stones except possibly piezoelectric qualities. The same safety measures are used to prevent burns (Box 12.5).

AROMATHERAPY

SECTION OBJECTIVES

Chapter objective covered in this section:

4. Safely integrate aromatherapy into the massage process.

Using the information presented in this section, the student will be able to perform the following:

- Define aromatherapy and essential oils.
- Explain the potential benefits of aromatherapy.
- Use essential oils safely.

Aromatherapy involves the use of essential oils, which are distilled extracts from aromatic plants. Aromatic plants and infusions prepared from them have been used in medicines and cosmetics for thousands of years, but the use of distilled oils dates back only 1000 years. Ancient civilizations used these oils to protect against disease, to ward off evil, and to aid spiritual healing. As various societies came in contact with each other and shared these oils, knowledge spread. The term *aromatherapy* was coined in the early 20th century and was recognized as a healing discipline (Tissarand and Balacs, 1995; Schnaubelt, 1998; Price and Price, 2006).

Essential oils can be directly inhaled or absorbed through the skin to achieve therapeutic effect. Massage can be combined with aromatherapy. This combination stems from the fact that essential oils, being lipids, are easily absorbed through the skin. Topical application also allows the client to benefit through inhalation for absorption through mucous membranes.

Medical aromatherapy is common in Europe, where physicians prescribe essential oils for the treatment of diseases and conditions. In the United States nurses and other health care providers often are trained in aromatherapy. Because essential oils have antiseptic, antibacterial, and antibiotic properties, they complement most forms of health care. Studies indicate the combined use of aromatherapy and massage supports pain and anxiety relief (Rivard et al., 2014; Wu et al., 2014). Recent systematic reviews and meta-analysis found no significant benefit of aromatherapy; however, the sample sizes were small

Box 12.5 Do No Harm and Avoid the Burn: Important Cautionary Note

Massage practitioners are rarely the target of lawsuits; however, incorrect use of hot stones, resulting in burns to the client, has produced a number of cases of litigation. Practitioners must be especially mindful to avoid burning a client by using stones that are too hot, especially when they are left in one place on the client's body.

Always place hot stones over a thick double-folded sheet or towel.

Do not place hot stones directly on the skin.

Frequently check the skin under the stone.

Do not leave large heavy hot stones at a temperature of 100 degrees in one place for more than a minute.

Do not use stones heated warmer than 100 degrees.

Heating stones in any device other than a unit specifically designed for this increases the risk of harm.

The hot stone should be able to be held in the therapist's bare hand for 5 seconds comfortably. Even with this safety test, the stone can still be too hot because the palm skin is thicker than skin on other body areas.

Prepare a bowl of iced water to lower stone temperature where required and place it for easy access during treatment.

Burns from hot stone massage most often occur when heated stones are placed on bare skin and left in this static position or placed underneath clients so that clients are laying on the stones. Burns occur when the stones are place over a thin sheet instead of a thicker towel. Also the elderly and children are more susceptible to being burned.

Be safe – make sure the client is safe. Evaluate risk versus benefit.

and of low quality (Ball et al., 2020; Rawal et al., 2022). Other studies and reviews suggest some physiological effects and encourage more research. Increasing experimental research in the pharmacology of essential oils suggests influence on neural pathways and oxidative stress as a reason for physiological and psychological effects (Abd et al., 2021 Singh, et al., 2021; Lizarraga-Valderrama 2021; Shah et al., 2021). Be cautious regarding unsubstantiated claims and assure safe use.

Aromatherapy training ensures that the practitioner is prepared to take a client history and can perform an assessment, recognize contraindications, and create essential oil blends designed to address the client's specific concerns. This approach would be considered a medical treatment. Essential oils can also be used for many spa applications (particularly in relation to skin care), such as cleansing and reducing the size of pores, soothing burns, treating sensitive or cracked skin, oil gland regulation, hair growth, and skin nourishment. These are common focuses in the spa setting.

Note: The client's consent should be obtained before essential oils are used.

Essential Oils

Essential oils are subtle, volatile chemicals distilled from plants, shrubs, flowers, trees, roots, bushes, and seeds. Essential oils are beneficial both through inhalation of the scent, which affects the limbic system, and through lipid absorption of the oil through the skin. Aromatherapy is an extensive study, and care and caution are advised in the use of essential oils. Only pure essential oils should be used, and they should be diluted in a carrier oil (e.g., olive, jojoba, grapeseed, or almond oil) before they are applied to the skin. Only three or four drops of essential oil are needed in 2 ounces of carrier oil. When a drop of oil is mixed with a small amount of salt (1/4 cup), it can be dissolved in a warm water immersion, such as a bath.

- Essential oils in the pure state should never be applied directly to the skin.
- Only use oils that are generally considered safe, such as the ones listed in this text.

Research on the efficacy of essential oils is lacking. The following are some of the claimed effects of essential oils:

- *Skin:* They can help remove dead surface cells, increase cell turnover, stimulate metabolism, improve texture, add softness, give radiance, stimulate, and tone.
- *Nervous system:* They can calm and soothe nerve endings, cause a sense of euphoria, and promote relaxation.
- *Glands:* They can have a soothing and sedating effect, or a toning and stimulating effect.
- *Muscles:* They can relieve fatigue, reduce soreness and stiffness, and improve the resilience and elasticity of muscle.

Additives for an aromatherapy bath or massage oil might include the following:

- Relaxing: lavender, clary sage, melissa, ylang-ylang, bergamot, chamomile
- Stimulating: rosemary, thyme, pine, cypress
- Soothing: chamomile, jasmine, geranium, rose
- Moisturizing: orange blossom, neroli, patchouli, lavender

Essential oils have hormone-like properties and are natural antiseptics. Each oil is thought to have a unique effect on the body and mind, but the oil also can be easily classified as antiseptic, analgesic, antiinflammatory, regenerating, stimulating, or sedating.

Essential oils are not oily; rather, they are more like water. They are generally transparent and can be an assortment of colors. Because essential oils are lipid (fat) based, they are soluble in alcohol, oils, and fats, but not water.

Degradation can be an issue with essential oils. Store them in dark glass bottles, away from heat and sunlight. Storage in a cool dark place, such as a refrigerator, is recommended. Use of stoppered caps helps prevent oxidation (which reduces efficacy or results in chemical changes). Never store essential oils in plastic, and make sure they are not within reach of children. Most essential oils should be used within 1 year of purchase, although refrigeration can at least double this life span. Some oils, such as orange, lemon, and lime, degrade more quickly and may last only 6 months without refrigeration.

Fragrance Oils

Essential oils are the organic constituents of fragrant plant matter and are extracted by distillation or cold pressing. They contain the true essence of the plant. Fragrance or perfume oils are blended synthetic aroma compounds diluted with carrier oils. These artificial oils are used most often in perfumes, cosmetics, and flavoring and are not therapeutically effective.

Because use of the terms *aromatherapy* and *therapeutic grade* are not regulated by the U.S. government, caution is required when using products. Many beauty and skin care preparations, candles, and other products are improperly labeled with the term *aromatherapy*, although the scent is actually artificial and derived from synthetic fragrance oils. As mentioned, fragrance oils do not offer the therapeutic value of pure high-grade essential oils.

Distillation is a primary determinant of high-grade status. The higher the pressure used in distillation, the higher the yield of oil; however, this also causes unnecessary fractionation of the oil molecules as a result of the higher temperatures created by increasing the pressure. Flavor and fragrance companies produce their oils this way because they are interested in the scent or flavor applications for food, soft drinks, and other beverages, at the lowest possible cost. Oils produced by high-pressure distillation work fine for flavor and fragrance. Oils produced under lower pressure preserve their molecular structures with the highest integrity.

Carrier Oils

As mentioned, essential oils are mixed with a carrier oil. Carrier oils are high-quality, fresh vegetable oils that are used to dilute essential oils. Carrier oils also have their own therapeutic properties. The most popular carrier oils are listed in Table 12.3. Make sure all carrier oils are fresh.

Benefits of Aromatherapy

The physiologic effect of essential oils is primarily chemical. The chemistry of essential oils is complex. Hundreds of components, such as terpenes, aldehydes, and esters, make up the oils. Lavender, for example, has antiseptic, antibacterial, antibiotic, antidepressant, analgesic, decongestant, and sedative properties. Essential oils also reach the bloodstream through inhalation. When inhaled, they pass through the tiny air sacs to the surrounding blood capillaries by the process of diffusion. Once in the bloodstream, the aromatic molecules interact with the body's chemistry.

In addition to their medicinal properties, essential oils have the ability to uplift the client's spirits through inhalation. The sense of smell is interrelated with the limbic system, an area of the brain primarily concerned with emotion and memory. This influence of aromas on the psyche has led many aromatherapists to practice a form of aromatherapy called *psychoaromatherapy*, in which essential oils are used to enhance the client's mood and emotions. The massage therapist needs to be

Table 12.3 Common Carrier Oils

Oil	Uses
Apricot kernel oil *(Prunus armeniaca)*	Extremely moisturizing; use to help revitalize dry skin, delicate skin, mature skin, and sensitive skin and to help soothe minor skin inflammations.
Avocado oil *(Persea americana)*	Rich in vitamins A, B1, and B2; excellent for cases of extremely dry skin (e.g., calluses on the feet). Use on dry, cracked, chapped, and irritated skin and for eczema and psoriasis.
Corn oil	Soothing for all skin types.
Evening primrose oil *(Oenothera biennis)*	Reduces the appearance of wrinkles; also beneficial for sluggish skin, scarring, inflammation, eczema, acne, and minor skin irritations.
Grapeseed oil *(Vitis vinifera)*	Used in most cosmetics as a base oil; use for thin skin around the eyes and for normal to combination skin as a light moisturizer.
Hazelnut oil *(Corylus avellana)*	Helps tone and tighten skin and to restore elastin to the skin; use to help promote cell regeneration; apply on oily and combination skin.
Hemp seed oil *(Cannabis sativa)*	Penetrates the skin to moisturize, stimulate, and repair cells damaged by the elements, sun, wind, and ultraviolet light; useful for any skin type.
Jojoba golden *(Simmondsia chinensis)*	Similar to sebum (the oil human skin produces). Skin absorbs it very quickly, and no oily residue is left on the surface; good for dry, chapped, and cracked skin.
Olive oil	A heavy oil used in cosmetics and soaps; for massage, it is best blended with a lighter vegetable oil.
Rose hip seed *(Rosa mosqueta)*	Has the highest natural vitamin C content of all the carrier oils and is a renowned cell-renewal agent. Use for scars, stretch marks, wrinkles, cracked skin, dry skin, and sunburn and to support collagen in the skin.
Sesame oil *(Sesamum indicum)*	Nourishes damaged skin. Use on dry, chapped, discolored, flaky, sun-damaged, and burned skin.
Soybean oil	Use on mature skin.
Sunflower oil *(Helianthus annuus)*	Has excellent healing properties. Use as a treatment for acne on the body and for accelerating the healing of wounds and insect bites.
Sweet almond oil *(Prunus dulcis)*	A favorite of massage therapists because of its nutritive and moisturizing qualities. Great for sensitive skin and high in vitamins A, B1, B6, and E. Use for dry skin, itchiness, and irritated and inflamed skin.
Wheat germ oil *(Triticum vulgare)*	Known for its high content of vitamins E and C. Use on mature skin, wrinkles, sun damage, dark spots, eczema, psoriasis, stretch marks, and skin showing signs of premature aging.

cautious of the scope of practice and ethical boundaries when oils are used for specific treatment of physical or mental disorders.

When an essential oil is inhaled, the chemicals in it stimulate the olfactory center, which receives the odor and carries it to the limbic system. The signal passes between the pituitary and pineal glands, targeting the amygdala (memory center for fear and trauma). These areas of the brain influence mood, and the hippocampus and amygdala are specifically related to emotion and memory. Scent memory is longer than visual memory. The experience is one of déjà vu; that is, feeling as if the current experience is familiar and seems to be triggered by memory.

An aromatherapy massage can help a person deeply relax and let go of worries, even if only for a short time. Relaxation is powerful enough to activate the body's self-healing ability. Combining the physical and emotional effects of massage with the medicinal and therapeutic properties of essential oils can alleviate stress and improves a person's mood.

Essential oils may help with moderate anxiety and depression, insomnia, digestive disorders, headaches, upper respiratory conditions, and muscle aches and pains.

Safety Guidelines for the Use of Essential Oils

As mentioned, essential oils are highly concentrated, volatile substances that, if used correctly, might have therapeutic benefit. Although many oils are useful, some are not safe to use at all, and proper safety guidelines must always be followed when using essential oils. Practitioners should receive advanced training in the use of essential oils before offering aromatherapy massage.

Massage therapists need to be concerned of over exposure to essential oils. This can occur when oils are frequently used as an adjunct to the massage. The massage therapist absorbs and inhales the oils during application to the client.

Note: The following cautions and information do not in any way replace medical and professional advice and may not include all cautionary information available:

- *Never* ingest (take internally) essential oil.
- *Never* apply undiluted oils on the skin.
- *Always* dilute essential oils in a carrier oil to prevent skin irritation and burning. Experienced aromatherapists may break with this rule, but without extensive training, it is important to work with these substances with caution.
- *Always* test for sensitization and irritation. When using a new oil on your client, it is important to patch test. To patch test, apply a small amount of the diluted oil to the client's skin and leave for 24 to 48 hours to determine whether a reaction occurs. Even if working with an oil that does not commonly cause irritation, the patch test is important as a measure of safety.
- Be familiar with essential oils that are contraindicated during pregnancy or for clients with diseases and illnesses such as asthma and epilepsy.
- Only small amounts of essential oils are needed, and you should use the smallest amount possible for effective treatment. If an additional drop is not necessary, do not use it.
- Many essential oils are not appropriate for use in aromatherapy. Do not assume that every essential oil can be used safely. Some oils, such as wormwood, onion, bitter almond, pennyroyal, camphor, horseradish, wintergreen, rue, and sassafras, should only be used by a qualified aromatherapist. Some oils should not be used at all.
- Keep essential oils out of children's reach. These oils can be tempting, because the scents are appealing and children may think they are lotions or even candy or sweet drinks (e.g., citrus oil). Treat these oils as medicines or poisons when considering storage.
- Keep essential oils away from animals.
- Essential oils are flammable. Store them properly and keep them away from fire hazards.
- Keep oils away from the eyes. If a drop or so of oil accidentally gets in the eye, put some vegetable oil (e.g., almond oil) in the eye; the vegetable oil will absorb the essential oil, and a tissue then can be used to remove the oil. Do not use water, which will spread the oil. If burning or itching occurs, seek medical treatment.
- Do not use the same oils for a prolonged period.
- Use photosensitizing oils cautiously (i.e., bergamot, verbena, lime, angelica root, bitter orange, lemon, and grapefruit). Advise the client to avoid sun exposure and the use of tanning beds for 12 hours after application of these oils. Photosensitization occurs when oils containing furanocoumarin compounds are applied to the skin and the skin is immediately exposed to sunlight or ultraviolet (UV) light. Furanocoumarin compounds allow the UV rays to penetrate the skin more readily, resulting in abnormal skin pigmentation or mild to severe burns. Remember, UV rays are present even on cloudy days.
- Store essential oils away from light and heat and keep the caps tightly closed. Essential oils are volatile and evaporate readily.

Some aromatherapy experts believe that certain essential oils should not be used unless administered by qualified aromatherapists, and some oils should not be used even by qualified practitioners. Box 12.6 provides a list of potentially hazardous essential oils; do not assume that an oil is safe to use if it is not included in the box. This information is for general educational purposes only and is not considered complete, nor is it guaranteed to be accurate.

Aromatherapy Applications

Essential oils can be used in various ways in combination with hydrotherapy and massage:

- *Aromatic compress:* Put 3 to 5 drops of oil into 1 to 2 cups of hot or cold water, depending on the need for a compress. Fold a clean cloth and submerge it in the water, then squeeze the excess water from the compress into the basin. Apply immediately to the treatment area.
- *Aromatic facial steam:* Use 1 to 2 drops of oil per 1 cup of boiling water. Place the oil in the bowl or basin after the water has boiled. Stir the water to disperse the oil. Immediately place a towel over the head and place the face as close as possible to the aromatic steam without causing any discomfort.

Box 12.6 Potentially Hazardous Essential Oils

Oils that should *not* be used on any client include the following:
Bitter almond
Boldo leaf
Calamus
Camphor (yellow)
Horseradish
Jaborandi leaf
Mugwort
Mustard
Pennyroyal
Rue
Sassafras
Savin (Juniperus sabina)
Southernwood
Tansy
Thuja
Western red cedar *(Thuja plicata)*
Wintergreen
Wormseed
Wormwood

Oils that should *not* be used on pregnant clients include the following:
Aniseed
Basil
Cinnamon
Clary sage
Cypress
Fennel
Hyssop
Jasmine
Juniper
Marjoram
Myrrh
Origanum
Peppermint
Rose
Rosemary
Sage
Thyme

Oils that should *not* be used on or by individuals with epilepsy include the following:
Camphor
Fennel
Hyssop
Sage

- *Environmental and room fragrance:* Electronic diffusers are an easy, effective way to fragrance a room for esthetic and therapeutic purposes. Use only pure essential oils or synergies of pure essential oils. Never use essential oils cut with carrier oils in diffusers because this clogs the diffuser.
- *Aroma lamps:* Aroma lamps are great for adding environmental fragrance. Add 10 drops of essential oils to 1 teaspoon of water and place in the designated receptacle on the lamp. The heat of the light disperses the fragrance.
- *Inhalation:* An effective and simple way to inhale essential oils is to place a couple drops of an oil or blend on a handkerchief or cotton cloth and inhale throughout the day. This is a nice gift for the person who just received the massage.
- *Aromatic spray:* Mix about 100 drops of essential oil (a single oil or a blend of oils) with 4 ounces of vodka or witch hazel. This creates a concentrate that can be added to water to create the aromatic spray. Add about 100 drops of the concentrate to 2 ounces of distilled water and shake well. To create a spritzer for the face or body, use only water and essential oils. For the body, add about 20 to 30 drops of essential oil or a blend to 4 ounces of distilled water. For the face, add 8 to 10 drops to 8 ounces of water. Do not allow spray to contact the eyes.
- *Massage:* Use a dilution of about 1% to 2.5% of essential oil to carrier oil when preparing the massage oil. This means approximately 5 to 15 drops of essential oil per 2 ounces (1/4 cup, 4 tablespoons, 60 ml) of carrier oil. If you are using more than one essential oil, blend them first and then add no more than 15 drops of the blend to the carrier oil. Remember, when creating a massage blend, less is more, and in fact the desired result can be achieved with very low dilutions.

Choosing Essential Oils to Complement Massage

A number of factors can affect the selection of essential oils to be used for massage. The choice can be based on the therapeutic quality of the oil or oils (Table 12.4), the client's emotional well-being (Table 12.5), or the presence of a specific condition (Table 12.6):

- Offer a selection of oils you, the massage therapist, can tolerate since you will be exposed to the oil as well as the client (no more than 10).
- Let the client sniff each oil; have the person choose one or two they like most and then one they like least. Look up the characteristics of the oils with the client (see Table 12.4) and see how they relate to the client's current condition.
- Create a unique blend for the client with 3 drops of the oil the client likes the most and 2 drops of the oil the client likes next for a total of 5 drops. If the client only chooses one, then use 5 drops of that oil. Next add 1 drop of the least favorite oil (blend no more than three oils). Then blend the mixture into 1 ounce (2 tablespoons) carrier oil chosen according to the client's skin type and the qualities of the carrier oil.

FOCUS ON PROFESSIONALISM

Products applied to the skin or inhaled may have benefits but there are also risks. Not only essential oils and carrier oils are a concern. Cannabis-based products such as CBD oils are sometimes included in massage application. All of these products need to be carefully evaluated on risk vs benefit. Remember, the client has a limited exposure during the massage session, but the massage therapist is exposed over and over if these types of products are used frequency during massage sessions. The massage therapist can become over-exposed and sensitized to the active ingredients. It may be more prudent to become educated in the potential benefits and risks to be a source of information for clients so they can rub essential oil (diluted in carrier oil) or CBD products on themselves.

Table 12.4 Therapeutic Qualities of Individual Essential Oils

Oil	Therapeutic Qualities
Bergamot	Skin conditioner, soothing agent, antiseptic, phototoxic
Cajeput	Stimulating agent, mood enhancer, antiseptic
Cardamom	Muscle relaxant, skin conditioner, soothing agent
Carrot seed	Muscle relaxant, soothing agent, skin conditioner
Cedarwood	Antiseptic, skin conditioner, deodorant, soothing agent
Clary sage	Skin conditioner, astringent, soothing agent, muscle relaxant. Do not use if client is pregnant or drinks alcohol
Eucalyptus	Antiseptic, soothing agent, skin conditioner, sinus clearing
Frankincense	Skin conditioner, soothing agent
Geranium	Skin refresher, muscle relaxant
Ginger	Astringent
Grapefruit	Soothing agent, astringent, skin conditioner
Jasmine absolute	Emollient, soothing agent, antiseptic
Juniper	Skin detoxifier, astringent, soothing agent; flammable
Lavender	Muscle relaxant, skin conditioner, soothing agent, astringent
Lemon	Soothing agent, antiseptic
Lemongrass	Skin conditioner, soothing agent, muscle relaxant, antiseptic
Lime	Soothing agent, skin conditioner, astringent
Mandarin	Soothing agent, skin conditioner, astringent
Myrrh	Antiinflammatory, emollient, antiseptic; use in moderation if client is pregnant
Neroli	Antiseptic, emollient
Nutmeg	Antiseptic, muscle relaxant; soothes irritated skin
Orange	Astringent, soothing agent, skin conditioner
Peppermint	Emollient, antiseptic, muscle relaxant
Pine	Antiseptic
Roman chamomile	Muscle relaxant, skin conditioner
Rose absolute	Skin conditioner
Rose otto	Astringent
Rosemary	Antiseptic, muscle relaxant, soothing agent, skin conditioner; do not use if client is pregnant or has high blood pressure
Rosewood	Muscle relaxant
Sandalwood	Antiseptic, emollient, soothing agent, skin conditioner
Spearmint	Emollient, astringent, soothing agent; use sparingly
Tea tree	Antiseptic, acne fighter, dandruff fighter
Ylang-ylang	Reduces stress and tension

Table 12.5 Oils for Emotional Well-Being

Condition	Treatment Oils
Anger	Bergamot, jasmine, orange, patchouli, rose, ylang-ylang
Anxiety	Clary sage, frankincense, geranium, lavender, mandarin, rose, sandalwood
Confidence	Bergamot, grapefruit, jasmine, orange, rosemary
Depression	Bergamot, clary sage, frankincense, geranium, grapefruit, jasmine, lavender, lemon, mandarin, neroli, orange, rose
Fatigue, exhaustion, and burnout	Bergamot, clary sage, frankincense, grapefruit, jasmine, lemon, peppermint, rosemary, sandalwood
Fear	Clary sage, frankincense, grapefruit, jasmine, lemon, neroli, orange
Grief	Frankincense, neroli, rose
Happiness, peace	Frankincense, geranium, grapefruit, lemon, neroli, orange, rose sandalwood, ylang-ylang
Insecurity	Frankincense, jasmine, sandalwood
Irritability	Lavender, mandarin, neroli, Roman chamomile, sandalwood
Loneliness	Bergamot, clary sage, frankincense, rose
Memory, concentration problems	Lemon, peppermint, rosemary
Stress	Bergamot, clary sage, frankincense, geranium, grapefruit, jasmine, lavender, mandarin, neroli, Roman chamomile, rose sandalwood, ylang-ylang

Data from Aromatherapy for Emotional Well-Being, Aroma Web, LLC, at http://www.aroma.com/articles/emotional/wellbeing.asp.

IMPLEMENT-ASSISTED MASSAGE: SAFETY FIRST

SECTION OBJECTIVES

Chapter objective covered in this section:

5. Describe the safe use of implements and kinesiology tape during a massage session.

Using the information presented in this section, the student will be able to perform the following:

- Safely use implements during massage .

An **implement** is some sort of device that is used to augment the massage application. The device can roll, press, scrape, or suction. The two main reasons for using an implement are as follows:

- The device reduces the effort required to apply massage, making massage application easier for the massage therapist.
- The device can apply mechanical force to the soft tissue more effectively than the massage therapist's hands, forearms, or other part of the body used to apply massage methods.

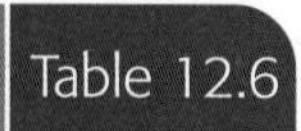

Table 12.6 Essential Oils for Common Physical Conditions

Condition	Treatment Oils
Abdominal cramps	Lavender, clary sage
Acne	Bergamot, chamomile, geranium, lavender, patchouli, sandalwood, tea tree
Aging skin	Carrot seed, frankincense
Arthritis	Chamomile, eucalyptus, ginger
Athlete's foot	Tea tree
Brain fog	Grapefruit, lemongrass, lime, orange
Colds, flu, bronchitis	Cajeput, eucalyptus, frankincense, ginger, lavender, peppermint, tea tree
Corns, warts	Lemon, tea tree
Bruises	Chamomile, lavender
Burns	Lavender
Children's stomach upsets	Mandarin, tangerine
Cold sores	Eucalyptus, tea tree
Coughs	Eucalyptus, ginger, tea tree
Dandruff	Lavender
Dermatitis	Chamomile, lavender
Dry skin	Geranium (especially skin with oily patches), sandalwood
Dysmenorrhea (painful periods/menstrual cramps)	Chamomile, clary sage, cypress, lavender
Edema	Carrot seed, grapefruit
Fevers	Eucalyptus, lemongrass
Flatulence	Lime
Headache	Chamomile, lavender, peppermint
Herpes	Tea tree
High blood pressure (hypertension)	Lavender, ylang-ylang
Indigestion	Chamomile, orange
Inflammation	Chamomile, lavender
Insect bites and stings	Chamomile, lavender, tea tree
Insect repellent	Lemongrass, lavender
Insomnia	Chamomile, lavender
Laryngitis, sore throat	Ginger, lavender, thyme
Muscle aches and pains	Chamomile, eucalyptus, ginger, grapefruit, lavender, rosemary
Nausea	Chamomile, lavender
Nervous exhaustion, fatigue	Peppermint, rosemary
Nervous tension, stress	Chamomile, clary sage, frankincense, lavender, sandalwood
Neuralgia	Chamomile
Poor circulation	Ginger, rosemary
Premenstrual syndrome (PMS)	Geranium, lavender
Scars	Frankincense, lavender
Sinusitis	Eucalyptus, pine
Sprains, strains	Chamomile, eucalyptus, lavender
Stretch marks	Mandarin, lavender
Vertigo	Lavender, peppermint

Remember that massage methods apply mechanical forces to deform soft tissue and that mechanical forces are a push or a pull. Any devices incorporated into massage should assist this process. There are many implements that can be used to push into tissue. In general, these devices are used to create compression stress. Rollers, balls, knobs, etc. are made in a variety of designs and made from materials including metal, plastic, and wood. The stones used in hot and cold stone massage are implements.

The main safety concerns are compression injury to soft tissue and sanitation. The various tools must be disinfected after every use. Compression injury is called a contusion. A contusion (bruise) is an injury to the soft tissue often produced by a blunt force resulting in pain, swelling, and discoloration. Nerves are especially susceptible to compression injury.

Traction devices pull. Traction is the act of applying a mild stretch at constant force to the body tissues, especially muscles and ligaments, around jointed areas. Most often implements that assist the massage therapist in performing traction are straps and bands.

The main safety concern from the strap is skin damage. There is also a potential for traction application to be too aggressive when a strap is used to assist with the traction method.

Implements can also be used for percussion and vibration. Bundled sticks, usually bamboo or rattan, and soft head mallets are examples of tools that can be used to replace the hands when performing percussion methods. The main safety concern related to percussion implements is the tissue damage that could occur with aggressive percussion. The tissue can be bruised, and depending on the implement (e.g., bundled sticks), the skin could be cut.

An implement that can apply vibrations is a tuning fork. When the tuning fork is hit with a rubber hammer, the tines begin to vibrate. The end of the tuning fork is placed on the body. Research on the mechanisms of vibrational effect is categorized into hemodynamic, neurological, and musculoskeletal (Bartel and Mosabbir, 2021). Tuning forks present a low risk of harm, and because vibration performed by the massage therapist is fatiguing, they may be a valuable tool.

Electric Devices. Electric devices can create percussion and vibration to augment massage application. A percussion device moves in-out and up-down like hammers or pistons. A vibration device moves back and forth. The use of handheld percussion and vibration devises as an adjunct to the massage session has increased in recent years. One reason is based on replacing labor intensive methods with electronic handheld equipment. There are ergonomics and biomechanics safety concerns for massage practitioners using electrical devices. Exposure to hand-arm vibration (HAV) can cause damage to arms, hands, and fingers, and lead to health risks ranging from musculoskeletal, vascular, neurological, osteoarticular, or any combinations thereof (Lindenmann et al., 2021; Faizan and Khan, 2022; Vihlborg et al., 2022).

Justification for Application

Vibration and percussion approaches provided by electrical devices may be indicated for pain, autogenic muscle inhibition, delayed onset muscle soreness, and to improve muscle strength and proprioception. The transmission of high- and low-intensity mechanical signals simulates physiological stimuli encountered in daily life, alters the interaction between the vibrated muscle and its antagonists, increases motor coordination, improves joint performance, decreases muscle stiffness, and stimulates blood and lymph circulation (Konrad et al., 2020; Alam et al., 2021; Paolucci et al., 2021). Overall, vibration therapy is a safe, inexpensive, and accessible form of treatment with many benefits (Lupowitz, 2022).

Contraindications

Use caution or avoid the area for stress fractures, neuropathy, fibromyalgia epilepsy, pregnancy, recent surgery or joint replacement, metal pins or plates, pacemakers, areas with skin rash or open wounds, and in individuals with hypertension or those at risk for clotting (Lupowitz, 2022).

How to use

- To alleviate pain, improve tissue extensibility, and reduce the potential for delayed onset muscle soreness, use lower frequency and amplitude coupled with longer duration (30+ seconds).
- To support physical performance or mimic exercise activity, use higher frequency and amplitude coupled with short duration usage (< 30 seconds).

Instrument-Assisted Soft Tissue Manipulation (IASTM)/Scraping

Gua sha, also called coining, spooning, or scraping, is an instrument assisted soft tissue method that has been used throughout Asia for centuries. Gua means "to rub" or "press stroke." *Sha* is a term that describes the marks caused by friction from the instrument scraping on the skin. The scraping causes capillaries to break open and leak blood into the skin.

Justification for Application

Evidence for the use of scraping-based methods is very low-quality and does not support the efficacy of IASTM in individuals with or without various pathologies on function, pain, and range of motion in the management of upper body, lower body, or spinal conditions (Nazari et al., 2023). It is hypothesized that the skin, the nervous system, and immune system interact to generate a cascade of physiological responses to the scraping, which may result in therapeutic benefits. Counterirritation is considered part of the potential therapeutic response (Chu et al., 2021). An increase in microcirculation in the treated area may have positive effects. Unidentified pain-relieving biomechanisms likely reduce pain intensity (Checketts, 2018). There may be increases in mobility and antiinflammatory responses when scraping methods are appropriately applied (Cheatham et al., 2016; Yuen et al., 2017). The main theory regarding the benefit of this type of application is that through controlled reinjuring of the body, inflammation and first-stage healing is reinitiated (Kim et al., 2017; Shin, 2022). The use of novel soft tissue and neuromuscular techniques for immediate short-term improvement seems to improve functional capacity even if the mechanisms are not understood (Angelopoulos et al., 2021).

Contraindications

- Do not scrape over any mole, pimple, or mark on the skin; also stay away from varicose veins, skin disorders, or open wounds and scratches.
- Do not use the approach on people who are very frail or are too weak to tolerate the treatment.
- Do not use on people with bleeding disorders, or for people who are taking anticoagulant medication such as like warfarin (Nielsen, 2014).

Again, the primary safety concerns are tissue damage and sanitation. Often the implement causes discomfort during the procedure and bruising afterward. Because the method causes controlled reinjury, extreme caution is necessary. Implements must be disinfected after each use.

Tools/Instruments

Arya Nielsen, author of Gua sha: A Traditional Technique for Modern Practice (Copyright 2013 Elsevier Ltd.), recommends plastisol lined caps as one-use disposable Gua sha/scraping instruments. Other tools can be used but must be disinfected after each use. Tools can be complex and designed in different ways or as simple as a spoon or butter knife with dull edges (Fig. 12.6).

Procedure Recommendations

- Apply ointment or oil to the skin in the intervention area.
- The instrument should be held somewhere between a 30- and a 45-degree angle to the area to be treat.
- Scrape in one direction—down, away from the head, or laterally away from the spine—never scrape downwards and then draw back upwards on the same spot.
- Start with gentle scraping for the first few strokes, then apply a little more pressure as required. Try to keep the pressure consistent, neither going too deep and hard, nor too soft. If it's painful for the client the pressure is too intense.
- Each stroke should be performed between 10 and 30 times before proceeding to the next area.
- Once the area is treated, cover it immediately with a towel to keep it warm.

Clients can be taught to use a simple tool like a spoon and use scraping as a self-help activity on their own between massage sessions.

Cupping/Vacuum/Negative Pressure Therapy

Multiple terms are used for an approach that uses suction to create a negative pressure on the superficial tissues. Terms include *vacuum therapy*, *negative pressure cupping*, and *myofascial decompression therapy*. Vacuum therapy is a noninvasive massaging technique that helps lift superficial tissue using a mechanical device equipped with suction cups.

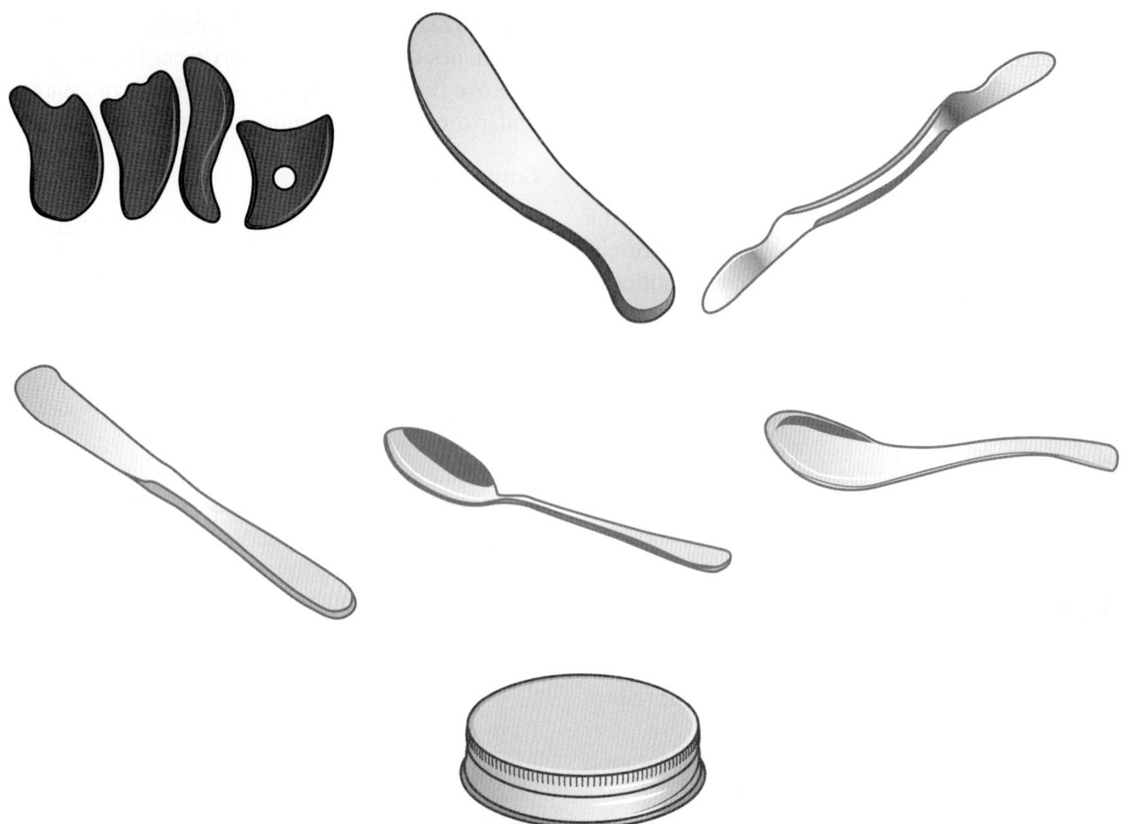

FIG. 12.6 Scraping tools.

Cupping therapy is a multicultural traditional and complementary medicine practice. There are numerous types of cupping therapy, such as wet, dry, massage, flash, magnetic, and water cupping. Cupping types can be classified according to five categories: technique, power of suction, method of suction, added therapy, and condition/area treated (Al-Bedah et al., 2018) (Fig. 12.7).

Justification for Application

The strongest evidence for cupping therapy's benefit is for the treatment of pain, particularly musculoskeletal pain, migraine, or tension headache (Furhad and Bokhari, 2022). There is weak evidence supporting vacuum manual therapy benefiting pain-related conditions and muscle stiffness (Hou et al., 2021; Jan et al., 2021; Mohamed et al., 2022). Suction may affect skin blood flow, biomechanical properties, and temperature of the skin, causing increased pressure pain thresholds in the treated areas (Liu et al., 2023). A logical and biologically plausible theory of action is called *Diffuse Noxious Inhibitory Controls (DNIC)* which is inhibition of nociceptive spinal neurons triggered by a second, noxious stimulus. DNIC is thought to underlie the principle of counter-irritation to reduce pain. Also, local damage of the skin and capillary vessels induced by suction may cause a nociceptive stimulus that activates DNIC.

The suction on the skin may produce analgesic effect by stimulating nerves that are sensitive to mechanical stimulation. The microenvironment is changed when stimulating the surface of the skin, and physical signals transform into biological signals. The signaling might activate the neuroendocrine-immune system, which produces the therapeutic effect (Guo et al., 2017; Li et al., 2017; Ma et al., 2018).

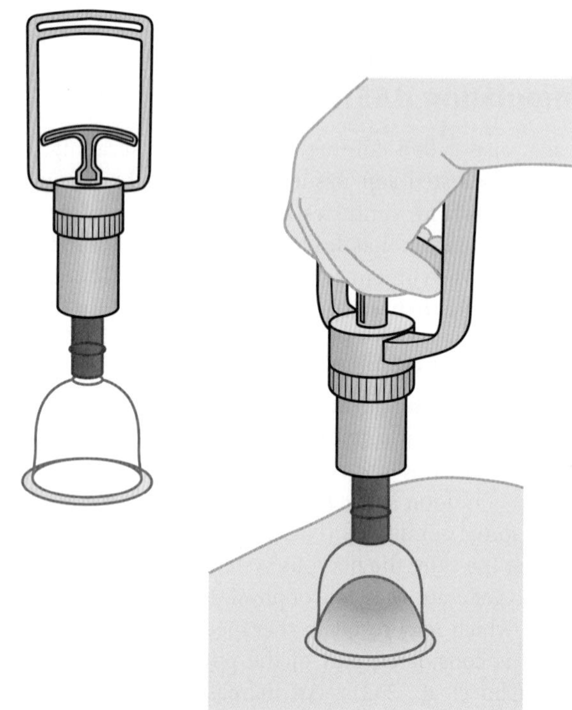

FIG. 12.7 Vacuum/suction devised vacuum manual therapy/suction/cupping.

Recent investigation of suction/negative pressure methods focused on managing lymphedema showed promising results (Lampinen et al., 2021; Dresing et al., 2021).

Contraindications and Cautions

Various adverse effects may occur related to too much suction and/or leaving the suction devise in one place for too long (Kim et al., 2014). The most common adverse side effects include erythema, edema, and ecchymosis. Other reported adverse events include headache, pruritus (itching), muscle tension, dizziness, tiredness, nausea, anemia, small hematoma, severe pain, and bullae (large fluid-filled blisters on the skin) (Alam and Abbas, 2021). Suction is contraindicated directly on surface veins, arteries, nerves, skin inflammation, any skin lesion or open wound, body orifices, eyes, lymph nodes, varicose veins, bone fractures, and sites of deep vein thrombosis (Aboushanab and AlSanad, 2018).

Because of the capillary breakage caused by the suction, the skin can become marked with dark red or purplish areas in the shape of the suction devise. These areas are not bruising which is tissue damage caused by compression. The discoloration can be reduced or avoided by moving the suction devise or only leaving it stationary for short periods such as 15 seconds.

- Massage therapists should not provide fire cupping where the suction is created by burning a swab inside the cup to remove air.
- Massage therapists should not perform wet cupping where the skin is pricked to promote bleeding prior to the suction applied.

Types of Application

Stationary technique: The suction cup is held still on the spot

Lift and twist technique: The suction cup is lifted and twisted

Sliding technique: The suction cup is slid softly over the skin using a lubricant

- Identify specific points or areas for suction.
- A suction tool of a suitable size is placed on the selected site and the air inside the device is removed by manual suction.
- Use the largest cup size that will fit the target area.
- The device can be left stationary or moved as follows:
  - The device can be left in place for up to 2 minutes which will typically result in suction marking.
  - The device can be left stationary (which can result in suction marking) and the adjacent joint actively or passively moved resulting in movement of the tissues around the device.
  - The device can be moved over the skin after attached. Apply oil or lotion to facilitate smooth movement. Suction marking is reduced with this approach.
- During movement, the edge of the cup can be used to add a scraping action in addition to the suction.

The main safety concern involves the marks and blisters left from the suction. The capillaries can be broken and bleed into the interstitial space. This bleeding forms a bruise-like mark. Fluid-filled blisters are created when the epidermis lifts up from the dermis, which is called *suction blistering*. If this occurs the potential for infection increases and a hazard for blood/body fluid–borne disease transmission exists. The cups must be disinfected after each use.

A variety of suction devises can be purchased inexpensively. Clients can be taught simple suction methods for self-help. There are many online videos for instruction.

Recommendations for Implement-Assisted Soft Tissue Manipulation

Implement-assisted massage can have both advantages and concerns. Because the device separates the massage therapist from direct contact with the client, extra caution is required to prevent injury. Also, devices should only be used because they perform methods more effectively than the therapist and/or make the massage easier to perform.

Suction implements such as silicone cups can be helpful in lifting superficial fascial. However, caution is required to prevent the capillary damage by keeping the cup moving and not leaving it in one spot.

The tools used to apply compression still require using the hands, so whether or not the tools create an advantage is questionable. The extended use of electronic percussion and vibration devices poses a risk of damage to the massage therapist. A tuning fork to apply vibration is safer for the massage therapist than an electrical vibration tool. Tools that are used to scrape the skin and push and pull superficial fascia create inflammation. Because controlled tissue damage is the outcome, caution is required; it is easy to do too much, resulting in undesirable levels of inflammation. It is likely that the desired outcome can be achieved more safely without using these types of tools.

The cost of the tools used to assist the massage therapist is a factor as well. Other than the electrical devices, implements should be inexpensive. Because the devices are typically economical, the massage therapist can recommend simple tools for client self-help and teach the client how to use the tools safely.

KINESIOLOGY TAPING

Kinesiology tape was developed in the 1970s by a chiropractor named Dr. Kenzo Kase, DC. Dr. Kase is from Japan and trained in chiropractic in Chicago. The specialized tape developed by Dr. Kase is a lightweight, hypoallergenic elastic tape made with cotton. The thinness and elasticity of kinesiology tape is different from rigid athletic tape. Athletic tape restricts movement. Kinesiology tape encourages normal movement. There are now many brands of this type of tape on the market. The tape is designed to be left in place for up to 3 days.

JUSTIFICATION FOR APPLICATION

There are many different theories about how kinesiology tape works. However, mode of action is unknown, and the physiological mechanisms that have been postulated are speculative. Theories include:

- Delivering continual proprioceptive input or by correcting alignment while movement is taking place (Malhotra et al., 2022).

- The tape can change the proprioception input of the sensory nervous system in the muscles, joints, and skin. The addition of kinesiology tape in weight bearing exercises can improve proprioception in active conditions (Binaei et al., 2021).
- The tape can lift to create negative pressure in an area, similar to suction, but is more subtle and can be left in place longer than suction devices.
- The tape is thought to improve the interaction between the skin and underlying structures, thus affecting the nervous system.
- The tape creates a sensation on the skin causing Diffuse Noxious Inhibitory Controls acting as a counter-irritant. Diffuse noxious inhibitory controls (DNIC) or conditioned pain modulation (CPM) is when responses from painful stimuli are inhibited by other noxious stimuli; this concept is known as "pain inhibits pain" (Ramaswamy and Wodehouse, 2021).
- Tape application may decrease edema in a local area, but research is weak and mixed (Hung et al., 2021; Yong et al., 2022).

Overall research is of low quality and mixed related to benefits, risks, and mechanism of action (Nunes, et al., 2015; Walsh et al., 2018; Alotaibi et al., 2018; Kasawara et al., 2018; de Freitas et al., 2018; Lietz-Kijak et al., 2018; Hosp et al., 2018; Alghamdi and Shawki, 2018; Cimino et al., 2018; Wang C et al., 2019; Wang Y. et al., 2018; Li, et al., 2018; Ouyang et al., 2018; Uzunkulaoğlu et al., 2018; Bagheri et al., 2018; Nunes et al., 2021; Kim and Kim 2022).

CONTRAINDICATIONS AND CAUTIONS

- Allergic reactions to adhesive tape
- Open wounds and burns
- Infection
- Diabetes peripheral neuropathy

Allergy and skin irritation from the tape adhesive is the most serious safety concern. Before using tape, the client should have a patch test where a small piece of tape is applied on the inner forearm and left for 24 hours to see if there is a reaction. Also, in situations with frail or thin skin the tape can lift the skin and pull it away when removed. Do not apply kinesiology tape on any skin surface that is damaged including scrapes, cuts, burns, sunburn or any type of rash or irritation.

GENERAL RECOMMENDATIONS FOR USING KINESIOLOGY TAPE

There a many internet videos available to demonstrate using this type of tape. The manufactures of the different brands also have instructions. Watch a series of different videos and read a variety of tape brand instructions. Then practice. There are many patterns of application that can be used. It is likely that the pattern is not as important for benefit as some resources indicate (Choi and Lee, 2018a,b; Li et el., 2022). However, there may be psychological influences related to appearance, intricacy of application, and color (Fig. 12.8).

Preparing the Skin

- Skin should be completely dry and clean. Wipe the entire area with rubbing alcohol.
- Body hair may affect the ability for the tape to adhere. Do not shave the hair but clip it close to the skin if needed.

Preparing and Applying the Tape

- The tape is single use. Avoid touching the adhesive side of the tape.
- The ends of each strip should be applied with no stretch.
- Make sure all ends are applied to skin, not to other pieces of tape.
- Cut the length of tape and round the corners to prevent ends from peeling.
- The clients body is positioned so the skin of the applied area is taut; this avoids pinching and allows for even application.
- Tear the backing 2-3 inches from one end to create an "anchor," which is the first part that will be applied. Apply the anchor end with no stretch in the tape, leaving the rest of the backing intact.
- Continue peeling the backing away in small segments as you stretch and apply the tape to the area.
- Generally, use a 50% stretch on the tape.
- As the end of the tape is reached stop stretching the tape and attach to the skin.
- After applying, rub tape briskly from the center to the ends to activate the adhesive.

Removing the Tape

- Apply a lotion or oil over the taped are a few minutes prior to removal.
- Remove tape in the direction of hair growth.
- Press the skin at the end of the taped area while gently peeling tape back.

Like so many methods, the research does not provide clear answers or recommendations. There is enough evidence to suggest some limited benefits. The massage therapist works from a position of biological plausibility and provides realistic information to clients. The risk is low as long as safety precautions are followed. The tape is relatively inexpensive, and the procedures are easy to learn.

The tape is available in many places for purchase. Brands and types of tape are made with varying intensities of elasticity and adhesive. Just as with hydrotherapy, essential oils, scraping and suction methods the client can learn to safely use kinesiology tape as a self-help method.

ADAPTIVE MASSAGE TARGETING LYMPH, BLOOD, AND CIRCULATION

SECTION OBJECTIVES

Chapter objective covered in this section:

6. Modify massage application to support beneficial blood and lymph movement in the body.

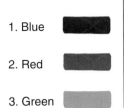

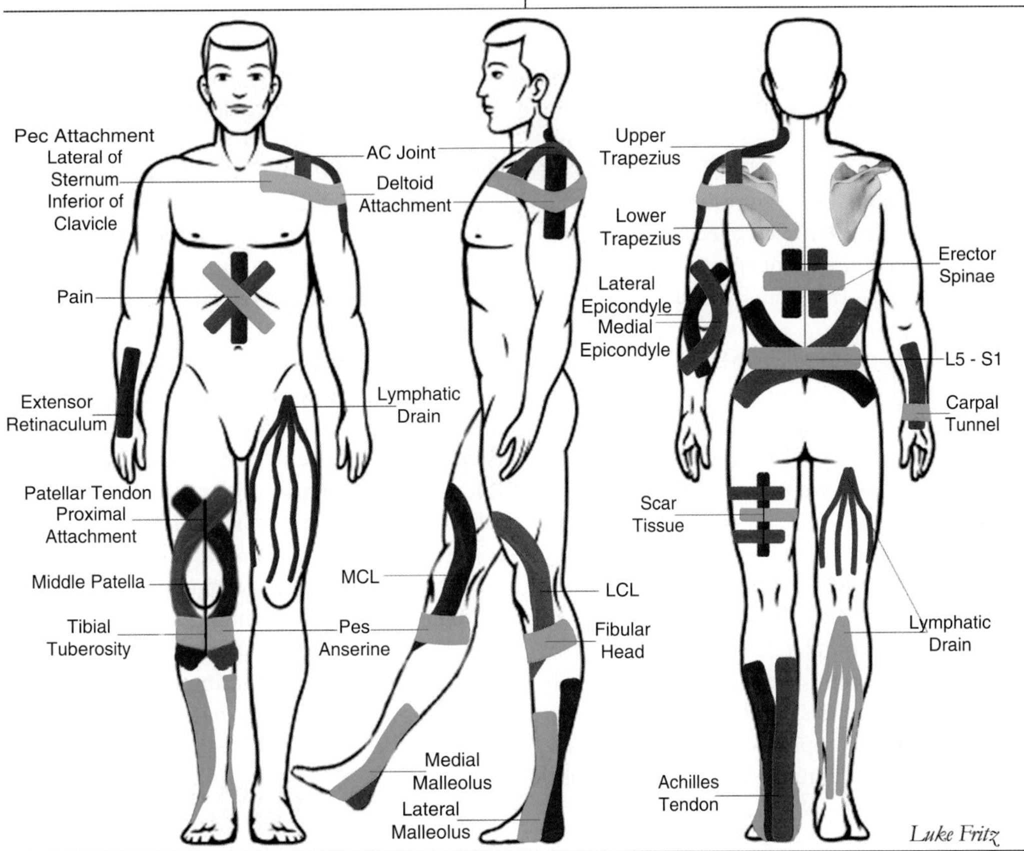

FIG. 12.8 Patterns of application for kinesiology tape.

Using the information presented in this section, the student will be able to perform the following:

- Explain the general effects of adaptive massage targeting lymphatic and circulation function.
- Identify indications for and contraindications to lymphatic drainage massage.
- Incorporate the principles of lymphatic and circulation focused massage into a general massage session.

Massage that targets normal fluid flow in the body should not be considered an adjunct but instead an adaptation. The reason this topic is covered in this chapter is because methods specifically targeting lymphatic movement have been developed into what some consider a unique application. Stimulation of the lymphatic and circulatory systems was once considered a well-documented benefit of massage.

Edema is the result of too much fluid being released from the capillaries into the tissue and overwhelming the capacity of the lymphatic system. Edema is common and ranges in severity for each person diagnosed with the condition based on the cause. Normally a mild edema with a logical cause will resolve. Edema could be a sign of an underlying health condition and early diagnosis and treatment could lead to the best prognosis.

Various pathological conditions related to fluid accumulation are considered system and regional contraindication for massage therapy. The two most serious noncancerous conditions are lymphedema and lipedema. *Lymphedema* refers to tissue swelling caused by an accumulation of protein-rich fluid that's usually drained through the body's lymphatic system. Lymphedema differs from edema. In lymphedema the lymphatic system is compromised. The arterial capillaries continue to function normally and continue to release their fluid in the interstitial spaces, but that fluid is not being drained away from the site because of pathology in the lymphatic system. Severe cases of increase the risks of skin infections and sepsis and can lead to skin changes. Treatment may include compression bandages, a specific massage adaptation, compression stockings, sequential pneumatic pumping, careful skin care and, rarely, surgery to remove swollen tissue or to create new drainage routes.

Lipedema is a condition that causes excess fat to accumulate in the lower part of the body. Lipedema most often involves the buttocks, thighs, and calves. The upper arms can also be affected. The condition does not affect the hands or feet. As more fat accumulates, it can block the lymphatic pathway. This causes a build-up of fluid called lymph known as secondary lymphedema or lipo-lymphedema. Lipedema is sometimes confused with lymphedema, but these are different conditions. However, lipedema can lead to lymphedema.

Manual lymphatic drainage (MLD) is a very light, rhythmic, and superficial massage technique focused on increasing the activity of the lymphatic system. Manual techniques first contact and tighten the skin, then relax the contacted area until the skin returns to the initial position. This skin stretching and resting combination promotes variations in interstitial pressures, effecting lymph collectors and local smooth muscles to increase the frequency of contraction of the lymphangion and raise lymphatic transport capacity (Koelmeyer et al., 2021).

The term *manual lymphatic drainage* (MLD) is somewhat inaccurate. Primarily, massage itself promotes movement of interstitial fluid into the lymph capillaries. Maybe a more accurate term would be *tissue fluid movement* or *interstitial fluid movement*. Regardless, the most common term used currently is MLD.

Methods used to support lymph drainage include medication called diuretics and decongestive therapy. The primary medical treatment for generalized edema is cautious use of diuretics to remove the fluid. Complete/complex decongestive therapy (CDT) is beyond the scope of massage therapy and is an intensive program that combines bandaging, compression garments, external pneumatic pumping sleeves that rhythmically compress the area, manual lymphatic drainage, exercise, and self-care.

Justification for Massage Adaptation for Fluid Movement

Research focuses primarily on fluid movement methods of manual lymphatic drainage (MLD). There is mixed data about the effectiveness of massage and fluid movement (Huang et al., 2013; Liang et al., 2020; Thompson et al., 2021; Wanchai and Armer 2021; De Vriezeet al., 2022; Haesler and Wounds 2022).

Not all interstitial fluid is taken up by lymphatic capillaries. Interstitial fluid microflow occurs along perivascular structures, adventitia (the outer layer of fibrous connective tissue surrounding an organ) located around neurovascular bundles. This fluid transport is different than the vessels found in the lymphatic and cardiovascular system (Kong et al., 2022). How these findings will influence strategies for supporting fluid flow in the body is unclear but does challenge some of the concepts of manual lymphatic drainage.

Current evidence from research supports the use of MLD in preventing or treating lymphedema when combined with other methods (Jeffs et al., 2018; Müller et al., 2018; Thompson et al., 2021; Liu and Yin 2022). Compression bandaging is weakly supported by research (Zasadzka et al., 2018; Kendrová et al., 2020).

Interestingly, methods such as manual lymphatic drainage have been shown to have an influence on physiological processes that have little to do with fluid movement including effects on the nervous, cardiovascular, respiratory, and musculoskeletal systems (Río-González et al., 2020). Massage methods typical in manual lymph drainage show reduced passive tissue stiffness and improved muscle extensibility. Since tissue stiffness relates to fluid volume these findings are biologically logical (Kablan et al., 2021).

The research is somewhat better for the use of pneumatic compression devises. Pneumatic compression devices consist of inflatable garments for limbs and electrical pneumatic pumps which fill the garment with compressed air. The garment is intermittently inflated and deflated with cycle times and pressures that vary between devices. These devices are expensive, but home use equipment is coming onto the market increasing access (Lerman et al., 2018; Martin et al., 2018; Rockson et al., 2018; Tessari et al., 2018; Mosti and Cavezzi 2019). Kinesiology taping may be beneficial for localized simple edema (Tremback et al., 2018; Cai et al., 2021

Research strongly supports exercise effects on lymphatic system function to prevent fluid build-up in tissues and interstitium. Peripheral muscle exercises such as walking and bicycling induce not only musculoskeletal contractions but also breathing alterations, arterial pulsations, varied skin tensions, and postural changes. These biological adaptions help activate the lymphatic system and promote lymph propulsion throughout the body, leading to a reduction of systemic fluid overload in interstitial spaces. Massage practitioners need to educate clients about the importance of exercise when fluid movement is the massage outcome (Fu et a; 2022).

Manual Techniques Addressing the Lymphatic System: Origins and Development

There are different types of complete/complex decongestive therapy (CDT) and manual lymphatic drainage (MLD) techniques including the Vodder, Leduc, Földi, Casley-Smith, and Godoy techniques. Most of the methods have a foundation based on the work by Dr. Vodder and the Vodder School in Austria. Godoy maneuvers slide over the skin while Vodder maneuvers only produce a traction of the skin. Changes in vital signs related to MLD techniques may result from affecting the autonomic nervous system; the smooth and rhythmic manual technique inhibits the sympathetic nervous system. There is a long history of manual methods in osteopathic medicine that target the lymphatic system. In the late 1800s Taylor Still, DO, proposed the initial principles of manual lymphatic drainage techniques (MLDTs) as part of osteopathic manipulative techniques. The osteopathic medical profession has designed a set of osteopathic manipulative techniques (OMT), called lymphatic pump techniques (LPT), to enhance the flow of lymph through the lymphatic system (Box 12.7). There is some validating research for the osteopathic methods. Osteopathic researchers performed the thoracic and abdominal pump technique (explained later) on dogs. Changes in thoracic and abdominal pressures are used to propel lymphatic flow from the abdomen into and through the thoracic duct. The pumps can be applied to the thoracic cage, abdomen (splenic and liver pumps), and feet and legs (pedal pumps) (Chikly, 2005; Hodge, 2012; Yao et al., 2014).

Manual Edema Mobilization (MEM), formalized in the mid-1990s, is a system evolved from European and Australian lymphedema treatment methods (Howard and Krishnagiri, 2001; Artzberger and Rodrick, 2002). MEM consists of massage in a proximal to distal then distal to proximal direction, pump point stimulation, a home exercise program, and low-stretch bandaging (Miller et al, 2017; Iannello and Biller, 2019). The adaptive massage approach for normal fluid movement described in this textbook is consistent with the principles of MEM.

There is a specific certification process for complete/complex decongestive therapy (CDT) and manual lymphatic drainage (MLD) techniques. The Lymphology Association of North America®, LANA®, is a nonprofit corporation specializing in the certification of health care professionals who diagnose and/or treat lymphedema and related disorders. Having recognized the need for a national certification examination for lymphedema therapists, LANA® tests knowledge considered fundamental in the management of lymphedema. This section in the chapter only provides an overview of the lymphatic system with suggestions for the biologically plausible modification in massage therapy application to support lymphatic function.

A logical, reality-based justification process can be used to make a case for the influence of massage on the movement of lymphatic fluid, even though we do not totally understand the mechanisms and research findings are conflicting. A logical, reality-based justification process is based on understanding normal function and using massage to mimic normal physiologic function. The management of simple edema as part of a general massage seems to be within the scope of practice. However, if pathology does exist, focused treatment by a massage therapist without supervision of a physician, nurse, or physical therapist may be outside the scope of practice. The following section presents biologically plausible adaptations to the massage approach that would be most likely to affect the movement of the lymph and blood in the body.

An Evidence-Informed Biologically Plausible Approach

MLD methods use a gentle skin/superficial fascia stretching technique or massage designed to move the skin/superficial fascia in specific directions based on the underlying structure and physiology of the lymphatic system. The intent of the various interventions is draining lymph already in the lymph vessels (collectors) and stimulating the formation of lymph by increasing the flow of interstitial fluid to the lymphatic capillaries (initial lymphatics). The working hypothesis (educated guess) for the manual methods is to support more normal fluid flow by creating spaces in the tissues and then massaging fluid into these spaces by external tissue compression.

Box 12.7 Modified Protocol Osteopathic Manipulative Techniques (OMT) and Lymphatic Pump Techniques (LPT)

Protocol

The modified OMT protocol for massage application consists of a mix of lymphatic and pump treatments:

The subject is positioned on their back on a treatment table.

The practitioner places both hands on both sides of the client's anterior aspect of the chest with fingers pointing toward the client's feet and heel of the practitioner's hands just below the inferior border of the clavicles. Rhythmic compressions are applied to the chest for approximately 2 minutes.

The practitioner then moves to the client's left thoracic cage and applies rhythmic compressions to the lateral thoracic cage while holding the left upper extremity in approximately 60 degrees of abduction for approximately 2 minutes.

Next the practitioner moves to the right thoracic cage and repeats this procedure for another 2 minutes.

The practitioner then returns to the upper thoracic cage and repeats the bilateral upper rib compression.

The subject is instructed to inhale deeply and then exhale fully and slowly. While the individual exhales, the practitioner applies oscillatory compressions. At the third inhalation, the practitioner instructs the client to inhale deeply against the practitioner's resistance to the inhalation. This is repeated three times against gentle resistance to inhalation. After the third exhalation, the practitioner quickly releases the resistance at the midpoint of the next forced inhalation, allowing the client to suddenly expand the chest.

With the client lying supine, the practitioner holds the client's ankles, and gentle pressure is repeatedly applied using the leg as a "lever" to rock the pelvis.

Then, while standing at client's feet, the palms of the practitioner's hands are placed on the ball of the foot and the ankles are rhythmically flexed and extended. Effective rhythm causes a rhythmic "sloshing" of the belly.

Next the hands are placed on the abdomen, and repeated rhythmic compression of the abdominal contents is applied toward the diaphragm.

Then, standing at the client's head, the practitioner reaches forward and grasps the pectoral muscles at the axillary fold and leans back, putting a stretch on the muscles and opening the chest. The client is instructed to take deep breaths. On inhalation, the muscles are pulled on, and with exhalation, tension is held. Repeat three to four cycles.

View a video that uses some of these methods: Yao S, Hassani J, Gagne M, et al: Osteopathic manipulative treatment as a useful adjunctive tool for pneumonia, *J Vis Exp*. 87, 2014, https://doi.org/10.3791/50687. Retrieved from http://www.jove.com/video/50687/osteopathic-manipulative-treatment-as-useful-adjunctive-tool-for.

From Walkowski S, Singh M, Benencia F: Osteopathic manipulative therapy induces early plasma cytokine release and mobilization of a population of blood dendritic cells, *PLoS One* 9:e90132, 2014. https://doi.org/10.1371/journal.pone.0090132. Retrieved from http://www.ncbi.nlm.nih.gov/pmc/articles/PMC3948629/.

The massage-like skin stretching used in MLD and the rhythmic rocking, shaking and compression described in the osteopathic approach are methods used for therapeutic massage.

Lymphatic System

The lymphatic system is a specialized component of the circulatory system that is responsible for waste disposal and immune response. The lymphatic system plays an important role in balancing fluid compartments in the body. The lymphatic system transports fluid from around the cells through a system of filters. Lymph and blood are similar except that lymph does not have red blood cells or platelets. Lymph has slightly higher protein content than blood, and it carries large molecules, such as proteins, lipids, bacteria, and other debris. Lymph begins as interstitial fluid (i.e., the fluid that surrounds the cell). It is generated when plasma is forced out of the blood capillaries and into cellular spaces to bathe and nourish the cells (Fig. 12.9).

The lymphatic system permeates the entire tissue structure of the body in a one-way drainage network of vessels, ducts, nodes, lacteals, and lymphoid organs such as the spleen, tonsils, and thymus.

The spleen, the largest organ of the lymphatic system, filters the blood. It manufactures lymphocytes, stores red blood cells, releases blood to the body in cases of extreme blood loss, and removes foreign substances and dead red blood cells. The spleen contains red and white pulp. The white pulp contains white blood cells and surrounds arteries that enter the spleen, and the red pulp surrounds veins that leave the spleen. Macrophages in the red pulp remove foreign substances and worn-out or dead red blood cells.

The tonsils form a ring of lymphatic tissue that surrounds the opening to the digestive and respiratory tracts, an area where harmful substances can easily enter the body. The three pairs of tonsils are the pharyngeal, palatine, and lingual tonsils.

The thymus forms antibodies in newborns and is involved in the initial development of the immune system. Lymphocytes

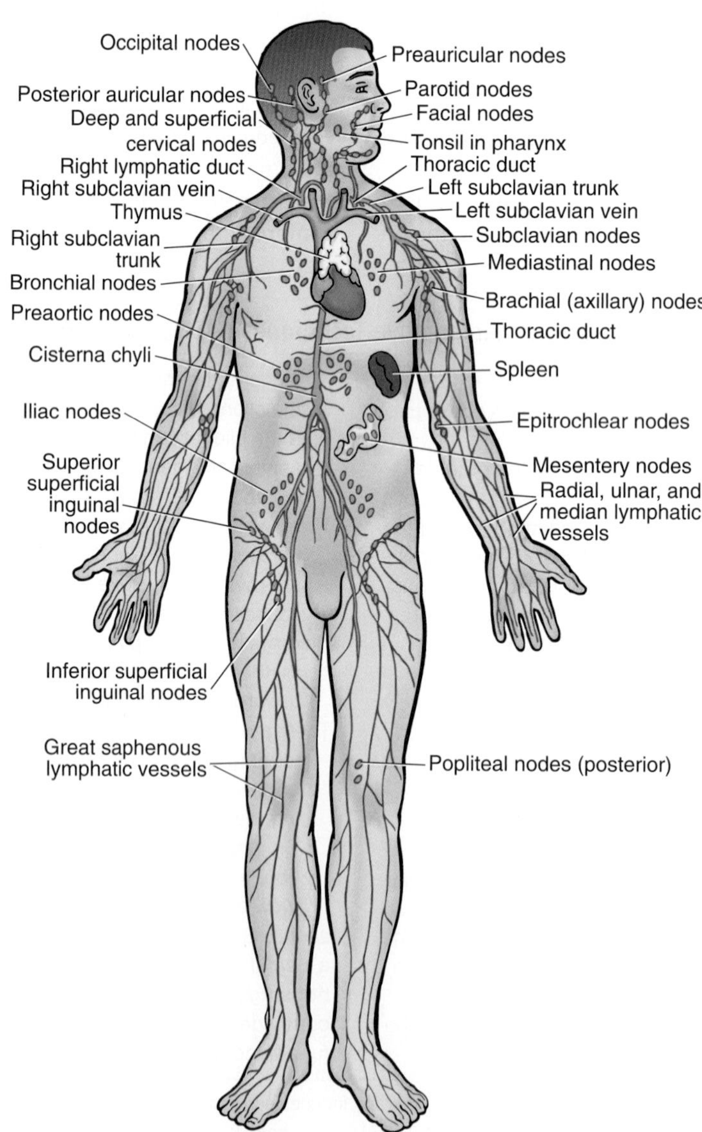

FIG. 12.9 The lymphatic system and lymphatic drainage pathways throughout the body.

produced in the red bone marrow migrate to the thymus, where they develop into T cells. The thymus also produces the hormone thymosin. The activity of the thymus gland declines with age.

Aggregated lymph nodules are collections of lymphatic tissue in mucous membranes that are continuous with the skin; examples of these nodules include the tonsils, the bronchi of the respiratory tract, the small intestine, and the appendix. Aggregated lymph nodules respond to antigens in those areas and create antibodies.

To get an idea of the extensive lymph network, visualize the roots on a plant. Tiny lymph vessels, known as *lymph capillaries*, are distributed throughout the body, except in the eyes, brain, and spinal cord. Fluid collects in the lymph capillaries in a manner somewhat similar to the way water is drawn up into a plant's roots. Segments of lymph capillaries are divided by one-way valves and a spiral set of smooth muscles called *lymphangions*. This system moves fluid against gravity in a peristalsis-type undulation.

The lymphatic tubes merge until major channels and vessels are formed. These vessels run from the distal parts of the body toward the neck, usually alongside veins and arteries. Valves in the vessels prevent the backflow of lymph.

Lymph nodes are enlarged portions of the lymph vessels that generally cluster at the joints. This arrangement assists movement of the lymph through the nodes by means of the pumping action from joint movement. These nodes filter the fluid and produce lymphocytes. An alternative term used instead of lymph node bed is *catchments* because they catch and slow lymph flow to filter and carry out immune processes; therefore, clearing the catchments can improve lymph flow.

All of the body's lymph vessels converge into two main channels: the thoracic duct and the right lymphatic duct. Vessels from the entire left side of the body and from the right side of the body below the chest converge into the thoracic duct, which in turn empties into the left subclavian vein, situated beneath the left clavicle. The right lymphatic duct collects lymph from the vessels on the right side of the head, neck, upper chest, and right arm. It empties into the right subclavian vein beneath the right clavicle. Waste products then are carried by the bloodstream to the spleen, intestines, and kidneys for detoxification.

Lymph moves along a pressure gradient from areas of high pressure to areas of low pressure. It moves from the interstitial space (high pressure) into the lymph capillaries (low pressure) through a pressure mechanism exerted by respiration, peristalsis of the large intestine, the compression of muscles, and the pull of the skin and fascia during movement. This action is especially prominent at the plexuses in the hands and feet. Major lymph plexuses are found on the soles of the feet and the palms of the hands. The rhythmic pumping of walking and grasping probably facilitates lymphatic flow. There is also a primary intrinsic pumping mechanism in the lymphatic system.

Lymph circulation involves two steps:

- First, plasma is forced out of blood capillaries and into the space around the cells. The fluid now located around the cells is called *interstitial fluid*. As fluid pressure increases between the cells, the cells move apart, pulling on the microfilaments that connect the endothelial cells of the lymph capillaries to tissue cells. The pull on the microfilaments causes the lymph capillaries to open like flaps, allowing interstitial fluid to enter the lymph capillaries. Once the fluid is in the lymph capillaries, it is called *lymph*.
- Next, the lymph moves through the network of contractile lymphatic vessels. The lymphatic system does not have a central pump like the heart, which performs that function for blood. Various factors assist the transport of lymph through the lymphatic vessels.

The *lymphatic pump* is the spontaneous contraction of lymphatic vessels as a result of the increased pressure of lymphatic fluid. These contractions usually start in the lymphangions adjacent to the terminal end of the lymph capillaries and spread progressively from one lymphangion to the next, toward the thoracic duct or the right lymphatic duct. The contractions are similar to abdominal peristalsis and are stimulated by increases in pressure inside lymphatic vessels. Contractions of the lymphatic vessels are not coordinated with the heart or breath rate. If the pressure inside the lymphatic vessels exceeds or falls below certain levels, lymphatic contractions stop.

Breathing is an essential part of lymphatic movement. During inhalation, the thoracic duct is squeezed, which pushes fluid forward and creates a vacuum in the duct. During exhalation, fluid is pulled from the lymphatics and into the thoracic duct to fill the partial vacuum.

Edema

Edema, which is an increase in interstitial fluid, can be caused by a variety of factors (See Box 12.8):

- *Lack of exercise.* Exercise, in which muscles alternately contract and relax, stimulates lymph circulation, and cleans muscle tissue. If the muscles stay contracted or flaccid, lymph circulation declines drastically inside the muscles, and edema can result.
- *Increase in exercise.* An increase in exercise can strain the lymph system by causing blood capillary permeability, resulting in an increase in fluid movement to the interstitial spaces. This is one cause of delayed onset of muscle soreness.
- *Salt consumption.* The body retains a specific ratio of salt to fluids. The more salt a person consumes, the more water is retained to balance it, resulting in edema.
- *Heart or kidney disease.* These diseases affect the blood and lymphatic circulations. Lymphatic massage stimulates the circulation of lymph. However, caution is indicated because the increase in fluid volume could overload an already weakened heart. In addition, because the kidneys regulate blood volume, an increase in blood volume could overload already weakened kidneys.
- *Menstrual cycle.* Water retention or a swollen abdomen (or both) are common before or during the menstrual cycle.
- *Lymphedema.* Limbs affected with this condition become very swollen and painful, resulting in difficulty moving the affected limb and disfigurement. Lymphedema can be life-threatening because the interstitial fluid is contaminated, injuries to the skin do not heal, and even small abrasions and sores can become infected.

Box 12.8 Assessment for and Treatment of Fluid Imbalance

1. Ask the client if tissue feels taut, distended, fat, or stiff. If the answer is no, palpate to confirm that edema is not present and then proceed with the general massage. If the answer is yes, ask for the history.
2. The history should include any injury, swelling, bruising, static position, and unusual increase in physical activity followed by extended inactivity. If the client answers yes to any of these, then observe.
3. Observe for a decrease in muscle definition, bruising, tissue distention, and changes in color. If any of these are found, palpate.
4. Palpate for increased muscle tone, specifically tissue tautness and an increase in fluid (pitting edema) or venous congestion. If these are noted, observe and palpate for signs of inflammation.
5. Palpate for heat and observe for redness. Ask about pain.
6. If the area is swollen, hot, red, and painful, refer the client to a medical professional. If inflammation is present, massage the area only after the reason for the condition has been determined.
7. If the area is not hot or red, determine whether the tissue is congested or swollen.
8. Congested tissue has increased blood in the veins and capillaries; the tissue feels dense and stiff but does not show pitting edema. Swollen tissue has increased interstitial fluid; this tissue pits when pressure is applied.
9. If the tissue is congested, massage methods that enhance venous return are indicated. Observe cautions for thrombosis, kidney disease, and heart disease.
10. If the tissue is swollen, lymphatic drainage is indicated. Observe cautions for infection, kidney disease, and heart disease.

- *Inflammation.* Increased blood flow to an injured area and the release of vasodilators, which are part of the inflammatory response, can cause edema in the localized area.
- *Other causes.* Medications, including steroids, hormones, and chemotherapy for cancer, may cause edema as a side effect. Scar tissue and muscle tension can cause obstructive edema by restricting lymph vessels.

Indications for Lymphatic Drainage Massage

Simple edema, with screening for contraindications, appears to respond to massage focused on the lymphatic system even though the research evidence is sparse. The following conditions may benefit from massage that focuses on the movement of lymph:

- Simple edema that results from inactivity (e.g., a long car ride, sitting at computer).
- Traveler's edema, which is the result of enforced inactivity, such as sitting in an airplane or a car for several hours (the same is true for anyone who sits for extended periods). Interstitial fluid (tissue fluid) responds to gravity, causing swelling in the feet, hands, and buttocks of a person who sits for extended periods. Lymphatic drainage massage can move the fluid and reduce the pain and stiffness caused by the edema. Caution is indicated because of the possibility of the formation of blood clots with prolonged inactivity.
- Exercise-induced, delayed-onset muscle soreness, which may be partly caused by increased fluid pressure in the soft tissues. Lymphatic drainage massage appears to be effective for reducing the pain and stiffness of this condition.
- Fluid retention caused by premenstrual hormonal changes.
- Residual edema in the later stages of the healing of strains, sprains, and other types of injuries.

Contraindications and Cautions for Lymphatic Drainage Massage

Edematous tissues have poor oxygenation, reduced function, and heal slowly after injury. Chronic edema results in chronic inflammation and fibrosis, which makes the edematous tissue coarse, thicker, and less flexible.

The massage style use to target fluid movement might lower blood pressure. If the client has low blood pressure, the concern exists that it may drop even farther, and the client may become dizzy on standing.

During a fever, white blood cells multiply more rapidly and bacteria and viruses multiply more slowly; fever, therefore, is part of the body's healing process. Because lymphatic drainage massage has been said to lower the body temperature, it should not be given to a client with a fever.

Lymphatic drainage adapted massage may affect the circulation of fluid in the body, which may strain an already compromised heart or kidneys. Caution is required (Box 12.9).

Principles of Lymphatic Drainage Massage

If massage does indeed affect the movement of lymph in the body, then somehow massage would need to mimic the natural mechanism of lymph movement.

The pressure provided by massage mimics the drag and compressive forces of movement and respiration and can move the skin to open the lymph capillaries. The pressure gradient from high pressure to low pressure is supported by creating low-pressure areas in the vessels proximal to the area to be drained. The depth of pressure, speed and frequency, direction, rhythm, duration, and drag are adjusted to support the lymphatic system.

Depth of Pressure

According to Vodder, the softer the tissue or the greater the edema, the lighter the pressure that should be used. Vodder estimated the proper pressure for lymphatic drainage to be 8 to 12 ounces per square inch, with the pressure in the peripheral lymphatics even lighter (less than 1-8 ounces per square inch). You can develop a sense of these levels of pressure by stroking the surface of a postage scale until you can easily keep the pressure within the recommended range. This pressure is just enough to move the skin and superficial fascia. The lymphatics are located mostly in superficial tissues, and surface edema occurs in those superficial tissues, not in the deep tissue.

Simple muscle tension puts pressure on the lymph vessels and may block them, interfering with efficient drainage. Massage can normalize this muscle tension. As the muscles relax, the lymph vessels open, and drainage becomes more efficient. Work on the areas of muscle tension first, using appropriate massage methods and pressure, then finish the area with light pressure focused on skin and superficial fascia movement.

Box 12.9 Massage Does Not Directly Affect Toxins in the Body

Massage therapy has many benefits; however, detoxification is not one of them. Some massage therapists and many clients think massage removes toxins. Massage therapists should avoid perpetuating this misinformation and educate clients. Another issue is that people use the words toxin and detoxification incorrectly. Here is what the words mean.

Toxin

1. A poisonous or harmful nonbiological substance, such as a pollutant.
2. Substances producing adverse biological effects of any kind.
3. May be chemical or physical in nature.

Detoxification

1. Recovery from the toxic effects of a drug.
2. Removal of the toxic properties from a poison.
3. Metabolic conversion of pharmacologically active principles to pharmacologically less active principles.

Various types of toxic substances occur and include those made in the body as part of physiologic processes and those from the environment that are ingested, injected, inhaled or absorbed.

Body Produced Waste

These waste products are processed by five detox organs: skin, lungs, kidneys, liver, and intestines. Our body knows how to handle these substances. Biotransformation is the process by which a substance changes from one chemical to another (transformed) by a chemical reaction within the body. Only when normal homeostatic processes break down do these types of substances accumulate and cause accumulation of toxins in the body. There are three main types of body produced wastes.

Catabolic waste remains after breaking down of large molecules into smaller ones for body processes and are removed from the body through the skin, kidneys, lungs, and intestines. Urea, ammonia, and uric acid are the three main wastes eliminated. Water is required to excrete these waste products. This is why we need to stay hydrated.

Metabolic waste is produced when a cell uses oxygen and nutrients to create energy. Carbon dioxide is the main waste product which is exhaled through the lungs. This why we need to exhale.

Digestive waste is what remains after the digestion and absorption of food and these solids are eliminated through the colon. This is why we need to have regular bowel movements.

The ongoing confusion and claims that massage can flush out toxins especially lactic acid persists.

Massage Does Not Flush Lactic Acid Out of the Muscles

Everything we do requires energy. This energy comes from glucose through a process called glycolysis. Glucose is broken down (metabolized) into a substance called pyruvate. When breathing does not supply sufficient oxygen, the body temporarily converts pyruvate into a substance called lactate, which allows glucose breakdown to continue. The working muscle cells can continue this type of anaerobic energy production for a few minutes but the lactate levels in the tissues increase. High lactate levels increase the acidity in the tissues resulting in the burning sensation experienced during heavy exertion. Once the body slows down, oxygen becomes available, and lactate reverts back to pyruvate and a shift back to aerobic metabolism occurs. This process takes only minutes. There never is an accumulation of lactic acid in the tissue.

Environmental Toxins

Toxins from the environment are considered poisons and are more difficult for the body to process and eliminate. Persistent Organic Pollutants (POPs) are chemicals that do not easily break down and can remain in the environment and the body. These substances can be found in plants, venom, produced by viruses, bacteria, fungi and protozoa, naturally occurring metals or synthetically manufactured substances such as pesticides, herbicides, fungicides, gasoline, fire retardants, and more. These toxic substances are found in the air, soil, water, as well as building materials, home furnishings, cleaning substances, cosmetics, and personal care products. We breathe, eat, and absorb some of these chemicals through the skin. Once these chemicals are in the body it can be excreted, stored, or biotransformed. Biotransformation is the chemical change the body makes in chemical substances so the substance can be used or eliminated. Digestion of food is a form of biotransformation. The liver is the primary biotransforming organ due to its large size and high concentration of biotransforming enzymes. The kidneys and lungs are next with 10–30% of the liver's capacity. The issue with POPs is that biotransformation processes do not efficiently or effectively change these substances into other chemicals that can be eliminated by normal processes; thus they become stored in the tissues. The primary sites in the body for accumulation of POPs are adipose tissue, bone, liver, and kidneys. Probiotic strains may offer a simple and effective way to counteract the negative effect of exposure to POP.

It would be fantastic if massage directly contributed to removal of these substances from the body; unfortunately, it does not.

Massage Does Not Detox Environmental Toxins

Research does indicate that sweating/diaphoresis (heavy perspiration) can help the body eliminate some (not all) POPs. Sweating can be considered a form of detoxification. Fluid excreted by the sweat glands consists of water containing sodium chloride and phosphate, urea, ammonia, sulfates, creatinine, fats, and other waste products. Regular sessions of induced perspiration can eliminate some of the environmental toxins stored in body tissue. Activities that create sweating include exercise and sauna. Water lost during sweating needs to be replaced. Drinking clean water would be a good idea.

Client Education

Explain that massage does not remove toxins stored in the body. Educate clients about potential benefits of activities that cause sweating if they are attempting to remove these types of toxic substances. We can recommend clients discuss the safe and beneficial use of exercise and sauna with their physician.

If massage therapy is going to be respected as a valid health service, then we must not perpetuate misinformation. Massage certainly has value for supporting health and well-being. Environmental toxin exposure is a growing public health concern and creates additional stain on our bodies. The body will be better able to maintain homeostasis when relaxed and rested. Massage therapy can help people relax and rest. That is a good thing.

Resources

Medical Dictionary for the Health Professions and Nursing. 2012. Farlex. 11 Dec. 2017 https://medical-dictionary.thefreedictionary.com/detoxification.

Continued

Box 12.9 Massage Does Not Directly Affect Toxins in the Body—cont'd

Genuis, Stephen J., Kevin Lane, and Detlef Birkholz. "Human Elimination of Organochlorine Pesticides: Blood, Urine, and Sweat Study." BioMed Research International (2016): 1624643. PMC. Web. 11 Dec. 2017. https://www.ncbi.nlm.nih.gov/pmc/articles/PMC5069380/.

Sears, Margaret E., Kathleen J. Kerr, and Riina I. Bray. "Arsenic, Cadmium, Lead, and Mercury in Sweat: A Systematic Review." Journal of Environmental and Public Health (2012): 184745. PMC. Web. 11 Dec. 2017. https://www.ncbi.nlm.nih.gov/pubmed/22505948.

Sears, Margaret E., and Stephen J. Genuis. "Environmental Determinants of Chronic Disease and Medical Approaches: Recognition, Avoidance, Supportive Therapy, and Detoxification." Journal of Environmental and Public Health (2012): 356798. PMC. Web. 11 Dec. 2017. https://www.ncbi.nlm.nih.gov/pmc/articles/PMC3270432/.

Kuan, Wen-Hui, Yi-Lang Chen, and Chao-Lin Liu. "Excretion of Ni, Pb, Cu, As, and Hg in Sweat under Two Sweating Conditions." International Journal of Environmental Research and Public Health 19, no. 7 (2022): 4323.

Średnicka, Paulina, Edyta Juszczuk-Kubiak, Michał Wójcicki, Monika Akimowicz, and Marek Roszko. "Probiotics as a biological detoxification tool of food chemical contamination: A review." Food and Chemical Toxicology 153 (2021): 112306.

Pop, Oana Lelia, Ramona Suharoschi, and Rosita Gabbianelli. "Biodetoxification and Protective Properties of Probiotics." Microorganisms 10, no. 7 (2022): 1278.

Disagreement exists about the intensity of the pressure used. Some schools of thought recommend light pressure, such as that described by Vodder. Other methods, such as the technique described by Lederman, uses moderate to heavy pressure. Lederman holds that the stronger the compression used, the greater the increase in the flow rate of the lymph. Light pressure is used initially, and the pressure is methodically increased as the area is drained (Lederman 2005; Gott et al., 2018). Moving the skin moves the lymphatics. Stretching the lymphatics longitudinally, horizontally, and diagonally stimulates them to contract. Negative pressure produced by suction may provide similar results.

Speed and Frequency

The greater the amount of fluid in the tissue, the slower the massage movements. Massage gliding to move superficial tissue is repeated at a rate of approximately 10 repetitions per minute in an area, the approximate rate at which the peripheral lymphatics contract.

Direction

The lymph is moved toward the closest cluster of lymph nodes, which are predominately located in the neck, axilla, and groin. Massage near nodes first and then move fluid toward them, working proximally from the swollen area toward the nodes. Massage the unaffected side first and then the obstructed side. For instance, if the right arm is swollen because of scar tissue from a muscle tear, massage the left arm first.

Rhythm

Slow, rhythmic repetition of the massage movements stimulates pulses in the lymph fluid similar to intestinal peristalsis (e.g., a pump).

Duration

Full-body lymphatic drainage massage lasts about 45 minutes. Focus on local areas for about 5 to 15 minutes.

Drag

Drag on the tissue pulls open the terminal ends of the lymphatic capillaries (flap), allowing interstitial fluid to enter. Drag moves the superficial tissues (skin and superficial fascia) into and out of bind. The intensity and intention of the drag is to only move tissue to the first sensation of tissue bind (movement barrier) and then allow the tissue to return to the start position.

When possible, position the area being massaged above the heart so that gravity can assist the lymph flow.

Because lymph capillary plexuses are present on the bottoms of the feet, rhythmic compression on the soles may also enhance lymph flow.

Rhythmic, gentle, passive, and active joint movement reproduces the body's normal means of pumping lymph.

The client helps the process by deep, slow breathing, which stimulates lymph flow in the deeper vessels.

Massage Application Modified to Support Lymphatic Function

The massage approach described next specifically targets the lymphatic system, incorporates elements of the various theories about manual lymphatic movement, and is appropriate for clients who are generally healthy. People commonly develop a somewhat sluggish lymphatic flow. The usual culprits are inactivity, consumption of junk food and beverages, and reduced water intake. All these factors stress the lymphatic system. General massage with a focus as presented in this section, coupled with corrective action by the client (i.e., appropriate water intake, increased activity, and reduced junk food intake) can reverse the problem. Additional training and medical supervision are required for professionals who intend to work with clients with pathologic lymphatic conditions (Proficiency Exercise 12.2).

PROFICIENCY EXERCISE 12.2

1. Fill a long balloon with water. Leave an air bubble in it. Use short gliding strokes with a drag component to move the bubble. Notice the level of pressure that moves the bubble most effectively.
2. Design a lymphatic self-massage. Incorporate deep breathing, movement and compression action at the joints, palms, and soles of the feet.

Procedure for Lymphatic Function: Targeted Massage

Pumping action on the thorax and abdomen increases lymphatic drainage through the lymph ducts by lowering intrapleural pressure and exaggerating the action of inhalation and exhalation.

1. Begin the massage session with a pumping action on the thorax.
2. Place both hands on the anterior surface of the thoracic cage.
3. As the client exhales completely, allow your hands to passively follow the movements of the thorax.
4. When the client starts to inhale, resist the movement of the thorax with counterpressure for 5 to 7 seconds.
5. Repeat this procedure four or five times.
6. Place hands on abdomen just under ribs.
7. Rhythmically compress and then release the abdominal tissues in a pump-like fashion. Compression should be sufficient to change the shape of the abdomen but should not be uncomfortable for the client.
8. Repeat abdominal pump four or five times.
9. Repeat thorax compressions.
10. The client helps the process by deep, slow breathing, which stimulates lymph flow in the deeper vessels.

Massage Application

With lymphatic-targeted massage, generally light pressure is indicated initially, which increases to a moderate level (including kneading, compression, and gliding) during repeated application to the area to reach the deep lymphatic vessels; the technique then returns to lighter pressure over the area. Drag is necessary to affect the microfilaments and to open the flaps at the ends of the capillary vessels.

1. Tissue drag and release. The massage application consists of a combination of short, light, pumping, gliding strokes beginning close to the torso at the node cluster and directed toward the torso; the strokes methodically move distally. The stroke does not slip but rather drags the tissue to bind. The focus of the initial pressure and finishing strokes is the dermis, just below the surface layer of skin, and the layer of tissue just beneath the skin and above the muscles. This is the superficial fascial layer, which contains 60% to 70% of the lymphatic circulation in the extremities.
2. The phase of applying pressure and drag is longer than the phase of pressure and drag release. The releasing phase cannot be too short because the lymph needs time to drain from the distal segment. Therefore the optimal duration of the pressure and drag phase is 6 to 7 seconds; for the release phase, it is about 5 seconds. Traditionally, this application was described as stationary circles, which essentially produces a bind/release movement.
3. This pattern is followed by long surface gliding strokes with a bit more pressure to influence deeper lymph vessels. The direction is toward the drainage points.
4. Repeat tissue drag and release.
5. A pumping, rhythmic compression on the soles and palms supports lymph movement.
6. Rhythmic, gentle passive and active joint movement reproduces the body's normal means of pumping lymph. When possible, position the area being massaged above the heart so that gravity can assist lymph flow.
7. Rhythmic rocking and shaking of the area move the skin and superficial fascia.
8. Repeat. This approach is methodical and repetitious (see the combined fluid movement protocol).

Lymphatic drainage to address pathologic lymphedema is a therapeutic method requiring specialized training that combines specific manual techniques and compression bandaging. The following information and suggested applications may be beneficial for the lymphatic system in general and for nonpathologic simple edema that occasionally occurs. As with all methods of massage, we need to appreciate the anatomy and physiology of body functions that are the target of the massage.

Adaptive Massage Targeting Blood Circulation

Research related to massage effects on circulatory function is mixed. A study in the Archives of Physical Medicine and Rehabilitation (Franklin et al., 2014) seems to support that massage therapy improves general blood flow and alleviates muscle soreness after exercise. The study also showed that massage improved vascular function in people who had not exercised, suggesting that massage has benefits for people regardless of their level of physical activity. Studies have also shown that massage in one body area alters microcirculation in the massaged area as well as other parts of the body via a reflex response (Rocha et al., 2017; Silva et al., 2018; Monteiro et al., 2020).

Massage duration of two to five minutes was found to reduce local tissue stiffness and promoted increased blood flow in the massaged tissue. Cumulative effects of repeated sessions indicate a dose-response affect (Schroeder et al., 2021; Matsuda et al., 2021).

Blood pressure may be affected and related to multiple mechanisms from reduced sympathetic arousal to effects on nitric oxide vasodilation (Nelson, 2015).

As with lymphatic massage, specific application for circulatory disease is out of the scope of practice for the massage professional unless the massage is performed under appropriate supervision. In this situation, massage may be beneficial as part of the overall treatment plan.

Clients who are not ill can benefit from increased efficiency in the circulatory system. Aerobic exercise (see Chapter 15) is possibly the best way to support circulation.

Circulatory System

The circulatory system is a closed system composed of a series of connected tubes and a pump. The heart's pumping action provides pressure to move the blood through the body via the arteries and eventually into the small capillaries, where blood gas and nutrient exchange happens. Microcirculation is the blood flow through the smallest vessels in the circulatory system (i.e., arterioles, venules, shunts, capillaries). The blood returns to the heart by way of the veins. Venous blood flow is not under pressure from the heart. Rather, it relies on muscle compression against the veins to change the interior venous pressure. As in the lymphatic system, backflow of blood is prevented by a valve system.

Massage Methods for the Circulatory System

Logically massage to encourage blood flow to the tissues (arterial circulation) is different from massage to encourage blood flow from the tissues back to the heart (venous circulation). Because the veins and lymph vessels have a valve system, deep, narrow-based stroking over these vessels from proximal to distal (from the heart outward) is contraindicated. A small chance exists of breaking down the valves if this is done. Compression, which does not slide, as does gliding or stripping, is appropriate for stimulating arterial circulation.

1. Compression is applied over the main arteries, beginning close to the heart (proximal), and moving systematically toward the tips of the fingers or toes (distal).
2. The manipulations are applied with a pumping action at a rhythm of approximately 60 beats per minute, or at a rhythm that matches the client's resting heart rate.
3. Compressive force changes the internal pressure in the arteries, stimulates the intrinsic contraction of arteries, and encourages the movement of blood out to the distal areas of the body.
4. Compression also begins to empty venous vessels and forms an arteriovenous pressure gradient, encouraging arterial blood flow.
5. Rhythmic, gentle contraction and relaxation of the muscles encourages arterial blood flow. Both active and passive joint movements support the transport of arterial blood.
6. The squeezing action of compression and kneading helps empty the capillary beds, allowing them to refill with arterial blood, thus supporting venous return.

PROFICIENCY EXERCISE 12.3

1. Hook up a hose to a faucet and barely turn on the water; this simulates the heart pump. Use compression to facilitate the movement, or "circulation," of the water in the hose.
2. Obtain a 3-foot piece of clear, soft plastic tubing. As if sucking on a straw, draw up a small amount of water into the tubing. Massage the water to the other end of the tube; this is similar to venous return massage.

After compression, the next step is to assist venous return flow. This process is similar to lymphatic massage in that a combination of short and long gliding strokes is used in conjunction with movement. The difference is that lymphatic massage is done over the entire body and the movements usually are passive (Proficiency Exercise 12.3).

1. With venous return flow massage, the gliding strokes move distal to proximal (from the fingers and toes to the heart) over the major veins, and the strokes actually slide somewhat like a squeegee washing a window.
2. The gliding stroke is short, only about 3 inches long; this enables the blood to move from valve to valve.
3. Long, gliding strokes carry the blood through the entire vein. Both passive and active joint movements encourage venous circulation.
4. Placing the limb or other area above the heart uses gravity in your favor.

See the fluid movement protocols for a visual demonstration of these methods.

FLUID MOVEMENT PROTOCOL

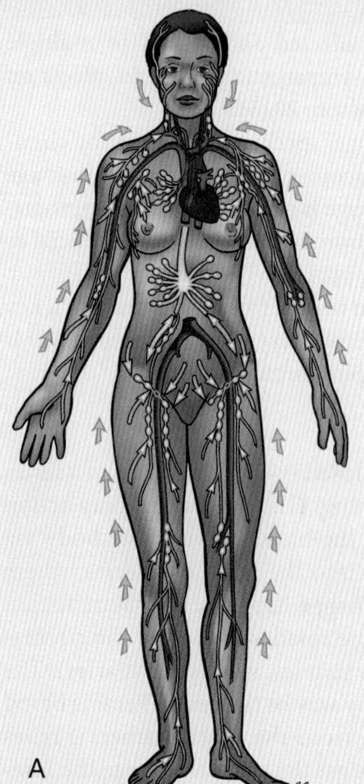

A. Direction of strokes for facilitating lymphatic flow.

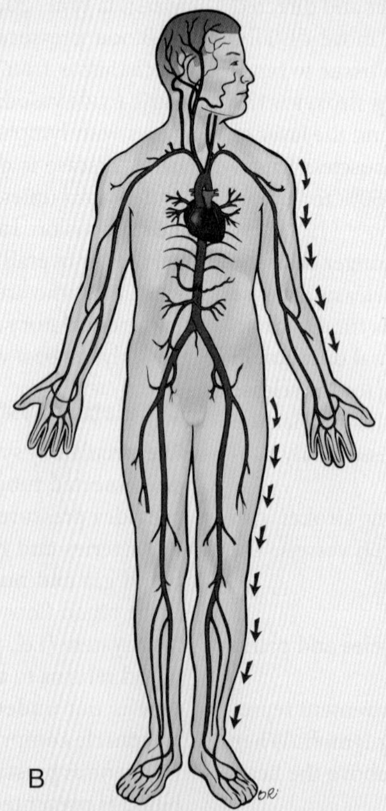

B. Direction of compression over arteries to increase arterial flow.

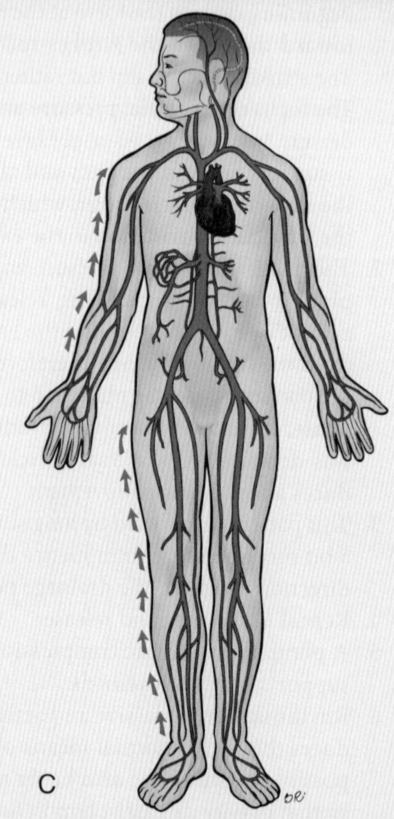

C. Direction of gliding strokes to facilitate venous flow.

FLUID MOVEMENT PROTOCOL: LYMPHATIC DRAINAGE AND VENOUS RETURN

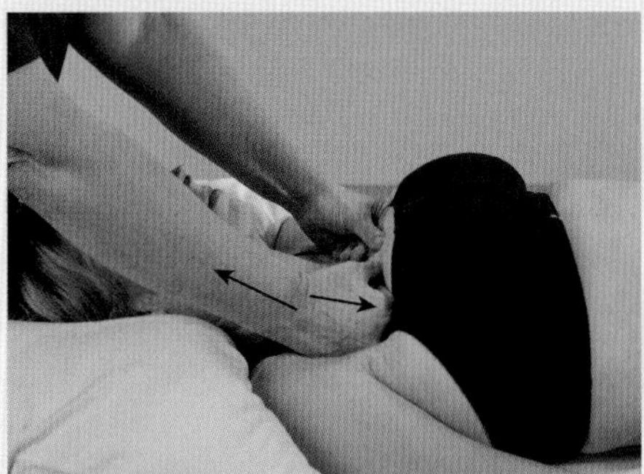

1. Pumping the thorax to support lymph drainage.

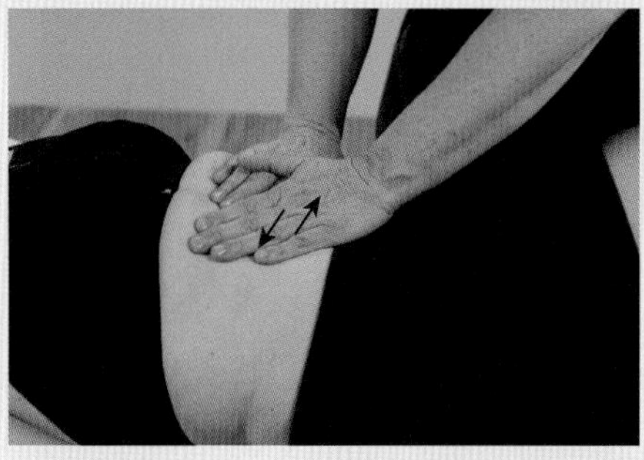

2. Pumping the abdomen to support lymph drainage.

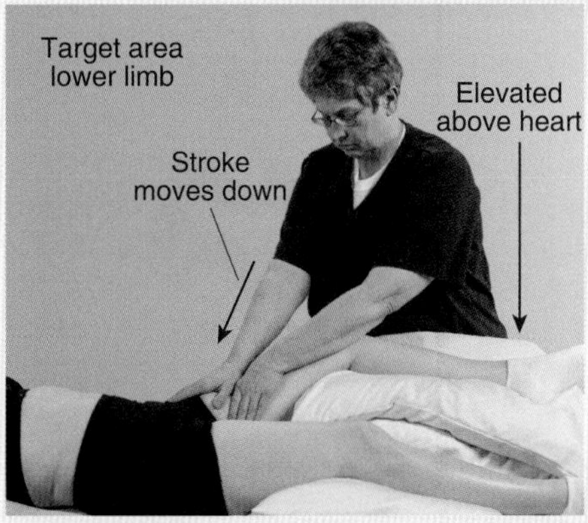

3. Elevate the area to be drained above the heart to support both lymph and venous flow. Begin close to the torso.

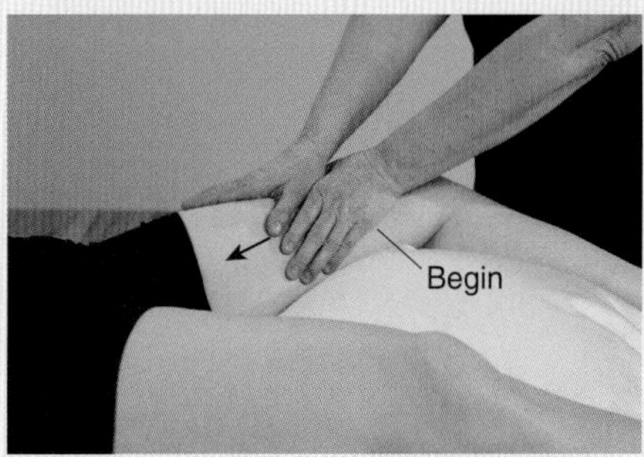

4. For specific focus on lymphatics, do not let the hands slip on the skin while moving tissue into and out of bind.

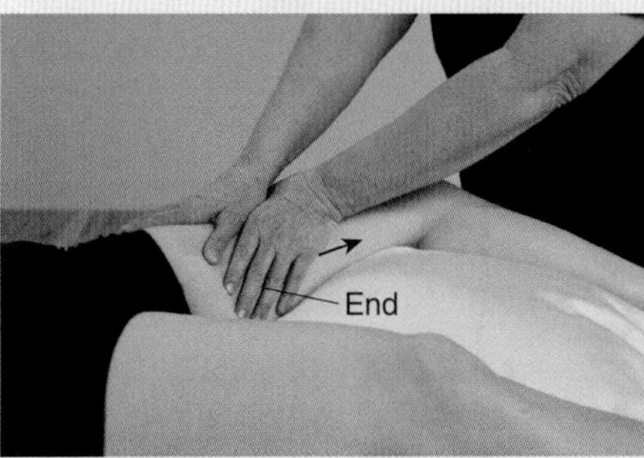

5. Do not let the hands slip on the skin as each area is moved into and out of bind.

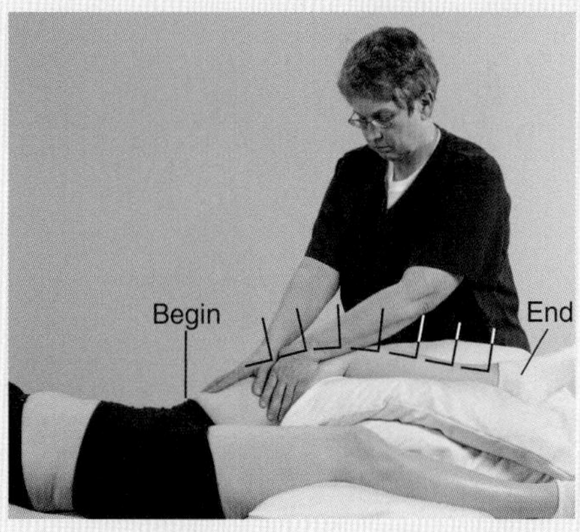

6. Move tissue into and out of bind as you travel slowly down the area.

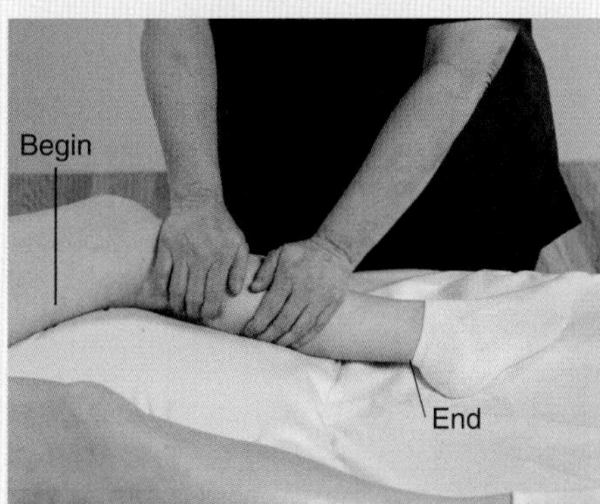

7. Knead tissue.

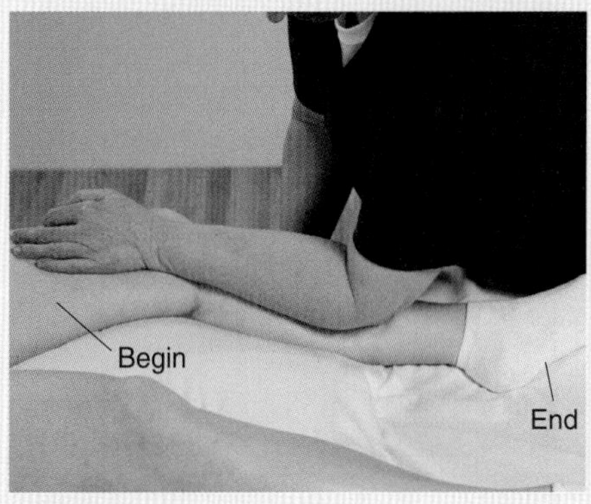

8. Compress tissue.

Continued

FLUID MOVEMENT PROTOCOL: LYMPHATIC DRAINAGE AND VENOUS RETURN—cont'd

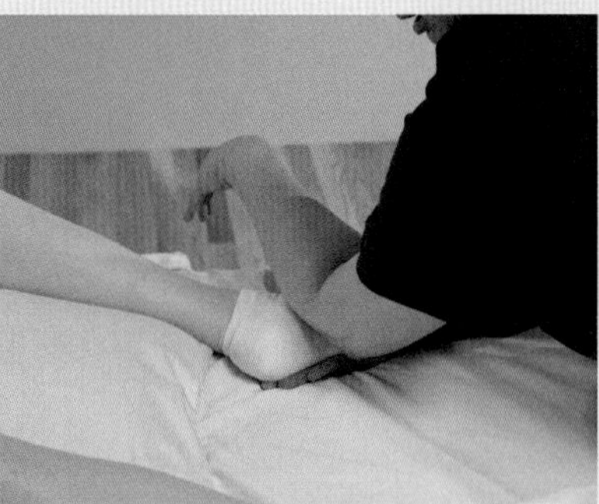

9. Compress the plexus in the foot.

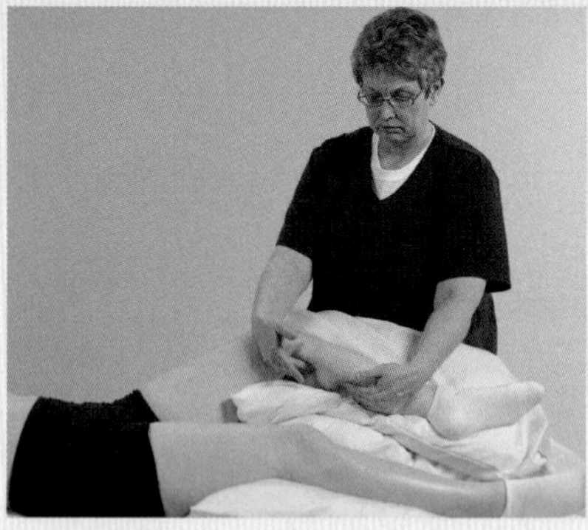

10. When shaking, flip the tissue back and forth rhythmically.

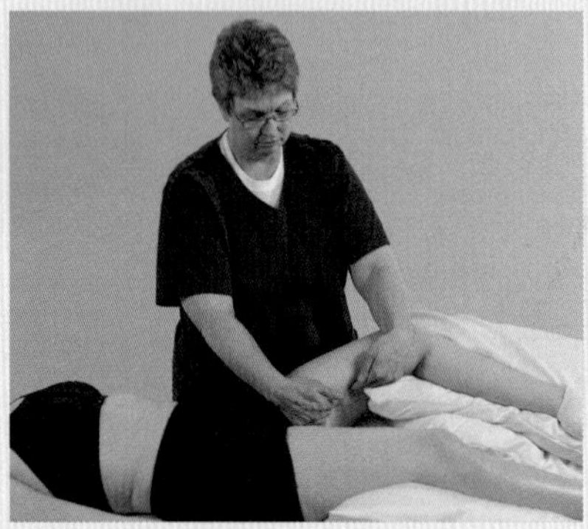

11. Move up the area being drained and flip the entire area rhythmically.

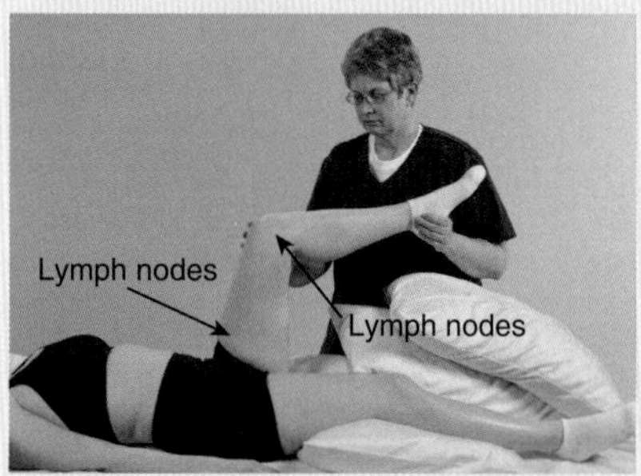

12. Move the limb to compress areas of lymph nodes.

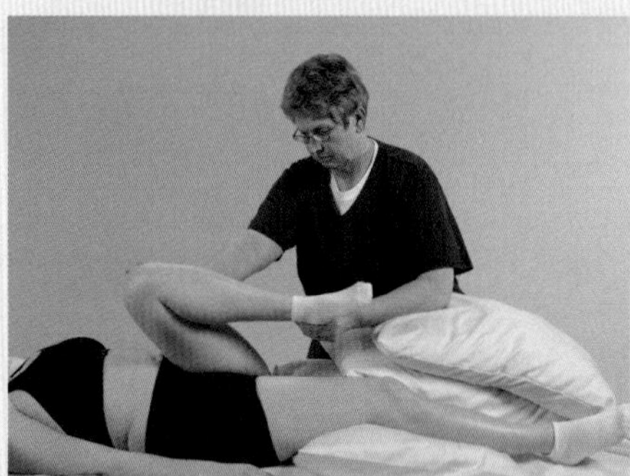

13. Move rhythmically back and forth to create a pumping action on the lymph nodes.

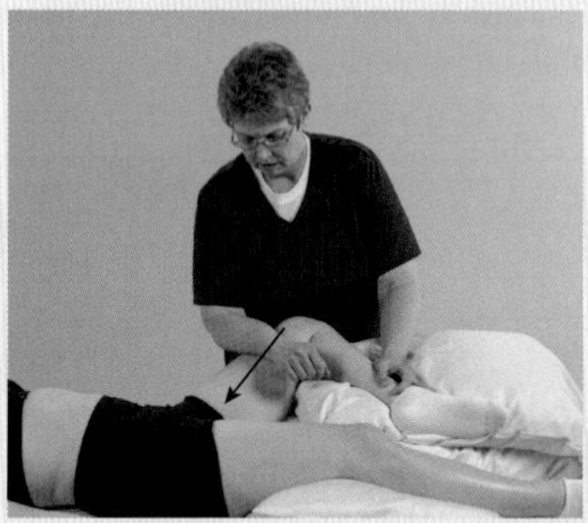

14. Reposition for venous return. Glide over veins moving distal to proximal with broad-based compression strokes about 3 inches long. Then use long strokes following the whole vein.

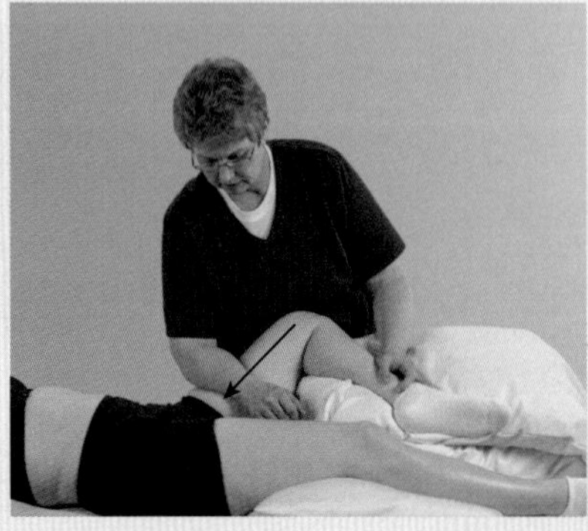

15. Repeat gliding.

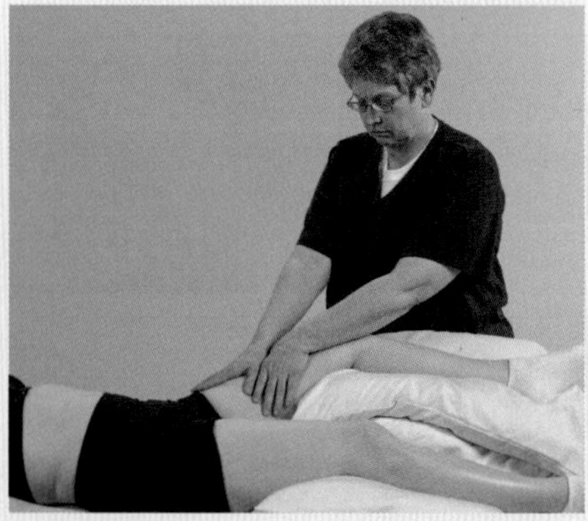

16. Repeat sequence.

FLUID MOVEMENT PROTOCOL: ARTERIAL CIRCULATION

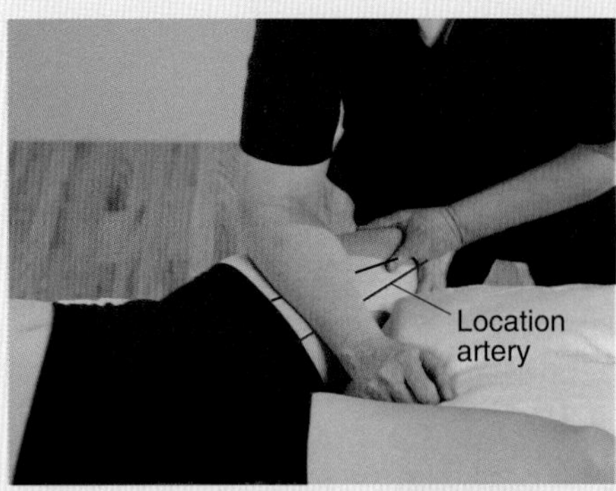

1. To support arterial circulation, begin with the area positioned below the heart. Focus compression over the arteries.

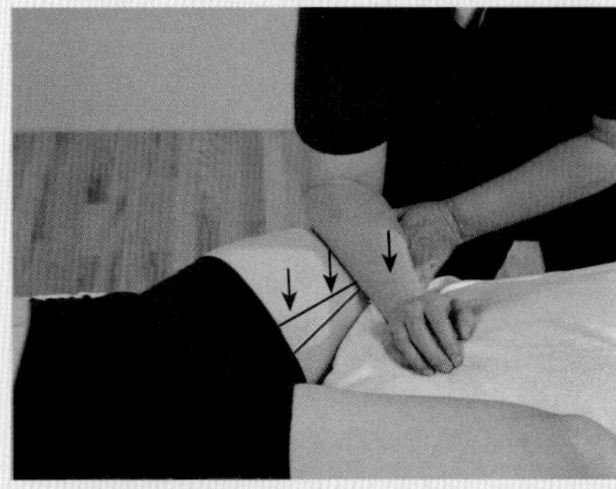

2. Move the compression down (away) from the heart at about one compression per second.

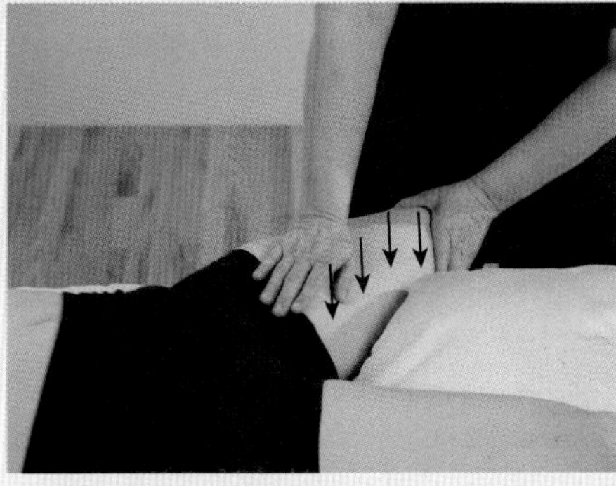

3. Repeat.

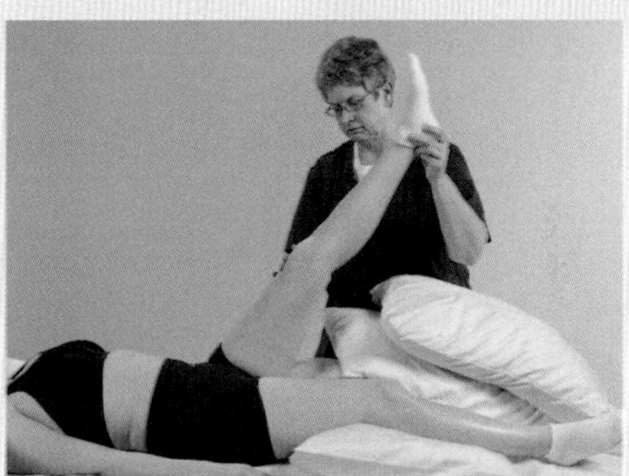

4. Move area and reposition for lymphatic drainage and venous return.

FLUID MOVEMENT PROTOCOL: INTEGRATED SEQUENCE

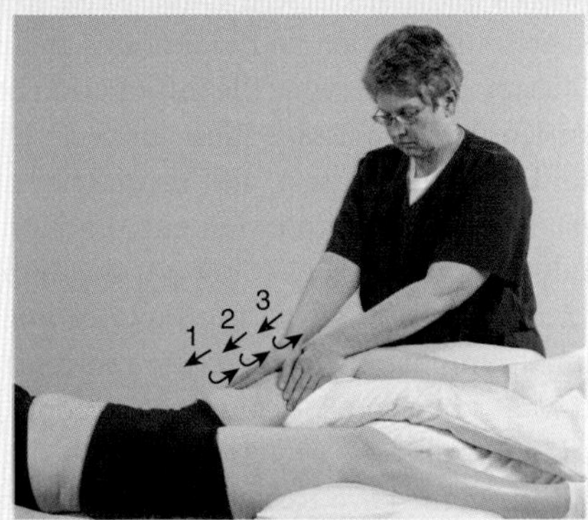

1. Begin lymphatic drainage.

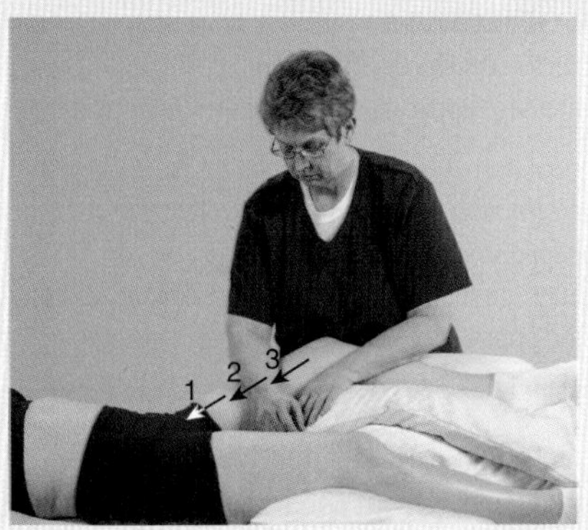

2. Switch to venous return.

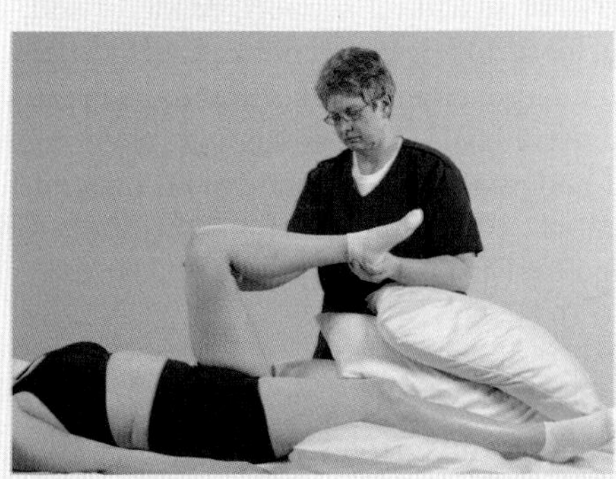

3. Rhythmically move area to support both lymph and venous flow.

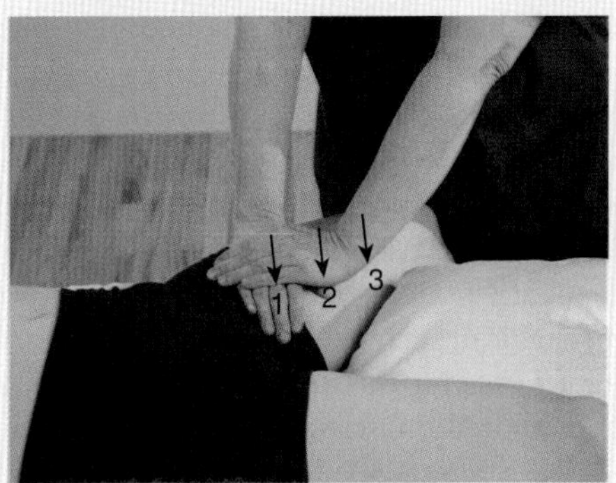

4. Reposition and begin arterial support.

Continued

FLUID MOVEMENT PROTOCOL: INTEGRATED SEQUENCE—cont'd

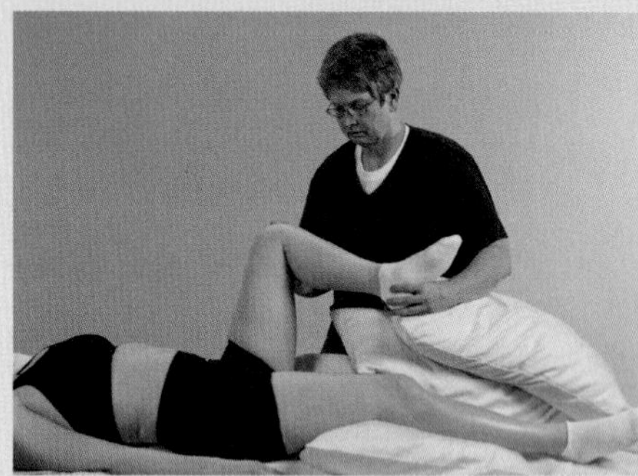
5. Move area again and reposition.

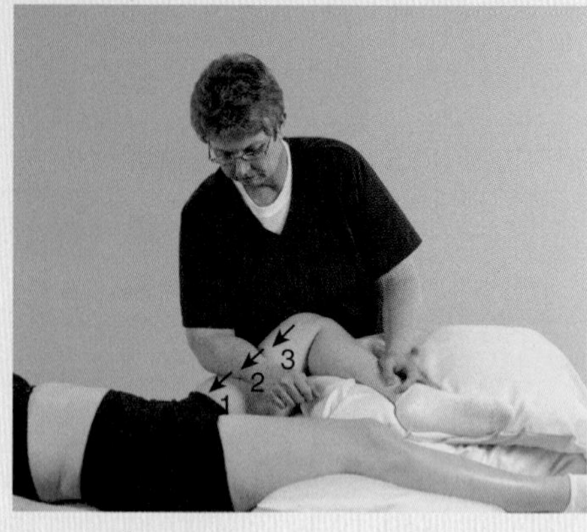

6. Target venous flow again.

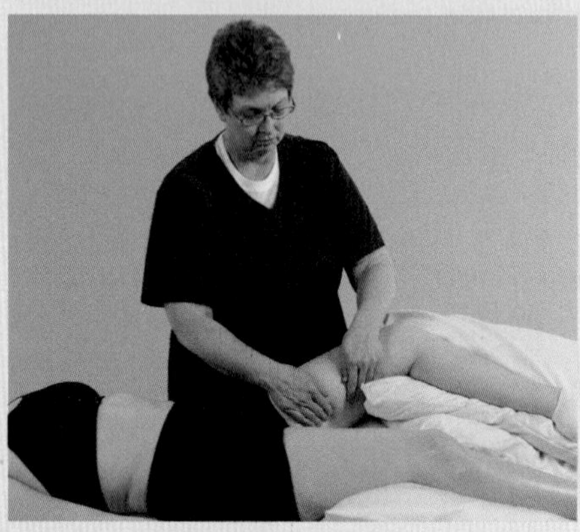
7. Shake tissue.

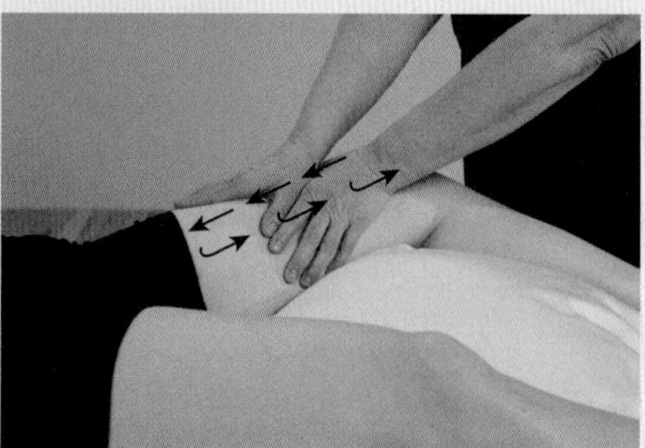
8. Resume lymphatic drainage.

CONNECTIVE TISSUE APPROACHES

SECTION OBJECTIVES

Chapter objective covered in this section:

7. Modify massage application to target the connective tissues of the body.

Using the information presented in this section, the student will be able to perform the following:

- Modify massage methods to address the connective tissue specifically.
- Explain the principles of transverse friction massage.

Methods that affect the connective tissue of the body have been discussed throughout the text, and research is mixed and either does not support or only weakly supports the benefits of connective tissue massage (Laimi et al., 2018; Wu et al., 2021). Yet again, with highly specialize applications, the massage therapist needs to be cautious about claims made for benefit and consider biological plausibility for methods used.

Connective tissue techniques use manually guided forces in numerous strain directions to treat injuries and somatic dysfunctions. Connective tissue bodywork styles range from the very subtle, light work of some types of myofascial release to the very mechanical, such as Dr. James Cyriax's friction massage. Current terms for this approach are transverse friction massage or cross friction massage (Pitsillides and Stasinopoulos, 2019).

This section provides introductory information about myofascial approaches and transverse friction. Refer to Chapters 5 and 6 for research information and indications and contraindications, and Chapter 10 to review the information on how mechanical forces created by massage affect connective tissue.

Superficial fascia, deep fascia, and myofascial tissues have both specific anatomy and physiologic function. Massage adapted to address these tissues is not a true adjunct method but instead a modification in massage application. However, as with manual lymphatic drainage, the modifications have evolved into what some consider a unique system.

The definition of *fascia* is evolving. Fascia is the soft tissue component of the connective tissue system that permeates the human body, forming a whole-body continuous three-dimensional matrix of structural support. Made of soft, collagen-containing, loose and dense fibrous connective tissue, the fascial system interpenetrates and surrounds all organs, muscles, bones, and nerve fibers, creating a unique environment which enables all body systems to operate in an integrated manner (Adstrum et al., 2017; Bordoni et al., 2018a,b,c; Kirchgesner et al., 2018; Zügel et al., 2018).

Nature of the Fascia

Fascia in some form surrounds and separates almost every structure and cell in the body. It forms the interstitial space (the space between individual cells). Fascia is involved in structural and visceral support and in separation and protection; it therefore influences respiration, elimination, metabolism, fluid flow, and the immune system. Fascia is stress responsive; it becomes stiffer in response to real or perceived threats and any other activation of the sympathetic autonomic nervous system.

Because the body is a tensegrity structure, an injury at any given site often begins as long-term strain in other parts of the body. The injury manifests where it does because of inherent weakness or previous injury, not purely and always because of local strain or a direct effect. Discovering these points of tension and easing chronic strain in the body help facilitate restoring balance in the structure and tend to prevent future injuries.

Transmission of tension through a tensegrity array provides a way to distribute forces to all interconnected elements and at the same time to tune the entire system mechanically as one. Creating a balance across the bones, myofascial component, and, further, across the entire fascial net could have profound implications for health, both cellular and general (Stecco and Stecco, 2014; Boghdady et al., 2021; Sharkey, 2021; Tomchuk and Anderson 2021; Armstrong 2021). The goal for massage is to support balance in the myofascial systems.

Location of the Fascia

Anatomically, fascia can be classified as superficial (subcutaneous) fascia or deep fascia; however, it is really one interconnected structure. Superficial fascia lies between the skin and the muscles. Deep fascia surrounding the muscles weaves diagonally through the body, creating fascial sheaths. Subserous fascia lies between the deep fascia and the membranes lining the body cavities. A deep level of fascia interconnects the cranium, spine, and sacrum, joining the connective tissue coverings of the central nervous system with the unity of the body. The body also has three or four transverse fascial planes. These are located in the cranial base, cervical thoracic area, diaphragm, and lumbar and pelvic floor areas. Transverse planes also exist for joints. Myofascia (muscle fascia) can be described as the intertwined muscle tissue and connective tissue comprising the main components of anatomic muscles (Stecco, 2004; Bordoni and Zanier, 2014).

These classifications of fascial layering are artificial. As previously described, the tensegrity of fascia composes one large, interconnected, three-dimensional microscopic dynamic grid structure that connects everything with everything (Ajimsha et al., 2020; Della Posta et al., 2022). Through the fascial system, if you pull on the little toe, you affect the nose, and if the structure of the nose is dysfunctional, it can pull anywhere in the body, including the little toe.

Although fascia generally orients itself vertically in the body, it orients in any directional stress pattern. For example, scar tissue may redirect fascial structures, as can trauma, repetitive strain patterns, and immobility. This redirection of structural forces is caused by compensation patterns associated with stress patterns (Schleip et al., 2013). During physical assessment, the body appears "pulled" out of symmetry or stuck.

Components of the Fascia

Fascia is a type of connective tissue. It contains fluid, fibers, sensory receptors, and other nerves and contractile cells called myofibroblasts (think mini muscles). The fluid can be thick and jelly-like to thin and watery. The fluid is slippery. The fibers are strong and ropelike, elastic and stretchy, or fluffy and spongy.

Fluid

The fluid part of connective tissue is the ground substance. Ground substance is found in all spaces between the fibers and cells of connective tissues. Water is a main component of ground substance, but the water is bound to sugar- and protein-based molecules (proteoglycans) to make it stiff like gelatin. Proteoglycans are responsible for the viscous character of the ground substance. Hyaluronan (or hyaluronic acid) is the dominant substance in connective tissues. Hyaluronan is the most abundant glycosaminoglycan (GAG) in the body. Glycosaminoglycan molecules are responsible for viscosity and are located primarily on the surface of cells or in the extracellular matrix (ECM). Along with the high viscosity of GAGs comes low compressibility, which makes these molecules ideal for a lubricating fluid in the joints. At the same time, their rigidity provides structural integrity to cells and provides passageways between cells, allowing for cell migration. Hyaluronan serves as a "backbone" for the assembly of other glycosaminoglycans in connective and skeletal tissue. Hyaluronan is also a major component of the synovial fluid, which fills joint cavities, and the vitreous body of the eye (Ugwoke et al., 2022). Fascia allows continuity of nerves, blood, and lymph vessels between the sliding tissues. With trauma to a tissue the overlying fascia no longer produces an adequate sliding layer of hyaluronan (Stecco et al., 2018). Restoring this natural sliding mechanism is an important outcome for massage application.

When considering the fluid aspect of connective tissue and fascia it is also important to include the imbedded interstitial fluid, and blood and lymph in the vessels. The interstitium (fluid filled spaces within connective tissue throughout the body) reflects this fluid fiber interface (Bordoni et al., 2018a; Bordoni et al., 2018b; Armstrong, 2020).

What Can Go Wrong? What Might Massage Do?

Ground substance in fascia should be pliable and slippery. Tissues need to slide against each other. However, when the ground substance becomes stiff and sticky, there is a change in the amount of hyaluronan. Factors related to the changes are overuse and lack of use; systemic inflammation; stress related to sympathetic autonomic nervous system overactivation; and physical factors, such as cold and wind, which reduce the ground substance viscosity and can allow the fibers to become tangled. Fascia allows continuity of nerves, blood, and lymph vessels between the sliding tissues. With trauma to the muscle, the overlying fascia no longer produces the sliding layer of hyaluronan. Restoring this natural sliding mechanism becomes an important task for the manual therapist. *Densification* is now the term being used to describe thick, sticky tissue. The term *dense* relates to the compactness of a substance.

Modified massage can help restore the pliability and slip of the ground substance. In general, variable pressure is applied at differing angles with consistent drag on the tissues, producing shear, tension, and torsion stress. This variation of pressure causes hyaluronan to flow near the edges of the fascial area where the tissue load is applied, resulting in greater lubrication. There is a space (fluid gap) between fascial layers that is filled with ground substance and is slippery because tissue layers are meant to slide over each other. When the mechanical force is applied, it causes the fluid gap to increase because the fluid pressure of hyaluronan increases as fascia is deformed. As the jelly-like ground substance is pushed, it creates a little mound in front of the contact point that separates the layers and increases the slipperiness. As a result, tissues are able to slide more normally (Roman et al., 2013; Harper et al., 2019; Langevin, 2021).

Fibers

Connective tissue is composed to two basic types of fibers which work together to provide strength (collagen) and pliability (elastin). Large ropelike collagen fibers give rigidity to tissues and organs, while small wavy elastin fibers give elasticity. Elastin is the protein that allows the connective tissues to stretch and then recoil to their original positions. The elastin chain cannot be pulled too far during connective tissue work because the companion collagen fibers limit the stretching of the elastin fibers (Box 12.10). Reticular fibers are fibers in connective tissue that are composed of collagen and form an intricate network with other similar fibers to serve as a supporting mesh (spongy) in soft tissues.

When tissue is strained unequally (think a snag in the fibers of a sweater), human fibroblasts respond with increased secretion of proinflammatory chemicals, resulting in increased cell proliferation, distinct changes in cellular structure, and a delayed inflammatory response. For example, delayed-onset muscle soreness may take up to 3 days to manifest and is associated with inflammation and cytokine induction, among other possible causes. The inflammatory response triggers abnormal collagen secretion and may lead to fibrosis, reducing the tissue's elasticity and ability to slide (Klyne et al., 2021).

Fibrosis is the formation of excess fibrous tissue or scar tissue, usually because of injury or long-term inflammation. When fibrosis occurs in response to injury, the term *scarring* is used. Fibrosis can also occur with overuse syndromes, such as tendonitis, which then becomes tendinosis. Massage can create mild inflammation in the fibrotic tissue and trigger an active acute, but controlled and productive, healing process. There is usually ground substance densification in areas of fibrosis; therefore increasing pliability and sliding is typically included as a massage outcome (Kwong and Findley, 2014). Physical scar management is a collective name for all the noninvasive scar treatments that make use of physical interventions such as massage to act on the scar. There is a wide variety of noninvasive treatment options that make use of mechanomodulation to improve various scar symptoms, including but not limited to manual scar massage, vacuum massage, pressure therapy. Moderate intensity and frequency of mechanical stimuli are indicated in physical scar management (Van Daele et al., 2022).

Both direct and indirect connective tissue methods have been shown to reverse the inflammatory effects in cells that have been strained repetitively. A direct technique moves the restricted tissue into the barrier caused by binding. An indirect technique moves the tissue away from the restrictive barrier to a point of ease. Changing the strain pattern in cells (indirect, away from the bind; or direct, toward the bind) may result in improvement in symptoms. It may take only 60 seconds for changes to occur (Meltzer and Standley, 2007; Standley and Meltzer, 2008; Cao et al., 2013).

If triggering a productive inflammatory response is the goal, then the tissue will need to be stressed by applying mechanical force to the fibrotic tissue for 1 to 3 minutes and possibly longer (Ajimsha et al., 2015).

Box 12.10 Tissue Responses to Massage

When a mechanical force (e.g., massage) is applied to the body, two tissue responses can occur:

The tissue can plastically deform and remain in its new shape. This happens in lax ligament syndrome, in which the ligaments have been overstretched. The massage practitioner may attempt to permanently change the shape of short tissues, such as a scar.

The tissue can behave elastically (as does a rubber band or bungee cord), changing shape and then returning to its original shape. This is normal behavior in most fascial types, including bone, which is more elastic than it appears.

A combination of these responses is also possible.

Sensory Receptors and Nerves

Microscopic study has shown that in many places in the fascia, a vein, an artery, and a nerve perforate (poke through) tissue layers. Called neurovascular bundles, these points are in the same location as most of the trigger points and acupuncture points. It is hypothesized that, these points become densified during injury, affecting the muscle nerve receptors and creating dysfunctions in fascial tone and mechanical strain in the fascial system.

The fascia is imbedded with sensory receptors that report the presence of pain (nociceptors), change in movement (proprioceptors), change in pressure and vibration (mechanoreceptors), change in the chemical milieu (chemoreceptors), and fluctuation in temperature (thermoreceptors). Deep fascia responds to sensory input by contracting; by relaxing; or by adding, reducing, or changing its composition through the process of fascial remodeling.

The deep fascia is a highly vascular structure with a superficial and a deep layer, each with an independent rich vascular network of capillaries, venules, arterioles, and lymphatic channels. Myofibroblasts are present, suggesting contractile ability. Any active contraction would need to be controlled by a nerve supply, and myelinated and unmyelinated nerve axons and Schwann cells are found in these deep fascial layers. Electron microscopy and special staining procedures demonstrate that fascia is populated by sensory neural fibers, suggesting that fascia contributes to proprioception and nociception and may be responsive to manual pressure, temperature, and vibration.

Many encapsulated endings found in fascia are mechanoreceptors that respond to mechanical pressure or deformation, and include Golgi receptors, lamellated (Pacinian) corpuscles, and bulbous (Ruffini) corpuscles (Kumka and Bonar, 2012).

In addition, connective tissue may function as a whole-body communication system. The loose connective tissue type (think spiderweb) has a language of tiny tugs and pulls that communicates mechanical messages throughout the body because of the principle of tensegrity (Langevin, 2006; Swanson, 2013).

The common location of the neurovascular bundles, myofascial trigger points, and places where the fascial fibers interconnect may explain how dysfunction in these focal points can cause body-wide disturbance. Massage application that normalizes these areas may result in a productive body-wide response (Remvig et al., 2008; Bordoni and Zanier, 2014). Sympathetic autonomic nervous system (ANS) activation is perceived as stress. Massage that reduces the fight-or-flight response (sympathetic dominance) and supports relaxation (parasympathetic dominance) may be analogous to getting out of too-tight clothes and getting into loose, soft pajamas.

It is also possible that the endocannabinoid system inside the deep fasciae is stimulated during manipulative treatments and exercises. Targeted massage potentially stimulates fascial fibroblasts, influencing the endocannabinoid system and anti-inflammatory responses (Fede et al., 2016).

Myofibroblast

The fascia has contractile cells, which respond to the application of mechanical force, and smooth muscle cells, which are controlled by the autonomic nervous system. The fascial tonus (tone) may be influenced and regulated by the state of the autonomic nervous system. Any intervention targeting the fascia is also an intervention on the autonomic system and vice versa (Schleip, 1998; Chaitow, 2014). Smooth muscle cell contraction is most likely controlled by the sympathetic aspect of the autonomic nervous system, but confirming research is sparse. If the sympathetic nervous system is the regulator, then activation would increase the overall fascial tension (Klingler et al., 2004). A comparison would be clothes shrinking while being worn.

Connective Tissue Dysfunctions

People can develop several basic connective tissue dysfunctions. Connective tissue may shorten, lose fluidity, and adhere, causing binding, pulling, and restricted movement. Another common problem is overstretched connective tissue at the joint, resulting in laxity and destabilization of the joint. This sets the stage for protective muscle spasms, which reduce joint space.

Normalization of connective tissue may allow the joint to function properly; however, this process may become problematic. One important function of the connective tissue is to stabilize; stabilization may require that the joint remain out of optimum alignment. For example, if the medial collateral ligament of the knee is lax due to repeated sprains, then the medial attachment of the gastrocnemius muscle may shorten and become fibrotic, increasing flexion of the joint a small amount. The knee is more stable but the relationship of the femur to the tibia is different.

As explained by Dr. David Gurevich, a Russian physician, the pattern of degeneration usually begins with dystonia, or disruption of motor tone. Sometimes direct trauma to a joint may cause misalignment, rather than increased or decreased muscle tension pulling joints out of alignment. Bones are designed to fit at the joint in a specific way. When this fit is disrupted, the next step is a protective muscle spasm, followed by connective tissue reorganization to stabilize the area. Areas of disruption in joint play or joint alignment eventually include a connective tissue component in the dysfunction (Kreighbaum and Barthels, 1995). Data suggest that the stiffness of lumbar fascia and the severity of low back pain are linked. Decreased stiffness after myofascial release can reduce low back pain (Ahmed et al., 2021; Tamartash and Bahrpeyma, 2022).

Treatment of Dysfunctions

Gurevich taught the treatment sequence is first massage, including connective tissue approaches; then mobilization (movement of jointed areas within a comfortable range of motion); and finally joint manipulation. Massage and mobilization are within the scope of bodywork practice, whereas joint manipulation is not. The services of a chiropractor, osteopath, or other professional trained in joint manipulation are needed for problems that require direct manipulation of the joint.

Professional experience suggests that the longer the problem has existed, the more mechanical the techniques required initially. Mechanical force application during massage pushes and pulls the connective tissue in multiple directions. Methods used include gliding, kneading, friction, compression, and movement to elongate, drag, and pull tissue. Slow sustained application is needed because connective tissue responds relatively slowly (30 seconds to 3 minutes) (Ercole et al., 2010; de Almeida et al., 2021; Stecco et al., 2023). It is often necessary to load the tissues multiple times, in multiple directions, using a variety of massage methods (Wheatly 2022; Simon and Zidi 2022).

Myofascial Approaches

Recall the definition of myofascia (muscle fascia) as intertwined muscle tissue and connective tissue which make up the main components of anatomic muscles. Most methods classified as **myofascial approaches** more specifically address the superficial fascia. For example, Bindegewebmassage, developed by Elizabeth Dickie, consists of light strokes without oil that focus on the superficial fascial layer (between the skin and muscles). The method involves movement of the superficial fascial layer in a specific pattern related to the neurologic dermatome distribution. The results are both neurochemical and mechanical. The depth of pressure is sufficient to move the superficial fascia on top of the muscle layer (Fig. 12.10).

Rolfing, developed by Ida Rolf, and its various offshoots, such as Hellerwork, are methods of structural integration focused to bring the physical structure of the body into an efficient relationship with the perpendicular alignment of the body in gravity. The focus is normalization and redirection of the deeper fascial components of muscles and fascial sheaths.

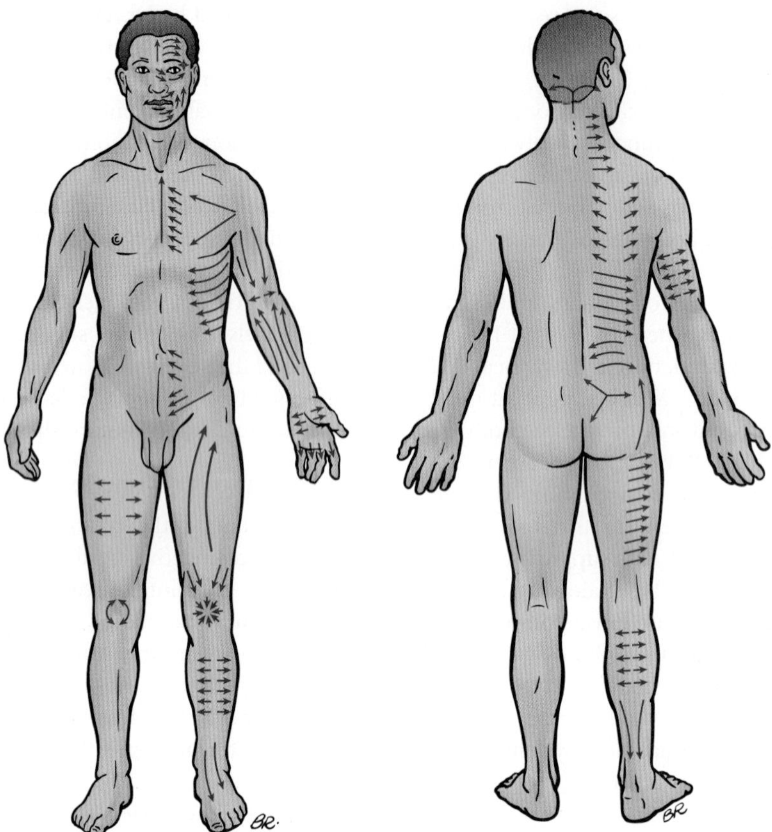

FIG. 12.10 Application of connective tissue massage, modified from Bindegewebmassage. This system primarily introduced the mechanical forces of tension, bend, shear, and torsion into the soft tissues. The arrows indicate the directions in which the massage application most efficiently targets connective tissue structures.

Osteopathy and physical therapy theory and practice contribute to the body of knowledge for myofascial approaches.

These styles of bodywork are often called soft tissue manipulation or myofascial release. Typically these methods are targeting superficial fascia while only indirectly addressing the muscle fascia complex or myofascia. Again, the terminology is frustrating.

Massage Methods Modified to Target Superficial Fascia, Deep Fascia, and Myofascia

In most cases a lubricant is not used because the drag quality on the tissue is necessary to produce results, and lubricant reduces drag. Methods that affect primarily the ground substance and specifically address densification require a quality of slow, sustained pressure and agitation. Most massage methods can soften the ground substance if the application is not abrupt. Tapotement/percussion and abrupt compression are less effective than slow gliding methods that have drag quality. Kneading and skin/superficial fascia rolling that incorporate a slow pulling action also are effective. The appropriate application introduces one or a combination of the mechanical force stresses of tension, compression, bend, shear, and torsion into the tissues at multiple angles multiple times to achieve results.

The fiber component may be affected by elongation methods by freeing and unraveling of fibers or a small therapeutic (beneficial and controlled) inflammatory response that signals for change in the fibers. The acute inflammation resolves with specialized pro-resolving mediators called resolvins. Resolvins are synthesized during the initial phases of acute inflammation and may be a factor in how introducing an acute inflammatory process can help resolve a chronic inflammatory condition (Abdolmaleki et al., 2020; Panigrahy et al., 2021; Das and Kulkarni 2022; McAphee et al., 2022).

The important consideration for all connective tissue massage methods is that variable pressure and multidirectional forces must actually move the tissue enough to create tension, torsion, shear, or bend stress (Chen et al., 2022). Additionally, the duration of the mechanical force application must last long enough for energy to build up, soften the ground substance, and influence the smooth muscle bundles. Research has shown that this process occurs in 10 to 30 seconds, and any change that will occur happens within that period (Findley, 2009). Fibrosis is addressed with transverse friction for up to 3 minutes.

The development of adaptive and maladaptive connective tissue changes is highly individualized; therefore, systems that follow a precise protocol and sequence often are less effective for dealing with these complex patterns (Proficiency Exercise 12.4).

PROFICIENCY EXERCISE 12.4

1. Make some gelatin using only half the specified amount of water. Let it set. Massage it into liquid form. Pay attention to the type of massage you use.
2. Twist and wad some plastic wrap into a ball. Then smooth it out. What methods did you need to use?
3. Take the same plastic wrap and pull it. Take out all the slack and telescope and elongate the tissue. What did you have to do to accomplish the stretch?

Tissue Movement Methods Specific to the Superficial Fascia Densification

To apply the more subtle connective tissue approaches, the practitioner must develop the skill to follow tissue movement related to fascial glide:

1. Make firm but gentle contact with the skin.
2. Increase the downward (vertical) pressure slowly until resistance is felt (bind); this barrier is soft and subtle.
3. Maintain the downward pressure at this point; now, add horizontal force until the resistance barrier (bind) is felt again.
4. Sustain the horizontal force and wait.
5. Follow the movement; stay at bind.
6. Slowly and gently release first the horizontal force and then the vertical force.

Fascial Restriction Method for Increased Fascial Tone and Densification

Fascial restriction involves an area larger than a small, localized spot. A restricted area is palpated as a barrier or an area of immobility (bind) within the tissue. The area is worked initially using routine massage techniques; if it does not soften, the pressure must be more specific. You can achieve this the following ways:

1. Stabilize the tissue with one hand.
2. With the fingers of the other hand, pull the tissue in the direction of the restriction.
3. Use the heel of the hand or the arm to separate the tissue.
4. Maintain pressure until softening occurs.

Twist-and-release kneading and compression applied in the direction of the restriction also can release these fascial barriers. See the connective tissue/myofascial protocol for a demonstration.

Transverse Friction Massage

In chronic conditions, it is important to induce a small inflammatory response in the dysfunctional area. This process initiates the reorganization of tissue by stimulating tissue repair mechanisms (Lederman, 2005; Chaitow and Delany, 2008, 2011).

The most specific localized example of connective tissue work is Cyriax's cross-fiber frictioning method, or **transverse frictioning**. This method is especially effective for fibrosis. Transverse frictioning is always a specific rehabilitation intervention; it introduces therapeutic inflammation through the creation of a specific and controlled reinjury of the tissues. A similar type of frictioning is incorporated into the *Fascial Manipulation Method* developed by the Steccos, who have refined the approach by developing an assessment process and to locate areas where back-and-forth force application of a compression friction-type massage is applied (Stecco and Stecco, 2009). Cyriax taught that the essential component of a transverse friction massage is the application of concentrated therapeutic movement over a small area. The key element is the use of friction to move the tissue against its grain (Cyriax and Coldham, 1984).

Although proficiency in this type of transverse friction is beyond the skill scope provided by this textbook, it is a valuable form of rehabilitative massage. Any massage practitioner working in a medical or sports setting should be trained in the techniques. The additional skills required are not so much in the delivery of the methods, which are fairly straightforward, but in the assessment of where to use friction and how to incorporate it into a comprehensive rehabilitation plan.

Proper rehabilitation after the massage is essential for the friction technique to be effective and to produce a mobile scar on rehealing of the tissue. The frictioned area must be contracted painlessly, without any strain put on the frictioned tissue. This is done by fixing the joint in a position in which the muscle is relaxed and then having the client contract the muscle as far as it will go. This is sometimes called a broadening contraction (Fig. 12.11).

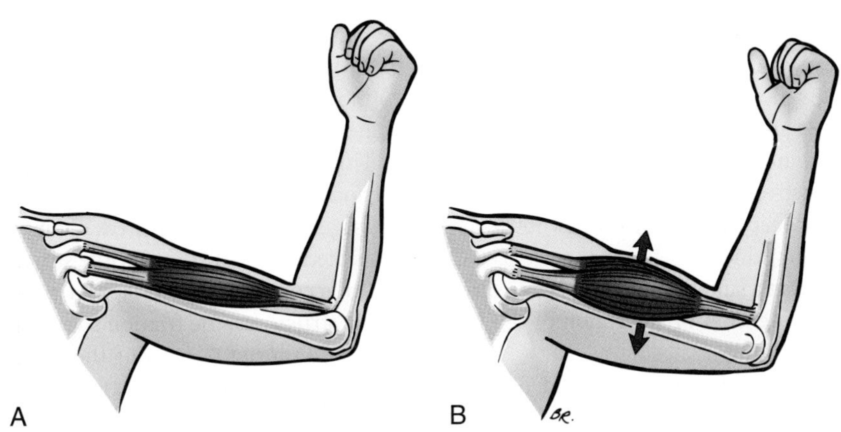

FIG. 12.11 **Broadening contraction. A,** Beginning point. **B,** Contract the muscle by flexing the joint.

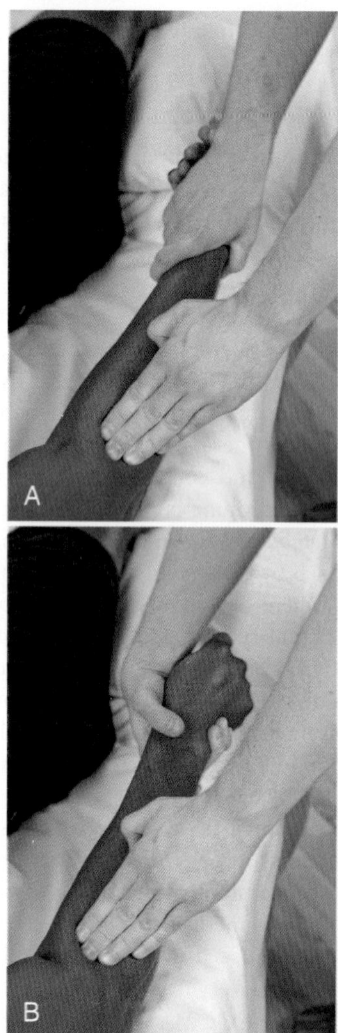

FIG. 12.12 A, B, Friction/compression with movement.

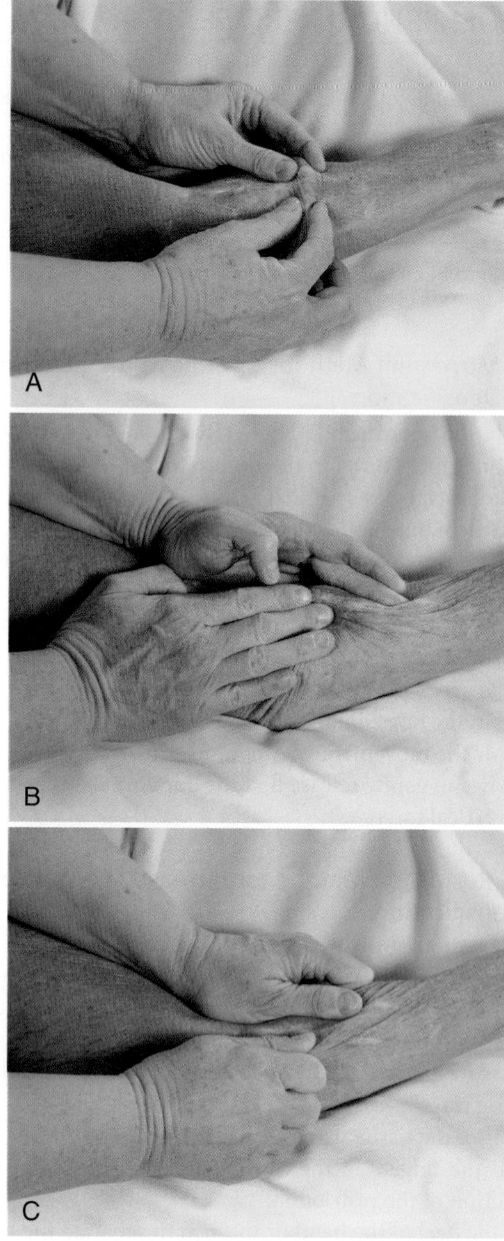

FIG. 12.13 Using connective tissue methods to increase the pliability of scar tissue. A, Application of bending to lift scar tissue. **B,** Application of shear. **C,** Application of tension.

Methods of Transverse Frictioning for Fibrosis

Cyriax teaches that when massage is given to a muscle, tendon, ligament, or joint capsule, the following principles must be observed (Fig. 12.12):

1. The right spot must be found.
2. The therapist's fingers or forearm and the client's skin must move as one. Care must be taken not to cause a blister. The client must understand that friction massage can be painful.
3. The friction must be given across the fibers composing the affected structure.
4. The friction must be given with sufficient sweep. Pressure only accesses the tender area; it does not replace the friction. Circular friction is not recommended. Only a back-and-forth friction is effective.
5. The friction must reach deep enough. If it does not reach the fibrotic area, it is of no value.
6. The client must be placed in a suitable position that ensures the appropriate degree of tension or relaxation of the tissues to be frictioned.
7. Muscles must be kept relaxed while being frictioned. Because the connective tissue of the muscle is affected, the massage must penetrate into the muscle and not stay on the surface.
8. Tendons with a sheath must be kept taut during friction massage.
9. Broadening contractions are used between sessions to promote circulation and mobile scar development during the healing process.

Using Cyriax's principles, this textbook introduces a modified version of these methods that can be incorporated into a general massage session for small areas of fibrotic tissue using transverse movement to mobilize soft tissue structures (Fig. 12.13).

To accommodate the lack of precise location of the anatomic structures, the friction suggested is done over a broader area for a shorter time using the following procedure:

1. Locate the area to be frictioned.
2. Place the tissue in a relaxed position.
3. Provide friction as described in Chapter 10.

CONNECTIVE TISSUE PROTOCOL

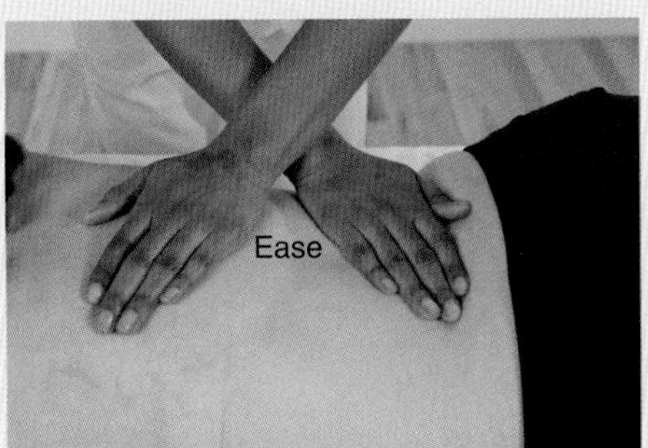

1. Place crossed hands over tissue and meld hands to the skin.

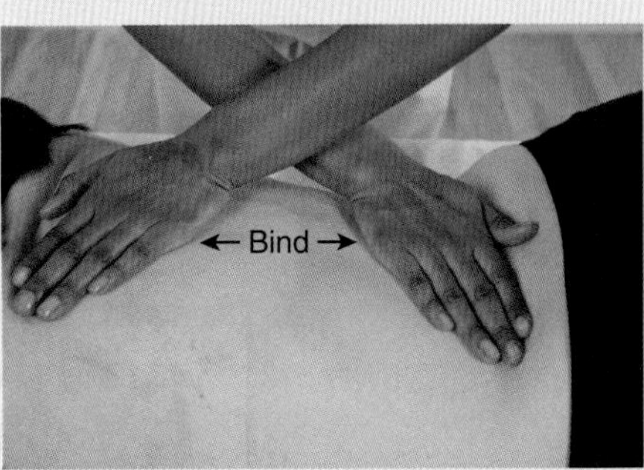

2. Separate hands moving tissue to and just into bind. Do not slip.

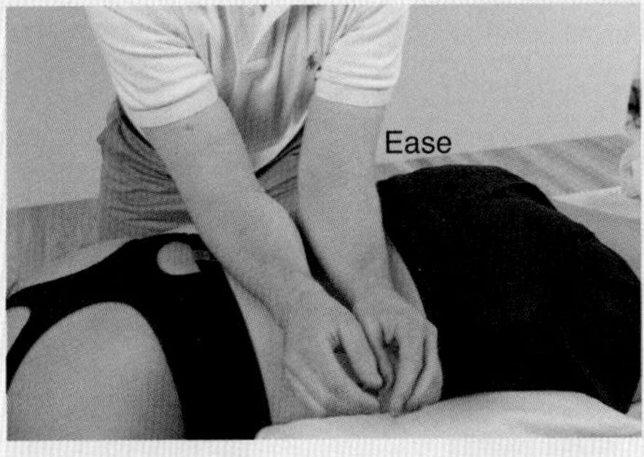

3. Forearms can be used. Place on the tissue and meld to it.

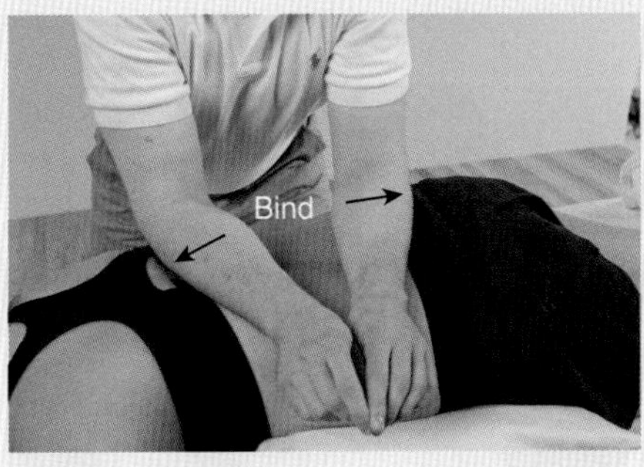

4. Separate arms moving tissue to and just into bind.

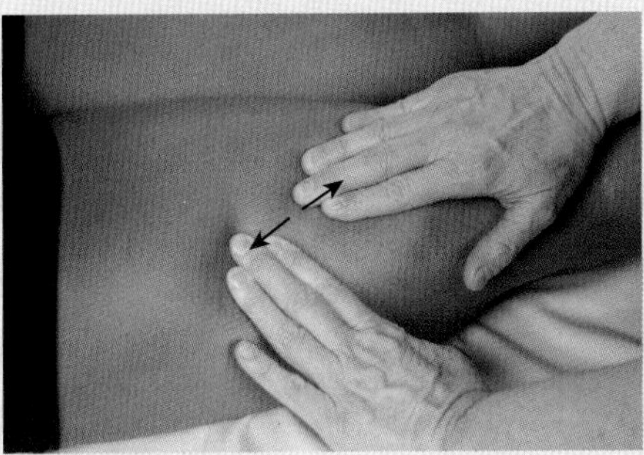

5. Small areas of tissue can be stretched by placing the short tissue between the fingers of both hands. Then, without slipping, separate tissues into the bind.

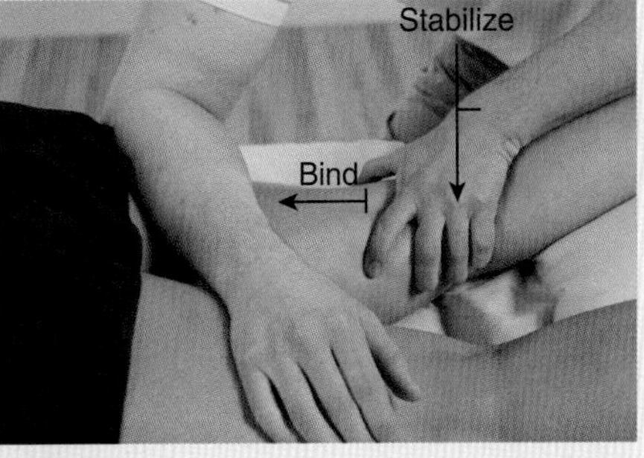

6. Stabilize tissue at one end of the target area and hold fast. Then, at the other end of the target area, slowly glide to separate tissues, with drag maintaining tension on the tissues at all times.

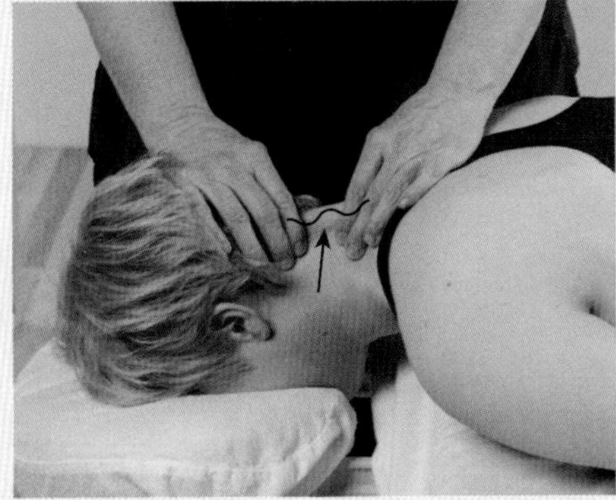

7. Use shear methods to move tissue in and out of bind.

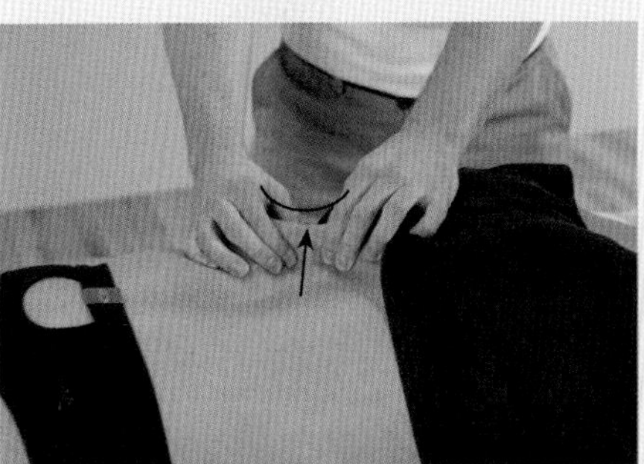

8. Use bending methods to move tissue into bind (skin rolling).

Continued

CONNECTIVE TISSUE PROTOCOL—cont'd

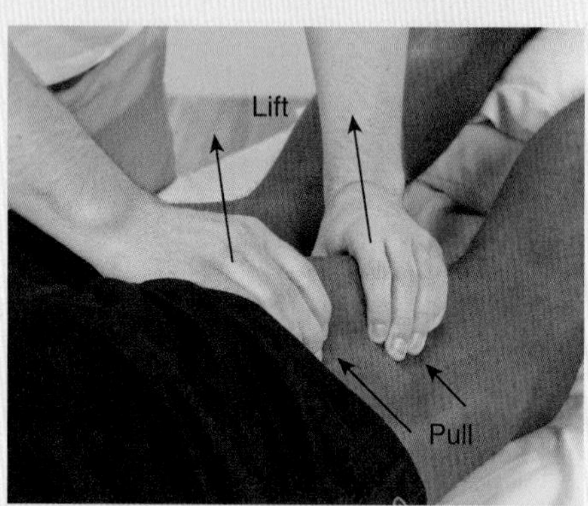

9. Grasp, lift, and pull to create combined loading to move tissue into and out of bind.

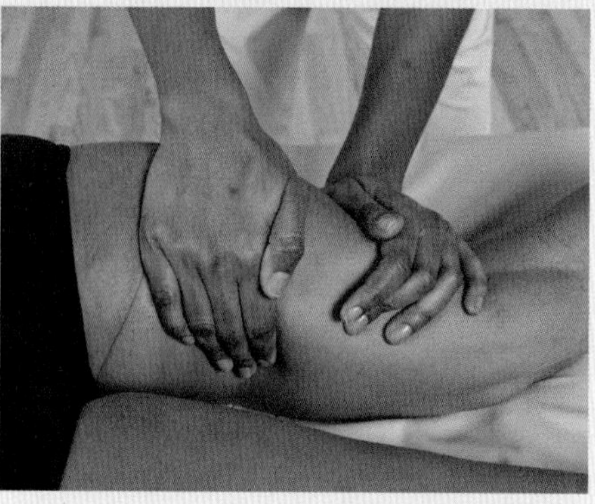

10. Use torsion methods to twist tissue into and out of bind.

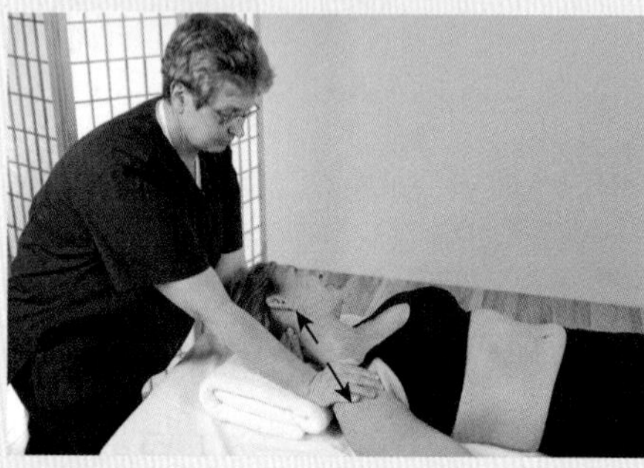

11. Elongation/stretching methods take tissue into bind. Hold at the ends of the area to be stretched and move away to create tension stress.

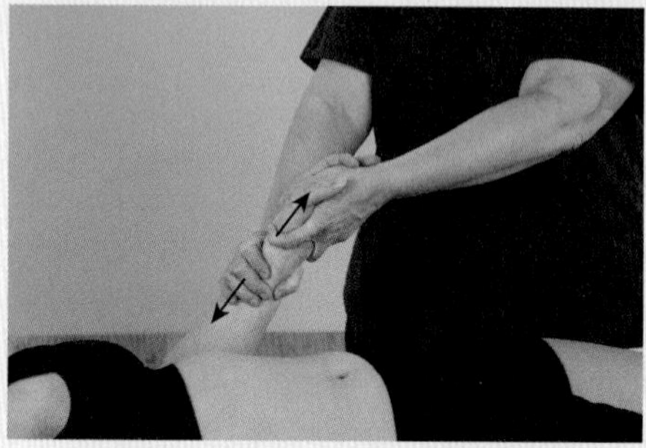

12. Traction applies tension load to the tissues surrounding a joint. Grasp firmly above and below the joint and move hands apart to create tension into bind.

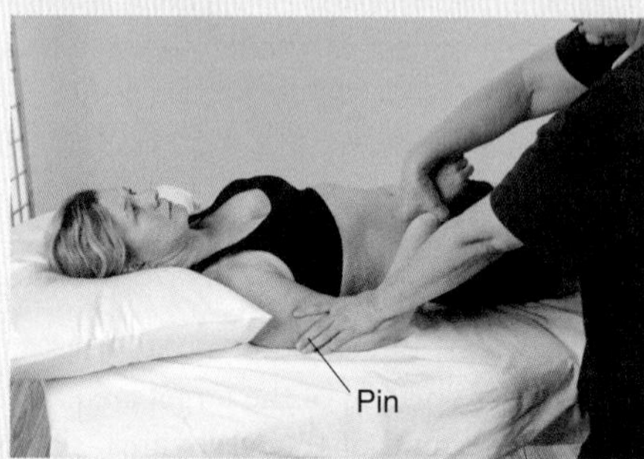

13. Pin and stretch variation. Move target tissue from ease position toward bind and hold in place.

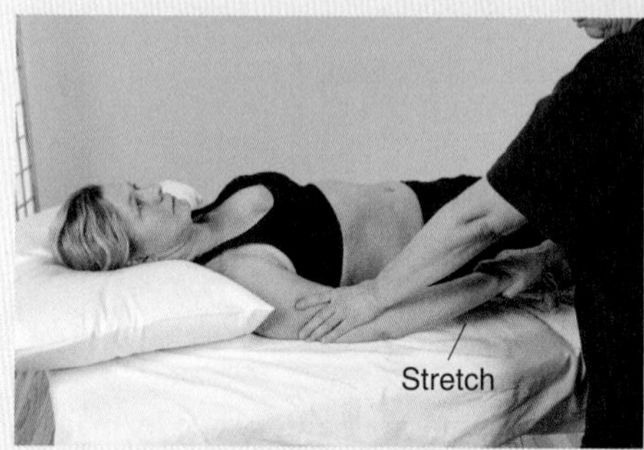

14. As the target tissue is held fixed, move the joint area to create the tension load into the bind.

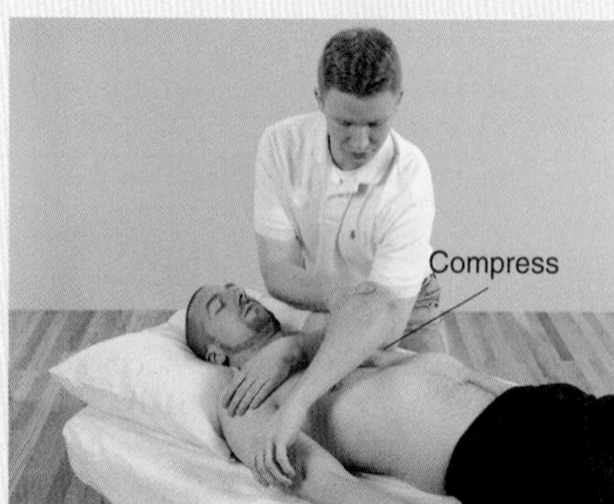

15. Active release variation. Compress target tissue while in ease and then move from ease to bind position.

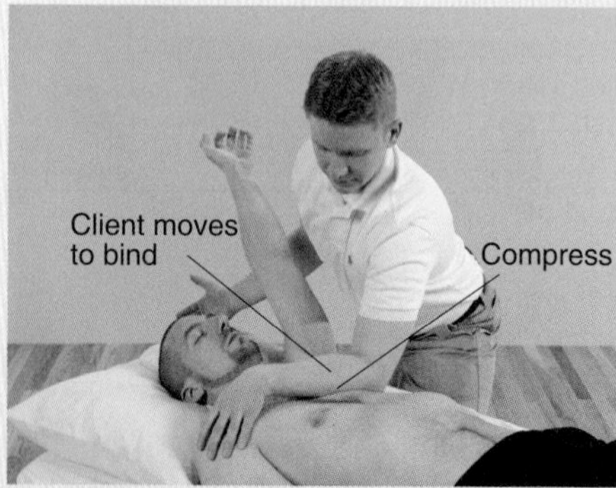

16. Client moves the jointed area away while the tissue is fixed to create the tension stress as the tissue moves into bind. The compressed and pinned tissue is held in place while the client moves away from the pinned tissue.

TRIGGER POINT INTERVENTION APPROACHES

SECTION OBJECTIVES

Chapter objective covered in this section:

8. Identify and effectively use massage to address trigger points.

Using the information presented in this section, the student will be able to perform the following:

- Describe a trigger point.
- Locate a trigger point.
- Use two methods to massage a trigger point.
- Implement trigger point treatment methods as part of a larger, neuromuscular therapy system.

Some confusion exists about the synonymous use of the terms *neuromuscular therapy* and *trigger point therapy.* **Neuromuscular therapy** is an umbrella term that encompasses a variety of treatment approaches, many of which can be used for addressing trigger points (TrPs).

Definition of a Trigger Point

Definitions of a trigger point are based on a hypothesis. The classic definition of a trigger point is an exquisitely tender spot in a discrete taut band of dense muscle tissue that produces local and referred pain, among other symptoms (Fernández-de-las-Peñas and Dommerholt, 2017). The most common definition of a **trigger point** is an area of local nerve facilitation of a muscle that is aggravated by multiple types of stress that affect the body or mind. The common theory of what causes trigger point formation involves an interaction of calcium and adenosine triphosphate (ATP) on myofascial tissues that have been stressed in some way. This causes the tissue to shorten in a localized area, producing a taut band and a nodule. The taut band/nodule generates localized and uncontrolled metabolic activity in the area and a localized acidic fluid environment, which makes the nerve endings hyperirritable; the result is pain. As this process persists, the ongoing inflammation in the area can cause connective tissue changes, and the tiny microfilaments in the muscles start to stick together (adhesions) (Gerwin, 2008; Shah et al., 2008). However, as the reader will find, multiple theories are emerging related to trigger points and myofascial pain syndromes.

When discussing the trigger point controversy, there are other scientific explanations such as referred pain, either of peripheral nerve or somatic origin or muscle spindle dysfunction (Quintner et al., 2014). It is possible that the pain of myofascial pain syndrome is due to the stimulation of sensory nerves by a pain producing substance in the inflammatory environment and the compression of inflammatory edema on tissues. It is thought that residual tension produced by the persistent static force of long-term awkward posture causes a blood circulation disorder irritating the peripheral nerve endings, causing sensory nerve dysfunction including referred pain, hyperalgesia, and allodynia. Sympathetic autonomic nervous system stimulation causes vasoconstriction of skin blood vessels and decreases blood flow, forming a vicious cycle (Cao et al., 2021).

Other theories involve fascial changes (discussed previously). Fascia can adapt to various states by reversibly changing biomechanical and physical properties. Myofibroblasts play a role in sustained myofascial tension (Plaut, 2022).

Unifying findings in most theories about the trigger point phenomenon is persistent inflammation and that a trigger point is a chronic and mild muscle injury. Studies have shown that chronic inflammatory cell infiltration promotes fibroblast proliferation, resulting in extracellular matrix (ECM) deposition and tissue fibrosis interfering with the tissue repair process (Yu et al., 2021).

The terms *contracture knot* and *trigger point* have been used interchangeably. Recent studies on animal models support the idea that contracture knots are collections of smaller trigger points with an increased proliferation of afferent nerves (Meng et al., 2015; Liu et al., 2019; Ball et al., 2022).

Currently there is no standard criteria for the diagnosis of trigger points, but advancements are occurring (Gerwin, 2018; Elbarbary et al., 2022). Controversy exists related to trigger point concepts and causes. There are no definitive answers but research continues (Birinci et al., 2018; Grabowski et al., 2018; Moraska et al., 2018; Ribeiro et al., 2018; Perreault et al., 2022; Guzmán-Pavón et al., 2022; Lu et al., 2022; Menon 2023).

A trigger point is a condition, not a method. Many different methods can be used to address trigger point-related dysfunction and pain. Hydrotherapy, acupuncture, dry needling, therapeutic exercise, massage, and nutrition are just a few possibilities. It is important to understand that with any altered physiology, such as the development of trigger points or connective tissue changes, these adaptive responses may constitute resourceful compensation and should *not* be changed. Knowing when to apply massage specifically and when *not* to is the hallmark of a professional. It is simple to find points on the body that are painful when pressed and then press on them. The individual may even feel better after the intervention; however, feeling better and being better are not the same thing. Assessment using the general massage approach as a sequence for palpation and joint movement is performed to identify potential tender points. Clinical reasoning skills are then used to determine what these points are and what should be done.

Trigger points can lead to alteration in the central nervous system processing of sensation. *Central sensitization* can be

MENTORING TIP

Many experts in the field recognize the ambiguity of the trigger point phenomenon. The debate goes round and round about the existence of trigger points, the cause of trigger points, and the location of trigger points. If you put all the experts on trigger points in a room and asked them whether they truly know what a trigger point is and what causes trigger points, they would honestly have to say no. The same can be said for those experts who say trigger points do not exist: they also do not truly know. Systems and teaching based solely on trigger points are likely flawed. This does not mean that the method should be totally dismissed. Something likely is occurring. But what is one to do? An old Russian doctor gave these words of wisdom: "Where there is pain, I rub."

defined simply as an increased sensitivity to stimulation resulting in a hypersensitive central nervous system (CNS) response. The stimulation does not need to be strong enough to cause pain, but it is processed as pain. Sometimes after an injury, a typically painless stimulation may recruit activity in these same central neurons, and the CNS interprets the sensory data as pain. This is actually a form of learned behavior, but it is not conscious behavior. The person with pain related to central sensitization is experiencing real pain, but the pain is no longer related to tissue damage. If this is one of the mechanisms of trigger point pain, then just pushing on these points actually may reinforce the pathway. On the other hand, pressure on the point may reset the abnormal sensitivity back to normal. The question you may be asking as you read is, "So do you apply compression to trigger points or not?" The answer is, "It depends. Sometimes yes and sometimes no."

Dr. Janet Travell did extensive research on myofascial pain involving trigger points and was considered the foremost authority in this area (Travell and Simons, 1999). Although some of her early research now is considered obsolete, most of her findings remain relevant. The work of Dr. Leon Chaitow provided additional information about trigger point therapy (Chaitow, 2014; Chaitow and Delany, 2008, 2011).

Integrating Trigger Point Intervention Into Massage Application

A simple working definition of trigger points is small areas of hyperirritability within muscles (Box 12.11). These areas are often located near motor nerve points. Motor nerve points are where nerve stimulation initiates contractions in small, sensitive muscle fiber bundles which in turn activates the entire muscle. Hyperirritability of these points may cause referred pain (Travel and Simons, 1999; Chaitow and Delany, 2011).

Any of the more than 400 muscles in the body can develop trigger points. The development of trigger points is accompanied by the characteristic referred pain pattern and restricted motion associated with myofascial pain. With classic trigger points, the referred pain pattern can be traced to its site of origin. The distribution of the referred trigger point pain does not usually follow the entire distribution of a peripheral nerve or dermatome segment (Fig. 12.14) (Travell and Simons, 1999; Chaitow and Delany, 2008).

Perpetuating Factors

The development of trigger points can be perpetuated by reflexive, mechanical, and systemic factors. Reflexive perpetuating factors include the following:

- Skin sensitivity in the area of the trigger point
- Joint dysfunction
- Visceral dysfunction in the viscerally referred pain pattern
- Vasoconstriction
- A facilitated nerve segment

Mechanical perpetuating factors include the following:

- Standing postural distortion
- Seated postural distortion
- Gait distortion

Box 12.11 Theory of Trigger Point Formation

The following progression has been proposed to explain the formation of trigger points:

1. Dysfunctional endplate activity occurs, commonly associated with a strain, overuse, or direct trauma.
2. Stored calcium is released at the site as a result of overuse or of tearing of the sarcoplasmic reticulum.
3. Acetylcholine (Ach) is released excessively at the synapse because of calcium-charged gates.
4. High calcium levels at the site keep the calcium-charged gates open, and the release of Ach continues.
5. Ischemia develops in the area, resulting in an oxygen and nutrient deficit.
6. A local energy crisis develops.
7. Because adenosine triphosphate (ATP) is no longer available, the tissue is unable to remove the calcium ions, and Ach continues flowing.
8. Removal of the superfluous calcium requires more energy than sustaining a contracture; therefore, the contracture remains.
9. The contracture is sustained not by action potentials from the spinal cord but by the chemistry at the innervation site.
10. The actin/myosin filaments slide to a fully shortened position (a weakened state) in the immediate area around the motor endplate (at the center of the fiber).
11. As the sarcomeres shorten, a contracture knot forms.
12. The contracture knot is the "nodule," a palpable characteristic of a trigger point.
13. The remainder of the sarcomeres of that fiber are stretched, creating the usually palpable taut band that also is a common trigger point characteristic.
14. Attachment trigger points may develop at the attachment sites of these shortened tissues (periosteal, myotendinous) where muscular tension provokes inflammation.

From Chaitow L, Delany J: *Clinical application of neuromuscular techniques, Vol 1: The upper body,* 2002, Churchill Livingstone.

- Immobilization
- Vocational stress
- Restrictive or ill-fitting clothing and shoes
- Furniture

Systemic perpetuating factors include the following:

- Enzyme dysfunction
- Metabolic and endocrine dysfunction
- Chronic infection
- Dietary insufficiencies
- Psychological stress

Assessment for Trigger Points

Determining whether a tender spot is really a trigger point, a point of fascial adhesion requiring friction, a motor point, or some other irritable reflex point, including active acupuncture points, can be difficult. However, elongation of the tissue housing the trigger point is essential to effective treatment; therefore, if doubt exists about the nature of the point, it should be treated as a trigger point.

The massage therapist usually finds trigger points during palpation or general massage using both light and deep

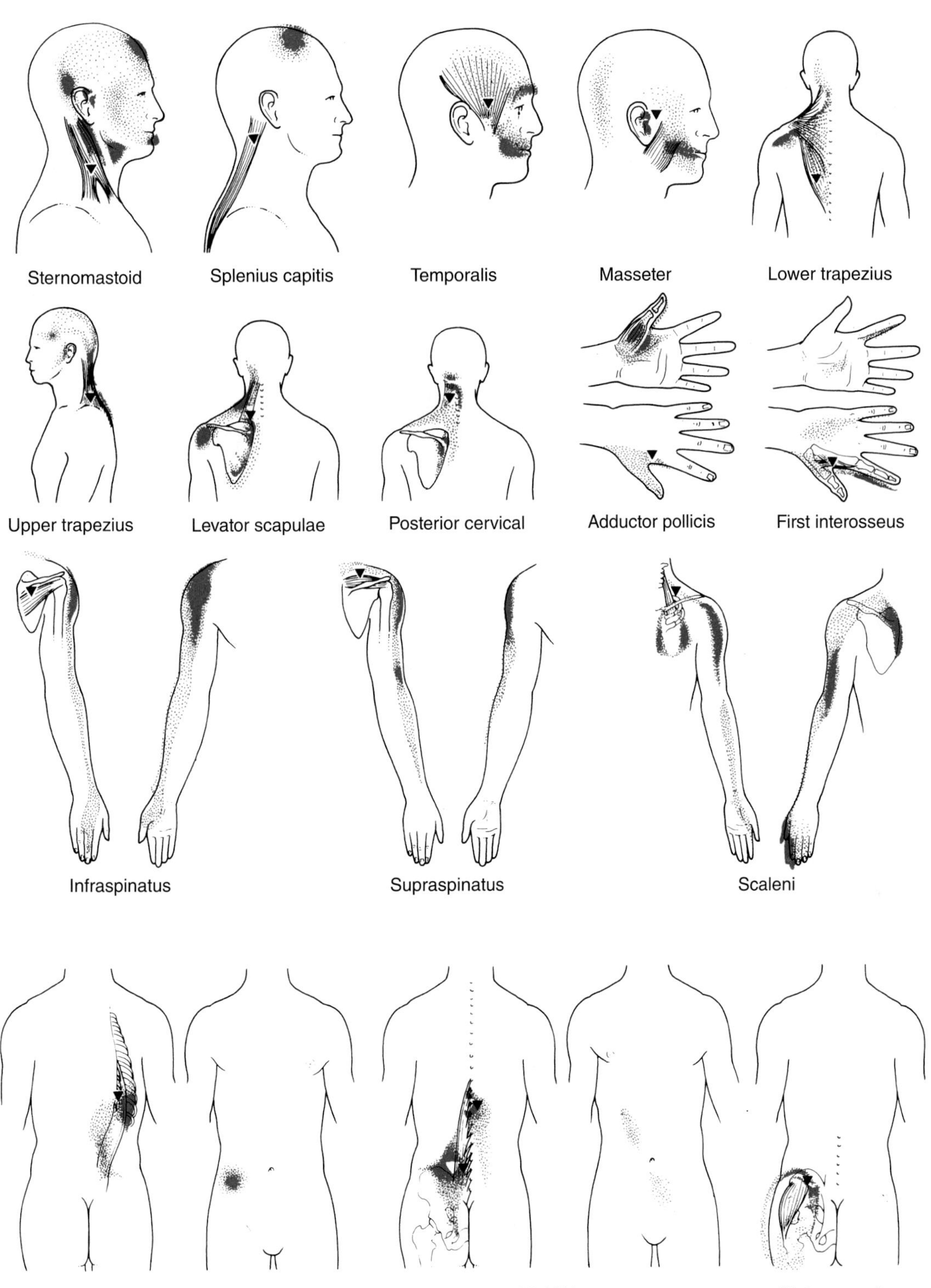

FIG. 12.14 Common trigger points. From Chaitow L: *Modern neuromuscular techniques*, ed 2, Edinburgh, 2003, Churchill Livingstone.

palpation consisting of gliding strokes (Box 12.12). Chaitow recommended that gliding strokes cover a region of 2 to 3 inches at a time.

Travell and Chaitow agreed that some pain is elicited during assessment and treatment; however, the pain elicited during treatment should be well within the client's comfort zone, so that the client is aware of the trigger point but does not initiate protective mechanisms such as guarding (tightening up), breath holding, or flinching. The muscle must be relaxed to be examined effectively. If the pressure is too great, severe local pain may overwhelm the referred pain sensation, making accurate evaluation impossible. Trigger points that are so active that referred pain is already produced have no need of exaggerated pressure.

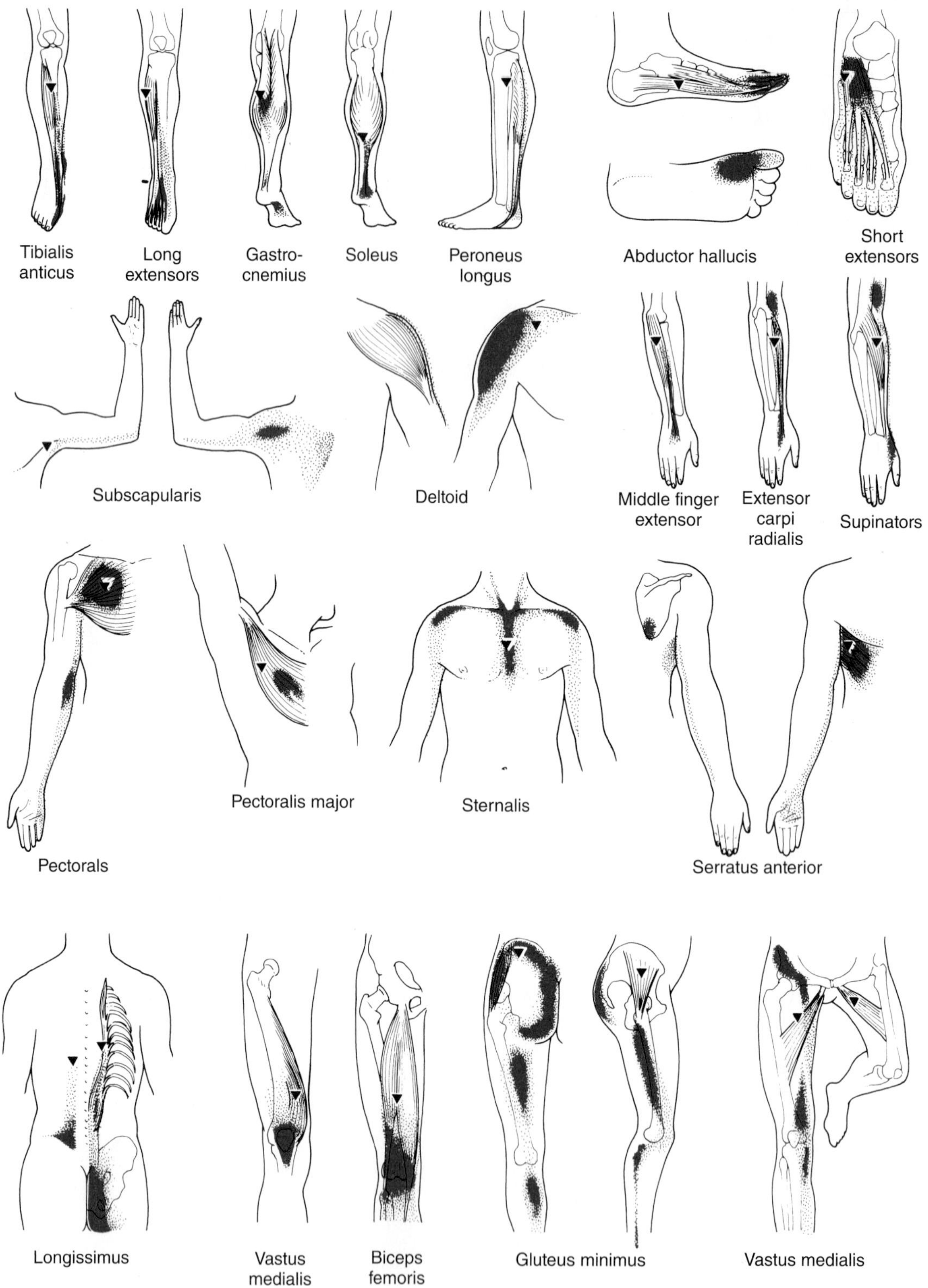

FIG. 12.14, cont'd

Only muscles which will be treated during the same visit should be examined. Palpation for trigger points can aggravate their referred pain activity; therefore, only areas intended for treatment should be palpated. In addition, development of contraction knots and trigger points may be resourceful compensation especially in individuals with hypermobility (Carvalho et al., 2022).

Methods of Treating Trigger Points

Research is lacking to support massage and manual therapy methods for trigger point treatment (Denneny et al., 2019). Therefore, caution is needed to avoid over-treating and causing discomfort if benefits are not supported. If you press hard enough and long enough on any spot it will hurt. Do not assume all tender areas are trigger points.

Box 12.12 Palpation for Trigger Points

In performing light palpation, the therapist may notice trigger points from the following responses.

Skin changes: The skin may feel tense and show resistance to gliding strokes. It may be slightly damp as a result of perspiration from sympathetic facilitation, causing the therapist's hand to stick or drag.

Temperature changes: The temperature in a local area increases with acute dysfunction but decreases with ischemia, which indicates fibrotic changes in the tissues.

Edema: Edema is an impression of fullness and a spongy feel in the tissues. With chronic dysfunction, edema gradually is replaced by fibrotic (connective tissue) changes.

Deep palpation: During deep palpation, the therapist establishes contact with the deeper fibers of the soft tissues and explores them for any of the following:

Immobility
Tenderness
Edema
Deep muscle tension
Fibrotic changes
Interosseous changes

Assessment and intervention related to trigger points must not be done for extended periods. Because of the nature of the syndrome and the irritation involved, 10 minutes is sufficient time to spend on trigger points and intervention should be incorporated into a more general approach, such as full-body massage.

Methods used to treat trigger points should progress from the least invasive (i.e., doing nothing specific) to the most invasive (i.e., deep transverse friction). This condition can be addressed in many ways. One approach is to do nothing specific to the trigger point but instead to use the symptom intensity of the trigger point as pre-assessment and post-assessment. Because trigger points are a condition, if the reasons for their development are removed, the trigger point activity should decline.

All the basic neuromuscular techniques, including muscle energy techniques (see Chapter 10) deal effectively with trigger points if the hyperirritable area within a muscle is manipulated and then lengthened, and connective tissue in the area is softened. Positional release with the appropriate lengthening is one of the most effective ways to treat trigger points.

Positional release with lengthening is the least invasive and gentlest method, often as effective as deep pressure and friction (Basu et al., 2018; Jain et al., 2020). Integrated muscle energy methods (Chapter 10) are more aggressive than positional release or direct manipulation but less aggressive than pressure or pinching methods. Gentler methods should be used first.

As a reminder, positional release consists of identifying the painful point and positioning the body in the easiest position that reduces the pain at the point. Positional release is the first step in the integrated muscle energy method, which then introduces muscle contraction before lengthening (see Chapter 10).

If the trigger point remains after the less invasive methods have been attempted, pressure techniques (i.e., inhibitory pressure) should be tried. Pressure techniques can end the hyperirritability by mechanical disruption of the sensory nerve endings mediating the trigger point activity. Pressing-based interventions can alleviate chronic inflammation, inhibit fibrosis, and promote skeletal muscle repair (Jaing et al., 2021; Rodríguez-Jiménez et al., 2022). The pressure may take the form of direct pressure, in which the trigger point is pressed against an underlying hard structure (bone), or pinching pressure, in which no bony tissue lies underneath, as in the "squeezing" of the sternocleidomastoid muscle.

When using the direct pressure technique, the therapist must hold the compression long enough to stimulate the spindle cells.

Done the pressure technique is done properly, the client usually senses referred pain within 10 seconds of the pressure application; therefore, the practitioner need not maintain pressure longer than 10 seconds when trying to locate the trigger point.

After the trigger point has been located, the time of applied pressure is different from the time used to locate the trigger point. Chaitow recommended a procedure of gradually intensifying pressure, building up to 8 seconds, and then repeating the process for up to 30 seconds or as long as 2 minutes. The procedure should end when the client reports that the referred pain has stopped or when the therapist feels a "release" in the trigger point tissue.

Chaitow also recommended variable pressure, rather than constantly held pressure from beginning to end, to prevent further irritation of the trigger area. Learners should not misinterpret this idea of variable pressure; it is not a "bouncing" in and out of the tissue, but providing a careful change of pressure for a specific purpose, reflecting the therapist's sensitivity to what is happening as the tissue responds. The therapist applies more pressure as the tissue relaxes, thus accepting more pressure. When the therapist senses increased tension, pressure is reduced.

As an alternative, transverse frictioning over the trigger point can be effective, followed by lengthening. This method is beneficial if the massage therapist suspects that the connective tissue around the trigger point has become dense and/or fibrotic.

Travell recommended that after treating the trigger point with pressure methods, the practitioner should stimulate circulation to the local area with circular friction, kneading, and/or vibratory massage techniques. Localized treatment of the muscle should always end with lengthening, whether passive or active, of the affected muscle.

Travell and Chaitow agreed that gradual, gentle lengthening to reset the normal resting length of the neuromuscular mechanism of a muscle must follow interventions. Incomplete restoration of the full length of the muscle means incomplete relief of pain. Failure to lengthen the area results in the eventual return of the original symptoms. Muscle energy approaches are more effective than passive stretching in achieving the proper response. They enable the muscle to "learn" that it can now return to a fuller resting length and more complete range of motion. Trigger points in deep layers of muscle or in a muscle that is difficult to lengthen by moving the body are addressed with local bend, shear, and torsion techniques.

After treating a trigger point, the practitioner should search the target (referred) area to uncover and deal with satellite or embryonic trigger points. Immediately after treatment, moist heat (a hot towel) over the region is soothing and useful. The area requires rest for a few days and avoidance of all stressful activity (C. Fernández-de-las-Peñas in Chaitow, 2014, pp. 253-260).

Deciding Which Trigger Points to Treat

Trigger points in the muscle belly usually are found in short, concentrically contracted muscles. Trigger points located near the attachments usually are found in eccentrically long, inhibited muscles acting as antagonists to overly facilitated muscles. Muscle contractions may serve compensation responses. The best course is to address trigger point activity in the short tissues first and see if trigger points in the long muscles and attachments resolve. The goal is balanced normalization of muscle posture interactions. A **latent trigger point** is one that exists but does not refer pain actively. Latent trigger points can influence muscle activation patterns, resulting in poorer muscle coordination and balance, exaggerated sensations of stiffness, restricted movement, and weakness. The sequence for addressing trigger points is as follows:

1. Those that are most painful and that reproduce familiar symptoms (active trigger points)
2. Those most medial
3. Those in the short tissue
4. Those in the muscle belly
5. Those in the surrounding tissue (latent trigger points)

As seen with the previous skills, the actual application of trigger point intervention methods is fairly basic. Increased proficiency is required related to assessment, analyzation of appropriateness and intensity of treatment, and choice of methods. As with myofascial methods, intervention application is deceptively simple, especially when the client's condition is multifaceted and complex. Often more than one method is required in these cases. Trigger point treatment is a good example of integration of multiple methods. Effective intervention involves use of several treatment protocols, massage manipulations, muscle energy techniques, stretching methods, and hydrotherapy applications (Fig. 12.15) (Proficiency Exercise 12.5).

Neuromuscular Therapy

Before ending this grouping of approaches, let's review the concept of neuromuscular therapy. A distinction must be made between the terms *neuromuscular techniques* and *neuromuscular therapy*. All massage methods can be used as neuromuscular techniques. Neuromuscular therapy (NMT) is a specialized form of manual therapy within the scope of practice of massage therapy. The European version continues to be practiced as originally developed. An alteration of that system is called the American version. Neuromuscular therapy enhances the function of joints, muscles, and the general arthrokinematics of the body. It covers six basic elements that cause pain:

- Postural distortion
- Biomechanical dysfunction
- Trigger points
- Nerve compression/entrapment
- Ischemia
- Postural distortion

These six areas are addressed using massage as described in this textbook, especially in Chapters 10 and 11 and this chapter. It is difficult to make a distinction between a massage therapist using neuromuscular techniques and a neuromuscular therapist aside from general massage therapy not being used in a neuromuscular therapist's treatment. Those that use the title "neuromuscular therapist" are typically licensed as massage therapists.

ASIAN BODYWORK METHODS

SECTION OBJECTIVES

Chapter objectives covered in this section:

9. Explain the fundamental concepts of Asian bodywork and incorporate the simple application of acupuncture and acupressure methods into massage therapy.
10. Compare shiatsu and Thai massage and incorporate mat methods into massage.

Using the information presented in this section, the student will be able to perform the following:

- Explain the basic physiology of acupuncture points and the effects of acupuncture.
- Locate an acupuncture point.
- Use simple methods to normalize acupuncture points.
- Compare the theory of shiatsu to the meridian theory of traditional Chinese medicine.
- Compare the application of shiatsu to the application of Thai massage.
- Integrate mat methods from shiatsu and Thai massage into a massage session.

The richness of Asian health theory and the unity of its body-mind-spirit connection are based on the energy of life. Life force, called *chi* (or *qi/ri*) energy, flows through the body in interconnected pathways like the streams, rivers, lakes, and oceans of the earth. When *chi* energy flows freely and unobstructed, all of life's processes are balanced. However, if obstruction or stagnation develops, dysfunction and disease result.

The Tao, or "Way," supports the balanced functioning of all the senses and teaches a lifestyle of moderation that avoids both deprivation and excess. *Chi* energy is the vital force of life, and Tao is the path or way to sustain the *chi* energy.

Some people are concerned about taking pieces from the totality expressed in the Tao. Western science has lifted techniques from this simultaneously simple and complex, all-encompassing system. Very often, a technique separated from its theoretical basis is less effective. Although techniques can stimulate physiologic functions, they cannot support the human experience. The small section presented in this textbook is based on an extremely limited part of the total Asian medicine system. As you begin to develop an understanding of these methods, be mindful and respectful of the larger body of knowledge from which they have been taken (Masunaga and Ohashi, 1977; Gunn, 1992; Ohashi, 1993; Wiseman and

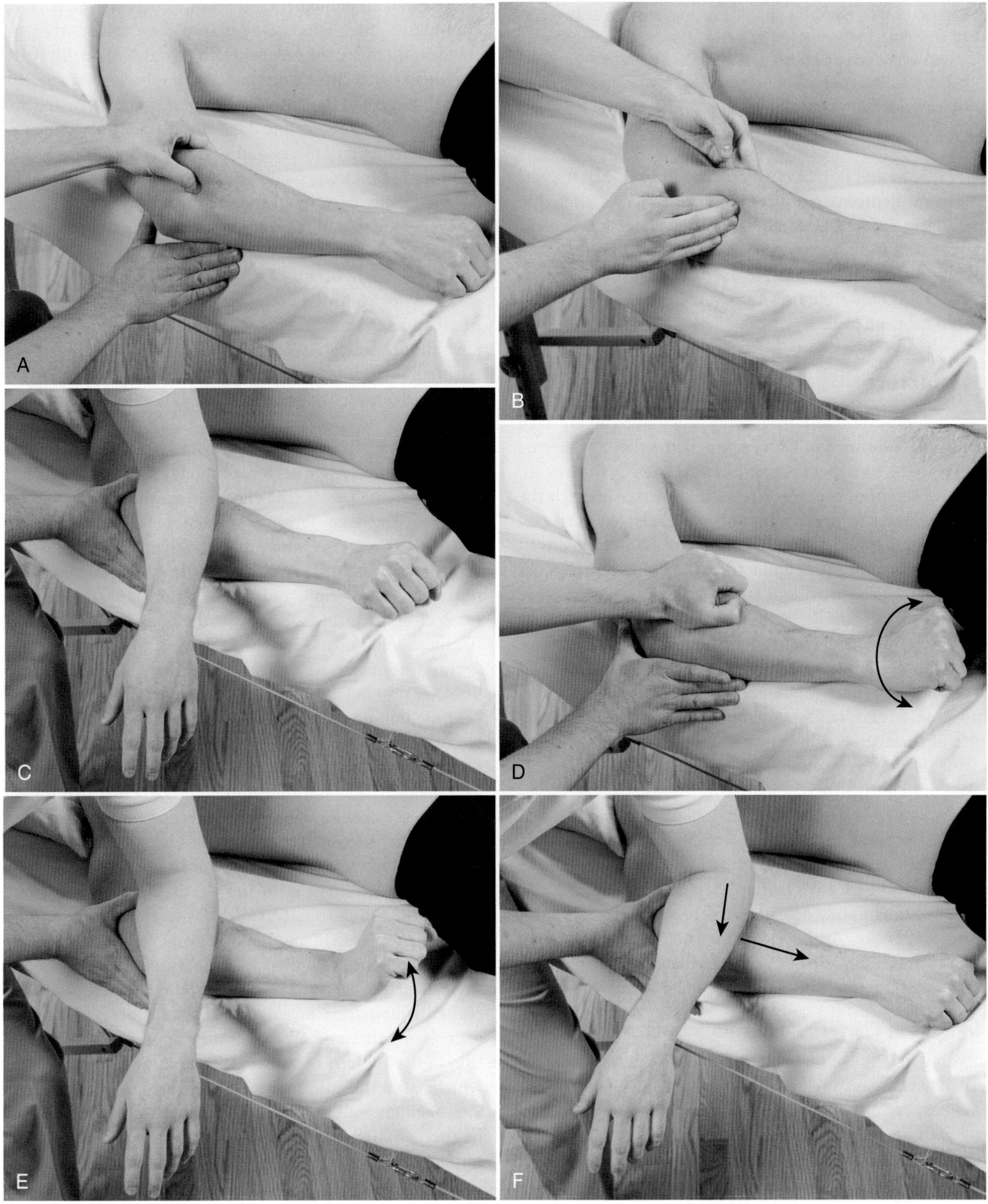

FIG. 12.15 Treatment sequence in a trigger point. A, Location of a trigger point. **B,** Holding at ease. **C,** Broad-based compression to area. **D,** Pinching/squeezing compression with movement active or passive. **E,** Active release. **F,** Direct pressure, then glide.

PROFICIENCY EXERCISE 12.5

1. Place a dried pea under a 0.5-inch piece of foam. Locate the pea with light and deep palpation.
2. Working with a partner, use light palpation to locate an area of suspected trigger point activity. After an area has been found, use deep palpation to find the exact area of the trigger point. Then use the methods described in this section to normalize the area.

Feng, 1997; Yu and Rose, 1999; Veith and Rose, 2002). Aspects of Asian medicine systems are similar to concepts related to homeostasis. Comparisons are helpful in understanding the wide varieties of massage approaches. Often techniques and application are similar, while philosophies of justification differ. Rarely is there a right or wrong way. Central is the positive intent to help and heal.

Acupuncture

Acupuncture is increasingly gaining acceptance by Western science. It is a branch of Chinese medicine that has proved effective in the treatment of many diseases and dysfunctions. The exact origin of acupuncture is unknown. Although the process remains a mystery in some respects, Western science is close to validating its phenomena. Whatever physiologic factors underlie acupuncture, the beneficial changes that occur clearly provide a sound basis for acupuncture treatment.

Acupuncture can be defined as the stimulation of certain points with needles inserted along meridians (channels) and *ah shi* (meaning "ouch") points outside the meridians. Interestingly, *ah shi* and traditional acupuncture points have a high degree of correlation with trigger points. The purpose of acupuncture is to prevent and modify the perception of pain (analgesia) or to normalize physiologic functions.

Acupressure is a modified version of acupuncture that substitutes pressure for needle insertion. The results of acupressure are not as dramatic as those of acupuncture, but the technique is still effective if frequency and pressure is sufficient. The human body has hundreds of acupuncture points. Approximately 360 of the most used points are located on 12 paired and 2 unpaired central meridians. These meridian patterns are similar to the meridians used in shiatsu.

Meridians in Chinese Bodywork Systems

According to Chinese theory, the meridians are internally associated with organs and externally associated with the surface of the head, trunk, and extremities. **Meridians** seem to correlate with nerve tracts located within fascial grooves (Cunningham, 2002; Dorsher, 2009). The primo-vascular system is gaining attention as a possible physical aspect of the meridian system. The primo-vascular system is a circulatory system composed of very tiny vessels in and around nervous tissue, organs, fascia, and blood and lymph vessels. These tiny vessels may facilitate numerous interconnected functions, including how some cancers metastasize (Lim et al., 2013; Soh et al., 2013; Kovich, 2019; Kim, 2022).

Yin and Yang

The Chinese perspective considers body functions in terms of balance between complementary forces. These complements, which often are thought of as opposites, actually are parts of a continuum. A circle is a good example; no matter where you stand, you can see the other side. In this idea of duality, we often forget that a circle is one concept; it is broken into sections only through the limitation of our perceptions. *Yin* and *yang* are representations of this concept. *Yin* and *yang* functions are complementary pieces of the whole. When all parts of the continuum function equally and in harmony, the natural balance of health exists in all areas of the body, mind, and spirit. Conversely, if part of the continuum becomes out of sync with the rest, stress is put on the entire circle. Thus, imbalances and symptoms might occur.

Physiologically, the body is a closed system. There cannot be areas of "too much" energy in the body without reciprocal areas of "not enough" energy. Just as muscles work in pairs and facilitate and inhibit each other, so do meridians. The body has *yin* meridians, or channels, and *yang* meridians, or channels (Fig. 12.16).

Yin meridians are associated with parasympathetic autonomic nervous system responses and the solid organs essential to life (e.g., the heart). The energy is considered "female" and a "negative" charge. Terminology and metaphor become confused with the terms *female* and *negative*. In this context, the terms mean that the functions draw in energy of sustenance, nurturing, restoration, and reproduction. *Yin* meridians are located on the inside soft areas of the body and flow outward (Chinese anatomic position with the arms lifted into the air).

Yang meridians are associated with sympathetic autonomic nervous system responses and the hollow organs which support life but are not essential (e.g., the stomach). The energy is considered "male" and a "positive" charge. In metaphor these terms mean the energy functions in short bursts related to transformation and transportation. *Yang* meridians are located on the outside areas of the body and flow inward.

Chinese philosophy teaches that a balance must exist between the forces of *yin* and *yang* for health to exist. This balance changes according to the weather, seasons, and other rhythms of nature (Box 12.13).

The patterns that acupuncture points make on the body's surface have been charted by practitioners of acupuncture for centuries. They have been grouped together in lines (called *channels* or *meridians*) and have been allocated to organs or functions on which they appear to act. In addition to the 12 pairs of bilateral meridians are two meridians which lie on the anterior and posterior midline of the trunk and head, as well as various extra meridians. Other points in the ear surfaces, the hands, and the face have specific reflex effects.

The 12 Main Meridians

The 12 main meridians are bilateral, symmetrically distributed lines of acupuncture points with affinity for or effects on the functions or organs for which they are named (Box 12.14).

Abundant evidence indicates the existence of reflex links between acupuncture points and specific organs and func-

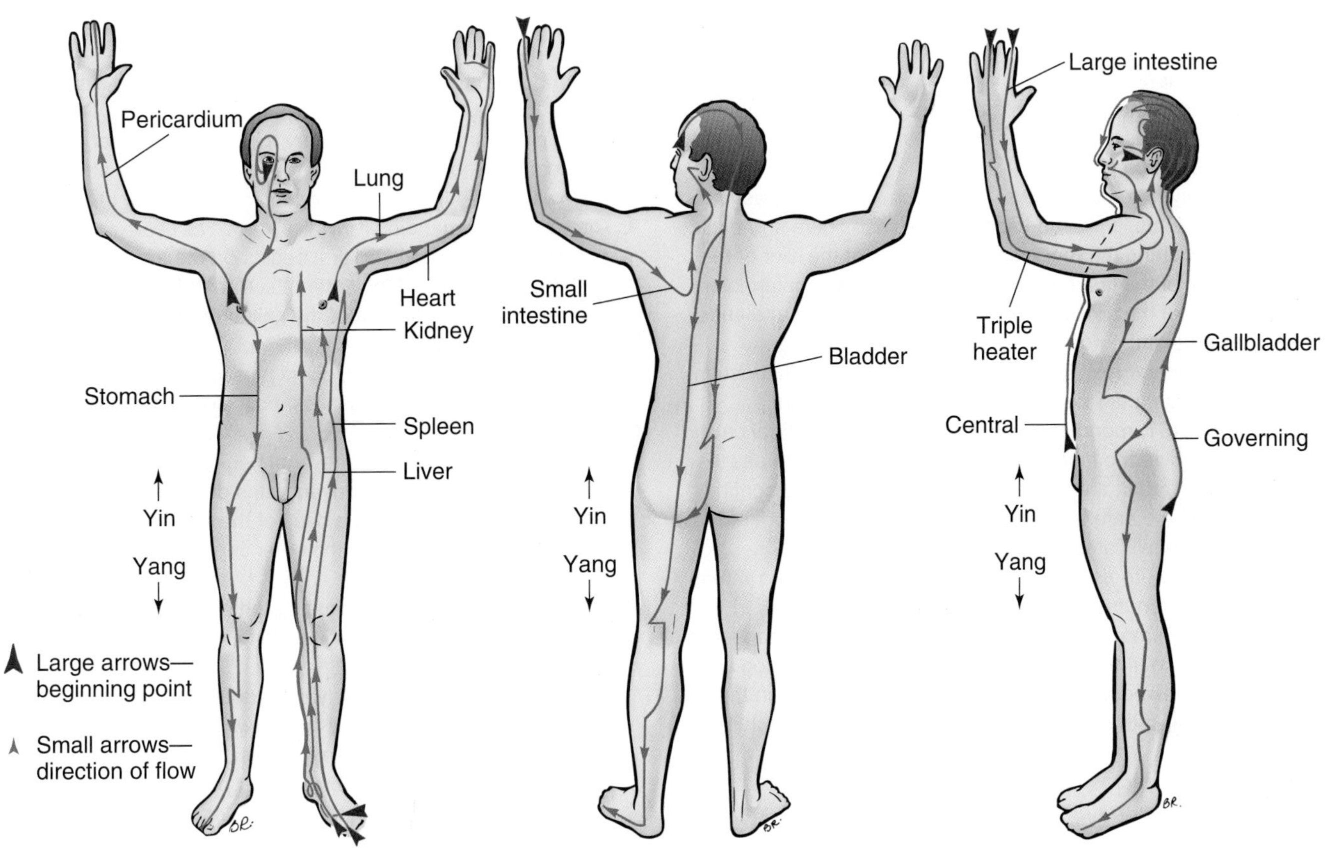

FIG. 12.16 Typical location of meridians. Meridians tend to follow nerves.

Box 12.13 Yin and Yang Meridians

Yin Meridians	Yang Meridians
Pericardium	Triple heater
Liver	Gallbladder
Kidney	Bladder
Heart	Small intestine
Spleen	Stomach
Lung	Large intestine

tions. However, nobody really knows what an acupuncture point is. Information derived from thousands of years of practice exists about acupuncture points, including their nature, structure, function, interrelationships, and interactions. Nevertheless, reliable authorities in Chinese medicine agree acupuncture points are mysterious. Acupuncture points are components of a system and have reflexive characteristics related to this system. They reflect information, energy, states of being, and existence related to the whole and its component parts, including body and mind. The system that comprises the acupuncture points is likewise a reflexive system of information generation and conveyance. In traditional Chinese medicine, this system is known as *jing luo*, usually translated into English as either "meridians" or "channels and network vessels."

The system of acupuncture points can be visualized as a matrix that passes through the body, connecting all its parts and serving as an energy and communications grid that generates, propagates, stores, and releases information and force related to the body and its various components. All parts of the body permeate and connect by means of the *jing luo* system, which is, in short, the fundamental infrastructure of Chinese anatomy and physiology. The similarity between this description and current research on fascial and primo-vascular systems is exciting.

The Chinese word-concept that we translate into English as "acupuncture point" is composed of elements conveying the sense of "body transport (of communication) hole." It is written *shu xue*. Functionally, acupuncture points seem to have two most basic functions: they open and they close. The names of the many points include words that mean "gate," "pass," or "door." In opening, they release information and energy. In closing, they store it.

Channels contain and convey *chi* and *xue* (blood). The basic nature of *chi* is the manifestation of transformation. From the Chinese viewpoint, everything sensed or experienced is a form of *chi*.

Yin-yang theory is one of the oldest doctrines in Chinese culture. The words *yin* and *yang* originally were pictographic representations of the shady and sunny sides, respectively, of a mountain or a hill. They came to represent two primordial forces that were the fundamental constituents of the universe and everything in it. *Chi* is the result of the interplay between *yin* and *yang*. *Yin* and *yang* mix together, and *chi* issues forth; when *yin* and *yang* were separated from the singularity at the beginning of existence, the resulting potential gave rise to *chi*.

Box 12.14 The 12 Main Meridians and Associated Acupuncture Points

1. **Lung (L) meridian** (yin) begins on the lateral aspect of the chest, in the first intercostal space. It passes up the anterolateral aspect of the arm to the root of the thumbnail (11 acupuncture points).

Pathologic symptoms: Fullness in the chest, cough, asthma, sore throat, colds, chills, and aching in the shoulders and back.

2. **Large intestine (LI) meridian** (yang) starts at the root of the fingernail of the first finger. It passes down the posterolateral aspect of the arm over the shoulder to the face and ends at the side of the nostril (20 acupuncture points).

Pathologic symptoms: Abdominal pain, diarrhea, constipation, nasal discharge, pain along the course of the meridian.

3. **Stomach (ST) meridian** (yang) starts below the orbital cavity and runs over the face and up to the forehead, then passes down the throat, the thorax, and the abdomen and continues down the anterior thigh and leg to end at the root of the second toenail (lateral side) (45 acupuncture points).

Pathologic symptoms: Bloating, edema, vomiting, sore throat, pain along the course of the meridian.

4. **Spleen (SP) meridian** (yin) originates at the medial aspect of the great toe. It travels up the internal aspect of the leg and thigh to the abdomen and thorax, where it finishes on the axillary line in the sixth intercostal space (21 acupuncture points).

Pathologic symptoms: Gastric discomfort, bloating, vomiting, weakness, heaviness of the body, pain along the course of the meridian.

5. **Heart (H) meridian** (yin) begins in the axilla and runs up the anteromedial aspect of the arm to end at the root of the little fingernail (medial aspect) (9 acupuncture points).

Pathologic symptoms: Dry throat, thirst, cardiac area pain, pain along the course of the meridian.

6. **Small intestine (SI) meridian** (yang) starts at the root of the small fingernail (lateral aspect) and travels down the posteromedial aspect of the arm and over the shoulder to the face, where it terminates in front of the ear (19 acupuncture points).

Pathologic symptoms: Pain in the lower abdomen, deafness, swelling in the face, sore throat, pain along the course of the meridian.

7. **Bladder (B) meridian** (yang) starts at the inner canthus, then ascends and passes over the head and down the back and leg to terminate at the root of the nail on the little toe (lateral aspect) (67 acupuncture points).

Pathologic symptoms: Urinary problems, mania, headaches, eye problems, pain along the course of the meridian.

8. **Kidney (K) meridian** (yin) starts on the sole of the foot, ascends the medial aspect of the leg, and runs up the front of the abdomen to finish on the thorax just below the clavicle (27 acupuncture points).

Pathologic symptoms: Dyspnea, dry tongue, sore throat, edema, constipation, diarrhea, motor impairment and atrophy of the lower extremities, pain along the course of the meridian.

9. **Circulation (C) meridian** (yin) (also known as heart constrictor or the pericardium) begins on the thorax lateral to the nipple, runs up the anterior surface of the arm, and terminates at the root of the nail of the middle finger (9 acupuncture points).

Pathologic symptoms: Angina, chest pressure, heart palpitations, irritability, restlessness, pain along the course of the meridian.

10. **Triple heater (TH) meridian** (yang) begins at the nail root of the ring finger (ulnar side) and runs down the posterior aspect of the arm, over the back of the shoulder, and around the ear to finish at the outer aspect of the eyebrow (23 acupuncture points).

Pathologic symptoms: Abdominal distortion, edema, deafness, tinnitus, sweating, sore throat, pain along the course of the meridian.

11. **Gallbladder (GB) meridian** (yang) starts at the outer canthus and runs backward and forward over the head, passing over the back of the shoulder, and down the lateral aspect of the thorax and abdomen. It passes to the hip area and then down the lateral aspect of the leg to terminate on the fourth toe (44 acupuncture points).

Pathologic symptoms: Bitter taste in the mouth, dizziness, headache, ear problems, pain along the course of the meridian.

12. **Liver (LIV) meridian** (yin) begins on the great toe, runs up the medial aspect of the leg, up the abdomen, and terminates on the costal margin (vertically below the nipple) (14 acupuncture points).

Pathologic symptoms: Lumbago, digestive problems, retention of urine, pain in the lower abdomen, pain along the course of the meridian.

Midline Meridians

The body has two midline meridians:

The conception (or central) vessel (CV) meridian (yin) starts in the center of the perineum and runs up the midline of the anterior aspect of the body to terminate just below the lower lip (24 acupuncture points); it is responsible for all yin meridians.

The governor vessel (GV) meridian (yang) starts at the coccyx and runs up the center of the spine and over the midline of the head, terminating on the front of the upper gum (28 acupuncture points); it is responsible for all yang meridians.

The Five Elements

Chinese medical thinking is based on the relationship of the human being with nature. The five elements of nature become a basis for examination, diagnosis, and treatment to support health and relieve disease. The concepts of health parallel natural occurrences of life force energy as represented in the five elements. The five elements are wood, fire, earth, metal, and water. Each organ is represented by an element, and each element has qualities of colors, sounds, smells, fluid secretion, anatomy, emotions, time, seasons, numbers, flavor, foods, planets, moon phases, dreams, and more (Fig. 12.17 and Table 12.7).

The human being reflects the universe, and the five elements become a metaphor for the life processes of people. The qualities of the five elements become the basis for life, and in Chinese medicine are the basis for examination, diagnosis, and treatment. Each element is a *yin-yang* relationship of two meridians.

- Earth—spleen/stomach
- Metal—lung/large intestine

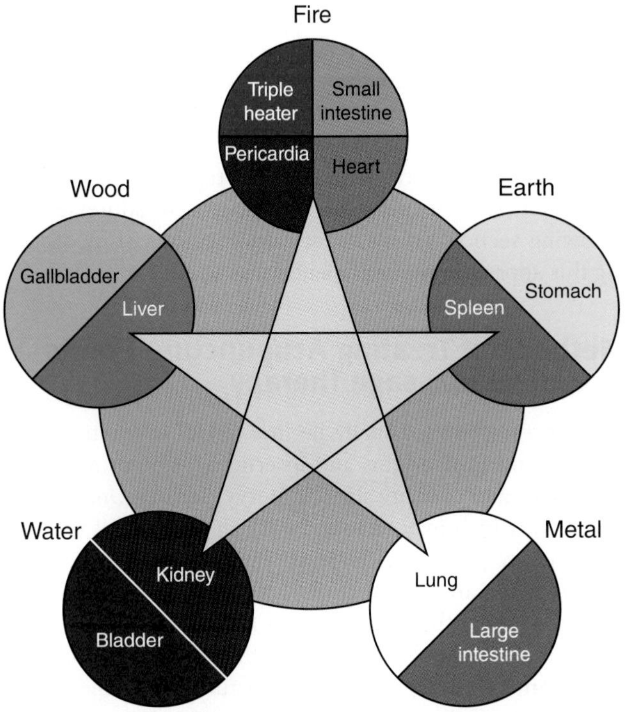

FIG. 12.17 The wheel illustrates the relationships connecting the five elements and the organs of the body. The center star depicts the *ko*, or control cycle. Wood controls earth by covering it or holding it in place with roots. Earth controls water by damming it or containing it. Water controls fire by dousing or extinguishing it. Fire controls metal by melting it. Metal controls wood by cutting it. The next set of lines that form a circle depict the sheng, or creative cycle. Water engenders wood. Wood fuels fire. Fire creates earth (ashes). Earth engenders metal. Metal engenders water. The five circles indicate the solid (*yin*) on the inside and hollow (*yang*) organs on the outside that are associated with the elements. Movement around the wheel (Fire-> Earth-> Metal-> Water->Wood-> Fire->) is the flow or support cycle, the clockwise movement from one element to the next.

- Water—kidney/bladder
- Wood—liver/gallbladder
- Fire—heart/small intestine, pericardium/triple heater

The outside circle of the five-element figure represents the *sheng*, or creative cycle. The metaphor is as follows: during the birth phase of the universe, wood came to represent all that grows. Wood can be fuel for fire and the ash matures as earth. As continued breakdown occurs, the metal, or inorganic, separates from the organic, with water representing death and rebirth of wood, and so the cycle continues. On the inside, a five-pointed star represents the *ko*, or control cycles. The dynamic balance between creation and control is representative of homeostatic mechanisms in Western science and is explained in the metaphor as follows:

- Wood controls earth by penetrating it with roots.
- Earth controls water by containing it (a pond or lake).
- Water controls fire by extinguishing it.
- Fire controls metal by melting it.
- Metal controls wood by chopping it.

These elegant metaphors in relation to the natural world are easy to understand and become the basis for understanding health and well-being, in addition to methods for assessment and treatment. If processes become disturbed in either the creative or the control cycle, homeostasis is disrupted.

Like *yin* and *yang*, the five elements are categories of quality and relationship, seen as phenomena in the universe as the products of movement and mutation. These elements represent qualities that relate to each other in specific ways, and metaphorically provided images ancient theorists used to organize their thinking about the physical world (Veith and Rose, 2002).

Table 12.7 Qualities of the Five Elements

Element					
Phase	Metal	Earth	Fire	Water	Wood
Yin	Lung	Spleen	Heart	Kidney	Liver
Yang	Large intestine	Stomach	Triple heater	Bladder, small intestine	Gallbladder
Sense	Smell	Taste	Speech	Hearing	Sight
Organ	Nose	Mouth, lips	Tongue	Ears	Eyes
Liquid	Mucus	Saliva	Sweat	Urine	Tears
Color	White	Yellow	Red	Blue/black	Green
Expression	Weeping	Singing	Laughing	Groaning	Shouting
Extreme emotion	Grief, anxiety	Worry, reminiscence	Shock, overjoyed	Fear	Anger
Balanced emotion	Openness, receptivity	Sympathy, empathy	Joy, compassion	Resolution, trust	Assertion, motivation
Taste	Pungent, spicy	Sweet	Bitter, burned	Salty	Sour
Season	Fall	Indian summer	Summer	Winter	Spring
Related activity	Releasing	Thinking	Inspiration	Willpower and intimacy	Planning and decision making
Times	Lung, 3–5 AM Large intestine, 5–7 AM	Stomach, 7–9 AM Spleen, 9–11 AM	Heart, 11 a.m.–1 PM Small intestine, 1-3 PM	Bladder, 3–5 PM Kidney, 5–7 PM Triple heater, 9–11 PM	Gallbladder, 11 PM–1 AM Pericardium, 7–9 PM Liver, 1–3 AM

The assessment process leading to a diagnosis then influences the treatment plan. *Si zhen* is the term for the *four methods of diagnosis:*

- *Wang zhen* is diagnosis by observation, which includes observation of the patient's complexion, skin color, physical build, development, nutrition, and tongue
- *Wen zhen* is diagnosis by hearing and smelling
- *Wen zhen* is diagnosis by interrogation
- *Qie zhen* is pulse-taking and palpation

The four examinations provide the raw data for diagnosis. It is essential that the data from all four examinations be correlated to arrive at a complete diagnosis.

Tui na is a general name for massage. The word *tui* means "push, push forward, promote." The word *na* means to "hold, to grasp." *Tui na* thus means pushing and holding (i.e., massage).

An mo is another general term for massage. The word *an* means "press, push down, keep one's hand on (something)." The word *mo* means "to rub, scrape, touch." *An mo* is a method of preventing and treating diseases using various massage techniques and methods and of undertaking manipulation and adjustment of the joints and the extremities. More specifically, *an mo* is one of the eight manipulations used in bone setting to relax muscle tissue, dissipate blood stasis, and reduce swelling.

Health Preservation and Exercise

An important part of Chinese medicine is the discipline of preserving health and extending life. Foremost among the various methods that fall in this category are exercise and disciplines aimed at cultivating the inborn treasures of the body, mind, and spirit.

- *Qi gong*, or breathing exercise, refers to a variety of traditional practices consisting of physical, mental, and spiritual exercises. The regulation of the breath (*qi*) is a common feature of such exercise methods. The word *gong* means "achievement, result; skill; work; exercise." It is composed of two radicals. The radical on the left is also pronounced *gong* and means "work." The radical on the right is the word *li* and means "strength or force." *Qi gong* can be understood as exercise designed to strengthen and harmonize the *chi*, regulate the body and mind, and calm the spirit.
- *Tai ji quan (tai chi)* is both a martial and a meditative art. It therefore has complementary aspects that combine in a comprehensive discipline of physical culture and mental and spiritual discipline. The word *quan* means "fist; boxing; punch."
- *Dao yin*. This discipline involves meditation and breathing exercises that seek to develop the ability to lead and guide the *chi* throughout the body for the benefit of the spirit, mind, and body. *Dao yin* exercises have a long history in China. They consist of bending, stretching, and otherwise mobilizing the extremities and the joints to free the flow of *chi* throughout the whole body. Like *Qi gong*, *dao yin* emphasizes control of the breath (*chi*). *Dao yin* also includes self-massage techniques that relieve fatigue and prolong life by activating and harmonizing the circulation of blood and *chi*. These techniques also stress the development of strength in the muscles and bones.

The vastness of the Asian medicine model and its elegance are far beyond the scope of this textbook; therefore, no attempt is made to present scaled-down versions of these systems. The learner is directed to the reference list for sources of further study. Learners who are drawn to these concepts are encouraged to explore them in depth as they continue their path of knowledge.

During the natural course of therapeutic massage, the physical aspects of meridians and points are addressed. The following section briefly investigates methods of incorporating this approach into therapeutic massage.

Methods of Treating Acupuncture Points as Part of Massage Therapy

Acupuncture points usually lie in a fascial division between muscles and near origins and insertions. A point feels like a small hole, and pressure elicits a "nervy" feeling. Unlike a trigger point, which may be found only on one side of the body, acupuncture points are bilateral (i.e., found on both sides of the body) and are located on the central, or governing, meridian. To confirm the location of an acupuncture point, locate the point in the same place on the other side of the body.

To stimulate a hypoactive acupuncture point (one with insufficient energy), use a short vibrating or tapping action. This method is effective if the area is sluggish or if a specific body function needs to be stimulated.

To sedate a hyperactive acupuncture point (one with too much energy) to reduce pain, elicit the pain response within the point itself. Use a sustained holding pressure until the painful energy dissipates, and the body's own natural painkillers are released into the bloodstream (Tappan and Benjamin, 2004). The pressure techniques are similar to those used for trigger points; however, an acupuncture point does not need to be lengthened and stretched after treatment.

As with other reflex points, if you are unsure whether the acupuncture point is hypoactive or hyperactive, alternately apply both techniques and allow the body to adjust to the intervention (Proficiency Exercise 12.6).

Asian methods work via physiologic reasons through the neuroendocrine and fascial systems. Particular effects can be demonstrated after acupuncture treatment. Some of these effects involve alteration of the function of organs or systems. An analgesic effect and an anesthetic effect also are seen. It is not necessary to hold that imbalance between *yin* and *yang* (the two equal and opposite forces of the universe, which act through *chi*) causes disease. Instead, the acupuncture benefit can be framed in terms of the body's homeostatic tendency, whereby a stable internal environment is maintained through the interaction of the various body processes and systems. For many years osteopaths and chiropractors have used reflex pressure techniques to assist the body in its efforts toward health. Many of the points used correspond with acupuncture points.

If one accepts that the body constantly strives for health, then one must agree that the body uses all helpful stimuli to that end. If this function can be assisted through acupuncture or manual pressure, the homeostatic interplay of organ systems will continue the work to the extent possible at that time (Fig. 12.18).

PROFICIENCY EXERCISE 12.6

1. Working with a partner, perform a massage that incorporates running the hand down each of the meridian grooves in the body. Stop at each depression/point you feel.
2. When you locate a point while performing this massage, decide whether the point needs to be stimulated with vibration or tapping or sedated with sustained direct pressure. How did you decide?

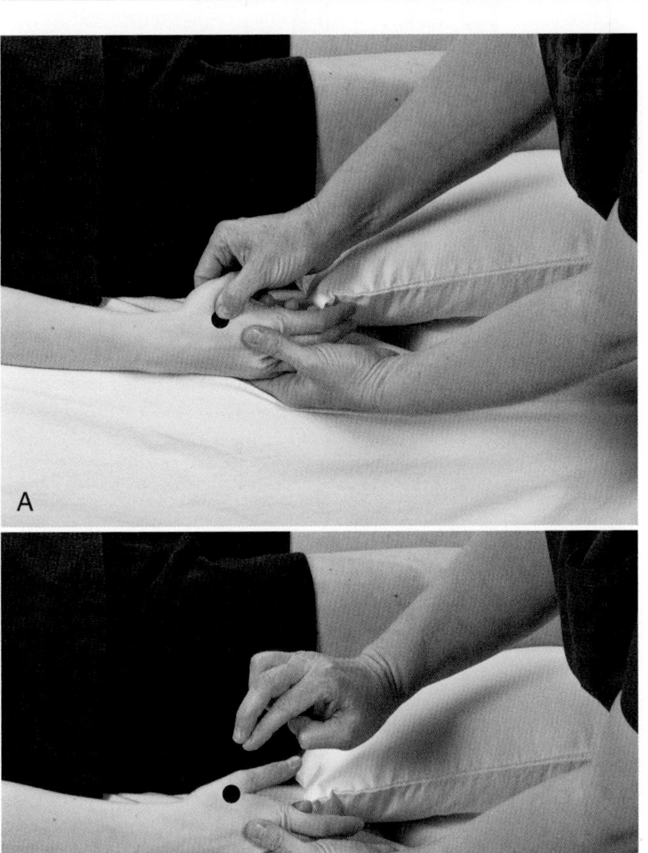

FIG. 12.18 Treatment of acupuncture points. A, Press, sedate. **B,** Tap, stimulate.

Acupuncture successfully induces the desired feeling of soreness and fullness that is a forerunner of the anesthetic effect (pain modulator). Electrophysiologic studies have shown that deep pressure applied to muscles and tendons has a definite inhibitory effect on the unit discharge of neurons in the nonspecific nucleus of the thalamus, which would support the claimed benefit of acupressure.

Pain relief may be the result of neutrally mediated changes in the brain's receptivity to nociceptive impulses, in addition to an effect of biochemical changes caused by the release of hormone-like substances both locally and generally.

Western research so far has produced no great breakthrough in our understanding of acupuncture, although Melzack and Wall have proposed the gate control theory and neuromatrix pain theory. Endogenous polypeptides that link to opiate receptors in the brain and central nervous system also offer an explanation for the acupuncture phenomenon. Regardless, skillful application of the method in beneficial and can easily be integrated into therapeutic massage.

Shiatsu

Shiatsu (finger pressure), which was developed in Japan, is one of the more familiar Asian bodywork systems. Shiatsu and acupressure sometimes are considered the same method. However, shiatsu is much broader in its application of methods and diagnosis. Shiatsu was recognized in Japan as a manipulative therapy about 70 years ago. Basically it is a form of massage in which the fingers are pressed onto particular points of the body to ease aches, pain, tension, fatigue, and symptoms of disease. These points, called *tsubo*, or acupuncture points, are located along the meridians described later in this section. One distinguishing method of shiatsu diagnosis is done through areas on the *hara* (abdomen or center) and the back. Pressure in these areas or along the meridians identifies energy flow (in Japanese, *ki*) as either *kyo* (under energy) or *jitsu* (over energy). Shiatsu restores balance by strengthening or stimulating (toning) the *kyo* and sedating the *jitsu*.

The traditional meridian system is the foundation of the shiatsu system (Figs. 12.19 and 12.20).

Thai Massage

Called Thai massage in the Western world, *nuad phaen boran* (the Thai term for the method) translates as "ancient massage" or "traditional massage." It can be traced to Thailand more than 2500 years ago from the Vajrayana or the Diamond Healing lineage of Tibet. It made its way to Thailand, where the Ayurvedic techniques and principles gradually became influenced by traditional Chinese medicine. For centuries, Thai massage was performed by monks as one component of Thai medicine. It combines elements of yoga, shiatsu, and acupressure, working with the energy pathways of the body and the therapy points located along these lines. Thai massage is believed to have been developed by Jivaka Kumar Bhaccha, physician to Buddha in India. The practice is deeply influenced by Indian Ayurveda and TCM.

Thai massage incorporates elements of mindfulness, gentle rocking, deep stretching, and rhythmic compression to create a singular healing experience. It uses assisted yoga *asanas* (yoga postures) to open the joints and relieve the tension in surrounding muscles, which allows *prana*, *chi*, or healing energy to move more freely through the body. Thai massage is also called Thai yoga massage because the therapist uses their hands, knees, legs, and feet to move the client into a series of yoga-like stretches. Thai massage is performed on a mat on the floor, and the client wears light, loose-fitting clothing. The session can last 1 to 3 hours or longer. The treatment style is slow, deliberate, and gentle. Thai massage is more energizing and rigorous than more classic forms of massage (Fig. 12.21).

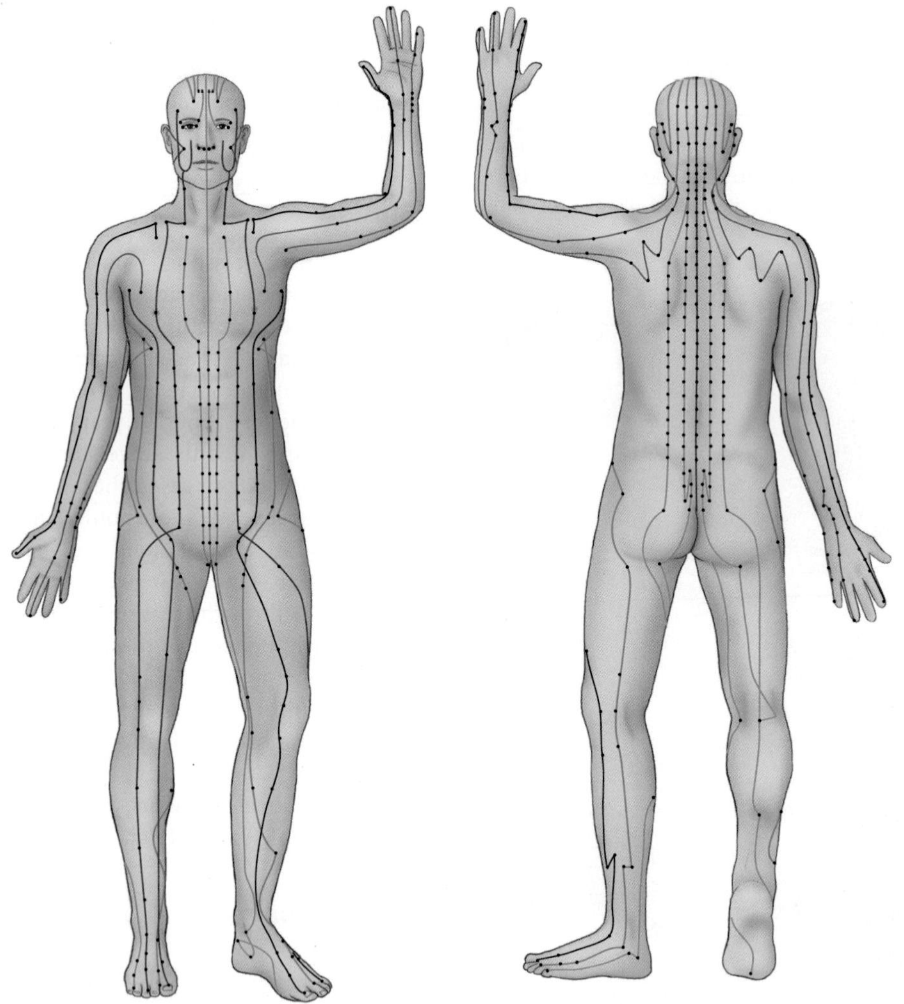

FIG. 12.19 The main meridian pathways of shiatsu. From Anderson SK: *The practice of shiatsu*, St. Louis, 2008, Mosby.

AYURVEDA

SECTION OBJECTIVES

Chapter objective covered in this section:

11. Explore the healing philosophy of Ayurveda.

Using the information presented in this section, the student will be able to perform the following:

- Identify and understand introductory Ayurvedic terminology.
- Locate the major chakras and explain the qualities of each.
- Explain and use color as a therapeutic element during massage.

Ayurveda is a system of health and medicine developed in India. The foundation of its theory base is similar to that of Asian systems. As with all the complementary systems presented in this chapter, Ayurveda is a distinct and rich body of knowledge. Massage professionals should be familiar with terms describing Ayurvedic principles of thought (Johari, 1996).

The word *Ayurveda* means "life knowledge" or "right living." Ayurveda is grounded as a body-mind-spirit system in the Vedic scriptures. The tridosha theory is unique to this system. A *dosha* is a body chemical pattern. When the doshas combine, they constitute the nature of every living organism. The three doshas are *vata* (wind), *pitta* (bile), and *kapha*

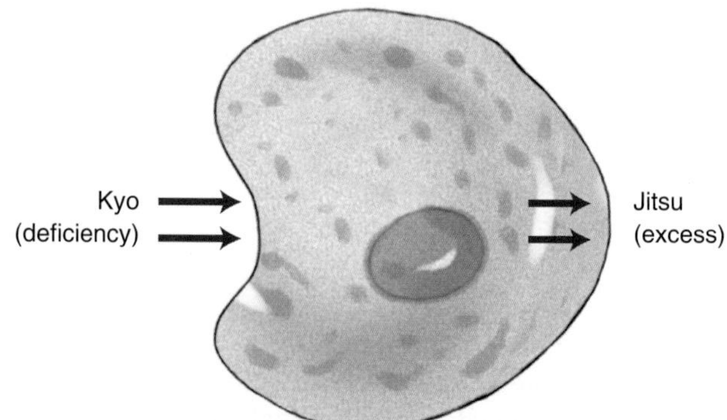

FIG. 12.20 Cell with kyo and *jitsu*. Every area of *jitsu* has a resulting area of *kyo*. Every area of *kyo* has a resulting area of *jitsu*. From Anderson SK: *The practice of shiatsu*, St. Louis, 2008, Mosby.

(mucus). These three combine to form the five elements (similar to Asian theory) of ether, air, fire, water, and earth.

Bones, flesh, skin, and nerves belong to the earth element. Semen, blood, fat, urine, mucus, saliva, and lymph belong to the water element. Hunger, thirst, temperature, sleep, intelligence, anger, hate, jealousy, and radiance belong to the fire

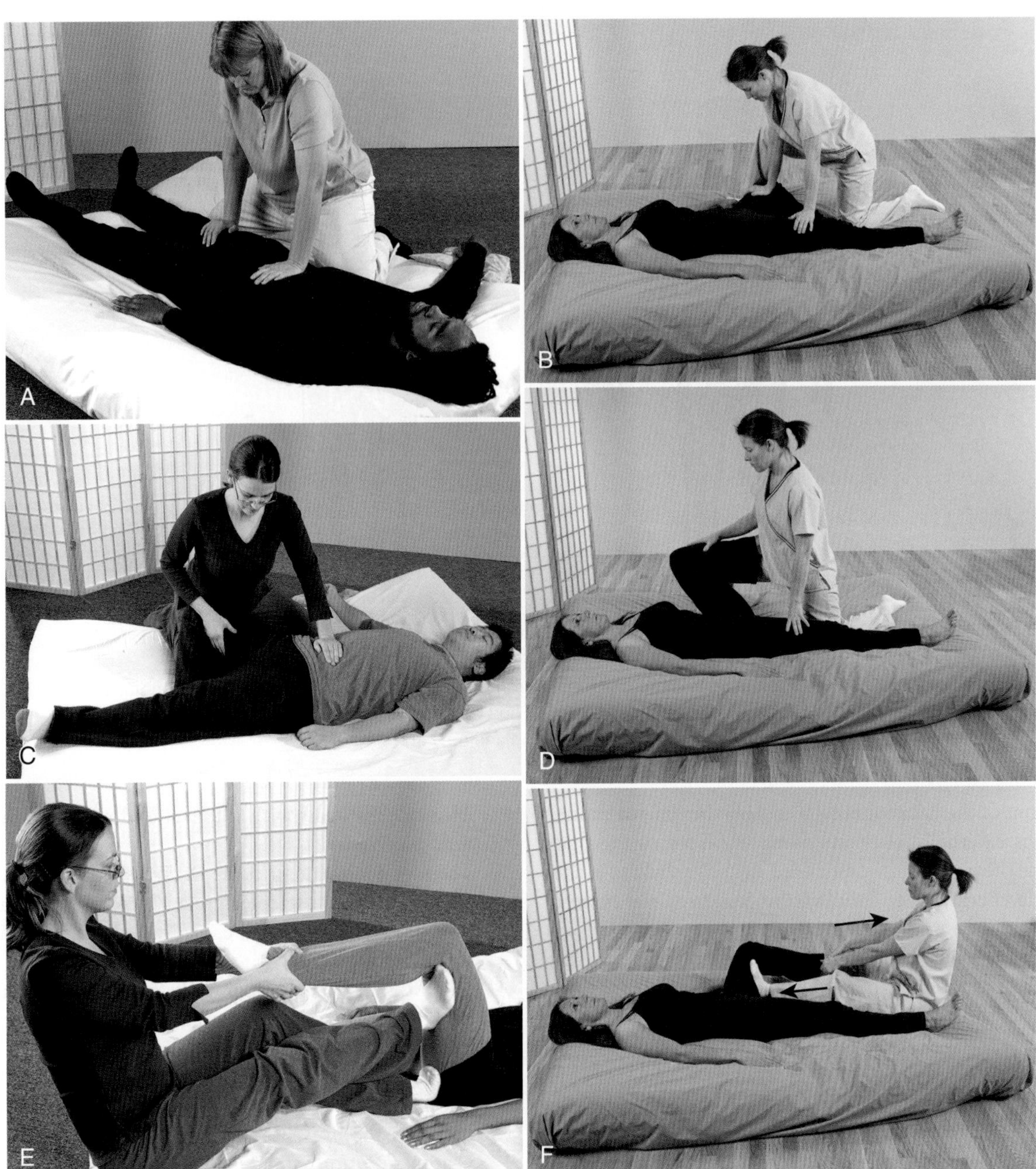

FIG. 12.21 Examples of shiatsu **A, C, E,** and Thai **B, D, F,** massage. **A, C,** and **E,** from Anderson SK: *The practice of shiatsu*, St. Louis, 2008, Mosby.

element. All movement, breathing, natural urges, sensory and motor functions, secretions, excretions, and transformation of tissues belong to the air element. Love, shyness, fear, and attachment belong to the ether element.

People display temperament based on the degree of influence or dominance of a particular dosha; this is considered an inherited genetic quality that influences a person through their entire life. The balance of function within the dosha system equates with health.

The points connected with this system are called *marmas*. There are about 100 marmas, which are concentrated at the junctions of muscles, vessels, ligaments, bones, and joints. In the Ayurvedic system these junctions form the seat of vital life force (in Hindi, *prana*). Marmas have a strong correlation with common trigger points and the location of the traditional meridians (Fig. 12.22).

In Ayurveda, chakras are considered the seven centers of the *prana*. They are located along the spinal column, interrelated with the nervous system and endocrine glands. These are subtle centers of consciousness that are the link between the universal source of intelligence and the human body. Chakras are wheels of energy, and they govern the various physical organs, in addition to etheric bodies, such as the emotional body (the feelings). Within every living body, although on the subtle rather than the gross or the physical level, there is said to be a series of energy fields or centers of consciousness, which in traditional Tantric teachings are called *chakras* (wheels) or *padmas* (lotuses). They are said to be located either along or

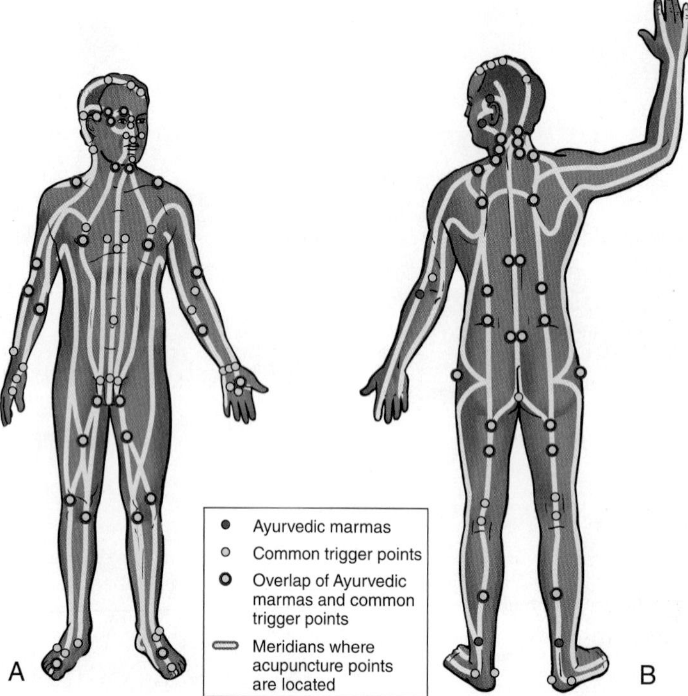

FIG. 12.22 Comparison of Ayurvedic *marmas*, common trigger points, and traditional meridians where acupuncture points are located. Anterior **A,** and posterior **B,** views of overlapping locations of various points suggest that the points have a common anatomy and physiology.

just in front of the backbone, even though they might express themselves externally at points along the front of the body (e.g., navel, heart, throat). Associated with the chakras is a latent subtle energy, called *kundalini* in Shaktism and *tumo* in Tibetan Buddhist Tantra.

The massage methods of Ayurveda are tapping, kneading, rubbing, and squeezing. The use of specialized oil preparations is integral to the systems (Johari, 1996).

Color and Chakra Therapy

Light can be used therapeutically. When the light spectrum is spread, a rainbow appears. Each color has a specific frequency that is thought to influence the body. Color can be incorporated into massage through uniforms, linens, or tinted lighting. The traditional Chinese medicine system also relies on color. Chakra therapy often is related to color. The following is a brief, basic discussion of various beliefs related to the individual chakras and color relationships (Fig. 12.23, Box 12.15):

- The chakras are numbered, beginning with the lowest vibration, which is the first chakra, or root chakra. Located at the base of the spine, the first chakra is associated with the color red. Energy is tied to the element of earth, grounding us, and connecting us to the physical plane. Glandular system: gonads.
- The second chakra, or sacral chakra, sits in the area of the reproductive organs and vibrates to the color orange. The sacral chakra controls emotions and sexuality. Glandular system: adrenal.
- The third chakra, or solar plexus chakra, is tied to the color yellow and is located just below the diaphragm. This chakra deals with intellect and ego. Glandular system: pancreas.
- The fourth chakra, or heart chakra, is located in the chest and is linked to the color green. It controls love and relationships, especially agape, or divine, love. Glandular system: lymphatic.
- The fifth chakra, or throat chakra, radiates blue and holds sway over expression, helping transmit the voice of the creative soul to the physical world. Glandular system: thyroid.
- The sixth chakra, or brow chakra, sits between and slightly above the eyes. Radiating indigo, it controls internal vision, intuition, and self-realization. Glandular system: pituitary.
- The seventh chakra, or crown chakra, lies directly atop the head and corresponds to the highest vibrations. It vibrates to the color purple and controls integration of the conscious and subconscious minds. Glandular system: pineal.

It is interesting to note that the color spectrum found in rainbows is the same as that found in the chakra system.

BIOFIELDS AND POLARITY THERAPY

SECTION OBJECTIVES

Chapter objective covered in this section:

12. Use the principles of polarity therapy as an energetic adjunct method.

Using the information presented in this section, the student will be able to perform the following:

- Explain the basic theory of polarity therapy and its relationship to biofields.

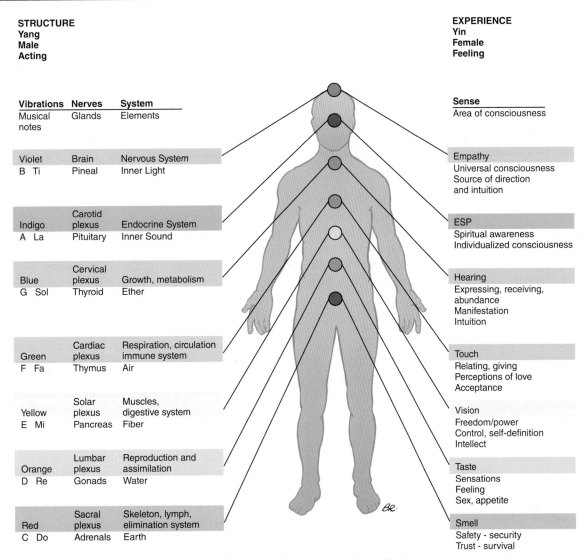

STRUCTURE
Yang
Male
Acting

EXPERIENCE
Yin
Female
Feeling

Vibrations / Musical notes	Nerves / Glands	System / Elements
Violet B Ti	Brain Pineal	Nervous System Inner Light
Indigo A La	Carotid plexus Pituitary	Endocrine System Inner Sound
Blue G Sol	Cervical plexus Thyroid	Growth, metabolism Ether
Green F Fa	Cardiac plexus Thymus	Respiration, circulation immune system Air
Yellow E Mi	Solar plexus Pancreas	Muscles, digestive system Fiber
Orange D Re	Lumbar plexus Gonads	Reproduction and assimilation Water
Red C Do	Sacral plexus Adrenals	Skeleton, lymph, elimination system Earth

Sense / Area of consciousness
Empathy Universal consciousness Source of direction and intuition
ESP Spiritual awareness Individualized consciousness
Hearing Expressing, receiving, abundance Manifestation Intuition
Touch Relating, giving Perceptions of love Acceptance
Vision Freedom/power Control, self-definition Intellect
Taste Sensations Feeling Sex, appetite
Smell Safety - security Trust - survival

FIG. 12.23 Names and locations of Major Chakras.

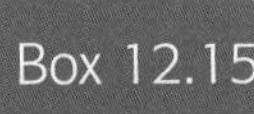

Color Therapy and Recognized Associations

Violet
Compassion, awareness of spiritual self, letting go
Indigo
Intuition, meditation, and spiritual awareness

Blue
Expression, relaxing, and serenity

Green
Feelings, healing, and love

Yellow
Mental energy, creativity, focus, and concentration

Orange
Joyfulness, warmth, and happiness

Red
Enthusiasm, passion, and vitality

Concepts of Energy Methods

Life force energy (e.g., *chi, qi,* and *prana*) has not been a popular subject of Western scientific research. The abstract quality and esoteric nature of the concept are still primarily held in the knowledge base of "spiritual truth." Many spiritual disciplines practice the "laying on of hands."

As with all methods of healing touch, something exists beyond the physiologic explanation for the benefit. This "something" is intangible but very real in the experience of it. Therein remains the mystery. The human biofield is a challenging concept that is not fully compatible with current biomedical research. The mechanisms behind this phenomenon are still unclear or unknown. However, some research and clinical effectiveness reports support further study (Matos et al., 2021; Feinstein 2022; Wahbeh et al., 2022).

The terms *subtle energy* or *biofield therapies* cover a wide range of techniques that affect the subtle electrical fields of the body. Some believe that massage and other forms of bodywork influence the energy component of the body by stimulating electrochemical, electromagnetic, and piezoelectric fields. The validity of the effectiveness of any method based on the reaction of the electrochemical, electromagnetic, or piezoelectric component of the body is controversial. The physiologic state of the practitioner while performing biofield-based therapies may be a factor (Baldwin & Hammerschlag, 2014). A quiet, calm, rhythmic, compassionate demeanor of the practitioner is a common factor in the application of biofield-based methods. Supportive therapeutic presence and compassionate interaction may be the basis of proposed benefits. The concept of body energy is not new and has been studied since the 1940s (Box 12.16).

Cell biologists now recognize that nuclear, cytoplasmic, and extracellular matrices form a continuous and interconnected communication system that plays a key role in the integration of functions, including immunity and injury repair. Mechanosensitive ion channels such as PIEZO1 are molecular transducers of mechanical force. These molecular structures are activated by mechanical stimuli exerted on cellular membranes and convert these stimuli into electrical, osmotic, and/or chemical signals. The exact mechanisms of mechanosensitive ion channels are currently unknown but may be an aspect of biofields (Lin et al., 2019; Ridone et al., 2019).

Tensegrity concepts may explain the various forms of energy absorbed and conducted throughout the framework of the body, affecting all cells. Crystalline components of the living matrix, such as the collagen arrays in tendons, ligaments, and bones and the arrays of lipids in cell membranes, may function as coherent, resonant molecular broadcasting systems.

Entrainment is the coordination or synchronization of rhythms. Internal rhythms of organisms synchronize with external rhythms, such as repetitive stimuli as found in music. Vibrating molecules throughout the body may become cooperatively entrained with the brain rhythms. As more molecules in the crystalline living matrix become vibrationally entrained, the fields become stronger. In the body, biologic oscillators such as the heart and the thalamus regulate the rhythmic occurrence of certain biochemical, physiologic, and behavioral events, such as sleep, hunger, and so forth. Synchronization of the heart rate, respiratory rate, and thalamus activity supports the entrainment process, and the other, more subtle body rhythms follow. Synchronization of the rhythms of the heart, respiration, and digestion promotes balance, or homeostasis, which supports a healthy body. A balance between the sympathetic and parasympathetic divisions of the ANS influences the heart and the vascular systems, modulating the heart rate and blood pressure. Nasal reflexes, which are stimulated by the movement of air through the nose, rhythmically interact with the heart, lungs, and diaphragm (Szirmai, 2010; Tavano et al., 2022).

Through entrainment, activities using repetitive motion or sound quiet or excite the nervous system (depending on the speed and pace of the rhythm), thereby altering physiologic processes of the body. Sometimes body rhythms are disrupted when exposed to discordant stimuli such as loud crowds, flashing lights, or the humming of machinery. People often become fatigued or out of sorts in these disharmonic environments.

The body most easily entrains to natural rhythms, such as the sounds of a babbling brook, ocean waves, or the rustling of leaves in the breeze. Studies have shown that the rhythmic physiologic patterns of a dog's or cat's breathing or heart rate can be beneficial to the elderly. Music with a regular 4/4 beat at 60 beats per minute or slower tends to order rhythms and calm the body. A tempo faster than 60 beats per minute seems to excite physiologically, but if the rhythm is even, the body can achieve a focused, alert state. Many forms of classical music provide resourceful entrainment rhythms. Music therapy is one of the main sources of entrainment research (Wang et al., 2002; Wu et al., 2022). Music is a common addition to massage and provides an external entrainment rhythm for the practitioner and the client.

When a person experiences positive emotional states, the biologic rhythms naturally tend to begin to oscillate together or entrain. Body entrainment processes also can be enhanced by techniques that shift the consciousness to breathing patterns and heart rate. Most meditation processes or relaxation

Box 12.16 Body Energy Is Not a New Idea

What is life? This is the main problem of biology. Many have asked this question, but nobody has answered it. Science is based on the experience that nature answers intelligent questions intelligently, so if she is silent, there may be something wrong about the question.

Think boldly, don't be afraid of making mistakes, don't miss small details, keep your eyes open, and be modest in everything except your aims.

—Albert Szent-Györgyi

Albert Szent-Györgyi (1893–1986), a Hungarian-born biochemist, was the first to isolate vitamin C, and his research on biologic oxidation provided the basis for an understanding of the Krebs citric acid cycle. His discoveries about the biochemical nature of muscular contraction revolutionized the field of muscle research. His later career was devoted to research in "submolecular" biology, applying quantum physics to biologic processes. He was especially interested in cancer and was one of the first to explore the connections between free radicals and cancer. Szent-Györgyi won the Nobel Prize in 1937 for Physiology or Medicine for his work in biologic oxidation and vitamin C, and the Lasker Award in Basic Medical Research in 1954 for contributions to an understanding of cardiovascular disease through basic muscle research.

Albert Szent-Györgyi proposed that electrons could propagate through crystalline structures both within and between molecules, forming semiconducting currents entirely separate from the movement of ions, previously assumed to be the only possible basis for bioelectricity. Said Szent-Györgyi in 1941, "The study of crystals and metals, however, has revealed the existence of a different state of matter. If a great number of atoms is arranged with regularity in close proximity, as for instance, in a crystal lattice, the terms of the single valency electrons may fuse into common bands. The electrons in this band cease to belong to one or two atoms only and belong to the whole system."

From U.S. National Library of Medicine, Bethesda, MD, National Institutes of Health, Department of Health & Human Services. Retrieved from http://profiles.nlm.nih.gov/WG/. Profiles in Science National Library of Medicine's Profiles in Science.

methods create an environment for entrainment by reducing external influences and focusing on internal rhythms, such as breathing. Many disciplines, such as yoga and *qi gong*, quiet the mind and body during meditation, centering attention on body areas with known biologic oscillators. The location of the chakra system correlates with biologic oscillators. Singing, chanting, and movement in religious and social rituals interact with biologic patterns, calming, exciting, organizing, or disrupting body rhythms.

Connective Tissues

A body-wide signaling network was recognized by ancient cultures. The role of tensegrity in the connective tissue structures may be an aspect of this signaling network. It also has been studied by authors such as Helenne Langevin, who made the connection between connective tissue planes and meridians (Langevin et al., 2004, 2006). The major stimulus for bone and cartilage formation is piezoelectric signals generated when bone or cartilage is subjected to tension or compression. This knowledge is widely used today in orthopedics (Oschman, 2008; Smit, 2008). The connective tissues form a mechanical three-dimensional network or matrix continuum, extending throughout the body, even into the innermost parts of each cell. All movement, of the body as a whole or of its smallest parts, is created by tensions carried through the connective tissue structure. The living matrix is the continuous molecular fabric of the organism, consisting of fascia, the other connective tissues, extracellular matrices, integrins, cytoskeletons, nuclear matrices, and DNA. The extracellular, cellular, and nuclear biopolymers or ground substances constitute a body-wide reservoir of charge that can maintain electrical homeostasis and "inflammatory preparedness" throughout the organism (Oschman, 2009).

Each force introduced to or generated by the body causes the crystalline lattice of the connective tissues to generate piezobioelectric signals that are precisely characteristic of those tensions, compressions, and movements. Stimulation of a piezomaterial causes either generation of electrical currents or a vibration. The connective tissue fabric is a semiconducting communication network that can carry bioelectronic signals between every part of the body (Wan et al., 2021).

The nervous system is an energy system in the body. Researchers study its operation by measuring electrical fields generated during the transmission of nerve impulses. Because electrical currents always give rise to magnetic fields, the nervous system is also a source of some biomagnetic fields in and around an organism. Moreover, the nervous system regulates all muscular movements and therefore is one of the keys to the conversion of thoughts into energetic actions (Kim et al., 2021).

Neurophysiologists, who focus most of their attention on the "classic" nervous system (composed of the neurons that conduct information from place to place as electrical impulses), maintain that all functions of the nervous system result from the activities of the neurons. Hence integration of brain function, memory, and even consciousness has been assumed to arise from the interconnectivity of neurons. This is a partial view, because it neglects another energetic and informational system consisting of the perineural connective tissue system, which constitutes more than half of the cells in the brain (the prefix *peri-* means about, around, encircling, or enclosing). Perineural cells surround each neuron in the brain and follow each peripheral nerve to its termination. Robert O. Becker was a pioneer in the exploration of the functions of the perineural system and its relationship with the semiconducting matrix that forms and surrounds it. To document the properties of this system, Becker refers to a "dual nervous system" consisting of the classic digital nerve network, which controls movement and body function, and the perineural analog network, which regulates wound healing and tissue repair. Dr. Becker was also a pioneer in the field of regeneration and its relationship to electrical currents in living things. He found clues to the healing process in the long-discarded theory of the 18th-century vitalists, that electricity is vital to life processes. Becker, an orthopedic surgeon, explored the relationship between human physiology and electricity. For 30 years he investigated the healing of bone, organs, and nerve tissue. He proved that electrical stimulation with direct current can promote healing in bone and other tissue. He went on to prove that some body parts can even be encouraged to regenerate.

Pulses of electrical and magnetic energy, called anticipatory fields, begin in the brain before any movement occurs. Anticipatory fields are an important phenomenon, and they are being investigated for their application in training for athletic events, dance, theater, music, etc. A benefit is derived from mental rehearsals or internal imaging without the individual physically doing anything. Many athletes, performers, and therapists of various kinds have described the profound experience of being totally prepared, present, and focused. In such a state, sometimes referred to as being "in the zone," extraordinary accomplishments take place. Many schools emphasize the importance of this phenomenon but call it intention; that is, the practitioner focuses in advance on the desired goals for a particular client. This approach is based on the frequent experience that a vivid image of expectations facilitates change in that direction. Intention also seems all the more effective when the client participates, as in directed movement therapies or image-based cancer treatments.

With the information presented thus far we can begin to visualize the energy systems in the living body. Current knowledge about the roles of electrical, magnetic, elastic, acoustic, thermal, gravitational, and photonic energies in living systems shows that, most likely, no single "life force" or "healing energy" exists. Rather, the living body seems to have many energy systems, and there seem to be many ways of influencing those systems. The concepts of "living state" and "health" encompass all these systems, both known and unknown, functioning collectively and synergistically. The debate over whether or not healing energies or life forces exist is being replaced by the study of ways biologic energy fields, structures, and functions interact.

Scientific discoveries in energy systems are complemented by a long history of experiential evidence and clinical techniques developed by therapists of various modalities. The growing popularity of bodywork, energy, and movement therapies is leading us to a synthesis of ideas that will benefit all. Scientific consensus has gone from certainty that weak environmental energies have no influence on living systems to agreement that such influences deserve study to determine the precise mechanisms involved. Collectively, the discoveries of modern researchers tell a story of biologic sensitivity that coincides with the daily experiences of energy therapists ranging from medical doctors using imaging techniques to acupuncturists, polarity therapists, Reiki practitioners, herbalists, aroma therapists, and so on.

Biofield therapies show some evidence for reducing pain intensity in pain populations and moderate evidence for reducing pain intensity in hospitalized and cancer populations (Aslan et al., 2023). Moderate evidence exists for reduction of negative behavioral symptoms in dementia and for decreasing anxiety for hospitalized patients. Evidence supports the effects of biofield therapies in improving fatigue and quality of life in cancer patients, for improving comprehensive pain outcomes and effects in pain patients, and for reducing anxiety in cardiovascular patients. The resulting relaxation experienced when receiving biofield therapies is likely the foundation for benefit. As always, further high-quality studies are needed in this area (Engebretson and Wardell, 2007; So et al., 2007; Fazzino et al., 2010; Jain and Mills, 2010; Van Kanegan and Worley, 2018; Matos et al., 2021).

Having an open mind to the potential of energy-based healing methods does not require us to abandon our sophisticated understandings of physiology, biochemistry, or molecular biology. The definition of living matter is being expanded, not replaced. Nerve impulses and chemical messengers are contained within the individual, whereas energy fields radiate indefinitely into space and therefore affect others who are nearby. For millennia, energy therapists have had a practical appreciation of these phenomena, which are finally open to scientific research (McCraty and Abdulgader, 2021).

Our culture has become accustomed to innumerable tasks being handled by invisible currents and beams flowing through and from technology. It is reasonable to consider and explore how subtle energies affect the mind and body.

The lack of sufficient Western scientific validation of the ancient energy flows (*chi*, *prana*, meridians, chakras, auras, etc.) causes us to represent this area of bodywork to the public carefully. Until validity of energy techniques is proven, it is important to represent these methods simply, professionally, and without false expectations and mysticism. It is also important not to discount the power of the placebo effect. If touch or positive intention can activate it, why not use it?

Polarity Therapy

The polarity system will be used as a representative method of a biofield-targeted approach. Another system called *Reiki* has become popular. Reiki is a Japanese technique for stress reduction and relaxation that promotes healing. The word *Reiki* is from two Japanese words. Rei, which means spirit, miraculous, divine; and Ki, which means life force energy. The approach is based on the idea that "life force energy" is what enlivens us. If one's "life force energy" is low, that may be unhealthy; if it is high, then the experience of life is happy and healthy.

Polarity Therapy reflects previously described Asian and Ayurvedic cultural healing systems in this chapter. The American Polarity Therapy Association (APTA) was officially launched in 1984 and held its first conference in 1986. The Certification Governing Council (CGC) was established in 2016 as a standing committee within APTA. In establishing the CGC, the Board has empowered and authorized the CGC to function independently regarding the development and administration of the APTA Board Certified Polarity Practitioner (BCPP) certification program. For more information, see the website at https://polaritytherapy.org.

Polarity therapy was developed by Dr. Randolph Stone in the mid-1900s. It is an eclectic, multifaceted system. Polarity therapy is also a respectful, compassionate, and intentional laying of the hands on the body. The bodywork principles of polarity blend easily with massage. The intention of the touch is the same as the themes of therapeutic massage presented throughout this text (see Chapters 1 and 2). Nothing is ever forced. The experience belongs to the client. The practitioner offers the methods not by protocol but through a practiced development of decision making guided by intuition. When the professional feels no attachment to the outcome for their own sense of achievement, the methods become "free" to influence the experience of the client.

As with the other methods discussed in previous sections of this chapter, the application of polarity methods is simple. However, for those interested in pursuing advanced learning, the goal is to develop the ability to deliver the methods in a purposeful and individualized way, detached from expectation but fascinated with the outcome. Eventually the practitioner learns that the more complex the client situation, the simpler the methods used. The simplicity of polarity makes it one of the gifts to bodywork.

Principles and Applications of Polarity Therapy

The purpose of polarity therapy is to locate blocked energy and release it, using the principles outlined here. When blocked energy is released, body systems and organs can function normally, and healing can take place naturally. Scientific inquiry has been unable to identify or explain the energetic body or the concept of blockages. Polarity therapy does not treat illness or disease; it affects the body (life) energy, which is said to flow in invisible electromagnetic currents through the body's organs and tissues. Polarity is used to stimulate inactive energy in a diseased body part. The following principles apply:

1. The head and spinal column form the central neutral (0) energy axis of the body.
2. Long vertical currents of energy travel from head to foot on the right side of the body, flowing down the front and up the back. Positive (1) outward energy is expressed through the right side. The right side represents the following:
   - Warmth
   - Expanding
   - Sun
   - Yang
   - Positive, expanding energy

3. On the left side of the body, the vertical currents flow up the front and down the back. Negative (2) inward energy is expressed through the left side. The left side represents the following:
   - Cooling
   - Contracting
   - Moon
   - Yin
   - Negative, receptive energy
4. Five electromagnetic currents are present on each side of the body. Each current is related to an element. The elements are ether, air, fire, water, and earth. Each current relates to the organs and functions of its area (Fig. 12.24).

The Five Major Body Currents

As mentioned, the five major body currents are ether, air, fire, water, and earth:

- *Ether* is associated with hearing, the voice, the throat, and the quality of nothingness. The core current of the torso flows from north to south (head to pelvis to back). The ether element represents pure vibration and responds to gentleness and love. Characteristics of the ether element are as follows:
  Color: Sky blue
  Sense: Hearing
  Food: Pure air
- *Air* is associated with respiration, circulation, the heart, the lungs, and speed. It flows from east to west (from front to back in a circular pattern). With a balanced air element, we are calm and relaxed. Characteristics of the air element are:
  Color: Emerald green
  Sense: Touch
  Food: Fruits and nuts
- *Fire* is associated with digestion, the stomach, the bowels, warmth, and the heat of the body. A diagonal current found on both sides of the body, it starts at the shoulders and goes to the opposite hip. It is part of the figure-eight energy and is activated by touch, food, and exercise. Characteristics of the fire element are:
  Color: Yellow
  Sense: Sight
  Food: Grains

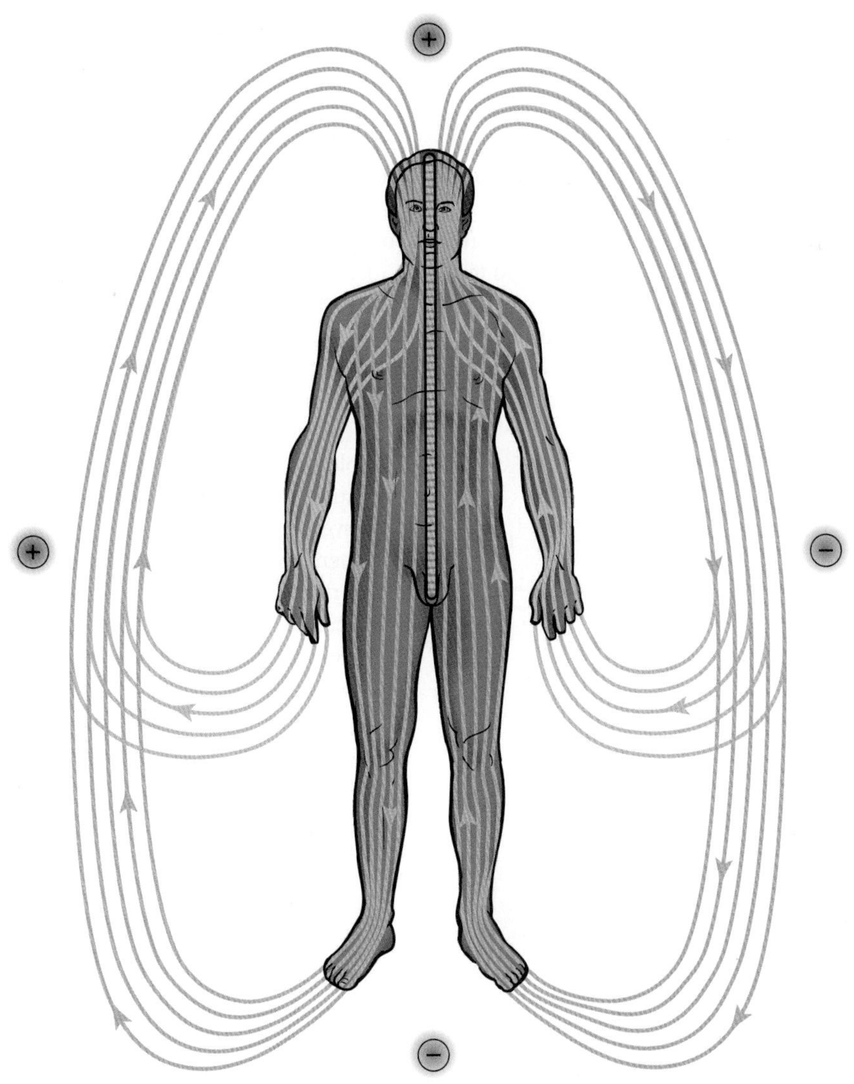

FIG. 12.24 Electromagnetic currents traveling vertically on the body.

- *Water* is associated with generative power, creativity, the pelvic organs, sexuality, glandular secretions, emotional drive, equilibrium, and balance. A long current that splits the body in half, it extends from the head to the foot, including the arms and legs. The right side moves clockwise, the left side counterclockwise. Characteristics of the water element are:
  Color: Orange
  Sense: Taste
  Food: Leafy green vegetables, seaweed, watery foods
- *Earth* is associated with the elimination of solids and liquids, the bladder, the rectum, the formation of bone, structure, and support. A zigzag current is formed by solid straight lines from one side to the other. Characteristics of the earth element are:
  Color: Red
  Sense: Smell
  Food: Tubers, meat, dairy

The polarity (positive [+] or negative [−]) of these electromagnetic currents is shown in Fig. 12.24. Positive and negative are opposites. However, the use of positive and negative labels is only relative; it is a way of showing relationships. Each of the five electromagnetic currents passes through a corresponding finger and toe, giving its name to the finger and toe (e.g., the middle, or fire, finger) (Fig. 12.25).

The right side of the body is positive (+), whereas the left side of the body is negative (−). The head is positive, whereas the feet are negative. The front of the body is positive, whereas the back is negative. The top is positive, whereas the bottom is negative. Each joint is neutral and is a crossover for energy currents, which change polarity at the crossover. The neutrality of the joints allows them to be flexible. Each finger and toe has its own individual polarity (see Fig. 12.25).

Blocked energy usually registers as soreness, tenderness, or pain. A simple way to bring energy to an area where it is blocked is to place your left hand on the pain and your right hand opposite that area, on the back, front, or side of the body.

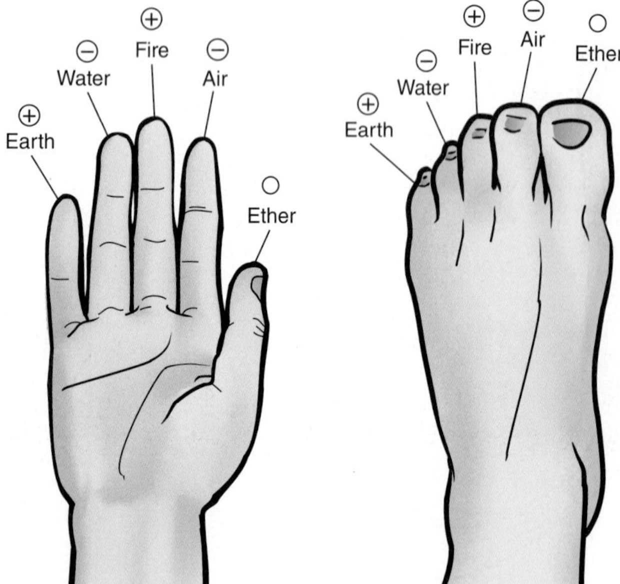

FIG. 12.25 Finger and toe chart.

Reflexes

Reflexes are points along an energy current that connect with other points along that current. When stimulated, a reflex point can affect the other reflexes on the same energy path. Manipulations that stimulate the foot and hand poles use the reflex principles located there (Fig. 12.26).

Positive and Negative Contacts

Because all polarity contacts are bipolar, both hands must be in contact with the body so that energy can move from one hand to the other through the blockage. If the energy blockage is on the front of the body, place the left hand over the painful, blocked area and the right hand on the back of the body directly opposite the left hand. This double contact draws energy through the body from front to back, side to side, and top to bottom.

In practice, a positive contact (e.g., the right hand or fire finger) activates and gives energy. The opposite is also true; a negative contact (e.g., the left hand or air finger) is relaxing and receives energy.

Fig. 12.26 shows the foot reflexes as they relate to the rest of the body. In addition to the feet, reflexes are present in the hands, arms, legs, and head. Alternately stimulating a reflex and then its corresponding body part can free blocked energy and allow normal functioning. The negative poles of the body are most frequently obstructed. The negative pole is stimulated first, then the positive pole, to send currents over the entire body.

The use of diagonal contacts on the body activates the serpentine brain-wave currents shown in Fig. 12.27.

Applying a Polarity Method

1. With most procedures, stimulate the area (rub briskly) for a few minutes, then hold and feel the energy.
2. Hold for 30 to 60 seconds. If you feel no energy after stimulating for 2 minutes, hold for 1 minute longer and then move on.
3. When possible, keep the client's body centered between your hands.
4. Be careful not to cross your hands on your client's body.
5. When stimulating points, use the fleshy pads of your fingers.
6. Be gentle; never force. Forcing creates tension, which blocks energy. A light, gentle touch moves energy.
7. When you feel the energy, the blocked energy is released. Life energy has intelligence. After it is moving, it knows what to do and where to go.
8. People heal at different rates; do not expect a physical result after completion of a procedure. Be neutral when working with a client. Do not let your expectations be a part of the energy.
9. If the manipulations are ineffective, place your hands on your client's body and send love. Visualize energy flowing through your hands to your client (Proficiency Exercise 12.7).

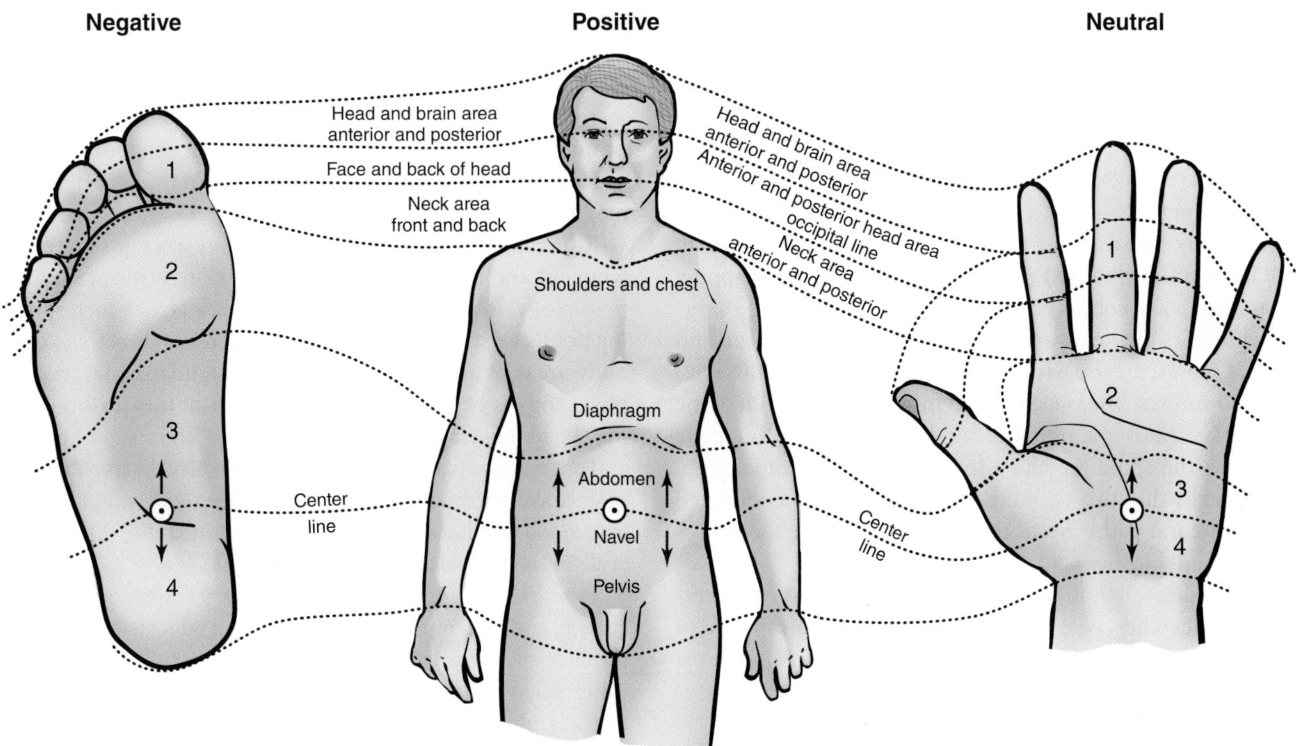

FIG. 12.26 Reflex relationships among the hand, foot, and body.

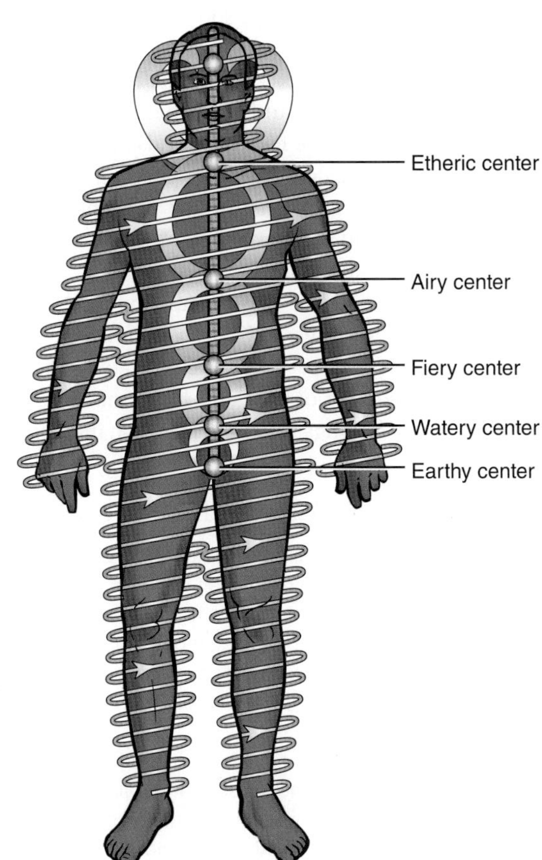

FIG. 12.27 Brain-wave currents crisscrossing the spine from the brain to the coccyx. These currents resemble the caduceus, the ancient Greek symbol for medicine. Each crossover point is known as a chakra, or energy center.

PROFICIENCY EXERCISE 12.7

1. Design 3 original massage sessions that incorporate a principle from each topic covered in this chapter.
2. Exchange massage with three learners using one of the massage sessions developed in this chapter.
3. While giving 3 general massages to "practice" clients, mentally note each time you use one of the methods in this chapter.
4. Using professional journals and massage school catalogs, find a continuing education opportunity for each method discussed in this chapter. The Internet can be a resource for finding this information.

REFLEXOLOGY

SECTION OBJECTIVES

Chapter objective covered in this section:

13. Modify foot massage to incorporate the philosophy of reflexology.

Using the information presented in this section, the student will be able to perform the following:

- Explain the physiologic benefits of foot and hand massage.
- Incorporate the principles of reflexology into a general massage session.

Reflexology is the stimulation of areas beneath the skin to improve the function of the whole body or of specific body areas away from the site of the stimulation. Eunice Ingham has been credited with formalizing the system in the West, based on the theory that certain points in the foot and hand affect other body organs and areas. Historically, the approach seems to have originated in China. Foot reflexology is the most popular type of reflexology.

Another approach to reflexology is referred to as *zone therapy.* This method is based on the theory that 10 zones run through the body, and reflex points for stimulation are located within these zones.

Reflexology applies the stimulus/reflex principle to healing the body. The foot has been mapped to show the areas to contact to affect different parts of the body. Charts mapping these areas vary somewhat (Fig. 12.28). Typically, the large toe represents the head, and the junction of the large toe and the foot represents the neck. The next toes represent the eyes, ears, and sinuses. The waist is about midway on the arch of the foot, with various organs above and below the line. The reflex points for the spine are along the medial longitudinal arch. It is thought that this stimulus-response reflex is conducted through neural pathways in the body that initiate the body's electrical and biochemical activities.

The medical definition of reflexology is "the study of reflexes." Reflexotherapy is treatment by manipulation applied to an area away from the disorder. In physiologic terms, a reflex is an involuntary response to a stimulus.

Reflexology Association of America (https://reflexology-usa.org/) defines reflexology as an integrative health practice which maps a reflection of the body predominately on the feet, hands, and outer ears. It uses unique manual techniques to deliver pressure to neural pathways assisting the body to function optimally. To qualify as a professional member, the Reflexology Association of America has set the requirement at 300 hours of training in reflexology. To be eligible to sit for national certification in reflexology, the American Reflexology Certification Board requires at least 110 hours of classroom instruction in reflexology. The American Reflexology Certification Board® (ARCB®) is a nonprofit independent testing agency, setting the standard of excellence in the field of Reflexology (https://www.arcb.net/).

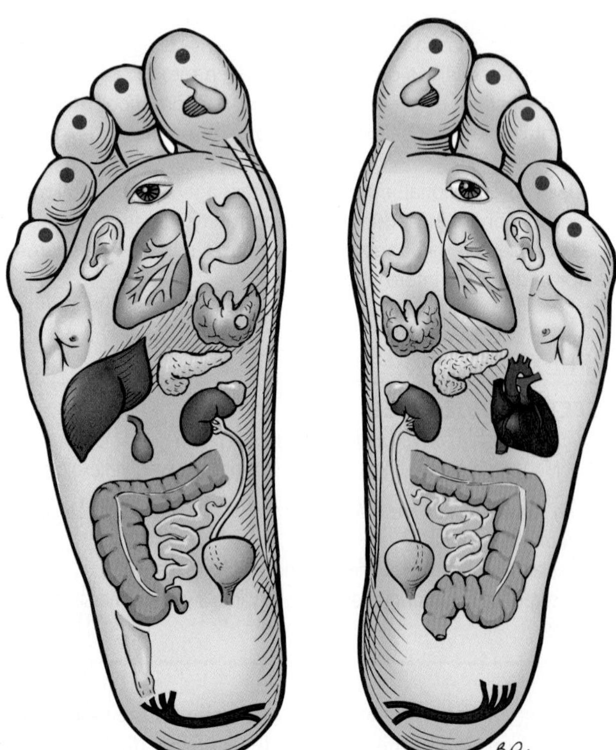

FIG. 12.28 In traditional reflexology, thumb pressure is typically used. However, the thumb cannot withstand this amount of compressive force. Instead of using the thumbs to apply pressure, use a knuckle.

This chapter's discussion of reflexology attempts to explain why foot and hand massage is beneficial in terms of standard physiology; it avoids the issue of whether actual corresponding points exist on the foot or hand that relate directly to other body areas. An explanation based on standard anatomy and physiology is better suited to the format of this textbook and may be better accepted by the public.

Foot massage is a non-invasive and convenient intervention with positive short-term effects on vital signs, sleep quality, and reducing fatigue and pain (Artioli et al., 2021; Mohammed et al., 2022; Huang et al., 2021; Jing et al., 2022; Liang et al., 2023).

Research to support reflexology theory is sparse and inconclusive, and it is important to inform and educate clients about the lack of Western-based scientific validation. At the same time, when methods such as reflexology have extensive historical and cultural foundations, it is wise not to fully discount the methods. General relaxation and stress management outcomes to support well-being are the most supported effects of focused foot massage. Biological plausibility is a key concept; it is likely that focused hand and foot massage is beneficial rather than stimulation of specific spots (Chandrababu et al., 2018; Yilar et al., 2018; Sayari et al., 2021; Whatley et al., 2022).

The foot is a complex structure. The ankle and foot consist of 34 joints, with many joint and reflex patterns (Box 12.17). The nerve distribution to the feet and hands is extensive. The position of the foot sends considerable postural information from the joint mechanoreceptors through the central nervous system. The sensory and motor centers of the brain devote a large area to the foot and hand.

It seems logical to assume that stimulation of the feet activates body-wide responses, such as gait reflexes and the autonomic nervous system. This outcome alone is helpful in explaining the benefits of foot and hand massage. In addition, many nerve endings on the feet and hands correlate

Box 12.17 Reflexes Associated With the Foot

Achilles tendon reflex: Plantar flexion/extension of the foot, resulting from contraction of the calf muscles after a sharp blow to the Achilles tendon; similar to the knee-jerk reflex.

Extensor thrust: A quick, brief extension of a limb after application of pressure to the plantar surface.

Flexor withdrawal: Flexion of the lower extremity when the foot receives a painful stimulus.

Mendel-Bekhterev reflex: Plantar flexion of the toes in response to percussion of the dorsum of the foot.

Postural reflex: Any reflex involved in maintaining posture.

Proprioceptive reflex: A reflex initiated by movement of the body to maintain the position of the moved part; any reflex initiated by stimulation of a proprioceptor.

Rossolimo's reflex: Plantar flexion of the second to fifth toes in response to percussion of the plantar surface of the toes.

with acupressure points, which when stimulated trigger the release of endorphins and other endogenous chemicals. In addition, major lymph system plexuses are located in the hands and feet. Rhythmic compressive forces in these areas stimulate lymphatic movement. Foot massage may also affect various neurochemicals such as oxytocin (Li et al., 2019).

Reflex Phenomena

Reflex phenomena must be put into perspective. Reflex points are located body-wide, including the hands, head, ears, and torso. If you consider all the reflexology points, acupuncture points, neurolymphatic points, motor points, and other reflex points, the body itself can be seen as one big point. Because of the reflexive nature of the body and its inherent ability to self-regulate in response to stimulation, it is often not necessary to overly focus on specific system names and uses for points.

More important is the ability to identify these various points during assessment procedures and to choose effective treatment for them. Assessment usually indicates an area tender to palpation if a point is hypersensitive or if the reflex structure associated with the particular point is hyperreactive. The opposite is true if the point area feels empty, numb, or disconnected from the surrounding tissue.

There are two basic treatment processes:

- If a reflexive point is tender and therefore likely to be overactive, relaxation and sedating methods are used.
- If the point is underactive, stimulation methods are applied.

If you are not sure which application is appropriate, trust the innate balancing ability of the body. Alternately, you can use both approaches, allowing the body to choose.

Massage for the Foot

An excellent way to massage the foot is to apply pressure and movement systematically to the entire foot and ankle complex. The pressure stimulates circulation, nerves, and reflexes. Moving all the joints stimulates large-diameter nerve fibers and joint mechanoreceptors, initiating hyperstimulation analgesia. The result is a shift in proprioceptive and postural reflexes. The sheer volume of sensory information flooding the central nervous system has significant effects in the body. The usual result is parasympathetic dominance.

Foot massage is usually boundary safe; that is, most people accept foot or hand massage when the idea of removing the clothing is objectionable. Hand and foot massage is likely to be the most effective form of self-massage. The hand and foot have similar motor cortex distribution patterns. Stimulation of the hands during self-massage does not override sensations to the feet being massaged. The hands are massaged while they massage the feet (Proficiency Exercise 12.8).

Often essential oils are applied to the feet (see the Aromatherapy section of this chapter). The sole of the foot is highly vascular and therefore is thought to absorb lipids (fat) in essential oils. The foot is also a safe place to apply essential oils because the oil is not easily spread into potentially irritable mucus membrane areas (e.g., the nose or eye). See reflexology techniques demonstrated in the foot massage/reflexology protocol.

PROFICIENCY EXERCISE 12.8

1. Exchange foot massages with another learner or visit a professional reflexologist for a foot massage. Compare the effects with those of a full-body massage.
2. Using a skeletal model, move each of the joints of the foot. Then move each of the joints of your foot.

FOOT MASSAGE/REFLEXOLOGY PROTOCOL

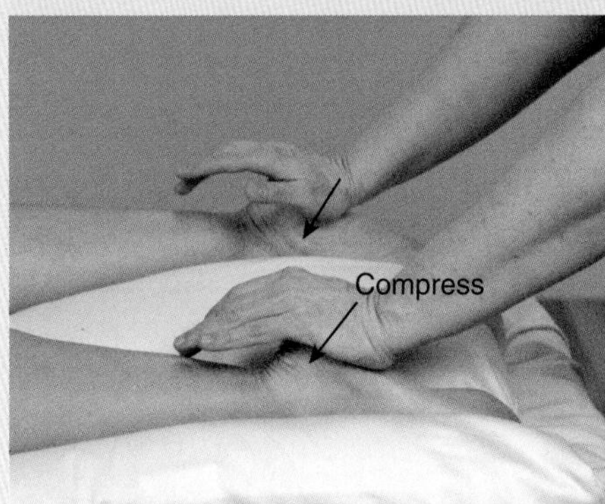

1. Prone compression.

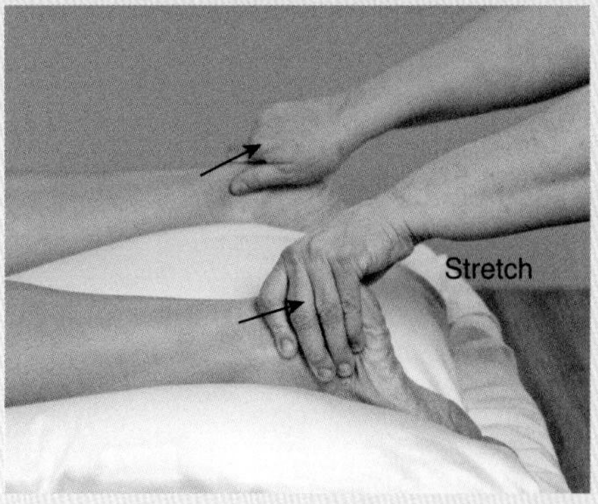

2. Prone stretch.

Continued

FOOT MASSAGE/REFLEXOLOGY PROTOCOL—cont'd

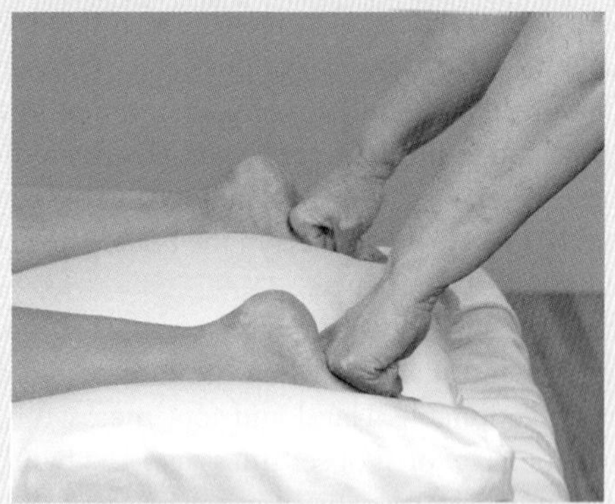

3. Fist compression.

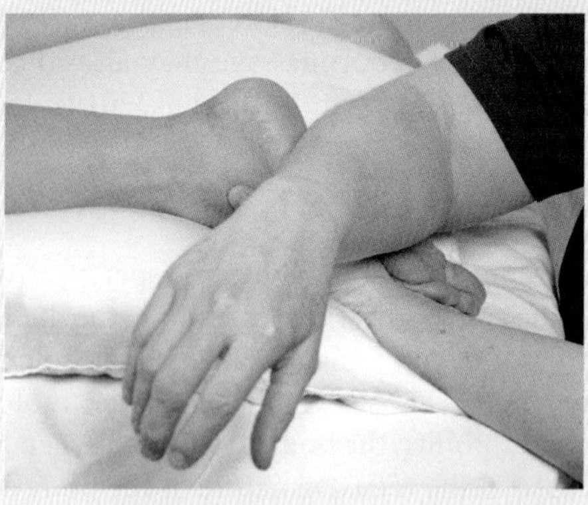

4. Forearm compression.

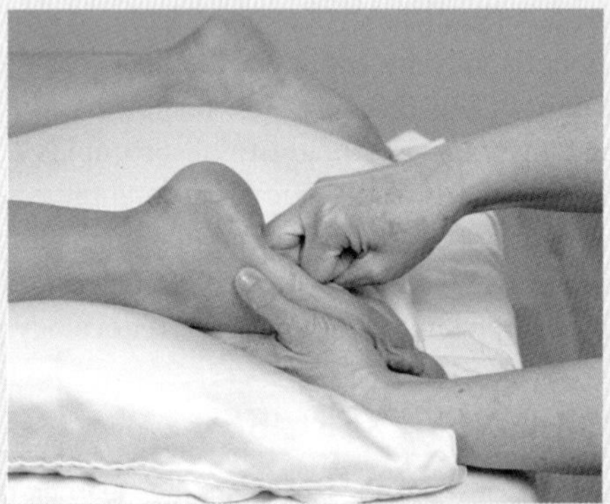

5. Knuckle used to compress specific reflexology points.

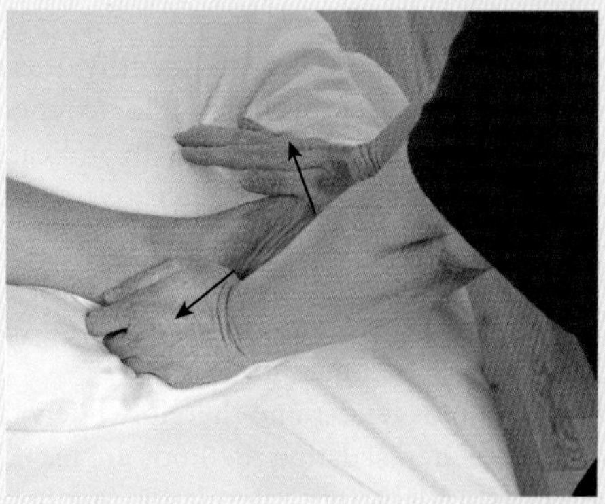

6. Side-lying stretch.

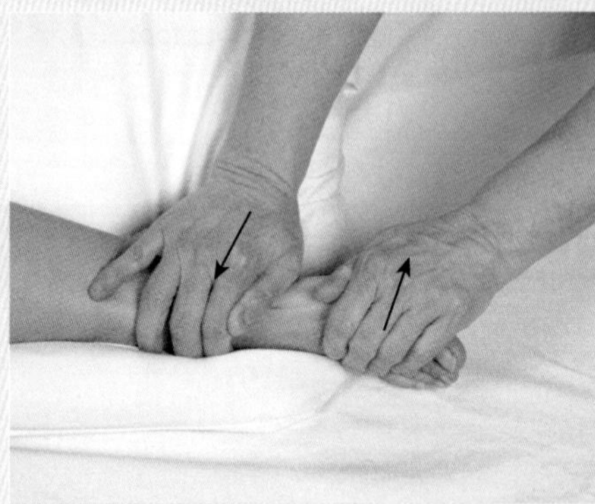

7. Stretch for foot, dorsal.

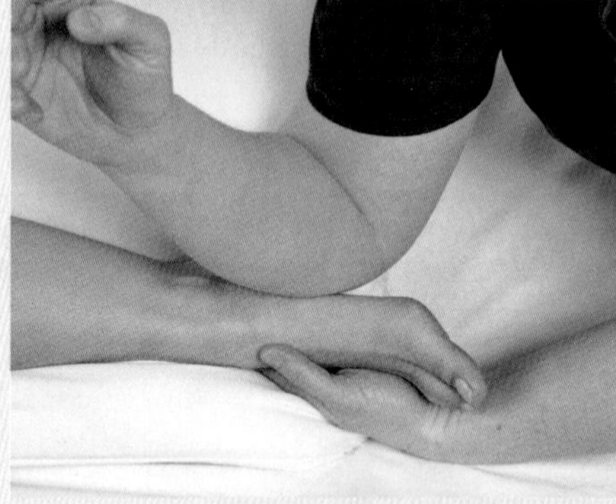

8. Side-lying forearm compression.

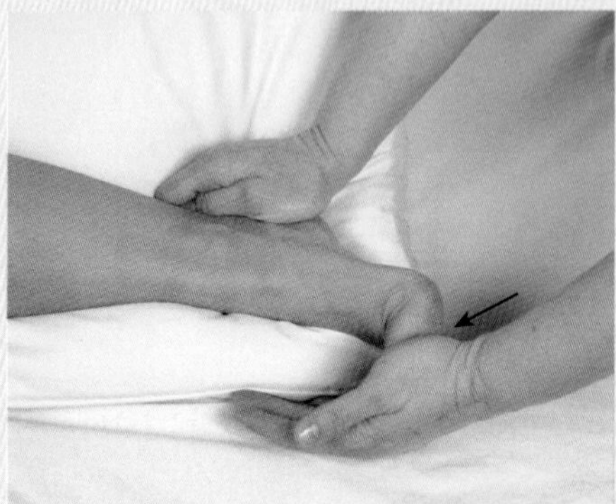

9. Arch and toe stretch.

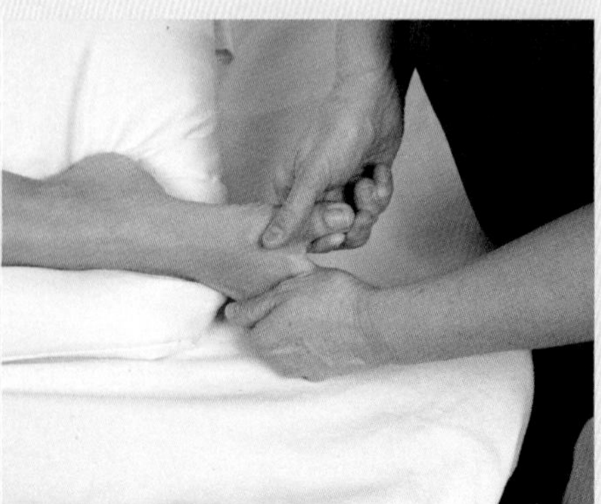

10. Individual toe stretch.

Foot in the Door

The foundation and staple of a successful massage therapy practice is the moderate pressure, basic, full-body massage used for assessment and to provide general relaxation outcomes. The infinite variations in pressure levels, speed, direction, and other qualities of touch make massage valuable, in and of itself, for helping clients reach their outcome goals. However, to get your foot in the door in many massage practice settings, the ability to provide variations on the theme is an asset. It can be satisfying to incorporate various thermotherapy and hydrotherapy methods before, during, or after the massage. An intentional and intuitive approach to your professional practice makes a profound difference in the client's experience. The pleasing scents of essential oils add to the massage experience when used safely. When you can explain to potential employers or clients how you can blend aspects of adjunct methods into the massage, they can factor into your qualifications the ability to offer a variety of stress-reducing methods.

Remember to describe your skills in complementary and adjunct bodywork methods ethically. Each of these systems has a unique base of knowledge and skills. Just because you can incorporate concepts of reflexology into foot massage does not mean you can claim to be a reflexologist.

SUMMARY

Each bodywork system is complete within itself; however, extensive overlap exists in both the application of techniques and physiologic effects. Massage can be adapted to address a physiologic function such as fluid movement or a tissue type like fascia. Although further study of the methods presented will benefit the massage professional, the ability to become proficient in the application of any of the systems, including therapeutic massage, is a lifelong study. Just as studying a foreign language tends to improve proficiency in a person's primary language, the study of bodywork systems complementary to therapeutic massage improves the understanding and technical application of massage methods. All bodywork systems are forms of structured professional touch that complement, rather than replace, each other.

Massage professionals who add these methods to their skills can provide a more specific focus during the massage. For example, a client might enjoy a relaxing foot bath and some hot tea while waiting for the appointment. The client and the massage therapist may drink a glass of water together after the session as a farewell ritual.

Adjunct and focused massage methods also can be integrated into a massage session in many other ways:

- A cold compress could be placed on the back of the neck, the forehead, or other area of the body during the massage.
- Safe use of an implement to assist with the massage application adds variety.
- Essential oils can be used as a room fragrance or added to the massage lubricant.
- Gliding could be focused to move lymph and veinous blood, or it could be specifically applied in the grooves of the body to stimulate the fascia and meridians.
- Compression could be applied moving down the arteries to stimulate arterial blood flow.
- Compression, vibration, and tapping of the acupuncture points may normalize body function.
- Drag can be increased to push and pull the superficial fascia supporting normal sliding function.
- Kneading, stretching, and friction methods applied slowly and deliberately to drag, pull, and elongate might soften and normalize the connective tissue.
- The occasional trigger point might be treated with direct pressure or frictioning, with a hot compress or stone applied afterward. An ice pack sometimes may be a better choice after frictioning to help control inflammation.
- Every joint in the hands and feet may be moved, and attention may be given to compression on the bottoms of the hands and feet to stimulate the flow of lymph. The client can be instructed in deep breathing to further encourage lymph movement.
- The compassionate "laying on of hands" becomes part of every technique. Warm stones or seed bags can be placed on the traditional energy centers.

As a result of the massage interaction, the client should experience a pleasant, relaxed, and alert state in response to the physiologic shifts in the body.

LEARN MORE ON THE WEB

MEDLINEPLUS is one of the most useful websites for massage therapists and massage therapy students interested in learning more about the techniques described in this chapter. Visit the site and use the search term *burns*, *hydrotherapy*, and *hot stone massage*, for example. The U.S. Food & Drug Administration has some content on essential oils, and the Evolve site provides links to articles related to connective tissue and aromatherapy.

Evolve

Visit the Evolve website: http://evolve.elsevier.com/Fritz/fundamentals/

Evolve content designed for massage therapy licensing exam review and comprehension of content beyond the textbook.

Evolve content includes:

- Content Updates
- Science and Pathology Animations
- Body Spectrum Coloring Book
- MBLEx exam review multiple choice questions

FOR EACH CHAPTER FIND:

- Answers and rationales for the end-of-chapter multiple-choice questions
- Electronic Workbook and Answer Key
- Chapter multiple choice question Quiz
- Quick Content Review in Question Form and Answers
- Technique Videos when applicable
- Learn More on the Web

REFERENCES

Abd Rashed A, Abd Rahman AZ, Rathi DNG. Essential oils as a potential neuroprotective remedy for age-related neurodegenerative diseases: a review. *Molecules*. 2021 Feb 19;26(4):1107. doi:10.3390/molecules26041107.

Abdolmaleki F, Kovanen PT, Mardani R, Gheibi-Hayat SM, Bo S, Sahebkar A. Resolvins: emerging players in autoimmune and inflammatory diseases. *Clin Rev Allergy Immunol*. 2020;58(1):82–91. doi:10.1007/s12016-019 08754-9

Aboushanab T, AlSanad S. A quality model to select patients in cupping therapy clinics: a new tool for ensuring safety in clinical practice. *J Acupunct Meridian Stud*. 2018;11(5):269–272. doi:10.1016/j.jams.2018.06.002.

Aboushanab TS, AlSanad S. Cupping therapy: an overview from a modern medicine perspective. *J Acupunct Meridian Stud*. 2018;11(3):83–87. doi:10.1016/j.jams.2018.02.001.

Absinta M, Ha SK, Nair G, et al. Human and nonhuman primate meninges harbor lymphatic vessels that can be visualized noninvasively by MRI. *eLife*. 2017;6:e29738.

Adstrum S, Hedley G, Schleip R, Stecco C, Yucesoy CA. Defining the fascial system. *J Bodyw Mov Ther*. 2017;21(1):173–177.

Ahmed J, Anwar K, Sajjad AG. Effects of strain counter strain technique in treatment of chronic mechanical low back pain: a randomized controlled trail. *Rehman J Health Sci*. 2021;3(2):85–91.

Ajimsha MS, Al-Mudahka NR, Al-Madzhar JA. Effectiveness of myofascial release: systematic review of randomized controlled trials. *J Bodyw Mov Ther*. 2015;19(1):102–112.

Ajimsha MS, Shenoy PD, Gampawar N. Role of fascial connectivity in musculoskeletal dysfunctions: a narrative review. *J Bodyw Mov Ther*. 2020;24(4):423–431.

Alam M, Abbas K. The role of Cupping Therapy (CT) in pain tackling, an insight into mechanism therapeutic effects and its relevance in current medical scenario. *Int J Curr Sci Res*. 2021;4(7)732–739.

Alam MM, Khan AA, Farooq M. Effects of vibratory massage therapy on grip strength, endurance time and forearm muscle performance. *Work*. 2021;68(3):619–632. doi:10.3233/WOR-203397.

Al-Bedah AMN, Elsubai IS, Qureshi NA, et al. The medical perspective of cupping therapy: effects and mechanisms of action. *J Tradit Complement Med*. 2018;9(2):90–97. doi:10.1016/j.jtcme.2018.03.003. Published 2018 Apr 30.

Alghamdi A, Shawki M. The effect of kinesio taping on balance control and functional performance in athletes with chronic ankle instability. *MOJ Orthop Rheumatol*. 2018;10(2):114–120.

Almassmoum SM, Balahmar EA, Almutairi ST, Albuainain G, Ahmad R, Naqvi AA. Current clinical status of hydrotherapy; an evidence based retrospective six-years (2012-2017) systemic review. *Bali Med J*. 2018;7(3)578–586. doi:10.15562/bmj.v7i3.1159.

Alotaibi M, Ayoub A, King T, Uddin S. The effect of kinesio taping in reducing myofascial pain syndrome on the upper trapezius muscle: a systematic review and meta-analysis. *Eur Sci J*. 2018;14(6):336. doi:10.19044/esj.2018.v14n6p336.

An J, Lee I, Yi Y. The thermal effects of water immersion on health outcomes: an integrative review. *Int J Environ Res Public Health*. 2019;16(7):1280.

Angelopoulos P, Mylonas K, Tsepis E, Billis E, Vaitsis N, Fousekis K. The effects of instrument-assisted soft tissue mobilization, tissue flossing, and kinesiology taping on shoulder functional capacities in amateur athletes. *J Sport Rehabil*. 2021;30(7):1028–1037.

Archanah T, Shashikiran HC, Shetty P, Chandrakanth KK. Effect of a hydrotherapy based alternate compress on osteoarthritis of the knee joint: a randomized controlled trial. *Inter J Res Med Sci*. 2018;6(4):1444–1449.

Armstrong C. The architecture and spatial organization of the living human body as revealed by intratissular endoscopy – an osteopathic perspective. *J Bodyw Mov Ther*. 2020;24:138–146.

Armstrong C. Unity, Continuity, Structure, and Function. The Ongoing Search for a Deeper Understanding of the Many Roles Attributed to Fascia in the Living Human Body-An Osteopathic Perspective. *OBM Integr Complement Med*. 2021;6(3):1–18.

Artioli DP, Tavares A, Bertolini GRF. Foot reflexology in painful conditions: systematic review. Braz J Pain. Published online 2021. doi:10.5935/2595-0118.20210022.

Artzberger S, Rodrick J. הרקב לופיטו ינשדח תקצבב/Manual Edema Mobilization: a new concept in subacute hand edema reduction. IJOT: The Israeli Journal of Occupational Therapy/*קוסיעב יופירל ילארשי תע בתכ*. 2002:E37–E63.

Bagheri R, Pourahmadi MR, Sarmadi AR, Takamjani IE, Torkaman G, Fazeli SH. What is the effect and mechanism of kinesiology tape on muscle activity? *J Bodyw Mov Ther*. 2018;22(2):266–275.

Baldwin AL, Hammerschlag R. Biofield-based therapies: a systematic review of physiological effects on practitioners during healing. *Explore (NY)*. 2014;10:150.

Ball EL, Owen-Booth B, Gray A, Shenkin SD, Hewitt J, McCleery J. Aromatherapy for dementia. *Cochrane Database Syst Rev*. 2020;8(8):CD003150. doi:10.1002/14651858.CD003150.pub3. Published 2020 Aug 19.

Ball A, Perreault T, Fernández-de-Las-Peñas C, Agnone M, Spennato J. Ultrasound confirmation of the multiple loci hypothesis of the myofascial trigger point and the diagnostic importance of specificity in the elicitation of the local twitch response. *Diagnostics (Basel)*. 2022;12(2):321. doi:10.3390/diagnostics12020321. Published 2022 Jan 27.

Barker CA. *Does Hydrotherapy Improve Health-Related Quality of Life (HR-QoL) in Adult Men and Women with Multiple Sclerosis (MS)?* Philadelphia College of Osteopathic Medicine; 2018.

Bartel L, Mosabbir A. Possible mechanisms for the effects of sound vibration on human health. *Healthcare (Basel)*. 2021;9(5):597. doi:10.3390/healthcare9050597. Published 2021 May 18.

Basu S, Jharna M, Palekar TJ, Vinaya Chitgopkar. EFFECT of positional release technique versus deep transverse friction massage on gluteus medius trigger point in mechanical low back pain–a comparative study. *Global J Res Ana*. 2018;6:5.

Bayülgen MY, Gün M. Effect of complementary and integrative treatments on fatigue symptoms in hemodialysis patients: a systematic review. *Holist Nurs Pract*. 2022;36(1):17–27. doi:10.1097/HNP.0000000000000489.

Benias PC, Wells RG, Sackey-Aboagye B, et al. Structure and distribution of an unrecognized interstitium in human tissues. *Sci Rep*. 2018;8:4947. http://dx.doi.org/10.1038/s41598-018-23062-6.

Binaei F, Hedayati R, Mirmohammadkhani M, Taghizadeh Delkhoush C, Bagheri R. Examining the use of kinesiology tape during weight bearing exercises on proprioception in participants with functional ankle instability. *Percept Mot Skills*. 2021;128(6):2654–2668.

Birinci T, Mustafaoglu R, Mutlu EK, Ozdincler AR. FRI0690 Comparison of effectiveness of different stretching exercises combined with pressure release technique on latent trigger points in the pectoralis minor muscle. *Ann Rheum*. 2018;77:864.

Boghdady CM, Kalashnikov N, Mok S, McCaffrey L, Moraes C. Revisiting tissue tensegrity: biomaterial-based approaches to measure forces across length scales. *APL Bioeng*. 2021;5(4):041501. doi:10.1063/5.0046093. Published 2021 Oct 1.

Bordoni BB, Zanier E. Clinical and symptomatological reflections: the fascial system. *J Multidiscip Healthc*. 2014;7:401–411.

Bordoni BA, Marelli F, Morabito B, Castagna RA. A new concept of biotensegrity incorporating liquid tissues: blood and lymph. *J Evid Based Integr Med*. 2018b;23 2515690X18792838.

Bordoni BB, Marelli F, Morabito B, Castagna R, Sacconi B, Mazzucco P. New proposal to define the fascial system. *Complement Med Res*. 2018a;25(4):257–262.

Bordoni BC, Lintonbon D, Morabito B. Meaning of the solid and liquid fascia to reconsider the model of biotensegrity. *Cureus*. 2018c;10(7):e2922.

Buccellato FR, D'Anca M, Serpente M, Arighi A, Galimberti D. The role of glymphatic system in Alzheimer's and Parkinson's disease pathogenesis. *Biomedicines*. 2022;10(9):2261.

Buchman DD. *The Complete Book of Water Therapy: 500 Ways to Use Our Oldest Natural Medicine*. Dutton; 1977.

Cao TV, Hicks MR, Campbell D, et al. Dosed myofascial release in three-dimensional bioengineered tendons: effects on human fibroblast hyperplasia, hypertrophy, and cytokine secretion. *J Manipulative Physiol Ther*. 2013;36:513.

Cao QW, Peng BG, Wang L, et al. Expert consensus on the diagnosis and treatment of myofascial pain syndrome. *World J Clin Cases*. 2021;9(9):2077–2089. doi:10.12998/wjcc.v9.i9.2077.

Carvalho HC, Machado NCSS, Yáñez-Silva A, et al. Autonomic nerve regulation in joint hypermobility patients with myofascial trigger points by Musculoskeletal Interfiber Counterirritant Stimulation (MICS). *Med Eng Phys*. 2022;109:103903. doi:10.1016/j.medengphy.2022.103903.

Cenaj O, Allison DHR, Imam R, et al. Evidence for continuity of interstitial spaces across tissue and organ boundaries in humans. *Commun Biol*. 2021;4(1):436. doi:10.1038/s42003-021-01962-0. Published 2021 Mar 31.

Chaitow L, Delany J. *The Clinical Application of Neuromuscular Techniques: Volume 1: The Upper Body*. 2nd ed. Churchill Livingstone; 2008.

Chaitow L, Delany J. *The Clinical Application of Neuromuscular Techniques: Volume 2: The Lower Body*. 2nd ed. Churchill Livingstone; 2011.

Chaitow L. *Fascial Dysfunction: Manual Therapy Approaches*. Handspring; 2014:118–119.

Chaitow L. *Hydrotherapy: Water therapy for health and beauty*. Collins & Brown; 2016.

Chaitow L. Workshop notes. *Trigger Point Assessment and Treatment*. Lapeer, MI; 1988 1991, 1992, 1993.

Chandrababu R, Rathinasamy EL, Suresh C, Ramesh J. Effectiveness of reflexology on anxiety of patients undergoing cardiovascular interventional procedures: a systematic review and meta-analysis of randomized controlled trials. *J Adv Nurs*. 2019;75(1):43–53.

Cheatham SW, Lee M, Cain M, Baker R. The efficacy of instrument assisted soft tissue mobilization: a systematic review. *J Can Chiropr Assoc*. 2016;60(3):200.

Checketts AB. *Instrument assisted soft tissue mobilization in the treatment of achilles tendinopathy*. 2018. https://digitalrepository.unm.edu/dpt/142.

Chen PC, Wei L, Huang CY, Chang FH, Lin YN. The effect of massage force on relieving nonspecific low back pain: a randomized controlled trial. *Int J Environ Res Public Health*. 2022;19(20):13191. doi:10.3390/ijerph192013191. Published 2022 Oct 13.

Chikly BJ. Manual techniques addressing the lymphatic system: origins and development. *J Am Osteopath Assoc*. 2005;105:457.

Choi BK, Hwang SH, Kim YI, Singh R, Kwon BS. The hyaluronic acid-rich node and duct system is a structure organized for innate immunity and mediates the local inflammation. *Cytokine*. 2019;113:74–82. 201p.

Choi IR, Lee JH. Effect of kinesiology tape application direction on quadriceps strength. *Medicine (Baltimore)*. 2018a;97(24):e11038.

Choi IR, Lee JH. The effect of the application direction of the kinesiology tape on the strength of fatigued quadriceps muscles in athletes. *Res Sports Med*. 2018b:1–10.

Chu ECP, Wong AYL, Sim P, Krüger F. Exploring scraping therapy: contemporary views on an ancient healing - a review. *J Family Med Prim Care*. 2021;10(8):2757–2762.

Cimino SR, Beaudette SM, Brown SH. Kinesio taping influences the mechanical behaviour of the skin of the low back: a possible pathway for functionally relevant effects. *J Biomech*. 2018;67:150–156.

Cunningham S. *Cunningham's Encyclopedia of Crystal, Gem and Metal Magic*. Llewellyn Publications; 2002.

Cyriax J, Coldham M. *The Textbook of Orthopaedic Medicine Treatment by Manipulation Massage and Injection*. 11th ed. Vol. 2. Bailliere Tindall; 1984.

Das S, Kulkarni P. Updated review on overview of dry needling. Int J Health Sci (IJHS). Published online 2022:5127-5140. doi:10.53730/ijhs.v6ns1.5991.

de Almeida TCC, Paes V, Soares M, de Freitas Fonseca G, Lima M, Silva JG. Acute effect of different duration times of application of myofascial release on quadriceps femoris strength: a randomized clinical trial. *J Bodyw Mov Ther*. 2021;27:233–238.

de Freitas FS, Brown LE, Gomes WA, Behm DG, Marchetti PH. NO effect of kinesiology tape on passive tension, strength or quadriceps muscle activation of during maximal voluntary isometric contractions in resistance trained men. *Int J Sports Phys Ther*. 2018;13(4):661.

Della Posta D, Branca JJV, Guarnieri G, Veltro C, Pacini A, Paternostro F. Modularity of the human musculoskeletal system: the correlation between functional structures by computer tools analysis. *Life (Basel)*. 2022;12(8):1186.

Denneny D, Frawley HC, Petersen K, et al. Trigger Point Manual Therapy for the Treatment of Chronic Noncancer Pain in Adults: A Systematic Review and Meta-analysis. *Arch Phys Med Rehabil*. 2019;100(3):562–577. doi:10.1016/j.apmr.2018.06.019.

De Vrieze T, Gebruers N, Nevelsteen I, et al. Manual lymphatic drainage with or without fluoroscopy guidance did not substantially improve the effect of decongestive lymphatic therapy in people with breast cancer-related lymphoedema (EFforT-BCRL trial): a multicentre randomised trial. *J Physiother*. 2022;68(2):110–122. doi:10.1016/j.jphys.2022.03.010.

Dorsher PT. Myofascial referred-pain data provide physiologic evidence of acupuncture meridians. *J Pain*. 2009;10:723.

Dorsher PT, da Silva MAH. Acupuncture's neuroanatomic and neurophysiologic basis. *Longhua Chin Med*. 2022;5:8. doi:10.21037/lcm-21-48.

Dresing K, Fischer AC, Lehmann W, Saul D, Spering C. Perioperative and posttraumatic anti-edematous decongestive device-based negative pressure treatment for anti-edematous swelling treatment of the lower extremity - a prospective quality study. *Int J Burns Trauma*. 2021;11(3):145–155.

Elbarbary M, Sgro A, Goldberg M, Tenenbaum H, Azarpazhooh A. Diagnostic applications of ultrasonography in myofascial trigger points: a scoping review and critical appraisal of literature. *J Diagn Med Sonogr*. 2022;38(6):559–573. doi:10.1177/87564793221102593.

Engebretson J, Wardell DW. Energy-based modalities. *Nurs Clin North Am*. 2007;42:243.

Ercole B, Stecco A, Day JA, Carla S. How much time is required to modify a fascial fibrosis? *J Bodyw Mov Ther*. 2010;14(4):318–325.

Faizan MD, Khan AA. Ergonomic assessment of log bucking operation using a chain saw. In: *Ergonomics for Improved Productivity*. Springer; 2022:87–95.

Fazzino DL, Griffin MT, McNulty RS, et al. Energy healing and pain: a review of the literature. *Holist Nurs Pract*. 2010;24:79.

Fede C, Albertin G, Petrelli L, et al. Expression of the endocannabinoid receptors in human fascial tissue. *Eur J Histochem*. 2016;60(2):2643.

Feinstein D. The energy of energy psychology. *OBM Integr Complement Med*. 2022;7(2):1.

Fernández-de-las-Peñas C, Dommerholt J. International consensus on diagnostic criteria and clinical considerations of myofascial trigger points: a Delphi study. *Pain Med*. 2017;19(1):142–150.

Findley T. Fascia research congress and scientific background; 2009. Retrieved from: http://structuralintegration.net/si_news/2009%20Fascia%20Research%20Congress.pdf

Franklin NC, Ali M, Robinson AT, et al. Massage therapy restores peripheral vascular function after exertion. *Arch Phys Med Rehabil*. 2014;95:1127.

Fu MR, Li Y, Conway C, Masone A, Fang J, Lee C. The effects of exercise-based interventions on fluid overload symptoms in patients with heart failure: a systematic review and meta-analysis. *Biomedicines*. 2022;10(5):1111. doi:10.3390/biomedicines10051111. Published 2022 May 11.

Furhad S, Bokhari AA. Cupping therapy. *StatPearls [Internet]*. StatPearls Publishing; 2022.

Gerwin RD. The taut band and other mysteries of the trigger point: an examination of the mechanisms relevant to the development and maintenance of the trigger point. *J Musculoskelet Pain*. 2008;15(suppl 13):115.

Gerwin R. Trigger point diagnosis: at last, the first word on consensus. *Pain Med*. 2018;19(1):1–2. doi:10.1093/pm/pnx219.

Gomes LR, Leão P. Recent approaches on signal transduction and transmission in acupuncture: a biophysical overview for medical sciences. *J Acupunct Meridian Stud*. 2020;13(1):1–11.

Gott FH, Ly K, Piller N, Mangion A. Negative pressure therapy in the management of lymphedema. *J Lymphedema*. 2018;13:43–48.

Grabowski PJ, Slane LC, Thelen DG, Obermire T, Lee KS. Evidence of generalized muscle stiffness in the presence of latent trigger points within infraspinatus. *Arch J Phys Med Rehabil*. 2018;99(11):2257–2262.

Gunn C. *Reprints on Pain, Acupuncture and Related Subjects*. Seattle: University of Washington; 1992.

Guo Y, Chen B, Wang DQ, et al. Cupping regulates local immunomodulation to activate neural-endocrine-immune worknet. *Complement Ther Clin Pract*. 2017;28:1–3.

Guzmán-Pavón MJ, Cavero-Redondo I, Martínez-Vizcaíno V, Torres-Costoso AI, Reina-Gutiérrez S, Álvarez-Bueno C. Effect of manual therapy interventions on range of motion among individuals with myofascial trigger points: a systematic review and meta-analysis. *Pain Med*. 2022;23(1):137–143.

Harper B, Steinbeck L, Aron A. Fascial manipulation vs. standard physical therapy practice for low back pain diagnoses: a pragmatic study. *J Bodyw Mov Ther*. 2019;23(1):115–121.

Haesler E. Evidence summary: single modality treatment of lymphoedema: manual lymphatic drainage. *Wound Pract Res*. 2016;24(2):116–118.

Hodge LM. Osteopathic lymphatic pump techniques to enhance immunity and treat pneumonia. *Int J Osteopath Med*. 2012;15:13.

Hongmei C, Wang W, Wang W, Zhou X. Kinesiology taping combined with manual lymph drainage reduces postoperative lymphedema related to breast cancer. *Chin J Tissue Eng Res*. 2021;25(14):2247.

Hosp S, Csapo R, Heinrich D, Hasler M, Nachbauer W. Does Kinesiology tape counter exercise-related impairments of balance in the elderly? *Gait Posture*. 2018;62:167–172.

Hou X, Wang X, Griffin L, Liao F, Peters J, Jan YK. Immediate and delayed effects of cupping therapy on reducing neuromuscular fatigue. *Front Bioeng Biotechnol*. 2021;9:678153. Published 2021 Jul 1.

Howard SB, Krishnagiri S. The use of manual edema mobilization for the reduction of persistent edema in the upper limb. *J Hand Ther*. 2001;14(4):291–301.

Huang H-C, Chen K-H, Kuo S-F, Chen I-H. Can foot reflexology be a complementary therapy for sleep disturbances? Evidence appraisal through a meta-analysis of randomized controlled trials. *J Adv Nurs*. 2021;77(4):1683–1697.

Huang TW, Tseng SH, Lin CC, et al. Effects of manual lymphatic drainage on breast cancer-related lymphedema: a systematic review and meta-analysis of randomized controlled trials. *World J Surg Oncol*. 2013;11:15.

Hung BL, Sun CY, Chang NJ, Chang WD. Effects of different kinesio-taping applications for delayed onset muscle soreness after high-intensity interval training exercise: a randomized controlled trial. *Evid Based Complement Alternat Med.* 2021;2021:6676967. doi:10.1155/2021/6676967. Published 2021 Jun 21.

Iannello C, Biller MK. Management of edema using simple manual lymphatic drainage techniques for hand and upper extremity patients. *J Hand Ther.* 2020;33(4):616–619.

Ilkkaya NK, Ustun FE, Sener EB, et al. The effects of music, white noise, and ambient noise on sedation and anxiety in patients under spinal anesthesia during surgery. *J Perianesth Nurs.* 2014;29:418.

Jiang Q, Feng X, Liu D, et al. Pressing intervention promotes the skeletal muscle repair of traumatic myofascial trigger points in rats. *J Pain Res.* 2021;14:3267–3278.

Jain NM, Zore L, Kumar A. Comparison of active release technique and positional release therapy for gastrosoleus trigger point release in recreational runners. *Int J Health Sci Res.* 2020;10(7):35–41.

Jain S, Mills PJ. Biofield therapies: helpful or full of hype? A best evidence synthesis. *Int J Behav Med.* 2010;17:1.

Jan YK, Hou X, He X, Guo C, Jain S, Bleakney A. Using elastographic ultrasound to assess the effect of cupping size of cupping therapy on stiffness of triceps muscle. *Am J Phys Med Rehabil.* 2021;100(7):694–699.

Jeffs E, Ream E, Taylor C, Bick D. Clinical effectiveness of decongestive treatments on excess arm volume and patient-centered outcomes in women with early breast cancer-related arm lymphedema: a systematic review. *JBI Database System Rev Implement Rep.* 2018;16(2):453.

Jing Y, Liu S, Pan C, Jian Y, Wang M, Ni B. The effects of foot reflexology on vital signs: a meta-analysis of randomized controlled trials. *Evid Based Complement Alternat Med.* 2022;2022:4182420.

Johari H. *Ayurvedic Massage: Traditional Indian Techniques for Balancing Body and Mind.* Healing Arts Press; 1996.

Joicy MS, Shetty GB, Sujatha KJ, Shetty P. Effect of neutral immersion bath with epsom salt on hypertensive individuals. *Indian J Integr Med.* 2021:39–43.

Kablan N, Alaca N, Tatar Y. Comparison of the immediate effect of petrissage massage and manual lymph drainage following exercise on biomechanical and viscoelastic properties of the rectus femoris muscle in women. *J Sport Rehabil.* 2021;30(5):725–730.

Kang KA, Maldonado C, Perez-Aradia G, et al. Primo vascular system and its potential role in cancer metastasis. In: Oxygen Transport to Tissue. Vol. XXXV. New York: Springer; 2013:289–296.

Kasawara KT, Mapa JMR, Ferreira V, et al. Effects of Kinesio Taping on breast cancer-related lymphedema: a meta-analysis in clinical trials. *Physiother Theory Pract.* 2018;34(5):337–345.

Kendrová L, Mikuľáková W, Urbanová K, Andraščíková Š, Žultáková S, Takáč P, Peresta Y. Comprehensive decongestive therapy as a treatment for secondary lymphedema of the lower extremity and quality of life of women after gynecological cancer surgery. *Med Sci Monit.* 2020;26:e924071.

Kim TH, Jeon WY, Ji Y, Park EJ, Yoon DS, Lee NH, Park SM, et al. Electricity auto-generating skin patch promotes wound healing process by activation of mechanosensitive ion channels. *Biomaterials.* 2021;275:120948.

Kim KJ, Kim JH. Comparison of the immediate effects of kinesio taping on the dynamic balance of stable ankle and functional ankle instability among young adults in their twenties: a preliminary study. *J Korean Soc Integr Med.* 2022;10(1):73–79.

Kim J, Sung DJ, Lee J. Therapeutic effectiveness of instrument-assisted soft tissue mobilization for soft tissue injury: mechanisms and practical application. *J Exerc Rehabil.* 2017;13(1):12.

Kim HG. Achievements of PVS (Primo Vascular System) research from a historical perspective. *J Acupunct Meridian Stud.* 2022;15(1):50–60).

Kim TH, Kim KH, Choi JY, Lee MS. Adverse events related to cupping therapy in studies conducted in Korea: a systematic review. *Eur J Integr Med.* 2014;6(4):434–440.

Kirchgesner T, Demondion X, Stoenoiu M, et al. Fasciae of the musculoskeletal system: normal anatomy and MR patterns of involvement in autoimmune diseases. *Insights Imaging.* 2018:1–11.

Klingler W, Schleip MA, Zorn A. Structural integration: European fascia research project report. *J Rolf Institute.* December; 2004. Retrieved from: http://www.fasciaresearch.de/ProjectInterimReport04.pdf.

Klyne DM, Barbe MF, James G, Hodges PW. Does the interaction between local and systemic inflammation provide a link from psychology and lifestyle to tissue health in musculoskeletal conditions? *Int J Mol Sci.* 2021;22(14):7299.

Koelmeyer LA, Thompson BM, Mackie H, Blackwell R, Heydon-White A, Moloney E, Gaitatzis K, Boyages J, Suami H. Personalizing conservative lymphedema management using indocyanine green-guided manual lymphatic drainage. *Lymphat Res Biol.* 2021;19(1).

Kong Y, Yu X, Peng G, Wang F, Yin Y. Interstitial fluid flows along perivascular and adventitial clearances around neurovascular bundles. *J Funct Biomater.* 2022;13(4):172.

Konrad A, Glashüttner C, Reiner MM, Bernsteiner D, Tilp M. The acute effects of a percussive massage treatment with a hypervolt device on plantar flexor muscles' range of motion and performance. *J Sports Sci Med.* 2020;19(4):690.

Koul R, Dufan T, Russell C, et al. Efficacy of complete decongestive therapy and manual lymphatic drainage on treatment-related lymphedema in breast cancer. *Int J Radiat Oncol Biol Phys.* 2007;67:841.

Kovich F. A new definition of an acupuncture meridian. *J Acupunct Meridian Stud.* 2019;12(1):37–41.

Krafft HS, Raak CK, Martin DD. Hydrotherapeutic heat application as support in febrile patients: a scoping review. *J Integr Complement Med.* 2022.

Kreighbaum E, Barthels KM. *Biomechanics: A Qualitative Approach for Studying Human Movement.* 4th ed. New York: Benjamin Cummings; 1995.

Kumka M, Bonar J. Fascia: a morphological description and classification system based on a literature review. *J Canadian Chiropr Assoc.* 2012;56:179.

Kuo PH, Stuehm C, Squire S, Johnson K. Meningeal lymphatic vessel flow runs countercurrent to venous flow in the superior sagittal sinus of the human brain. *Tomography.* 2018;4(3):99.

Kwong EH, Findley TW. Fascia—Current knowledge and future directions in physiatry: narrative review. *J Rehabil Res Dev.* 2014;51(6).

Laimi K, Mäkilä A, Bärlund E, et al. Effectiveness of myofascial release in treatment of chronic musculoskeletal pain: a systematic review. *Clin Rehabil.* 2018;32(4):440–450.

Lampinen R, Lee JQ, Leano J, Miaskowski C, Mastick J, Brinker L, Topp K, Smoot B. Treatment of breast cancer-related lymphedema using negative pressure massage: a pilot randomized controlled trial. *Arch Phys Med Rehabil.* 2021 Aug;102(8):1465–1472.e2. doi:10.1016/j.apmr.2021.03.022 Epub 2021 Apr 16. PMID: 33872573.

Langevin HM, Konofagou EE, Badger GJ, et al. Tissue displacements during acupuncture using ultrasound elastography techniques. *World Fed Ultrasound Med Biol.* 2004. Retrieved from: http://www.med.uvm.edu/neurology/TB1+BL.asp?SiteAreaID=518.

Langevin HM. Connective tissue: a body-wide signaling network? *Med Hypotheses.* 2006;66:1074.

Langevin HM. Fascia mobility, proprioception, and myofascial pain. *Life.* 2021;11(7):668.

Lederman E. *Fundamentals of Manual Therapy: Physiology, Neurology, and Psychology.* 2nd ed. New York: Churchill Livingstone; 2005.

Lee BS, Lee BC, Park JE, et al. Primo vascular system in human umbilical cord and placenta. *J Acupunct Meridian Stud.* 2014;7:291.

Lerman M, Gaebler JA, Hoy S, et al. Health and economic benefits of advanced pneumatic compression devices in patients with phlebolymphedema. *J Vasc Surg.* 2018.

Leutualy V, Madiuw D, Tasijawa FA, Sumah DF, Manuhutu F, Maelissa S. Non-pharmacology interventions on pain in critically ill patient: a scoping review. *Open Access Maced J Med Sci.* 2022;10:182–189 no. F.

Li JQ, Guo W, Sun ZG, et al. Cupping therapy for treating knee osteoarthritis: the evidence from systematic review and meta-analysis. *Complement Ther Clin Pract.* 2017;28:152–160.

Li P, Wei Z, Zeng Z, Wang L. Acute effect of kinesio tape on postural control in individuals with functional ankle instability following ankle muscle fatigue. *Front Physiol.* 2022:1785.

Li Q, Becker B, Wernicke J, et al. Foot massage evokes oxytocin release and activation of orbitofrontal cortex and superior temporal sulcus. *Psychoneuroendocrinology.* 2019;101:193–203.

Li X, Zhou X, Howe Liu NC, et al. Effects of elastic therapeutic taping on knee osteoarthritis: a systematic review and meta-analysis. *Aging dis.* 2018;9(2):296.

Liang M, Chen Q, Peng K, Deng L, He L, Hou Y, Zhang Y, Guo J, Mei Z, Li L. Manual lymphatic drainage for lymphedema in patients after breast cancer surgery: A systematic review and meta-analysis of randomized controlled trials. *Medicine (Baltimore).* 2020;99(49):e23192.

Liang X, Wu S, Li K, et al. The effects of reflexology on symptoms in pregnancy: A systematic review of randomized controlled trials. *Heliyon.* 2023;e18442.

Lietz-Kijak D, Kijak E, Krajczy M, Bogacz K, Łuniewski J, Szczegielniak J. The impact of the use of kinesio taping method on the reduction of swelling in patients after orthognathic surgery: a pilot study. *Med Sci Monit.* 2018;24:3736–3743.

Lim CJ, Yoo JH, Kim Y, et al. Gross morphological features of the organ surface primo-vascular system revealed by Hemacolor staining. *Evid Based Compl Altern Med.* 2013;12. Retrieved from: http://www.hindawi.com/journals/ecam/2013/350815/.

Lindenmann A, Uhl M, Gwosch T, Matthiesen S. The influence of human interaction on the vibration of hand-held human-machine systems–The effect of body posture, feed force, and gripping forces on the vibration of hammer drills. *Appl Ergon.* 2021;95:103430.

Lin YC, Guo YR, Miyagi A, Levring J, MacKinnon R, Scheuring S. Force-induced conformational changes in PIEZO1. *Nature.* 2019;573(7773):230–234.

Lupowitz L. Vibration therapy–a clinical commentary. *Int J Sports Phys Ther.* 2022;17(6):984–987.

Liu X, Wang Y, Wu Z. Infrared thermal imaging-based skin temperature response during cupping at two different negative pressures. *Sci Rep.* 2022;12(1):1–12.

Liu J, Di C, Yin X. Effect of manual lymphatic drainage combined with vacuum sealing drainage on axillary web syndrome caused by breast cancer surgery. *Int Wound J.* 2023;20(1):183–190.

Liu QG, Huang QM, Liu L, Nguyen TT. Structural and functional abnormalities of motor endplates in rat skeletal model of myofascial trigger spots. *Neurosci Lett.* 2019;711:134417.

Lizarraga-Valderrama LR. Effects of essential oils on central nervous system: focus on mental health. *Phytother Res.* 2021;35(2):657–679.

Lu W, Li J, Tian Y, Lu X. Effect of ischemic compression on myofascial pain syndrome: a systematic review and meta-analysis. *Chiropr Man Ther.* 2022;30(1):1–11.

Ma SY, Wang Y, Xu JQ, Zheng L. Cupping therapy for treating ankylosing spondylitis: the evidence from systematic review and meta-analysis. *Complement Ther Clin Pract.* 2018;32:187–194.

Malhotra D, Sharma S, Chachra A, Dhingra M, Alghadir AH, Nuhmani S, Jaleel G, et al. The time-based effects of kinesio taping on acute-onset muscle soreness and calf muscle extensibility among endurance athletes: a randomized cross-over trial. *J Clin Med.* 2022;11(20):5996.

Manjuladevi T, Mooventhan A, Manjunath NK. Immediate effect of hot chest pack on cardio-respiratory functions in healthy volunteers: a randomized cross-over study. *Adv Integr Med.* 2018;5(2):63–68.

Martin JS, Martin AM, Mumford PW, Salom LP, Moore AN, Pascoe DD. Unilateral application of an external pneumatic compression therapy improves skin blood flow and vascular reactivity bilaterally. *PeerJ.* 2018;6:e4878.

Masunaga S, Ohashi W. *Zen Shiatsu: How to Harmonize Yin and Yang for Better Health.* New York: Japan Publications; 1977.

Matos LC, Machado JP, Monteiro FJ, Greten HJ. Perspectives, measurability and effects of non-contact biofield-based practices: a narrative review of quantitative research. *Int J Environ Res Public Health.* 2021;18(12):6397.

Matsuda Y, Nakabayashi M, Suzuki T, Zhang S, Ichinose M, Ono Y. Evaluation of local skeletal muscle blood flow in manipulative therapy by diffuse correlation spectroscopy. *Front Bioeng Biotechnol.* 2021;9.

McAphee D, Bagwell M, Falsone S. Dry needling: a clinical commentary. *Int J Sports Phys Ther.* 2022;17(4):551.

McCraty R, Abdulgader AA. Consciousness, the human heart and the global energetic field environment. *Cardiol Vasc Res.* 2021;5(1):1–19.

Meltzer KR, Standley PR. Modeled repetitive motion strain and indirect osteopathic manipulative techniques in regulation of human fibroblast proliferation and interleukin secretion. *J Am Osteopath Assoc.* 2007;107:527.

Meng F, Ge HY, Wang YH, Yue SW. Myelinated afferents are involved in pathology of the spontaneous electrical activity and mechanical hyperalgesia of myofascial trigger spots in rats. *Evid. Based Complement. Altern. Med.* 2015;2015:404971.

Menon NA. Myofascial Pain: A Review of Diagnosis and Treatment. *Indian Journal of Physical Medicine & Rehabilitation.* 2023; 33(1):2–7.

Mohamed AA, Zhang X, Jan Y-K. Evidence-based and adverse-effects analyses of cupping therapy in musculoskeletal and sports rehabilitation: a systematic and evidence-based review. *J Back and Musculoskelet Rehabil.* 2022:1–17 Preprint.

Mohammed AAE, Ayed MMA, El-Sayed Ali A. Effect of foot massage on physiological indicators, fatigue, and pain among children undergoing chemotherapy. *Egypt J Health Care.* 2022;13(4)26–39.

Monteiro RL, Rocha C, Ferreira HT, Silva HN. Lower limb massage in humans increases local perfusion and impacts systemic hemodynamics. *J Appl Physiol.* 2020;128(5):1217–1226.

Mooventhan A, Nivethitha L. Scientific evidence-based effects of hydrotherapy on various systems of the body. *N Am J Med Sci.* 2014;6:199.

Moraska AF, Hickner RC, Rzasa-Lynn R, Shah JP, Hebert JR, Kohrt WM. Increase in lactate without change in nutritive blood flow or glucose at active trigger points following massage: a randomized clinical trial. *Arch Phys Med Rehabil.* 2018;99(11)2151–2159.

Mosti G, Cavezzi A. Compression therapy in lymphedema: between past and recent scientific data. *Phlebology.* 2019;34(8):515–522.

Müller M, Klingberg K, Wertli MM, Carreira H. Manual lymphatic drainage and quality of life in patients with lymphoedema and mixed oedema: a systematic review of randomised controlled trials. *Qual Life Res.* 2018;27:1403–1414.

Miller LK, Jerosch-Herold SL. Effectiveness of edema management techniques for subacute hand edema: a systematic review. *J Hand Ther.* 2017;30(4):432–446.

Nazari G, Bobos P, Ze Lu S, et al. Effectiveness of instrument-assisted soft tissue mobilization for the management of upper body, lower body, and spinal conditions. An updated systematic review with meta-analyses. *Disabil Rehabil.* 2023;45(10):1608–1618.

Nelson NL. Massage therapy: understanding the mechanisms of action on blood pressure. A scoping review. *J Am Soc Hypertens.* 2015;9(10):785–793.

Nielsen A. *Gua sha-E-Book: A Traditional Technique for Modern Practice.* Elsevier Health Sciences; 2014.

Nunes GS, Vargas VZ, Wageck B, dos Santos Hauphental DP, da Luz CM, de Noronha M. Kinesio Taping does not decrease swelling in acute, lateral ankle sprain of athletes: a randomised trial. *J Physiother.* 2015;61(1):28–33.

Nunes GS, Feldkircher JM, Tessarin BM, Bender PU, Medeiros da Luz C, de Noronha M. Kinesio taping does not improve ankle functional or performance in people with or without ankle injuries: systematic review and meta-analysis. *Clin Rehabil.* 2021;35(2):182–199.

Ohashi W. *Do-it-Yourself Shiatsu: How to Perform the Ancient Japanese Art of Acupuncture Without Needles.* New York: Penguin Books; 1993.

Oschman JL. Charge transfer in the living matrix. *J Bodyw Mov Ther.* 2009;13:215.

Oschman JL. Perspective: assume a spherical cow—the role of free or mobile electrons in bodywork, energetic and movement therapies. *J Bodyw Mov Ther.* 2008;12:40.

Ouyang JH, Chang KH, Hsu WY, Cho YT, Liou TH, Lin YN. Non-elastic taping, but not elastic taping, provides benefits for patients with knee osteoarthritis: systemic review and meta-analysis. *Clin Rehabil.* 2018;32(1):3–17.

Page P. Making the case for modalities: the need for critical thinking in practice. *Int J Sports Phys Ther.* 2021;16(5):28326.

Panigrahy D, Gilligan MM, Serhan CN, Kashfi K. Resolution of inflammation: an organizing principle in biology and medicine. *Pharmacol Ther.* 2021;227:107879.

Paolucci T, Agostini F, Bernetti A, Paoloni M, Mangone M, Santilli V, Pezzi L, Bellomo RG, Saggini R. Integration of focal vibration and intra-articular oxygen–ozone therapy in rehabilitation of painful knee osteoarthritis. *J Int Med Res.* 2021;49(2):0300060520986705.

Parker R, Higgins Z, Mlombile ZN, Mohr MJ, Wagner TL. The effects of warm water immersion on blood pressure, heart rate and heart rate variability in people with chronic fatigue syndrome. *S Afr J Physiother.* 2018;74(1):1–7.

Perreault T, Ball A, Dommerholt J, Theiss R, Fernández-de-las-Peñas C, Butts R. Intramuscular Electrical Stimulation to Trigger Points: Insights into Mechanisms and Clinical Applications—A Scoping Review. *J Clin Med.* 2022;11(20):6039.

Pitsillides A, Stasinopoulos D. Cyriax friction massage—suggestions for improvements. *Medicina (Mex).* 2019;55(5):185.

Plaut S. Scoping review and interpretation of myofascial pain/fibromyalgia syndrome: an attempt to assemble a medical puzzle. *PLoS One.* 2022;17(2):e0263087.

Price S, Price L. *Aromatherapy for Health Professionals.* London: Churchill Livingstone; 2006.

Quintner JL, Bove GM, Cohen ML. A critical evaluation of the trigger point phenomenon. *Rheumatology (Oxford).* 2014;54(3):392–399.

Rafferty P, McMahon K, Arrigale M, Carpenter A. Cyrotherapy reduces macrophage infiltration and inflammatory mediators following muscle injury. *FASEB J.* 2018;32(suppl 1):588–629.

Ramaswamy S, Wodehouse T. Conditioned pain modulation—a comprehensive review. *Neurophysiol Clin.* 2021;51(3):197–208.

Rawal R, Read J, Chesterman E, Walters K, Schrag A, Ambler G, Armstrong M. The effectiveness of aromatherapy in neurodegenerative disorders: a systematic review and meta-analysis. *Neurodegener Dis Manag.* 2022;12(5):253–265.

Remvig L, Ellis RM, Patijn J. Myofascial release: an evidence-based treatment approach? *Int Musculoskel Med.* 2008;30:29.

Ridone P, Vassalli M, Martinac B. Piezo1 mechanosensitive channels: what are they and why are they important. *Biophys Rev.* 2019;11(5):795–805.

Río-González Á, Cerezo-Téllez E, Gala-Guirao C, González-Fernández L, Conde RD-M, de la Cueva-Reguera M, Guitérrez-Ortega C. Effects of different neck manual lymphatic drainage maneuvers on the nervous, cardiovascular, respiratory and musculoskeletal systems in healthy students. *J Clin Med.* 2020;9(12):4062.

Ribeiro DC, Belgrave A, Naden A, Fang H, Matthews P, Parshottam S. The prevalence of myofascial trigger points in neck and shoulder-related disorders: a systematic review of the literature. *BMC Musculoskelet Disord.* 2018;19(1):252.

Rivard R, Crespin D, Finch M, et al. Effectiveness of therapeutic massage in conjunction with aromatherapy for pain and anxiety relief of hospitalized patients. *J Altern Compl Med.* 2014;20:A125.

Rocha C, Silva H, Frazão I, Castelão V, Ferreira H, Rodrigues LM. Exploring the impact of massage on peripheral microcirculation with the wavelet transform. *J Vasc Res.* 2017;54:34 Allschwilerstrasse 10, CH-4009 Basel, Switzerland: Karger.

Rockson SG. Intermittent pneumatic compression therapy. In: *Lymphedema.* Cham: Springer; 2018:443–448.

Rodríguez-Jiménez J, Ortega-Santiago R, Bonilla-Barba L, Falla D, Fernández-de-Las-Peñas C, Florencio LL. Immediate effects of dry needing or manual pressure release of upper trapezius trigger points on muscle activity during the craniocervical flexion test in people with chronic neck pain: a randomized clinical trial. *Pain Med.* 2022.

Roman M, Chaudhry H, Bukiet B. Mathematical analysis of the flow of hyaluronic acid around fascia during manual therapy motions. *J Am Osteopath Assoc.* 2013;113:600.

Sayari S, Nobahar M, Ghorbani R. Effect of foot reflexology on chest pain and anxiety in patients with acute myocardial infarction: a double blind randomized clinical trial. *Complement Ther Clin Pract.* 2021;42:101296.

Schleip R, Findley TW, Chaitow L, et al. *Fascia: The Tensional Network of the Human Body: The Science and Clinical Applications in Manual and Movement Therapy.* Edinbourgh: Elsevier Health Sciences; 2013.

Schleip R. An interview with Prof. Dr. Med J. Staubesand, Rolf Lines. 1998;26:35. Retrieved from: http://www.somatics.de/somatics-06.html.

Schnaubelt K. *Advanced Aromatherapy: The Science of Essential Oil Therapy.* Rochester, VT: Healing Arts Press; 1998.

Schroeder J, Wilke J, Hollander K. Effects of foam rolling duration on tissue stiffness and perfusion: a randomized cross-over trial. *J Sports Sci Med.* 2021;20(4):626.

SevgiÜnal Aslan K, Çetinkaya F. The effects of Reiki and hand massage on pain and fatigue in patients with rheumatoid arthritis. Explore (NY). 2023;19(2):251–255. doi:10.1016/j.explore.2022.06.006.

Shah JP, Danoff JV, Desai MJ, et al. Biochemicals associated with pain and inflammation are elevated in sites near to and remote from active myofascial trigger points. *Arch Phys Med Rehabil.* 2008;89:16.

Shah M, Murad W, Rehman Ur N, Halim SA, Ahmed M, Rehman H, Zahoor M, Mubin S, Khan A, Nassan MA, Batiha GE, Al-Harrasi A. Biomedical applications of scutellaria edelbergii Rech. F.: in vitro and in vivo approach. *Molecules.* 2021;26(12):3740. https://doi.org/10.3390/molecules26123740.

Sharkey J. Fascia and tensegrity the quintessence of a unified systems conception. *Int J Anat Appl Physiol.* 2021;7(02):174–178.

Shin JY, Ji JO, Choi DW, et al. Expression of genes in primo-vasculature floating in lymphatic endothelium under lipopolysaccharide and acupuncture electric stimulation. *J Acupunct Meridian Stud.* 2019:3–10.

Shin S. Effectiveness of instrument assisted soft tissue mobilization on range of motion: a systematic review and meta-analysis. *Ann Med Health Sci Res.* 2022;12:8–11.

Silva H, Ferreira HA, da Silva HP, Rodrigues LM. The venoarteriolar reflex significantly reduces contralateral perfusion as part of the lower limb circulatory homeostasis in vivo. *Front Physiol.* 2018;9: 123.

Simon C, Zidi M. Regional variation in the mechanical properties of the skeletal muscle. *J Mech Behav Biomed Mater.* 2022;136:105521.

Singh B, Singh JP, Kaur A, Yadav MP. Insights into the chemical composition and bioactivities of citrus peel essential oils. *Food Res Int.* 2021;143:110231.

Ślaga J, Gizińska M, Rutkowski R, Rąglewska P, Balkó Š, Straburzyńska-Lupa ANNA. Using hydrotherapy at different temperatures for promoting recovery in professional athletes. *Trends Sport Sci.* 2018;2(25):57–67.

Smit AA. *Movement and the Matrix: The Importance of Biomechanical Signals in Matrix Remodeling. Baden-Baden.* Germany: Verlegt Durch: International Academy for Homotoxicology; 2008.

So PS, Jiang Y, Qin Y. Energy-based modalities. *Nurs Clin North Am.* 2007;42:243.

Soh KS, Kang KA, Ryu YH. 50 years of Bong-Han theory and 10 years of primo vascular system. *Evid Based Compl Altern Med.* 2013;2013:587827. Retrieved from: http://www.hindawi.com/journals/ecam/2013/587827.

Standley PR, Meltzer K. In vitro modeling of repetitive motion strain and manual medicine treatments: potential roles for pro- and anti-inflammatory cytokines. *J Bodyw Mov Ther.* 2008;12:201.

Stecco A, Lorenza B, Chiara GF, Carla S, Carmelo P. The Effect of Mechanical Stress on Hyaluronan Fragments' Inflammatory Cascade: Clinical Implications. Life. 2023;13(12):2277.

Stecco L, Stecco C. *Fascial Manipulation for Internal Dysfunctions.* Padua, Italy: Piccin; 2014:33–43.

Stecco L, Stecco C. *Fascial Manipulation. Practical Part.* Padua, Italy: Piccin; 2009:56–65.

Stecco L. *Fascial Manipulation for Musculoskeletal Pain.* Padova Itilay: Piccin; 2004.

Stecco C, Fede C, Macchi V, et al. The fasciacytes: a new cell devoted to fascial gliding regulation. *Clin Anat.* 2018;31(5):667–676.

Stefanov M. Primo vascular system: before the past, bizarre present and peek after the future. *J Acupunct Meridian Stud.* 2022;15(1):61–73.

Sujatha KJ, Vasant V, Shetty P: Comparative study on naturopathic treatments cold and hot spinal bath on autonomic and respiratory variables in healthy volunteers. 2018;5(7) Iaetsd journal for advanced research in applied sciences

Swanson RL. Biotensegrity: a unifying theory of biological architecture with applications to osteopathic practice, education, and research—a review and analysis. *J Am Osteopath Assoc.* 2013;113:34.

Szirmai I. How does the brain create rhythms? *Ideggyogy Sz.* 2010;63:13.

Tamartash H, Bahrpeyma F. Comparative effect of lumbar myofascial release with electrotherapy on the elastic modulus of lumbar fascia and pain in patients with non-specific low back pain. *J Bodyw Mov Ther.* 2022;29:174–179.

Tappan F, Benjamin P. *Tappan's Handbook of Healing Massage Techniques: Classic, Holistic, and Emerging Methods.* 4th ed. New York: Appleton & Lange; 2004.

Tavano A, Maess B, Poeppel D, Schröger E. Neural entrainment via perceptual inferences. *Eur J Neurosci.* 2022;55(11-12):3277–3287.

Tessari M, Tisato V, Rimondi E, Zamboni P, Malagoni AM. Effects of intermittent pneumatic compression treatment on clinical outcomes and biochemical markers in patients at low mobility with lower limb edema. *J Vasc Surg Venous Lymphat Disord.* 2018;6(4):500–510.

Thompson B, Gaitatzis K, de Jonge XJ, Blackwell R, Koelmeyer LA. Manual lymphatic drainage treatment for lymphedema: a systematic review of the literature. *J Cancer Surviv.* 2021;15(2):244–258.

Tick H, Nielsen A, Pelletier KR, et al. Evidence-based nonpharmacologic strategies for comprehensive pain care: the consortium pain task force white paper; 2018.

Tissarand R, Balacs T. *Essential Oil Safety.* New York: Churchill Livingstone; 1995.

Tomchuk D, Anderson BE. Biotensegrity is needed in athletic training professional education. *Athl Train Educ J.* 2021;16(2):150–158.

Travell JG, Simons DGMyofascial Pain and Dysfunction: The Trigger Point ManualVol. 2. Baltimore: Williams & Wilkins; 1999.

Tremback-Ball A, Harding R, Heffner K, Zimmerman A. The efficacy of kinesiology taping in the treatment of women with post–mastectomy lymphedema: a systematic review. *J Womens Health Phys Therap.* 2018;42(2):94–103.

Ugwoke CK, Cvetko E, Umek N. Pathophysiological and therapeutic roles of fascial hyaluronan in obesity-related myofascial disease. *Int J Mol Sci.* 2022;23(19):11843.

Uzunkulaoğlu A, Aytekin MG, Ay S, Ergin S. The effectiveness of Kinesio taping on pain and clinical features in chronic non-specific low back pain: a randomized controlled clinical trial. *Turk J Phys Med Rehabil.* 2018;64(2):126–132.

Van Daele U, Meirte J, Anthonissen M, Vanhullebusch T, Maertens K, Demuynck L, Moortgat P. Mechanomodulation: physical treatment modalities employ mechanotransduction to improve scarring. *Eur Burn J.* 2022;3(2):241–255.

Van Kanegan G, Worley J. Complementary alternative and integrative treatment for substance use disorders. *J Psychosoc Nurs Ment Health Serv.* 2018;56(6):16–21.

Veith I, Rose K. *The Yellow Emperor's Classic of Internal Medicine.* Berkeley: University of California Press; 2002.

Vihlborg P, Pettersson H, Makdoumi K, Wikström S, Bryngelsson L, Selander J, Graff P. Carpal tunnel syndrome and hand-arm vibration:

a swedish national registry case–control study. *J Occup Environ Med.* 2022;64(3):197.
Walsh J, Walsh T, Heazlewood IT, et al. Growth in public interest and scientific research on kinesiology taping. *Inter J Sci Cult Sport.* 2018;6(3):389–398.
Wahbeh H, Speirn P, Yount G. Extended perception corroboration: a pilot study with energy medicine practitioners. *PsyArXiv.* 2022. https://noetic.org/publication/energy-medicine/.
Wan Q-Q, Qin W-P, Ma Y-X, Shen M-J, Li J, Zhang Z-B, Chen J-H, Tay FR, Niu L-N, Jiao K. Crosstalk between bone and nerves within bone. *Adv Sci.* 2021;8(7):2003390.
Wanchai A, Armer JM. Manual lymphedema drainage for reducing risk for and managing breast cancer—related lymphedema after breast surgery: a systematic review. *Nurs Womens Health.* 2021;25(5):377–383.
Wang SM, Kulkarni L, Dolev J, et al. Music and preoperative anxiety: a randomized, controlled study. *Anesth Analg.* 2002;94:1489. Retrieved from: http://www.medscape.com/medline/abstract/12032013.
Wang CK, Fang YHD, Lin LC, et al. Magnetic resonance elastography in the assessment of acute effects of kinesio taping on lumbar paraspinal muscles. *J Magn Reson Imaging.* 2019;49(4):1039–1045.
Wang Y, Gu Y, Chen J, et al. Kinesio taping is superior to other taping methods in ankle functional performance improvement: a systematic review and meta-analysis. *Clin Rehabil.* 2018;32(11):1472–1481.
Whatley J, Perkins J, Samuel C. Reflexology: exploring the mechanism of action. *Complement Ther Clin Pract.* 2022;48:101606.
Wheatley BB. Investigating passive muscle mechanics with biaxial stretch. *Front Physiol.* 2020;11:1021.
Wiseman N, Feng Y. *A Practical Dictionary of Chinese Medicine.* Brookline, MA: Harcourt; 1997.
Wu JJ, Cui Y, Yang YS, et al. Modulatory effects of aromatherapy massage intervention on electroencephalogram, psychological assessments, salivary cortisol and plasma brain-derived neurotrophic factor. *Compl Ther Med.* 2014;22:456.
Wu Z, Kong L, Zhang Q. Research progress of music therapy on gait intervention in patients with Parkinson's disease. *Int J Environ Res Public Health.* 2022;19(15):9568.
Wu Z, Wang Y, Ye X, Chen Z, Zhou R, Ye Z, Huang J, Zhu Y, Chen G, Xu X. Myofascial release for chronic low back pain: a systematic review and meta-analysis. *Front Med.* 2021;8:697986.
Yao S, Hassani J, Gagne M, et al. Osteopathic manipulative treatment as a useful adjunctive tool for pneumonia. *J Vis Exp.* 2014;87:e50687. http://dx.doi.org/10.3791/50687.
Yılar Erkek Z, Aktas S. The effect of foot reflexology on the anxiety levels of women in labor. *J Altern Complement Med.* 2018;24(4):352–360.
Yong J-H, Lim J-S, Moon I-Y, Yi C-H. Effects of kinesio taping on edema control in patients with musculoskeletal injuries: a literature review. *Phys Ther Korea.* 2022;29(3):171–179.
Yu HZ, Rose K. *Who can Ride the Dragon?* Brookline, MA: Harcourt; 1999.
Yu S, Su H, Lu J, Zhao F, Jiang F. Combined T2 mapping and diffusion tensor imaging: a sensitive tool to assess myofascial trigger points in a rat model. *J Pain Res.* 2021;14:1721.
Yuen JWM, Tsang WWM, Tse SHM, et al. The effects of Gua sha on symptoms and inflammatory biomarkers associated with chronic low back pain: A randomized active-controlled crossover pilot study in elderly. *Complement Ther Med.* 2017;32:25–32.
Zasadzka E, Trzmiel T, Kleczewska M, Pawlaczyk M. Comparison of the effectiveness of complex decongestive therapy and compression bandaging as a method of treatment of lymphedema in the elderly. *Clin Interv Aging.* 2018;13:929.
Zügel M, Maganaris CN, Wilke J, et al. Fascial tissue research in sports medicine: from molecules to tissue adaptation, injury and diagnostics. *Br J Sports Med.* 2018;52(23):1497.

MULTIPLE-CHOICE QUESTIONS FOR DISCUSSION AND REVIEW

The answers, with rationales, can be found on the Evolve site.

Use these questions to stimulate discussion and dialog. You have to understand the meaning of the words in the question and possible answers. Each question provides ability to review terminology, practice critical thinking skills and improve multiple-choice test-taking skills. Answers and rationales are on the EVOLVE site. It is just as important to know why the wrong answers are wrong as why the correct answer is correct.

1. An element added to the massage session but is not an essential aspect of massage therapy is called an____?
   a. Adjunct
   b. Implement
   c. Adaptation
   d. Infusion
2. Hydrotherapy applications to manage pain are called ______.
   a. Analgesic
   b. Antipyretic
   c. Antispasmodic
   d. Antiedemic
3. The secondary effect of a local cold application is ______.
   a. Sedative
   b. Increased localized circulation
   c. Diaphoretic
   d. Decreased systemic circulation
4. Reflexology can be beneficial because ______.
   a. The complex structure of the foot is highly innervated and sensitive to changes in pressure and position, making it highly responsive to massage manipulation
   b. The flexor withdrawal mechanism of the foot is inhibited with pressure to the foot, and this inhibits neural activity in the dorsal horn of the spinal cord
   c. The specific mapped areas of reflex activity in the foot to organs have a direct relationship to visceral/cutaneous responses
   d. Stimulation of the zone therapy points on the bottom of the foot activates meridian energy movement in the chakra system
5. Myofascial methods are focused most specifically on change in the ______.
   a. Motor point
   b. Lymph nodes
   c. Gait control mechanism
   d. Tissue layer sliding
6. Which of the following is correct in application of trigger point therapy?
   a. 10-minute application in combination with tissue lengthening
   b. 45-minute application with hydrotherapy cold applications
   c. Limiting application to latent trigger points only
   d. Using pressure methods first and limiting lengthening
7. In shiatsu the points are called ______.
   a. Marmas
   b. Meridians
   c. Jitsu
   d. Tsubo
8. A client comes in for a massage session and the massage therapist notices circular areas of discoloration. What is the most logical reason for this situation?
   a. Instrument assisted scraping
   b. Kinesiology taping
   c. Cupping
   d. Frictioning

9. Which of the following is considered an implement for implement assisted massage application
   a. Spoon
   b. Lotion
   c. Hot pack
   d. Essential oil
10. Which of the follow adjunct methods is left in place following application?
   a. Hot stone
   b. Kinesiology tape
   c. Gua Sha
   d. Tuning Fork
11. A client has been receiving massage for a mild peripheral arterial circulation problem. Which of the following would be an appropriate self-help method to teach the client?
   a. Lymphatic drainage
   b. Skin rolling
   c. Alternating applications of hot and cold
   d. Frictioning
12. POLICE, MEAT and MCE applications for first aid are appropriate for _______.
   a. Primary care of abrasion
   b. Grade 2 and 3 sprains and strains
   c. Neural injury
   d. Shock
13. A client injured their right shoulder 3 years ago. Assessment indicates decreased mobility of the skin surrounding the shoulder coupled with a painful but normal range of motion. Which is the best treatment option for this client?
   a. Transverse friction
   b. Superficial myofascial release
   c. Compression
   d. Lymphatic drainage
14. An active trigger point that is left untreated for 6 months often will _______.
   a. Become an ashi point
   b. Become hot to the touch
   c. Have fibrotic changes
   d. Only elicit referred pain
15. When applying an intervention to trigger points, _______.
   a. Direct pressure methods and squeeze methods should be used first
   b. Positional release is an effective but gently approach
   c. Connective tissue stretching needs to accompany muscle energy application
   d. Lengthening of the tissue housing the trigger point is only effective with a local tissue stretch
16. In yin/yang theory, if yang is over energy, which is correct?
   a. Meridians are in balance.
   b. Stimulate yin and sedate yang.
   c. Sedate yin and stimulate yang.
   d. Apply acupressure to jitsu points.
17. Which is the most correct about the application of lymphatic drainage methods?
   a. The pressure levels are only sufficient to drag the skin.
   b. The direction is toward the heart.
   c. The rhythm is variable and moderate too fast.
   d. Pressure is variable applied slowly toward drain patterns.
18. A client has mild edema in their lower legs from a long plane fight the previous day. Which of the following is an appropriate treatment plan?
   a. Short, light gliding strokes focused on the legs. Compression to the soles of the feet. Active and passive joint movement for the ankle, knee, and hip. Placing the legs above the heart.
   b. Compression to the legs focused on the medial side from proximal to distal. Muscle energy and lengthening combined with stretching in the area of the most accumulation of fluid.
   c. Deep gliding strokes from proximal to distal on the legs. Placing the legs above the heart. Limiting movement to encourage drainage.
   d. Superficial and deep compression along the vessels in the lateral leg. Active resistive joint movement combined with shaking.
19. A client is getting ready to play a tournament tennis game in 60 minutes and wants to increase circulation and prepare muscles for the game. Which of the following treatment plans is the best option?
   a. Long gliding strokes from distal to proximal focused toward the heart combined with rocking. Duration of the massage: 45 minutes.
   b. Broad-based compression to the soft tissue of the limbs generally focused from proximal to distal combined with shaking and tapotement. Duration of the massage: 20 minutes.
   c. Full-body massage with muscle energy methods and lengthening. Duration of the massage: 45 minutes.
   d. Compression, superficial myofascial release, and trigger point work focused on the limbs combined with passive joint movement and shaking. Duration of the massage: 15 minutes.
20. Which of the following would be an indication for using lymphatic drainage during the massage?
   a. A client has edema in the lower extremities but no logical reason for the fluid retention.
   b. A client has premenstrual bloat and edema.
   c. A client has kidney disease although the client does not need dialysis.
   d. A client has a fever and is generally lethargic and achy.

Activity

Write at least three more multiple choice questions. Make sure to develop plausible wrong answers and be sure that the correct answer is clearly correct. Then write a rationale for each question. The more questions you write, the better you will understand the material. Exchange questions with fellow classmates or discuss in class. The questions from all the learners can be combined to create a review quiz.

Massage Career Tracks and Practice Settings

CHAPTER 13

http://evolve.elsevier.com/Fritz/fundamentals/

CHAPTER OBJECTIVES

After completing this chapter, the student will be able to perform the following:

1. Describe the history of the wellness center/spa/franchise industry and current trends.
2. Adapt massage for the wellness center/spa/franchise practice setting.
3. Define terms and identify types of products used in the wellness center/spa/franchise environment.
4. Identify cross-training recommendations for a career in the wellness/wellness center/spa industry.
5. Identify and demonstrate the skills and responsibilities necessary to practice in the medical care environment.
6. Explain how massage therapists behave and what skills are necessary to maintain compliance with the Health Insurance Portability and Accountability Act (HIPAA), health insurance, record keeping, and confidentiality in the medical care environment.
7. Use basic pharmacology information to practice massage safely in the medical care environment.
8. Practice massage therapy as part of integrative medical care.
9. Identify cross-training recommendations for a career in the health care environment.
10. Identify and demonstrate the skills and responsibilities necessary for massage therapy practice in the sports and fitness environment.
11. Describe and adapt massage for the sport and fitness practice setting.
12. Identify cross-training recommendations for a career in the sports and fitness industry.

CHAPTER OUTLINE

KEY TERMS

Best practice
Biopsychosocial model of medicine
Complementary and alternative medicine (CAM)
Franchise
Integrative medicine
Pharmacology
Recovery massage
Rehabilitative massage
Remedial massage
Salon
Wellness center/spa

The three main career tracks for massage can be categorized as follows:

- Health and wellness center/spa/franchise
- Medical care (clinical/medical)
- Sports performance and fitness

These career tracks typically are defined by where the massage is provided, common outcomes requested for the massage, and parameters that define a specific population.

The current kaleidoscope of massage practice can create confusion for the massage student, the massage therapist, potential employers, and the consumer. The trend is for all the outcomes, environments, and populations to overlap. Consider the following examples:

- Scar tissue management for cosmetic surgery may be combined with general full-body massage in a medical center/spa; this appears to be a case of clinical/medical massage, but it takes place in the wellness center/spa setting.
- Restorative massage with essential oils, soft music, and lighting may be done to support relaxation and sleep for athletes after a competition; this appears to be wellness center/spa/franchise focused, but the population derives from sports and fitness.
- Massage to increase flexibility, improve posture and gait, and provide lymphatic drainage may be done to address soreness after exercise for participants in a cardiac rehabilitation program; this appears to be sports and fitness targeted, but the massage is provided in the clinical/medical setting.

Think of the career situation in massage as something like a sandwich. The "filling" is always the same (i.e., the information presented in this text and in *Mosby's Essential Sciences for Therapeutic Massage*); however, each massage therapist may choose different "bread" (i.e., wellness center/spa/franchise, clinical/medical, or sports/fitness environments). When you graduate from a well-designed, well-implemented massage curriculum, you should have the filling in this professional sandwich; this chapter provides an overview of the bread.

What determines the focus of the massage? The most obvious answers are the practice setting and individual client outcomes. The wellness concept to support well-being and quality of life is the main practice focus for massage therapy, regardless of the practice setting.

The practice types can vary from the self-employed sole practice to employment in multiple types of wellness centers/spas and franchise centers, large interdisciplinary health centers, hospitals, medical clinics, long-term care facilities, gyms, sports teams, and fitness centers. The variety of options and practice settings can be confusing to the new graduate of massage education.

In brief, a general description of practice settings includes the following:

- *Wellness Center/Spa:* The wellness center/spa environment is extremely varied; it includes local day spas and chains, wellness centers, spas in various resorts, hotel chains, and cruise ships. The franchise model of independently owned massage businesses is often categorized under the wellness center/spa environment. Many self-employed massage therapists frame their private practice as wellness focus and spa services.
- *Medical care:* The medical environment consists of health care professionals who work in various settings, such as hospitals, physical therapy clinics, and specialty centers (e.g., cancer treatment or dialysis); as private practice physicians; and in hospice and long-term care.
- *Sports/fitness:* The sports and fitness environment consists of fitness centers, academic sports facilities (e.g., for high school track or collegiate gymnastics), and centers for professional or semiprofessional athletes (e.g., golfers, football players, soccer players, baseball players). These facilities are staffed by professionals such as exercise specialists, athletic trainers, and coaches. In addition, the needs of individuals who exercise for fitness as well as recreational and mature athletes must be addressed.

Each of these three main environments has specific roles that require various professionals and specific ways for massage to fit into and support multidisciplinary care. Regardless of the environment, each client must be addressed according to their unique situation. The adaptations needed for individual clients with specific conditions are discussed in depth in Chapter 14. In each of the practice settings, the massage therapist can practice as a self-employed professional or as an employee (see Chapter 3) (Focus on Professionalism 13.1).

FOCUS ON PROFESSIONALISM 13.1

When we provide massage in a specific environment and interact with other professionals, it is necessary to understand what they do and to help them understand what we do. We are all engaged in a team effort. For example, if a massage therapist is working in a pain clinic and, during a massage, identifies a rash on a client or patient's skin, the therapist should report this to the supervisor, usually a nurse. If this same massage therapist is in private practice and self-employed, the therapist would inform the client and refer the individual to the client's physician for diagnosis and treatment. If a massage therapist works in a fitness setting and a client seeks advice about a specific exercise protocol, it is ethical to refer that client to the exercise staff at the center rather than specifically advise the client about what to do. However, if that same client complains of shoulder stiffness to the exercise staff, those professionals should refer the client for massage.

In the wellness center/spa/franchise setting, if a client specifically asks about a skincare product, referral to the staff esthetician is advisable. However, if the therapist is working in private practice, it would be out of the scope of practice for the massage therapist to recommend a skincare product.

In a specific practice setting, the scope and focus of the massage are influenced, and in many cases limited, by the setting. For example, it is less likely that a client would request a relaxation/well-being–based massage in a physical therapy department. However, that same client on a cruise ship may be seeking a massage with the goal of being pampered by receiving a pleasurable, outcome-based session. When a massage therapist has a private practice and is not attached to a specific environment, the practice can be much more varied. The client base can include those with specific orthopedic concerns or chronic illness and others seeking general relaxation or improved recovery time after a sports competition.

THERAPEUTIC MASSAGE IN THE HEALTH AND WELLNESS CENTER/SPA/FRANCHISE ENVIRONMENT

SECTION OBJECTIVES

Chapter objectives covered in this section:

1. Describe the history of the wellness center/spa industry and current trends.
2. Adapt massage for the health and wellness center/spa practice setting.
3. Define terms and identify types of products used in the wellness center/spa environment.
4. Identify cross-training recommendations for a career in the wellness center/spa industry.

Using the information presented in this section, the student will be able to perform the following:

- Describe various wellness center/spa and franchise settings.
- Describe the unique aspects of massage in the wellness center/spa/franchise environment, such as brand image, safety, etiquette, and the responsibilities of the massage therapist.
- Alter fundamental massage training to the specific requirements of the wellness center/spa/franchise career pathway.

The wellness center/spa/franchise industry is becoming the largest and the fastest-growing career option for massage therapists. This environment targets fitness, stress management, pain management, peace of mind, quality of life, and health and wellness. The wellness center/spa environment, as a place of health and healing, can be confused with the salon environment. A **salon** is a business that provides beauty treatments related to hair, skin, and nails. The wellness center/spa/franchise environment may also provide salon-based services, and vice versa.

The massage skills required to be successful in this practice setting are the most varied, requiring a broad and thorough education. Various styles of massage therapy and adjunct approaches related to the physical effects of hydrotherapy, safe use of essential oils, the use of adjunct implements, products, and methods such as kinesiology taping are found in this textbook. Much of this information was presented in Chapter 12. Understanding how these methods are combined to create the signature massage style offered by the wellness center/spa/franchise is important. Many variations on the wellness center/spa/franchise theme are available (Box 13.1). Therapeutic massage is one of the unifying services found in wellness center/spa/franchise environments. Massage therapists pursuing this career pathway need to be able to address all evidence-informed outcomes: relaxation, stress management, pain management, and functional mobility.

A **brand** is a collection of services and products created and marketed for a specific business identity. Standardization in service delivery is essential, which is why most of these businesses train staff (massage therapists etc.) to the brand standard regardless of their background.

Box 13.1 Types of Spas

- *Resort spas* are located on the property of a hotel, normally in a resort where other activities are offered in addition to the spa program. Spa and hotel guests intermingle.
- *Amenity spas* are similar to resort spas in that the actual goal of management is to add the spa as an amenity to the hotel. The spa is not necessarily viewed as a profit center as seriously as some resort spas.
- *Destination spas* are hotel properties geared specifically to the spa guest and spa program. Outside guests are not normally part of the program. Everything is geared toward the spa and its program.
- *Blended spas* are low- to high-priced spas that emphasize physical fitness, nutrition, beauty, and relaxation.
- *Luxury spas* are high-priced spas with posh surroundings that offer an array of state-of-the-art facilities and services.
- *Weight-loss spas* cater specifically to those interested in losing weight and incorporate a variety of methods, such as medically supervised dieting, behavioral modification, exercise, detoxification, and fasting.
- *Medical/wellness spas* enlist the services of physicians to assist guests in achieving optimum health and well-being. The emphasis in these spas is on prevention and lifestyle changes rather than on treatment of acute illness. Programs include back care, sports medicine, physical therapy, lifestyle education, stress management, risk reduction, smoking cessation, and heart-healthy regimens.
- *Self-awareness spas* provide a wide range of alternatives to more traditional spas and focus on elements such as spiritual awareness, the body/mind connection, holistic health, yoga, vegetarianism, acupuncture, aromatherapy, reflexology, tai chi, and transcendental meditation.
- *Adventure spas* focus on customers interested in various outdoor activities such as hiking, rafting, mountain biking, skiing, mountain climbing, and fishing.
- *Mineral spring spas* are built around naturally occurring hot or cold water springs rich in minerals. In addition to mineral springs, some of these spas offer mud and thalassotherapy (seawater treatments), herbal wraps, saunas, and a host of other services typically found in spas.
- *Day (or urban) spas* offer a 1-day service. The client spends the day receiving various spa treatments, breakfast and lunch are provided, and activities such as aerobics and yoga are included. These are local, "in and out" spas.

The History of the Spa

Although the popularity of wellness centers/spas seems recent, people have been visiting spa-like environments for thousands of years. The word "spa," rooted in Latin, is short for *salus per aquam*, meaning "health from water." Using water therapeutically can be traced back to early civilizations (see Chapter 12). Indigenous people around the world discovered medicinal waters and used them for physical regeneration and spiritual health. Throughout history, different time periods brought different meanings and purposes for baths or spas. Many ancient cultures used social bathing for health and to treat pain and disease. The natural hot springs in Bath, England, were used by the Romans and are recognized for their therapeutic properties. This mineral water contains numerous elements, such as magnesium, potassium, sulfur, and calcium.

Today, hot water is common; in previous centuries, hot water in nature was rare, and the process of heating water was time consuming and labor intensive. Eventually, baths and spas became more than just places near hot springs; they evolved into modern-day resorts. During the 18th and 19th centuries, spas began to be staffed by medical professionals who prescribed and carefully monitored the treatments given to each visitor. The treatments primarily consisted of either soaking in the water or drinking it.

With the medical discoveries of the early 20th century, hospitals replaced spas with health care, while spas changed focus and began offering luxury accommodations. Many eventually turned into vacation locations or clinics concentrating on weight loss or catering to the wealthy.

Current trends in the wellness center/spa environment include interesting combinations of ancient traditions from many cultures and modern scientific research, such as technology now facilitating various water therapies (e.g., a hot tub replaces the hot spring).

In recent years, the value of prevention, healthy lifestyles, and relaxation has been rediscovered, and the wellness center/spa

Box 13.2 Wellness Environment

Healing environments encompass the senses of sight, smell, hearing, taste, and touch. Examples include the following:

Sight: Color and light
Smell: Essential oils and flowers
Hearing: Music and wind chimes
Taste: Herbal teas and juice drinks
Touch: Massage, facials, and body wraps

Signature wellness center/spa services feature unique combinations to target the five senses:

- Product related
  Smell: Product fragrance
  Touch: Texture and application of product
- Hydrotherapy related
  Sight: Scenery (e.g., mountain view)
  Smell: Scented oils and scrubs
  Hearing: Waterfall, fountain
  Taste: Mineral waters, flavored waters
  Touch: Whirlpool, showers
- Culture related
  Sight: Plants, ethnic dress
  Smell: Local flowers, incense
  Hearing: Ethnic music
  Taste: Ethnic food and drinks
  Touch: Cultural-based bodywork (i.e., shiatsu, Lomi Lomi)

Wellness center/spa services and environments are targeted to populations based on the following:

- Geography (e.g., rural, agricultural, urban, resort)
- Desired outcome: Pampering, fitness, skincare, detoxification, longevity, vacation
- Age: Adolescents, middle-aged clients, elder adults

is returning to its roots as a location uniquely qualified to address these needs of healing and well-being (Box 13.2).

Evolution of the Spa-Integrative Health and Wellness Centers

Integrative health centers incorporate all aspects of wellness, including body therapies, fitness, yoga, meditation, nutrition, and spirituality. Guest-centered approaches, rooted in education, proactive wellness, and prevention, are the cornerstones of programs addressing the whole person. Comprehensive programs blending Eastern traditions and Western scientific advances provide guided approaches to personal well-being. Under physician guidance, highly trained staff can create customized programs based on the needs of the individual for optimum health and wellness. Such centers use multidisciplinary approaches with medical teams trained in complementary and integrative medicine (CAM) and specialized service providers in preventive medicine and fitness. Massage is an important aspect of this multidisciplinary and interdisciplinary health and wellness center concept.

A variation on this model is the medical spa. A medical spa is a facility that operates under the full-time, on-site supervision of a licensed health care professional. The facility operates within the scope of practice of its staff (e.g., dermatology, cosmetic surgery, weight loss) and offers traditional, complementary, and alternative health practices and treatments in a spa-like setting. Treatments at medical spas include herbal therapies, chiropractic treatments, self-help imagery, hypnosis, homeopathy, biofeedback, acupuncture, massage, and energy healing. Medical spas are becoming popular as adjuncts to plastic surgery, dentistry, chiropractic, dermatology, and antiaging medical practices. Medical cosmetic procedures include cellulite treatments; Botox injections; laser hair removal; microdermabrasion; waxing and sugaring; permanent makeup application; electrolysis; hydrotherapy; sclerotherapy/vein therapy; collagen injections and fillers; chemical peels; and photo rejuvenation that uses several types of low-level lasers to treat stretch marks and remove scars. Cosmetic surgical procedures such as facelifts, tummy tucks, and hair restoration are offered at some medical spas.

Massage Therapy Franchises

The number and styles of franchise-based massage businesses are expanding and will likely become the main employment opportunity for graduates of massage therapy education. The massage therapy-based franchise is quickly evolving into the wellness center concept. The franchise model is primarily focused on massage therapy as the main offering, with skincare and limited hydrotherapy available. Recall from Chapter 3 that a **franchise** is a business contract through which an individual (the franchisee) purchases the rights to sell or market the products or services (or both) of a large group that has developed a brand (the franchisor). The franchisee receives training and marketing support from the franchisor and pays a fee for ongoing support. Franchisees typically are small business owners. All massage therapists who work for the franchise are employees.

When the massage therapy franchise, as a business, model, emerged in the early 2000s, there was misunderstanding and resistance from the massage therapy community. At that time, most massage therapists were self-employed. Much confusion is related to how management and ownership of franchises works, massage therapists being hired as employees, and how employee wages are calculated. Unfortunately, this confusion and resistance continue to influence my understanding of this career pathway. There are now 3000+ franchise locations in the United States employing up to 50,000 massage therapists in a variety of fulfilling careers.

Massage Therapy in the Wellness Center/Spa/Franchise

Those who are knowledgeable and skillful in concepts provided in this textbook, and anatomy and physiology are prepared for employment in wellness centers/spas upon graduation from a 500- to 1000-hour therapeutic massage program. Although this text does not present specific wellness center/spa procedures, the information prepares you to be easily and effectively trained in the signature treatments provided at individual wellness centers, spas, and franchises. Typically, clients choose from a variety of services and treatments. Some services may be performed by the massage practitioner; others may fall under the scope of practice of a physician, cosmetologist, or esthetician. Clients often ask questions about various services and treatments. The massage therapist needs to understand all services offered, whether they perform them or not, to educate clients and support business sales (Box 13.3).

Because many wellness centers/spas develop signature approaches and sell a variety of products, those working in this sector should be provided in-house training and extensive orientation in equipment use, treatments, and products.

Retail sales are an important source of business income. The massage therapist needs to understand the reason a product is used and how various ingredients in the product work. Products can include pain relieving ointments and CBD products. Skincare products basically include cleansers, exfoliants, and moisturizers (Box 13.4).

Massage therapists employed in the wellness center/spa/franchise industry should be licensed by the appropriate government agency. A therapist's expertise is determined by the number of school hours attended to obtain a license, the number of total years in practice, cross-trains, and the extent of continuing education obtained after graduation (Fig. 13.1).

Pay Scales for Massage Therapists in the Wellness Center/Spa/Franchise Environment

Wellness centers, spas, and franchises typically pay fair wages and can be a lucrative career pathway (see Chapter 3). Most hire all staff as employees and calculate wages on base hourly rate plus commission for massage hours performed. Another common method to calculate wages is at a per massage hour rate, which can be confusing, since employee wages must conform to Department of Labor regulations and minimum hourly wages. This was explained in detail in Chapter 3.

Several operating expenses of wellness centers/spas/franchises must be considered. For example, the ambiance of the environment is extremely important, and facility management is expensive. Marketing and advertising are essential aspects of the business plan. As a result, the overhead costs for a wellness center/spa or massage franchise are high, typically at least 50% of gross income. Compensation for staff in this setting must be figured on the remaining 50% of gross receipts. Also, the owner needs to make a profit. The wellness center/spa/franchise environment is in the service sector. Therefore gratuities are common. Although not guaranteed, an average tip for a service is between 10% and 25% of the fee. Massage therapist income potential varies in this environment related to the demographics of the business location, overhead costs, fees charged, and how much retail income influences business gross. Remember, massage therapists are employees in this career pathway. Income comparison to other business models such as self-employment needs to be based on a similar volume of clients and income numbers that are subject to income tax. Gratuities can conservatively add 15% to the income potential. Demographics can increase income potential by up to 20/%. Following are examples of conservative income calculations:

Box 13.3 Bodywork Terms, Descriptions, and Treatments Commonly Used in the Wellness Center/Spa Setting

- *Bodywork exfoliation:* Exfoliation is the process by which the skin is rubbed, polished, or scrubbed, or enzymes are used to remove dead skin cells, rancid oils, dirt, and debris.
- *Dry brush:* Dry brushing involves the use of a loofah, brush, washcloth, or sponge to exfoliate dead surface skin. After this process, lotion is applied. The main purpose is to stimulate circulation.
- *Salt glow:* Special salt is mixed with oil or liquid soap to exfoliate the entire body or just an area for a spot treatment. Afterward, lotion is used on the client. A dry brush tool, such as a loofah, may be used with the salt mixture for added exfoliation. If salt is used, the client should not shave for 1–2 days before the treatment.
- *Body polish:* Salt or any abrasive substance or granular scrub can be used as a body polish. The product used has a cream base with granules of the abrasive substance added to exfoliate and condition or soften the skin at the same time.
- *Full-body seaweed mask:* Seaweed powders normally are mixed with water to a consistency resembling pancake batter. The mixture is applied over a conditioning lotion. The entire body may be covered, or the stomach, breasts, and buttocks may be not treated, depending on the client's wishes. Essential oils are often added to full-body seaweed masks to achieve different effects on the body. The full-body seaweed mask treatment normally takes about 60 minutes.
- *Full-body mud mask:* Sea-based muds and clay muds, depending on the particular type, are said to cleanse and draw out impurities, condition and mineralize the body, or just soften and hydrate the skin. The mud is applied thickly to the body, which is then wrapped in plastic or foil. The client rests for 20–30 minutes. A full mud treatment normally takes about 60 minutes.
- *Herbal body wrap:* Linen or muslin sheets are heated and soaked in an appliance called a *hydrocollator,* in which the temperature is 150–175°F. Herbal pouches or bags of herbs and essential oil essences are placed in the hydrocollator to achieve the desired effects. The body is first covered with towels or rubber sheets, and the linen or muslin sheets are laid over this. The body then is wrapped in sheets and blankets, and the client is allowed to rest for 20 minutes. A cool, wet cloth is applied to the client's forehead during the treatment and changed often. This treatment can be done in 30 minutes.
- *Paraffin body wrap:* When applied to the body, paraffin forms a mask with heat. This helps the body perspire, and the trapped moisture is absorbed into the skin, along with nutrients that either are put on the skin first or are in the oils in the paraffin. The paraffin may be used alone, or it may be mixed with mud or seaweed. Paraffin can be painted on the body with a paintbrush. Also, large gauze strips can be dipped in the paraffin and molded to different parts of the body. Several layers are applied, because the more layers there are (i.e., three to five), the greater the heat and the longer it lasts. The body then is wrapped with foil or plastic, and the client is allowed to rest for 15–20 minutes. Paraffin commonly is used for the hands, feet, and face.

Box 13.4 Common Terminology for Wellness Center/Spa Products

Allantoin: A substance derived from comfrey root that is believed to aid the healing of damaged skin by stimulating new tissue growth.

Aloe vera: A regenerating, soothing, softening, and reparative substance with antimicrobial and antiinflammatory properties. It is rich in more than 200 nutrients and is very healing and moisturizing.

Alpha-hydroxy acids (AHA): These acids, which include lactic acid and glycolic acid, often are used as peeling agents. Most are fruit acids. At higher concentrations they also have a descaling or keratolytic action, thinning the stratum corneum.

Alpha-lipoic acid: A powerful water- and oil-soluble antioxidant, alpha-lipoic acid is 400 times more potent than vitamin C as an antioxidant. It also increases the level of glutathione, the body's most important antioxidant, and is a powerful antiinflammatory.

Bentonite: A substance that brightens dull, lifeless skin and gives it a fresh, renewed texture.

Borax: A cleansing agent that helps blend water and oil. A mild alkali, it cleanses without drying the skin.

Clay, kaolin: This substance draws out impurities and is used as a deep pore cleanser. It removes excess oil, dirt, and grime.

Cleanse: To clean and remove impurities from the skin's surface.

Cleansers: Products used to remove makeup and impurities on the skin's surface. They also remove sebum (oily secretions produced by the sebaceous gland) and dead skin cells.

Cream: A cream is a more occlusive, thicker barrier on the skin. Those that contain dimethicone are particularly useful for hand dermatitis.

Emollient: An ingredient that softens and soothes the skin. Emollients are used in moisturizers to correct dryness and scaling of the skin.

Emulsion: A substance made by blending oil and water in the right proportions with an *emulsifier,* an agent that prevents the oil and water from separating.

Exfoliant: An agent used in scrubs and wraps and in some facials to remove dead skin cells from the skin's surface.

Glycerin: A humectant and emollient obtained from plants. It absorbs moisture from the air and helps keep moisture in creams and other products.

Glyceryl stearate: A substance that helps produce a neutral, stable emulsion. It is also a solvent, humectant, and consistency regulator in water-in-oil and oil-in-water formulations. It is derived from palm kernel or soy oil for cosmetic use. It also is found naturally in the body.

Humectant: A substance that increases the water-holding capacity of the stratum corneum. It is particularly important in the management of ichthyoses (inherited or acquired scaly disorders of the skin).

Lanolin: A sebum-like product obtained from washing sheep's wool. It acts as an emollient and a humectant for the skin.

Lotion: A substance that is more occlusive than an oil. Lotions are best applied immediately after bathing to retain the water in the skin and should be used at other times, as necessary.

Mask: A mask draws impurities to the skin's surface. Masks also slough off dead skin cells and stimulate blood circulation, leaving the skin feeling smoother and softer. Masks are applied after cleansing but before toning and can be used once or twice a week.

Moisturizers: Products that use advanced humectants to help the skin retain water; they also provide a protective barrier to prevent the evaporation of the skin's natural moisture.

Night creams: Creams that contain a higher concentration of nutrients that assist in the rebuilding of the molecular structure of the skin's underlying tissues. They also improve the skin's ability to retain moisture.

Ointments: Pure oil preparations (e.g., equal parts white, soft, and liquid paraffin or petroleum jelly), which are prescribed for drier, thicker, more scaly areas. Many clients find them too greasy.

Phospholipid: A substance derived from plants that reduces moisture loss from the skin and acts as a carrier for deep penetration.

Retinol: A vitamin A carotenoid with antioxidant and skin-renewing properties.

Rubefacient: A local irritant that reddens the skin.

Salicylic acid: A substance that softens the keratinized barrier cells has antibacterial properties and helps eliminate clogged pores.

Salt: A substance that is good for drying, cleansing, drawing, and soothing. It also can be used as an exfoliant. It dilates pores, allowing the skin to absorb trace minerals, and it encourages the skin to secrete its natural oil. It soothes irritated skin and aching muscles.

Serum: An intense concentration for exceptional revitalization of aging skin.

Shea butter: A moisturizing, soothing emollient fat that has cellular renewal properties.

Silicone: A substance derived from silica, a naturally occurring mineral, which has a softening effect on the skin.

Skin lighteners: Products that help reduce the production of melanin, which causes coloration of the skin. These products are used to lighten the complexion. Skin lightening regimens include their own cleansers, masks, toners, moisturizers, and serums.

Sodium bicarbonate: A highly alkaline, gentle substance that cleans, soothes, and softens the skin. It also is deodorizing, and it draws out oil and impurities.

Toner: A substance that removes any residue left by cleansers and returns the skin to its proper pH by maintaining the skin's natural acidic balance. Toners and lotions prepare the skin for the application of a moisturizer.

- Full-time income
  Entry level: $32,000–$35,000 subject to income tax per year
  3–5 years of experience: $40,0000 to $45,000 subject to income tax per year
- Three-quarter time income (most common)
  Entry level: $26,000–$28,000 subject to income tax per year
  3–5 years of experience: $30,000 to $33,750 subject to income tax per year
- Half-time income
  Entry level: $18.000–$19,000 subject to income tax per year
  3–5 years of experience: $20,000 to $22,500 subject to income tax per year

Cross-Training Recommendations

If you are considering a career in the wellness center/spa/franchise industry, it may be beneficial to cross-train as a cosmetologist or

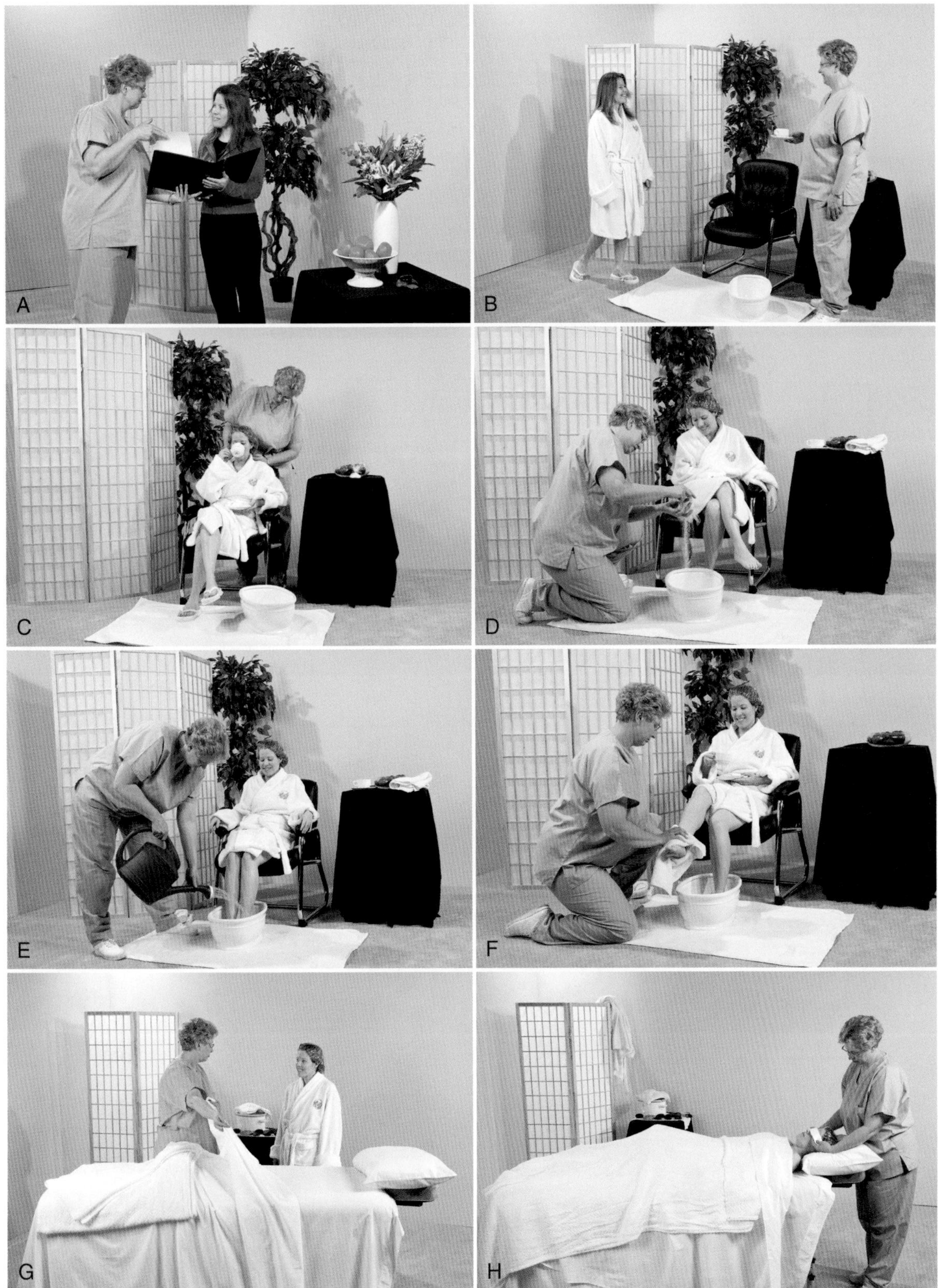

FIG. 13.1 A day at the wellness center/spa. A, The client is greeted warmly. The intake interview is conducted, and the client is presented with a wellness center/spa menu. **B,** The client changes and then is offered a cup of tea. **C,** The client's hair is protected with a cap. **D,** Signature aromatherapy oils and bath salts are used for the treatments. **E,** The client is encouraged to enjoy the hydrotherapy treatment. **F,** The client's feet are gently dried and then given a reflexology treatment. **G,** The client is given a relaxation-based, full-body signature massage. **H,** A compress can be placed over the client's eyes.

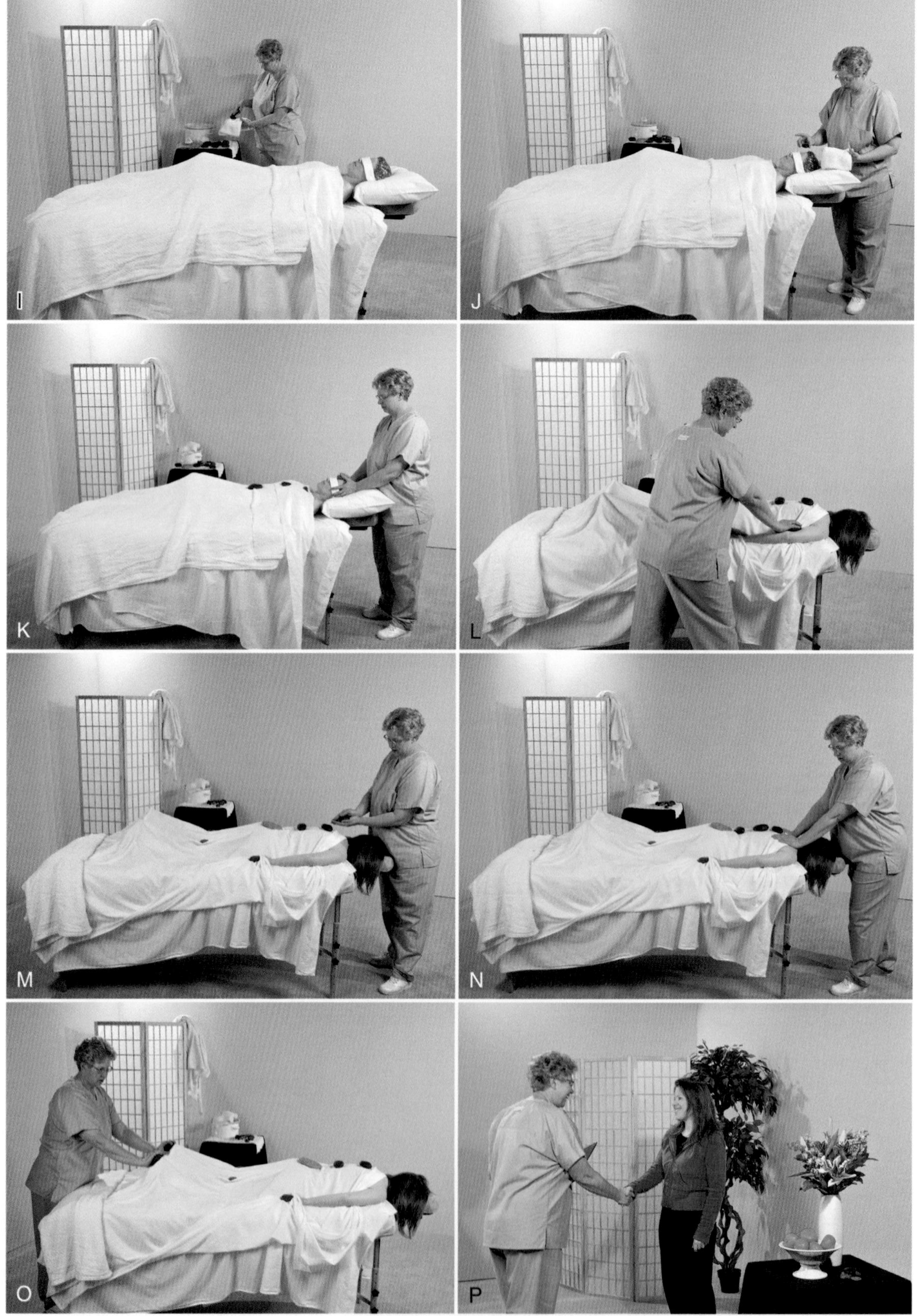

FIG. 13.1, cont'd I, Hot stones are prepared for a treatment. **J,** The temperature of the stones is tested, and then they are gently placed at nodal points. **K,** A few stones can be placed on the chakras with focused energy intention. **L,** Massage can be performed with a hot stone. **M,** The massage therapist can warm the hands with the stone. **N,** The massage is given with warm hands'. **O,** The massage therapist finishes and focuses (compassionate energy). **P,** The therapist says goodbye and encourages the client to visit again soon.

esthetician. Cosmetologists assist customers with their physical appearance. They include hairstylists who can cut, style, and color a client's hair. Some cosmetologists also are trained to provide manicures, pedicures, scalp treatments, and facials; maintain hairpieces; and give makeup analysis. Formal training and education are required. These classes are available at various community colleges, technical schools, and cosmetology schools. The length of the programs varies; most last 9–24 months. Cosmetologists must be licensed, and state education requirements vary from 1200 to 2100 school hours. Most are 1500–1800 hours.

Estheticians are not cosmetologists. An esthetician is a skincare specialist who performs cosmetic skin treatments, such as facials, light chemical peels, body treatments, and waxing. All estheticians must be licensed in the state in which they work. Training takes 250–600 hours, depending on the state.

THERAPEUTIC MASSAGE IN THE MEDICAL CARE ENVIRONMENT

SECTION OBJECTIVES

Chapter objectives covered in this section:

5. Identify and demonstrate the skills and responsibilities necessary to practice in the medical care environment.
6. Explain how massage therapists behave and what skills are necessary to maintain compliance with the Health Insurance Portability and Accountability Act (HIPAA), health insurance, record keeping, and confidentiality in the health care environment 7. Use basic pharmacology information to practice massage safely in the medical care environment.
7. Practice massage therapy as part of integrative medical care.
8. Identify cross-training recommendations for a career in the health care environment.

Using the information presented in this section, the student will be able to perform the following:

- Explain why it is important for massage practitioners to work under supervision in the medical care setting using best practices.
- Describe the written and verbal communication necessary for working in the medical care environment.
- Perform necessary record keeping for compliance with HIPAA and health insurance billing.
- Adapt massage based on prescribed medications.

Health care is much broader than medical care. Health care includes the maintenance and improvement of physical and mental health. Most states license massage therapists as health care professionals. This section differentiates between the more general concept of health care and the more focused medical approach. Medical care can be considered the diagnosis and treatment of health issues by providing medical services to identify and treat illness and injury. The medical environment consists of facilities such as clinics, hospitals, long-term care facilities, as well as homecare mobile services. In this environment, staff includes physicians; Doctor of Osteopathic Medicine DO, Doctor of Medicine MD, Doctor of Chiropractic (DC), Doctor of Physical Therapy (DPT), Doctor of Naturopathic Medicine (ND), Doctor of Nursing Practice DNP, Nurse Practitioner (NP), nurses, and various allied health professions and support staff.

Allied health is a term used to describe the broad range of health professionals who are not doctors, dentists, or nurses.

Massage therapists working in this environment are usually employees. Self-employed massage therapists can be part of referral networks with medical professionals.

Therapeutic massage has much to offer in the medical care environment. Clients are stressed, and relaxation-based massage approaches support other medical interventions and the healing process in general. Massage before surgery can help with anxiety. Comfort or palliative care before and after a person undergoes an invasive medical procedure can ease discomfort somewhat. Massage provided during drug rehabilitation programs supports the recovery process. Massage for medical staff promotes their ability to serve effectively because health care staff are often stressed and overworked. Increasingly, research is validating the effects of massage, making its inclusion in medical care possible. Just as the wellness center/spa environment is evolving toward health maintenance and management of chronic health conditions, the medical environment is moving toward integrative whole-person care. The overlap of environments is occurring now. The possibilities for massage in the medical care environment are numerous.

For massage practitioners, the medical care environment is a unique place requiring specific skills and professional behaviors. The massage therapist who pursues a career in medical care must understand all the aspects of therapeutic massage provided as part of an integrated medical practice. Increasingly, massage and other complementary therapies are being integrated into the medical environment. Methods and knowledge overlap significantly in the broad category of career tracks covering health care, sports and exercise, and wellness. All these methods are solidly grounded in the theory and practice of therapeutic massage. The challenge for massage therapists who want to work in this environment is how to work effectively with other medical professionals serving the patient, not how to work with specific diseases. The biopsychosocial model of medicine broadens the scope of intigrative clinical practice. Multiple health professionals work together to address the whole person with an individual/life experience and not a patient with a disease that has deviated them from normal functioning.

Various terms are used to describe therapeutic massage in the medical care environment, most commonly *clinical massage* or *medical massage*. This text is based on the premise that all massage is therapeutic and that the terms *clinical massage* and *medical massage* can be used interchangeably. Both describe massage offered within the medical care environment to serve people who have diagnosed medical conditions and are being treated at some level by a medical professional. In the medical setting, massage typically focuses on systemic illnesses (e.g., cancer, multiple sclerosis, diabetes) and on soft tissue dysfunctions that affect the general population.

Clinical/Medical Massage

The massage community has not reached an agreement on the knowledge base and scope of practice that define a career path in clinical/medical massage. Best practices are the working standards or ethical guidelines that provide the best course(s) of action in a given situation. Best practice quideline for massage therapy are not formalized but are an expectation in the medical care setting. This situation creates scope of practice confusion. Clinical/medical massage terminology is often used to describe a specialized focus on pain management and functional mobility outcomes. Self-employed massage therapists can frame professional practice as clinical/medical, indicating more focus on addressing health dysfunction rather than health enhancement within the wellness sector. Interface, consultation, and oversight from medical professionals are indicated for working with clients experiencing acute and complex medical conditions.

For the purposes of this textbook, *clinical/medical massage* (or simply *massage* in the remainder of the text) is an outcome-based treatment specifically targeted to address conditions that have been diagnosed by an appropriate medical care professional. Massage is included as an aspect of a total treatment program.

In clinical/medical massage, the focus is not on what kind of massage methods to use but on massage application based on the diagnosis, the prescribed treatment, and the determined outcomes for the patient. Special considerations arise for massage therapists who work with clients in a medical care environment (e.g., a hospital, rehabilitation center, extended care facility, or mental health facility). A principal factor to consider is that massage therapists must be willing to work in situations involving an increased risk of disease transmission. Even if clients do not have a contagious disease, if they are in a hospital setting or have a chronic condition, the risk of infection may be greater (e.g., methicillin-resistant *Staphylococcus aureus* [MRSA]).

Also, because people increasingly are being cared for in their homes by visiting nurses and home health workers, the massage professional in these situations functions as part of a medical care team and works to meet the objectives of a comprehensively designed treatment plan. The overall treatment plan is supervised by a medical professional, usually a physician. The massage therapist often is supervised directly by a physician's assistant, nurse, physical therapist, occupational therapist, or some other qualified medical care professional.

Becoming Part of the Medical Care Team

In 1994, the Bureau of Health Professions released the findings of a task force that studied the use of interdisciplinary teams in medical care. Task force members identified five characteristics of successful interdisciplinary teams:

- Team members provide care to a common group of patients.
- Team members develop common goals for performance outcomes and work together toward these goals.
- Appropriate roles and functions are assigned to each team member.
- Members understand and respect the roles of others.
- All members contribute and share essential information about both tasks and group processes.

The team also establishes a means of ensuring that plans are implemented, services are coordinated, and the performance of the team is evaluated. The interdisciplinary medical team functions as a whole and requires the understanding and involvement of all team members. Individual tasks may lend themselves to one team member or another with specialized skills, but the outcome is a team effort. Deciding on the diagnostic and therapeutic criteria that must be met for optimum patient management is a job that typically falls to the physician.

The expectations and responsibilities of the massage therapist as part of an interdisciplinary team are still being determined. The massage therapist's role will become clearer as massage therapy becomes more fully integrated into medical care. The massage therapist must know the scope of practice of each of the members of the interdisciplinary team and must be able to explain their own role. The massage therapist must develop an understanding of various treatments used by the integrated team and must be able to adapt massage application to contribute to the patient's care.

If you pursue a massage career in the medical care setting, you must understand the indications, necessary adaptations, and potential contraindications to massage methods in relation to each medical care intervention proposed and implemented. You also must be able to adapt to the varied medical care environments, equipment, and rules and regulations.

Professionalism

Professionalism is vital in the medical setting. Some characteristics of professionalism include loyalty, dependability, courtesy, initiative, flexibility, credibility, confidentiality, and a positive attitude. Behaving in a professional manner in the medical environment creates trust. Trust is one of the most crucial factors in preventing medical professional liability lawsuits.

Dress, attitude, and appearance all influence the credibility of the massage therapist. Appearance will be generally neat and clean and include scrubs; flat shoes with closed toes and rubber soles; little or no jewelry or makeup; short, clean, unpolished fingernails; no fragrances; and a modest hairstyle pulled away from the face. Visibility of tattoos and other forms of body art may need concealment.

Responsibilities of the Massage Therapist

Both health care and medical care are provided in many settings, and the massage therapist must be able to adapt to various locations. Massage is offered in hospitals, physical therapy practices, private physicians' practices, mental health facilities, chiropractic clinics, long-term care facilities, hospice care, and home health care (Fig. 13.2). Each setting has policies to sup-

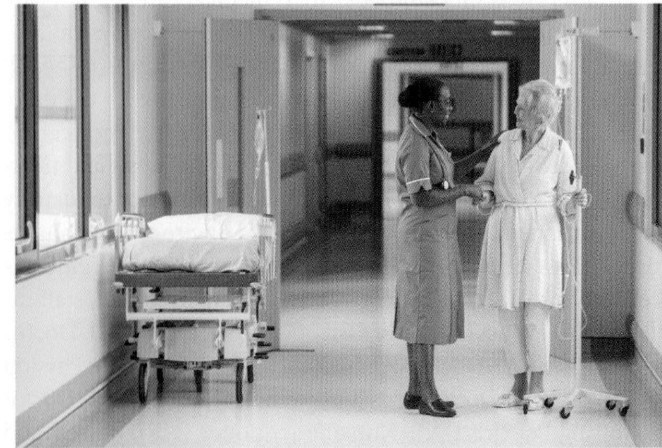

FIG. 13.2 Working in a medical setting requires understanding the roles of other staff members and how to adapt to the unique environment. (iStock.com/spotmatik.)

port quality care. These policies generally involve HIPAA compliance, Standard Precautions, professional conduct, supervisor hierarchy, and incident reporting procedures. Typically, all professionals working in a medical setting participate in an orientation process that presents this material. Massage therapists must pay close attention to instructions, always ask clarifying questions, and seek assistance if unsure of any activity involving patients and staff. Because the medical staff members are busy, be clear and concise during all communications; however, never be afraid to ask relevant questions so that you can be a supportive team member and maintain the safety of the patients.

Massage therapists who want to work in the medical care setting must be skilled and knowledgeable in the following areas:

- Infection control
- Sanitation measures
- Clinical reasoning and problem solving
- Preparation of justifications for treatment
- Setting qualifiable and quantifiable goals
- Medical terminology
- Pathology
- Medications
- Assistive and medical devices
- Assessment
- Development of treatment plans
- Analysis of the effectiveness of methods used
- Charting/documentation and record keeping, especially electronic medical records systems
- Effective communication of information
- Third-party insurance reimbursement requirements

Massage therapists also must have a basic understanding of various medical tests, procedures, and treatments so that they can make safe, beneficial decisions on ways to use massage to complement the medical treatments the patient is receiving (Box 13.5).

For professionals who already have medical care training, it is unrealistic to expect that simple exposure to massage is sufficient to enable them to work effectively with the vast knowledge base of massage. It is just as unrealistic to believe that a massage professional with an entry-level education can function independently in the medical care environment. Supervision by a medically trained professional, such as a nurse, is necessary to support the entry-level massage therapist. Of course, massage therapists do not diagnose; rather, they typically work from a "prescription," following treatment orders.

Massage therapists who choose to develop a career in the medical care setting must be willing and able to be a team player, accept supervision and instruction from medical professionals, follow orders and relay information accurately (both written and verbal), and contribute to the patient's care. Agreeing to work in this area means deference to the supervising physician, nurse, and other health/medical care providers. They have a more comprehensive education than the typical massage therapist, and they also shoulder the responsibility for the serious and even life-and-death decisions made during medical care.

Choosing a career in the medical care environment requires understanding the responsibility of providing service to those who face health challenges. This is not a decision that should be made lightly. Maintaining appropriate professional boundaries is important. The more complex a patient's condition and life circumstances are, the harder you must work to achieve a balance between empathic dedication to service and remaining neutral and objective in professional practice. Massage in the medical care environment is the most restrictive practice setting due to the complex nature of the client/patient and the importance of supervision by the medical team. This is not the environment for independent decision making, and treatment orders must be followed.

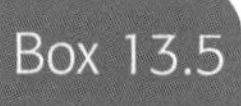

Consensus Views on Competencies and Teaching Methods for an Interprofessional Curriculum on Complementary and Integrative Medicine

COMPETENCY 1–Value and Ethics for Interprofessional Practice

General Competency Statement: Work with individuals of other professions to maintain a climate of mutual respect and shared values

COMPETENCY 2–Roles and Responsibilities

General Competency Statement: Use the knowledge of one's own role and those of other professions to appropriately assess and address the health care needs of the patients and populations served.

COMPETENCY 3–Interprofessional Communication

General Competency Statement: Communicate with patients, families, communities, and other health professionals in a responsive and responsible manner that supports a team approach to the maintenance of health and the treatment of disease

COMPETENCY 4–Teams and Teamwork

General Competency Statement: Apply relationship-building values and the principles of team dynamics to perform effectively in different team roles to plan and deliver patient-/population-centered care that is safe, timely, efficient, effective, and equitable.

COMPETENCY 5–Evidence-informed Practice

General Competency Statement: Explain, evaluate, and apply scientific evidence in the context of practitioner experience and patient preferences and apply evidence-informed decision making in integrated health care delivery.

COMPETENCY 6–Institutional Health Care Culture and Practice

General Competency Statement: Prepare practitioners who were not principally educated in mainstream/conventional academic, hospital, and outpatient delivery environments to work in such settings and systems.

(Data from Homberg A, Krug K, Klafke N, Glassen K, Mahler C, Loukanova S. Consensus views on competencies and teaching methods for an interprofessional curriculum on complementary and integrative medicine: a Delphi study. *J Integr Med*. 2021;19(3):282–290. https://doi.org/10.1016/j.joim.2021.03.001).

Communication Within the Medical Care Team

Precise and concise information exchange is important between the massage therapist and other medical care professionals. Most communication is done electronically through treatment orders and charting. The massage professional must have effective documentation skills in the medical care environment. Medical care professionals, especially physicians, are busy, and likely unable to speak at length about a particular client. Balance must exist between professional exchanges of information, with each team member carrying out their part of the treatment plan and expectations for extensive face-to-face communication.

Highly trained massage therapists can discuss treatment plans intelligently with various medical professionals. They provide valid input, and if disagreement arises, they can state their position accurately and professionally and use evidence-informed practice to justify their recommendations to supervising personnel.

Guidelines and Competencies for Integrated Care Systems

Health care is evolving, and an emerging trend is the biopsychosocial model of medicine. This approach to health care is like the body/mind/spirit model of wellness. For the sake of clarity, medical practices currently derived from a biomedical western scientific model are referred to as conventional health care. Many conventional health care professionals are frustrated and concerned about the inability to treat lifestyle-related illnesses effectively, particularly those that are chronic, with standard approaches using medication and surgery (Peters et al., 2001; Sharp et al, 2018; Vranceanu et al., 2022).

The term *complementary* refers to approaches or therapies that are used in addition to conventional medical treatments—for example, the use of acupuncture or massage with physical therapy.

The term *alternative* refers to approaches or therapies that are used instead or in place of conventional medicine—for example, the use of homeopathy and homeopathic remedies instead of pharmaceuticals.

Integrative Medicine

Combining conventional and complementary approaches to health care has become more accepted because the intent is to emphasize care in a wider context of body/mind/spirit interconnectedness and the importance of supporting health and wellness in addition to treating pathological conditions. This is called *integrative medicine* (Box 13.6).

Box 13.6 A Model for Clinical Massage in a Health/Medical Setting

Veterans Health Administration (VHA) (https://www.va.gov/health/)

Clinical massage therapy is one of the evidence-based, complementary, and integrative health (CIH) approaches within the VHA Whole Health System of care.

VHA Definitions

Integrative Health: A comprehensive approach in the delivery of health care that considers each patient from a whole person perspective, considering not only what is needed to treat and clinically manage the disease but also what may be needed proactively or beneficial, considering the full spectrum of available health care services, to optimize the patient's health and sense of well-being. (This term also subsumes the definition of Integrative Medicine.)

Integrative Medicine: The practice of medicine that reaffirms the importance of the relationship between practitioner and patient, focuses on the whole person, is informed by evidence, and makes use of all appropriate therapeutic approaches and health care professionals and disciplines to achieve optimal health and healing.

Practitioner: A practitioner is an individual who has training and expertise in the delivery of a CIH; who is licensed or certified by a state; whose licensure or certification permits the individual to provide such CIH; and whose VA Scope of Practice (SOP) (aligned with their VA credentialing and privileging) permits them to deliver such service to consenting patients

Treatment Guidance

Currently in VA, massage therapy is recommended primarily for pain conditions for which there is an evidence base. An evidence map of massage therapy was developed by the US Department of Veteran Affairs Health Services Research & Development. This systematic review provides a visual map of the evidence for massage therapy. Massage therapy appears to have very few risks when used appropriately and when provided by a professionally qualified Massage Therapist. Treatment for a variety of conditions can usually be accomplished between 3–12 weeks with 4–8 visits/treatments within that timeframe.

HEALTH TECHNICIAN/MASSAGE THERAPY: Job Description, Educational Standards, and Criteria for Advancement.

Standards for VA employees and community care professionals practicing massage therapy as part of their position fall under Qualification Standard GS-0640 series guidelines:

- The provider has adequately passed the requirements for basic or advanced training in Massage Therapy
- The provider maintains license/credentials as required for Massage Therapy

1. COVERAGE. The following are requirements for appointment as a Health Technician (Massage Therapy) in the Veterans Health Administration (VHA). The requirements apply to all VHA Health Technicians employed in the GS-0640 series.

Massage Therapy is the practice of manual assessment and manipulation of the superficial soft tissues of skin, muscle, tendon, ligament, fascia, and the structures that lie within the superficial tissues.

The Health Technician (Massage Therapy) occupation provides clinical services that address a vast array of problems impacting the health and function of a diverse patient population. The work requires the application of knowledge of therapeutic massage concepts, principles and practices, and encompasses a large variety of modalities from Western and Eastern traditions. Massage Therapy promotes the circulation of blood and lymph, relieves muscle tension, and can induce a general relaxation response, alleviate pain and anxiety, promote sleep, reduce stress, and enhance the general sense of wellness. Employees in this occupation may utilize appropriate tools and external

Box 13.6 A Model for Clinical Massage in a Health/Medical Setting–cont'd

applications of water, heat, and cold to enhance therapeutic benefits. Employees in this occupation incorporate knowledge of various systems of anatomy, physiology, and pathology to apply a plan of care for those with a variety of soft tissue dysfunctions, stress-related conditions, and imbalances.

Eligibility

(1) Candidates must be currently licensed, registered, or certified to practice as a massage therapist in a state, territory, or Commonwealth of the United States, or the District of Columbia. Acceptable credentials must have required successful completion of a minimum 500-hour massage therapy education program and pass the Massage and Bodywork Licensing Examination or equivalent state-issued examination.

OR,

(2) Candidates must possess and maintain a board certification from the National Certification Board for Therapeutic Massage and Bodywork (NCBTMB).

Level of Practice

Health Technician (Massage Therapy), GS-5 - Entry Level

(1)
- (a) Education, Experience, and Licensure. None beyond the basic requirements
- (b) Assignment. Health Technician (Massage Therapy) at this level performs basic massage therapy services under close supervision. The technician functions independently in applying basic massage services. Basic massage therapy includes, but is not limited to effleurage (stroking), petrissage (kneading), tapotement/percussion, friction, vibration, passive and active stretching, and draping. The Health Technician (Massage Therapy) is responsible for changing linen between clients, refilling oils, cleaning the massage table/chair/armrest, and providing a clean, calm environment. The Health Technician (Massage Therapy) promotes and educates patients on the health and wellness benefits of massage and develops therapeutic relationships with patients/family/significant others by demonstrating sensitivity and respect for a patient's personal beliefs. Deviations from regular procedures, unanticipated problems, and unfamiliar situations are referred to the supervisor for a decision or assistance. Any unusual patient interactions are documented and immediately reported to the supervisor.

(2) Health Technician (Massage Therapy), GS-6 - Developmental Level
- (a) Education, Experience, and Licensure. In addition to the basic requirements, candidates must possess one year of experience equivalent to the GS-5 grade level and demonstrate all the KSAs below.
- (b) Demonstrated Knowledge, Skills, and Abilities:
  - i. Skills to provide massage techniques including draping, using the appropriate tools, supplies, and equipment based on the needs of the patient;
  - ii. Knowledge of anatomy, physiology, pathology, therapeutic effects, and evidence-based practice of massage therapy;
  - iii. Ability to collaborate with an interdisciplinary team in a health care setting;
  - iv. Knowledge of all patient safety procedures, rules, and regulations as they pertain to a clinical environment;
  - v. Ability to effectively communicate verbally/non-verbally and in writing (through a variety of modalities).
- (c) Assignment. Employees at this grade level serve as developmental Health Technicians (Massage Therapy) and perform treatments that are routine and standardized in nature. The Health Technician (Massage Therapy) provides treatments in various inpatient and outpatient settings, in accordance with applicable policies and procedures. Health Technicians (Massage Therapy) perform a substantially full range of duties but receive guidance and directions regarding unfamiliar or unusual situations for more complex patient issues.

(3) Health Technician (Massage Therapy) GS-7 - Full Performance Level
- (a) Education, Experience, and Licensure. In addition to the basic requirements, candidates must possess one year of specialized experience equivalent to the GS-6 grade level performing massage therapy and demonstrate all the KSAs below:
- (b) Demonstrated Knowledge, Skills, and Abilities:
  - i. Ability to assess the physical and mental status of patients (including history and physical assessment), interpret the appropriate information to identify each patient's population-specific needs, identify indications/contraindications for massage, develop the plan of care, and monitor their response to treatment;
  - ii. Ability to use various communication techniques to encourage and educate individuals and groups to enhance massage therapy outcomes;
  - iii. Skill in developing and maintaining strong interpersonal relationships;
  - iv. Ability to advise staff and students in massage therapy practices.
- (c) Assignment. At the full performance level, Health Technicians (Massage Therapy) independently assess the physical and mental status of patients. The Health Technician (Massage Therapy) takes a complete patient history and performs a physical assessment. The Health Technician (Massage Therapy) interprets relevant clinical information to identify each patient's population-specific needs, identify indications/contraindications for massage, and develop the plan of care. Health Technicians (Massage Therapy), at this level, are responsible for performing massage therapy services with complexity higher than the developmental level. The Health Technician (Massage Therapy) performs duties with limited supervision and seeks assistance from the supervisor in urgent or emergent circumstances. The Health Technician (Massage Therapy) evaluates patient responses to treatment and documents responses to treatment, by maintaining accurate records in an electronic environment. The Health Technician (Massage Therapy) coordinates follow-up massage therapy as necessary. Health Technicians (Massage Therapy), at this level, serve as consultants to the health care team in the evaluation and treatment of the patient. Under routine academic oversight, the Health Technician (Massage Therapy) assists with clinical supervision of massage therapy students.

Continued

Box 13.6 A Model for Clinical Massage in a Health/Medical Setting–cont'd

(4) Health Technician (Massage Therapy) GS-8 - Advanced Clinical Level
  (a) Experience. In addition to meeting the basic requirements, candidates must possess one year of progressive experience equivalent to the GS-7 grade level. In addition, the candidate must demonstrate all the following KSAs:
  (b) Demonstrated Knowledge, Skills, and Abilities
    i. Skill in providing advanced massage techniques using the appropriate tools, supplies, and equipment based on the needs of the patient;
    ii. Knowledge of anatomy, physiology, and pathology relevant to massage therapy within specialty population(s);
    iii. Ability to modify massage therapy techniques based on an understanding of specialty populations, and various clinical/environmental settings;
    iv. Knowledge of teaching methods and learning principles;
    v. Ability to conduct research and quality improvement activities, related to massage therapy;
    vi. Knowledge of complementary integrative health, and holistic health principles.
  (c) Assignment. For all assignments above the full performance level (GS-7), the higher-level duties must consist of significant scope, complexity (difficulty), and variety, and be performed by the incumbent at least 25% of the time. At this level, the Health Technician (Massage Therapy) provides a full range of complex treatment procedures and modalities, which may include, but are not limited to reflexology, injury rehabilitation, lymphatic drainage, neuromuscular therapy, myofascial release, and/or craniosacral work. The Health Technician (Massage Therapy) is responsible for providing massage therapy services for specialty areas, such as pain management, poly-trauma, surgery, traumatic brain injury, palliative care, neurology, orthopedics, geriatrics, cardiology, pulmonary, rheumatology, spinal cord injury, mental health, and oncology. The Health Technician (Massage Therapy) assists other staff through education and as a member of an interdisciplinary health care team. The Health Technician (Massage Therapy) is a subject matter expert responsible for mentoring other Health Technicians (Massage Therapy) who participate in educational and research activities. The Health Technician (Massage Therapy) provides education in massage techniques to patients, caregivers, and employees. The Health Technician (Massage Therapy) contributes to identifying, collecting, and analyzing aggregate patient care information, to ensure safety and quality of care.

(5) Lead Health Technician (Massage Therapy), GS-8
  (a) Experience. In addition to meeting the basic requirements, candidates must possess one year of progressively complex experience equivalent to the GS-7 grade level. In addition, the candidate must demonstrate all the following KSAs:
  (b) Demonstrated Knowledge, Skills, and Abilities
    i. Ability to delegate tasks and responsibilities;
    ii. Ability to manage staffing requirements, workload priorities, and coordinate the work of the unit;
    iii. Ability to provide staff development and training;
    iv. Ability to review and monitor data to ensure all records and reports are complete and accurate.
  (c) Assignment. For all assignments above the full performance level, the higher-level duties must consist of significant scope, complexity (difficulty), and variety, and be performed by the incumbent at least 25% of the time. The Lead Health Technician (Massage Therapy) monitors workload, provides input on performance, resolves daily workplace issues, and maintains efficient workflow. Assignments at this level include but are not limited to ensuring coverage of all areas of responsibility, conducting clinical reviews to assess the quality of work, providing input to staff that includes changes in policies and procedures, creating and maintaining employee work schedules, orienting and providing on-the-job training for new and current Health Technicians (Massage Therapy), and ensuring all training requirements are met. The Lead Health Technician (Massage Therapy) reviews and analyzes aggregate patient care data, to ensure safety and quality of care.

(6) Supervisory Health Technician (Massage Therapy), GS-9
  (a) Experience. In addition to meeting the basic requirements, candidates must possess one year of progressively complex experience equivalent to the GS-8 grade level. In addition, the candidate must demonstrate all the following KSAs:
  (b) Demonstrated Knowledge, Skills, and Abilities
    i. Ability to provide the full range of administrative and supervisory duties which include, but are not limited to: assignment of work, performance evaluations, selection of staff, and recommendation of awards and/or advancements;
    ii. Advanced knowledge of massage therapy across multiple areas of practice, and the demonstrated ability to provide guidance to staff massage therapists;
    iii. Knowledge of how massage therapy integrates with other health care disciplines;
    iv. Ability to assist in matters related to policy development, equipment requests, and workload analysis;
    v. Ability to delegate authority, evaluate and oversee people and programs, accomplish program goals, and adapt to changing priorities.
  (c) Assignment. For all assignments above the full performance level, the higher-level duties must consist of significant scope, complexity (difficulty), and variety, and be performed by the incumbent at least 25% of the time. The Supervisory Health Technician (Massage Therapy) is responsible for the supervision, administrative management, and direction of Health Technicians (Massage Therapy). The Supervisory Health Technician (Massage Therapy) has full administrative and professional responsibility for planning and directing the activities for the service or equivalent unit. Typical duties include making work assignments, monitoring the staff's clinical performance, conducting performance appraisals, and other clinical and administrative responsibilities, as assigned, to ensure that the mission of the service and the medical center has been satisfied. The Supervisory Health Technician

Box 13.6 A Model for Clinical Massage in a Health/Medical Setting–cont'd

(Massage Therapy) develops policies and procedures for the work unit and contributes to the promotion of complementary and integrative health services. The Supervisory Health Technician (Massage Therapy) is responsible for reviewing aggregate patient care data and taking appropriate actions to ensure the safety and quality of care.

https://www.va.gov/WHOLEHEALTH/professional-resources/Massage_Therapy.asp

VA Handbook 5005/108 March 12, 2019, VHA established the profession of Massage Therapy to be covered under 38 U.S.C. §7401(3) and associated qualification standards for Massage Therapists to be able to provide this service. (VHA DIRECTIVE 1137(2 2021)

Lifestyle illnesses (diseases of longevity) are increasing as a result of stress, fatigue, poor nutritional choices, obesity, and similar factors. Many people come to recognize the overwhelming need to change their lifestyle and turn to integrative medicine as a means of change. Integrative medicine reaffirms the importance of the relationship between practitioner and patient, focuses on the whole person, is evidence informed, and makes use of all appropriate therapeutic and lifestyle approaches, health care professionals, and disciplines to achieve optimal health and healing.

The Veterans Administration's health/medical care model for inclusion of massage therapy will likely become a model for how massage can be provided in medical settings. Extensive research and planning went into the job descriptions and pay scales for in-house care. The Veterans Administration and its medical care network have implemented programs that embrace integrative health care principles. Details of the Whole Health program can be found at va.gov using the search term *Whole Health*. Hospital and inpatient care and referral-based community care options are available.

All approaches provided in the Whole Health program are based on evidence. Massage Therapy was supported by a report compiled by researchers at the Veterans Administration called *Evidence-Based Synthesis Program (ESP) Massage for Pain: An Evidence Map 2016.*

The job descriptions and criteria for advancement for employment in VA hospitals and medical centers have been well researched and will likely become a model for employment in the medical setting. Massage therapy for the VA is classified as a health technician (massage therapy) occupation. Details are available in the Department of Veterans Affairs VA Handbook 5005/108, Washington, DC, 20420, Transmittal Sheet March 12, 2019. National Center for Complementary and Integrative Health (NCCIH) is the Federal Government's lead agency for scientific research on complementary and integrative health approaches. The mission of NCCIH is to determine, through rigorous scientific investigation, the fundamental science, usefulness, and safety of complementary and integrative health approaches and their roles in improving health and health care.

NCCIH's new strategic plan for Fiscal Years (FY) 2021–2025 expands the definition of integrative health to include whole person health, that is, empowering individuals, families, communities, and populations to improve their health in multiple interconnected domains: biological, behavioral, social, and environmental. The plan has been informed and shaped by an effort to better define and map a path to whole-person health by expanding and building on current activities while advancing new research strategies and ideas.

The growing acceptance of complementary therapies coincides with an increased interest in lifestyle change, health promotion, and low-technology treatments. These approaches, integrated into conventional medical care, might provide inexpensive, safe ways to address conditions that currently do not respond well to conventional care.

Conventional medicine can be the best treatment for trauma and acute care, providing effective treatment for many common conditions, such as acute bacterial infection, congestive heart failure, and glaucoma. Complementary and alternative methods or adjunctive treatments within an interdisciplinary structure support this care. Accepted modalities currently available in medical care (e.g., nursing, physiotherapy, specialist referral, counseling, and medications) do not necessarily meet the needs of patients whose problems are not "fixable." Other people have long-term relapsing structural or functional disorders, for which medical treatment often is less than satisfactory. People with conditions that do not respond to conventional medical care alone might have better outcomes with the combined approach used in multi-professional and multidisciplinary integrated health care.

The biggest hurdles to integrating massage into conventional health care are (1) finding appropriately trained massage therapists and (2) identifying the source of funds to pay for massage. Currently, health insurance does not routinely cover therapeutic massage. Further research must be done to show that massage treatment is more cost effective than conventional medical treatment for various conditions and that it has the same or better benefits without increased risk to the patient. Research can also document whether conventional medical treatment achieves better outcomes when combined with complementary methods. When this has been shown (and the massage community is confident that it will be), the final hurdle will be overcome for full integration of massage into the health/medical care community.

Massage therapists are unlikely to work and bill health insurance companies independently. More likely, qualified massage therapists will be directly supervised by medical care providers who can bill for the massage session.

The Health Insurance Portability and Accountability Act of 1996

The Health Insurance Portability and Accountability Act of 1996 covers a multitude of the regulatory aspects of the health care environment. As described in Chapter 2, the massage therapist should receive in-service training about procedures relating to HIPAA requirements and how they are implemented in the specific health care environment.

Medical and other health information is private and must be protected. HIPAA's Privacy Rule gives individuals rights over their health information and specifies who can look at and receive health information. The Privacy Rule applies to all forms of an individual's protected health information (PHI), whether electronic, written, or oral. The Security Rule protects health information in electronic form. It requires entities covered by HIPAA to ensure that electronic PHI is secure. Protected information includes the following:

- Information physicians, nurses, and other health care providers put in a medical record
- Conversations the physician has about a patient's care or treatment with nurses and others
- Information about an individual in a health insurer's computer system
- Billing information about a patient

HIPAA also seeks to limit administrative costs by supporting the use of electronic transfer of information, and it establishes guidelines for preventing fraud and abuse.

Health Insurance

Health insurance is a type of third-party payer system. This means that the consumer pays for insurance; then, when medical expenses occur, the costs are billed to and potentially covered by the insurance. Numerous third-party payers base reimbursement on what is referred to as the allowable charge, which has been influenced by managed care organizations and the government. *Managed care* is a broad term used to describe a variety of health plans developed to provide health care services at lower costs.

Health insurance is available to people in many ways. People can buy individual policies, but most get health insurance by being a member of a group that pools resources to purchase health insurance. Examples of groups that provide health insurance are employees in a business (sometimes the employer offers health insurance as a benefit) or a chamber-of-commerce arrangement, through which small business owners can get coverage.

Insurance policies have many coverage options, from minimal coverage to maximum coverage. Some may include alternative and complementary care coverage, whereas others do not. In group coverage situations, the types and amount of coverage a person is eligible to receive may not be amendable to include certain types of treatment, such as massage therapy.

Major third-party payers with which the massage therapist should become familiar include major medical group insurance, Aetna, Blue Cross/Blue Shield, Medicaid, Medicare, CHAMPVA, TRICARE, and workers' compensation. Medicare, the largest third-party insurer in the United States, makes quality health care affordable for elder adults and other select groups. Medicaid is another US government–sponsored health care plan for individuals who qualify for these benefits based on income limitations or disability. Workers' compensation covers employees who are injured or who become ill because of accidents or adverse conditions in the workplace. Disability programs reimburse individuals for monetary losses incurred because of an inability to work for reasons other than those covered under workers' compensation.

Health Insurance Reimbursement

Reimbursement for services by health insurance companies is a widespread practice in medical care. Lack of reimbursement for many complementary methods, such as massage, is one of the main obstacles to their inclusion in the medical care process. This situation probably will improve as more research identifies a positive risk/benefit/cost value for massage services to justify reimbursement.

In the medical care environment, the infrastructure already exists for billing insurance companies for payment for services rendered. Large facilities, such as hospitals, have designated departments for health insurance billing. Small medical practices usually have one person responsible for health insurance billing. Fortunately, a major advantage of employment in the medical care environment is that the massage therapist is paid a salary or fee for each massage, regardless of insurance reimbursement.

The massage therapist with a career in medical care needs to understand enough about health insurance and reimbursement to support the billing specialist (the insurance biller and coder). The massage therapist's responsibility is to maintain appropriate records to justify insurance reimbursement and to follow the preauthorized treatment plans as presented by the supervisory medical care professional.

Although some massage therapists work in areas that bill directly to insurance for payment, this is not common practice. In some situations, a massage therapist may receive health insurance reimbursement outside the traditional medical care setting, in the context of private practice. A physician's referral and preauthorization may be required.

Integrating Massage Into the Medical Care Setting

Most massage applications in the health care setting are general in nature, targeting restorative mechanisms, maintenance of homeostasis, and palliative care. Massage related to soft tissue dysfunction targets common conditions such as headaches, neck and shoulder pain, low back pain, tendinitis, bursitis, and arthritis. Pain management also is an important consideration. In addition, you must understand how the inflammatory response is connected to seemingly unrelated diseases (see Chapters 5 and 6).

Massage care is supportive, not curative, for those who are ill or injured. Massage effectively supports various forms of medical intervention (including mental health) and the body's innate ability to heal. The intent is that diseases and injuries are cured with the medical intervention. This is especially true of acute care situations. However many people are not necessarily cured with medical care interventions such as medication or surgery; instead, their condition is managed, a situation that puts a major strain on the medical care delivery system. Because most medical conditions are managed and therefore require long-term care, treatment is expensive. Massage offers benefits for the management of many chronic medical conditions in a potentially cost-effective manner.

Some health benefits of massage have been validated by research (see Chapter 5); others are based on clinical experience or are historically supported by many cultures over centuries of practice. The main focuses of massage in the medical care environment are as follows:

- Breathing effectiveness
- Circulation support (blood and lymph)
- Comfort and pleasure
- Edema and fluid imbalance management
- Enhanced parasympathetic dominance
- Pain management
- Reduced sympathetic dominance
- Support for sleep and reduction of fatigue
- Soft tissue normalization (neuromuscular and myofascial)

These outcomes can overlap. For example, reducing sympathetic dominance should improve breathing, support sleep, and increase pain tolerance. Reducing edema could ease pain and increase circulation to an area. Neuromuscular balance allows for effective movement, and myofascial balance supports mobility and stability; together they support effective, efficient movement that encourages circulation, increases comfort, and supports productivity.

In this text, massage application is presented as an outcome-based process, which is necessary to develop and follow treatment plans and work effectively in the medical care setting (Box 13.7). Best practices to consider when offering massage in the medical care environment include the following key points.

Box 13.7 Basic Pharmacology for the Massage Therapist

Pharmacology is the science of drugs. It encompasses the development of drugs, explanations of their mechanisms of action, and descriptions of their conditions of use. Pharmacists are the medical professionals who specialize in pharmacology. The terms *medication* and *drugs* often are used interchangeably. However, medication is specific to pharmaceutical agents used in the treatment of disease, whereas drugs can encompass a broader scope of chemical use, including substances such as cocaine and over-the-counter (OTC) medications. The following discussion typically uses the term *drug*. The focus of the section is the possible interaction of massage and these chemicals. Because drugs are a major treatment factor in the health care setting, it is essential that the massage therapist working in this environment understand the fundamentals of pharmacology.

Pharmacodynamics

Pharmacodynamics is the study of the effects of a drug on the body and the mode of the drug's action. The chemicals in the drug are distributed throughout the body by the blood and other fluids of distribution. Once they arrive at the proper site of action, they act by binding to receptors, usually located on the outer membrane of cells, or on enzymes located within the cell.

Various drugs are designed to target specific receptors to elicit a specific response. Receptors are like biological "switches" that turn on and off when stimulated by a drug that binds to the receptor and activates it. For example, narcotic pain relievers such as morphine bind to receptors in the brain that sense pain and reduce the intensity of that perception. Non-narcotic pain relievers, such as aspirin, ibuprofen (e.g., Motrin), and acetaminophen (e.g., Tylenol), bind to an enzyme located in cells outside the brain, close to where the pain is localized (e.g., the low back), and reduce the formation of biologically active substances known as prostaglandins, which cause pain and inflammation. These peripherally acting (i.e., acting outside the central nervous system) analgesics (pain modulators) also may reduce the sensitivity of the local pain nerves, meaning fewer pain impulses are sensed and transmitted to the brain.

In some instances, a drug's site of action, or receptor, may be something in the body that is not anatomically a part of the body. For example, for antacids such as Tums or Rolaids, the site of action is the acid in the stomach, which these drugs chemically neutralize. Antibiotics are another example of drugs that bind to a receptor that is not part of the body. Antibiotics bind to portions of bacteria that are living in the body and causing disease. Most antibiotics inhibit an enzyme inside the bacteria, which causes the bacteria either to stop reproducing or to die from the inhibition of a vital biochemical process.

As medical science has learned more about how drugs act, pharmacologists have discovered that the body is full of different types of receptors that respond to many different types of drugs. Some receptors are selective and specific, whereas others lack such specificity and respond to several different types of chemical molecules.

The massage therapist must understand the action of a medication and then must use clinical reasoning skills to adapt the massage appropriately (see Appendix C). All chemicals taken into the body, whether medications, OTC drugs, drugs of abuse, environmental pollutants, food, vitamin supplements, herbs, or manufactured food ingredients (e.g., artificial sweeteners, colorings, and preservatives), have the potential to influence the body in both beneficial and negative ways.

Drug Interactions

Certain foods, herbs, and vitamins can affect the action of drugs. This interaction can be supportive or detrimental. For example, patients who take certain medications (e.g., statins, which lower cholesterol) should not eat grapefruit. Serious side effects can occur if a patient taking a selective serotonin reuptake inhibitor (SSRI), such as Zoloft or Paxil, also takes St. John's wort, SAMe, or 5-HPT. Vitamins typically are best when taken with food; however, the absorption of some medications is inhibited if the drug is taken with food. The entire potential interaction process can be extremely complicated.

Using a Drug Reference

It is helpful to have a drug reference available so you can look up a particular medication to learn how it is used and the possible side effects. Then, when you apply what you know about the effects of massage on the body (see Chapters 5 and 6), you can make informed, intelligent decisions about how to adapt the massage based on the medication or medications your client is taking.

A good drug reference to add to either your book or electronic library is *Mosby's Drug Reference for Health Professions*. The MedlinePlus website has an excellent section on drugs, herbs, and supplements. Additional information is found on the Evolve site.

Key Points

- Typically, the target population is ill or injured; however, preventive care is increasing in popularity.
- The more severely injured or ill the patient, the more general the massage application.
- Massage should support, not interfere with, medical treatment.
- Healing is a body, mind, and spirit process that requires a multidisciplinary approach; this honors the roles of various professionals and respects each one's scope of practice.
- Healing does not necessarily mean a cure. Successful coping is a healing process.
- Living well with hope and compassion, regardless of circumstances, is an important goal of healing.
- Massage is targeted to the body, and the appropriate scope of practice must be maintained; therefore the massage therapist respects and honors but does not cross over into the mind and spirit aspects of treatment.
- Respect for the patient and the medical care team is paramount.

Regardless of the setting, the following guidelines apply:

- Standard Precautions and other sanitation procedures must be followed precisely.
- The massage therapist often must work around various types of equipment and devices, such as intravenous lines.
- The massage often must be modified because the client is unable to assume the classic position of lying on a massage table.
- Many clients are confined to a bed or wheelchair.
- Privacy often is compromised, and interruptions are common.
- The environment may be noisy and busy with other activity.
- Various medications and their interaction with the effects of the massage must be considered.
- The effects of medical tests or preparation for tests can affect massage interventions.

Pay Scales for Therapeutic Massage in the Medical Care Environment

The Veterans Administration job descriptions and pay scales reflect realistic income expectations for massage therapists in the medical environment including chiropractic, physical therapy clinics, hospitals, etc. Massage therapy is classified as Health Technician GS-5 - Entry Level. GS-5 is the 5th paygrade in the General Schedule (GS) pay scale, which is the pay scale used to determine the salaries of most civilian government employees. The GS-5 pay grade generally marks an entry-level position. The pay range is $17–$20 per hour. The pay scale is reviewed yearly and factored related to demographics (https://www.federalpay.org/gs/2022/GS-5, https://www.federalpay.org/gs/calculator).

Cross-Training Recommendations

If the medical care setting is your career path of choice, it may be prudent also to train as a certified nursing assistant/patient care technician, licensed practical/vocational nurse, or EMT. The education in these areas will provide specific information about procedures and conduct in the medical care setting and indicate that you have the skills to function in the medical setting safely as a massage therapist.

Patient care technicians, also called certified nursing assistants or nurse's aides, perform basic care procedures in hospitals, clinics, and nursing homes. Most programs take 1 year or less to complete and prepare learners for state certification examinations. EMT training usually is achieved through a 6-month to 2-year certificate, diploma, or associate degree program, depending on the level of certification. Most licensed practical/vocational nurse training programs take 1 year to complete, and a licensing examination is required.

THERAPEUTIC MASSAGE IN THE SPORTS AND FITNESS ENVIRONMENT

SECTION OBJECTIVES

Chapter objectives covered in this section:

9. Identify and demonstrate the skills and responsibilities necessary for massage therapy practice in the sports and fitness environment.
10. Describe and adapt massage for the sport and fitness practice setting.
11. Identify cross-training recommendations for a career in the sports and fitness industry.

Using the information presented in this section, the student will be able to perform the following:

- Provide massage in various sports and fitness environments.
- Explain remedial, rehabilitative, medical, and orthopedic massage in the sports and fitness environment.
- List common goals and outcomes in the sports and fitness environment.
- Describe the elements of practice for a sports event.

Sports, fitness, and rehabilitation professionals are turning to massage as part of the treatment or management of various conditions. There is no such thing as "sports massage," only the appropriate massage application for each client. Whether the client is a runner; bowler; swimmer; surfer; golfer; baseball, basketball, football, or soccer player, or simply a person who has just finished a treadmill stress test, this individual still needs a treatment plan designed for their needs (Fig. 13.3).

Clients of sports- and fitness-focused massage present a range of diverse needs. Some clients are undergoing physi-

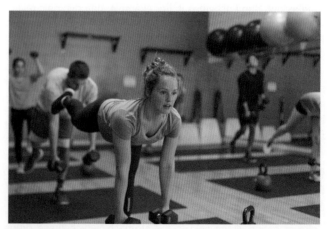

FIG. 13.3 Adapting to the fitness practice setting. It is important to understand how the various activities may influence massage outcomes. (iStock.com/FatCamera.)

cal rehabilitation that requires an exercise program (e.g., cardiovascular and cardiorespiratory rehabilitation or physical therapy for an orthopedic injury). Other clients are taking up exercise as part of a comprehensive fitness and wellness program, including weight management. Still other clients are recreational athletes or competitive athletes, both amateur and professional.

Typically massage therapists with advanced training have some athletic clients as part of their professional practice and will modify massage for the athlete (see Chapter 14). Many massage practitioners who are interested in sports massage want to work with professional athletes. The reality is, those jobs are rare because there are not that many professional or Olympic athletes. The National Basketball Association (NBA) has fewer than 400 players, and the National Football League (NFL) has fewer than 2500. Other team sports fall somewhere between those numbers. Individual professional athletes, such as tennis players, golfers, and bowlers, are also a small community. Most massage therapists interested in sport and fitness massage will serve high school, collegiate, amateur, or semi professional athletes and, even more, those undergoing rehabilitation or striving to maintain fitness.

Another common misconception is that professional athletes make many millions of dollars; the truth is only a few make it into that category. Most make far less, and amateurs generate no athletic income at all. Therefore justifying the cost/benefit of therapeutic massage, compared with the expense and regularity of use, is an ongoing issue. More commonly, sports fitness and rehabilitation cost money, often lots of it. If a person is going to use massage regularly, the fees must be manageable.

Additional demands are placed on professionals who work with athletes or in physical rehabilitation because of the extraordinary circumstances of these clients. The environment of competitive sports or physical rehabilitation makes for bigger-than-life moments. There is the drama of win or lose, the trauma of injury, and the career-determining or even life-or-death situations of surgery and rehabilitation. Working in the sports and fitness environment can be like a roller-coaster ride, but with a lot of monotony between the highs and lows.

Massage therapists in this field must be skilled in the massage applications appropriate for the sport or fitness activity of their individual clients. Beyond the necessary massage skills is a requirement for a host of less obvious skills: motivation, maturity, reliability, compassion, tenacity, tolerance, stamina, flexibility, commitment, perseverance, humbleness, self-esteem, little need for personal glory, the ability to work behind the scenes, and the ability to improvise and, above all, to problem-solve.

Remedial, Rehabilitative, Medical, and Orthopedic Massage in the Sports and Fitness Environment

The terms *remedial massage, rehabilitative massage, medical massage,* and *orthopedic massage* are all interrelated. Remedial massage is used for minor to moderate injuries. Methods used in remedial massage include all those presented in this text. Rehabilitative massage is used for more severe injuries or as part of the post-surgical intervention plan; if the injury or surgery is related to bones or joints, this type of massage can be considered orthopedic massage.

The massage methods used in rehabilitation vary. Immediately after injury or surgery, the techniques used generally are more nonspecific and focus on reducing stress and promoting healing. Attention is given to the entire body while the area of injury or surgery heals. If immobility, use of crutches, or changes in posture or gait are factors during recovery, compensation patterns are likely to develop. Massage can manage these compensation patterns while the physician, physical therapist, and athletic trainer focus on the injured area. During active rehabilitation, massage can become part of the total treatment plan for recovery when supervised by an appropriately qualified professional.

Common Goals and Outcomes for Massage in Sports and Fitness

Two primary goals of sports massage are to assist the athlete in achieving and maintaining peak performance and to support the healing of injuries. Many factors contribute to mechanical injuries or trauma in this environment. In sports, *trauma* is defined as a physical injury or wound, produced by an external or internal force sustained as the result of a sports endeavor. Healing mechanisms manifest as the inflammatory response and resolution of the inflammatory response. Different tissues heal at different rates. For example, the skin heals quickly, whereas ligaments heal slowly. Stress can influence healing by slowing the repair process. Sleep and proper nutrition are necessary for proper healing.

A massage professional should be able to recognize common sports injuries and refer the athlete to appropriate medical professionals. Once a diagnosis has been made and the rehabilitation plan developed, the massage professional can support the athlete with general massage application and appropriate methods to enhance the healing process.

Massage professionals who intend to work with athletes benefit from additional training. Many specialized training programs for sports massage are available. Such training should include the physiological and psychological functions of an athlete, overuse and repetitive use syndromes, the biomechanics of specific sports, the use of hydrotherapy methods, injury repair and rehabilitation, and education in training regimens.

There is a dangerous misconception that sports massage involves intense, deep, aggressive massage application. These types of methods, along with aggressive stretching; heavy, deep transverse friction in broad tissue areas; and any other methods that create inflammation, are especially contraindicated in massage for the general recovery of the athlete. The client should not be sore or stiff 12–24 hours after the massage. If this occurs, the massage creates inflammation instead of helping the body resolve inflammation (Proficiency Exercise 13.1).

PROFICIENCY EXERCISE 13.1

Research information about each of the three career pathways and develop a pro and con list related to your career focus.

The Sporting Event as a Practice Option

Early in the 1980s, the concept of sports massage was used as a public awareness and promotional activity. Representatives of massage schools and massage organizations often were present at amateur sporting events. The work was primarily based on a volunteer model, not a career setting. At that time, the AMTA offered specific sports massage testing and certification. Also during that time, sports massage was categorized by when it was given and the reasons for the massage. Some of those categories are discussed in the next paragraphs. However, if outcome-based goals are used, these categories become irrelevant. For example, if massage is used to assist a pre-exercise warm-up, it should focus on those goals.

Pre-Event (Warm-Up) Massage

The pre-event, or warm-up, massage is a stimulating, superficial, fast-paced, rhythmic massage that lasts 10–15 minutes. The emphasis is on the muscles used in the sporting event, and the goal is to help the athlete feel that their body is perfectly prepared. Uncomfortable techniques should be avoided. The pre-event massage is given in addition to the physical warm-up; it is not a substitute. This style of massage can be used from 3 days before the event until just before the event. The massage therapist should focus on enhancing circulation and should be careful not to overwork any area. The sports pre-event massage should be general, non-specific, light, and warming. Neither friction nor deep, heavy strokes should be used. Massage techniques that require recovery time or that are painful are strictly contraindicated. Preferably, only massage therapists who work on a continual basis with a particular athlete should give the person a pre-event massage.

Intercompetition Massage

Intercompetition massage, given during breaks in sports events, concentrates on the muscles being used or those about to be used. The techniques are short, light, and focused.

Recovery/Post-Event Massage

Recovery massage focuses primarily on athletes who want to recover from a strenuous workout or competition and have no injuries. The method used to help an athlete recover from a workout or competition is similar to a generally focused, full-body massage, and incorporates methods that support homeostasis.

Promotional (Event) Massage

Promotional massages usually are given at events for amateur athletes. The massages are offered as a public service to provide educational information about massage. The sports event massage is quick paced and lasts about 15 minutes. In this type of public, promotional environment, following a sports massage routine is important. The use of lubricants is optional, and the massage practitioner may choose not to use them because of the risk of allergic reaction, staining an athlete's uniform, or other factors.

If a massage professional is doing promotional work at a sports event and is working with many unfamiliar athletes, the best course is to do post-event massage, because the effects of any neurological disorganization caused by the massage are not significant. No connective tissue work, intense stretching, trigger point work, or other invasive work should be done with an athlete at a sporting event. The massage should be superficial and supportive and should be focused more on enhancing circulation. It is important to watch for swelling that may indicate a sprain, strain, or stress fracture; if any of these are noted, the athlete should be referred to the medical tent for immediate evaluation. It also is important to watch for evidence of thermoregulatory disruption, such as symptoms of hypothermia or hyperthermia; if these are noted, the massage therapist should refer the individual immediately without using any diagnostic terms or unduly alarming the person.

It is important to have written documentation of informed consent from each person who wants to receive a massage at these events (Box 13.8). One way to do this is to provide an informed consent statement on the top of a sign-in sheet and have each participant read and sign it before receiving a

Box 13.8 Sample Informed Consent Form for Use at Sporting Events

Name: ____________________

Sporting event: ____________________

Date: ____________________

I have received, read, and understand informational literature concerning the general benefits of massage and the contraindications for massage. I have disclosed to the massage practitioner any condition I have that would be contraindicated for massage. Other than to determine contraindications, I understand that no specific needs assessment will be performed. The qualifications of the massage practitioner and reporting measures for misconduct have been disclosed to me.

I understand that the massage given here is for the purpose of recovery and restoration. I understand that massage practitioners do not diagnose illness or disease, perform any spinal manipulations, or prescribe any medical treatments. I acknowledge that massage is not a substitute for medical examination or diagnosis, and it is recommended that I see a health care provider for those services.

I understand that an event sports massage is limited to providing a general, non-specific massage approach using standard massage methods but does not include any methods to address specifically soft tissue structure or function.

Participant's signature: ____________________ Date: __________

Participant's signature: ____________________ Date: __________

Participant's signature: ____________________ Date: __________

massage. Each participant should be given a short brochure or pamphlet explaining the benefits, contraindications, and cautions for sports massage. If the organizer of the event allows it, the brochure could include contact information to allow participating athletes to contact the massage professional at a later date.

The Sports Massage Team

Often a group of massage professionals and supervised learners work on an event as a team. A team leader who is familiar with the sport is usually in charge of the sporting event. All the participating massage practitioners follow a similar routine. Remember, each member of a sports massage team represents the entire massage profession. Ethical, professional behavior is essential. The organizer's permission is required if you intend to distribute marketing information at such an event.

Pay Scales for Therapeutic Massage in the Sport and Fitness Environment

Locations and potential employers who would provide opportunities to practice sport-specific massage include fitness centers, wellness centers/spas, sports clubs (e.g., tennis, golf, racquetball, and so on), sports training facilities (amateur and professional), gyms, sports medicine facilities, and individual athletic clients.

Because experience and additional training are necessary to work with the complexities of athletic performance, pay scales are somewhat higher than in the medical setting. Instead of being employed by the organization, most massage therapists who specialize in massage for athletes are self-employed. There are signs that employment opportunities will become more common. It is likely that the wellness center approach will begin to specifically serve this population. Also, sports medicine is a medical specialty and massage therapy is likely to expand in that setting as well. Both are employee-based environments and pay scales would be similar.

Cross-Training Recommendations

In the sports and fitness setting, two main options exist for a massage practitioner interested in an advanced education that includes additional skills. The option most often chosen is serving as a personal trainer. A personal trainer helps people exercise. The training for this job can be obtained in a formal school format or through a series of courses, and a certification process is available. Almost all personal trainers work in physical fitness facilities, health clubs, and fitness centers, mainly in the amusement and recreation industry or in civic and social organizations.

The second option is working as an athletic trainer. Athletic training involves preventing, diagnosing, and providing interventions for emergency, acute, and chronic medical conditions involving impairment, functional limitations, and disabilities. The AMA recognizes athletic training as a health care profession. To practice, individuals must complete an athletic training degree program (bachelor's degree or entry-level master's degree) that is accredited by the Commission on Accreditation of Athletic Training Education.

Foot in the Door

What type of door do you want your foot in? Massage therapy is a unique career opportunity because of the spectrum of places massage can be offered. Be it a wellness center/spa, franchise, hospital, chiropractor's office, hospice, pain clinic, fitness center, sports team, or multiple other options, you can build a career specialization. Each career track has potential cross-training options. You may put your foot in the door to an additional training program and learn to become an esthetician, a certified nursing assistant, or a personal trainer. It is necessary for career success to be adaptable to various practice settings. This requires ongoing learning, whether gained through formal methods (such as cross-training) or through practical experience in the practice setting. Remember to keep your feet moving toward continuing education for career success.

SUMMARY

The three main career tracks described in this chapter are related to the environment in which massage is offered. Each practice setting requires professional behavior and the ability to provide excellent massage; however, the culture of the environment influences the knowledge, skills, and abilities needed to be successful in that setting. Massage practitioners newly graduated from an entry-level program can work in the wellness center/spa/franchise setting if they are committed to expanding their skills with continuing education. This practice environment offers the most flexible career pathway. Medical care and sports/fitness settings typically require education beyond entry-level; therefore if you set your sights on a career in these areas, you should pursue advanced education.

MENTORING TIP

Career focus changes as experience is gained. Sometimes massage therapists begin to feel limited or discontented by the environment in which they practice. Often individuals begin to dislike the practice setting and begin to degrade the value of massage offered in a particular environment. These feelings indicate that the massage therapist has outgrown and is no longer challenged by the type and focus of massage in that practice setting. Instead of complaining or becoming frustrated, the therapist is encouraged to get additional training and move on.

LEARN MORE ON THE WEB

The website *healthcare.gov* explains the law and provides resources for finding health insurance and understanding the benefits provided under the Affordable Care Act.

Evolve

Visit the Evolve website: http://evolve.elsevier.com/Fritz/fundamentals/

Evolve content designed for massage therapy licensing exam review and comprehension of content beyond the textbook. Evolve content includes:

- Content Updates

- Science and Pathology Animations
- Body Spectrum Coloring Book
- MBLEx exam review multiple choice questions

FOR EACH CHAPTER FIND:

- Answers and rationales for the end-of-chapter multiple-choice questions
- Electronic Workbook and Answer Key
- Chapter multiple choice question Quiz
- Quick Content Review in Question Form and Answers
- Technique Videos when applicable
- Learn More on the Web

RESOURCES

Spa Industry Association
https://dayspaassociation.com/
allan@spaindustryassociation.com
480-350-7075

International Spa Association
https://experienceispa.com/
2365 Harrodsburg Road, Suite A325
Lexington, Kentucky 40504 USA
Email: ispa@ispastaff.com
Phone: 1.859.226.4326
Toll Free: 1.888.651.ISPA(4772)

REFERENCES

Peters D, Chaitow L, Harris G, et al. *Integrating Complementary Therapies in Primary Care*. Edinburgh: Churchill Livingstone; 2001.

Sharp D, Lorenc A, Feder G, et al. Trying to put a square peg into a round hole: a qualitative study of healthcare professionals' views of integrating complementary medicine into primary care for musculoskeletal and mental health comorbidity. *BMC Complement Altern Med*. 2018;18(1):290.

Vranceanu AM, Bakhshaie J, Reichman M, Ring D; International Musculoskeletal Mental and Social Health Consortium (IMESH). A Call for Interdisciplinary Collaboration to Promote Musculoskeletal Health: The Creation of the International Musculoskeletal Mental and Social Health Consortium (I-MESH). *J Clin Psychol Med Settings*. 2022;29(3):709–715.

MULTIPLE-CHOICE QUESTIONS FOR DISCUSSION AND REVIEW

The answers, with rationales, can be found on the Evolve site.

Use these questions to stimulate discussion and dialogue. You must understand the meaning of the words in the question and possible answers. Each question provides you with the ability to review terminology, practice critical thinking skills, and improve multiple choice test-taking skills. Answers and rationales are on the Evolve site. It is just as important to know why the wrong answers are wrong as why the correct answer is correct.

1. Which of the following describes the shift in the American spa concept?
   a. Including performance-specific training
   b. Evolving into a wellness center
   c. Incorporating more rehabilitation service
   d. Increasing offerings in salon services
2. What is the main difference between a wellness center, massage franchise, and spa concept?
   a. Focus on massage therapy as the main service
   b. Inclusion of fitness services
   c. Privately owned business
   d. Self-employment versus employment
3. In which practice setting would the massage therapist have the most autonomy for massage style and care plans?
   a. Chain wellness center/spa
   b. Hospital
   c. Franchise
   d. Fitness center
4. In which practice setting is it least likely for massage therapists to receive gratuities?
   a. Wellness center/spa
   b. Franchise
   c. Chiropractic office
   d. Fitness center
5. In what setting would hydrotherapy be most integrated into the offerings?
   a. Physician's office
   b. Destination wellness center/spa
   c. Runners club
   d. Franchise
6. In which practice setting would massage therapists find themselves collaborating with an occupational therapist?
   a. Medical outpatient clinic
   b. Golf league
   c. Medical wellness center/spa
   d. Wellness clinic
7. In which environment would the massage therapist need to receive HIPAA training?
   a. Senior center
   b. Dialysis center
   c. Wellness center
   d. Fitness center
8. In what way is the Veterans Administration leading the way for the integration of massage therapy?
   a. Providing cross-training
   b. Using a collaborative model
   c. Addressing acute care
   d. Offering practice oversight
9. In the sports and fitness environment, which of the following is a common occurrence encountered by the massage therapist?
   a. Illness
   b. Joint surgery
   c. Soft tissue injury
   d. Infection
10. Which of the following career pathways has the fewest opportunities for non-degree cross-training?
    a. Wellness center/spa
    b. Medical environment
    c. Franchise
    d. Sports environment
11. A 3-year-old has undergone many surgical procedures to improve function from a heart defect. What role could massage play in the treatment of this child to reduce anxiety?
    a. Specific scar tissue management
    b. Rehabilitation
    c. Breathing training
    d. Retraining so that touch is pleasurable

12. Which of the following would be the definition for approaches or therapies that are used instead of or in place of conventional medicine?
    a. Alternative
    b. Complementary
    c. Hierarchy
    d. Quackery
13. Integrated medicine refers to ___________.
    a. Alternative methods that replace conventional medical care
    b. Complementary therapies combined into the structure of conventional medical care
    c. A system in which mainstream medical care and complementary therapies are separated
    d. Claims that are made by a person or group on society, a group, or an individual
14. Which of the following is NOT accurate when working in the health care setting?
    a. Typically the target population is ill or injured; however, preventive health care is increasing, as reflected in wellness programs and medical wellness centers/spas.
    b. The more injured or ill the patient, the more intense and specific the massage application.
    c. Massage should support, not interfere with, medical treatment.
    d. Healing is a body, mind, and spirit process requiring a multidisciplinary approach.
15. Which of the following attributes needs to be cultivated in the health care environment?
    a. Respect for cultural diversity
    b. Conflict avoidance
    c. Individual exclusionism
    d. Accreditation
16. Which of the following statements indicates why athletes may benefit from massage as much or more than the general population?
    a. Normal physiological mechanisms inhibit the tendency to function at the body's anatomical and physiological limits.
    b. Most people usually do not run as fast as possible or exert all available energy to complete a task.
    c. Most people back off when the body signals fatigue, pain, or strain, which indicates that the anatomical or physiological limits have been reached.
    d. Athletes often strive to exceed normal physical and mental functioning.
17. Which of the following is NOT an action of prescribed medication?
    a. Stimulate a body process
    b. Support pathogen invasion
    c. Inhibit a body process
    d. Replace a chemical in the body
18. Which of the following stress management strategies most involves the massage therapist?
    a. Coping skills
    b. Education
    c. Anger management
    d. Pain management
19. Which types of medication have the LEAST amount of synergistic interaction with massage?
    a. Muscle relaxants
    b. Non-steroidal antiinflammatories
    c. Opioids
    d. Antidepressants
20. Decisions about what career environment is the best fit for a massage therapist are best made based on ________.
    a. Pay scale
    b. Critical thinking
    c. Past experience
    d. Level of education

CHAPTER

14 Adaptive Massage

http://evolve.elsevier.com/Fritz/fundamentals/

CHAPTER OBJECTIVES

After completing this chapter, the student will be able to perform the following:

1. Explain the benefits of massage for animals and adapt massage for cats and dogs.
2. Describe indications, cautions, and contraindications for massage, and appropriately adapt massage for athletes.
3. Describe and apply appropriate massage in the breast area.
4. Adapt for massage during pregnancy.
5. Adapt massage for infants, children, and adolescents.
6. Explain the aging process and adapt massage for the geriatric population.
7. Describe gender-affirming interventions and adapt massage as needed.
8. Recognize acute care situations and adapt massage appropriately.
9. Describe the mechanisms of chronic illness and adapt massage for those with chronic conditions.
10. Adapt massage to support clients undergoing oncology care.
11. Adapt massage for integration into the various medical settings.
12. Communicate effectively, and appropriately adapt massage for individuals with physical impairments.
13. Communicate effectively, and appropriately adapt massage for individuals diagnosed with psychological conditions.

CHAPTER OUTLINE

KEY TERMS

Abuse
Acute illness
Acute injury
Anxiety
Athlete
Chronic illness
Depression
Dissociation
Gender diversity
Hospice
Mental impairment
Obesity
Pain and fatigue syndromes
Panic
Physical disability/impairment
Post-traumatic stress disorder (PTSD)
Reenactment
Specialization
State-dependent memory
Tactical athletes
Trauma

In this chapter we examine ways massage professionals can show respect for and accommodate those who benefit from various adaptations of the massage application. The intent is to help massage professionals focus on the benefits of therapeutic massage for clients with specific needs. Each section offers a general description of the adaptive situation, the application for massage, and directions for obtaining further training and information.

Specific methods or protocols do not exist. There is no such thing as sports massage, prenatal massage, or hospital massage. Critical thinking and evidence informed practice are fundamental to determine adaptation of massage therapy for each client. Thought-out responses based on principles, information, and the complexities of the situation are based on whole person care in a client centered approach. Effective decision making requires a person to:

- Define the situation or problem: Identify the client's outcomes and what unique factors influence the decision-making process.
- Consider the facts of what occurred or would influence the situation: Conduct a client history and assessment. Perform a literature search to gather information.
- Generate possible solutions or courses of action: What does the client recommend? How have other massage therapists addressed the issues? What are other similar situations that could provide ideas?
- Evaluate the logical consequences of cause and effect (pros and cons) and the effect on people regarding each potential solution or course of action: The client needs to be actively involved in this aspect of critical thinking. The massage therapist needs to evaluate possible courses of action based on scope of practice, practice setting, other professionals involved, their individual skills and experience, access to supervision, peer support and mentoring.
- Decide about what to do: This is a cooperative approach between the client and the massage therapist and other professionals involved in integrated care plans.
- Create a plan: The decision achieved between the client and massage therapist is formalized into a care/treatment plan and becomes the platform for informed consent and how the massage therapist conducts the massage sessions.
- Implement the plan.
- Evaluate the results and adapt as needed.

Each decision is evidence informed and unique. Evidence-informed decisions are based on:

- Client's wants and needs
- Best available evidence
- Expert opinion consensus
- Logical, plausible, and justifiable strategies
- Massage therapist's knowledge and skills

Individuals (or animals) with diverse needs that require adaptation can be seen in any massage environment in which you may practice. The fundamental skills presented in this textbook seldom change when applied in these unique situations and sometimes unique environments. Gliding and kneading for a person (or animal), regardless of the need for adaptation, is still gliding and kneading. The difference is the recipient of treatment, and the way treatment is done. Working with diverse populations requires additional knowledge about the specific situations or conditions addressed. The practitioner also must keep in mind the effects of any training protocols, developmental stages, medical treatments, accommodations (e.g., barrier-free access), or counseling in conjunction with the therapeutic massage.

In the exploration of each situation, it is important always to see the individual as a person first. Language used and the approach to care focus on each individual person first, then on their unique needs. There are no visually impaired, hearing impaired, sick, or abused people; there are people who have visual or hearing impairments, who deal with various illnesses, or who have experienced trauma. Factors related to cultural competency and respect are important. Ongoing monitoring of personal and professional biases is essential. Basic massage skills are sufficient to serve all people because they promote general health and well-being. Certainly, specific rehabilitative massage requires additional education, but the most common application of therapeutic massage, in conjunction with diverse situations, is general, nonspecific support.

The massage professional's responsibility is to learn as much as possible about the client's situation and the environment in which the massage is provided. If you are working with an individual experiencing post-traumatic stress disorder (PTSD), then learn about PTSD; if you are working with children with attention deficient disorder (ADD), then you must understand ADD and its treatment protocols. If you are working with a horse in a stall, you need to understand horses. Using the clinical reasoning model, a massage professional can develop intervention plans and justifications for the benefits of therapeutic massage as part of a comprehensive care program, regardless of the circumstances.

The best way to obtain information about a client's adaptive needs is to ask the person directly. It is important to clearly understand the action plans required for various environments. It is necessary to expand skills and knowledge in response to real practice challenges. There is no way a school or textbook can prepare you for every conceivable situation you may encounter in professional practice. Various research avenues are available, and the internet is an especially helpful source of information. When the practitioner understands the client's particular situation, the physiological effects of massage that provide the most benefit can be identified, and massage therapy care plans can be developed.

Massage can be an effective way to reduce stress, promote well-being, and enjoy a respite from the daily challenges of life. The ability to respond successfully and provide massage in any environment, be it the rushed and hectic setting of an airport or the sacred space of the deathbed, expands access to the benefits of massage to anyone, anywhere.

FOCUS ON PROFESSIONALISM

This chapter introduces the idea of **specialization**. This means using massage skills that specifically target a common group of occurrences shared by individuals. For example, some factors are commonly related to age (e.g., infants and elder adults). When we begin to specialize, it is necessary to learn more about the identified commonalties. However, each individual will need a unique adaptation. Increased knowledge can guide you in adapting the massage process, helping you meet the goals for each specific client. For example, if you are interested in specializing in clients with amputations, there is a learning curve that includes several concerns, such as how to adapt the environment to support clients using assistive devices, how a prosthesis is fitted and used, how the body compensates, and so forth. Massage is massage—you serve your clients by using your knowledge to individualize each application.

ANIMAL MASSAGE

SECTION OBJECTIVES

Chapter objective covered in this section:

1. Explain the benefits of massage for animals and adapt massage for cats and dogs.

Using the information presented in this section, the student will be able to perform the following:

- Identify the difference between massage, grooming, and petting.
- Explain the benefits of massage both for well animals and for those receiving veterinary care.
- List necessary components of specific animal massage education.
- Adapt a massage based on outcomes and the animal's size and species.
- Recognize pain behavior and adapt massage to target pain management.

Just as it is with humans, massage for animals is a complementary therapy that encourages the animal's own healing and wellness processes (Box 14.1). Therapeutic massage works in animals for the same reasons it works in humans. Animals are important in people's lives. Care for an animal companion can promote well-being and quality of life. Understanding how to adapt massage for companion animals is a way to interact with clients in a productive way.

It is important to note that *massage is more than petting.* Petting is less focused and much more general than massage. Petting animals is pleasurable and beneficial to both the animal and the person. However, massage is a deliberate, focused technique of touching. It is the manipulation of soft tissue to promote well-being at both a physical and an emotional level. The desired effect for an individual animal can be achieved by applying various mechanical forces to different areas of the body.

Each animal is assessed and treated as an individual. What works for one animal might not be right for another. Determining factors include species, age, size, activity level, injuries, and medications. Assessment identifies target areas, contraindications, and outcomes. The history is based on information from the person responsible for the animal's well-being.

The various methods used for human massage are also used for animal massage. The anatomy and physiology of animals are similar to those of humans. However, before working with a particular species, the massage therapist should review the anatomy unique to that species (Fig. 14.1).

Massage therapists who work with animals are likely to find themselves in the role of teacher. They often must demonstrate massage techniques and instruct the caretaker in their use for the specific animal. The massage therapist must be confident and comfortable with the particular animal, or the massage application will be stressful for both the massage therapist and the animal. Although massage can be adapted for many kinds of animals, this chapter focuses on massage for dogs, cats, and horses, which more commonly receive massage.

Box 14.1 Veterinary Care and Massage

The specialist in the health care of animals is the veterinarian. Methods such as massage should never be substituted for proper veterinary care. The American Veterinary Medical Association (AVMA) has offered the following guidelines for massage therapy in conjunction with medical care:

Massage therapy on nonhuman animals should be performed by a licensed veterinarian with education in massage therapy or, where in accordance with state veterinary practice acts, by a graduate of a licensed massage school who has been educated in nonhuman animal massage therapy. When performed by a person who is not a veterinarian, massage therapy should be performed under the supervision of or referral by a licensed veterinarian who is providing concurrent care.

Body of Knowledge for Animal Massage

Formal training for animal massage is varied, and opinions on the correct methods are inconsistent. A massage professional who is interested in obtaining specific education in animal massage should thoroughly investigate any provider of animal massage training to make sure the individual is qualified to teach. Massage therapists who want to work with animals may obtain training in animal grooming, animal training, or some sort of veterinary assistant education. Legislative scope of practice regarding which individuals can legally practice massage therapy on animals are state dependent, and full regulations are found through the International Association of Animal Massage & Bodywork/Association of Canine Water Therapy (IAAMB/ACWT). https://iaamb.org/resources/laws-by-state/.

Credentialing for this area of specialization exists through the National Board of Certification for Animal Acupressure and Massage. https://www.nbcaam.org/.

Before providing massage to any animal on a professional basis, the massage therapist should obtain additional training in the following areas (Proficiency Exercise 14.1):

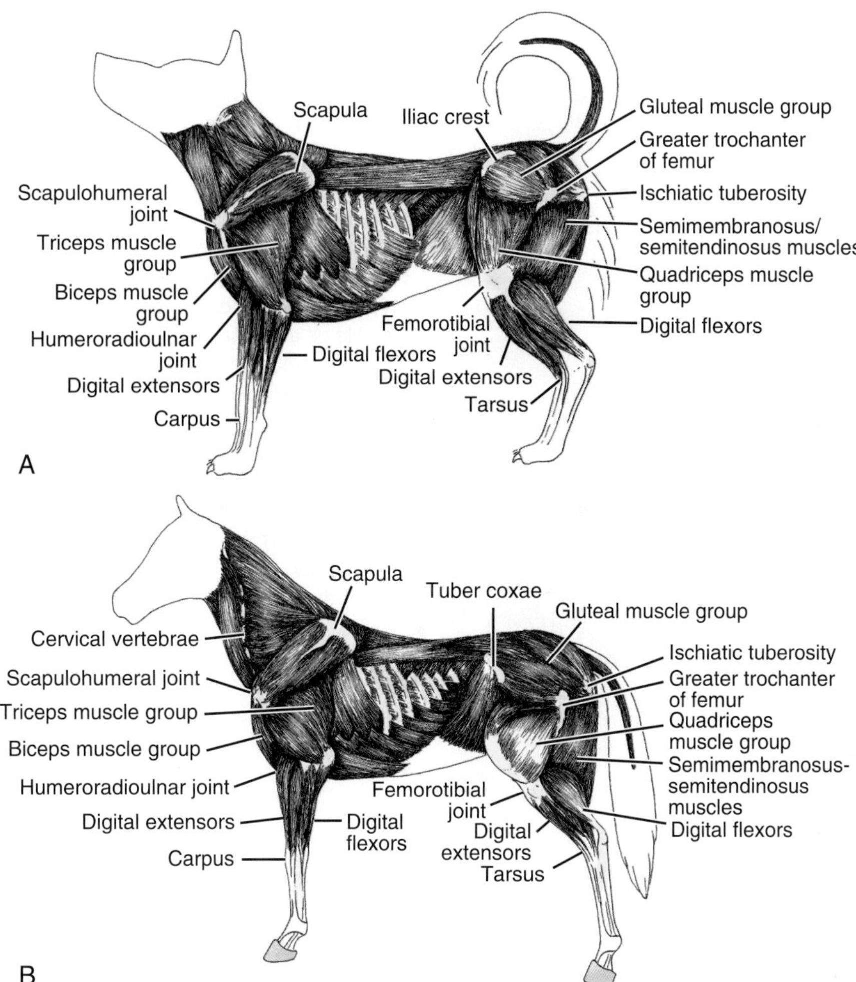

FIG. 14.1 A, Canine musculature. **B,** Equine musculature. From Chistenson DE: *Veterinary medical terminology,* ed 2, 2009, Saunders.

PROFICIENCY EXERCISE 14.1

1. Discuss with a groomer or veterinary technician what it is like to work with animals.
2. Spend time at the local Humane Society or animal rescue shelter and massage the animals to support socialization.

- *Animal behavior and handling:* Animal behavior, handling, breed characteristics, developmental periods, proper socialization, basic health routines, disease prevention, and animal communication
- *Training tools:* Clickers, collars, leashes, housetraining aids, chewing deterrents, interactive toys, and safety devices
- *Anatomy and physiology specific to the animal:* Anatomical terms, the musculoskeletal system, and comparative anatomy and physiology
- *Kinesiology and biomechanics:* Joint movements, physical structures, and gait
- *Massage training:* Continuing education as an aspect of massage education above entry-level requirements in a qualified and valid education program
- *Pathology:* Animal health, common ailments, and emergency care

Learning grooming procedures, especially for large animals such as horses, provides the necessary skills for safety, sequence, and flow for the massage, which would follow grooming patterns and provide information about animal behavior.

Communication

With animals, just as with infants and young children, body language is an important communication process. The massage professional must not be tentative or afraid of the animal and must work with each animal client with confidence and respect while continually being aware of subtle communication from the animal.

Animals generally are good communicators if you take the time to observe and to learn how they communicate with you. Animals tend to interpret our movements and gestures as if we were one of them. Therefore we should not assume that animals always understand our words and gestures the way we mean them. Some rules for dealing with unfamiliar animals include the following:

- Do not approach or reach for an unfamiliar animal.
- Do not make quick movements toward an animal; quick movements can be frightening or threatening to the animal.

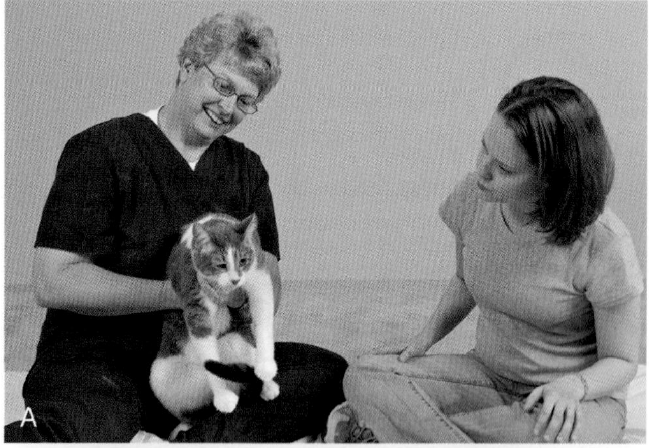

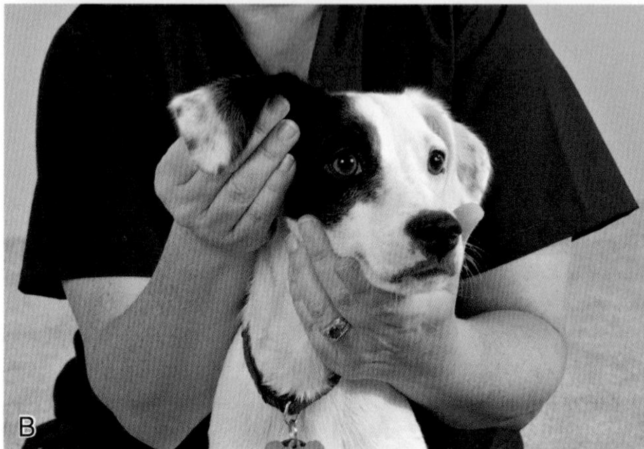

FIG. 14.2 Examples of animal massage.

- Do not stick out a hand for an animal to smell.
- Do not make direct eye contact; this is threatening to many species of animals.
- Do not stand over most animals; this is also threatening to them.
- Do not speak loudly or sharply to animals; this can frighten them.
- Speak softly in a gentle tone; dogs, for example, may interpret deep voices as growls.

The best advice is to become familiar with the gestures and signals of the animals you are going to massage. Do not risk interacting with the animal if you are uncertain how it will respond. Just as with infants and children, it is important to approach animals at their level. For small animals (dogs and cats), sit down on the floor and wait for the animal to approach you. For large animals (horses), stand still, look down, and wait for the animal to approach you. Rely on the human caregiver to comfort the animal and stay by its side (Fig. 14.2). Never force an interaction (Estep and Hetts, 2011).

Typical outcomes for animal massage are support, bonding, stress reduction, relaxation and pleasure, pain relief, and increased performance (Porter, 2005; Coppola et al., 2006; Kathmann et al., 2006; Riley et al., 2021). Massage can enhance muscle function and efficiency and reduce recovery time. The available research for massage specific for animals is sparse. Initially animals may be used for massage-related research for human benefit. Therefore it seems logical that the massage benefits for animals are similar to those for humans (Formenton et al., 2017). Many veterinarians and respected research scientists believe that massage can assist an animal's body in the healing process. It can be used in conjunction with prescribed veterinary care and to augment that care. (Box 14.2) (Memon et al., 2016; Dybczyńska et al., 2022; Bergh et al., 2022).

Box 14.2 Benefits of Massage for Animals

- Improves circulation, increasing the supply of blood and nutrients to muscles and bone
- Aids elimination of waste and toxins from the body
- Increases the flexibility and function of the joints
- Helps maintain posture and body balance
- Stimulates the metabolism, aiding weight loss
- Improves muscle tone
- Enhances range of motion and gait function
- Promotes a healthy skin and coat
- Helps alleviate age-related problems and assists in recovery from injury or surgery
- Helps reduce muscle atrophy resulting from inactivity or disuse
- Relieves muscle tension, soreness, and spasms
- Aids the elimination and prevention of muscular adhesions and connective tissue changes
- Shortens the time required for rehabilitation of soft tissue injuries
- Reduces chronic pain and discomfort caused by arthritis, hip dysplasia, and other conditions
- Calms hyperactive, anxious, and nervous animals
- Counteracts the effects of stress and anxiety
- Builds trust and acceptance of being touched
- Supports bonding

Animals That Benefit From Massage

Many types of animals can benefit from massage:

- Working animals, such as dogs and horses (e.g., guide and service dogs, police horses, farm horses)
- Entertainment and education animals
- Athletic animals (e.g., racehorses or greyhounds)
- Older animals
- Infant and adolescent animals
- Shy or recently adopted animals
- Animals recovering from injury or undergoing postoperative rehabilitation (Box 14.3)

Human Benefit

Animal massage bestows some important benefits on the person doing the massage. Teaching those who are anxious, lonely, or depressed to massage animals can be a productive aspect of the person's treatment and care. Research has shown that when stroking an animal, people relax, their oxytocin increases, and their blood pressure drops (Handlin et al., 2011; Beetz et al., 2012; Gee et al., 2021; Hunt, 2022).

Pain Management

A major outcome for animal massage is pain management. Animal behavior changes in response to pain, particularly persistent pain (Monteiro et al., 2022). The changes that occur

Box 14.3 Rehabilitative Massage for Animals

Rehabilitation therapy is any measure taken to restore maximum function after an injury, an illness, or surgery. Conditions for which rehabilitative massage may be used include:

- Arthritis
- Hip dysplasia
- Fractured limb (after repair)
- Cruciate ligament injury
- Intervertebral disk disease
- Muscle sprains and strains
- Scar tissue management after surgery

Rehabilitative massage for an animal should be supervised by a veterinarian or an experienced animal handler as part of a total treatment program.

depend on the degree of pain, the animal's tolerance of it, species type, the situation in which the pain occurs, the animal's stress level, and a variety of other factors. Acute pain may produce aversive reactions in animals. A normally compliant, friendly animal may attempt to bite a person who is causing it pain, or the animal may try to flee from the pain cause.

Chronic or long-term pain (e.g., arthritis) is likely to produce more subtle behavioral changes. Animals, just like people, react to pain through coping mechanisms that are both internal and external. Descending pathways from the brain to the spinal cord inhibit neuronal activity and reduce the sensation of pain. In addition, compounds are released that have opioid effects (e.g., endorphins and enkephalins) (Cantwell, 2010; Machin et al., 2020).

Animals in pain often withdraw from their social group, choosing instead to remain alone, to be less active, and less responsive to external stimuli. Persistent pain sometimes causes an animal to traumatize the area that hurts, typically by excessively scratching, rubbing, biting, or licking the site. This behavior may be an attempt at pain management through counterirritation. Abnormal postures, such as a hunched back or a tiptoe gait, may also indicate pain. Food and water intake often alters, regardless the source of pain.

Grooming is an important activity for animals, and failure to groom is an early sign of pain. The hair or fur may be standing up rather than lying down smoothly. It may be dull rather than shiny, and it may be matted or clumped, particularly around the face, mouth, anus, and genitals.

Pain Behavior in Dogs, Cats, and Horses

Dogs

Dogs in pain generally appear quieter, less alert, and withdrawn. Their body movements are stiff, and they are unwilling to move. A dog in severe pain may lie still or adopt an abnormal posture to minimize discomfort. With less severe pain, the dog may appear restless because the immediate response to acute but low-intensity pain may be increased alertness. Shivering and increased respiration with panting may occur. Spontaneous barking is unlikely; the dog is more likely to whimper or howl, especially if left unattended. It may growl without apparent provocation. A dog may lick or scratch painful areas of its body, and the tail often is between the legs. Penile protrusion and frequent urination also may occur. A dog in pain may have an anxious look, and it may seek a cold surface on which to lie. When handled, the dog may be abnormally apprehensive or aggressive.

Cats

Cats in pain generally are quiet and have an apprehensive facial expression. The forehead may appear creased. The cat may cry or yowl, and it may growl and hiss if approached or made to move. Cats in pain tend to hide or separate from other cats. The posture usually becomes stiff and abnormal, varying with the site of pain. A cat with head pain may keep its head tilted. If the pain is generalized in the thorax and abdomen, the cat may be crouched or hunched. With thoracic pain alone, the head, neck, and body may be extended. With abdominal or back pain, the cat may lie on its side with the back arched. If the animal is standing or walking, the back is arched, and the gait is stilted. Incessant licking is sometimes associated with localized pain. With pain in one limb, the cat usually limps or holds up the affected limb.

A cat in severe pain may show frantic behavior and make desperate attempts to escape. Touching or palpating a painful area may produce an instant and violent reaction. The animal may pant, and the pulse rate may be increased, and the pupils dilated. A cat in chronic pain may have an ungroomed appearance and may show a marked change from its normal behavior. The limbs are tucked, the head and neck are hunched, the ears are flattened, and the animal utters a distinctive cry or hissing and spitting sound. Cats in pain show fear of being handled and may cringe.

Horses

Periods of restlessness are typically observed in horses experiencing pain or distress. Food is held in the mouth uneaten. The horse exhibits an anxious appearance, with dilated pupils and glassy eyes. Other signs include increased respiration and pulse rate, flared nostrils, profuse sweating, and a rigid stance. With prolonged pain, the animal's behavior may change from restlessness to depression, with the head lowered. With pain associated with skeletal damage, the limbs may be held in unusual positions, the head and neck are "fixed," and the horse may be reluctant to move. Pain-induced tachycardia may be seen.

With abdominal pain, a horse may look at, bite, or kick its abdomen; it may get up and lie down frequently, walk in circles, or roll. When near collapse, the horse may stand very quietly and appear rigid and unmoving. Horses in pain generally show a reluctance to be handled.

Pain Medication for Animals

Opioid Agonists

Opioids used in veterinary medicine include morphine, meperidine, fentanyl, oxymorphone, etorphine (M99), and carfentanil. They are all effective analgesics that work through the central nervous system (CNS).

Implications for Massage

The side effects of the opioid-based medication in animals are like those in humans. These medications can depress the CNS and affect breathing and levels of consciousness. It is important to observe these effects and immediately report them to the veterinarian.

Nonsteroidal Antiinflammatory Drugs

Nonsteroidal antiinflammatory drugs (NSAIDs) produce analgesia by reducing inflammation and peripheral sensitization. Unlike opiates, they typically do not act on the central nervous system.

Side effects of NSAIDs include gastric ulcers and interference with platelet function, anticoagulative action, and kidney function. Because cats metabolize NSAIDs slowly and toxicity can quickly occur, these pain medications are not typically used in cats. NSAIDs commonly used in dogs are aspirin and naproxen.

Implications for Massage

The side effects of NSAIDs are like those seen in humans: altered pain perception and a tendency for increased bleeding and bruising, which would influence the amount of compressive force delivered during massage. Kidney failure is a serious condition. Signs of kidney failure include decreased appetite, increased water consumption and urination, increased sleeping, lethargy, itching, and a change in the smell of the breath. If these behaviors are noticed, the animal should be immediately referred to the veterinarian for emergency care.

Local Anesthetics

Pain relief can be obtained by using local anesthetics, which can be injected around specific nerve trunks that supply a surgical or injury site or infiltrated into the muscular and subcutaneous tissue layers around the area.

Implication for Massage

Do not massage over the area where local injections are given.

Topical Analgesics

Various ointments that act as counterirritants can be used for local pain. It is important to make sure that the ingredients are nontoxic because animals typically lick areas that are painful.

Implications for Massage

Massage can be used to apply the ointment and to enhance its action using tactile stimulation to increase the counterirritant effects.

Providing Massage for Animals

The methods of massage application presented in this text can all be adapted to animals; there are no unique modalities. However, animals generally have a more well-developed sense of smell than humans. Avoid using any scented products.

Animals constitute a population, just as do infants, elder adults, and athletes. Animals can be babies, toddlers, adolescents, parents, middle aged, and elderly. Each of these life stages presents unique circumstances that must be considered. In general, recommendations for humans can be translated to animals. For example, baby animals and baby humans act similarly, except that animals go through the stages much faster. They may be babies for only a few weeks, and then become rambunctious toddlers, and then independent adolescents. Nursing parents can be protective of their babies, and elderly animals have characteristics of human elders.

Humans become attached to their animal companions. Pets are part of the family, and the massage therapist who works with animals must be able to communicate and respect humans as much as the animal.

History and Assessment

A history and assessment are required for an animal, just as they are for a human client. The massage therapist should obtain answers to the following questions from the animal's caretaker:

- What is the animal's name?
- Does the animal have any medical problems?
- Is the animal used to being handled?
- Does the animal bite?
- Is the animal easily frightened?

The massage therapist should meet the animal and become familiar with it and its human companion. Once the animal feels comfortable with the massage therapist, the next step is to perform a visual and physical assessment to make sure the animal does not have any open wounds or sores that would contraindicate massage or require referral to a veterinarian.

Massage therapists need to be alert for problems indicated by body temperature, texture of skin and muscle fibers, tenderness of certain areas, and tension. The outcome for massage needs to be determined and a treatment plan established.

Massage Application

The qualities of touch previously described in this textbook also apply to massage for animals.

- *Pressure:* Just as with humans, it is important to be sure that the pressure applied is effective in achieving the determined outcomes but does not cause unnecessary pain or tissue damage. Animals do not like to be poked, prodded, or dug into. Animals will communicate when the pressure is inappropriate. Animals can vocalize, attempt to move away, and nip (not bite). If the pressure is appropriately intense, the animal typically vocalizes but does not attempt to move away from the pressure and may even lean into it. Pressure varies with the size of the animal (e.g., a ferret does not need as much pressure as a horse).
- *Drag:* Hair, fur, and feathers make it difficult to apply drag to the skin surface. The superficial fascia and deeper tissues can be worked by lifting the skin (which may be quite loose) and then moving the tissues into ease and bind.
- *Direction:* The direction of massage application, which is similar to that in human massage, varies according to the desired outcome (e.g., fluid movement or changes in muscle motor tone).
- *Duration:* The duration of a massage depends on the animal's acceptance and condition. The first session typically is an introductory meeting to allow the massage practitioner to become more familiar with the animal, to learn about its history, and to help the animal build trust and acceptance

of being touched. The first session lasts about 1 hour; the massage itself lasts 15–20 minutes, depending on the animal. Some animals accept a 60-minute, full-body massage at the first session, and others may take multiple sessions to learn to enjoy massage. The massage therapist works with the specific needs of each animal and teaches the person responsible for care how to perform the massage.

- *Frequency:* Therapeutic massage can be given daily for 10–30 minutes for healthy animals. If a disease or injury is involved, massage of different areas of the body every other day is recommended. However, the needs of each animal vary. For animals and people, a weekly massage provided as part of a well-balanced maintenance plan is recommended.

Special Considerations for Horses

Massage for horses, or equine massage, is popular. Because horses are large animals, the potential for harm to the massage therapist is greater. The following suggestions are important when massaging a horse or any large animal:

- Do not jump around or move suddenly, do not wear shiny or noisy jewelry or strongly scented products, and do not behave nervously around horses. All these result in a nervous horse that is unsafe to work around.
- Wear hard-toed shoes or boots when working around horses. One of the most common horse-related injuries is having a foot stepped on.
- Always let the horse know what you intend to do. Quick, sudden movements startle horses and should be avoided.
- Keep all equipment away from the work area unless it is being used at the moment. This prevents the horse from stepping on it, playing with it, or chewing on it; it also prevents the massage therapist from accidentally tripping over it.
- Start massaging on the left side of the neck and work toward the rear of the horse. Then repeat on the right side. This pattern follows the standard grooming process for horses. Areas that have few muscles and bones near the surface, such as the face, legs, and hips, should be massaged carefully and gently. Stand near the horse during the massage and use fluid, rhythmic movements (instead of quick, jerky movements).
- When changing sides, walk far enough away to avoid getting kicked. Never step over the lead rope or crossties. This puts you in a dangerous position should the horse panic and pull back on the rope. Never crawl under the horse's belly. Even the most docile horse can spook and step on you.
- Be aware that some horses are ticklish and may become fidgety. During fly season, particularly, a horse often thrusts its hind leg forward to chase flies from the abdomen; therefore it is wise to keep your head and body out of striking range when working in that area.
- When massaging the legs, bend at the hips or remain in a squat position. Do not sit on the ground or rest one or both knees on the ground. These are committed positions, which means that once you are in them, it takes longer than a split second to get out of them. In committed positions, if the horse should become frightened, the time taken to move away and chances of becoming seriously injured increases. It always helps to have your free hand resting on the horse's body while working on the legs so you can feel if muscles suddenly tense and be warned the horse is about to panic.

Key Points

- Each animal is assessed and treated as an individual.
- Massage adaptation factors include species, age, size, activity level, injuries, and medications.
- Massage therapists who work with animals are likely to find themselves in the role of teacher.
- Grooming procedures provide the necessary skills for safety, sequence, and flow for the massage.

ATHLETES

SECTION OBJECTIVES

Chapter objective covered in this section:

2. Describe indications, cautions, and contraindications for massage, and appropriately adapt massage for athletes.

Using the information presented in this section, the student will be able to perform the following:

- List the experts in the care and training of athletes.
- Identify factors to consider when adapting massage for athletes.
- Identify common athletic injuries.

An **athlete** is a person who participates in sports as either an amateur or a professional. **Tactical athletes** are individuals in service professions who have significant physical fitness and performance requirements associated with their work. Tactical athletes include individuals in military service, law enforcement, and first responders such as firefighters and emergency medical technicians. Military service workers can be enrolled in active duty, in the reserves, or in the National Guard, or be veterans.

Athletes require precise use of their bodies and train their nervous system and muscles to perform in specific ways. Often activities involve repetitive use of one muscle group more than others, which may result in hypertrophy; changes in strength and movement patterns; connective tissue formation; and compensation patterns in the rest of the body. These factors contribute to soft tissue difficulties often found with athletes. Fitness (see Chapter 15) is necessary for everyone's wellness, but physical activities of athletes go beyond fitness and are also performance based.

Massage can be beneficial for athletes if the professional performing the massage understands the biomechanics required by the sport or activity. If the specific biomechanics are not understood, massage can impair optimum function in the athletic performance. Because of the intense physical activity involved in sports, an athlete may be more prone to injury.

The experts for athletes are sports medicine physicians, physical therapists, athletic trainers, exercise physiologists, and sports psychologists. It is especially important for athletes to work under the direction of these professionals to ensure proper sports form and training protocols. The professional athlete is more likely to have access to these professionals. Amateur athletes may not have the financial resources to hire training personnel and can be injured by inappropriate training protocols.

If a massage professional plans to work with an athlete on a continuing basis, it is important that the practitioner becomes part of the entire training process.

Massage Adaptation

Typical adaptations for athletes include support for training effects, alternating the massage style for both pre- and post-competition application, avoiding tissue damage, and complementing or considering the effects of medications.

Training Effect

Athletes depend on the effects of training and the resulting neurological response for precise functioning. Because they use their bodies in specific ways to achieve performance, athletes create functional alterations in their bodies. For example, they may have increased mobility in one body area and increased muscle mass in another. It is important to understand the reasons for these changes, so that the massage can be adapted to support performance and manage problems that may occur because of the body changes based on training.

Pre-competition

Adaptation of massage is especially important before competition. Without the proper training and experience, massage therapists might disorganize the neurological responses if they do not understand the patterns required for efficient functioning in the sport. The effect is temporary, and unless the athlete is going to compete within 24 hours, it usually is not significant. However, if nonadapted massage is given just before competition, the results could be devastating. Any type of massage before a competition must be given carefully. Even when the massage therapist has experience with a specific athlete, caution is necessary 24 hours before competition.

Massage that focuses on supporting circulation is appropriate (see Chapter 12). Avoid aggressive stretching, transverse friction, specific myofascial release, and extensive trigger point work.

Tissue Damage

An athlete often pushes the body to its limits. Although this extreme function may increase performance, it also increases the potential for tissue damage. Tissues have relative abilities to resist a particular load (force). A *load* can be one or a group of outside or internal forces acting on the body. Recall that a *force* can be defined as a push or pull. The resistance to a load is called *mechanical stress,* and the internal response is a *deformation,* or change in dimensions. Deformation also is defined as a mechanical strain. The stronger the tissue, the greater magnitude of load it can withstand.

All human tissues have viscous and elastic properties, allowing for deformation. Tissues such as bone are brittle with fewer viscoelastic properties than soft tissue, such as muscle. The loads applied to bone and soft tissues that can cause injury are tension, compression, bend, shear, and torsion. When tissue is deformed to the extent that its elasticity is almost fully exceeded, a yield point has been reached. This is what can occur during athletic performance. When the yield point has been exceeded, mechanical failure occurs, resulting in tissue damage.

Care needs to be taken not to cause tissue damage during massage or increase tissue damage related to an existing injury. Methods with the potential to damage tissue are aggressive stretching, overpowering a client's resisting muscle contraction force, transverse friction, and methods often called *deep tissue massage* that involve heavy focused pressure or stripping of tissue. These same methods can increase the extent of an injury. The goal is to support healing and performance. Too often massage applied aggressively results in tissue injury. If any client is sore and stiff during movement or experiences increased pain in general or in a specific area 24–48 hours after a massage, tissue has been damaged and performance compromised.

The same mechanical forces that can cause tissue damage are applied therapeutically during massage to encourage tissue repair. The type of force that offers the most therapeutic value should be used during massage. In general, during the stage 1 acute and stage 2 subacute phases, the massage therapist should not use the same force as that which loaded the tissue and produced the injury. For example, if a sprain occurs from a torsion load, then kneading, which applies a torsion stress, may not be the best choice until healing progresses and stability restores in the area. For old injuries that have not healed optimally, the massage therapist, during the massage, may need to carefully introduce the same type of tissue load that caused the injury to achieve results.

Medications

Athletes commonly use medications, particularly analgesics for pain and antiinflammatory drugs. The effects of these drugs must be considered in the development of a care plan. Pain medication reduces pain perception so that the athlete may continue to perform before healing is complete. This interferes with successful healing. Antiinflammatory drugs may slow the healing process. When adapting massage, the practitioner must consider changes in sensory feedback if pain medication is used. Massage also can cause inflammation if tissue damage occurs. If the athlete uses antiinflammatory medication, healing occurs more slowly, interfering with performance potential.

Common Sports Injuries

Massage professionals working with athletes should be able to recognize common sports injuries and should refer the athlete to the appropriate medical professional. The massage therapist adapts the massage application using appropriate methods to enhance the healing process once a diagnosis has been made and the rehabilitation plan developed. Understanding sports injuries and massage application requires knowledge of tissue susceptibility to trauma and the mechanical forces involved.

Many factors contribute to mechanical injuries or trauma in sports. In sports, **trauma** is defined as a physical injury or wound sustained in a sport that was produced by an external or internal force. Healing mechanisms manifest as the inflammatory response and resolution of the inflammatory response.

Different tissues heal at different rates. Skin heals quickly, whereas ligaments heal slowly. Stress can influence healing by slowing the repair process. Sleep and proper nutrition are necessary for proper healing.

Skin Injuries

Numerous mechanical stresses and strains can adversely affect the skin's integrity, such as friction (rubbing), scraping, compression (pressure), tearing, cutting, and penetration.

Wounds are classified according to the mechanical load that caused them:

- *Friction blister:* Continuous rubbing over the surface of the skin causes a collection of fluid below or within the epidermal layer; this is called a *blister.*
- *Abrasions:* Abrasions commonly arise from conditions in which the skin is scraped against a rough surface. The epidermis and dermis are worn away, exposing numerous capillaries.
- *Skin bruise:* When a blow compresses or crushes the skin surface and causes bleeding under the skin, the condition is identified as a bruise (aka *contusion*).
- *Laceration:* A laceration is a wound in which the flesh has been irregularly torn.
- *Skin avulsion:* Skin torn by the same mechanism as a laceration, to the extent that avulsion occurs, meaning tissue is completely ripped from its source.
- *Incision wound:* An incision is a wound in which the skin has been sharply cut.
- *Puncture wound:* A puncture is a wound caused when a pointed object penetrates the skin.

Skin injuries are a regional contraindication to massage. Sanitation is essential, and care must be taken to prevent infection.

Muscle Injuries

Overexertion Muscle Problems

Overexertion is a problem that arises in physical conditioning and training. Even though the pattern of gradually overloading the body is the best way to achieve ultimate success, many athletes and training personnel still believe the old adage, "no pain, no gain."

Overtraining is reflected by muscle soreness, decreased joint flexibility, and general fatigue 24 hours after activity. Four specific indicators of possible overexertion are acute muscle soreness, delayed-onset muscle soreness, muscle stiffness, and muscle cramps and spasms.

Acute Muscle Soreness

Overexertion in strenuous exercise often results in muscular pain. At one time or another, most people have experienced muscle soreness, usually because of some physical activity to which the person is unaccustomed. The older a person gets, the more easily muscle soreness seems to develop. Acute muscle soreness accompanies fatigue. This muscle pain is transient and occurs during and immediately after exercise. It is caused by a lack of oxygen to the muscles and the buildup of metabolic waste from anaerobic functions. This type of soreness dissipates as oxygen is restored and metabolic waste is removed from muscle tissue.

Delayed-Onset Muscle Soreness

Delayed-onset muscle soreness becomes most intense after 24–48 hours and then gradually subsides; usually the muscle tissues become symptom free after 3 or 4 days. This type of pain is described as a syndrome of delayed muscle pain leading to increased muscle tension, swelling, stiffness, and resistance to stretching. Delayed onset muscle soreness is thought to result from several potential causes. It may arise from very small tears (microtrauma) in the muscle tissue, which result in an inflammatory process and seem to be more likely with eccentric or isometric contractions. Delayed onset muscle soreness may also arise from disruption of the connective tissue that holds muscle tendon fibers together. Another contributor is increased interstitial fluid, which results in pressure on pain-sensitive structures.

Muscle soreness can be prevented by beginning exercise at a moderate level and gradually increasing intensity over time. Treatment of muscle soreness usually involves general massage with a focus on fluid movement. Antiinflammatory drugs should be avoided, if possible, because they delay healing. Ice can be used for pain control after the acute healing phase.

Muscle Stiffness

Muscle stiffness does not produce pain. It occurs when a group of muscles has been worked hard for a long period. The fluids that collect in the muscles during and after exercise are absorbed into the bloodstream slowly. As a result, the muscles become swollen, shorter, and thicker and therefore resist stretching. Light exercise, lymphatic drainage-type massage, and passive mobilization help reduce stiffness. Stiffness also results with decreased pliability of connective tissue. This occurs when the ground substance thickens as part of enzyme processes during sympathetic dominance. If the condition continues, it may progress to densification. Massage to restore connective tissue pliability (slow, sustained compression and kneading) helps reduce the stiffness.

Muscle Cramps and Spasms

Muscle cramps and spasms can lead to muscle and tendon injuries. A cramp is a painful, involuntary contraction of a skeletal muscle or muscle group. Cramps often occur because of lack of water or other electrolytes, muscle fatigue, or interruption of the appropriate neurological interaction between opposing muscles. A spasm is a reflex reaction caused by trauma of the musculoskeletal system. The two types of cramps and spasms are the clonic type, with alternating involuntary muscular contraction and relaxation in quick succession, and the tonic type, with rigid muscle contraction that lasts a period of time.

Cramps can be temporarily reduced with firm pressure on the belly of the cramping muscle. Cramps and spasms respond to proper hydration and rest.

Muscle Guarding

When an injury occurs, the muscles that surround the injured area contract to splint the area, thus minimizing pain by limiting movement. Often this splinting is incorrectly referred to as a muscle spasm; however, *muscle guarding* is a more appropriate term for the involuntary muscle contractions that occur in response to pain after musculoskeletal injury. Muscle guarding is appropriate during the acute and subacute healing processes and massage application should not attempt to reduce it.

Contusion

A bruise, or contusion, arises from a sudden traumatic blow to the body. Contusions can range from superficial injuries to injuries involving deep tissue compression and hemorrhage (Fig. 14.3).

A contusion can penetrate to the skeletal structures, causing a bone bruise. The extent to which an athlete may be hampered by this condition depends on the location of the bruise and the force of the blow. The speed with which a contusion heals, as with all soft tissue injuries, depends on the extent of tissue damage and internal bleeding. Caution is necessary when providing massage over contusions. Compressive force and depth of pressure must be modified to prevent further injury. Lymphatic drainage-type applications are usually appropriate.

Cautions. A brain contusion is a concussion; this is a serious condition. If the client history indicates a potential for concussion, caution and referral are necessary.

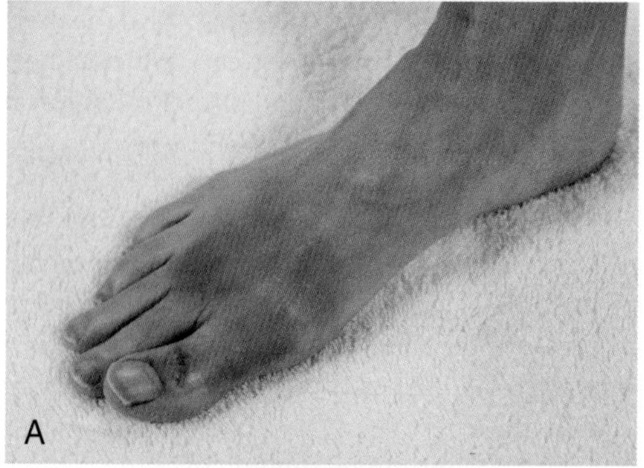

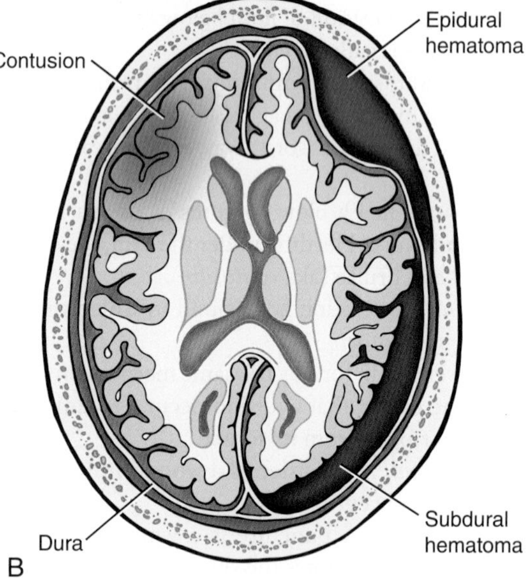

FIG. 14.3 A, A bruised foot. **B,** Example of a brain contusion, also known as a *concussion.* The epidural and subdural hematomas are masses of clotted blood, resulting from broken blood vessels.

Strain

A *strain* is a stretch, tear, or rip in the muscle or adjacent tissue, such as the fascia or muscle tendons (Fig. 14.4). The cause of muscle strain frequently is not clear. Often a strain is produced by an abnormal muscular contraction during reciprocal coordination of the agonist and antagonist muscles. Possible explanations for the muscle imbalance may be a mineral imbalance caused by profuse sweating, the collection of fatigue metabolites in the muscle itself, or a strength imbalance between agonist and antagonist muscles. Synergistic dominance of firing patterns is also crucial.

A strain may range from a tiny separation of connective tissue and muscle fibers to a complete tendinous avulsion or muscle rupture (grade 1, grade 2, or grade 3). The resulting pathological condition is similar to a contusion or sprain, with capillary or blood vessel hemorrhage. The three types of strain are:

- *Grade 1 (mild) strain:* Local pain that is increased by tension of the muscle and minor loss of strength; mild swelling and local tenderness.
- *Grade 2 (moderate) strain:* Similar to a mild strain but with moderate signs and symptoms and impaired muscle function.
- *Grade 3 (severe) strain:* Severe signs and symptoms with loss of muscle function and, commonly, a palpable defect in the muscle.

Muscle strain usually causes muscle guarding. The guarding should not be reduced by massage because it protects the area from further injury. Gentle massage over the area to encourage fluid movement may support healing. During the acute and subacute phases, the soft tissue should be massaged in the direction of the fibers and crowded toward the site of the injury to promote reconnection of the ends of

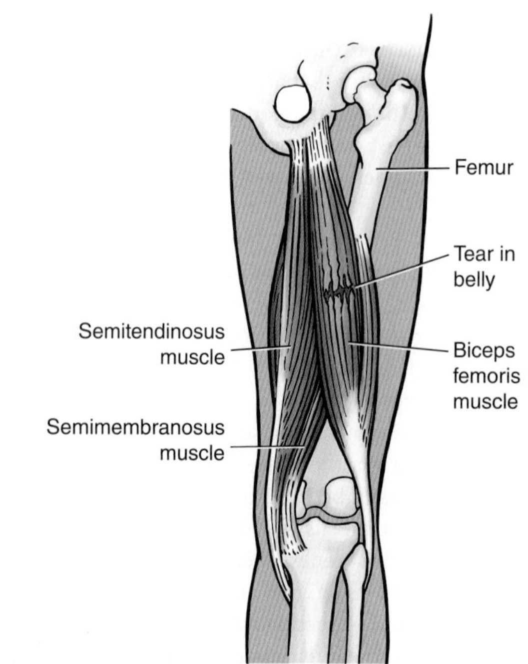

FIG. 14.4 This example of muscle strain is located in the biceps femoris muscle of the hamstring group (in this case, a tear in the midportion of the belly of the muscle).

the separated fibers. Depth of pressure, duration, and intensity all need to be adjusted during the healing phase. Once the acute phase of healing is complete, the methods that support mobile scar formation can be introduced, including moving the tissue away from the injury site and massaging across the fibers (Cummings et al., 2009; Abd-Elsayed et al., 2022).

Tendon Injuries

Tendons have wavy, parallel, collagenous fibers that are organized in bundles surrounded by a gelatinous material that reduces friction. A tendon attaches a muscle to a bone and concentrates a pulling force in a limited area. When a tendon is loaded by tension, the wavy collagenous fibers straighten in the direction of the load; when the tension is released, the collagen returns to its original wavy shape. In tendons, collagen fibers break if the physiological limits are exceeded. A breaking point is reached after a 6%–8% increase in length. Because a tendon usually is double the strength of the muscle it serves, tears most commonly occur in the muscle belly, musculotendinous junction, or bony attachment.

Tendon injuries usually progress slowly over a prolonged period. Often repeated acute injuries can lead to a chronic condition. Constant irritation caused by poor performance techniques or constant stress beyond physiological limits eventually can result in a chronic condition. These injuries often are attributed to overuse microtrauma.

Myositis/Fasciitis

In general, the term *myositis* means inflammation of muscle tissue. More specifically, it can be considered a fibrositis, or connective tissue inflammation. A fascia that supports and separates muscle can also become chronically inflamed after injury. A typical example of this condition is plantar fasciitis.

Tendinitis

Tendinitis is marked by a gradual onset, degenerative changes, and diffuse tenderness caused by repeated microtrauma. Obvious signs of tendinitis are swelling and pain.

Tenosynovitis

Tenosynovitis is inflammation of the synovial sheath surrounding a tendon. In the acute stage, rapid onset of pain, articular crepitus, and diffuse swelling are seen. In chronic tenosynovitis, the tendons become locally thickened, and pain and articular crepitus are present during movement (Fig. 14.5).

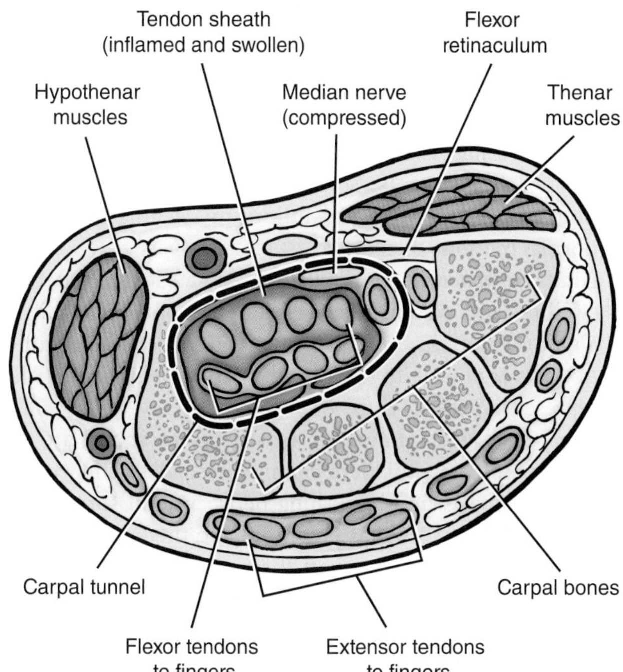

FIG. 14.5 Tenosynovitis and carpel tunnel syndrome in a cross-section view of the wrist.

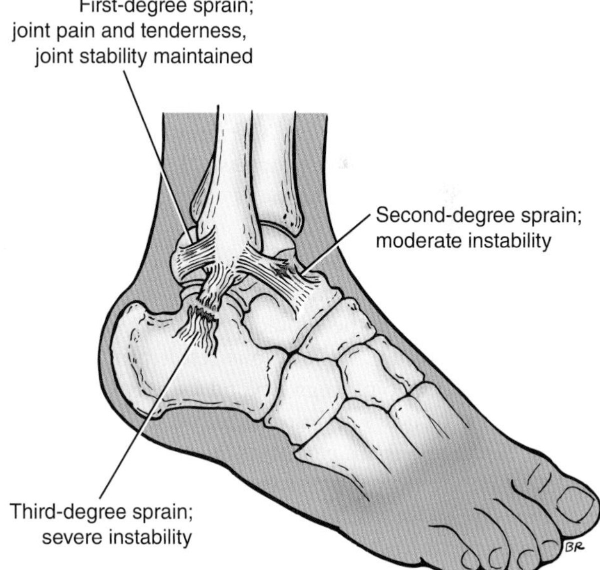

FIG. 14.6 A sprain was the mechanism of injury to the lateral ligament complex of this ankle.

Tendinosis

Tendinosis occurs when an inflamed or irritated tendon (tendonitis) fails to heal, and the tendon degenerates. Tendinosis is also linked to ligament laxity. A weakened or lax ligament leads to an unstable joint, which means the tendon has no static support and would be stressed.

Synovial Joint Injuries

The major injuries affecting the synovial joints are sprains, subluxations, and dislocations. Sprains are among the most common and disabling injuries seen in sports. A sprain is a traumatic twisting of the joint that results in stretching or complete tearing of the stabilizing connective tissues (Fig. 14.6). Ligaments, the articular capsule, and the synovial membrane all are injured.

Sprains

A sprain causes the effusion of blood and synovial fluid into the joint cavity, producing joint swelling, a local temperature increase, pain or point tenderness, and skin discoloration. Ligaments and capsules, like tendons, can experience forces that completely rupture them or that produce an avulsion fracture. Ligaments and joint capsules heal slowly because of their relatively poor blood supply; however, they are plentifully supplied with nerves, and injury to these structures often causes a great deal of pain.

Like muscle strains, sprains are classified into one of three grades according to the extent of injury:

- *Grade 1 (mild) sprain:* Some pain, minimum loss of function, mild point tenderness, little or no swelling, and no abnormal motion when tested.
- *Grade 2 (moderate) sprain:* Pain, moderate loss of function, swelling, and in some cases slight to moderate instability.
- *Grade 3 (severe) sprain:* Extreme pain, major loss of function, severe instability, tenderness, and swelling; may also represent a subluxation.

The joints most vulnerable to sprains in sports are the ankles, knees, and shoulders. Sprains occur less often to the wrists and elbows. Distinguishing between joint sprains and tendon or muscle strains is often difficult; therefore the massage professional should expect the worst possible condition and manage it accordingly. Repeated joint twisting eventually can result in chronic inflammation, degeneration, and arthrosis. Once the proper diagnosis has been made, the massage therapist can provide general full-body massage to reduce compensation patterns from changes in gait function and posture. In addition, lymphatic drainage massage can manage swelling outside the joint capsule. Massage methods that support circulation enhance healing, and hyperstimulation and counterirritation methods reduce pain. Care must be taken not to disrupt the healing tissue in the acute phase. Once the inflammation has diminished, mobilization of the soft tissue promotes mobile scar formation. The duration and intensity of massage increases as healing progresses. Ligaments can take 3–6 months or longer to heal fully.

Dislocations and Diastasis

Dislocations are second to fractures in terms of disabling the athlete. The fingers and the shoulder joint have the highest incidence of dislocation. Dislocations result primarily from forces that cause the joint to go beyond its normal anatomical limits. The two classes of dislocations are subluxations and luxations. *Subluxations* are partial dislocations in which two articulating bones are separated incompletely. *Luxations* are complete dislocations, or a total disunion of bone apposition between the articulating surfaces.

Two types of diastases are seen: a disjointing of two bones parallel to each other (e.g., the radius and ulna or the tibia and fibula) and the rupture of a "solid" joint, such as the symphysis pubis. A diastasis commonly occurs with a fracture.

Several factors are important in recognizing dislocations:

- Limb function is lost. The athlete usually complains of having fallen or of having received a severe blow to a particular joint and then suddenly being unable to move that part.
- Deformity is almost always apparent. Because the deformity often can be obscured by heavy musculature, it is important that the injured site be evaluated by the appropriate medical professional.
- Swelling and point tenderness are immediately present.

As with fractures, x-ray examination of the dislocation sometimes is the only absolute diagnostic measure.

The massage practitioner needs to be aware of any history of dislocation. Increased muscle tension and connective tissue formation may occur around the dislocated joint as an appropriate stabilization process. Care must be taken to maintain joint stability while supporting mobility.

Chronic Joint Injuries

Like other chronic physical injuries or problems that arise from sports participation, chronic synovial joint injuries stem from microtrauma and overuse. The two major categories in which they fall are osteochondrosis and traumatic arthritis (*osteoarthritis,* or inflammation of surrounding soft tissues, such as the bursal capsule and the synovium). A major cause of chronic joint injury is failure of the muscles to control or limit deceleration during eccentric function. Athletes can avoid such injuries by avoiding chronic fatigue, by not training when tired, and by wearing protective gear to enhance the active absorption of impact forces (Fig. 14.7).

Traumatic arthritis arthrosis usually is the result of accumulated microtrauma. With repeated trauma to the articular joint surfaces, the bone and synovium thicken, and pain, muscle spasm, and articular *crepitus* (grating on movement) occur. Joint wear leading to arthritis can come from repeated sprains that leave a joint with weakened ligaments. Misalignment of the musculoskeletal structure, which stresses joints, can be a factor, or arthritis can arise from an irregular joint surface or be caused by repeated articular chondral injuries. Loose bodies that have been dislodged from the articular surface can also irritate the joint and produce arthritis. Athletes with joint injuries that are improperly immobilized or who are allowed to return to activity before proper healing has occurred eventually may be afflicted with arthritis. The condition often becomes degenerative joint disease. Massage applications for chronic joint injury involve palliative care to control pain. More focused massage application combined with therapeutic exercise and education related to joint function capacity and adaptation are indicated. While results may be short term, the participation in regular supportive care can be helpful in maintaining quality of life (Skillgate et al., 2019).

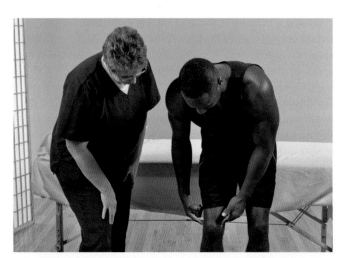

FIG. 14.7 Joint injuries are common among athletes.

Bursitis

A *bursa* is a fluid-filled sac that is found in places where friction might occur in body tissues. Bursae provide protection between tendons and bones, between tendons and ligaments, and between other structures where friction occurs. Sudden irritation can cause acute bursitis. Overuse of muscles or tendons in addition to constant external compression or trauma can result in chronic bursitis. The signs and symptoms of bursitis include swelling, pain, and some loss of function. Repeated trauma may lead to calcific deposits and degeneration of the internal lining of the bursa.

Bursitis in the knee, elbow, and shoulder is common among athletes. Massage can be used to lengthen the shortened structures, reducing friction. Ice applications and rehabilitative exercise are indicated. Short-term use of antiinflammatory medication may be helpful. Steroid injections at the site are a common treatment. Massage is contraindicated in the area of steroid injection until the medication has been fully absorbed by the body. Five to 7 days is a safe waiting period, after which massage may be resumed.

Bone Injuries

Because of its viscoelastic properties, bone can bend slightly. However, bone generally is brittle and a poor shock absorber because of its mineral content. This brittleness increases under tension forces more than under compression forces. Bone trauma generally can be classified as acute bone fractures and stress fractures.

Acute Bone Fractures

A bone fracture can be a partial or a complete interruption of the bone continuity. It can occur without external exposure or can extend through the skin, creating an external wound (open fracture). As a result of normal remodeling, a bone may become vulnerable to fracture during the first few weeks of intense physical activity or training. Weight-bearing bones undergo bone reabsorption and become weaker before they become stronger. Fractures also can result from direct trauma; that is, the bone breaks directly at the site where a force is applied. A fracture that occurs some distance from the point where force is applied is called an *indirect fracture*. A sudden violent muscle contraction or repetitive abnormal stress to a bone also can cause a fracture. Fractures are one of the most serious hazards of sports and should be routinely suspected in musculoskeletal injuries.

Stress Fractures

The exact cause of stress fractures is unknown, but a number of possibilities are likely: an overload caused by muscle contraction, altered stress distribution in the bone because of muscle fatigue, a change in the ground traction force (e.g., moving from a wood surface to a grass surface), or rhythmically repetitive stress.

Early detection of a stress fracture may be difficult. Because of their frequency in a wide range of sports, stress fractures always must be suspected in susceptible body areas that fail to respond to the usual management. The major signs of a stress fracture are swelling, focal tenderness, and pain. In the early stages of the fracture, the athlete complains of pain when active but not at rest. Later, the pain is constant and becomes more intense at night. Percussion (i.e., light tapping on the bone at a site other than the suspected fracture) produces pain at the fracture site. The most common sites of stress fractures are the tibia, fibula, metatarsal shaft, calcaneus, femur, lumbar vertebrae, ribs, and humerus (Fig. 14.8).

The management of stress fractures varies with the individual athlete, the injury site, and the extent of injury. Stress fractures that occur on the concave side of bone heal more rapidly and are managed more easily than those on the convex

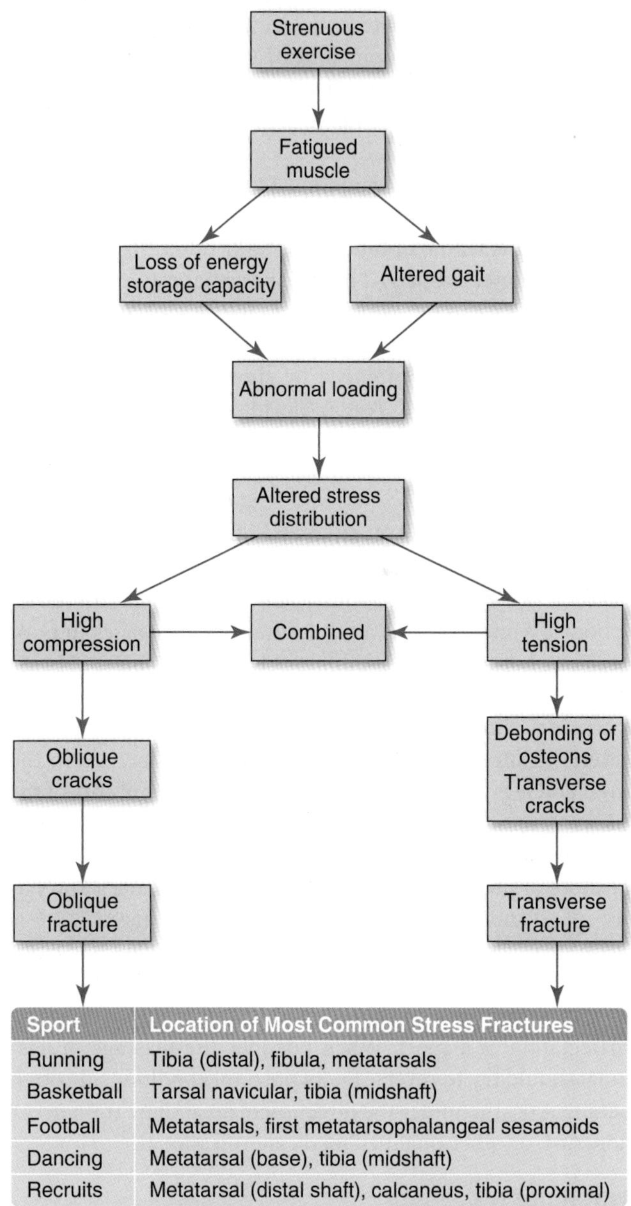

Sport	Location of Most Common Stress Fractures
Running	Tibia (distal), fibula, metatarsals
Basketball	Tarsal navicular, tibia (midshaft)
Football	Metatarsals, first metatarsophalangeal sesamoids
Dancing	Metatarsal (base), tibia (midshaft)
Recruits	Metatarsal (distal shaft), calcaneus, tibia (proximal)

FIG. 14.8 Sequence of events leading to stress fractures. Loss of the muscle's energy storage capacity (fatigue) leads to microscopic bone failure (stress fracture). In the text with green shading, the locations of the most common sport-specific stress fractures are listed. From Malone T, McPoil T, Nitz AJ. *Orthopedic and sport physical therapy,* 3rd ed. 1997, Mosby; and Miller MD, Cooper DE, Warner JJP, et al. *Review of sports medicine and arthroscopy,* 2nd ed, 2002, Saunders.

side. Stress fractures on the convex side can quickly produce a complete fracture. The massage practitioner needs to be aware of the potential for stress fractures and refer the athlete if necessary. The main massage approach during fracture healing is support for the whole body with general massage and methods to reduce compensation from changes in gait and reduced activity.

Nerve Injuries

The two main stresses that cause major nerve injury are compression and tension. As with injuries to other tissues in the body, nerve injury may be acute or chronic. Any number of traumatic experiences that directly affect nerves can also produce a variety of sensory responses, including pain. For example, sudden stretching or pinching of a nerve can produce both muscle weakness and a sharp, burning pain that radiates down a limb. Neuritis, a chronic nerve problem, can be caused by a variety of forces that usually have been repeated or continued for a prolonged period. Symptoms of neuritis can range from minor nerve problems to paralysis.

Pain that is felt at a point in the body other than its actual origin is known as *referred pain.* A potential cause of referred pain is a trigger point, which occurs in the muscular system. Massage applications for nerve injuries are palliative to reduce pain. If the nerve is impinged by short muscles and fascia, massage can be used to restore normal pliability and length, increase tissue sliding, and reduce pressure on the nerve.

Postural Changes

Postural deviations often are a major underlying cause of sports injuries. Postural misalignment may arise from unilateral (one side of the body) muscle and soft tissue asymmetries or bony asymmetries. As a result, the athlete engages in poor mechanics of movement (pathomechanics). Many sports activities, such as weightlifting, are unilateral and thus lead to asymmetries in body development. For example, a consistent pattern of knee injury may be related to asymmetries in the pelvis and legs (short leg syndrome) or reduced mobility of the ankles. A number of postural conditions are genuine hazards for athletes, making them prone to specific injuries. Some of the more important conditions are foot, ankle, and leg anomalies; spinal anomalies; and various stress syndromes.

Unfortunately, not much in the form of remedial work is usually performed. As a result, an injury often becomes chronic, sometimes to the point that the athlete must stop participating in a sport. When possible, the massage professional should try to reverse faulty postural conditions through therapy, working under the direction of an athletic trainer, orthopedist, or other qualified medical professional.

Heat Illnesses

Exercising in a hot, humid environment can cause various forms of heat illness, including heat rash, heat syncope, heat cramps, heat exhaustion, and heatstroke.

Heat Rash

Heat rash, also called *prickly heat,* is a benign condition associated with a red, raised rash that is accompanied by sensations of prickling and tingling during sweating. It usually occurs when the skin is continuously wet with unevaporated sweat. The rash generally is localized to areas of the body covered with clothing. Massage is regionally contraindicated.

Heat Syncope

Heat syncope, or *heat collapse,* is associated with rapid physical fatigue during overexposure to heat. It is usually caused by standing in the heat for lengthy periods or by not being accustomed to exercising in the heat. It is caused by peripheral vasodilation of superficial vessels, hypotension, or a pooling of blood in the extremities, which results in dizziness, fainting, and nausea. Heat syncope is quickly relieved by having the athlete lie down in a cool environment and replacing fluids.

Heat Cramps

Heat cramps are extremely painful muscle spasms that occur most commonly in the calf and abdomen, although any muscle can be involved. The occurrence of heat cramps is related to excessive loss of water and several electrolytes or ions (sodium, chloride, potassium, magnesium, and calcium), which are essential elements in muscle contraction. Profuse sweating results in the loss of large amounts of water and small amounts of electrolytes, which destroys the balance in concentration of these elements in the body. This imbalance ultimately results in painful muscle contractions and cramps. The person most likely to develop heat cramps is one who is in good condition but simply overexerts in the heat.

Heat cramps can be prevented by adequate replacement of sodium, chloride, potassium, magnesium, calcium, and, most important, water. Ingestion of salt tablets is not recommended. Sodium can be replaced by simply salting food a bit more heavily; bananas are particularly high in potassium; and calcium is present in green, leafy vegetables, milk, cheese, and dairy products. The immediate treatment for heat cramps is ingestion of large amounts of water with added electrolytes and mild stretching, with ice massage of the muscle in spasm. An athlete who experiences heat cramps generally is not able to return to practice or competition that day because cramping is likely to recur. Massage is contraindicated and will not relieve heat cramps. Rest and hydration are indicated.

Heat Exhaustion

Heat exhaustion results from inadequate replacement of fluids lost through sweating. Clinically, the victim of heat exhaustion collapses and has profuse sweating, pale skin, a mildly elevated temperature (102°F [39°C]), dizziness, hyperventilation, and a rapid pulse.

It sometimes is possible to spot athletes who are having problems with heat exhaustion. They may begin to develop heat cramps. They may become disoriented and light-headed, and their physical performance is not up to their usual standards. In general, people in poor physical condition who attempt to exercise in the heat are most likely to suffer from heat exhaustion.

Immediate treatment of heat exhaustion requires ingestion and eventually intravenous replacement of substantial amounts of water. Massage is contraindicated.

Heatstroke

Unlike heat cramps and heat exhaustion, *heatstroke* is a life-threatening emergency. The specific cause of heatstroke is unknown. It is characterized clinically by sudden collapse with loss of consciousness; flushed, hot skin with less sweating than would be seen with heat exhaustion; shallow breathing; a rapid, strong pulse; and, most important, a core temperature of 106°F (41°C) or higher. In the heatstroke victim, the body's thermoregulatory mechanism has broken down because of an excessively high body temperature; the body loses the ability to dissipate heat through sweating.

Heatstroke can occur suddenly and without warning. The athlete usually does not experience signs of heat cramps or heat exhaustion. The possibility of death from heatstroke can be reduced significantly if the body temperature is lowered to normal within 45 minutes. The longer the body temperature is elevated to 106°F (41°C) or higher, the higher the mortality rate. Death is imminent if the body's core temperature rises to 107°F (41.7°C) or higher.

Every first aid effort should be directed toward lowering the body temperature. Get the athlete into a cool environment, strip off all clothing, sponge the person down with cool water, and fan the individual with a towel. Do not immerse the athlete in cold water. It is imperative that the heatstroke victim be transported to a hospital as quickly as possible. The replacement of fluid is not critical in initial first aid. Massage is contraindicated.

Hypothermia

Cold weather is a common condition in many outdoor sports in which the sport itself does not require heavy protective clothing; consequently, the weather becomes a pertinent factor in the athlete's susceptibility to injury. In most instances the activity itself enables the athlete to increase the metabolic rate sufficiently to function normally and dissipate the resulting heat and perspiration through the usual physiological mechanisms. If an athlete fails to warm up sufficiently or becomes chilled because of relative inactivity for varying periods, the individual is more prone to injury.

Dampness or wetness further increases the risk of hypothermia. An air temperature of 50°F (10°C) is relatively comfortable, but water at the same temperature is intolerable. The combination of cold, wind, and dampness creates an environment that easily predisposes the athlete to hypothermia.

A relatively small drop in the body's core temperature can induce shivering sufficient to materially affect an athlete's neuromuscular coordination and performance. Shivering stops when the body temperature drops below 85°F–90°F (29.4°C–32.2°C). Death is imminent if the core temperature drops to 77°F–85°F (25°C–29.4°C). Treatment involves warming and drying the athlete.

Ongoing Care of the Athlete

For athletes, regular massage may benefit performance especially based on perception of benefit, accelerated recovery time, and may help discomfort related to delayed-onset muscle soreness (Kennedy et al., 2018; Moseley et al., 2018; Vavken, 2018; Zhang et al., 2022). There are no specific protocols for massage targeting athletes. The basic massage process presented in Chapter 10, coupled with appropriate assessment procedures (see Chapter 11) and the addition of various aspects of hydrotherapy, implement assisted massage, cupping, kinesiology tape, fluid movement, connective tissue application, and trigger point interventions (see Chapter 12), can address the needs of this population (Angelopoulos et al., 2021).

Massage therapy is beneficial as part of musculoskeletal and sports rehabilitation because it decreases pain level and increases pain threshold with few adverse effects. In addition, massage may improve blood flow to the affected area (Mohamed et al., 2023). Massage provides a small benefit in reducing symptoms of delayed onset muscle soreness (DOMS) and results in a small but significant improvement in flexibility (Davis et al., 2020). The psychological effects of massage are as beneficial as any physical affects (Shamsi et al., 2021).

Key Points

- Working with athletes can be demanding. Their schedules may be erratic, and their bodies change almost daily in response to training, competition, or injury.
- Athletes in training have reduced adaptive capacity. *Do not* over massage, cause tissue damage, or assume that athletes require an aggressive approach.
- Most athletes require varying depths of pressure, from light to firm; consequently, the massage practitioner must make sure to use effective body mechanics.
- Athletes can become psychologically dependent on massage; therefore commitment by the massage professional is necessary.

BREAST MASSAGE

SECTION OBJECTIVES

Chapter objective covered in this section:

3. Describe and apply appropriate massage in the breast area.

Using the information presented in this section, the student will be able to perform the following:

- Determine when breast massage is appropriate.
- Consider ethical principles in deciding when breast massage is performed.

Note: Massage of the female breast is a controversial issue. A conservative approach is taken in this textbook. Although a body area is not a population, the topic needs to be addressed because many have breast health issues.

Anatomically the breast is part of the integumentary system. It becomes a functional part of the female reproductive system only during lactation. The breast is considered an erogenous zone. An erogenous zone is an area of the body where sexual tension concentrates and can be relieved through stimulation. Other erogenous zones are the mouth, genitals, and anus. These areas usually have some sort of erectile tissue that engorges with blood when stimulated. In the breast, the nipple is this erectile tissue. The controversy over the appropriateness of massage of the female breast centers on the breast as an erogenous area.

Considerations for Breast Massage

Breast massage can be appropriate for certain conditions, such as the development of scar tissue after surgery.

Types of Breast Surgery

Breast Cancer

Surgery for breast cancer may involve either removal of only the cancerous tissue or a mastectomy. Often reconstructive surgery is performed. The massage practitioner must attend to contraindications and cautions in connection with treatments given after surgery. For example, radiation over the area can weaken the bones, predisposing them to fracture.

Breast Implants and Reduction

Breast implants are another consideration. Care must be taken to apply gentle pressure over the implants while still addressing the connective tissue changes that can occur when implants are used.

Breast reduction surgery is performed for both cosmetic and health reasons. The same attention is paid to scar tissue development and healing as is given in other surgical procedures.

Gender-Affirming Surgery

Top surgery is surgery that removes or augments breast tissue and reshapes the chest to create a more masculine or feminine appearance for people as part of gender transition.

Massage Adaptation

As for any surgery or area of healing, unless specifically trained, focused massage to the area is not provided during the acute phase. After the initial healing is complete, gentle massage that mobilizes the tissue around the surgical area can be performed. After 4 weeks, if healing is progressing well, the scar itself can be gently massaged. The most common method used is a gentle form of superficial fascia movement involving moving the affected and adjacent tissue into ease and then into bind as explained in Chapter 12. After 3 months, more specific connective tissue methods can be used.

Scar Tissue

When the therapist works with existing scar tissue, the work progresses slowly and deliberately. Most scar tissue tends to be less pliable than surrounding tissue. It also tends to shorten and pull. Breast surgery can result in a pulling forward of the shoulder and discomfort from taut, long tissue in the midback.

Methods that target connective tissue (see Chapter 12) are effective for managing scar tissue. More generalized massage manipulations, such as gliding, kneading, and compression, prepare the tissue for more specific work.

Positioning the Client

Soft tissue under the breast tissue can be accessed effectively by placing the client in the side-lying position, in which the breast tissue falls away from the chest wall toward the table. In the supine position the breast tissue usually falls to the side, allowing massage over the sternum and intercostal area. These two positions provide adequate access to the soft tissue of the chest wall. Therefore there is no reason to massage through the breast tissue proper to reach these areas (Fig. 14.9).

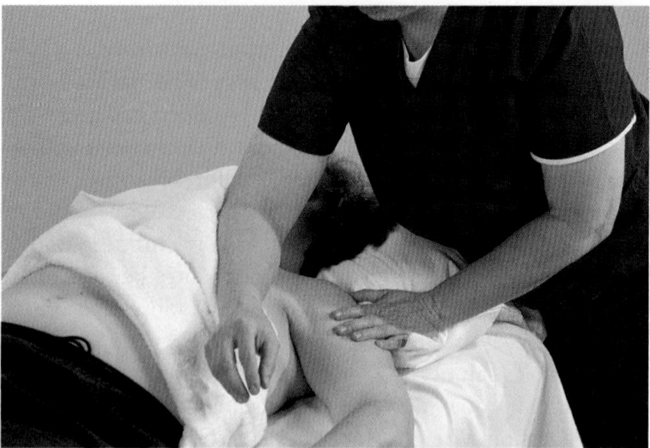

FIG. 14.9 Using the forearm to massage around the breast tissue.

Ethical Considerations

The ethical principles discussed in Chapter 2 serve as the basis for decision making regarding the appropriateness of breast massage for any gender. The massage professional should particularly consider the following:

- *Proportionality:* The benefit must outweigh the burden of treatment.
- *Nonmaleficence:* The practitioner must do no harm and must prevent harm from occurring.
- *Beneficence:* The treatment must contribute to the client's well-being.

Other health care professionals adequately undertake breast examination and the teaching of breast self-examination. It is not necessary for the massage professional to provide such services.

Breast massage as part of a general massage serves no specific physiological purpose that cannot be achieved in ways other than breast massage; therefore the concerns may outweigh the benefit (Proficiency Exercise 14.2).

PROFICIENCY EXERCISE 14.2

Investigate the surgical procedure for breast cancer, breast augmentation with implants, or breast reduction. Write an intervention plan and justification statement for the use of therapeutic massage. For guidance, check out the example on the Evolve site.

Example: Therapeutic massage for ______________

1. Gather facts to identify and define the situation.
   Key questions: What is the problem? What are the facts?
2. Brainstorm possible solutions.
   Key questions: What might I do? What if ...?
3. Evaluate possible interventions logically and objectively; look at both sides and at the pros and cons.
   Key question: What would happen if ...?
4. Evaluate the effect on the people involved.
   Key question: How would each person involved feel?
5. Develop an intervention plan and justification statements.

Key Points

If breast massage for a specific condition is deemed appropriate by a health care professional and the client is referred to the massage professional, the following measures are recommended:

- Work with specific written informed consent for breast massage.
- Work with another professional in the room, much as a male gynecologist has a female nurse present during examinations. If this is not possible, male therapists should refer a female client to a female therapist.
- Use careful draping. Do not expose the entire breast unless absolutely necessary. Do not expose both breasts.
- Work gently, professionally, and confidently.
- Avoid the nipple area.

PREGNANCY

SECTION OBJECTIVES

Chapter objective covered in this section:

4. Adapt for massage during pregnancy.

Using the information presented in this section, the student will be able to perform the following:

- List the three stages of pregnancy and describe the physical and emotional changes associated with each one.
- List common disorders of pregnancy and determine the need for referral.
- Design a general massage session to meet the needs of a person who is pregnant.
- Teach a support person the basic massage methods to use during labor.

Pregnancy is divided into three distinct segments: the first, second, and third trimesters. An individual who is pregnant undergoes extensive physical and emotional changes during each of these stages. Research indicates that healthy individuals with uncomplicated pregnancies may receive massages during the entire course of the pregnancy. Massage therapy during the first trimester of normal pregnancy is safe.

Unfortunately, some practitioners believe that stimulation of certain acupressure points or reflexology points during pregnancy may induce labor. THIS IS NOT TRUE! There are no scientific indications to support this claim. No effects on the onset of labor could be determined as a result of acupressure. Individuals who were pregnant and received foot reflexology treatments during pregnancy had no adverse side effects that affected the pregnancy (Fogarty et al., 2019; Mueller and Grunwald, 2021; Smith et al., 2022). Research results indicate that massage therapy during pregnancy is effective in reducing anxiety and discomfort while improving sleep quality (Santi et al., 2021).

First Trimester

During the first 3 months (the first trimester), the body must adjust to tremendous hormonal changes, which are likely to cause mood swings. This is also a vulnerable time for the developing baby. The following changes are common during the first trimester:

- *Nausea,* or the sensation of feeling sick, and vomiting are commonly referred to as *morning sickness.* Morning sickness tends to be most severe in the early morning but can occur in the evening and may last all day and night. Symptoms usually diminish by the 10th week of pregnancy and usually are gone by the end of 14 weeks. Only rarely does this last through the entire pregnancy.
- *Frequent urination* occurs because of the presence of the hormone progesterone, which causes relaxation of the smooth muscle of the bladder. This tendency diminishes by the second trimester. The therapist should offer the use of the restroom to the client before beginning the massage as well as during the massage session.
- *Constipation* occurs because the hormone progesterone causes relaxation of the smooth muscle of the large intestine. This results in slow movement of the fecal matter through the system and increased water absorption from the colon. Constipation may continue throughout the pregnancy. Mechanical pressure from the enlarging uterus contributes to the problem.
- *Blood pressure* often falls in early pregnancy, specifically the diastolic pressure. This is also the result of the presence of progesterone, which relaxes the muscular wall of the blood vessels. The expectant individual may be fatigued and may feel light-headed or faint, especially during prolonged standing. Blood pressure usually returns to normal during the 14th week of pregnancy. The therapist may want to offer to help the client off the massage table in case of dizziness when sitting up or standing.
- *Breast changes* begin during this stage, including a sense of increased fullness, tenderness, and heightened sensitivity. These changes may continue throughout the pregnancy.
- *Musculoskeletal changes* are caused by the influence of estrogen, progesterone, and relaxin. Relaxin is produced as early as 2 weeks into the pregnancy and is at its highest levels in the first trimester; it then falls 20% and remains at that level until labor. During the first trimester, relaxin helps promote the embryo's implantation into the uterine wall and encourages the growth of the placenta. Relaxin works to inhibit uterine contractions during early pregnancy to help prevent early childbirth. Relaxin affects the composition of collagen in the joint capsules, ligaments, and fascia to allow greater elasticity. This enables more movement in the joints and creates more yield in the abdomen. Although all joints are affected, the most vulnerable are those of the pelvis, such as the symphysis pubis and sacroiliac joint, and those that bear weight, such as the ankle and the joints of the foot.
- *Taste* and *smell* are altered in the early stages of the pregnancy. Certain smells and foods become disagreeable. The client should be asked before any scented oils or other fragrances are used.

Massage given during the first trimester is general wellness massage, which may help balance the physiological responses. Positioning is not a concern unless the breasts are tender. Deep work on the abdomen is avoided. Surface stroking of the abdomen can be pleasurable to the client (Box 14.4).

Box 14.4 Accurate Information to Dispel Myths About Massage During Pregnancy

- Therapeutic massage, when properly adapted, is safe during all stages of a normal pregnancy.
- General wellness massage in the first trimester *does not cause miscarriage.*
- Massage therapy provided appropriately *does not increase the risk of miscarriage.* Miscarriage in the first 12 weeks typically indicates a problem with the pregnancy.
- There are no points related to traditional Chinese meridians that can cause miscarriage in the first trimester or any time thereafter.
- There is no evidence that applying pressure to points on the feet or ankles will cause uterus contractions.
- Massage cannot cause labor to begin.
- Massage does not put the baby at risk to be poisoned by toxins released by massage because massage does not cause the body to release toxins.
- Massage does not affect the quality of breast milk, and there is no need to "pump and dump" breast milk post-massage.

Second Trimester

The second trimester usually brings a leveling of the hormones, and the individual feels better. During this time, they may start to "show" and feel the first movements of the baby. If the pregnancy was planned, this is a joyful time. If not, the physical evidence of the growing baby may cause additional stress.

Toward the end of the second trimester, the connective tissue, under the influence of relaxin, begins to soften to allow the pelvis to spread. The following are common considerations during the second trimester:

- *Joint looseness* develops because of the softening of the connective tissue, and the muscles of the legs, glutes, and hip flexors must provide joint stabilization and tension; as a result, pain can develop. Overstretching must be avoided.
- *Carpal tunnel syndrome*, caused by fluid retention, is common during pregnancy and may be perpetuated even after the birth because of caring for the infant.
- *Edema* is common at any time during pregnancy due to retention of fluid. The mechanical obstruction created by the uterus and its contents causes an increase in venous pressure distally, resulting in edema. Although edema may be caused by excessive weight gain, it may also be a symptom of preeclampsia. In the latter case, the midwife or physician should be informed.
- *Preeclampsia* is a serious complication that requires medical attention. The diagnosis of preeclampsia is made when the patient has elevated blood pressure, generalized edema, and a high concentration of protein in the urine. Some common elements that may predispose a person to preeclampsia are as follows:
    - First pregnancy
    - Multiple pregnancies
    - Chronic hypertension or long-term hypertension
    - Chronic renal disease
    - Malnutrition
    - Diabetes
- *Supine hypotension* occurs as the fetus grows and compresses the aorta and inferior vena cava against the lumbar spine. This may cause a person to feel faint when lying on their back. The side-lying position during massage is preferred.
- *Shortness of breath* is also common. This is the result of a combination of mechanical changes in the thorax and the position of the diaphragm and physiological changes.

During massage in the second trimester, support for the abdomen is important. The side-lying position is most comfortable and lying on the left side produces the least amount of abdominal congestion for the expanding uterus. Be attentive for strain in the back muscles during positioning. Keep the head in alignment with the spine. Using a support so the shoulder lies comfortably and does not fall forward or toward the ear is helpful. Support between the knees helps keep the hips in the neutral position and relieves stress in this area. A support under the top arm may also be comfortable. Allow the client to change position often. As in the first trimester, deep work on the abdomen must be avoided.

Third Trimester

During the last (third) trimester, weight of the growing baby, postural shifts, and movement of internal organs may cause discomfort. Because many internal organs are pushed up and back, the diaphragm works less efficiently. Neck and shoulder muscles are used to breathe, possibly causing discomfort or thoracic outlet symptoms. Breathing pattern disorders may develop. Massage offers temporary relief of these symptoms.

About 2 weeks before birth (in the first pregnancy), the baby turns head down and drops into the birth canal. This provides more space for the diaphragm to work, and breathing becomes easier; however, pressure on the bladder causes frequent urination. Impingement on lymph vessels may cause the legs and feet to swell. Edema or fluid accumulation may be a symptom of more serious complications, and the client should be referred to a physician immediately if these are noted. The low back may ache from postural shifts and massage therapy may provide temporary relief (Yuningsih et al., 2022). The breasts have enlarged in preparation for lactation. Fatigue and sleep disturbances may result. Massage is gentle, supports comfort, and assists circulation. If a comfortable position cannot be found, allow the client to change position often and use the restroom as needed. General massage may help the pregnant client feel better for a little while and support comfortable sleep.

Disorders of Pregnancy

Although pregnancy and delivery are considered normal physiological functions, problems can occur. Early recognition and referral are important (McKinney et al., 2017). Warning signs of a pregnancy at risk that require immediate referral include the following:

- Vaginal bleeding
- Severe, continuous abdominal pain
- Breaking of water (rupture of membranes)
- Preeclampsia, edema, dizziness, elevated blood pressure, severe headache

- Fever and frequent/painful urination (may indicate a urinary tract infection)
- Excessive vomiting of such severity and frequency that no food or fluids can be retained
- Excessive itching (occasionally may suggest liver or kidney dysfunction [cholestasis])
- Miscarriage is the loss of pregnancy before 20 weeks of pregnancy. The medical term for miscarriage is *spontaneous abortion.* An early miscarriage is the loss of a pregnancy in the first 12 weeks. Early miscarriages usually happen because the embryo is not developing as it should. Chromosome problems are thought to be the most common cause. The most common signs and symptoms of miscarriage are vaginal bleeding and strong period-type cramps.

Recommendations for Massage During Pregnancy

Unless specific circumstances or complications are involved, massage for pregnant clients should be a general massage (Fig. 14.10).

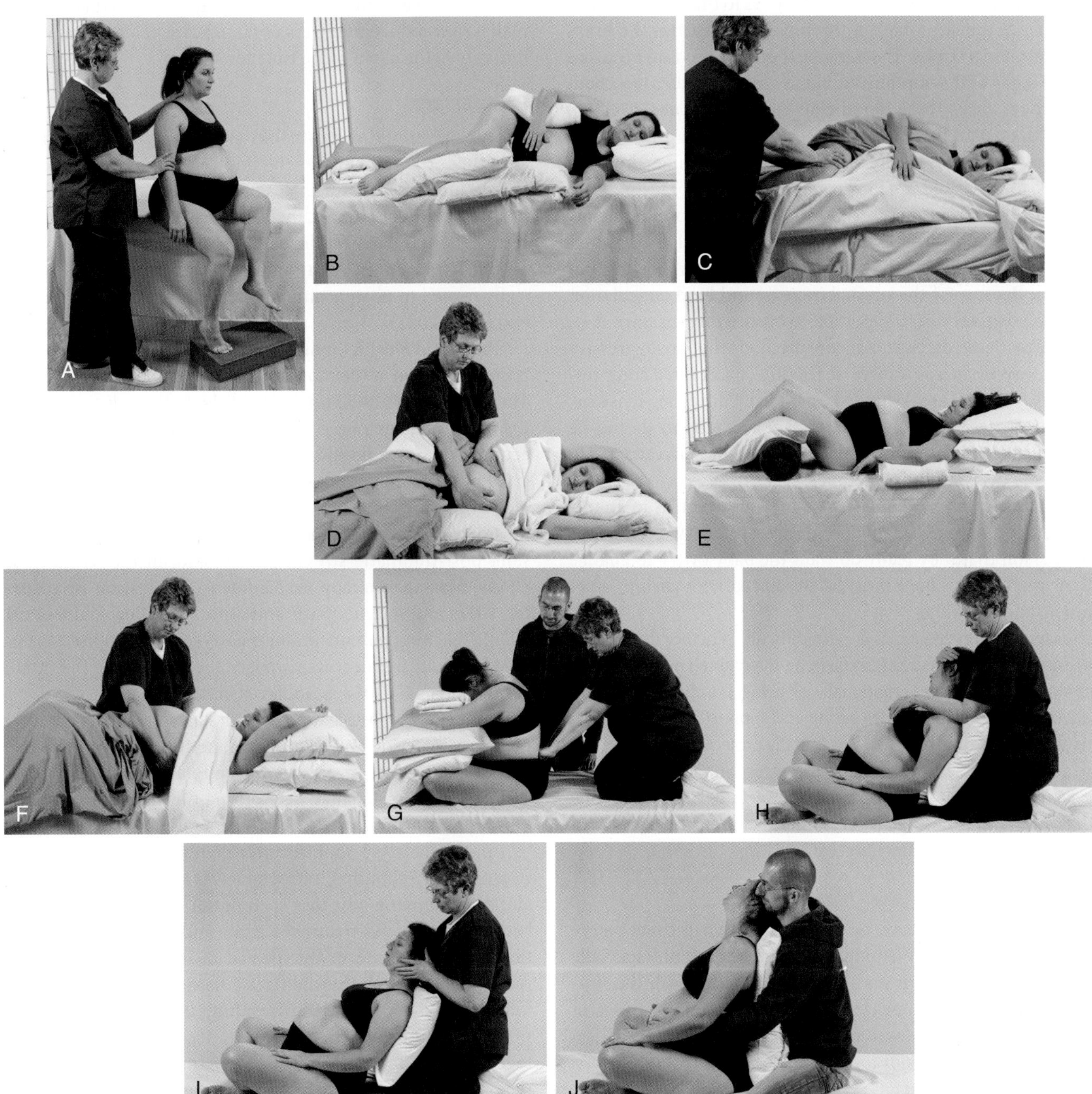

FIG. 14.10 Prenatal massage. A, Assist the client onto the table. **B,** Bolster. **C,** Perform the massage with the client in the side-lying position. **D,** Gentle massage of the baby. **E,** Client bolstered in the supine position. **F,** Massage of the lower back. **G,** Client in the seated position while support person is taught the technique. **H,** Effective seated positioning. **I,** Massage the face with focus and intention. **J,** Client's partner performs supportive massage.

Do not massage vigorously or extremely deep, do not overstretch, and do not massage the abdomen other than with gentle superficial pressure. Watch for fever, edema, varicose veins, and severe mood swings. Pregnancy is typically considered a hypercoagulable state, meaning that blood clots more readily than normal and predisposes a person to deep-vein thrombosis or other clot-related conditions. Keep in mind that blood clots during pregnancy are rare but are serious conditions that may become life-threatening if the blood clot dislodges from the formation site. The blood clot can become stuck in smaller blood vessels in the lung, a condition known as *pulmonary embolism*. If the thrombus or blood clot goes to the heart, one will experience a heart attack; a thrombus that reaches the brain may result in a stroke. The massage therapist needs to be aware of the signs and symptoms of blood clots and refer the client for proper care. These blood clots usually produce swelling, redness, or pain in one part of the client's body, especially in the legs. The pain typically increases during walking. The veins may be more visible and look larger than normal. During massage, it is important to screen for the potential for blood clots as the pregnancy progresses. The tendency for clot formation increases during the third trimester and early postpartum period. Because of the normal increase in blood coagulation during pregnancy, it is important to ensure that massage does not cause tissue damage, and any methods that are aggressive and invasive (such as transverse friction or sustained compression over a small area) should be avoided. During leg massage, caution is necessary, and the massage application should be adapted using a light to moderate, broad-based contact. Do not apply deep stripping methods.

In some cases pregnancy is not a joyous event, as in an unwanted pregnancy. The practitioner must not try to convince the person that they really do want the baby or try to change their mood. The client must be supported with caring, quiet touch, and listening.

Interrupted pregnancies are also difficult. Whether the cause is an induced abortion or miscarriage, an interrupted pregnancy is a strain on the body and emotional well-being. If a client has had an interrupted pregnancy, extra caring and support are helpful, particularly at the time the birth was initially projected.

Giving a general relaxation and stress management massage to a pregnant person can be a rewarding experience, one that allows the massage professional to watch the miracle of life develop (Proficiency Exercise 14.3).

Labor

Labor occurs as the baby moves down the birth canal before birth. Education and birthing classes are important, especially for first pregnancies. It may be appropriate to teach the support person some massage techniques before the onset of labor. Massage given by the support person helps them feel useful and involved with the pregnancy and birthing process.

PROFICIENCY EXERCISE 14.3

Locate a pregnant dog or cat. While giving the animal a massage, gently palpate the abdomen and observe the response.

Massage of the lower back and stroking of the abdomen may provide comfort and a point of focus during labor. Massaging the feet is often helpful. Massage can relax the body and divert the attention of the nervous system, thereby providing distraction during early labor. Labor proceeds easier and faster if they are relaxed.

During a phase of labor called *transition,* the person often does not want to be touched. Transition occurs just before the second stage of labor, with the actual movement of the baby down the birth canal. The contractions at this time are intense and have not yet been replaced by the urge to push.

After delivery, massage may help the body return to normal; it may reduce the stress of taking care of a new baby; and it may give the client some time for self-care.

Postpartum

The postpartum (or postnatal) period begins immediately after the birth of a child as the body, including hormone levels and uterus size, returns to a nonpregnant state. After birth, postpartum depression can become a serious problem for some. There is some evidence to support massage therapy as a strategy to help move through the postpartum period, especially related to postpartum fatigue (Mathew et al., 2018; Icke and Genc, 2021).

The World Health Organization (WHO, 2014) describes the postnatal period as the most critical and yet the most neglected. The postpartum period can be divided into three distinct stages: the initial or acute phase, 6–12 hours after childbirth; the subacute postpartum period, which lasts 2–6 weeks, and the delayed postpartum period, which can last up to 6 months.

During the subacute postpartum period, psychological disorders may emerge. Among these are post-partum depression, post-traumatic stress disorder, and, in rare cases, psychosis. Massage therapy may influence depression by reducing stress and fatigue (Sarli and Sari, 2018; Pusparatri et al., 2022). Teaching parents infant massage is also helpful to support bonding and decrease anxiety about handling the infant (Midtsund et al., 2018; Stoodley et al., 2022).

The delayed postpartum period starts after the subacute postpartum period and lasts up to 6 months. During this time, muscles and connective tissue return to a prepregnancy state, and general massage may help during this transitional phase. Urinary incontinence may be problematic.

Approximately 3 months after giving birth (typically between 2 and 5 months), estrogen levels drop and postpartum alopecia involving hair loss is common. Hair typically grows back normally, and treatment is not indicated. Other conditions that may arise in this period include postpartum thyroiditis. Postpartum thyroiditis is inflammation of the thyroid following delivery of a baby, resulting in hyperthyroidism at first and eventually hypothyroidism. It is important the massage therapist be aware of symptoms and refer the client to a medical professional if necessary.

If the client is breast-feeding, the positions used to hold the baby can cause neck, shoulder, arm, and low back discomfort. Stress can interfere with the milk letdown response, which is related to oxytocin. Because the hormonal changes that accompany lactation are modulators of mood and can influence the emotions and behavior, a small percentage of those breastfeeding experience feelings of depression, anxiety, or agitation beginning immediately before their milk lets down and lasting only a few minutes. Called dysphoric milk ejection reflex (D-MER), the condition is a physiological response related to a decrease in dopamine immediately before milk letdown. Should the client share this information with you, it is appropriate to educate and refer the client to her physician.

Key Points

- Each trimester of pregnancy typically requires unique massage adaptation.
- Pregnancy is not an illness, but disorders occur, and the massage therapist needs to monitor for referral.
- Massage can be helpful during labor.
- The postpartum period is when the body returns to a nonpregnant state. Massage is indicated in the postpartum period.

PEDIATRICS

SECTION OBJECTIVES

Chapter objective covered in this section:

5. Adapt massage for infants, children, and adolescents.

Using the information presented in this section, the student will be able to perform the following:

- Explain the importance of adapting massage to the physical and emotional state of the infant, child, and adolescent.
- Teach parents to massage their babies.
- Understand the importance of a confident touch when working with children.
- Apply general massage methods to ease growing pains.
- Train family members in massage techniques for use at home.

Pediatric Age Ranges

The term *pediatric* is from the Greek *pais* meaning "children" and *iatros* meaning "healer." Pediatrics is considered the branch of medicine that deals with the health and medical care of infants, children, and adolescents from birth up to the age of 18. Age categories for this population are as follows:

Newborn: 0–28 days
Baby/infant: 1–12 months
Toddler: 1–3 years
Preschooler: 3–5 years
Grade schooler: 5–12 years
Adolescent: 12–18 years

Research supports massage therapy for the pediatric population (Field, 2019; de Britto et al., 2021; Ririn and Israyati, 2021; Bernstein et al., 2021; Mrljak et al., 2022). An important legal consideration is that one or both parents or guardians must provide informed consent for the massage of a minor and must be present during any professional interaction.

Baby/Infant (1–12 Months)

Protection, nutrition, connection, bonding, stimulation, and soothing acceptance are crucial for human infants. Infants are born with a need for sociability, along with the more basic needs for food, shelter, and so forth. People of most cultures massage their babies. Although this practice has been almost lost in the westernized world, it is being revived. Massage provides an organized, logical approach to sensory stimulation, which is important for infants because part of their growth is learning to sort and organize sensory stimulation. By 12 months of age, the baby can move independently from place to place but still is utterly dependent on the protection of a parent or family group (Fig. 14.11).

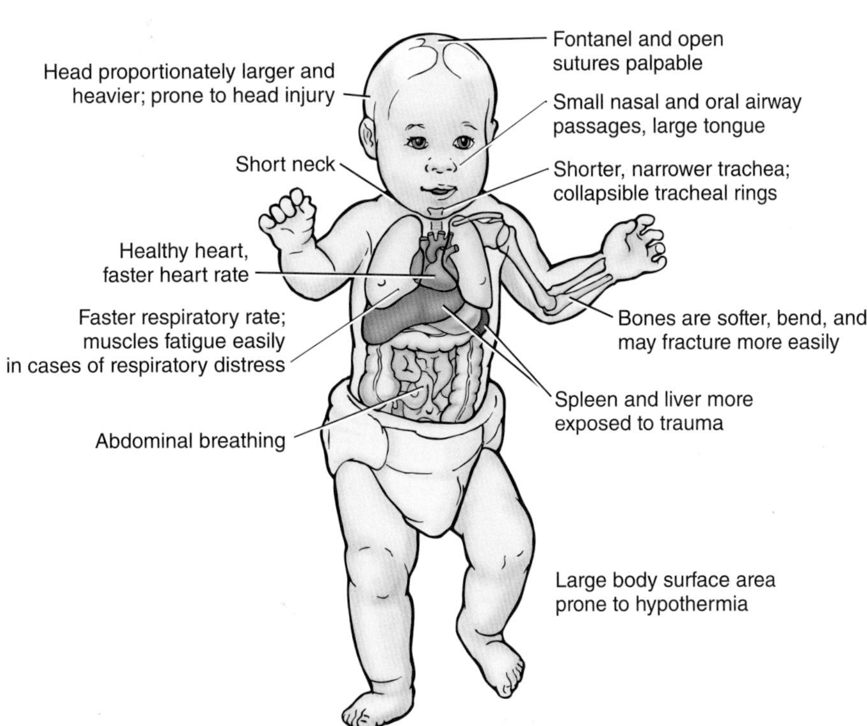

FIG. 14.11 The unique anatomical and physiological features of infants and young children.

A parent or massage practitioner who expects the infant to settle into the massage immediately may be disappointed. Relaxing takes time. Repetitive long strokes and rhythmic movement of the limbs can initiate a calming response in an infant (Fig. 14.12). Bilateral (on both sides) pressure is calming. Swaddling provides this type of consistent, even pressure that reduces neural activity. If the baby stiffens with the massage, the tactile stimulation most likely is too intense, too light, uneven, or painful. The infant nervous system is sensitive. Confining the massage to the feet or rhythmic rocking may be preferable to stroking for infants who seem highly tactile sensitive. In well-baby care, a shorter massage of 15–30 minutes is sufficient. A confident touch is important; babies can detect nervousness immediately. To them this is not a "safe" touch,

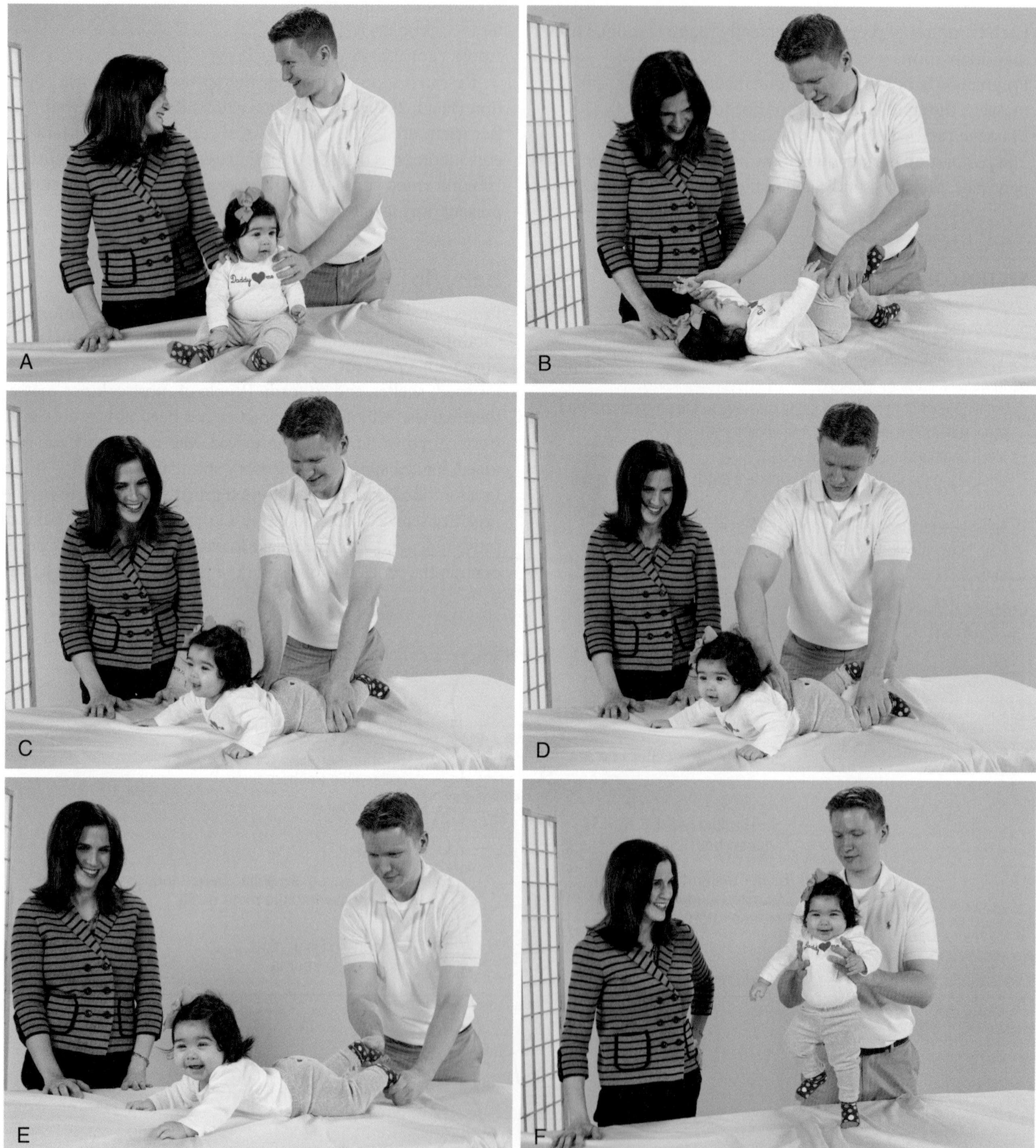

FIG. 14.12 Massage for infants and older babies. A, Establish a rapport with the parent, and prepare to teach. **B,** Connect with the infant while performing assessments. **C,** Make sure the massage is pleasurable to the baby. **D,** Even babies have tender points; keep alert for changes in expression. **E,** After treating tender points, return to pleasurable massage. **F,** A happy baby and an educated mom.

and they will not respond and/or potentially withdraw. When just the right combination of methods is found, the infant responds calmly to the touch.

Teaching parents to massage their own babies is appropriate. Massage may be especially helpful for parents who have trouble bonding with their infants. Bonding is the attachment process that occurs between parent and child. Although bonding is considered primarily an emotional response, it is theorized that some biochemical and hormonal interactions support the process. The hormone oxytocin is present in males and females and may be a factor in the bonding process. Massage, through skin stimulation, increases the oxytocin level.

Other than in a hospital-type setting, the massage practitioner is unlikely to develop a clientele of infants. However, teaching infant massage can be an exciting career addition. Classes and various books and videos are available to help the massage therapist develop infant massage classes for caregivers. Learning massage is an excellent way for parents to become confident with their touch (Fig. 14.13).

The nervous system of infants born to individuals addicted to drugs or alcohol is especially challenged. Research is under way to determine whether the gentle, organized, tactile approaches of massage can help these special babies. The initial findings are promising. Remember, each baby is different. "Listen" to these little bodies and structure the massage to best meet the baby's needs (Proficiency Exercise 14.4).

Toddler (1–3 Years)

Children in this age group are still babies, even though we consider them toddlers. Three-year-olds are quite different in both function and body form. By the time a child can control bladder and bowel functions reliably (about age 3), cognitive functions are better able to be organized. When learning the meaning of *no,* picking up toys, and sharing, the infant is ready to pass into childhood (Stiles and Jernigan, 2010; Tau and Peterson, 2010).

Understanding the limitations of these walking babies is important. How many 2-year-olds have been punished for not sharing toys or putting toys away, when physically and developmentally they are incapable of understanding the concept? Touch then develops a negative connotation. Lots of hurts happen at this age. The parents' expectations can be too high, resulting in frustration on the part of both parents and child. These wonderful and challenging twos are a great time to incorporate massage-breaks. If approached appropriately, this can be calming for both the parent and the child, reinforcing touch as a positive experience.

A 2-year-old in a tantrum is caught up in the physiological process. It takes time for both the nervous and endocrine systems to calm down. When verbal skills are not sufficient to express the problem, crying may be a way to burn off internal agitation that has built up through the day.

Toddlers may not want someone other than the parents to provide massage. This is the age range when they are becoming aware of social structure, who is familiar and who is not, and may not interact with the massage therapist. Again, teaching the parent and other caregivers how to provide basic massage is recommended. Demonstrating massage on a stuffed toy or doll would likely be interesting to the toddler, who may actually attempt to mimic the massage.

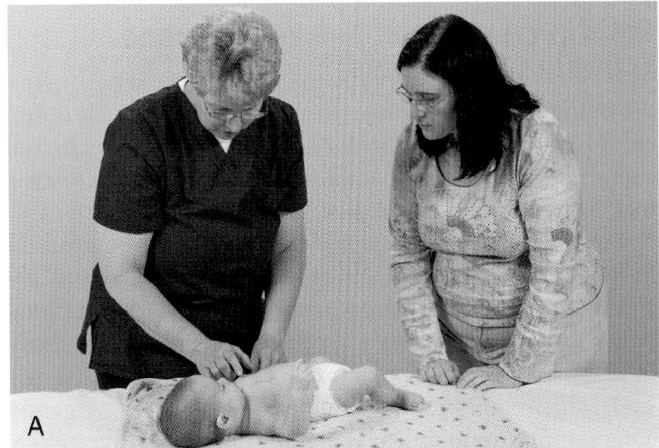

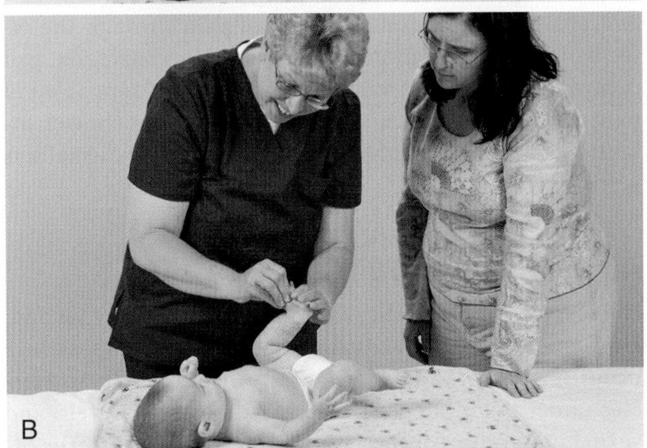

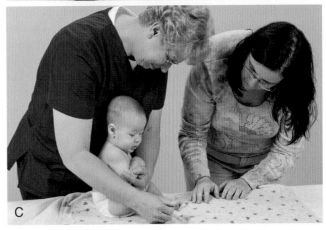

FIG. 14.13 Massage for an ill or injured infant. A, Assess the infant, and explain to the parent or caregiver what you intend to do. Always follow the treatment plan provided by a physician. **B,** Take time to connect with the baby. **C,** Showing care and concern, teach the parent or caregiver how to massage the baby.

PROFICIENCY EXERCISE 14.4

1. Using professional journals, investigate resources to expand your knowledge of infant massage.
2. Find a litter of puppies or kittens and massage these "babies."

Child (Preschooler: 3–5 Years/Grade Schooler: 5–12 Years)

Providing massage services for children is not much different from providing massage for adults. Children love physical contact. It is interesting that the horsing around and wrestling that occur during play look a lot like massage.

From age 3 to puberty, physical growth is seen mostly in height. Both physical and emotional growing pains are common. Physical growing pains occur because the long bones grow more rapidly than the muscle tissue, resulting in a pull on the periosteum (bone covering connective tissue), which is pain sensitive. Massage can help by gently lengthening the muscles, softening the connective tissue, and providing symptomatic relief of pain through the effects of counterirritation, hyperstimulation analgesia, gait control, and release of various neurochemicals involved in pain modulation. Because children may have shorter attention spans than adults, a 30-minute massage usually is sufficient.

Adolescent (12–18 Years)

Adolescents live in bodies that are changing every second. Hormone levels fluctuate constantly, and mood swings occur regularly. At adolescence, growth in height accelerates under the influence of increased hormone levels, and sexual maturation occurs. Natural sleep-wake patterns often are disrupted. It is common for a teenager to be up all night and want to sleep all day. Massage may help an adolescent become more comfortable with this ever-changing body. It certainly helps with physical growing pains. Use special caution when working with adolescent boys. The reflexive physical sexual response is sensitive, and almost anything can trigger an erection. The therapist should be sensitive to this by not using a taut or smoothed sheet over the groin area when working with male adolescents. Instead, keep the sheet bunched in this area to disguise any physical response.

Massage Adaptation

Massage application for the pediatric population involves adapting to the size of the baby, child, or adolescent. The massage may be performed over clothing. Generally 30 minutes is sufficient. It also is important that the practitioner never work with children or adolescents unless a parent or guardian is present. Part of the massage time can be used to teach the parent or guardian some massage methods to help the child and to teach the child some massage methods for use on the parent. Massage provides a structured approach to safe touch. It may help families stay connected during both good and challenging times (Fig. 14.14 and Proficiency Exercise 14.5).

Key Points

- The permission of a parent or guardian is required to work with minors.
- Parents can be taught to massage their infants and children.

GERIATRICS/OLDER ADULTS

SECTION OBJECTIVES

Chapter objective covered in this section:

6. Explain the aging process and adapt massage for the geriatric population.

Using the information presented in this section, the student will be able to perform the following:

- Provide a rationale for the benefits of massage for older adults.
- Describe the physical, mental, and emotional changes associated with the aging process and adapt massage methods accordingly.
- Understand the need for fee and time adjustments when working with older adults.

In industrialized societies, the fastest growing segments of the population are those over age 65. Although the massage methods are no different, older adults do present specific concerns, and appropriate adjustments are required in massage application. The demographic span for senior/older adults is generally considered to be 65 years to 85 years. Elder adults are 85 years old and up.

The physiological age is more ambiguous. Some 65-year-olds have the problems of the aged, and some 85-year-olds are in better physiological condition than some 65-year-olds. For this reason, the wiser course with people over age 65 is to consider the physiological condition rather than the chronological age. Specific care for the aging population is called *geriatrics*.

Massage practitioners who plan to work with older adults may need more training to learn about the special needs of this population. In most cases, a general massage session using the skills presented in this text and an attentive, caring attitude are sufficient for interacting professionally with those 65 years and older (Fig. 14.15 and Proficiency Exercise 14.6).

Massage Adaptation

Physical Effects of the Aging Process

The aging process is normal. Muscle tissue diminishes, as do fat and connective tissues. Connective tissue becomes less pliable, reproduces more slowly, and forms fibrotic tissue more easily. Bones are not as flexible and are more prone to breaking. Joints are worn, and osteoarthritis and osteoarthrosis are common. The skin is thinner, circulation is not as efficient, and fluid in the soft tissue is reduced.

The body tends to collapse a bit during aging. The spaces provided for the nerves are reduced, and bones and soft tissue structures can put pressure on the nerves, resulting in sciatica and thoracic outlet syndrome. Feet hurt because the intricate joint structure of the foot has broken down. Circulation to the extremities is diminished, often resulting in a burning pain. These conditions are not life threatening, but they may cause a person to feel miserable. If only temporarily, massage can help ease the discomfort of these conditions.

Dehydration, lack of appetite, and weight loss can be problems with advanced age, but the parasympathetic stimulation produced by massage can increase appetite and improve digestion for older clients. Proper hydration is important. Sleep also can be improved. Many older adults have periods of insomnia

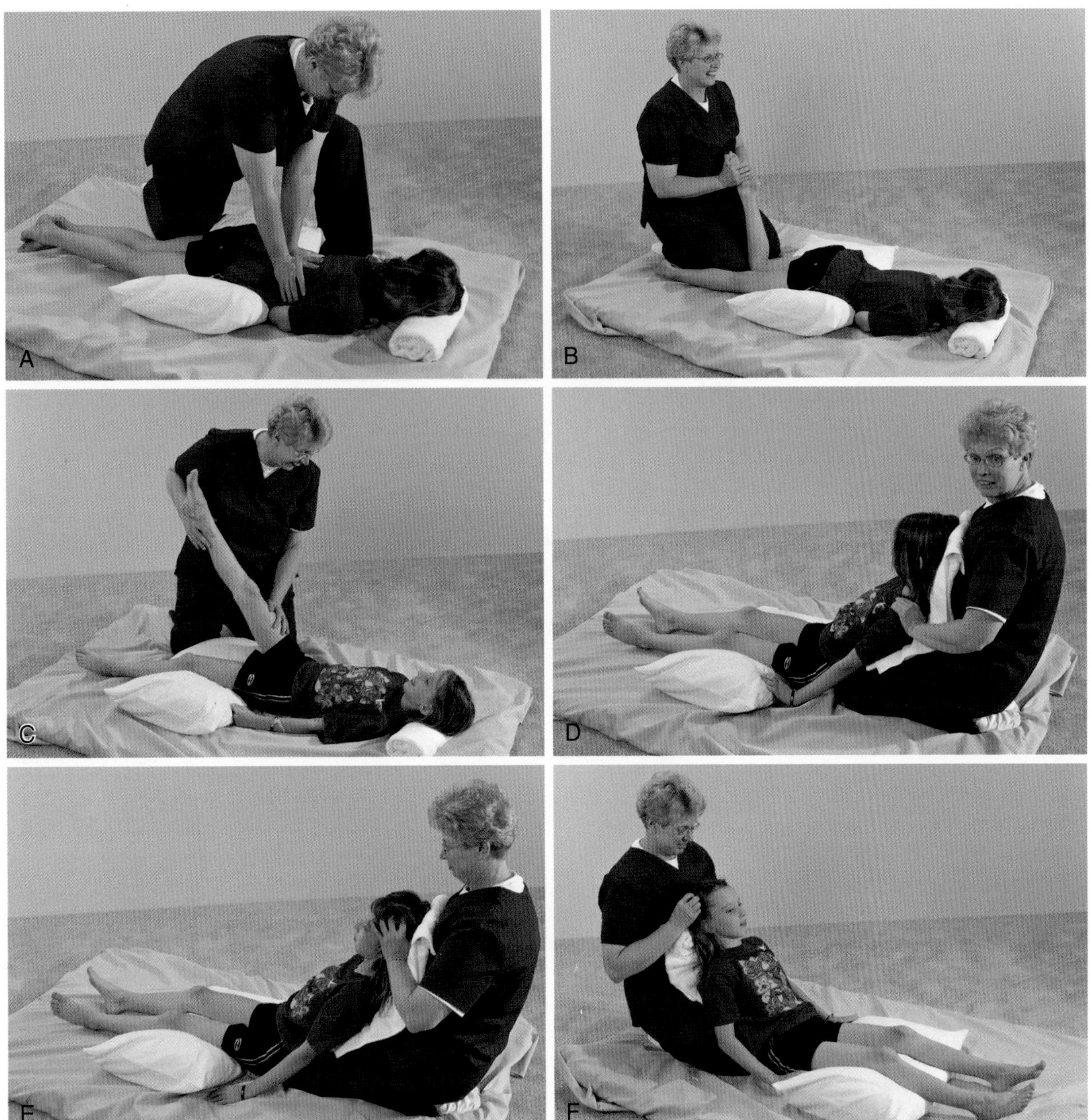

FIG. 14.14 Massage for children and adolescents. A, Most children prefer to keep their clothes on, and they often like a mat. **B,** Interact with the parent or guardian (not pictured). **C,** Maintain your focus on the child. **D,** Continue to connect with the parent or guardian, and explain your massage methods. **E, F,** Relax, nurture, and remember to teach the parent or guardian.

PROFICIENCY EXERCISE 14.5

1. Give massages to three children or adolescents of various ages. Make sure the parent or guardian is present.
2. Develop a one-page handout with five massage techniques that families can share.

or disrupted sleep patterns. Improved sleep supports restorative mechanisms and increases vitality (Cohen, 2022).

Medications

Many older adults take several medications. These individuals are also more sensitive to the dosage level of medication and less able to self-regulate homeostatic processes. The massage professional must be attentive to the physiological interactions between the effects of massage and the medications.

Depression and Dementia

Older and elder adults are sometimes depressed. This frequently is both a chemical depression and a situational condition. Massage stimulates neurochemicals that can lift mild depression temporarily. Dementia, such as Alzheimer's disease, has shown temporary improvement after massage (Suzuki et al., 2010; Alm, et al., 2018; Keshavarz et al., 2018; Leng et al., 2020; Liu et al., 2022).

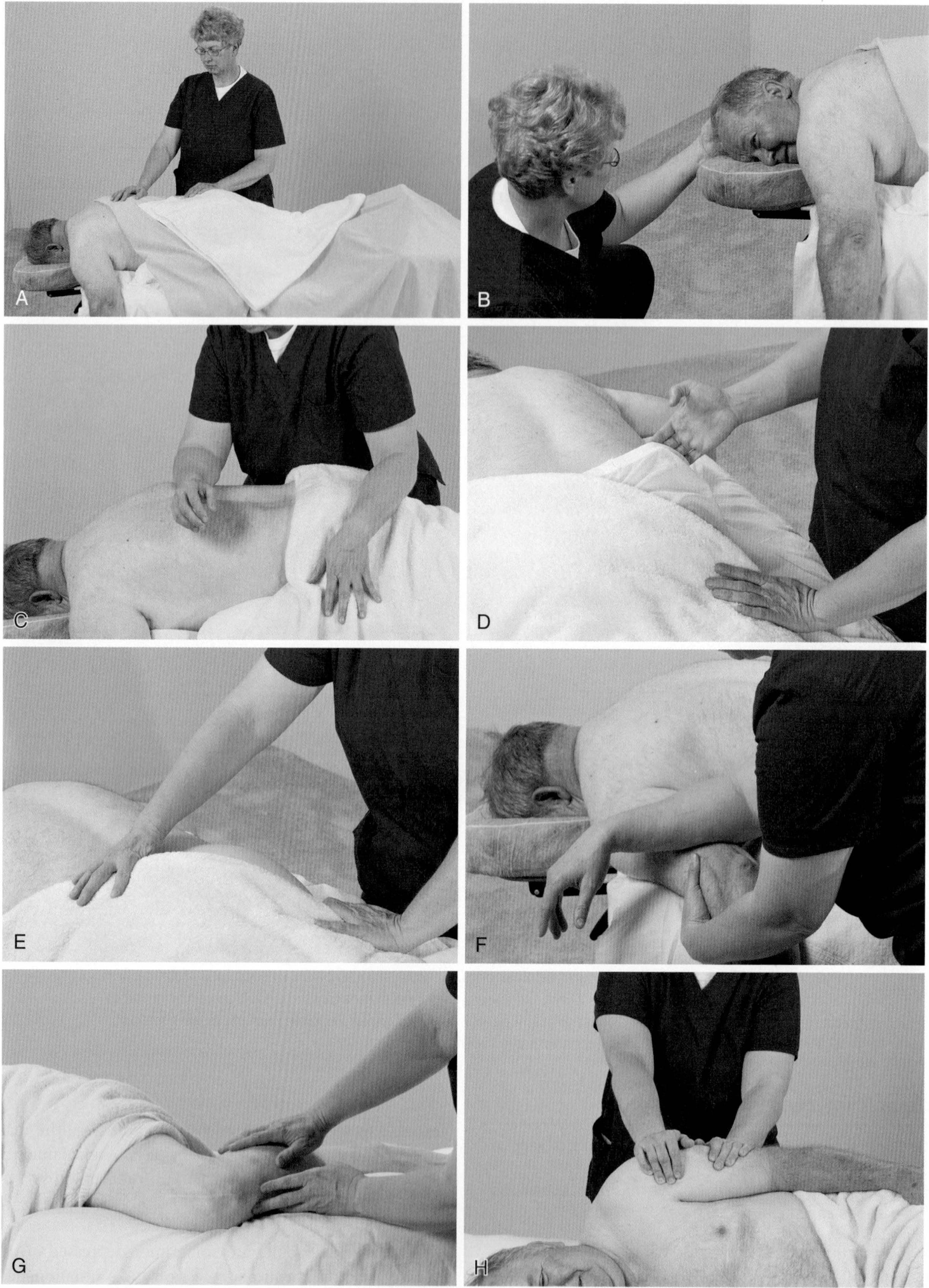

FIG. 14.15 Massage procedure for an older client. A, Drape the client for modesty and warmth. **B,** Interact appropriately with the client. **C,** Be cautious but confident in providing the massage. **D,** With consent, respectfully move underclothing. **E,** Maintain secure draping. **F,** Use broad-based contact, and be cautious about depth of pressure and degree of drag. Be vigilant in observing the client's reactions and adapt the massage as appropriate. (**G, H,**) The side-lying position often is most comfortable for older clients.

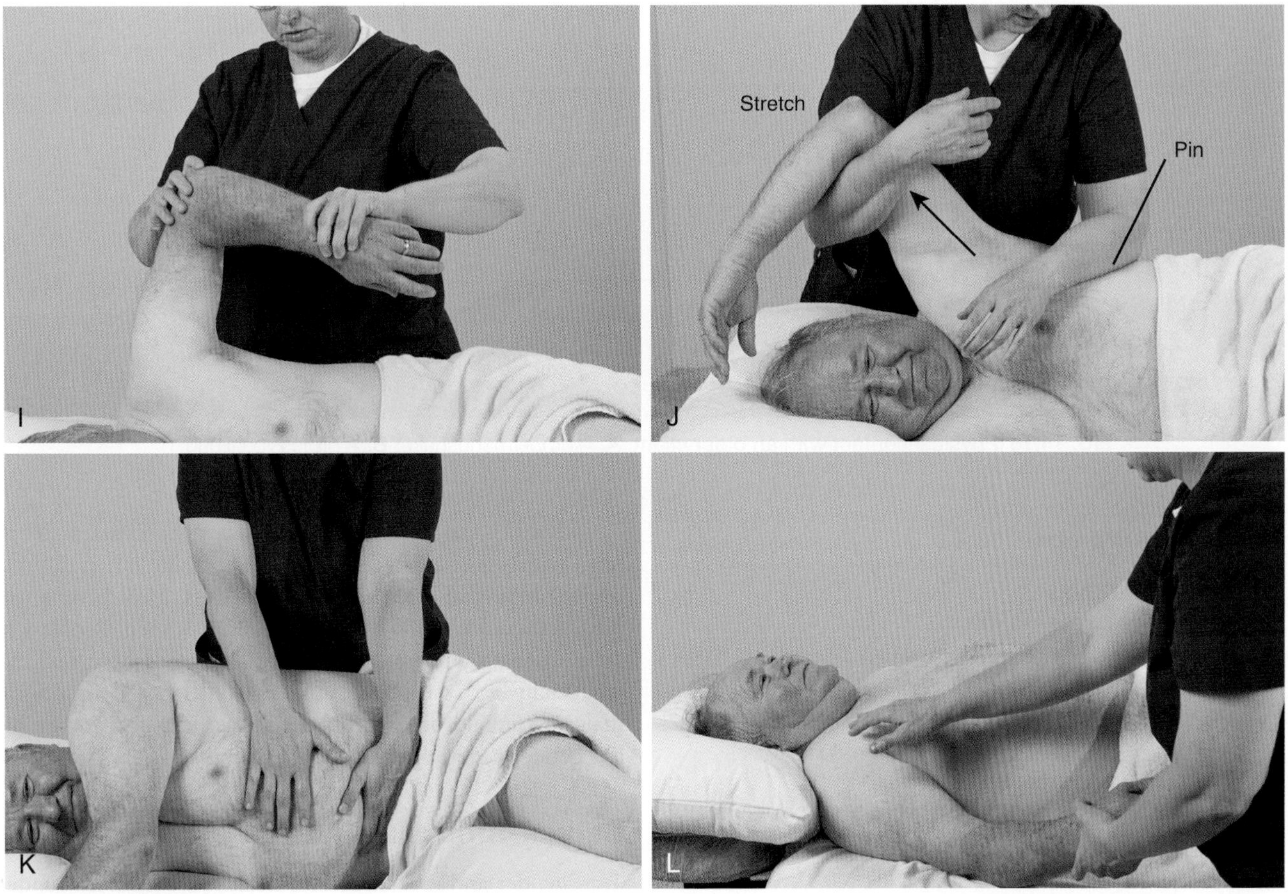

FIG. 14.15, cont'd **I,** Assess range of motion carefully; never force movement. **J,** Stretch cautiously; pin and stretch methods increase tension on tissue while protecting joints. **K,** Abdominal massage supports digestive and elimination functions. **L,** Gentle oscillation (shaking and rocking) is effective for supporting joint function.

PROFICIENCY EXERCISE 14.6

1. Volunteer to give massages at a local senior citizens center for at least 4 weeks or a total of 32 hours.
2. Contact a local long-term care facility and ask whether a resident who has few visitors might appreciate receiving a massage.

If a person does not have adequate cognitive functioning skills, they will be unable to give informed consent for the massage. The guardian, physician, or other health care professional must intervene to give the necessary permission.

Social Interaction

Many older and elder adults live alone. Their spouses may have passed away, and families busy with their own lives. We all need stimulation. If a person is not physically and emotionally stimulated, neurological function begins to deteriorate. The interaction with a massage therapist can provide both physical and emotional stimulation. If nothing else, the physical contact with another human being provides sensory stimulation, with beneficial results (Fig. 14.16).

Because some older clients are alone or have a limited income (or both), the massage therapist should take into consideration not only the fees charged but also the amount of time spent with the client. The social interaction of talking with an older and elder client may be just as important as the physical interaction of the massage. If the massage professional listens attentively, much can be learned from this population, who have many years of experience to share. The time should be given willingly. However, professional boundaries need to be maintained, including boundaries around the time spent for the appointment.

Additional information on aging is provided by the National Institutes of Health's National Institute on Aging.

Key Points

- The age range for the category of older adults is 65–85 years, and an elder adult is 85 years and older.
- Physiological age is a better indicator of function and capacity than chronological age.
- Adaptations are based on the physiological changes of aging, such as thinner skin, less efficient circulation, and sleep disturbances.
- Medication use is common in this population.
- Depression and dementia may interfere with the client's ability to provide informed consent for care.
- Massage therapy adaptation involves understanding the aging process.

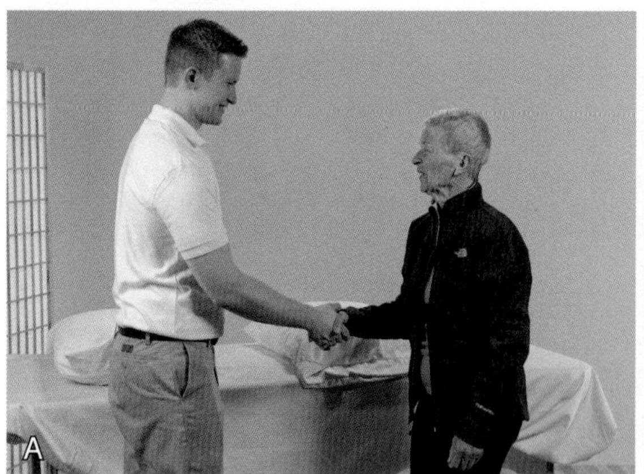
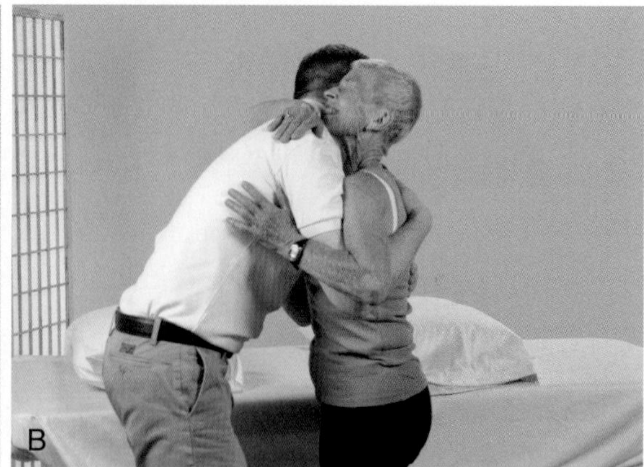

FIG. 14.16 Physical contact with an older client. A, A proper handshake. **B,** A professional hug.

GENDER DIVERSITY

SECTION OBJECTIVES

Chapter objective covered in this section:

7. Describe gender-affirming interventions and adapt massage as needed.

Using the information presented in this section, the student will be able to perform the following:

- Define the terms *transgender, gender diverse, gender transition, gender congruence,* and *gender affirmation*.
- Modify massage application based on gender-affirming practices and interventions.

The terms **transgender** and **gender diverse** (TGD) describe members of many varied communities of people with gender identities or expressions that differ from the sex assigned to them at birth. Gender identity and sexual orientation are not the same. Sexual orientation is an individual's emotional, sexual, and/or romantic attraction to others. Gender identity is the internal innermost concept of self.

Gender transition refers to any combination of social, medical, and legal changes a person makes in order to support their gender identity and congruence. Usually, this involves transitioning from one gender role to another or moving away from the gender assigned at birth. **Gender affirmation** is an umbrella term for the range of actions involved in living, surviving, and thriving as authentic gendered individuals. Gender affirmation practices are unique and based on what is personally affirming for the person and what feels safe to do, and what is accessible and available.

Most people, including most transgender people, identify as either male or female. But some people do not neatly fit into the categories of "man" or "woman," or "male" or "female." For example, some people have a gender that blends elements of being a man or a woman, or a gender that is different than either male or female. Some people do not identify with any gender. Some people's gender changes over time.

People whose gender is not male or female use many different terms to describe themselves, with *nonbinary* being one of the most common. Other terms include *genderqueer, agender, bigender,* and more. None of these terms mean exactly the same thing, but all speak to an experience of gender that is not simply male or female.

Intersex is an umbrella term that encompasses people born with sex characteristics that fall outside our traditional understanding of male and female bodies. Most people who are intersexed identify as either men or women. People who are nonbinary and transgender are not usually intersex; they are usually born with bodies that may fit typical definitions of male and female, but their innate gender identity is other. Just like gender is not binary, neither are bodies.

Gender-Affirming Care

Transgender and gender diverse health care involves gender-affirming interventions including endocrinology, surgery, voice and communication, dermatology, primary care, reproductive health, sexual health, and mental health disciplines. Gender-affirming interventions include puberty suppression, hormone therapy, and gender-affirming surgeries.

Gender-affirming hormone therapy (GAHT) is an essential part of gender affirmation for many transgender and gender-diverse individuals. Transmen (female sex assigned at birth, male gender identity) typically receive testosterone. Transwomen (male sex assigned at birth, female gender identity) often receive estrogens frequently combined with anti-androgens.

Feminizing hormone therapy using estrogens causes changes including breast growth, softening of the skin, reduced body hair, and changes in body shape and composition. In most cases, antiandrogen therapy is needed. In some cases, progesterone is used to effect breast development. Transgender women on estradiol therapy may have a higher risk of stroke and venous thromboembolism

Masculinizing hormone therapy using testosterone causes increased body and facial hair, deepening of the voice, menstrual suppression, and increased muscle development. Testosterone treatment may affect triglycerides and cause moderate-to-severe acne (T'Sjoen et al., 2019; Bhargava et al., 2021; Green et al., 2022; Coleman et al., 2022).

Massage Adaptation Supporting Gender Congruency

Massage therapists respect people and make appropriate clinical decisions about massage therapy care. No matter what a person's gender identity or sexual orientation is, everyone wants to feel valid and recognized for being themselves. Gender diversity is about acknowledging and respecting the many ways people identify outside of the male/female binary. Avoid making assumptions about people's gender. You cannot tell if someone is nonbinary or transgender based on appearance. Using correct names and pronouns for gender diverse people, as well as gender neutral language are reasonable expectations in the professional environment. Use the name a person asks you to use.

If you are not sure what pronouns someone uses, ask. Different nonbinary people may use different pronouns. Many nonbinary people use "they" while others use "he" or "she," and still others use other pronouns. Asking whether someone should be referred to as "he," "she," "they," or another pronoun may feel awkward at first, but is one of the simplest and most important ways to show respect for someone's identity.

Gender congruence is the feeling of harmony and being one's authentic self. Legal aspects of gender congruence include changing identification documents such as birth certificate, driver's license, or passport. Social congruence involves social identifiers such as clothing, hairstyle, gender identity, name and/or pronouns. Congruence also involves the use of medical approaches such as hormone therapy to promote physical, mental, and/or emotional alignment. Surgical procedures include the addition, removal, or modification of gender-related physical traits. Massage therapy adaptation would be related to various gender-affirming interventions. Gender-affirming practices might include chest binding, which may or may not be removed during massage application (Julian et al., 2021). Laser hair removal can cause temporary discomfort, redness and swelling, and is considered a local contraindication when skin irritation is present. Support for healing and scar tissue management are used for gender-affirming surgical procedures that do not involve the genitals since massage of this area is not part of massage therapy practice. Massage of the chest to support healing and scar tissue management would follow recommendations for breast massage described previously.

Key Points

- Gender identity is the innermost concept of self.
- Gender transition is any combination of social, medical, and legal changes a person makes in order to support their gender identity and congruence.
- Transgender and gender diverse health care involves gender-affirming interventions including endocrinology, surgery, voice and communication, dermatology, primary care, reproductive health, sexual health, and mental health disciplines
- Massage therapy adaptation would be related to various gender-affirming interventions

ACUTE CARE

SECTION OBJECTIVES

Chapter objective covered in this section:

8. Recognize acute care situations and adapt massage appropriately.

Using the information presented in this section, the student will be able to perform the following:

- Define acute illness and injury.
- Determine the appropriate massage application for the acute healing phase.
- Use a specific massage sequence to support wound healing.
- Adapt massage application to manage scar tissue.
- Adapt massage application to manage acute pain.

Acute care assumes that an individual has a current injury or illness. Combining pain management strategies and palliative care provides a framework for massage in acute care situations.

Acute Illness

The application of massage differs for acute illness and acute injury. **Acute illness** follows palliative massage care guidelines. One concern when working with individuals experiencing illness is whether the illness is contagious and how it is spread. If the individual is experiencing a fever, the body is actively involved in fighting the disease and adaptive ability is strained. It may be prudent to avoid massage or working only in a limited manner, such as providing foot massage. If massage is used during acute illness, a general approach should be used involving moderate pressure that is not painful, limited to 30–45 minutes.

Acute Injury

Acute injury indicates that damage to the body has occurred, such as a fracture, wound, sprain, strain, burn, or contusion. It is important to know both the cause and the outcome to understand the nature of the injury (e.g., a fracture caused by a fall in a person who has osteoporosis). Massage therapists working in the medical setting, especially hospitals, often encounter surgically created wounds, such as an incision site; surgical procedures may include several types of microsurgeries or minimally invasive surgery, in which tiny incisions are used to enable faster healing.

Wound Healing

Surgical incisions are performed in a sterile environment, which reduces the risk of infection. Wounds that occur from accidents are more prone to infection. With any type of wound, infection control is essential. Massage in the area of a wound in the acute stage is contraindicated, to prevent infection. Massage can occur once the protective skin barrier has healed.

Infection is not as much of a concern with forms of injury that do not involve wounds; however, the process of healing still needs to be understood so that massage supports healing. These types of injuries include sprains, strains, contusions, etc. (The prior section on athletes in this chapter describes care of these types of common injuries).

Box 14.5 lists recommendations for massage during various stages of healing. Massage during wound healing also targets functional scar development (Box 14.6). Methods to address problematic old scars are also described in Box 14.6.

Box 14.5 Massage Approach During Healing

Massage During the Acute Phase

- Manage pain
- Support sleep

Massage During the Early Subacute Phase

- Manage pain
- Support sleep
- Manage edema
- Manage compensation patterns

Massage During the Later Subacute Phase

- Manage pain
- Support sleep
- Manage edema
- Manage compensation patterns
- Support rehabilitative activity
- Support mobile scar development
- Support tissue regeneration process

Massage During the Remodeling Phase

- Manage irreversible compensation patterns
- Restore tissue pliability
- Support rehabilitation activity
- Encourage appropriate scar tissue development
- Manage adhesions
- Restore firing patterns, gait reflexes, and neuromuscular responses
- Eliminate reversible compensation patterns

Massage Adaptation

Massage is effective at managing acute and chronic pain and supports other pain treatments, such as medication, ultrasound, hydrotherapy, and so on. A common error is to think of massage targeting pain reduction as therapeutic change. In fact, it is palliative. Massage that is so aggressive it creates inflammation and excessive pain during application is incorrect, as is massage that produces inflammation and pain afterward, except in rare situations in which methods to introduce therapeutic inflammation are indicated. Pain management massage strategies are presented in Box 14.7.

Acute Pain Management

Acute pain is considered to last up to 7 days, the medical team manages Acute pain. The primary method is pharmacology. Medical guidelines support using multiple medications as well as adjunctive use of nonpharmacologic ice, heat, elevation, rest, immobilization, exercise, and massage therapy. Common medications used for acute pain are acetaminophen, nonsteroidal antiinflammatory medication, and opioids. Local anesthetics such as lidocaine are short-duration medicines used to temporarily numb small parts of the body before performing minor medical procedures.

Opioids remain the mainstay short-term treatment of moderate to severe acute pain. Opioids can be essential

Box 14.6 Therapeutic Massage Application for Wounds, Scars, Sprains, and Strains

Days 1 and 2

- Sanitation and prevention of infection are essential.
- Avoid the area during massage to protect the wound from contamination.
- Lymphatic drainage can be used above and below the wound; however, do not perform it if any signs of infection are present, such as heat, swelling, redness (especially any type of streaking), pus, or sour smell.

Days 3 and 4

- Use bend, shear, and tension forces around the wound far enough away to prevent any chance of contamination. The goal is to gently drag the skin in multiple directions to prevent adhesions from forming. The connective tissue formation is random at this time. The wound edges should not be disturbed.

Days 5 and 6

- Increase the intensity and depth of the forces in the area that has been treated and move closer to the wound. Reduce the intensity, and gently apply bend, shear, and stretch (tension) force to the tissue. The wound edges should not be disturbed.

Day 7

- Increase the intensity in the previously treated areas, and then move closer to the wound. At this point, the wound should be moving a bit from the forces loading the adjacent tissue, but the wound edges must not be disturbed. Progressively increase the intensity daily by moving closer and closer to the wound.
- As soon as the wound has healed completely (14 days is typical, but it can take longer), begin to bend and shear the scar tissue and stretch it using tension forces.
- To prevent infection, make sure the wound is completely healed before working on it directly. Before working on the scar formation in the healing tissue, work on the tissue surrounding the wound; this can be addressed after the acute phase has passed (usually after 2–3 days). Maintain attention to the scar for at least 6 months. These methods can be taught to the client or family member.

Old and Problematic Scars

- Old scars that have adhered to underlying tissue can be softened. Mechanical force application is used in multiple directions on the scar each session until the scar tissue and the tissue at least 1 inch away from the scar become warm and slightly red. The intensity should be enough that the client feels a burning, stretching sensation. A small degree of inflammation is desirable, and after the massage the area may be a bit tender to the touch but should not be painful to movement. Ideally the area would be treated every other day, allowing the tissue to recover on the alternate days. These methods can be taught to the client or family member.

Box 14.7 Massage Strategies for Pain Management

1. General full-body application with a rhythmic, slow approach for 45–60 minutes as often as feasible.
   Goal: Parasympathetic dominance and increased production of pain-modulating neurochemicals.
2. Typically a moderate pressure depth is used with enough pressure to move through the superficial fascia to deeper tissue using a broad-based application. No poking, frictioning, or application of pain-causing methods should be done. Light pressure should be used in some cases, especially in patients undergoing radiation therapy and those who are especially fragile.
   Goal: Support serotonin, gamma amino-butyric acid (GABA) and the cascade of neurochemical production and reduce substance P and adrenaline.
3. Drag is slight unless connective tissue is targeted. Drag is targeted to lymphatic drainage (unless contraindicated) and skin stimulation.
   Goal: Reduce swelling and create counterirritation through skin stimulation.
4. Nodal points (e.g., in the feet, hands, head, and along the spine) have high concentrations of neurovascular components because they are the locations of cutaneous nerves, trigger points, acupuncture points, and reflexology points. When these points are massaged with a sufficient depth of pressure that does not cause pain, a "good hurt" sensation is created without eliciting defensive guarding or withdrawal; this may help relieve pain.
   Goal: Elicit gate control response and release of endorphins and other pain-inhibiting chemicals.
5. Direction of massage varies but deliberately targets fluid movement unless contraindicated.
   Goal: Support circulation.
6. Mechanical forces to load tissues creating tension, shear, bend, and torsion stress are introduced with an agitation quality to affect the ground substance without creating inflammation.
   Goal: Increase tissue pliability, support fascia sliding, and reduce tissue density.
7. Mechanical forces to load tissues with shear, bend, and torsion stress are used to address adhesions or fibrosis; however, these forces must be specifically targeted and limited in duration.
   Goal: Reduce localized nerve irritation and support circulation.
8. Muscle energy methods and lengthening are applied rhythmically and gently and are targeted to shortened muscles.
   Goal: Reduce nerve and proprioceptive irritation and improve circulation.
9. Elongation to introduce tension stress is applied slowly, without pain, and targeted to shortened tissue areas.
   Goal: Reduce nerve and proprioceptive irritation.
10. Massage therapists are focused, attentive, and compassionate while maintaining appropriate boundaries.
    Goal: Develop therapeutic relationship and alliance. Provide a safe, nonthreatening environment.

medications for the management of pain; however, they carry considerable potential risk.

Acupuncture and acupressure may reduce postoperative pain. Adjunctive passive therapies of massage, other manual therapies, and thermotherapies can be helpful (Schug et al., 2020; Dowell, 2022).

Key Points

- Acute care assumes that the person has a current injury or illness.
- Acute care is managed by medical professionals.
- Massage therapy is a supportive adjunctive care.
- Pain management strategies and palliative care provide a framework for massage in acute care situations.

CHRONIC ILLNESS

SECTION OBJECTIVES

Chapter objective covered in this section:

9. Describe the mechanisms of chronic illness and adapt massage for those with chronic conditions.

Using the information presented in this section, the student will be able to perform the following:

- Explain the basic cause of chronic illness.
- Explain the difference between acute illness and chronic illness.
- Develop realistic expectations for working with people who have a chronic illness.

Chronic illness is defined as a disease, an injury, or a syndrome that shows either little change or slow progression. Acute illness or injury is a short-term condition that resolves through normal healing processes and, if necessary, supportive medical care. Compared with chronic illness, acute conditions can be dealt with relatively easily because healing produces measurable results. Dealing with chronic illness is difficult for the person who has it, for the physician and the health care team, and for the massage therapist. In many situations little can be done except to make day-to-day living with the illness more tolerable. Healing is an option in some situations, but even then, total recovery is a long process that requires work, commitment, and support.

The dynamics of family relationships, work situations, emotions, and coping skills play an important role. This process may be subconscious and therefore difficult for the client to recognize or change. The dynamics required to support chronic illness patterns reach far beyond the physiology of the disease, and professional counseling may be required.

Working with chronic illness does not often produce measurable improvements. More often a slowed deterioration or, at best, stabilization is seen. For this reason, the treatment of chronic illness does not easily fit into the current medical system, which is geared mostly toward acute illness, injury, and trauma care.

Chronic pain perception is a major challenge. Recall from Chapters 5 and 6 that chronic pain is nonproductive. Chronic pain is processed by the central nervous system as a multifaceted, flawed feedback loop. Multiple strategies are necessary to help individuals better understand the pain experience.

Massage Adaptation

Massage therapists who work with people with a chronic illness should understand as much as possible about the illness. By using this information and conferring with the physician and other health professionals involved in the client's care, the massage practitioner can integrate the effects of massage into the comprehensive treatment plan, helping the client achieve the highest quality of life possible.

Long-term debilitating diseases which respond well to the short-term symptomatic relief massage provides include Parkinson's disease, multiple sclerosis, systemic lupus erythematosus (SLE), rheumatoid arthritis, fibromyalgia, chronic fatigue syndrome, asymptomatic infection with the human immunodeficiency virus (HIV), acquired immunodeficiency syndrome (AIDS), and disk problems that may cause back pain. Massage can also reduce general stress, helping individuals cope better with the condition (see Chapters 5 and 6).

Treatment plans focus on therapeutic change, condition management, or palliative care. Because of the nature of chronic illness, the emotional factors involved, and possible secondary gain, the treatment most often chosen is condition management, with palliative care provided during acute episodes of the illness. This recommendation does not mean that an actual therapeutic change plan is not possible; it simply is not as common.

Often additional training is required to understand chronic illness patterns, the effects of the medications involved, and the skill necessary to work in conjunction with other health care professionals.

Medications

People with chronic illnesses usually are under a physician's care and may be taking medications. The massage practitioner must understand the effects of the various treatments and medications and how massage may interact with the treatment.

Chronic Illness Cycle

Chronic illness follows an uneven cycle, with good and bad periods. On good days, the person may overexert and deplete an already weakened energy source. The immune system may be compromised, making the person with a chronic illness more susceptible to infections, such as colds and influenza. Because most chronic illness patterns have good days and bad days, the intensity of massage sessions must be geared to the client's condition that day. When symptoms are more active, the better course may be to give massages more often for shorter periods.

Encouraging Hardiness and Resilience

One approach to rehabilitating chronically ill individuals is a hardening or toughening program. Hardiness is the physical and mental ability to withstand external stressors. Individuals with chronic illnesses often reduce their activity levels, isolate themselves, and become less hardy. Massage, hydrotherapy, thermotherapy, specially designed hardening programs, and exercise can increase a person's hardiness. Resilience is the ability to recover from setbacks, adapt well to change, and keep going in the face of adversity. People who are resilient identify the reality of their circumstances yet have the belief that life is meaningful and will cope and overcome using the ability to problem solve and improvise. People who feel and function better are able to be more resilient.

Integrative Approaches to Healing

Mind/body approaches, behavior modification, relaxation techniques, spiritual healing, and other types of interventions and alternatives may be helpful to those with chronic illnesses. These approaches tend to empower the client, rallying powerful internal resources. It is important not to discount methods a person uses for self-help.

Goals and Expectations for Massage

The Massage Therapist

The massage professional who wants to work with the chronically ill must have realistic expectations. Instead of developing a massage approach to bring about a cure for the illness, which is out of the scope of massage practice anyway, the focus should be on helping the client feel better for a little while. There is value in knowing that massage may be the only care of this type the client is receiving, that not getting worse is an improvement for the client, that some people need their illness to cope, and that massage eases suffering in the illness pattern.

Often the client's present situation is the best that can be achieved under the existing circumstances. If each pattern presented by a client is seen as a solution to a preexisting condition, it is easier to understand why approaches that relieve the symptoms and support healing often are met with resistance. For example, a client with a chronic fatigue syndrome pattern consumes four or five cups of coffee after noon and finds they cannot sleep at night. Massage has been ineffective in supporting sleep. Though the caffeine intake is likely the cause, the client will not stop drinking coffee in the afternoon because they need it to function at work. So, what does the massage therapist do? There is no easy answer, and survival mechanisms reinforce short-term solutions, even if the behaviors create long-term problems.

The Client

A resourceful goal for working with people with chronic illness is helping the client rediscover the fact that each person is in charge of their own life, and the illness is not. The illness may have been allowed to take over the person's life and personal power. "Healing" may be the act of reasserting control over one's life, not getting rid of the disease. The benefits of massage may provide enough relief to enable the client to find the necessary inner resources for dealing constructively with the effects of chronic illness, thereby enhancing the client's quality of life and the lives of those around them (Proficiency Exercise 14.7).

PROFICIENCY EXERCISE 14.7

1. Choose one chronic illness and investigate it thoroughly.
2. Develop an educational brochure explaining the benefits of massage as part of a plan for coping with the chronic illness you have investigated. Share the brochure with fellow learners.

Key Points

- Dealing with chronic illness is difficult for the person who has it and the health/medical care team.
- A clinical reasoning process is used to determine the type of care most beneficial for a client with a chronic illness.
- The massage practitioner needs to research and understand the effects of the various treatments and medications.
- Complementary and alternative forms of health care may be helpful to those with chronic illnesses.

ONCOLOGY CARE

SECTION OBJECTIVES

Chapter objective covered in this section:

10. Adapt massage to support clients undergoing oncology care.

Using the information presented in this section, the student will be able to perform the following:

- Define cancer and oncology.
- List the types of cancer treatments.
- Adapt massage application for patients undergoing cancer treatment.
- Describe the use of palliative-based massage as part of cancer treatment.

The treatment of cancer, called *oncology,* combines disease-specific scientific knowledge, public health awareness, and psychosocial sensitivity. *Cancer* refers to any one of a large number of diseases characterized by the development of abnormal cells that divide uncontrollably and could infiltrate (metastasize) and destroy normal body tissue. Tumors are cell masses that are either benign or malignant and cancerous. Not all tumors are cancerous, and not all cancers form tumors. For example, leukemia is a cancer that involves blood, bone marrow, the lymphatic system, and the spleen, but it does not form a single mass or tumor. Not only do cancerous cells invade and destroy normal tissue, but they also can produce chemicals that interfere with body functions. For instance, some lung cancers secrete chemicals that alter the levels of calcium in the blood, affecting nerves and muscles, causing weakness and dizziness.

Cancer occurs with increasing incidence throughout the middle years of life and later. The American Cancer Society (ACS) estimates that half of men and one-third of women in the United States will develop cancer during their lifetimes. The three most commonly diagnosed cancers in women are expected to be cancers of the breast, lung, and bronchus. Colon cancer and rectal cancer are expected to be the most commonly diagnosed cancers in men. The most common cause of cancer death among people is cancer of the lung and bronchus. The most common cause of death in patients with cancer is infection, followed by respiratory failure, hepatic failure, and renal failure. Usually, many months pass between the diagnosis of metastatic cancer and the development of these complications.

Treatment

Until recently, cancer was considered incurable. However, it is no longer an automatic death sentence. More than half the people diagnosed with cancer survive 5 years or longer after diagnosis. One key to survival is early detection of cancer, and many screening tests are available. Massage therapists should know the most common nonspecific symptoms, such as fatigue, pain, anorexia, insomnia, and nausea, indicating potential cancer development. Occasionally the massage therapist may find that a client has a palpable mass. It is important for the massage therapist to support regular physician screening care and to refer clients when symptoms indicate the need.

Once cancer has been diagnosed, the care begins with a detailed history and physical examination. Most people with cancer receive some type of therapy once a histological diagnosis has been made. Treatment for cancer can be curative or palliative. *Staging* is the process of finding out how much cancer there is in the body and where it is located. Accurate staging provides a basis to weigh individual benefits and risks associated with a treatment.

Whether treatment has a curative or a palliative intent, success depends on the disease stage and acceptance of the treatment plan. If the intent of therapy is curative, both the oncology team and the individual are more apt to accept the harshness and toxicities of treatment. Treatment advances, including therapies that target specific molecules in or on cancer cells, or in the tumor's immediate surroundings, are changing the treatment process in oncology. Massage intervention spans the time of treatment, recovery, and return to health.

Multidisciplinary Care

The value of multidisciplinary and integrative approaches to care and treatment of individuals with cancer has been increasingly recognized (Mao et al., 2022). It is common to use several treatment modalities together (concurrently) or in sequence with the goal of preventing recurrence. This is referred to as *multimodality treatment* of the cancer. In many health care environments, multidisciplinary cancer clinics offer people the opportunity to be evaluated by the medical oncologist, surgical oncologist, radiation oncologist, nutritionist, physical therapist, and social worker at the time of their first or second clinic visit. Therapeutic massage is fast becoming an important aspect of multidisciplinary care in these settings.

Other complementary therapies, such as meditation, yoga, and aromatherapy, are incorporated into the multidisciplinary care centers. The spiritual needs of individuals are also considered and supported. In multidisciplinary approaches to patient management, each discipline performs a complementary function. In this regard cancer care, like hospice care, is becoming a model for effective integrative medical care with many professionals working together to achieve the best possible outcome.

Surgery

Surgery is performed to diagnose cancer, determine its stage, and treat the cancer. The primary care physician most often refers the person to a surgeon for biopsy and pathological diagnosis; therefore the surgical oncology team often is the first to see an individual with a newly diagnosed or suspected cancer.

A biopsy involves taking a tissue sample from the suspected cancer for examination by a specialist in a laboratory. A biopsy often is performed in the physician's office or in an outpatient surgery center. A positive biopsy result indicates the presence of cancer; a negative biopsy result may indicate that no cancer is present in the sample.

When surgery is used for treatment, the cancer is typically removed along with some adjacent tissue. In addition to locally treating the cancer, surgery may yield information useful for predicting the likelihood of cancer recurrence and whether other treatment modalities will be necessary.

Radiation Therapy

Radiation therapy, or radiotherapy, uses high-energy rays to damage or kill cancer cells by preventing them from growing and dividing. Like surgery, radiation therapy is a local treatment used to eliminate or eradicate visible tumors. Radiation therapy may be delivered externally or internally. With external radiation, high-energy rays are delivered directly to the tumor site from a machine outside the body. Internal radiation, or brachytherapy, involves the implantation of a small amount of radioactive material in or near the cancer.

Radiotherapy has both curative and palliative indications in the treatment of cancer. Radiation often is given in conjunction with surgery and chemotherapy. Radiotherapy is an integral and indispensable modality for pain relief and palliation of other symptoms, such as metastatic disease to bone or obstructing bronchial lesions. Individuals undergoing radiation experience varied symptoms, most often related to the organs that are within the direct radiation field. Radiation dermatitis and skin breakdown can occur, and patients often have associated fatigue and nausea.

Patients receiving brain radiation, whether for a primary CNS tumor or a metastatic lesion, can experience many symptoms, including severe fatigue, disequilibrium, nausea, vomiting, confusion or short-term memory loss, and hair loss.

Chemotherapy

Chemotherapy is any treatment involving the use of drugs to kill cancer cells. More than half of all people diagnosed with cancer receive chemotherapy. For many this approach helps treat their cancer effectively, enabling them to enjoy full, productive lives. Although surgery and radiation therapy destroy or damage cancer cells in a specific area, chemotherapy works throughout the body. Chemotherapy can destroy cancer cells that have metastasized or spread to parts of the body far from the primary tumor.

More than 100 chemotherapy drugs are used in various combinations. Cancer chemotherapy may consist of single drugs or combinations of drugs. Chemotherapy can be administered through a vein, usually through a chemotherapy port, which is a vascular access device implanted under the skin. Chemotherapy may also be injected into a body cavity or delivered orally in the form of a pill. Chemotherapy is different from surgery or radiation therapy in that the cancer-fighting drugs circulate in the blood to parts of the body where the cancer may have spread, and they can kill or eliminate cancer cells at sites great distances from the original cancer. As a result, chemotherapy is considered a systemic treatment. Unfortunately, most chemotherapy drugs cannot distinguish between a cancer cell and a healthy cell. Therefore chemotherapy often affects the body's normal tissues and organs, which complicates treatments or results in side effects.

Side Effects of Chemotherapy

Side effects of chemotherapy cause inconvenience and discomfort and occasionally may be fatal. In addition and perhaps more important, side effects may prevent delivery of the prescribed drug dose at the specific time scheduled by the treatment plan. Because the expected outcome of therapy is based on the delivery of treatment at a prescribed dose and schedule, a change from the treatment plan may reduce the chance of achieving the optimum outcome. In other words, side effects not only cause discomfort and unpleasantness but also may compromise the chances of cure by preventing the delivery of therapy at its optimum dose and time.

All chemotherapy is associated with a wide variety of side effects. However, some side effects occur more frequently than others. How the individual receiving chemotherapy experiences side effects, which ones, and their severity depend on a variety of factors, including the type of cancer, the type of chemotherapy drug or regimen used, the person's physical condition and age, and other such factors. The following side effects typically associated with chemotherapy are most pertinent to the massage therapist's understanding and to the development of a massage treatment plan:

- Anemia
- Fatigue
- Infection/neutropenia
- Nausea/vomiting
- Mouth sores
- Hair loss
- Constipation
- Diarrhea
- Pain
- Reproductive/sexual dysfunction
- Low platelet count (thrombocytopenia)

Fortunately, a great deal of progress has been made in the development of treatments to help prevent and control the side effects of cancer therapy. Many side effects once associated with chemotherapy can now be easily prevented or controlled, allowing people to work, travel, and participate in many of their other normal activities while receiving chemotherapy. For example, modern drugs to prevent vomiting (called *antiemetics*) have reduced the severity of nausea and vomiting with chemotherapy. In addition blood cell growth factors can protect from infection, reduce fatigue associated with anemia, and ensure treatment can be delivered according to the planned dose and schedule.

Fatigue is one of the most common complaints of people with cancer and increases in some cancer survivors. Fatigue is difficult to describe, and patients express it in a variety of ways, using terms such as *tired, weak, exhausted, weary, worn out, heavy*, or *slow*.

For many people diagnosed with cancer, fatigue may become a critical issue in their lives. Fatigue may influence a person's sense of well-being, daily performance and activities of daily living, relationships with family and friends, and compliance with treatment. Therapeutic massage is beneficial for managing some side effects, such as fatigue and pain.

Advances in Cancer Treatment

Improved use of immunotherapy, tissue-agnostic therapies that target the tumor's genetics rather than location, newly approved drugs, and more innovative treatments are leading to effective treatment, longer survival rates, remissions, and cures. The prognosis for those diagnosed with cancer is improving.

Palliative Care

Clients with a cancer diagnosis are often concerned about the possibility of experiencing pain and discomfort during treatment for cancer. Palliative care is aimed at relieving suffering and improving quality of life in individuals undergoing treatment for the primary condition. Such care addresses physical symptoms, such as pain, shortness of breath, and nausea, but also non-physical causes of pain, such as sadness, depression, and anxiety. Palliative care is different from hospice, which provides end-of-life care for those who no longer want to pursue more aggressive therapy. A major priority is to incorporate the principles of palliative care into the care of all people with cancer from the time of diagnosis, not only in the setting of advanced or terminal disease. Palliative care focuses on the whole person, encompassing body and mind to enhance comfort and preserve dignity.

Massage Adaption

Massage is accepted as part of a multidisciplinary approach to cancer treatment. The benefits of massage are obvious: stress management, preoperative and postoperative pain management, management of treatment side effects, and more. There are no specific protocols for massage and cancer care. The person undergoing cancer treatment must be evaluated each session, and the massage treatment must be based on the individual's status at that time.

The concern massage increases metastasis is unfounded. However, it is prudent not to massage over any associated tissue masses. The areas of radiation treatment need to be avoided, because the skin is damaged by the treatment.

Cautions

- Avoid all sources of heat (hot water bottles, heating pads, and sun lamps) on the treatment field.
- Avoid exposing the treatment area to cold temperatures (ice bags or cold-water treatment).
- Avoid any form of saltwater treatment.
- Avoid the use of all lotions or oils on the skin in the treatment field and use only approved lotion during massage.
- Avoid direct massage of the treatment area, other than a light application of approved lotion

Bones under areas of radiation treatment can be brittle; therefore massage pressure levels need to be monitored carefully. Do not use any massage methods that may cause tissue damage because chemotherapy reduces the body's ability to repair tissues. The general protocol may be too intense during cancer treatment, but the modified, palliative protocol (discussed later in the chapter) can be used as an appropriate starting point for massage and then adapted specifically for each client.

Post-Treatment Issues

Many cancer survivors have ongoing health concerns because of the cancer or due to treatment. These may include fatigue, difficulty sleeping, neuropathy and other types of pain, depression, anxiety, and changes in cognitive function. Additionally, many experience changes in social, economic, and family dynamics, leading to stress. People are living with cancer as a chronic condition but with ongoing uncertainty of reoccurrence and posttreatment health issues. Massage therapists working with individuals who are undergoing post cancer treatment need to be aware of the complex physical and psychosocial issues that can occur.

Key Points

- Cancer treatment can be curative or palliative.
- Massage can be part of an oncology treatment plan that targets palliative care as part of symptom management, especially the side effects of treatment.
- Survival rates for cancer patients are steadily increasing because of early detection and advances in treatment.
- Cautions for massage typically arise from changes in the client's skin as a side effect of treatment.
- Caution is necessary for fatigue and limits in adaptive capacity.
- Care continues beyond treatment to assist with the stress of a return to a "new normal."

HOSPITAL, LONG-TERM CARE, AND HOSPICE PATIENTS

SECTION OBJECTIVES

Chapter objective covered in this section:

11. Adapt massage for integration into the various medical settings.

Using the information presented in this section, the student will be able to perform the following:

- Explain the importance of comfort measures.
- Adapt massage application based on the circumstances of hospital care.
- Adapt massage application for individuals in long-term medical care.
- Define hospice care.
- Adapt massage for end-of-life care.

The use of massage therapy in hospitals is becoming more common, for a variety of reasons:

- Pain management
- Relief for cancer patients
- Pregnancy massage
- Adjunct to physical therapy
- Mobility/movement training
- Palliative care

Box 14.8 Benefits of Massage for Hospital Patients

1. *Pain:* Through the use of massage, the subjective experience of pain is diminished, even when the use of analgesics is reduced.
2. *Anxiety:* Anxiousness caused by the hospital stay and fear of procedures is reduced.
3. *Nausea:* The subjective experience of nausea and the use of antiemetics are reduced.
4. *Stress:* Physiological indicators of stress (e.g., raised cortisol level) are diminished, and indicators of reduced stress (e.g., improved serotonin level) are increased.
5. *Sleep:* The ability to sleep more easily and for longer periods increases with massage.

A common theme in hospital-based massage is pain management. Massage is effective at managing acute and chronic pain and supports other pain treatments, such as medication, ultrasound, and hydrotherapy. As mentioned, although massage targeting pain reduction commonly is thought of as therapeutic change, in reality it is palliative (see Chapter 6). Massage for the hospital patient is not targeted specifically to the pathological condition or injury; rather, it is intended to provide comfort care and symptom management (Box 14.8; also see Box 14.7).

The Importance of Palliative Care

The purpose of palliative care is to reduce suffering and create comfort. Massage offers pleasure, comfort, and relief from aching, all of which can reduce suffering. The massage used in palliative care is based on pleasure and compassion, and the focus is on reducing discomfort and providing comfort. Gentle, nonspecific massage application is used. As a reminder, gentle does not necessarily mean light pressure. Gentle means slow, focused, and pleasurable. Pressure typically is not deep, but most patients enjoy a sense of pressure that feels good.

Recommendations for a gentle, soothing, palliative massage include the following:

- Make sure the client is in a comfortable position and is physically supported.
- Use lotion when massaging to reduce friction and add moisture to the skin.
- Target areas that have the most discomfort (i.e., have limited movement). Massage is helpful in areas of prolonged pressure from sitting or lying. Often the neck, shoulders, low back, and calves ache because of immobility.
- Determine what pressure or movement is the most helpful and adjust the level and focus of pressure in response to feedback.
- Provide a hand and foot massage, which can provide a sense of comfort and well-being. Gentle yet firm movements can be used.
- Encourage the person to continue to tell you what is most helpful and to let you know right away if any method causes discomfort.
- Maintain the intention of reducing suffering by focusing attention on what feels good to the client.

MENTORING TIP

In 2007, I had open heart surgery. That is me, your textbook author, in Figs. 14.17 and 14.18, the day after surgery, with my son and textbook coauthor, Luke, providing palliative massage. Palliative care massage is an especially important gift.

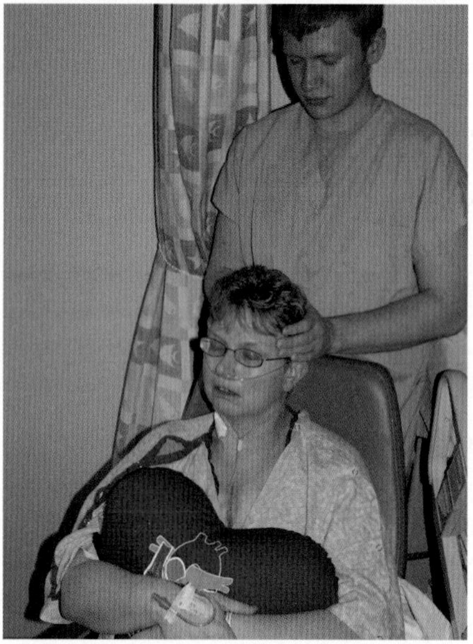

FIG. 14.17 Providing massage in a hospital chair. From Fritz S, Chaitow L, Hymel G: *Clinical massage in the healthcare setting,* 2007, Mosby.

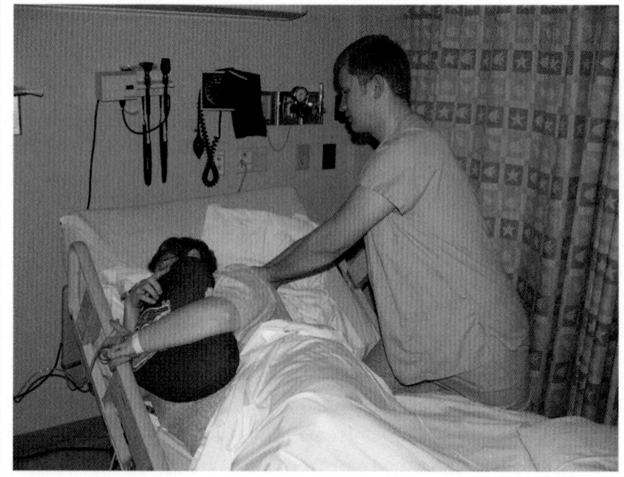

FIG. 14.18 Working around medical devices. From Fritz S, Chaitow L, Hymel G: *Clinical massage in the healthcare setting,* 2007, Mosby.

Typically the massage lasts no longer than 45 minutes, and 15–30 minutes in targeted areas may be sufficient. More frequent massage, such as daily or every other day, for a short duration (e.g., 15 minutes) may be helpful for comfort care.

Adapting to the Hospital Room

Maintaining Proper Body Mechanics

One of the biggest challenges massage therapists may face in a hospital or long-term care setting is providing massage when individuals are unable to lie on a massage table. Often massage is provided in the hospital bed or a standard chair (Fig. 14.17). In these situations, massage therapists must pay special attention to their body mechanics. Fortunately, deep pressure requiring a lot of leverage is not needed.

Maintain the basic principles of body mechanics as presented in Chapter 8 as much as possible. If the hospital bed can move up and down, adjust the height to a comfortable level. When possible, avoid reaching and instead stay as close to the patient as possible. If the patient's mobility is limited, placing one knee on the bed or sitting on the bed may be helpful. Before doing this, clear it with the individual who is supervising, but keep in mind that this may not be allowed in some cases. If you sit or kneel on the bed, use a clean towel as a sanitary barrier. Place it on the bed, and then sit or kneel on it. Do not get into uncomfortable positions and keep changing your position. It may not be possible to access all body areas.

Working Around Medical Devices

Working with individuals in hospital beds means that you must know how to operate the bed's controls. It also is important to be able to operate the nurse call buttons. Another challenge is working around various medical devices such as monitors and intravenous (IV) lines. Be cautious when moving around in the hospital room to avoid disturbing equipment (Fig. 14.18).

Avoid all areas where something enters or exits the body, such as IV lines, catheters, drains, respiratory devices, and so forth. Avoid all surgical sites. Do not disturb or remove any bandaging. If this should occur, inform the nurse so that infection control is maintained. Be cautious when working around monitoring leads, and do not dislodge them. If this should occur, call the nurse. Do not attempt to replace them because proper placement is required for accurate information. Use only the lotion provided or approved by the hospital. Do not add anything to the lotion.

The Massage Therapist's Responsibilities to the Patient and Medical Personnel

- Do not attempt to help a patient out of bed to use the restroom or for other activity. Do not assist a patient to move into various positions. It is better to let the person move because they will be protective of sensitive areas.
- Be courteous to other patients who may be sharing a hospital room. However, do not provide massage if asked unless authorized to do so.
- Leave the room when the physician, nurses, or other hospital personnel are providing care.
- Massage therapy is almost always provided in the hospital or similar medical setting as optional care. If a patient is sleeping or does not want a massage, do not insist. Report the situation to supervising personnel.

Long-Term Care

Although different from a hospital, a long-term care facility is similar due to its variety of medically based services that are provided to care for people with a chronic illness or disability. In addition long-term care helps meet personal needs. Most long-term care provides people with support services for activities such as dressing, bathing, and using the bathroom. Long-term care can be provided at home, in the community, in assisted living, or in nursing homes.

According to the World Health Organization, by 2030, 1 in 6 people in the world will be aged 60 years or over. By 2050, the world's population of people aged 60 years and older will double (2.1 billion). The number of persons aged 80 years or older is expected to triple between 2020 and 2050 to reach 426 million (https://www.who.int/initiatives/decade-of-healthy-ageing). According to the Centers for Medicare and Medicaid Services (CMS), by 2020, 12 million older Americans will need long-term care. A study by the US Department of Health and Human Services says that people who reach age 65 will likely have a 40% chance of entering a nursing home. About 10% of the people who enter a nursing home will stay 5 years or longer. The remaining elder adults will be cared for at home. The need for home-based, long-term care will increase as the elder adult population grows (CMS, 2022).

Assisted living facilities offer housing alternatives for individuals who may need help with dressing, bathing, eating, and toileting but who do not require the intensive medical and nursing care provided in nursing homes. Assisted living facilities may be part of a retirement community, nursing home, or senior housing complex or may be stand-alone facilities. Assisted living provides 24-hour supervision, assistance, meals, and health care services in a homelike setting. Residents of assisted living facilities usually have their own units or apartments.

Massage therapy can be integrated into long-term care services. The adaptations used for hospital patients also can be used for long-term care residents.

Terminal Illness, End-of-Life Care, and Hospice Care

When nothing further can be done to prolong life, care focuses more on comfort measures. **Hospice** is a philosophy of care, not a place. Hospice care can be provided in a hospital or long-term care setting, a specific residential hospice setting, or, most commonly, in the home (Box 14.9).

The experts in terminal illness are the dedicated hospice nurses and staff members who treat death with dignity. It has been said that the staff members of hospices are midwives to the dying.

To work successfully with those dealing with a terminal illness, the massage practitioner must be aware of their personal feelings about death. Massage professionals who want to work with clients during this very important, challenging, and special time of life are strongly encouraged to become hospice volunteers and to take the training that hospices offer.

No one knows when a person is going to die (Table 14.1). However, two powerful psychological forces influence living and dying: hope and the will to live. Attitudes about death vary. Adults usually have more fears about death than children do. They fear pain, suffering, dying alone, the invasion

Box 14.9 Providing Massage in the Home

It is important to move efficiently into and out of the area without disrupting the natural rhythm of the environment. It is important to respect the client's environment. Examples include removing shoes to protect the carpet and carrying special rubber-soled shoes to wear during the massage or cleaning up water splashes in the restroom after washing your hands. It is important to make sure the massage equipment and lubricants do not damage the client's floors or walls. Place a sheet on the floor under the massage table to protect the flooring.

Confidentiality is extremely important. The intimacy of the environment makes it more difficult to maintain professional boundaries and time management without seeming distant and hurried. It takes longer to enter and exit the onsite environment, not just because of the equipment setup and breakdown, but also because of the need to be respectful of the area and to be polite. The personal safety of the massage professional is a concern because the onsite massage environment has fewer safeguards than an office setting. Get to know those living in the home ahead of time, make sure someone else knows where you are, and check in with that person. Always carry a cell phone with you.

Table 14.1 Signs and Symptoms of the Final Stages of Death

Signs and Symptoms	Reason
Coolness, color, and temperature change in hands, arms, feet, and legs; mottling of the legs; perspiration	Peripheral circulation diminishes as blood shunts to vital organs. Patient may feel cool to touch, but core temperature is normal.
Increased sleeping	Conservation of energy, psychological withdrawal, medications.
Disorientation, confusion about time, place, person	Metabolic changes, medications, changing sleep/wake cycles, decreased oxygenation.
Incontinence of urine and/or bowel	Decreased muscle tone and consciousness.
Upper airway secretions; noisy respirations	Decreased cough reflex, inability to expectorate secretions or clear throat, relaxation of glottis, decreased muscle tone.
Restlessness	Metabolic changes and decrease in oxygen to the brain.
Decreased intake of food and fluids, nausea	Blood shunted away from gastrointestinal (GI) tract, causing decreased GI motility and anorexia; ketosis.

From Ebersole P, Touhy TA, Hess P, et al: *Toward healthy aging: needs and nursing response*, 7th ed, 2007, Mosby.

of privacy, loneliness, and separation from family and loved ones. They worry about who will care for and support those left behind. Elder adults usually have fewer of these fears than younger adults. They may be more accepting that death will occur and have had more experience with dying and death. Many have lost family members and friends. Some welcome death as freedom from pain, suffering, and disability.

Massage Adaptation

Massage has much to offer in comfort measures for the terminally ill. Being bedridden and immobile is painful. Massage can distract sensory perception, provide comfort and human contact, and give caregivers something constructive to do with their loved one.

Massage can become an important stress reduction method and a means of support for family members and caregivers. Caring for someone who is terminally ill can be stressful. The support person may require massage simply to have someone take care of them for an hour. Teaching simple massage methods to caregivers provides them with a means of meaningful and structured interaction with their loved one, in addition to a means of connecting with and supporting each other.

The massage professional should be an integral part of the team that works to make this time of passage as gentle as possible. This means that once the decision to work with someone who is terminally ill has been made, it is important to stay with the process until the client dies, if possible. The therapist probably will grow to care for the person and will mourn and grieve when death comes.

As always, it is up to the client to choose what they want and to give informed consent. A client who is dying needs to retain as much personal empowerment as possible. It should not be discouraging if all that is done during a massage session is to stroke a client's hands. At this time, it is especially crucial to "listen" and "allow" (Proficiency Exercise 14.8).

Key Points

- A major outcome for hospital patients is pain management.
- Adaptation for individuals in the hospital or other medical facility is required because of the presence of medical equipment (e.g., the hospital bed) and devices such as catheters and IV lines.
- Infection control is a priority.
- Clients receiving long-term care may require adaptations similar to those for patients in the hospital.
- Hospice care is a way of providing care, not a place where care is provided.
- Hospice is an integrated care approach.
- The goals of hospice care are to ensure that individuals needing care are as free of pain and symptoms as possible, yet still alert enough to enjoy the people around them and make important decisions for themselves (Proficiency Exercise 14.9).

PROFICIENCY EXERCISE 14.8

1. Plan your funeral or memorial service. List all plans and details regarding final arrangements.
2. Talk with an attorney about living wills.
3. Volunteer to provide massage for hospice staff members (devote a minimum of 32 hours to this responsibility).
4. Write about how you wish to be taken care of when it is your time to die. What level of intervention do you want? Do you want to die in a hospital or at home? When do you want hospice services?

PROFICIENCY EXERCISE 14.9

1. Obtain a course catalog from a college and compare your current massage education with the curriculum required for a nurse, a physical therapy assistant, an occupational therapist, a respiratory therapist, or another similar health care professional.
2. Discuss with a physician, nurse practitioner, chiropractor, physical therapist, or psychologist the skills they would want to see in a massage professional who would work with that person in the professional setting.

INDIVIDUALS WITH A PHYSICAL IMPAIRMENT

SECTION OBJECTIVES

Chapter objective covered in this section:

12. Communicate effectively, and appropriately adapt massage for individuals with physical impairments.

Using the information presented in this section, the student will be able to perform the following:

- Communicate more effectively with people who have a physical impairment.
- Become aware of subtle discrimination and implicit bias.
- Adjust the massage environment to better support those with a physical impairment.

According to the guidelines of the Americans with Disabilities Act, a **physical impairment** is any physiological disorder, condition, cosmetic disfigurement, or anatomical loss that affects one or more of the following body systems: neurological, musculoskeletal, special sense organs, respiratory (including speech organs), cardiovascular, reproductive, digestive, genitourinary, hemic and lymphatic, skin, and endocrine. Extremes in size and extensive burns also may be considered physical impairments (McGladre and Pullen, 1994). A **disability** is any mental or physical impairment or record or perception of a mental or physical impairment, that substantially limits one or more major life activities (e.g., ability to walk, talk, see, hear, breathe, learn, sleep, take care of oneself, or work).

People with physical impairments can benefit from massage for all the same reasons that any individual can. The client's body may develop compensation patterns in response to the disability. For instance, a person who uses a wheelchair could have increased neck and shoulder tension from moving the chair. In addition dealing with a physical impairment daily can make routine functions more stressful. The following sections present guidelines that may help the massage therapist provide services for clients with a variety of physical and sensory impairments.

A therapist must never presume to know, understand, or anticipate a client's need. *It is important to ask!* A concerned therapist does not try to pretend that the client's unique situation does not exist, but rather responds professionally. After the client has provided the necessary information about the disability, the therapist should accept the impairment as part of how the person functions.

Personal Awareness

Feeling uncomfortable is common in any new situation. This discomfort comes from not knowing what to do or say or from various other causes. Sometimes we are uncomfortable and cannot move beyond these feelings. The client will sense our discomfort. Simple disclosure of feelings allows communication and understanding. For some professionals communicating these types of feelings and accepting personal limitations may be difficult. Sometimes referral to a practitioner who is not affected by a particular situation is the best choice for both the massage professional and the client.

The impairment should not take precedent over the person. If the impairment is first in the massage therapist's mind, the person is not. Lack of knowledge is a factor in this form of subtle discrimination. Implicit bias occurs automatically and unintentionally and affects judgments, decisions, and behaviors. The massage professional is responsible for acting professionally and communicating effectively with all clients, including those who have disabilities. The best source of information is the person with the impairment:

- Ask your client to explain their situation.
- Ask what assistance, if any, might be needed.
- Ask how that assistance should be given if requested.

The practitioner should use good judgment when deciding whether to ask if assistance is needed and wait until the person accepts the offer before providing assistance. The client can give the best directions on how to proceed. For example, in offering assistance, it may be best to say, "If you need any assistance, I am glad to help. Tell me what you need." If the client declines, no offense should be taken. If another person is present, all remarks should be directed to the client and not to the companion.

Barrier-Free Access

All massage facilities must be barrier free. Commercial buildings usually are required by law to have barrier-free access and elevators, in addition to restroom facilities accessible to individuals with handicaps (Proficiency Exercises 14.10, 14.11, and 14.12).

Massage Adaptation

Supporting Clients Who Are Blind or Have Low Vision

Many people with a visual impairment have some type of sight. Comparatively few people have no vision at all.

The therapist should begin the conversation by using the client's name so that the person is aware of being addressed. The therapist then should state their name; they should not touch the client until the person is aware of their presence.

PROFICIENCY EXERCISE 14.10

Contact your local building department and speak with the person in charge of the barrier-free code requirements. Find out the requirements and the reason for each one.

When assisting a client with a visual impairment, the therapist should never push or pull on the person. Instead, if guiding is necessary, the therapist should stand just in front and a bit to the left of the client, who can then touch the therapist's right elbow when following.

Useful directions should also be given to a person with a visual impairment. If asked where something is, the therapist should not point and say, "Over there." Instead, terms such as *left, right, about ten steps,* and so on are much easier to follow. You may also use the example of time on a clock for some clients to indicate where things are located. For example, "The massage table is at 12:00, and a table for your belongings is at 3:00." It is not necessary to speak more loudly to individuals with a visual impairment, as they can usually hear without difficulty.

If a person with a visual impairment places anything anywhere, it should not be moved. If a door is opened, the direction of the opening (toward or away from the person) and the location of the hinges (left or right) should be explained. It is best to let the client open the door to become better oriented to its position.

If a service dog is harnessed and working, whether a guide dog or otherwise, the therapist must not pet, feed, or in any other way interact with the dog. This distracts the dog and makes its job difficult.

Supporting Clients Who Have a Speech Impairment

Understanding a person with a speech problem can be difficult. The therapist should ask the person to repeat anything that was unclear until it is understood and then should repeat what was said so that the person can clarify if necessary. If the therapist cannot understand what is being said, the client should be informed of this. If necessary, a notepad can be used to communicate in writing. Although speaking with an accent is not a speech impairment, it can make communication difficult. Not speaking the same language also hinders communication.

Supporting Clients Who Are Deaf or Have Hearing Loss

To gain the attention of a client who is deaf or has hearing loss, the therapist should lightly tap the person once on the shoulder or discreetly wave a hand. If no interpreter is present, all talking should be done in a normal tone and rhythm of speech.

If a client can lip read, the massage therapist should always face the person and not cover her own mouth when talking. A normal voice tone and speed should be used. If the therapist normally speaks quickly, the speed should be slowed a bit. If necessary, a notepad can be used to communicate in writing.

Hearing aids amplify sound; they do not make sound clearer. Reducing background noise helps those with a hearing impairment hear better. It may be wise to ask before using any music during the massage session. Getting too close to a hearing aid can cause the device to make high-pitched noises; take care when massaging near the ears.

Supporting Clients Who Have a Mobility Impairment

It is important for the massage therapist to ask questions to understand each individual situation. There are many types of mobility impairments and many reasons for them. For example, a person who uses a wheelchair may not be paralyzed.

When speaking to a client who uses a wheelchair, the therapist should do so from eye level, so sitting down or squatting may be the best option. Looking up strains the client's neck. A wheelchair must never be pushed unless the person gives permission. The individual will also give directions for pushing the wheelchair over barriers.

When a client must be transferred from a wheelchair to the massage table, the client can give the best directions on how to proceed. A transfer to a mat on the floor may be easier to accomplish, in which case the massage should be given there. The most efficient transfer is a lateral transfer to a table that is the same height as the wheelchair. This entails a shift in body mechanics by the massage therapist to accommodate a lower table unless a hydraulic or electronic massage lift table is used (Fig. 14.19).

Special care must be taken in giving a massage to a person with paralysis because normal feedback mechanisms are not functioning. The client's tissues can be injured by inappropriate pressure or drag. Clients with catheters or other equipment must instruct the therapist in the handling of the devices. In most cases the catheter can be ignored.

If the client has undergone amputation and uses a prosthesis, they may or may not want the device removed during the massage. Ask permission before massaging near the amputated area. If the client is comfortable with this, massage can be especially beneficial if a prosthesis is used. A client who is unable to shift and move their body throughout the day can become stiff and experience uncomfortable sensations related to immobility. Adapting massage to include a gentle range of motion and positional shifts when possible can relieve some discomfort.

Supporting Clients Who Have Brain Injuries

Brain injuries can result from external trauma, such as a blow to the head, or internal trauma, such as a cerebrovascular accident (CVA), loss of oxygen to the brain, or a tumor. Each individual who suffers a brain injury experiences different effects, depending on the part of the brain injured. Brain injury can cause cognitive, physical, behavioral, and personality changes. In addition the effects often change over time. Some impairments are permanent, whereas others improve slowly or may also fluctuate from day to day.

Depending on the client's needs, the massage therapist must adapt the massage. If the client has altered mobility, provide barrier-free access. Adapt communications skills to meet any cognitive, behavioral, and personality challenges presented by the client.

Supporting Clients Who Have Size Considerations

If the client is of short stature, a stool may be needed to help them reach the massage table, clothing hangers, or restroom fixtures. The massage professional should casually sit down to establish eye contact with the client so that the person does not have to look up, which strains the neck.

People who are tall (i.e., over 6 feet) also have challenges. They are not comfortable in the typical massage chair, and

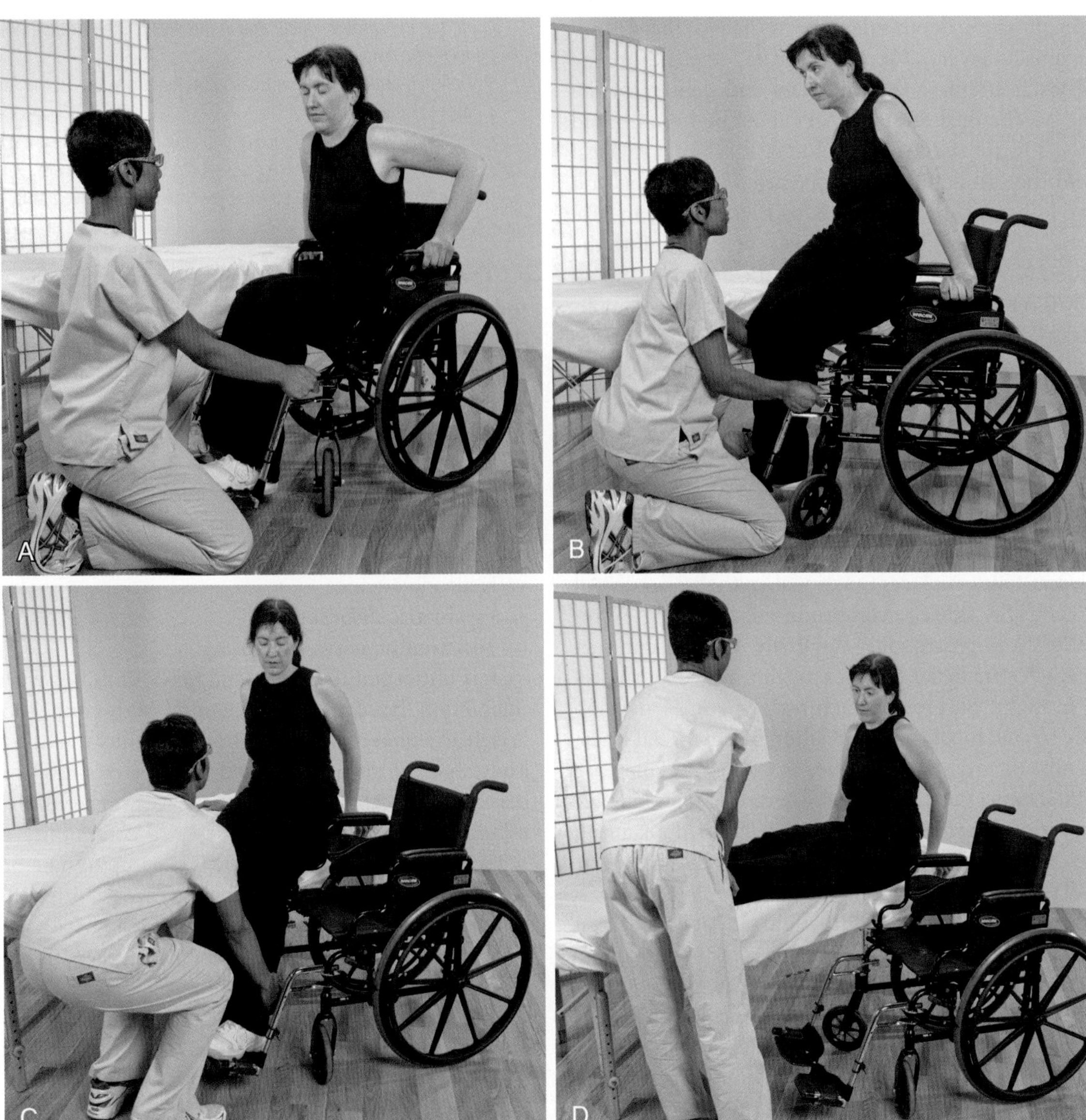

FIG. 14.19 Transfer of a client from a wheelchair to the massage table. A, Place the wheelchair close to the massage table, and stabilize the chair (i.e., lock the wheels). **B,** Carefully monitor the client's movements as they transfer to the table. **C,** After the client is seated on the table, prepare to assist by lifting the legs. **D,** Transfer the legs to the massage table.

their legs often extend beyond the massage table. The draping material is too short to cover the client's feet. Bolsters are too small. Adaptation during massage responds to these issues. It is advisable to have a set of draping materials that have extended length. It is easy to sew an additional piece of fabric to the sheets and blanket. A large towel can be wrapped around a bolster to make it larger.

Adaptations are appropriate for a person who is very thin. Someone can be thin by nature and still be healthy. Others may be underweight because of illness or medical treatment. The table will often require additional padding because the client does not have much soft tissue to cover bony prominences. It will not take as much mechanical force to access deeper tissues. It may be more difficult to use the forearm to provide massage, so the full hand can be used instead. The massage table may need to be positioned higher.

A large person (in height or weight or both) may not trust the massage table and may be more comfortable on a floor mat. However, getting up and down from the floor may be difficult. Sometimes seated massage is the better option. Ask the client what is preferable. If the practitioner is nervous about doing the massage on the massage table, the client must be told because the therapist's anxiety will affect the quality of the massage.

Obesity is a condition of having excessive body fat. It is different from being overweight, which means weighing too much. The weight may come from muscle, bone, fat, or body water. Massage adaptation for individuals who are obese primarily focuses on the comfort of the massage table, bolstering, draping materials, and positioning. The initial massage table height may need to be lower. In addition increased adipose tissue in superficial fascia can present challenges to delivering a pressure depth adequate to access the deeper fascia and muscle layers. The increased fat deposits in the superficial fascia increase the thickness and density of the tissue layer. Mechanical force delivery must be broad based and slow to allow for tissue displacement. It is better to use a forearm and the full hand during massage. Remember, you do not have to press hard into the tissue to access the muscle layers. Instead, compression on the surface penetrates into the deeper tissues. Narrow point contact with the fingers or the tip of the elbow is often uncomfortable; avoid these types of applications. Make sure you always have larger sheets on hand to accommodate larger clients. A step stool is also advisable because it is harder for larger clients to get up on the massage table.

Supporting Clients Who Have Burns and Disfigurements

People who have been burned may face an assortment of challenges, ranging from impaired mobility to disfigurement. As burns heal, scar tissue replaces functional epithelial tissue. All the functions of the skin are compromised, including excretion, sensation, and protection. Scar tissue tends to contract and pull, which can make the area of the healed burn feel shortened or tight. Severe contractures sometimes develop and must be treated medically. Elongation of superficial fascia and other connective tissue techniques can soften and increase sliding of the connective tissue. Massage of this type may reduce the effect of this shrinkage somewhat. It is important to learn more about burn types and treatment, including tissue grafting and scar tissue formation.

Many disfigurements tend to draw our attention because the mind is designed to notice differences. Although many disfigurements do not limit function in any way, they can create social difficulties. Attempting not to notice a disfigurement usually fails. The client recognizes that the situation exists and has various levels of comfort with the condition. Honest communication is effective in redirecting attention from the disfigurement to the person over time. The practitioner might offer a simple statement, such as "I can't help but notice (the particular disfigurement). I'm not uncomfortable, but the difference naturally draws my attention. Please be patient with me until I become more familiar with you."

Key Points

- Use people-first language when working with clients who have some sort of impairment.
- The client is the best source of information about what assistance, if any, and what accommodation, if any, may be needed.
- All massage facilities need to have barrier-free access.
- Do not interact with service animals.

INDIVIDUALS WITH A PSYCHOLOGICAL DIAGNOSIS

SECTION OBJECTIVES

Chapter objective covered in this section:

13. Communicate effectively, and appropriately adapt massage for individuals diagnosed with psychological conditions.

Using the information presented in this section, the student will be able to perform the following:

- Define mental impairment based on the provisions of the Americans with Disabilities Act.
- Understand the importance of verifying informed consent when working with individuals who have a psychological diagnosis.
- Structure a massage to support psychological interventions.

The Americans with Disabilities Act defines **mental impairment** as any mental or psychological disorder, such as developmental/intellectual impairments, organic brain syndrome, emotional or mental illness, and specific learning challenges. The conditions considered in this section include the following:

- Chemical addictions
- Chemical imbalances in the brain
- Intellectual impairment
- Cognitive differences
- Neurodivergence
- Psychiatric disorders
- Post-traumatic stress disorder

It is important to understand how our minds work and the interaction that constitutes the mind/body connection. It now is well accepted in the scientific community that the mind, the body, and the spirit are linked to a person's health and well-being. A dedicated learner of massage will seriously consider taking some psychology courses at a community college or other educational center and will keep up to date on new research findings. Some mental health care facilities offer education to the public. Massage will continue to have a key place in mind/body medicine and treatments, along with other forms of mental health services.

The actual massage approach is no different when the therapist works with individuals with a cognitive or psychological diagnosis. The principal factor is the person receiving the massage. Practitioners who want to work with clients with psychological diagnoses need additional training to understand the physiology and psychology of various disorders and the challenges these clients face. An understanding of psychotropic pharmacology is important because massage and these medications affect the body in similar ways. A psychologist or psychiatrist (Box 14.10) should closely supervise this type of work.

Chemical Addictions

Individuals withdrawing from chemical and alcohol addictions may find that massage helps reduce stress levels. The type of chemical to which the person is addicted determines the

Box 14.10 The Importance of Informed Consent

Informed consent is an important concern when working with clients who have chemical imbalances or developmental disabilities, or who are under the influence of drugs (whether prescribed or not). Exceptional care must be taken to ensure that the client is able to provide informed consent. If doubt exists, the massage should not be given.

types of stressful experiences incurred. The massage therapist assesses the client to decide whether the massage could calm an anxious client or give a boost to a depressed client.

Chemical Imbalances in the Brain

Certain types of mental disorders arise from an imbalance of brain chemicals; bipolar (manic-depressive) disorder, schizophrenia, seasonal affective disorder, obsessive-compulsive disorder, and clinical depression are just a few chemical disorders of the brain.

Medications

Medication is important in helping these individuals. The massage professional should never make the client feel guilty for taking medication or suggest that medication is not necessary. A physician must carefully monitor medication, with the smallest effective dosage given to prevent side effects. Massage cannot replace medication, but in some situations regular massage may allow the client's physician to reduce the dosage and duration of some types of medications. In other situations, the side effects of certain medications can be managed with massage. It is important to collaborate with the client's physician and chart the client's response to the massage carefully.

Intellectual Diversity

Intellectual impairment is the limited capacity for performing cognitive tasks, functions, or problem solving and is exhibited by more than one of the following: a slower rate of learning; disorganized patterns of learning; difficulty with adaptive behavior; and/or difficulty understanding abstract concepts.

Massage effects those with intellectual impairments the same as everyone else. Care must be taken to communicate at the client's level of understanding, but not below the client's functioning level. Adults with intellectual impairments are not children and should not be treated as such. People with intellectual impairments may become frustrated and anxious during a day of challenges. If these clients accept massage, it can be soothing, calming, and beneficial. However, not everyone likes to be touched. All individual's needs must be respected.

Cognitive Differences

Cognition is the variety of mental processes involved in gaining knowledge and comprehension. These are higher-level functions of the brain that encompass language, imagination, perception, and planning. Cognitive skills, also called cognitive abilities, cognitive functions, or cognitive capabilities, are mental skills used in acquiring knowledge, manipulating information, reasoning, and problem solving.

Neurodiversity

The term *neurodiversity* describes normal, genetic, brain-based variations in behavior. Neurodiversity researchers now realize that attention deficit/hyperactivity disorder (ADHD), autism, and other cognitive conditions emerge through a combination of genetic predisposition and environmental interaction. These cognitive differences are not the result of disease or injury, and people with differences do not need to be cured; they need help and accommodation instead. Despite well-documented brain differences and functional challenges, these differences may or may not be considered a disorder. The assertion that the person is different—not defective—is a much healthier self-concept. Although neurodiversity is not necessarily an impairment, people who have atypical (neurodivergent) neurological development have no protections beyond the general ones afforded under the Americans with Disabilities Act. Therefore these conditions are often referred to as disorders. Having neurodiversity can be challenging because neurodiverse people, by definition, are not "just like everyone else." As a result, they may have challenges fitting in socially, behaving in expected ways, or easily adjusting to change.

Attention Deficit Disorder (ADD) and Attention Deficit/Hyperactivity Disorder (ADHD)

Most professionals agree that ADD/ADHD is a brain-based, or neurological, variation. This means the brains of people with ADD/ADHD seem to work a little differently than those of other people. For example, people with ADD/ADHD may produce less of the neurotransmitter dopamine while also having more dopamine receptors. Researchers suspect that low dopamine levels are related to ADD/ADHD symptoms. ADD/ADHD has a large genetic component with numerous gene variations in people with ADD/ADHD, when compared with people who do not have ADD/ADHD. Although ADD/ADHD is a serious challenge, it is also a condition that can be effectively managed. People with ADD/ADHD can be highly creative and intelligent. They can be exceptionally good at thinking outside of the box and seeing solutions where others would not. The main features of ADHD are the same for children and adults and include inattention, hyperactivity, and impulsivity. Those with ADD may not manifest the hyperactivity.

Autism Spectrum Condition

Autism spectrum condition (ASC) is believed to be characterized by impaired social interaction and communication and a restricted repertoire of interests that hurt the person's ability to function properly in school, work, and other areas of life. Although autism can be diagnosed at any age, it is said to be a "developmental disorder" because symptoms generally appear in the first 2 years of life. The American Academy of Pediatrics recommends that all children be screened for autism.

Autism is known as a "spectrum" condition because there is wide variation in the type and severity of symptoms people experience. Interventions and support services can improve a person's symptoms and ability to function. Although people with ASC experience many challenges, they may also have many strengths, including the ability to learn things in detail and remember information for long periods of time, excelling in math, science, music, or art. Contrary to popular belief, most children and adults with autism spectrum do want to be touched but may be upset by a slight change in a routine or being placed in a new or overstimulating setting. A reliable, structured touch with firm, consistent pressure is usually preferred. Massage applied in a deliberate way that the client accepts has been shown to increase social interaction somewhat and reduce anxiety.

Tourette's Syndrome

Tourette's syndrome is tic disorder starting in childhood that involves involuntary, repetitive movements and vocalizations.

Learning Differences

Learning differences, sometimes called learning disabilities are common. Difficulty with basic reading and language skills are most common. Learning differences are neurologically based processing problems that can interfere with learning basic skills such as reading, writing, or math. Neurological issues can also challenge organization ability, time planning, abstract reasoning, long- or short-term memory, and attention. Examples of these types of cognitive differences include auditory processing; dyscalculia, which is difficulty understanding numbers and math; dysgraphia, a learning disability that affects a person's handwriting ability and fine motor skills; and dyslexia, which affects reading and related language-based processing skills. Difficulties with processing sensory input, which occurs in some learning disorders, may be helped by the organized, systematic, sensory stimulation of massage. Having a learning difficulty is stressful, and stress from dealing with the environment aggravates the learning difficulty. Self-esteem is hard to maintain when a person has been made to feel inadequate in school because they could not write, spell, or read. Massage reduces their stress, thereby facilitating learning and enabling them to feel more positive about themselves. (NOTE: The author of this textbook, Sandy Fritz, functions quite well with dyslexia and dysgraphia.)

Chronic Traumatic Encephalopathy (CTE)

Chronic Traumatic Encephalopathy (CTE) is a progressive degenerative disease of the brain found in people with a history of repetitive brain trauma, including symptomatic concussions as well as asymptomatic subconcussive hits to the head. The repetitive trauma triggers progressive degeneration of the brain tissue, including build-up of abnormal tau proteins. These changes in the brain can begin months, years, or even decades after the last brain trauma. The brain degeneration is associated with memory loss, confusion, impaired judgment, impulse control problems, aggression, and depression.

Mild Cognitive Impairment (MCI)

Mild cognitive impairment (MCI) is a condition in which people have memory or other thinking problems greater than normal for their age or capability. The problems associated with MCI may be caused by certain medications, cerebrovascular disease which affects blood vessels that supply the brain, and other factors. Some of the problems brought on by these conditions can be managed or reversed. The main symptom is an impaired thinking skill other than memory loss, such as trouble planning and organizing or poor judgment.

Dementia

Dementia, also referred to medically as Major Neurocognitive Disorder (NCD), is the loss of cognitive functioning of thinking, remembering, and reasoning to such an extent that it interferes with a person's daily life and activities. Some people with dementia cannot control their emotions, and their personalities may change. Dementia ranges in severity from the mildest stage, when it is just beginning to affect a person's functioning, to the most severe stage, when the person must depend completely on others for basic activities of living.

There are several different forms of dementia, including Alzheimer's disease. A person's symptoms can vary depending on the type. Common is mixed dementia, caused by processes related to both Alzheimer's disease or other dementia types and vascular disease.

Massage Adaptation

When working with clients who have cognitive differences, the most common massage approach is general stress reduction. Attempting to adapt to expectations and environments is stressful and fatiguing. Massage affects the autonomic nervous system and brain chemicals by encouraging the release of serotonin, dopamine, endocannabinoids, and endorphins, which alter mood. It also affects the release of various hormones that influence mood. Massage has a strong normalizing effect on stress perception and response.

Psychiatric Disorders

Psychiatric disorders, such as anxiety, panic, depression, and eating disorders, interplay in a combination of autonomic nervous system functions and hormone neurotransmitters, neuropeptides, and other brain chemicals.

Anxiety, Panic, and Depression

Anxiety is an uneasy feeling usually connected with increased sympathetic arousal responses. **Panic** is an intense, sudden, and overwhelming fear or feeling of anxiety that produces terror and immediate physiological change that results in immobility or senseless, hysterical behavior. A panic attack is an episode of acute anxiety that occurs at unpredictable times with feelings of intense apprehension or terror. It may be accompanied by a feeling of shortness of breath that leads to hyperventilation, dizziness, sweating, trembling, and chest pain or heart palpitations. Most symptoms can be related to overactivation of the sympathetic autonomic nervous system.

Depression is characterized by a decrease in vital functional activity; mood disturbances of exaggerated emptiness, hopelessness, and melancholy; or unbridled periods of high energy with no purpose or outcome.

Anxiety and depressive disorders are commonly seen with fatigue and pain syndromes. **Pain and fatigue syndromes** are multicausal and often chronic, nonproductive patterns that interfere with well-being, activities of daily living, and productivity. Some syndromes are fibromyalgia, chronic fatigue syndrome, infection with the Epstein-Barr virus, sympathetic reflex dystrophy, headache, arthritis, chronic cancer pain, neuropathy, low back syndrome, idiopathic pain, somatization disorder, and intractable pain syndrome. Acute "episodes" of chronic conditions can be factors in these syndromes. Panic behavior, phobias, and the sense of impending doom, along with a sense of being overwhelmed or hopelessness, are common with these conditions. Symptoms of these conditions and syndromes include mood swings, breathing pattern disorders, sleep disturbance, concentration difficulties, memory disturbances, outbursts of anger, fatigue, and changes in habits of daily living, appetite, and activity levels.

A breathing pattern disorder often is a significant underlying factor with anxiety and panic. Massage can normalize the breathing muscles, which must be done to correct a breathing pattern dysfunction.

Eating Disorders

Eating disorders involve mood disorders, physiological responses to food, and control issues. They are complicated situations that usually require professional intervention. The job of the massage therapist is to be aware of the possibility of an eating disorder and refer the client. Any substantial weight loss must be referred to a physician. Individuals with anorexia nervosa (a starving disorder) lose a great deal of weight. Recognizing bulimia, which involves binge eating and purging using vomiting and laxatives, is more difficult. The teeth and gums are affected by the stomach acids, and the massage professional may notice this. Referral should be made because of symptoms, not because the therapist is attempting to diagnose the disorder.

Massage Adaptation

When working with clients who have psychiatric disorders, the most common massage approach is general stress reduction, which can be adjusted to be a little more stimulating or a little more relaxing. The key is to begin where the person is at the time of the massage. Someone who is anxious may initially resist long, slow strokes and instead do better with active joint movement and rapid compression; as they calm the massage can gradually shift to rocking and long, slow strokes. The person who is a little depressed may not initially want to actively participate in the massage. The work might begin with rocking and long, slow strokes and end with stimulating active joint movement, rapid compression, and tapotement.

Massage affects brain chemicals by encouraging the release of serotonin, dopamine, endocannabinoids, and the endorphins, which alter mood. It also affects the release of various hormones that influence mood. Massage has a strong normalizing effect on the autonomic nervous system and can support other interventions for psychiatric disorders.

Trauma and Post Traumatic Stress Disorder

Trauma results from an event, series of events, or set of circumstances that is experienced by an individual as harmful or life threatening. While unique to the individual, generally the experience of trauma can cause lasting adverse effects, limiting the ability to function and achieve mental, physical, social, emotional, or spiritual well-being. Trauma-informed practice is an approach to health care interventions which is grounded in the understanding that trauma exposure can impact an individual's neurological, biological, psychological, and social development. The purpose of trauma-informed practice is not to treat trauma-related difficulties, which is the role of trauma-specialist services and practitioners (US Department of Health and Human Services, 2014; Simons et al., 2022).

There are several types of trauma, including:

- Acute trauma: This results from a single stressful or dangerous event.
- Chronic trauma: This results from repeated and prolonged exposure to highly stressful events. Examples include cases of child abuse, bullying, or domestic violence.
- Complex trauma: This results from exposure to multiple traumatic events.

It is natural to feel afraid during and after a traumatic situation. Fear triggers split-second changes in the body to help defend against danger or avoid it. This "fight-or-flight" response is a typical reaction meant to protect a person from harm. Nearly everyone will experience a range of reactions after trauma, yet most people recover from initial symptoms naturally. Those who continue to experience problems may be diagnosed with PTSD. Post-traumatic stress disorder (PTSD) develops in some people who have experienced a shocking, scary, or dangerous event. People who have PTSD may feel stressed or frightened, even when they are not in danger. Symptoms include reexperiencing of flashback memory, in addition to state-dependent memory, somatization, anxiety, irritability, sleep disturbance, concentration difficulties, times of melancholy or depression, grief, fear, worry, anger, and avoidance behavior. Excessive stress can manifest as a number of disorders, such as cardiovascular problems, including hypertension; digestive difficulties, including heartburn, ulcer, and bowel syndromes; respiratory illness; susceptibility to bacterial and viral illnesses; endocrine dysfunction, particularly adrenal or thyroid dysfunction; delayed or diminished cellular repair; sleep disorders; and breathing pattern disorders, to mention just a few. PTSD can have long-term effects.

Abuse

People who have experienced various forms of **abuse** often experience PTSD. When people are abused, whatever the form of abuse, they must learn to survive as best they can at the time of the abuse. These survival mechanisms take many forms, such as dissociation, hypervigilance, aggressive behavior, learning to "disappear," low self-esteem, and withdrawal. As mentioned, PTSD is common. These patterns may generalize into many life situations.

If the abuse happens to a young child, the coping mechanisms develop around a twisted reality. The younger the child, the more difficult effective survival will be, and possibly the more magnified the inappropriate survival mechanisms that develop. The older we are, the more inner resources we have to support effective coping. The effects of the abuse should not be judged by their intensity or context.

Memory, Trauma, and Dissociative Behavior

State-dependent memory is a process of recalling an experience when a physiology occurs in the body that is similar to the one experienced when the event first occurred. State-dependent memory functions in all life experiences (Zarrindast and Khakpai, 2020). When a person gets ready to hit a baseball or drive a car, the individual assumes the appropriate position and the body remembers what is required. In a traumatic experience, this mechanism locks in the factors that coincide with the experience. In the future, this repressed memory may be triggered by any one of the sensations or physiological factors involved in the state-dependent memory. For example, smell can trigger a memory. With massage, the pressure, location of the touch, and position or movement of the client may trigger the client's memory.

A person who experiences trauma during the formative years may have difficulty sorting it all out in adulthood. The memories may be spotty or piecemeal, or only one of the sensations (e.g., smell, touch, position) may be encoded in the memory. It is important not to discount this memory pattern simply because all the pieces do not fit together to form a whole picture. It may be affirming to know that all the pieces do not have to fit together for the person to have enough information to resolve and integrate past experiences and develop more resourceful behavior for the present and future (Wolf and Nochajski, 2022).

Physical abuse (e.g., beatings, neglect) and emotional abuse (e.g., criticism, unrealistic expectations, brain washing, indoctrination) ravage a person's self-esteem. Sexual abuse is often laden with mixed signals, role confusion, and secrecy.

Some life experiences that may affect a person in a manner similar to deliberate abuse are illness, medical procedures, hospitalization, accidents, or other trauma, such as that experienced by military personnel or survivors of natural disasters. This process is also common in the training and development of athletes, dancers, and musicians. Developing these skills is difficult and often physically painful. The success of the individual's coping skills depends on the type of support received during and soon after the traumatic event, in addition to the dynamics surrounding the situation. A child who attempts to hide pain during a medical procedure to not upset the parents is being denied full emotional and physical expression in the situation. If the medical staff does not explain the procedure so that the child comprehends or if the child is too young to understand, this, too, may become a difficult situation to integrate into a person's life experiences. If a parent or support person is physically separated from or emotionally unavailable to a child or adult during a crucial time, this can have a lasting effect.

Abuse of an adult, such as occurs with rape, violent crime, stalking, spouse beating, and abuse of elder adults, also must be considered. Typically, adults feel powerless in the situation and may feel as though the abuse is deserved or that they somehow did something to cause it. If elder adults are also mentally impaired, such as with Alzheimer's disease, they may become childlike in their reasoning and survival mechanisms. Those who have experienced upheaval in their environment, such as those who live in war-torn areas or areas of disaster, can develop feelings of powerlessness and devastation even when the person is no longer in the environment and is now safe.

Often the client does not remember the details or recall who, what, where, when, or how. Instead, a vague uneasiness, or **dissociation** (i.e., detachment, discontentedness, separation, isolation), develops. One mechanism for surviving physical, sexual, and emotional trauma is to "leave the body" and therefore not feel the abuse or to believe that the abuse is happening to someone else.

Many types of appropriate dissociative coping mechanisms are valuable in times of performance, demand, emergency, or survival. This is sometimes called "entering the zone" or "zoning out." However, if the pattern of dissociation becomes repetitive and generalized, coping becomes strained. The massage professional should be aware of a client dissociating during a massage. It is not our job to change the dissociative pattern. More specialized training is required to deal effectively with all the ramifications of a client's shift in coping style. This frequently involves professional counseling.

The massage therapist can begin to recognize the pattern of the dissociation and the massage techniques or positions that seem to trigger the pattern. With this information the therapist can alter the approach to the massage, providing the client with the opportunity to stay with the body more easily.

For example, if the therapist notices that every time the client's left knee is bent the client's body becomes unresponsive, the eyes become distant, or the breathing shifts, it is best to work with the knee in a different position. Also, rather than moving the client, the practitioner can have the client move into the position, which is more empowering for the individual.

Some people may also self-abuse, which can take many forms, such as a destructive lifestyle, addictive processes, and self-inflicted trauma. Self-abuse may be calming for the person. Mood-altering chemicals are released during self-abuse. The mechanisms of counterirritation and hyperstimulation analgesia come into play. The massage professional may notice bruises, cuts, burns, or other injuries on the client's body. In a professional manner, the practitioner should bring these areas to the client's attention and note them in the client's record. Acknowledging an injured area to a person who abuses themself may cause the person to feel guilty or ashamed, tell a cover story, or ignore the question. This behavior indicates potentially serious underlying conditions, and referral is indicated.

Intrusive Experiences

A characteristic of PTSD is the intrusive experience, which is a sense of reliving the event in vivid visual images, along with physiological responses; it may include sounds and smells, all of which occur with an intense feeling of panic and fear as experienced in the distressing situation. An internal or external reminder of the event triggers these intrusive experiences, resulting in a sense of lack of control over their appearance.

Reenactment, or flashback, means reliving the event as though it were happening again right now. *Integration* is remembering the event but being able to remain in the present moment, with an awareness of the difference between then and now, to bring some sort of resolution to the event.

Reenactment does not necessarily provide the awareness and understanding necessary to integrate the physical response and emotions into the client's experience in an empowering way. Instead, with reenactment the client repeats an abusive pattern and feels disempowered and lost. The massage professional must be aware of the potential for harm to a client by deliberately triggering a reenactment response. Without the additional and necessary support of qualified counselors and other support personnel to provide for an integration process, a reenactment is undesirable.

Indications for Massage Therapy

Because therapeutic massage works well in normalizing the effects or physiological manifestations of stress on the body, it can be an effective tool in management of or recovery from PTSD. Several mechanisms justify the use of massage therapy for those who have experienced trauma including safety in the therapeutic relationship and the effects of massage on calming the nervous system. Moderate pressure massage increases activity in the parasympathetic nervous system, inducing the relaxation response. A plausible explanation for massage benefit is that 'pleasant-touch' responsive nerves, the c-tactile afferents (CT), account for the positive effects of touch to influence emotional regulation and the ability to perceive internal physiological sensations called interoceptive awareness. Touch that activates these fibers is processed in the brain, mainly in the insula, which is connected to several other brain structures involved in the processing of tactile information (McGreevy and Boland, 2022) (see Chapter 5).

Massage Adaption

Boundaries are important. Review the importance of respect for personal boundaries (see Chapter 2). The client may personalize the nurturing touch of the therapist (transference) and may want to involve the therapist in the experience. Referral for appropriate counseling is important. When a person is actively exploring personal trauma and its results, it is important that the massage therapist not take on the client's problems (countertransference).

Self-Abuse can be defined as any behavior that causes damage or harm to oneself. Individuals who self-harm do so to release painful emotions which can develop into a coping mechanism. People who engage in self-inflicted injury typically do so in an attempt to cope with distress, anger, and other painful emotions. Occasionally a client demands or requests very deep and painful massage when the soft tissue condition does not indicate the need for this type of invasive work. Self-abuse mechanisms may be involved in this situation. It is important not to become involved in a situation that perpetuates an abuse pattern. The therapist needs to trust their intuition about appropriate care but should not force the client to face the situation by confronting the person with the possibility of self-abuse mechanisms.

Emotional Responses

An emotion is a complex psychological state triggered by stimuli. Emotional responses are the reactions people have to stimuli that produces emotion in them. Behind every emotion is a process that starts with a stimulus, initiates an internal reaction, and results in a visible expression (Zych and Gogolla, 2021).

If a client should respond emotionally during the massage by crying, shaking, becoming ticklish, agitated, or fearful, or demonstrating another emotional pattern, it is important for the massage professional to pause the massage and maintain gentle contact. Be quiet and let the person experience the emotion. If needed, provide tissues in an unobtrusive way. Changes in breathing are common. For example, the client may cough, hold the breath, increase the breathing rate, or yawn. It is wise during these situations to avoid telling the client how to breathe. Breathing patterns are usually linked to experiences. Unless a client has high blood pressure and is holding their breath, the massage therapist should only observe the breathing and identify changes. The client should be asked no questions other than, "Do you want me to continue?" It is not necessary to know the client's story. Do not ask for a description of the past experience. The practitioner should be calm and accepting of the response and should never try to encourage or stop the response. It is important not to interfere with the person's experience by interjecting suggestions. The therapist needs to stay connected with the client but distanced from the client's experience. The emotional experience belongs to the client, not to the practitioner, who supports in a quiet, straightforward way. When the emotional response has dissipated, the massage can be continued. Similar explanations, as previously mentioned, help the client understand what happened. A client who seems unsettled and needs additional help coping should be referred to their physician, who can recommend a qualified mental health professional.

Trauma-Informed Care

Confidence, respect, and trust are necessary to provide massage which enhances the well-being of those who have been or are being traumatized. Always remember that confidentiality is a sacred trust; the therapist does not talk about clients or any experience with clients to anyone else. Additional training is needed to serve clients who have a history of trauma. The actual techniques of massage are no different, but an understanding of coping mechanisms requires additional study. Bodywork in some form may be a valuable tool for some individuals who want to resolve these issues, whereas for others it is not the best choice. Effective decision-making skills and support and supervision by qualified professionals determine the appropriateness of massage interventions for this population (Box 14.11).

PROFICIENCY EXERCISE 14.11

Based on the information presented in this section, choose one psychological challenge, and design an intervention plan and justification statement for the use of therapeutic massage.

Learner Note: Here is the clinical reasoning process again. If you have been practicing by doing the exercises in the beginning of this chapter, you should be starting to understand the process. For help, see the example on the Evolve site.

Example: Therapeutic massage for ________________

1. Gather facts to identify and define the situation.
   Key questions: What is the problem? What are the facts?
2. Brainstorm possible solutions.
   Key questions: What might I do? What if...?
3. Evaluate possible interventions logically and objectively; look at both sides and the pros and cons.
   Key question: What would happen if...?
4. Evaluate the effect on the people involved.
   Key question: How would each person involved feel?
5. Develop an intervention plan and justification statements.

PROFICIENCY EXERCISE 14.12

1. Read three books that address surviving trauma, or conduct research on PubMed (www.pubmedcentral.nih.gov) on the treatment of trauma.
2. Contact the child protection agency in your community and obtain information on recognizing signs of child abuse and reporting suspected cases.
3. Investigate methods used by the military to help soldiers deal with stress.
4. Describe an incident in which you felt abused, then describe an incident in which you feel you abused someone.
I felt abused when:
I abused someone when:

Prevent Re-traumatization

Key to trauma-informed care is avoiding any re-traumatization events for the client. Re-traumatization is the re-experiencing of thoughts, feelings, or sensations experienced at the time of a traumatic event or circumstance in a person's past. Re-traumatization is generally triggered by reminders of previous trauma which may or may not be potentially traumatic in themselves.

The decision to deal actively with an abusive history requires commitment and time from the client. Professional help or support groups often are needed. The practitioner must not suggest that a client was abused or that the client needs to deal with their situation. Our job is to honor, respect,

Box 14.11 Trauma-Informed Care Begins with Awareness

As part of an interdisciplinary care plan, massage therapy has much to offer in the experience of safe and compassionate touch. Trauma-informed care is not a type of intervention or treatment; rather, the focus is on safety and understanding.

Trauma is widespread, harmful, and occurs as a result of violence, traumatic experiences, abuse, neglect, loss, disaster, war, human trafficking, and other emotionally harmful experiences. Traumatic exposure cuts across age groups, gender, socioeconomic status, race, ethnicity, geography, and sexual orientation. Individual trauma results from an event, series of events, or set of circumstances that is experienced by an individual as physically or emotionally harmful or life-threatening that has long-term effects on the individual's functioning and mental, physical, social, emotional, or spiritual well-being. It is important to remember that what happened to the person is not nearly as important as what the trauma means to the individual.

A trauma-informed perspective views trauma-related symptoms and behaviors as an individual's best and most resilient attempt to manage, cope with, and rise above their experience of trauma.

Traumatic stress reactions can be understood as normal reactions to abnormal situations. In embracing the belief that trauma-related reactions are adaptive, you can begin relationships with clients from a hopeful, strengths-based stance that builds upon the belief that their responses to traumatic experiences reflect resilience, creativity, and self-preservation.

Biology of Trauma

Exposure to trauma leads to a cascade of biological changes and stress responses. These biological alterations include:

- Changes in limbic system functioning
- Hypothalamic–pituitary–adrenal axis activity changes with variable cortisol levels
- Neurotransmitter-related dysregulation of arousal and endogenous opioid systems

Hyperarousal

A common symptom that arises from traumatic experiences is hyperarousal (also called hypervigilance). Hyperarousal is the body's way of remaining prepared. It is characterized by sleep disturbances, muscle tension, and a lower threshold for startle responses. It can persist years after trauma occurs.

When Massage Therapy Can Help

Physical (somatic) symptoms are likely to occur in individuals with traumatic stress reactions, including PTSD; this is called somatization. Many individuals who present with somatization are likely unaware of the connection between their emotions and their physical symptoms. Common physical disorders and symptoms include sleep disturbances, gastrointestinal, cardiovascular, neurological, musculoskeletal, respiratory, and dermatological disorders, urological problems, and substance use disorders. It is common for these symptoms to be related to a breathing pattern disorder. The physical experiences are often related to physiological manifestations of hyperarousal. Physical symptoms must not be discounted, and medical examination is necessary to rule out any underlying conditions. At times, clients may remain resistant to exploring emotional content and remain focused on physical symptoms as a coping mechanism.

People from certain ethnic and cultural backgrounds may initially or solely present emotional distress via physical ailments or concerns. Various cultures approach emotional distress through the physical realm.

Some clients may insist that their primary problems are physical even when medical evaluations and tests fail to confirm ailments. In these situations, somatization may be a sign of a mental illness.

Trauma-Informed Care (TIC)

Trauma-informed care and trauma-informed systems function according to the following guidelines:

- Realize the prevalence of traumatic events and the widespread impact of trauma
- Recognize the signs and symptoms of trauma
- Respond by integrating knowledge about trauma into your work policies, procedures, and practices
- Seek to actively resist re-traumatization

The Five Principles of Trauma-Informed Care

Safety: Ensuring physical and emotional safety

Principles in Practice: Common areas are welcoming and privacy is respected

Choice: Individual has choice and control

Principles in Practice: Individuals are provided a clear and appropriate message about their rights and responsibilities

Box 14.11 Trauma-Informed Care Begins with Awareness—cont'd

Collaboration: Making decisions with the individual and sharing power

Principles in Practice: Individuals are provided a significant role in planning and evaluating services

Trustworthiness: Task clarity, consistency, and interpersonal boundaries

Principles in Practice: Respectful and professional boundaries are maintained

Empowerment: Prioritizing empowerment and skill building

Principles in Practice: Providing an atmosphere that allows individuals to feel validated and affirmed

Learn More

All massage therapists need to practice in a trauma-informed manner. A specific massage therapy focus as part of trauma-informed care and treatment is a specialization requiring additional education. Because of the complexity of the population, care is best provided by an interdisciplinary team.

References and Resources

Hansen KA, Walsh EG, Price C. A call to action: Adoption of trauma informed care in complementary and integrative health services. *J Altern Complement Med*. 2021;27(2):103–107.

Center for Substance Abuse Treatment (US). *Trauma-Informed Care: A Sociocultural Perspective*. Substance Abuse and Mental Health Services Administration; 2014. Available at https://www.ncbi.nlm.nih.gov/books/NBK207195/

US Department of Health and Human Services

Substance Abuse and Mental Health Services Administration

The Substance Abuse and Mental Health Services Administration (SAMHSA) is the agency within the US Department of Health and Human Services that leads public health efforts to advance the behavioral health of the nation. SAMHSA's mission is to reduce the impact of substance abuse and mental illness on America's communities.

https://www.samhsa.gov/

Agency for Healthcare Research and Quality

The Agency for Healthcare Research and Quality supports research to improve the quality, safety, efficiency, and effectiveness of health care for all Americans.

https://www.usa.gov/federal-agencies/agency-for-health-care-research-and-quality

The National Child Traumatic Stress Network

NCTSN is funded by the Center for Mental Health Services (CMHS), Substance Abuse and Mental Health Services Administration (SAMHSA), the US Department of Health and Human Services, and jointly coordinated by UCLA and Duke University.

https://nhttac.acf.hhs.gov/soar/eguide/respond/Trauma_Informed_Care

https://www.nctsn.org/what-is-child-trauma/trauma-types

Office for Victims of Crime Training and Technical Assistance Center is a component of the Office for Victims of Crime, Office of Justice Programs, US Department of Justice.

The US Department of Justice's Human Trafficking Task Force e-Guide provides practical information on how to respond in a trauma-informed way to the different types of needs for individuals who have experienced trafficking.

https://www.ovcttac.gov/TaskForceGuide/EGuide/

Office on Trafficking in Persons

https://www.acf.hhs.gov/otip

The SOAR training equips professionals with skills to identify, treat, and respond appropriately to human trafficking.

https://www.acf.hhs.gov/otip/training/soar-health-and-wellness-training

consider, regard, protect, defend, preserve, praise, value, safeguard, shelter, sustain, support, tolerate, appreciate, approve, recognize, understand, accept, and never harm.

Key Points

- An understanding of psychotropic pharmacology is important because massage and these medications affect the body in similar ways.
- Informed consent may be difficult to obtain.
- It is necessary to understand the signs, symptoms, and treatments for any condition a client may have.
- Trauma-informed care is foundational in massage therapy practice.
- A team approach for assisting those with psychological disorders is important.

SUMMARY

Respect is important in any interaction with another person or with an animal. In all situations, remember to see and address the client first and then accommodate the individual's specific needs by offering assistance and following directions provided by the client.

Foot in the Door

When you can adapt massage to meet the unique needs of individuals, your foot more easily gets into the doors of a variety of massage careers. Do you have a specific area of passion and compassion? For example, do you feel drawn to specialize in hospice care? Maybe you want to work with athletes or infants. Do you have a specific understanding of what it is like to be deaf or blind? Maybe you have cultural experience or are bilingual, which can help you better interact with a specific group of people. When you are competent and passionate about your career goals, others can begin to believe in you. What a terrific way to get your foot in the door, by serving a group of clients who share an experience, activity, condition, or time of life.

Massage therapists who want to focus their professional skills to best meet a client's specific needs will seek out training and information pertinent to the client's therapeutic needs. Often the knowledge required to provide massage to many diverse populations becomes too extensive, and specialization is necessary. When this is the case, such as when a massage professional obtains additional training for pregnancy, labor, and delivery massage, the information is integrated into the fundamentals of massage, and the additional training focuses on application of massage fundamentals for special situations.

The wise professional recognizes when less intervention is more appropriate. Considerable learning, great skill, and patiently developed empathy are required to therapeutically hold a person's hand.

LEARN MORE ON THE WEB

On the Evolve site you will find links relevant to the topics covered in this chapter. Whether you are interested in working with athletes, older adults, people with post-traumatic stress disorder, or any of the other topics, more information has been provided for you.

MedlinePlus is an excellent initial resource for learning about client conditions, medications, and other treatments. Use the search feature to locate information about specific topics, but also explore all the features on this government site. The Evolve site has topic-specific links. Other helpful sites include the National Center on Health, Physical Activity and Disability (NCHPAD) and the National Health Services (NHS) (United Kingdom). NHS Choices is the UK's biggest health website.

Evolve

Visit the Evolve website: http://evolve.elsevier.com/Fritz/fundamentals/.

Evolve content designed for massage therapy licensing exam review and comprehension of content beyond the textbook. Evolve content includes:

- Content Updates
- Science and Pathology Animations
- Body Spectrum Coloring Book
- MBLEx exam review multiple choice questions

FOR EACH CHAPTER FIND:

- Answers and rationales for the end-of-chapter multiple-choice questions
- Electronic Workbook and Answer Key
- Chapter multiple choice question Quiz
- Quick Content Review in Question Form and Answers
- Technique Videos when applicable
- Learn More on the Web

REFERENCES

Abd-Elsayed A, Pope J, Mundey DA, et al. Diagnosis, treatment, and management of painful scar: A narrative review. *J Pain Res*. 2022;15:925–937.

Alm AK, Danielsson S, Porskrog-Kristiansen L. Non-pharmacological interventions towards behavioural and psychological symptoms of dementia: an integrated literature review. *Open J Nurs*. 2018;8(07):434.

Angelopoulos P, Mylonas K, Tsepis E, Billis E, Vaitsis N, Fousekis K. The effects of instrument-assisted soft tissue mobilization, tissue flossing, and kinesiology taping on shoulder functional capacities in amateur athletes. *J Sport Rehabil*. 2021 Apr 9;30(7):1028–1037. doi:10.1123/jsr.2020-0200. PMID: 33837162.

Beetz A, Julius H, Turner D, et al. Effects of social support by a dog on stress modulation in male children with insecure attachment. *Front Psychol*. 2012;3:352. http://dx.doi.org/10.3389/fpsyg.2012.00352. eCollection 2012.

Bergh A, Asplund K, Lund I, Boström A, Hyytiäinen H. A systematic review of complementary and alternative veterinary medicine in sport and companion animals: soft tissue mobilization. *Animals*. 2022;12(11):1440.

Bernstein K, Karkhaneh M, Zorzela L, Jou H, Vohra S. Massage therapy for paediatric procedural pain: a rapid review. *Paediatr Child Health*. 2021;26(1):e57–e66.

Bhargava A, Arnold AP, Bangasser DA, Denton KM, Gupta A, Krause LMH, Mayer EA, et al. Considering sex as a biological variable in basic and clinical studies: an endocrine society scientific statement. *Endocr Rev*. 2021;42(3):219 258.

Cantwell SL. Traditional Chinese veterinary medicine: the mechanism and management of acupuncture for chronic pain. *Top Companion Anim Med*. 2010;25:53.

Centers for Medicare and Medicaid Services (CMS). What is long-term care? Available at: https://www.medicaidlongtermcare.org. Accessed November 2022.

Cohen Marill M: Is this normal aging or not? Available at: www.webmd.com/healthy-aging/features/normal-aging-changes-and-symptoms. 2022.

Coleman E, Radix AE, Bouman WP, et al. Standards of care for the health of transgender and gender diverse people, version 8. *Int J Transgend Health*. 2022;23(Suppl 1):S1–S259.

Coppola CL, Grandin T, Mark Enns R. Human interaction and cortisol: can human contact reduce stress for shelter dogs? *Physiol Behav*. 2006;87:537.

Cummings NH, Stanley-Green S, Higgs P. *Perspectives in Athletic Training*. Mosby; 2009.

Davis HL, Alabed S, Chico TJA. Effect of sports massage on performance and recovery: a systematic review and meta-analysis. *BMJ Open Sport Exerc Med*. 2020;6(1):e000614.

de Britto Pereira PAD, Mendes Abdala CV, Portella CF, Ghelman R, Schveitzer MC. Pediatrics massage evidence map. *Complement Ther Med*. 2021;61(102774):102774.

Dowell D. CDC clinical practice guideline for prescribing opioids for pain—United States, 2022. MMWR. *Recommendations and Reports*. 2022;71.

Dybczyńska M, Goleman M, Garbiec A, Karpiński M. Selected techniques for physiotherapy in dogs. *Animals (Basel)*. 2022;12(14):1760.

Estep D, Hetts S. Proper etiquette with animals. Available at: www.AnimalBehaviorAssociates.com. 2011. Accessed November 2022.

Field T. Pediatric massage therapy research: A narrative review. *Children (Basel)*. 2019;6(6):78.

Fogarty S, McInerney C, Stuart C, Hay P. The side effects and mother or child related physical harm from massage during pregnancy and the postpartum period: An observational study. *Complement Ther Med*. 2019;42:89–94.

Formenton MR, Pereira, MAA, Fantoni, DT. Small animal massage therapy: a brief review and relevant observations. *Top Companion Anim Med*. 2017 Dec;32(4):139-145. doi: 10.1053/j.tcam.2017.10.001.

Gee NR, Rodriguez KE, Fine AH, Trammell JP. Dogs supporting human health and well-being: A biopsychosocial approach. *Front Vet Sci*. 2021;8:630465.

Green AE, DeChants JP, Price MN, Davis CK. Association of gender-affirming hormone therapy with depression, thoughts of suicide, and attempted suicide among transgender and nonbinary youth. *J Adolesc Health*. 2022;70(4):643–649.

Guy J, Arcelus L, Gooren DT, Klink V. Endocrinology of transgender medicine. *Endocr Rev*. 2019;40(1):97–117.

Handlin L, Hydbring-Sandberg E, Nilsson A, et al. Short-term interaction between dogs and their owners: effects on oxytocin, cortisol, insulin and heart rate: an exploratory study source. *Anthrozoos*. 2011;24:301.

Hunt JD. Cism & canines: The bond that helps heal first responders. *Crisis, Stress, and Human Resilience*. 2022;4(1):16–25.

Icke S, Genc R. Effect of foot massages on postpartum comfort and pain level of mothers after vaginal delivery: a randomized trial. *Holist Nurs Pract*. 2021;35(3):140–149.

Julian JM, Salvetti B, Held JI, Murray PM, Lara-Rojas L, Olson-Kennedy J. The impact of chest binding in transgender and gender diverse youth and young adults. *J Adolesc Health*. 2021;68(6):1129–1134.

Kathmann I, Cizinauskas S, Doherr MG, et al. Daily controlled physiotherapy increases survival time in dogs with suspected degenerative myelopathy. *J Vet Intern Med*. 2006;20:927.

Kennedy AB, Patil N, Trilk JL. 'Recover quicker, train harder, and increase flexibility': massage therapy for elite paracyclists, a mixed-methods study. *BMJ Open Sport Exerc Med*. 2018;4(1):e000319.

Keshavarz S, Mirzaei T, Ravari A. Effect of head and face massage on agitation in elderly Alzheimer's disease patients. *Evidence Based Care*. 2018;7(4):46–54.

Leng M, Zhao Y, Wang Z. Comparative efficacy of non-pharmacological interventions on agitation in people with dementia: a systematic review and Bayesian network meta-analysis. *Int J Nurs Stud*. 2020;102(103489):103489.

Liu YC, Liao CN, Song CY. Effects of manual massage given by family caregivers for patients with dementia: A preliminary investigation. *Geriatr Nurs*. 2022;46:112–117.

Machin H, Taylor-Brown F, Adami C. Use of acupuncture as adjuvant analgesic technique in dogs undergoing thoracolumbar hemilaminectomy. *Vet J*. 2020;264:105536.

Mao JJ, Ismaila N, Bao T, et al. Integrative medicine for pain management in oncology: Society for Integrative Oncology-ASCO guideline. *J Clin Oncol*. 2022;40(34):3998–4024.

Mathew L, Phillips KF, Sandanapitchai P. Interventions to reduce postpartum fatigue: an integrative review of the literature. *GJ Health Science Nurs*. 2018;1:112.

McGladre Y, Pullen R. *The Americans with Disabilities Act (rev)*. Panel Publishers; 1994.

McGreevy S, Boland P. Touch: An integrative review of a somatosensory approach to the treatment of adults with symptoms of post-traumatic stress disorder. *Eur J Integr Med*. 2022;54(102168):102168.

McKinney ES, James SR, Murray SS, Nelson K, Ashwill J. *Maternal-Child Nursing*. 5th ed. Saunders; 2017.

Memon MA, Shmalberg J, Adair HS, et al. Integrative veterinary medical education and consensus guidelines for an integrative veterinary medicine curriculum within veterinary colleges. *Open Vet J*. 2016;6(1):44–56.

Midtsund A, Litland A, Hjälmhult E. Mothers' experiences learning and performing infant massage: a qualitative study. *J Clin Nurs*. 2018.

Mohamed AA, Zhang X, Jan YK. Evidence-based and adverse-effects analyses of cupping therapy in musculoskeletal and sports rehabilitation: a systematic and evidence-based review. *J Back Musculoskelet Rehabil*. 2023;36(1):3–19.

Monteiro BP, Lascelles BDX, Murrell J, Robertson S, Steagall PVM, Wright B. 2022 WSAVA guidelines for the recognition, assessment and treatment of pain. *J Small Anim Pract*. 2023;64(4):177–254.

Moseley GL, Baranoff J, Rio E, Stewart M, Derman W, Hainline B. Nonpharmacological management of persistent pain in elite athletes: rationale and recommendations. *Clin J Sport Med*. 2018;28(5):472–479.

Mrljak R, Arnsteg Danielsson A, Hedov G, Garmy P. Effects of infant massage: a systematic review. *Int J Environ Res Public Health*. 2022;19(11).

Mueller SM, Grunwald M. Effects, side effects and contraindications of relaxation massage during pregnancy: A systematic review of randomized controlled trials. *J Clin Med*. 2021;10(16):3485.

Pusparatri E, Sudarmiati S, Rejeki S. Nursing intervention for mother with postpartum fatigue: a literature review. *Jurnal Kebidanan*. 2022;11(1):1–8.

Porter M. Equine rehabilitation therapy for joint disease. *Vet Clin North Am Equine Pract*. 2005;21:599.vi.

Riley LM, Satchell L, Stilwell LM, Lenton NS. Effect of massage therapy on pain and quality of life in dogs: a cross sectional study. *Vet Rec*. 2021;189(11):e586.

Ririn Y, Ardhiyanti N. The effect of massage therapy in overcoming constipation in infants aged 7-12 months. *Science Midwifery*. 2021;9(2):228–231.

Santi LKS, Sudewi AAR, Duarsa DP, Lesmana CBJ. The relationship of pregnancy massage to the rate of anxiety depression and stress in pregnant women. *Int J Health Med Sci*. 2021;4(2):208–214.

Sarli D, Sari FN. The effect of massage therapy with effleurage techniques as a prevention of baby blues prevention on mother postpartum. *Inter J Advan Life Sci Res*. 2018;1(3):15–21.

Schug SA, Palmer GM, Scott DA, Alcock M, Halliwell R, Mott JF, APM/SE Working Group of the Australian and New Zealand College of Anaesthetists and Faculty of Pain Medicine (2020). *Acute Pain Management: Scientific Evidence* (5th edition), ANZCA & FPM, Melbourne.

Shamsi H, Okhovatian F, Khademi-Kalantari K. Physiological and neurophysiological effects of sports massage on the athletes' performance: a review study. *J Rehabil Med*. 2022;11(5):680–691. https://dx.doi.org/10.32598/SJRM.11.5.12.

Simons M, Kimble R, Tyack Z. Understanding the meaning of trauma-informed care for burns health care professionals in a pediatric hospital: A qualitative study using interpretive phenomenological analysis. *Burns*. 2022;48(6):1462–1471.

Skillgate E, Pico-Espinosa OJ, Côté P, et al. Effectiveness of deep tissue massage therapy, and supervised strengthening and stretching exercises for subacute or persistent disabling neck pain. The Stockholm Neck (STONE) randomized controlled trial. *Musculoskelet Sci Pract*. 2020;45(102070):102070.

Smith CA, Hill E, Denejkina A, Thornton C, Dahlen HG. The effectiveness and safety of complementary health approaches to managing postpartum pain: A systematic review and meta-analysis. *Integr Med Res*. 2022;11(1):100758.

Stiles J, Jernigan TL. The basics of brain development. *Neuropsychol Rev*. 2010;20(4):327–348.

Stoodley C, McKellar L, Ziaian T, Steen M, Fereday J, Gwilt I. The role of midwives in supporting the development of the mother-infant relationship: a scoping review. *BMC Psychol*. 2023;11(1):71.

Suzuki M, Tatsumi A, Otsuka T, et al. Physical and psychological effects of 6-week tactile massage on elderly patients with severe dementia. *Am J Alzheimers Dis Other Demen*. 2010;25:680.

Tau GZ, Peterson BS. Normal development of brain circuits. *Neuropsychopharmacology*. 2010;35(1):147–168.

T'Sjoen G, Arcelus J, Gooren L, Klink DT, Tangpricha V. Endocrinology of transgender medicine. *Endocrine Reviews*. 2019;40(1):97–117.

US Department of Health and Human Services. SAMHSA's concept of trauma and guidance for a trauma-informed approach. (2014): 1.

Vavken P. Evidence-based treatment of muscle Injuries. *Schweiz Z für Sportmedizin & Sporttraumatologie*. 2018;67(1).

Wolf MR, Nochajski TH. 'Black Holes' in memory: Childhood autobiographical memory loss in adult survivors of child sexual abuse. *Eur J Trauma Dissociation*. 2022;6(1):100234.

World Health Organization. *WHO Recommendations on Postnatal Care of the Mother and Newborn*. World Health Organization; 2014.

Yuningsih N, Kuswandi K, Rusyant S. The effect of effleurage massage on lowback pain in trimester iii pregnant women at mandala puskesmas, lebak regency in 2021. *Science Midwifery*. 2022;10(2):774–779.

Zarrindast MR, Khakpai F. State-dependent memory and its modulation by different brain areas and neurotransmitters. *EXCLI J*. 2020;19:1081–1099.

Zhang H, Zhao M, Wu Z, et al. Effects of acupuncture, moxibustion, cupping, and massage on sports injuries: A narrative review. *Evid Based Complement Alternat Med*. 2022;2022:1–10.

Zych AD, Gogolla N. Expressions of emotions across species. *Curr Opin Neurobiol*. 2021;68:57–66.

MULTIPLE-CHOICE QUESTIONS FOR DISCUSSION AND REVIEW

The answers, with rationales, can be found on the Evolve site. Use these questions to stimulate discussion and dialogue. You have to understand the meaning of the words in the question and possible answers. Each question provides you with the ability to review terminology, practice critical thinking skills, and improve multiple-choice test-taking skills. Answers and rationales are on the Evolve site. It is just as important to know why the wrong answers are wrong as why the correct answer is correct.

1. In which area would additional study be required when working with any population group to support appropriate adaptation?
   a. Massage methods
   b. Accommodation
   c. Psychology
   d. Relaxation methods
2. A massage professional has been working with an 86-year-old client. The client still lives independently with some outside support. Family lives in a nearby state. The client is unable to drive. In which way does this client most likely benefit from a weekly massage?
   a. Physical and emotional stimulation
   b. Increased circulation
   c. Friendship
   d. Spiritual support
3. A parent massaging an infant encourages ______.
   a. Hardiness
   b. Dissociation
   c. Developmental disorders
   d. Bonding

4. A massage therapist has just started a job at a family practice medical center. The center deals with many clients who exhibit stress-related symptoms. Which of the following professional skills will the massage therapist need to perfect?
   a. Muscle energy methods
   b. Restorative massage
   c. Charting and record keeping
   d. Lymphatic drainage
5. A client just began working with a massage professional who specializes in massage for those with physical impairment. Which of the following accommodations would the client likely notice?
   a. The building is barrier free.
   b. Special massage methods are used.
   c. All clients have guardians.
   d. All clients set quantifiable and qualifiable goals.
6. A massage therapist has developed a referral network with a group of physicians and physiologists treating patients with anxiety and panic disorders. Which of the following will they need to be effective in managing with massage?
   a. Exercise protocols
   b. Nutrition
   c. Support group interactions
   d. Breathing pattern dysfunction
7. A massage client is in the first trimester of their third pregnancy. Which of the following is contraindicated?
   a. Prone position
   b. Massage of the feet
   c. Deep abdominal massage
   d. Lymphatic drainage
8. A long-term client has just notified you that they have a terminal illness. Which massage approach is indicated?
   a. Therapeutic change
   b. Palliative care
   c. Remedial massage
   d. Rehabilitation massage
9. Which of the following is a medical emergency?
   a. Heat rash
   b. Heatstroke
   c. Capsulitis
   d. Heat cramp
10. A client discloses that they have dyslexia. What accommodation might this client need?
    a. A consistent environment and massage sequence
    b. Pressure depth related to medication
    c. Assistance with completion of intake forms
    d. A guardian providing informed consent
11. An adult client has many surgical scars on their chest and abdomen. History indicates that the client had surgical intervention as a child to repair congenital malformations. The client enjoys massage on the limbs and back in the prone position but appears distant and unsettled when turned to the supine position. What is the most logical explanation for this response?
    a. An abusive family history
    b. Intrusive thoughts
    c. Dissociation
    d. Integration
12. A college football player is seeking massage as part of a healing program for an injured knee that required surgical intervention. The athletic trainer is supervising the massage. The massage consists of general full-body massage that addresses any developing compensation caused by the gait change while the knee is healing. Specific applications of kneading and myofascial release are being used to maintain pliability in the soft tissue of the thigh and leg. What type of massage is being performed?
    a. Post-event massage
    b. Recovery massage
    c. Palliative massage
    d. Rehabilitation massage
13. In which of the following circumstances would anterior chest massage related to gender-affirming surgery be most appropriate?
    a. General massage
    b. Adjunct to breast cancer treatment
    c. Scar tissue management
    d. Examination for lumps
14. What would be the most challenging countertransference situation a massage professional faces when working with clients who have chronic illnesses?
    a. Understanding the combined effects of massage and medications
    b. Managing frustration with a client whose condition does not improve
    c. Maintaining boundaries with a client who sees massage as the answer to all physical problems
    d. Managing acute episodes of chronic illness
15. A massage practitioner has been asked by a group of mental health professionals to begin working at a residential facility. The practitioner would need to be most concerned over which of the following?
    a. Types of mental health issues
    b. Obtaining informed consent
    c. Learning specific massage protocols for each condition
    d. Frequency and duration of the massage
16. In which of the following circumstances would massage without supervision by a medical care professional best benefit a child?
    a. Growing pains
    b. Anxiety disorder
    c. Touch sensitivity
    d. Attention deficit disorder
17. Which of the following complaints by athletes can be addressed with fluid movement approach?
    a. Muscle guarding
    b. Laceration
    c. Delayed-onset muscle soreness
    d. Cramp
18. A massage therapist specializes in prenatal massage. Which of the following would they need to be aware of between the 24th and 30th week of pregnancy?
    a. Breast changes
    b. Constipation
    c. Preeclampsia
    d. Positioning

19. A massage professional has been working with a client who has chronic pain syndrome. The massage helps when combined with physical therapy, judicious use of pain medications, and support group attendance. Improvement in the condition began after 6 or 7 massage sessions. After 10–12 sessions, the client missed 3 or 4 sessions, and then returned for massage and indicated that they are right back where they started and do not feel like the situation will ever improve. What is the most logical explanation for this behavior?
    a. State-dependent memory
    b. Increase in hardiness
    c. Secondary gain
    d. Acute pain

20. Which of the following athletic injuries is addressed most effectively with massage?
    a. Grade 3 acute strain
    b. Dislocation
    c. Stress fracture
    d. Chronic tendinitis

Activity

Write at least three more multiple choice questions. Make sure to develop plausible wrong answers and be sure that the correct answer is clearly correct. Then write a rationale for each question. The more questions you write, the better you will understand the material. Exchange questions with classmates or discuss them in class. The questions from all the learners can be combined to create a review quiz.

CHAPTER 15

Wellness and Self-Care for the Massage Therapist and Client Education

http://evolve.elsevier.com/Fritz/fundamentals/

CHAPTER OBJECTIVES

After completing this chapter, the student will be able to perform the following:

1. List and describe challenges individuals encounter that interfere with wellness.
2. Describe the importance of diet to a wellness lifestyle and plan a healthy diet.
3. Explain physical exercise as part of a wellness program.
4. Identify and define relaxation and restorative activities.
5. Explain how the mind and body connection affects wellness.
6. Implement and respect the importance of an individualized spiritual approach to wellness.

CHAPTER OUTLINE

KEY TERMS

Aerobic exercise training
Challenge
Commitment
Control
Deep inspiration
Defensive measures
Denial
Endurance
Fitness
Forced expiration
Forced inspiration
Overload principle
Quiet expiration
Quiet inspiration
Salutogenesis
Stressors
Surrender
Training stimulus threshold

Individuals who seek massage therapy for health, wellness, and restorative outcomes as well as disease prevention and symptom management may be receptive to health promotion messages from their massage therapists. One reason massage therapists may be particularly helpful in health promotion efforts is that those who seek complementary and integrative care typically see those practitioners on multiple occasions, which may allow for more opportunities for health promotion messages to be presented and reinforced. Also, as described in Chapter 1, the definition of massage used in this textbook is as follows: Massage therapy consists of the application of massage and non-hands-on components, including health promotion and education messages, for self-care and health maintenance; therapy, as well as outcomes, can be influenced by therapeutic relationships and communication; the therapist's education, skill level, and experience; and the therapeutic setting (Kennedy et al., 2018).

Most massage therapy licensing that determines the scope of practice allows massage therapists to provide self-care information related to self-massage, general exercise, flexibility, sleep hygiene, pain management methods, and healthy lifestyle education.

Massage therapy is an important part of any wellness program because it supports self-regulation and homeostasis and provides a connection with other human beings. As a massage professional, you must understand the components of wellness. With this information, you can explain to clients how massage fits into the overall wellness plan.

In addition, you can use this same information to create your own wellness plan. This entire textbook is devoted to your success as a massage therapist. You have learned about professional boundaries, professional burnout and prevention, workplace safety, and (especially in Chapter 8), how to prevent work-related injury and fatigue.

Box 15.1 Elements of a Wellness Program

Body
Nutrition
Light and dark exposure
Sleep
Breathing
Physical fitness
Sensory stimulation

Mind
Relationships with oneself and others
Communication
Beliefs
Intellectual stimulation

Spirit
Sense of purpose
Connection
Faith
Hope
Love

We are considered well/healthy when the body, mind, and spirit are in ideal balance. We are not well when imbalance exists; when this occurs, balance must be restored.

Everyone would benefit from developing a personal wellness plan. Just as in designing a massage, there is no right or wrong way to formulate this plan. However, by following a few basic guidelines, we can discover what works best for us as individuals. Massage therapists must remember that massage alone cannot address all aspects of well-being. Wellness is about the whole person. The empathetic massage professional realizes that during a client's search for wellness, the time spent with the massage therapist provides focused attention, acceptance, and effective listening, which are as important as the massage methods used.

As with massage, often the simpler the overall wellness program is, the better. Box 15.1 provides attributes around which wellness programs can be built. A wellness program also needs to change as the individual changes. We are supposed to be well, and our bodies will recognize the best process for achieving wellness. Wellness has a domino effect. Commitment to only a few carefully considered lifestyle alterations can produce chain reactions throughout a person's life. When an effective wellness program is conducted, a person looks forward to getting back to living life to the fullest and, at the appropriate time, to dying with dignity.

OPPORTUNITIES AND CHALLENGES TO WELL-BEING

SECTION OBJECTIVES

Chapter objective covered in this section:

1. List and describe challenges individuals encounter that interfere with wellness.

Using the information presented in this section, the student will be able to perform the following:

- Explain the meaning of salutogenesis.
- List common stress responses.
- Explain the basic concept of stress management.
- Relate excessive demands to increased stress.
- Explain loss and how it relates to wellness.
- Describe the role of intuition and wellness.
- Explain the importance of qualified professional help and personal relationships for maintaining wellness.

Making changes leading to wellness takes determination. Letting go of behavioral patterns is difficult. It is hard to do this alone; therefore relationships with those who are supportive and believe in us (e.g., support groups, professional therapists) are helpful. Massage professionals can be important in supporting clients making wellness changes. However, as health professionals, we also need commitment to self-care.

Salutogenesis: Movement Toward Health

Salutogenesis is a theory/model of how and why people stay healthy. In contrast, the pathogenic model is illness-focused. Both models are needed, and each complements the other. Salutogenesis focuses on discovering the elements of health and identifying healthy or salutary factors and behaviors. *Salutary* means favorable to the health of the mind or body (Mittelmark and Bauer, 2017; Mittelmark et al., 2022). Pathogenesis focuses on understanding the causes of disease and identifying disease risk factors. Both support health and quality of life but from different perspectives (García-Moya and Morgan, 2016).

Aaron Antonovsky introduced salutogenesis as a model of health creation in his 1979 book, *Health, Stress and Coping*. An important aspect of salutogenesis is having a sense of coherence (SOC). SOC is built on optimism with the ability to realistically assess life situations and find and use resources to solve problems and adapt to life circumstances. According to Antonovsky, there is a mindset that works behind the phenomenon of salutogenesis (Manohar, 2016):

1. I can comprehend: a belief that things happen in an orderly and predictable fashion and a sense that you can understand events in your life and reasonably predict what will happen in the future.
2. I can manage: a belief that you have the skills or ability, the support, the help, or the resources necessary to take care of things, and that things are manageable and within your control.
3. There is meaning: a belief that things in life are interesting and a source of satisfaction, that things are really worthwhile, and that there is good reason or purpose to care about what happens.

A sense of coherence is a learning process and can be developed by assessing and understanding experiences from the past to move in a health-promoting direction. A strong sense of coherence helps us find and use resources to cope with stressors and manage tension successfully. We become resilient. Resilience is essential to well-being. Resilient people develop specific characteristics:

- Emotionally perceptive: understanding what they're feeling and why as well as what others are feeling and why; sometimes called emotional intelligence.

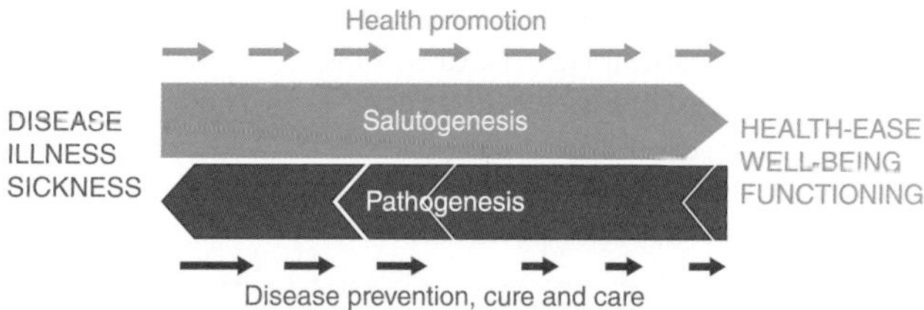

FIG. 15.1 Movement toward wellness.

- Intuitive: trusting instinctive collections of subconscious experiences and the gut feeling of non-conscious thinking.
- Perseverance: not giving up and learning from mistakes.
- Internal locus of control: finding meaning in life's challenges and believing that they are in control of their own lives rather than seeing themselves as victims.
- Optimistic: seeing the positives in most situations while being solution-oriented.
- Sense of humor: being able to laugh at life's difficulties and at themselves.
- Spirituality: being internally connected to faith and hope.

Developing a sense of coherence and focusing on the concept of salutogenesis is a process. By understanding that stressors and tension are normal, and seeing demands or expectations as appropriate challenges, we are better able to cope (Langeland et al., 2022). We are all somewhere between total wellness and total illness (Fig. 15.1).

Stress

Stress is our response to any demand on the body or mind to respond, adapt, or alter. It is a state of readiness to survive, one that requires hypervigilance by the body and mind. A person's emotional reaction to stress may be the difference between positive action and destructive breakdown, especially if many of the stressors seem beyond control (Chaitow, 1991; Williams et al., 2021; Selye, 1978).

The ancient Greek philosophers clearly recognized that regarding human conduct, the most important but perhaps also most difficult thing was "to know thyself." It takes great courage to attempt this honestly. Yet it is well worth the effort and humiliation because most of our tensions and frustrations stem from compulsive needs to act the role of someone we are not.

Before any wellness program can be developed, a person needs to at least "explore thyself." The next step is to analyze and explore the stressors that we all encounter in our daily lives. There are four major elements of stress:

- The stressor itself
- Coping strategies
- Defensive measures
- Mechanisms for surrender

Recall from Chapters 5 and 6 that **stressors** are any internal perceptions or external stimuli that demand a change in the body. Certain cognitive (thinking) and behavioral (doing) patterns are used to manage stressful situations and are known as *coping strategies*. Resourceful adaptive coping strategies include the following:

- Problem solving to eliminate the source of stress by altering the situation
- Cognitive restructuring (changing beliefs) to manage stressful situations by altering the meaning or reframing the event
- Social support to help manage stress by seeking and accepting help from others
- Expressing emotions constructively to those involved in the stress event or to a supportive listener
- Using massage therapy, meditation, yoga, and/or exercise as effective short-term strategies in which the person does not have to directly engage with the stressful event

Maladaptive coping has the potential to increase psychological distress, anxiety, and physiological symptoms such as chronic fatigue and pain, headache, and digestive and cardiovascular symptoms. Maladaptive coping involves the following:

- Ongoing problem avoidance
- Wishful thinking that draws attention away from the stressor
- Social withdrawal and avoidance of others
- Self-criticism
- Blaming or criticizing others
- Substance abuse

Generally, the higher one's perception of stress in their life the more likely it is that they will use unhealthy maladaptive coping strategies (Enns et al., 2018; Gupta et al., 2018; Slimmen et al., 2022).

Defensive measures are the ways our bodies defend against the stressor, such as the production of antibodies and white blood cells or behavioral and emotional defenses. However, sometimes defending is not the best way to deal with stress. It is important and resourceful to know when to quit or **surrender**. When we surrender, we give up the belief that we can make reality different than what it is. Surrender is the willingness to meet life as it is, to stop fighting with or trying to change the situation (Lasota and Mróz, 2021).

Hormonal and nervous stimuli encourage the body to retreat and ignore stressors. On an emotional level, this is sometimes called **denial**, which can be an important short-term method of coping with stress (Selye, 1978). Sometimes called avoidant coping, ignoring the stress-producing issue or event can provide relief.

Mental excitement and physical stressors cause an initial exhilaration followed by a secondary phase of depression. Certain chemical compounds, such as the hormones produced during the acute alarm reaction phase of the general adaptation syndrome (see Chapters 5 and 6), are able first to key up the body for action and then to cause depression (Box 15.2). Both effects may have protective value for the body. It is necessary to be "keyed up" for peak accomplishment, but it is equally important to relax and restore in the secondary phase of depression. This prevents us from carrying on too long at top speed. As Selye (1978) wrote:

> The fact is that a person can be intoxicated with their own stress hormones. I venture to say that this sort of drunkenness has caused much more harm to society than the alcoholic kind. We are on our guard against external intoxicants, but hormones are parts of our bodies; it takes more wisdom to recognize and overcome the foe that fights from within. In all

Box 15.2 Common Stress Responses

- General irritability, hyperexcitation, or depression
- Pounding heart
- Dry throat and mouth
- Impulsive behavior and emotional instability
- Overpowering urge to cry, run, or hide
- Inability to concentrate
- Weakness or dizziness
- Fatigue
- Tension and extreme alertness
- Trembling and nervous tics
- Intermittent anxiety
- Tendency to be easily startled
- High-pitched, nervous laughter
- Stuttering and other speech difficulties
- Grinding the teeth
- Insomnia
- Inability to sit still or physically relax
- Sweating
- Frequent need to urinate
- Diarrhea, indigestion, queasiness, and vomiting
- Migraine and other tension headaches
- Premenstrual tension or missed menstrual cycles
- Pain in the neck or lower back
- Loss of appetite or excessive appetite
- Increased use of chemicals, including tobacco, caffeine, and alcohol
- Nightmares
- Neurotic behavior
- Psychosis
- Proneness to accidents

These signs of stress are produced by fluctuations in the autonomic nervous system and resulting shifts in endogenous chemicals.

our actions throughout the day, we must consciously look for signs of being too keyed up, and we must learn to stop in time. Watching our critical stress level is just as important as watching our critical quota of cocktails and even more so. Intoxication by stress is sometimes unavoidable and usually insidious. You can quit alcohol, and even if you do take some, at least you can count the glasses; but it is impossible to avoid stress as long as you live, and your conscious thoughts often cannot gauge its alarm signals accurately. Curiously, the pituitary is a much better judge of stress than the intellect. Yet you can learn to recognize the danger signals fairly well if you know what to look for.

Stress Management

Stress has many causes, and many methods of stress management can be used. In general, if proportionately too much stress occurs in any physical or emotional area of the body, the energy needs to be diverted to a different area. If a person is thinking too much, then they should use the larger muscles of the body (e.g., work in the garden, take a brisk walk, exercise). If too much physical activity is causing stress, balance can be restored by reading a novel, watching a movie, or listening to soft music. If too much stress occurs in the body, rest is required.

Life Demands

Today many of the demands placed on us are outside the design of the body's coping ability: too much information, too much to know, too much to do, too much stuff, too much debt, too many responsibilities, and too many places to be. Our lives have become hurried, marked by a constant battle for time. We have too many options and too many choices, and it all costs too much.

Wellness often revolves around the simplification of a person's lifestyle. Simplification requires choices, boundaries, discipline, and "letting go" in many dimensions. For example, to simplify life it may be necessary to let go of a few volunteer activities and concentrate on only one or two that are especially meaningful. It may mean letting go of many acquaintances and instead cultivating a few supportive friends. Simplification may mean letting go of belief systems (e.g., family gatherings tend to be complex affairs) and cultivating easy relationships without fuss. Letting go may involve a sense of relief but also a feeling of loss that must be resolved.

Loss and Grief

Sometimes an event in life removes some part of us. It could be a body part, a body function, a relationship, a member of our family, or a job. Loss heals through grieving. Grief is a physiological response that includes stimulation of the sympathetic autonomic nervous system. The emotional response is alarm first, then disbelief and denial, progressing to anger and guilt. This process continues toward finding a source of comfort and finally adjusting to the loss. To heal, we need to reconstruct that part or learn to live resourcefully without it. We also need to give ourselves the time we need to work through the process of grieving.

Intuition: Recognizing When Wellness Is Off Balance

Many of us have been sick, or at the very least vertically ill. It may take extraordinary effort to reverse these situations. That is when we realize maybe we should have taken better care of ourselves in the first place. This realization does not always come at once, however. We all have that "voice in the back of our head" and that feeling when something "just isn't right." Learning to recognize our intuition and pay attention to it is a key component of maintaining wellness in our lives.

A balance exists between intuition and scientific research in wellness (i.e., what science knows and what we know we need). In developing a wellness program, it is important to consider these two important sources of information. Science and intuition are both needed to maintain wellness.

Seeking Help

Professional Help

Wellness training requires an extensive amount of information about diet, exercise, lifestyle, and behavior patterns. It is important to consult those with experience to obtain

PROFICIENCY EXERCISE 15.1

Identify something in your life that is interfering with your self-concept. For example, do you have an acquaintance who makes you feel inferior, or are you ashamed of a habit such as nail biting? Often the identification is the beginning of the process of change.

that information. Do not depend on only one information source. For each topic, talk with experts and read as many books or high-quality websites as possible (e.g., MedlinePlus or the website of the Centers for Disease Control and Prevention [CDC]) before making decisions about what could be done to benefit or improve your wellness. Remember, only a few symptoms combine to create a huge array of illness and disease patterns. Fortunately, a combination of only a few lifestyle changes is required to redirect a disease pattern toward a more resourceful and healing pattern (Proficiency Exercise 15.1).

Many professionals can help us with specific therapeutic interventions as the wellness program is developed. Physicians, counselors, other health and medical care providers, educators, and religious and spiritual advisors all play an important part in helping us become well again or maintaining our wellness. Ultimately, each of us must do the work and take responsibility for our lives, but it is important to use the help that is available. For example, if someone wants to increase wellness with exercise, a certified personal trainer might be helpful. Other examples include seeking education to better manage finances, becoming involved in a support group for addictive behaviors, and obtaining guidance from a spiritual advisor to walk a path of faith.

Supportive Relationships

Our sense of self in relation to others is also important. If this connection with others is not respected and nurtured, the wholeness of our lives is strained. This strain may interfere with our spiritual, emotional, and physical health.

When we have developed a healthy relationship with ourselves, we can also develop and sustain healthy relationships with others. Supportive relationships are important to wellness. If a relationship continues to generate stress in your life, maybe it is not a resourceful relationship. This does not mean that effort and concern are not required for family and friends or even global concern for a population. What is important is that we are empowered in a relationship and free to give and receive with a balance of energy exchanged. Sometimes one gives more and other times one receives more, but the total outcome is mutual support for one another's highest good that supports wellness and maximizes the quality of life for all. Review the quality-of-life domains presented in Chapter 4.

THE BODY: NUTRITION

SECTION OBJECTIVES

Chapter objective covered in this section:

2. Describe the importance of diet to a wellness lifestyle and plan a healthy diet.

Using the information presented in this section, the student will be able to perform the following:

- Describe the main food groups.
- Identify nutrition that supports wellness by planning a healthy diet.
- Explain the importance of proper hydration in the diet.
- List the components of an antiinflammatory diet.
- Explain how nutritional supplements and herbs influence wellness.

Our bodies are our dwelling places in this life. They are the most concrete aspects of our being. The care of our bodies is an important part of any wellness program.

According to the National Cancer Institute, poor nutrition is the reason three out of four people develop a disease or illness. Given these statistics, good nutrition means more than just choosing certain foods; it is about wanting to live a life without the complications of disease and illness. Therefore people need to educate themselves about proper nutrition.

Proper nutrition is easy to explain. However, because of our fast-paced lifestyle and influences including advertising, people do not always follow healthy nutritional recommendations. This is because nutrition involves more than just eating. Eating affects the mood, mood influences feelings, and behavior supports feelings. Food therefore becomes an emotional issue.

The Main Food Groups

Proteins

Proteins are the chief structural components of the body. Enzymes, some hormones, muscle tissue, and a substantial proportion of chromosomes are proteins. Proteins are essential components of the cell membrane. They break down into amino acids, which the body then absorbs and uses to meet its metabolic requirements, including growth and development. Important compounds such as epinephrine and acetylcholine are derived from amino acids. Dietary proteins include animal products and bean and grain combinations.

Carbohydrates

The term *carbohydrate* often means any food that is rich in either complex carbohydrates (starches, as found in grains such as brown rice) or simple carbohydrates (sugars, as found in candy, soda, and desserts). Carbohydrates (saccharides) are divided into four groups: monosaccharides, disaccharides, oligosaccharides, and polysaccharides. Monosaccharides and disaccharides are commonly referred to as sugars.

Carbohydrates perform many important jobs in the body, especially in storing and providing energy. Complex carbohydrates are long chains of glucose molecules, which are the main fuel for the manufacture of adenosine triphosphate in the cell. The liver converts sugars to glucose.

Fats

Fats, or lipids, are triglycerides that break down into fatty acids and glycerol. A fatty acid is a molecule consisting of a chain of carbons with no double bonds (saturated) or several double bonds (unsaturated). Unsaturated fats most closely resemble body fat and are more easily assimilated and used. Saturation (the addition of hydrogen molecules) makes fat a solid and less desirable in the diet. Linoleic acid is an example of a fatty acid that is essential to human nutrition. In addition to serving as a reservoir of stored energy, fats are essential components of many hormones, the cell membrane, and the myelin sheath of nerve fibers. Dietary fats are found in nuts, seeds, oils, and animal products.

Vitamins

Vitamins are growth factors needed in small amounts for daily body metabolism. They are classified as fat-soluble or water-soluble. Many vitamins function as enzyme activators (coenzymes). The fat-soluble vitamins are more likely to become toxic because excess amounts are stored in the fat tissue and are not excreted readily. Water-soluble vitamins are absorbed and excreted more easily, so there is less danger of overdosing.

Minerals

The body uses two kinds of minerals, macrominerals and trace minerals. It needs larger amounts of macrominerals than trace minerals. The macromineral group is made up of calcium, phosphorus, magnesium, sodium, potassium, chloride, and sulfur. The body needs just a tiny bit of each trace mineral. Trace minerals include iron, manganese, copper, iodine, zinc, cobalt, fluoride, and selenium.

Planning a Healthy Diet

The basics of balanced nutrition are explained in the Department of Agriculture's new guide to good eating. These newer recommendations have reconfigured the previous six-section MyPyramid guide into MyPlate (https://www.myplate.gov/) (Fig. 15.2). MyPlate supports a diet that is high in fruit, vegetables, whole grains, and low-fat milk and milk products, but that also includes lean meats, poultry, fish, beans, eggs, and nuts. Saturated and trans fats should be avoided, along with extra sodium and sugars.

MyPlate urges the public to make the most sensible choices from every food group, to find a healthy balance between food consumption and physical activity, and to understand the number of calories a food has and the effect this has on general calorie counts.

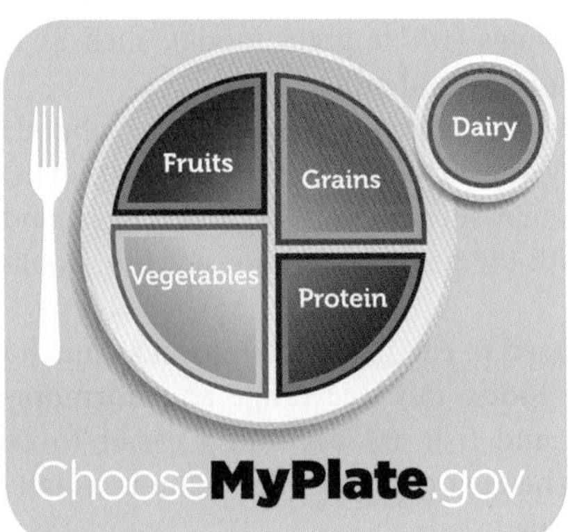

FIG. 15.2 MyPlate food guide symbol. MyPlate | US Department of Agriculture https://www.myplate.gov/.

Box 15.3 Functions of Water in the Human Body

- Provides a medium for chemical reactions
- Plays a crucial role in regulating chemical and bioelectric distributions within cells
- Transports substances such as hormones and nutrients
- Aids oxygen transport from the lungs to body cells
- Aids carbon dioxide transport from body cells to the lungs
- Dilutes toxic substances and waste products and transports them to the kidneys and liver
- Distributes heat around the body

From Fritz S: *Mosby's essential sciences for therapeutic massage: anatomy, physiology, biomechanics, and pathology.* 4th ed. 2013, Mosby.

Cycles of high and low blood sugar are produced by unbalanced diets, aggravated by improper spacing between meals, and promoted by substances such as coffee, alcohol, and soft drinks. These fluids stimulate the production of adrenaline, which forces the release of sugar into the bloodstream. The body then releases insulin to lower the sugar level again.

Adequate fiber and water in the diet promotes bladder and bowel habits that support wellness. Eating on a regular schedule is important to support body rhythms that in turn support wellness.

Hydration

Drinking appropriate amounts of clean plain water is important to a wellness program (Box 15.3). A healthy diet requires adequate hydration. The total amount required varies from person to person and depends on multiple factors, including the individual's physical condition, diet, age, activity level, and even where they live (Table 15.1).

Fruits and Vegetables

Fruits and vegetables reduce the risk of cardiovascular disease. Folic acid and potassium appear to contribute to this effect,

Table 15.1 Water Composition of Different Body Tissues

Tissue	Water Composition (%)
Blood	83.0
Kidneys	82.7
Heart	79.2
Lungs	79.0
Spleen	75.8
Muscle	75.6
Brain	74.8
Intestine	74.5
Skin	72.0
Liver	68.3
Skeleton	22.0
Adipose tissue	10.0

From Fritz S: *Mosby's essential sciences for therapeutic massage: anatomy, physiology, biomechanics, and pathology.* 3rd ed. Mosby.

which has been seen in several epidemiological studies. Inadequate consumption of folic acid also is responsible for a higher risk of serious birth defects, and a low intake of lutein (a pigment in green, leafy vegetables) has been associated with greater risks of cataracts and degeneration of the retina. Fruits and vegetables also are the primary source of many vitamins needed for good health; if these foods are eaten raw, the nutrients are not diminished, as occurs with cooking or processing. Only a few vegetables provide better nutrient absorption when cooked.

Red Meat

High consumption of red meat has been associated with an increased risk of coronary artery disease, probably because of meat's high saturated fat content. Excessive consumption of fatty red meat also increases the risk of type 2 diabetes and colon cancer, can aggravate the inflammatory response, and increases pain sensitivity. The elevated risk of colon cancer may be partly related to the carcinogens produced during cooking and the chemicals found in processed meats such as salami and bologna.

Poultry and Fish

Poultry and fish have less saturated fat and more unsaturated fat than red meat. Fish is also a rich source of essential omega-3 fatty acids. Eggs do not appear to increase the risk of heart disease (except among diabetics), probably because the effects of a slightly higher cholesterol level are counterbalanced by other nutritional benefits, especially with eggs from chickens fed special vegetarian diets to increase nutritional value.

Nuts and Healthy Fats

Many people avoid nuts because of their high fat content; however, the fat in nuts—including peanuts—is mainly unsaturated, and walnuts are a particularly good source of omega-3 fatty acids. Also, people who eat nuts are less likely to be obese. Perhaps because nuts are more satisfying, eating them seems to significantly reduce the intake of other foods (Proficiency Exercise 15.2).

PROFICIENCY EXERCISE 15.2

Keep a food diary for 2 days. If your diet is not well balanced, decide what it would take to achieve a well-balanced diet. Do you need to cut down on saturated fats or sugar? Do you eat the proper amount of vegetables, fruits, and grains? Are you drinking enough water?

Controlling Inflammation Through Diet

An important aspect of health maintenance is the management of inflammation; therefore eating a diet targeted to reduce inflammation is prudent. An antiinflammatory diet follows the recommendations just provided (Box 15.4). Foods especially high in antioxidants are also valuable.

Nutritional Supplements

Food sources of vitamins and minerals are compromised by depleted soil and artificial fertilizers and tainted by pesticides and other chemicals. The nutritional value of food also is compromised by long-term storage and preservation. Obtaining optimal nutritional value from the food we eat is difficult without extraordinary attention to our diet, which requires time, dedication, and discipline.

Box 15.4 Guidelines for an Antiinflammatory Diet

- Eat fruits, vegetables, whole grains, omega-3–containing eggs, fish, chicken, yogurt (unsweetened) with live cultures, extra virgin olive oil, and flaxseed oil.
- Avoid dairy (except yogurt, kefir, and some other fermented products), pork, beef, processed meat, refined grains and sugar, artificial food, and most fats and oils (especially hydrogenated oils).
- Some foods and herbs (e.g., ginger, turmeric, cumin, pineapple, and papaya) are especially valuable for controlling inflammation.

From Fritz S: *Sports and exercise massage: comprehensive care in fitness, athletics, and rehabilitation*, ed 2, St. Louis, 2013, Mosby.

People may use nutritional supplements to help achieve optimal nutrition. Experts disagree on the value of all vitamins but recommend a quality multivitamin. The US Food and Drug Administration (FDA) does not regulate the nutritional supplement industry, so caution should be exercised when choosing any nutritional supplement, including multivitamins. Choosing supplements verified by the US Pharmacopeia (USP) may help ensure safety. Herbs, which are powerful substances also not regulated by the FDA, should not be used as nutritional supplements or medicines without knowledge of their effects.

Physicians who have educated themselves on nutrition likely will order a nutrition panel for their patients with health concerns. Nutritional levels can be an indication of why the body is reacting in a certain manner.

Supplementation is a plausible answer to a lack of nutritional food. The only recommendation offered is that the closer a supplement is to "real food," the better the body is able to use it. Supplements usually are best taken with food to enhance absorption.

Key Points

- A healthy diet consists of appropriate portions of healthy fats, such as olive, grapeseed, and flaxseed oils, and healthy carbohydrates (whole grain foods), such as whole wheat bread, oatmeal, and brown rice.
- Vegetables and fruits should be eaten in abundance.
- A healthy diet includes moderate amounts of healthy sources of protein such as nuts, legumes, eggs, and fermented dairy, with the possible additions of fish, poultry, and lean meat.
- People need to eat clean, fresh food as much as possible. Organic foods and free-range and hormone-free meat, poultry, and fish are becoming easier to obtain. Even though the cost is higher, the value is usually worth the investment.
- A high-quality multiple vitamin that breaks down quickly in the digestive system is suggested for most people.

- A healthy diet minimizes the consumption of fatty red meat; refined grains, including white bread, white rice, and white pasta; and sugar. It eliminates foods made with trans fats, including fast food and most prepared food.

THE BODY: PHYSICAL FITNESS

SECTION OBJECTIVES

Chapter objective covered in this section:

3. Explain physical exercise as part of a wellness program.

Using the information presented in this section, the student will be able to perform the following:

- Describe the importance of exercise and flexibility.
- Explain aerobic exercise.
- Implement a self-care exercise program.
- Describe the physiological changes that occur with exercise.
- Explain the metabolic rate.
- Explain flexibility.
- Demonstrate safe stretching methods.

Fitness is a general term used to describe the ability to perform physical work. Performing physical work requires cardiorespiratory functioning, muscular strength and endurance, and musculoskeletal flexibility. To become physically fit, individuals must participate regularly in some form of physical activity that challenges all large muscle groups and the cardiorespiratory system and promotes postural balance.

Our bodies are designed for purposeful movement toward a goal, such as gathering food for the day or running for safety. The body still functions as though this were the reality, even though we do not need to work as hard to gather our food in the grocery store, and seldom do we have to run or fight for our lives. Providing a massage is a physical activity that can contribute to fitness. However, massage application also involves repetitive movement and does not challenge cardiovascular function enough to increase cardiovascular fitness. Moderate aerobic activity is needed on a regular basis.

Exercise and flexibility programs are important parts of any wellness program because they provide activities our body was designed for. Exercise is essential. However, fitness programs need to be appropriate; it is important to modify exercise systems and flexibility programs to fit the individual. Many resources are available for studying wellness-based movement programs.

Frequent 5-minute movement and breathing breaks should be built into everyone's day, especially those who spend prolonged periods in static positions. Such breaks may increase productivity, and people may feel less fatigue at the end of a busy day.

Any exercise and flexibility program must begin slowly. Activity levels can be increased gradually each week. It takes about 7–8 weeks for those new to these movements to reach a level of comfort. More activities may be added slowly once the body has adapted (Proficiency Exercise 15.3). However, too much of a good thing becomes a bad thing. Overexercise and aggressive programs can be detrimental instead of beneficial.

PROFICIENCY EXERCISE 15.3

Design a daily 15-minute relaxation program specifically for you.

Deconditioning

Deconditioning occurs with prolonged bed rest. Frequently seen in those recovering from extended illness, deconditioning is marked by a decrease in maximum oxygen consumption, cardiac output, and muscular strength, which occurs rapidly. These effects are also seen, although possibly to a lesser degree, in individuals who spend some time on bed rest without accompanying disease and individuals who are sedentary because of lifestyle or increasing age.

Aerobic Exercise Training

Aerobic exercise training is an exercise program that focuses on increasing fitness and endurance. A training response requires exercise of sufficient intensity, duration, and frequency to produce both cardiovascular and muscular adaptation in a person's endurance. This is different from training for a particular sport or event, by which the individual improves in specific exercise tasks but may not improve in other tasks or whole-body conditioning.

Adaptation

Adaptation increases the efficiency of body function and represents a variety of neurological, physical, and biochemical changes in the cardiovascular, neuromuscular, and myofascial systems. Performance increases because of these changes, and these systems adapt to the training stimulus over time. Significant changes in fitness can be measured in 10–12 weeks.

A person with a low level of fitness has more potential to improve than one who has a high level of fitness. This is reflected in the training stimulus threshold, or the stimulus that elicits a training response. Training stimulus thresholds vary, depending on the individual's health, level of activity, age, and sex. The higher the initial level of fitness, the greater the intensity of exercise needed to elicit a significant change.

Energy Expenditure

Energy is expended by individuals engaging in physical activity. Activities can be categorized as light or heavy by determining the energy cost. Most daily activities are light activities and are aerobic (oxygen-based) because they require little power but occur over prolonged periods. Heavy work usually requires energy supplied by both the aerobic and anaerobic systems (non–oxygen-based).

Conditioning

The rapid increase in energy requirements during exercise requires equally rapid circulatory adjustments. The adjustments are essential to meet the increased need for oxygen and nutrients; to remove the end products of metabolism, such as carbon dioxide and lactic acid; and to dissipate excess heat. The shift in body metabolism occurs through a coordinated activity of all the systems of the body: neuromuscular, respiratory, cardiovascular, metabolic, and hormonal.

Effective endurance training must produce a conditioning or cardiovascular response. Conditioning depends on three critical elements of exercise: intensity, duration, and frequency.

Intensity

The intensity of exercise is based on the **overload principle**; that is, to achieve improvement, stress on an organism must be greater than the one regularly encountered during everyday life. To improve cardiovascular and muscular endurance, an overload must be applied to these systems.

The exercise intensity load must be just above the training stimulus threshold for adaptation to occur. Once adaptation to a given load has occurred, the training intensity (exercise load) must be increased for the individual to achieve further improvement. Increasing intensity too quickly can result in injury.

Duration

The optimal duration of exercise for cardiovascular conditioning depends on the total work done, the intensity and frequency of the exercise, and the person's fitness level. The greater the intensity of the exercise, the shorter the duration needed for adaptation. The lower the intensity of the exercise, the longer the duration needed. A 20- to 30-minute session at 70% of the maximum heart rate is generally optimal. The maximum heart rate can be determined in a number of ways. For example, it can be estimated by subtracting a person's age from 220 (this is only an approximate guide). For most individuals, the maximum heart rate declines with age, and values usually are 100–170 beats per minute.

When the intensity is below the heart rate threshold, a 45-minute continuous exercise period may provide the appropriate overload. With high-intensity exercise, 10- to 15-minute exercise periods are adequate. Three 5-minute daily periods may be effective in someone who is deconditioned. Exercising for longer than 45–60 minutes increases the risk of musculoskeletal injury and soreness, and the risk does not justify the benefit.

Frequency

The optimal frequency for fitness training generally is three to four times a week. Frequency varies, depending on the person's health and age. If training is done at low intensity, greater frequency may be beneficial. A frequency of two times a week does not generally evoke cardiovascular changes, although individuals who are deconditioned initially may benefit from a program of that frequency. As frequency increases beyond the optimal range, the risk of musculoskeletal injury and soreness increases. The World Health Organization and the American Health Association recommend that adults aged 18–64 should do at least 150 minutes of moderate-intensity aerobic physical activity throughout the week or do at least 75 minutes of vigorous-intensity aerobic physical activity throughout the week or an equivalent combination of moderate- and vigorous-intensity activity. Aerobic activity should be performed in bouts of at least 10 minutes in duration. Muscle-strengthening activities should be done involving major muscle groups on 2 or more days a week. Thirty minutes a day, five times a week is an easy goal to remember. Benefits can be experienced with two or three segments of 10–15 minutes. Physical activity includes leisure- and work-related physical activity as well as a formal exercise program.

Maintaining Fitness

The frequency or duration of physical activity required to maintain a certain level of aerobic fitness is less than that required to improve it. The beneficial effects of exercise training are reversible. The process of deconditioning occurs rapidly when a person stops exercising. After only 2 weeks of reduced activity, significant reductions in work capacity can be measured, and improvements can be lost within several months.

The Exercise Program

Because the components of an exercise program can be accomplished in many ways, a person can engage in many activities that support health. One day you might walk for about an hour, and the next day you might strengthen the core muscles with activities on exercise balls or a movement program, such as tai chi. Yoga supports flexibility. Climbing stairs is a great exercise.

An appropriate exercise program can result in higher levels of fitness for a healthy individual, slow the decrease in the functional capacity of elder adults, and recondition those who have been ill or who have chronic disease or a sedentary lifestyle. The three components of an exercise program are (1) the warm-up, (2) aerobic exercise, and (3) the cool-down.

The Warm-Up

The purpose of the warm-up period is to enhance the numerous physiological adjustments that must take place before physical activity. Physiologically, a time lag exists between the onset of activity and the adjustments the body must make to meet the physical requirements.

A warm-up raises the muscle temperature. The higher temperature increases the efficiency of muscular contraction by reducing connective tissue viscosity and increasing the rate of nerve conduction. More oxygen is extracted from hemoglobin at higher muscle temperatures, which supports the aerobic process. Dilation of constricted capillaries, resulting in increased circulation, increases oxygen delivery to the active muscles and minimizes oxygen deficit and the formation of lactic acid. The venous return also increases. Adaptation in the sensitivity of the neural respiratory center increases the respiratory rate.

Warm-up activities include rhythmic movement of the large muscles of the body. An increasingly brisk walk is an excellent warm-up activity.

Aerobic Exercise

The aerobic exercise period is the conditioning part of the exercise program. Attention to the intensity, frequency, and duration determines the effectiveness of the program. In choosing a specific method of training, the exerciser's main consideration is intensity; it should do the following:

- Be sufficient to stimulate increased cardiac output
- Enhance local circulation
- Increase aerobic metabolism within the appropriate muscle groups
- Not cause injury
- Be weight-bearing to support bone health
- Exceed the threshold level to allow adaptation
- Not evoke fatigue symptoms

In aerobic exercise, a submaximal, rhythmic, repetitive, and dynamic exercise of large muscle groups is emphasized. The four types of training that condition the aerobic system are continuous, interval, circuit, and circuit-interval methods.

Continuous Training

Continuous training involves a submaximal energy requirement sustained throughout the exercise period. Once the steady state is achieved, the muscle obtains energy by means of aerobic metabolism. Stress is placed primarily on the slow-twitch muscle fibers. The activity can be prolonged for 20–60 minutes without exhausting the oxygen transport system. The work rate is increased progressively as training improvements are achieved; overload can be accomplished by increasing the exercise duration. In a healthy individual, continuous training is the most effective way to improve endurance. Brisk walking and swimming laps are excellent examples of continuous training.

Interval Training

In interval training, the exercise period is interspersed with relief or rest intervals. Interval training is generally less demanding than continuous training. In a healthy individual, interval training tends to improve strength and power more than endurance. The relief interval is either a rest relief (passive recovery) or a work relief (active recovery), and it ranges in duration from a few seconds to several minutes. Work recovery involves continuing the exercise but at a reduced level from the work period. During the relief period, the aerobic system replenishes a portion of the oxygen associated with myoglobin and the muscular stores of adenosine triphosphate (ATP, the energy source for muscle), both of which were depleted during the work period.

The longer and more intense the work interval, the more the aerobic system is stressed. With a short work interval, the duration of the rest interval is critical if the aerobic system is to be stressed. A rest interval equal to 1.5 times the work interval allows the succeeding exercise interval to begin before recovery is complete and stresses the aerobic system. An example would be a 5-minute work interval followed by a 7-minute rest interval.

A significant amount of high-intensity exercise can be achieved with interval or intermittent work if the work-relief intervals are spaced appropriately. Examples include lap swimming with rest periods or sprinting followed by periods of walking.

Circuit Training

Circuit training uses a series of exercise activities. At the end of the last activity, the individual starts from the beginning and again moves through the circuit. The series of activities is repeated several times. Several exercise modes can be used involving large and small muscle groups and a mix of static or dynamic effort. The use of circuit training can improve strength and endurance by stressing both the aerobic and anaerobic systems. Often a combination of aerobic activities and weight training is included in the exercise program. Core training that strengthens the postural muscles of the torso can be included in circuit training. Activities using assorted sizes of exercise balls promote postural balance and core strength.

Circuit-Interval Training

A combination of circuit and interval training is effective because of the interaction of aerobic and anaerobic production of ATP. In addition to the aerobic and anaerobic systems being stressed by the various activities, the relief interval allows a delay in the need for anaerobic processes and the production of lactic acid because the rest period allows blood oxygen levels to replenish.

The Cool-Down

A cool-down period is necessary after the aerobic exercise period. The cool-down period prevents pooling of the blood in the extremities because the exerciser continues to use the muscles to maintain venous return. The cool-down enhances the recovery period through the oxidation of metabolic waste and replacement of the energy stores, and prevents myocardial ischemia, arrhythmias, and other cardiovascular conditions.

The characteristics of the cool-down period are like those of the warm-up period. Total body exercises, such as calisthenics or brisk walking, which decrease in intensity are appropriate. The cool-down period should last 5–10 minutes and be followed by a flexibility regimen.

Physiological Changes That Occur With Exercise

Changes in the cardiovascular and respiratory systems and in muscle metabolism occur with endurance training. These changes happen at rest and with exercise. It is important to note that all the following training effects cannot result from one training program. A regular regimen of exercise with a variety of activities is necessary to achieve and maintain fitness.

Cardiovascular Changes

Changes at rest involve a reduction in the resting pulse rate with a decrease in sympathetic dominance and lower levels of norepinephrine and epinephrine. Parasympathetic restoration mechanisms increase and a decrease in blood pressure can occur. Blood volume and hemoglobin often increase; this facilitates the oxygen delivery capacity of the system.

Changes during exercise include an increase in the pulse rate and a decrease in norepinephrine and epinephrine. Cardiac function increases, as does the extraction of oxygen by the working muscle.

Respiratory Changes

Changes at rest include larger lung volumes because of improved pulmonary function. Changes during exercise occur as a result of a larger diffusion capacity in the lungs because of the larger lung volumes and a greater alveolar-capillary surface area. Breathing is deeper and more efficient.

Metabolic Changes

Muscle hypertrophy and increased capillary density are observed at rest and during exercise after endurance training. Also, the number and size of mitochondria increase significantly, thereby increasing the capacity to aerobically generate ATP. The rate of depletion of muscle glycogen decreases, and blood lactate levels during submaximal work are lower because of an increased capacity to mobilize and oxidize fat, in addition to an increase in fat-mobilizing and metabolizing enzymes (Box 15.5).

Other System Changes

Changes in other systems that occur with exercise training include decreased levels of body fat, blood cholesterol, and triglyceride levels, as well as increased levels of heat acclimatization and the breaking strength of bones, ligaments, and tendons.

Flexibility

Flexibility is the ability to move a single joint or series of joints through a normal, unrestricted, pain-free range of motion. Flexibility depends on the extensibility of muscle tissue, which allows muscles that cross a joint to relax, lengthen, and yield to an elongation action. The arthrokinematics of the moving joint and the ability of connective tissues associated with the joint to deform also affect the joint range of motion and an individual's overall flexibility.

Dynamic flexibility refers to the active range of motion of a joint. This aspect of flexibility depends on the degree to which a joint can be moved by a muscle contraction and the amount of tissue resistance met during the active movement.

Passive flexibility, the degree to which a joint can be passively moved through the available range of motion, depends on the extensibility of muscles and connective tissues that cross and surround a joint. Passive flexibility is a prerequisite for but does not ensure dynamic flexibility.

Stretching is a general term used to describe any therapeutic technique designed to increase flexibility. Stretching methods should not increase joint flexibility beyond the normal range of motion. Passive stretching involves an external force, applied either manually or mechanically, that lengthens the shortened tissues while the person is relaxed. Active inhibition uses various muscle energy methods in which the person participates in the stretching maneuver. The result is an increased tolerance to the sensation of stretch. Although it appears that stretching directly affects the soft tissue, most of the increase in motion is modulated through the nervous system.

Stretching methods should increase pliability and slide of fascia and not stretch ligaments unless some sort of contracture exists. Stretching should increase efficient mobility but not create instability or strain the joint. Increased tissue temperature increases fascial pliability and can make stretching more effective.

Many types of flexibility programs are available. It is important that a flexibility program is gentle. Too much flexibility can create hypermobility and joint instability. Maintain movements within normal joint range. Massage is an excellent way to support flexibility programs, especially if the methods used address both the elasticity and pliability of the soft tissue. When the body gets the movement it needs, relaxation activities are more effective (Fig. 15.3).

Box 15.5 Metabolic Rate

The metabolic rate is the rate of energy release. The basal metabolic rate (BMR) is not the minimum metabolic rate and does not indicate the smallest amount of energy that must be expended to sustain life. The BMR is the smallest energy expenditure that can sustain life and maintain the waking state and a normal body temperature in a comfortably warm environment. It is the rate of energy expenditure under basal conditions; that is, when the individual (1) is awake but lying down and not moving, (2) is in a comfortably warm environment, and (3) has not eaten a meal in 18–23 hours.

The BMR is not the same for all individuals because of the following factors:

- *Size:* The BMR is calculated from an individual's height and weight. A large individual has more surface area (and a higher BMR) than a small individual.
- *Sex:* Males oxidize food approximately 5%–7% faster than females. Therefore even if a male and a female are the same size, the male has a higher BMR. This sex difference probably results from the difference in the proportion of body fat determined by sex hormones. Females tend to have a higher percentage of body fat (and thus a lower total lean mass) than males. Fat tissue is less metabolically active than lean tissue, such as muscle.
- *Age:* The younger the individual, the higher the BMR for a given size and sex.
- *Thyroid hormones:* Thyroid hormones (triiodothyronine [T3] and thyroxine [T4]) stimulate the basal metabolism. Without a normal amount of these hormones in the blood, the body cannot maintain a normal BMR.
- *Body temperature:* An increase in body temperature increases the BMR. A decrease in body temperature (hypothermia) has the opposite effect.
- *Drugs:* Stimulants increase the BMR and depressants reduce the BMR.
- *Other factors:* Other factors such as emotions, pregnancy, and lactation (milk production) also influence basal metabolism.

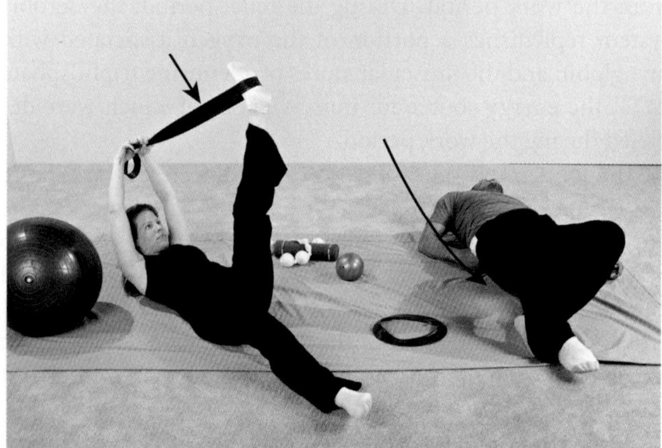

FIG. 15.3 Examples of flexibility self-care.

THE BODY: RELAXATION

SECTION OBJECTIVES

Chapter objective covered in this section:

4. Identify and define relaxation and restorative activities.

Using the information presented in this section, the student will be able to perform the following:

- Describe the relationship of relaxation to the autonomic nervous system.
- Define mindfulness.
- Describe the relationship of breathing to wellness.
- Explain the phases of breathing.
- Demonstrate relaxed breathing.
- Perform and teach basic breathing exercises.
- Explain the importance of restorative sleep to wellness.

Relaxation methods initiate a parasympathetic response. Because muscle tension patterns are habitual, most successful relaxation methods combine movement, stretching, and tensing and releasing of muscles (progressive relaxation). Heart and breathing rates synchronize while an individual focuses on quiet or neutral topics, events, or pictures (visualization). Slow, rhythmic music can benefit a relaxation program. Most meditation and deliberate relaxation processes are built around this pattern.

The focus of relaxation is to quiet the physical body, not necessarily to create a spiritual experience; however, many prayer systems use similar patterns, which also are beneficial for relaxation.

Almost any type of pleasurable, simple, repetitive activity that requires focused attention induces a relaxation response. Gardening, needlepoint, knitting, playing music, and watching fish in an aquarium or birds at a bird feeder are all forms of relaxation if there is no need to achieve, compete, or produce results in a specific period. Knitting a sweater for pleasure and having to finish one in a week are two different activities. Relaxation takes time, and when something is urgent, it usually interferes with the ability to relax.

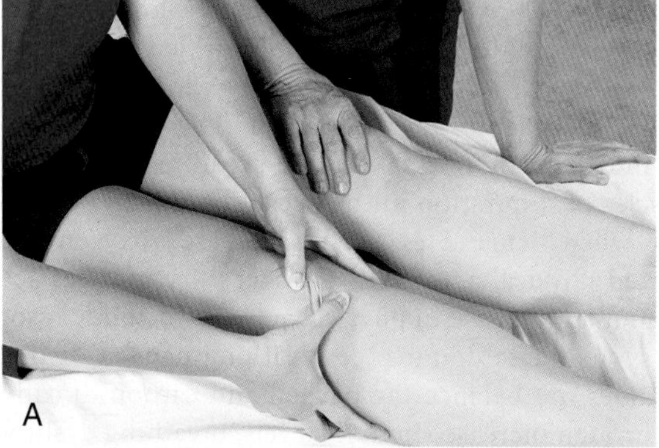

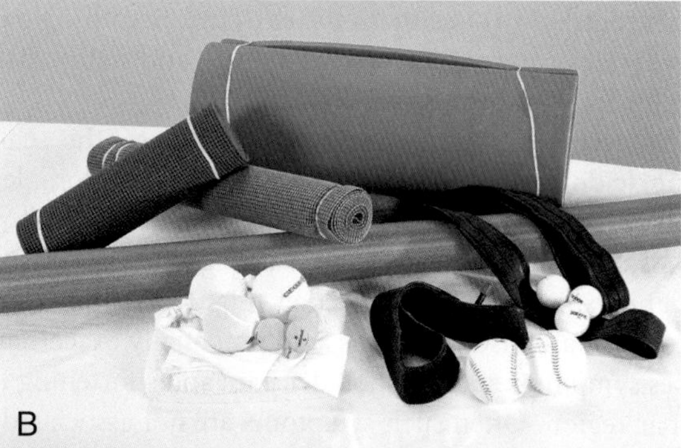

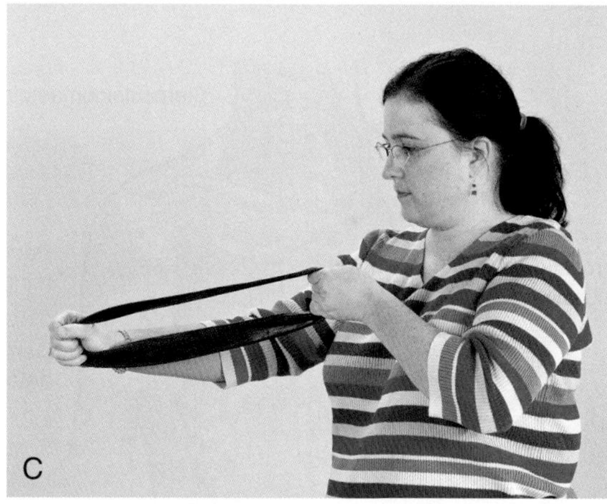

FIG. 15.4 Self-massage. A, Teaching self-massage to a client. **B,** Products for use in self-massage. **C,** Self-applied muscle energy technique using a resistance band.

Mindfulness

Mindfulness is a concept of relaxation. Mindfulness is being attentive to the moment, secure that we have learned from and let go of the past, and that we are planning for the future without worry.

Just as tension patterns are habitual, relaxation can become a habit. Typically, it takes 8–10 weeks of consistent reinforcement to build a habit pattern.

Unlike exercise, which can be varied to prevent boredom, a relaxation sequence needs to be the same each time to reinforce the conditioned response to the habit structure. It is important to use the same location, music, time of day, smells (e.g., essential oils), colors, position, and breathing pattern in the sequence. Any of the components of the relaxation program can soon become triggers to relaxation.

A person should experiment with relaxation methods until the right program is found and then consistently use it every day for at least 15 minutes (It takes this long for the physiology to make a shift from an aroused state to a relaxed one). Many audio programs provide progressive relaxation and self-hypnosis and pull together all the components of a relaxation program. Self-massage can also support relaxation (Fig. 15.4).

Breathing

Breathing provides us with essential air. Breathing patterns are a direct link to altering autonomic nervous system patterns, which in turn affect mood, feelings, and behavior. Almost every meditation or relaxation system uses breathing patterns. Other ways to modulate breathing are by singing and chanting.

Proper breathing is important, yet most of us do not breathe efficiently. For many, air quality is poor. Others may feel too hurried to breathe deeply. Slow, deep breathing takes time. Recall from Chapter 6 that the simple bellows breathing mechanism is a body-wide coordination of muscle contraction and relaxation. The shoulders should not move during normal relaxed breathing. The accessory muscles of respiration in the neck area should be activated only when demand exists for increased oxygen and increased physical activity. If the accessory muscles activate without an increase in physical activity, the body resorts to the sympathetic dominance breathing pattern. If the person does not balance the oxygen and carbon dioxide levels through increased activity levels, breathing dysfunction (hyperventilation) occurs in the extreme. Breathing pattern disorders can perpetuate anxiety states and many disturbing physical symptoms (see Box 15.5).

The accessory muscles of respiration (e.g., the scalenes, sternocleidomastoid, serratus posterior superior, levator scapulae, rhomboids, abdominals, and quadratus lumborum) may be constantly activated for breathing when forced inhalation and expiration are not needed (Fig. 15.5). This results in dysfunctional muscle patterns, and potentially exacerbates or causes symptoms such as shoulder pain and shortening in the lumbar region. Often such symptoms are not associated with

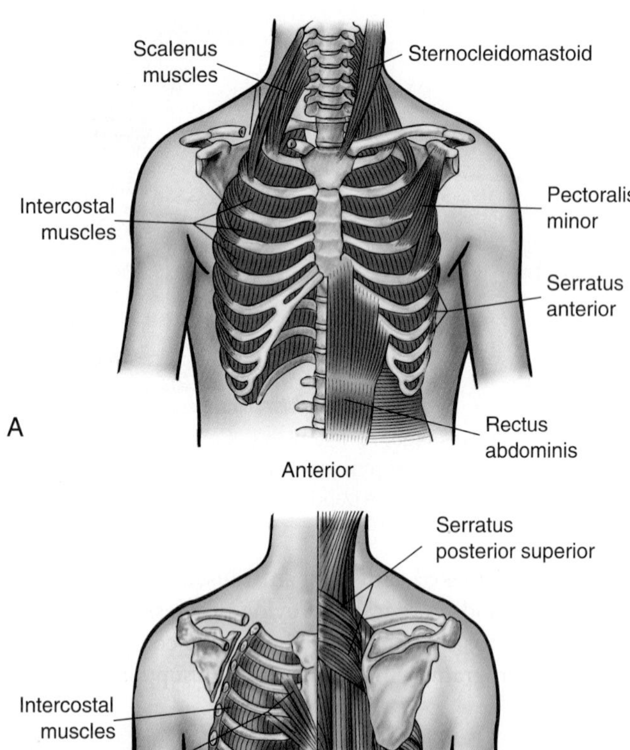

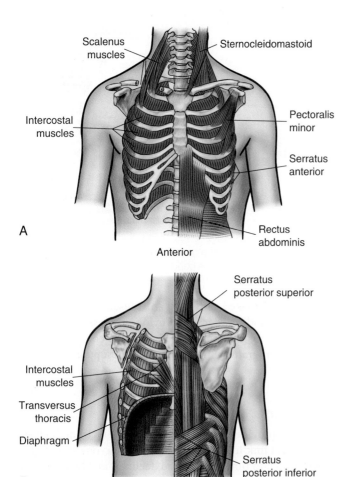

FIG. 15.5 Breathing muscles. Modified from Seidel HM, Ball JW, Dains JE, et al: *Mosby's guide to physical examination*, 5th ed. 2003, Mosby.

inefficient breathing. During assessment, the massage professional should stay alert to the secondary effects of breathing dysfunction.

Phases of Breathing

Breathing comprises three phases of inspiration (bringing air into the body) and two phases of expiration (moving air out of the body). **Quiet inspiration** takes place when an individual is resting or sitting quietly. The diaphragm and external intercostals are the prime movers. As **deep inspiration** occurs, the actions of quiet inspiration are intensified. When people need more oxygen, they breathe harder. Any muscles that can pull the ribs up are called into action. **Forced inspiration** occurs when an individual is working hard and needs a great deal of oxygen. Not only are the muscles of quiet and deep inspiration working, but also the muscles that stabilize or elevate the shoulder girdle to elevate the ribs directly or indirectly.

Quiet expiration is mostly a passive action. It occurs through relaxation of the external intercostals and the elastic recoil of the thoracic wall and tissue of the lungs and bronchi while gravity pulls the rib cage down from its elevated position. Essentially, no muscle action is involved. **Forced expiration** brings in muscles that can pull the ribs down and compress the abdomen, forcing the diaphragm upward.

Normal breathing consists of a shorter inhale in relation to a longer exhale. The ratio of inhale time to exhale time is one count inhale per two to four counts exhale. The ideal pattern is two to four counts for the inhale and at least eight counts for the exhale. The reverse of this pattern, in which the exhale is shorter and the inhale longer, is the basis for breathing pattern disorders. Bodywork and breathing retraining methods seek to restore normal breathing.

Massage to Support Breathing Function

Consider breathing mechanisms during assessment. One way to determine whether a client uses accessory muscles for relaxed breathing is to place your hands on the person's shoulders as they breathe; the shoulders should not move up and down (Fig. 15.6).

Another method to detect the use of accessory muscles is to observe the client. If the accessory muscles are used, movement is concentrated in the upper chest instead of the lower ribs and abdomen.

If the breathing pattern is dysfunctional, the accessory muscles show increased tension and a tendency to develop trigger points. These conditions can be identified through palpation. Also, connective tissue changes are common because breathing dysfunction is often chronic.

Therapeutic massage may normalize many of these conditions and support more effective breathing. Breathing well is difficult if the mechanical components are not working efficiently. Many who attempt breathing retraining become frustrated by their inability to accomplish the pattern. They may be more successful post-massage due to the normalized tone of accessory breathing muscles and/or effects related to parasympathetic dominance.

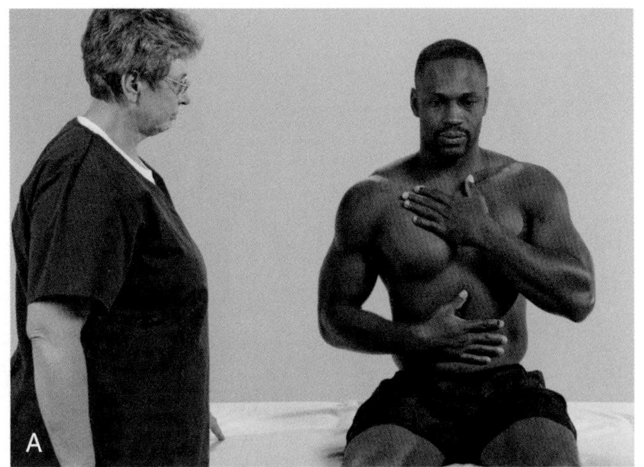

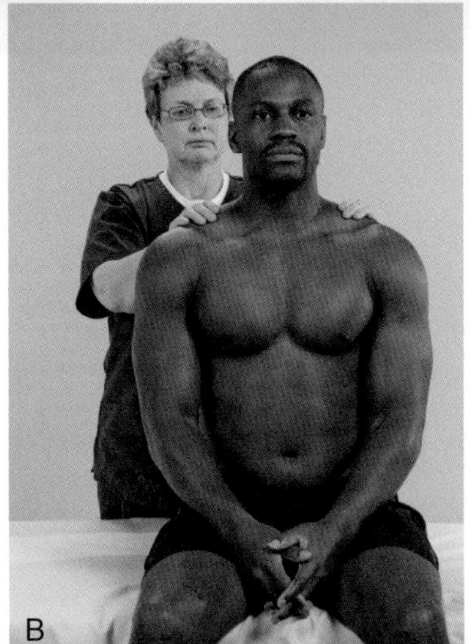

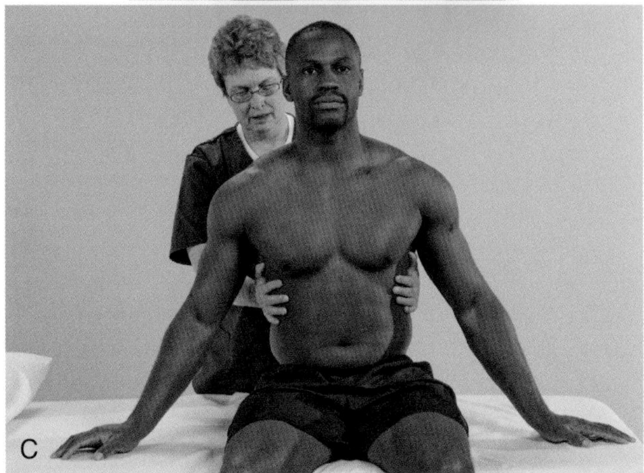

FIG. 15.6 Breathing assessment. A, Observe the client's breathing. **B,** Place your hands on the client's shoulders. They should not move up and down unless the client is using accessory muscles inappropriately during normal, relaxed breathing. **C,** Place your hands on the client's lower ribs. These areas should move if the client is breathing properly.

The breathing exercises presented in Box 15.6 can be taught to clients. Three common activities—yelling, crying, and laughing—can help normalize a breathing pattern because all three support an extended exhale. Each of these activities is sustained for 3–5 minutes and can be valuable in any breathing retraining program (Proficiency Exercise 15.4).

PROFICIENCY EXERCISE 15.4

1. This exercise helps you understand how normalizing breathing affects the entire body. Begin by doing a simple physical assessment: move yourself into forward trunk flexion, side-bending lateral trunk flexion, trunk extension, neck flexion, extension, and lateral flexion. Identify the areas of your body that seem most restricted. Now yell or howl as loud as you can for 1 minute. Next, pretend to cry and sob for 1 minute. Finally, belly laugh as hard and as long as you can. Now perform the simple physical assessment again. In the space provided, describe the results.
2. Develop a "how to breathe" handout to give to clients. Include at least three breathing patterns.

Sleep

Restorative sleep is necessary for wellness. Lack of quality sleep is becoming a major health concern. Many people do not get enough sleep. An absolute minimum of 6 hours of uninterrupted sleep is necessary, and most people require 8–9 hours.

During sleep, the body renews, repairs, and generally restores itself. Growth hormone is a key factor in this process, with more than half of its daily secretions taking place during sleep. If the deeper stages of sleep are not sustained, the body's restorative mechanisms are compromised. Sleep and dreaming are when we seem to repair, sort, and restore emotionally. Dreaming is still a mystery, but research indicates that it is essential for emotional well-being. Sleep disturbances are, in fact, a major factor in many chronic fatigue and pain syndromes.

Many things can interrupt sleep, such as pain that repeatedly awakens the person, external random noise (e.g., traffic noise), tending to infants and children, varied work schedules, a restless or snoring bed partner (including pets), sinus or other respiratory difficulties (e.g., coughing), and urinary frequency. Others have disrupted sleep patterns because of insomnia, sleep apnea, hormone fluctuations, high cortisol (stress hormone) levels, medications, and stimulant intake, such as caffeine. Regardless of the perpetuating factors, sleep is compromised, and the deep sleep stage is seldom achieved.

Light/dark cycles regulate sleep patterns. For effective sleep, we need adequate exposure to daylight, which stimulates serotonin. We also need adequate exposure to darkness. Absence of light supports the release of melatonin, a pineal gland hormone that is involved with the sleep pattern. With the advent of artificial lighting, we have spent less and less time in the dark, which disturbs sleep. Methods to support effective sleep are presented in Box 15.7 (Proficiency Exercise 15.5).

Box 15.6 Breathing Exercises

The following breathing exercises should be taught to clients in an instructional format that addresses the client's specific needs for better breathing.

Exercise 1 (Figures A and B)

1. Sit in a relaxed position.
2. Place your hands in your lap and interlace the fingers.
3. Firmly press your fingers and thumbs into the tops of your hands.
4. Hold this position as long as possible without discomfort as you breathe normally.

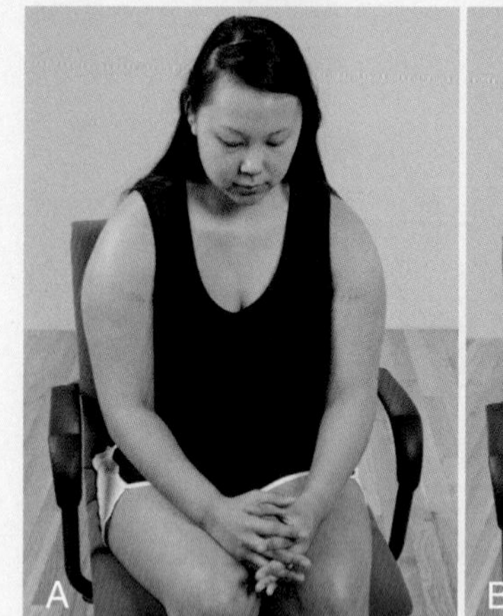

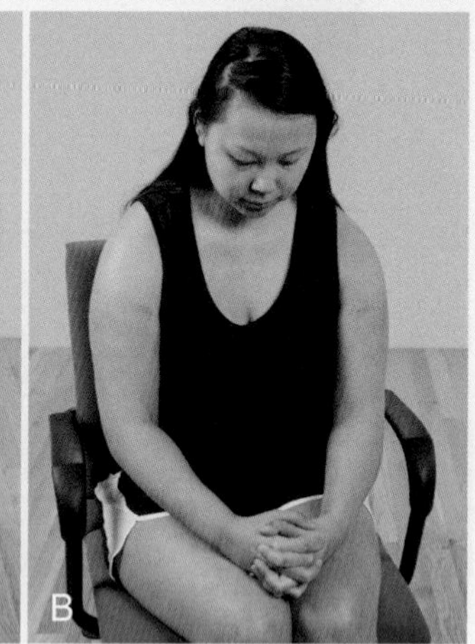

Exercise 2 (Figure C)

1. Place your hands behind your head.
2. Point your elbows up and back.
3. Hold this position as long as it is comfortable while breathing normally.

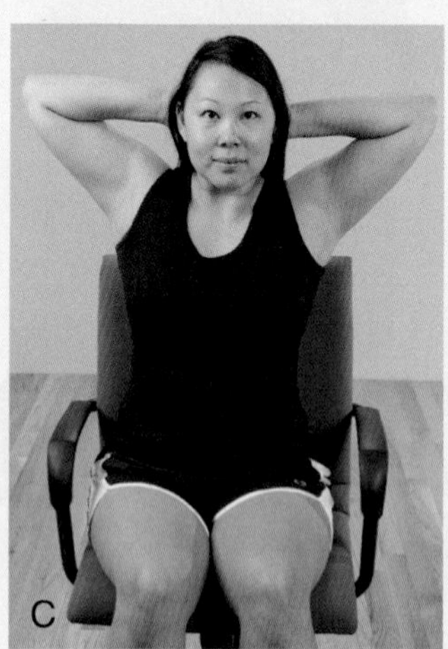

Exercise 3 (Figure D)

1. Interlace your fingers behind your back.
2. Pull your shoulder blades together.
3. Hold this position as long as possible while breathing normally.

These exercises inhibit the accessory breathing muscles. Essentially, in these positions the client cannot use the accessory muscles to breathe, and the intercostal muscles and diaphragm are supported in breathing function. Clients should do these exercises as often as possible throughout the day. They should try to accumulate 30 minutes of exercise per 24-hour period.

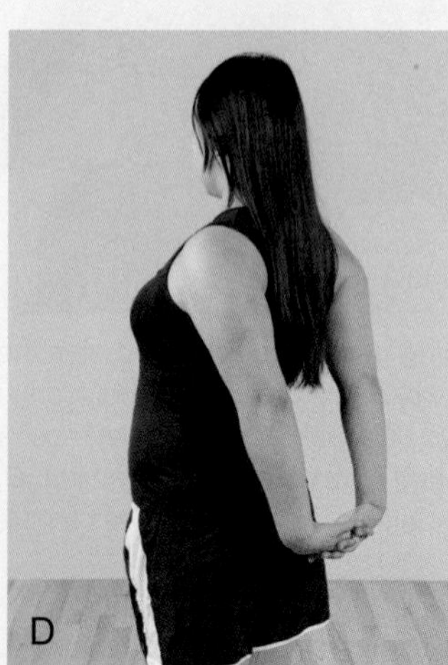

Box 15.6 Breathing Exercises—cont'd

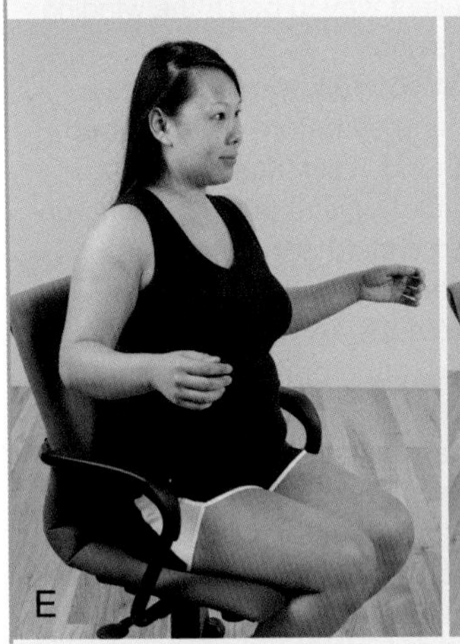

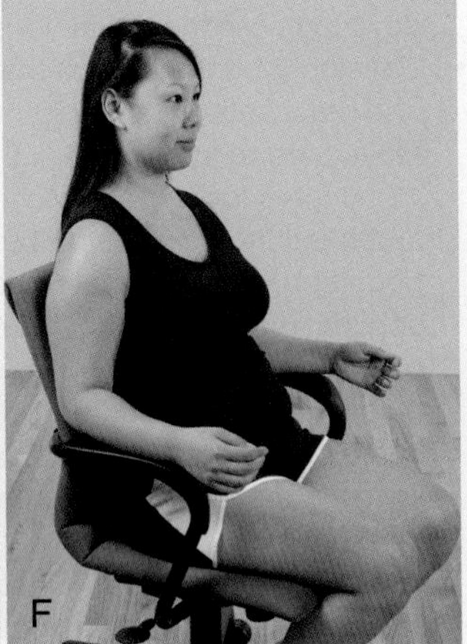

Exercise 4 (Figures E and F)

1. Sit in a relaxed, upright position in a chair with arms.
2. Place your arms on the arms of the chair.
3. Firmly press the parts of your forearms that are closest to the elbow into the arms of the chair.
4. Hold this position as long as it is comfortable and breathe normally.

Exercises for Controlled Breathing

1. Lift your chin into the air and relax your shoulders.
2. Slowly exhale through your mouth as if blowing out a candle; at the same time, pull in your abdomen. Then exhale until you have expelled as much air as possible without straining.
3. At the bottom of the breath (i.e., when no further air can be exhaled without strain), stop breathing. This is different from holding your breath, which requires effort. Remain in this resting phase for 3–5 seconds.
4. Before inhaling, relax all muscles, drop your chin to your chest, and keep your shoulders relaxed.
5. Inhale slowly through your nose until your lungs are comfortably full, allowing your abdomen to expand.
6. Stop breathing for 3–5 seconds. Then repeat the entire sequence, beginning with step 1.

The exhalation should take two to four times as long as the inhalation.

Many additional resources are available for retraining breathing patterns. Find one that is comfortable and use it regularly.

PROFICIENCY EXERCISE 15.5

In the space provided, analyze your personal sleep pattern using the information in this section. Identify three activities that support restorative sleep and three activities that can be improved.

My current sleep pattern is:

Three current activities that support sleep:

Three activities that could improve sleep:

THE MIND

SECTION OBJECTIVES

Chapter objective covered in this section:

5. Explain how the mind and body connection affects wellness.

Using the information presented in this section, the student will be able to perform the following:

- Define *mind.*
- Relate mind, emotions, feelings, and behavior as a pathway to stress or wellness.
- Define *emotions.*
- Explain how emotions relate to maladaptive learned behavior.
- Relate feelings to emotions.
- Describe how massage therapy interacts with the physiological feelings related to emotions.
- Explain addictive behavior.
- Describe a wellness expression of a full range of emotions.
- Define self-concept and self-worth.
- Define resourceful coping.

The mind is the part of us that is able to reason, understand, remember, think, and adapt. It coordinates the conscious and subconscious parts of us that influence and direct mental and physical behavior. The mind processes what we believe; it involves emotions and feelings, behavior, self-concept, and coping.

Although we can change our minds (beliefs) quickly, habitual belief patterns are difficult to overcome. Changes in beliefs need to be supported over time to be reflected in lifestyle and wellness programs. The body responds to mind changes, but more time may be required for the effects of that response to manifest in the organic form of the body's anatomy and physiology. Patience is required to objectively identify body changes in response to mind changes. This interaction between mind and body is the basis for current approaches to mind-body medicine.

Emotions

Emotions begin or end in our minds. Feelings, the actual physical sensations, can be caused by emotions, and feelings can in turn cause emotions. Physical sensations that occur in our body need to be understood. If our body experiences a sensation, our mind tries to understand the meaning. For example, if a medication is taken that increases the heart rate, the mind may interpret the increase in heart rate as a threat to safety and the person becomes fearful. Fear is an emotion. If a person is afraid, the heart rate increases, and the person feels anxious. The emotions lead to actions, representing the consequences of how we think and what we do. What we think and feel and how we live are all inextricably linked.

As human beings, we learn to be helpless, to be addictive, and to have low self-esteem. We learn to hate. The important point to remember is that if we learned the maladaptive behavior in the first place, we can also learn a more resourceful behavior. Emotions can be powerful. If used resourcefully, they can provide us with the empowerment to reach our goals.

Box 15.7 Supporting Restorative Sleep

Therapeutic massage supports restorative sleep in the following ways:

- It reduces the activity of the sympathetic autonomic nervous system and cortisol levels.
- It promotes parasympathetic autonomic nervous system dominance.
- It relieves or reduces pain and discomfort that may interrupt sleep.

Self-help measures for supporting restorative sleep include the following:

- Maintain a regular sleep-wake cycle. Get up and go to bed at the same time every day, including days off.
- Get at least 30 minutes of daylight exposure by being outside or by placing yourself in front of an open window.
- Exercise moderately on a regular basis, but do not exercise aerobically 4 hours before sleeping.
- Reduce stimulant intake substantially and ingest no stimulants 10 hours before sleeping. If you go to bed at 11:00 p.m., do not drink caffeinated beverages (e.g., energy drinks, colas, or coffee) after 1:00 p.m.
- Concentrate protein food intake 6 hours before going to sleep. Eat carbohydrates after this time. Do not eat a heavy meal before going to bed. Do not go to bed hungry. Eat a small snack of complex carbohydrates without sugar with some fermented dairy product (e.g., yogurt) 30 minutes before bed if hungry. Although a protein, turkey is high in tryptophan, which encourages sleep. A small turkey sandwich is a possible bedtime snack.
- Stretch gently for a few minutes 1 hour before bed. A slow, rhythmic pattern is best.
- Stay in a dark room or one with soft lighting (only enough light for safe movement) 1 hour before bedtime. Stretching in the dim light is an excellent way to begin the winding down process to prepare for sleep.
- Develop a bedtime ritual that you follow consistently. The ritual should begin 30 minutes before going to bed. Make sure to stay in dim lighting. This ritual should be 15 minutes long. It can include hygiene (e.g., washing up and brushing your teeth), but should not consist of full body application of water, because both hot and cold application can stimulate the body. (A warm bath 1 hour before sleep is relaxing.) Meditating or reading something that is gentle and can be finished in 5–10 minutes may be helpful. Listening to soft and gentle music is soothing. Drinking a cup of relaxing herbal tea is soothing. Meditate, pray, and review your day in a thankful way. After you develop this ritual, it needs to be reinforced. Do it the same way every night. Eventually, the ritual will signal the body into a sleep pattern.
- When drowsiness occurs, immediately relax into sleep. The drowsy pattern known as the *sleep window* lasts only about 15 minutes, and then a new body rhythm cycle begins, which lasts about 90 minutes.
- If you miss the sleep window, continue with calm activities until the sense of drowsiness again occurs. Then go back to bed.
- Sleep in the dark. Do not sleep with the television or computer on. Also avoid looking at bright screens from other electronic devices, such as smartphones and tablets.
- Get up at the same time every morning regardless of when you went to bed.
- Avoid long naps. A short nap (15–30 minutes) is usually okay for midday fatigue.

Many good things have come from an emotion turned into resourceful behavior.

Wellness encompasses a full range of emotions. Some pride themselves on not feeling certain emotions, but if we can experience an emotion in a resourceful way, it is not healthy to deny its expression. For example, if something as powerful as anger is turned inward, it does not lead to positive outcomes. However, if expressed resourcefully, to the person or in the situation involved, a sense of resolution takes place, and we can get on with our lives, free of anger.

Wellness comes from using the emotion instead of the emotion using us. Used resourcefully, emotions can provide the motivation to achieve wellness. When used in a negative manner, they can make us ill and be destructive to those who share our lives (Box 15.8).

Feelings

Feelings are the body's physical interpretation of emotions. They occur as a response to the effect of hormones, neurotransmitters, and other endogenous chemicals. Traits or behaviors such as the need to create crises, eating disorders, accident proneness, hypervigilance, panic, illness, pain, and codependent relationships generate the physical sensations we call feelings. Behaviors such as gentle caregiving, giving presents, and appreciating beauty generate feelings of compassion, nurturing, and belonging.

People use chemical substances such as food, nicotine, alcohol, and drugs to create or dampen feelings. Often if a person's physiology can be changed, their feelings can also be changed. The easiest way to change physiology is to move, as in exercising or breathing. A massage also changes physiology. This is perhaps why massage "feels" so good. Being touched in a resourceful way supports wellness. Sensory stimulation is essential for the body to thrive. Many people are deprived of touch, and many adults exchange touch only in the context of sexual relationships. Touch is essential for wellness. Touching generates and expresses feelings. The power of touch was explored at the beginning of this text.

When feelings are detrimental to wellness, an opposing response must be activated to restore balance. For example, if you are weighed down with too much thinking, moving around and pulling some weeds in the garden creates a balance. If you feel angry, find a way to laugh. If you feel down, help someone. If you feel anxious and alone, get a hug or a massage (Proficiency Exercise 15.6).

Behavior

Behavior is what we do in response to emotion, to trigger thoughts and feelings, and occasionally to avoid feelings. Resourceful behavior results in feeling good about what has

Box 15.8 Immunity and the Mind

The immune system is controlled directly by the mind. The science of psychoneuroimmunology has clearly established that unresolved emotions and thought patterns of hate, fear, anger, and jealousy reduce the efficiency of the body's defenses (Chaitow, 1991).

In 1975, Dr. Robert Ader (1932–2011) conditioned rats to dislike sweetened water by injecting them with a chemical to make them feel ill whenever they drank it. After the injections had been stopped for some time, some rats began dying. On investigation, Ader found that the chemical he had used was a suppressor of immune function. The rats not only had become conditioned to feeling ill whenever they drank sweet water, but they also were mimicking the chemical's other effects and depressing their immune systems. This ability to depress the immune function was proof of nervous system control over the immune system. Many subsequent studies have confirmed this finding in human beings, supporting the growth and validity of mind/body-based interventions.

From Ader R, Cohen, N: Behaviorally conditioned immunosuppression, *Psychosom Med* 37:333–340, 1975; Hadamitzky M, Sondermann W, Benson S, Schedlowski M: Placebo effects in the immune system, *Int Rev Neurobiol* 138:39–59, 2018; Colloca L: The fascinating mechanisms and implications of the placebo effect, *Int Rev Neurobiol* 138:xv, 2018.

PROFICIENCY EXERCISE 15.6

Honestly identify two personal behaviors that have a repetitive pattern; one resourceful and one unresourceful. What feelings are generated by these behaviors? Regarding unresourceful behavior, identify one alternative resourceful behavior to generate similar feelings.

Example

Resourceful behavior: Watching uplifting human interest movies
Feelings: Empowerment, security, connectedness
Unresourceful behavior: Overeating at night
Feelings: Being connected, fulfilled, cared for
Replacement behavior: Playing with my dog

Your Turn

- Resourceful behavior:
  Feelings:
- Unresourceful behavior:
  Feelings:
- Replacement behavior:
- Resourceful behavior:
  Feelings:
- Unresourceful behavior:
  Feelings:
- Replacement behavior:

happened. Detrimental behavior still results in a good feeling (or we would not do it), but often we feel bad about what happened or others feel bad.

Addictive Behavior

Addictive behavior creates physical sensations that feel pleasant and bypass the conscious experience of emotion. A person who is addicted to food, drugs, alcohol, exercise, pain, crisis, or loss develops a lifestyle that both protects and supports the substance or behavior of choice. Addictions require a great deal of time and energy. Addictive behavior throws the balance of wellness off course. It takes hard work and lots of support to change an addictive behavior. Sometimes a less damaging addiction is replaced by a more damaging one, and vice versa. For example, a person may use a food habit to bypass the emotion of loneliness and then alter the food habit by creating an exercise dependency. Whichever is the more damaging addiction needs to be evaluated. Behavior changes that are at least steps in the resourceful direction should not be discouraged. To truly alter behavior, a person must evaluate their sense of self.

Self-Concept

What we think about ourselves and how we talk to ourselves are aspects of self-concept. They are especially important contributors to wellness. Most of us want inner peace or peace of mind, purpose, and a sense of achievement, success, and self-confidence.

A positive self-concept is achievable when we stop comparing ourselves to others. Misjudging our worth threatens our well-being. Rather than basing personal value on external standards, healthy people develop internal standards of self-worth. Everyone is good at something; no one is good at everything. Measure success and self-worth by how good you feel about your accomplishments instead of by money or fame. Especially with massage, an inner sense of accomplishment is important. Massage is a quiet, unpretentious profession. It does not usually receive a lot of public glory. Massage is an important and needed service, and its benefits often cannot be measured objectively.

Coping

An aspect of wellness is the ability to live each day and feel we did our jobs well. How we lived that day influences our mind's perception of how we feel, and sometimes the simplest things can be effective. For example, when we are stressed and preoccupied with our responsibilities in the day, stopping for a moment to notice the sun shining and feeling the warmth on our faces may be a simple way to regain our balance and cope with that stress. This mind exercise is an example of a resourceful coping mechanism. Resourceful coping consists of commitment, control, and challenge.

Commitment

Commitment is the ability and willingness to be involved in what is happening around us and to have a purpose for being. This purpose is more than what we do; it is how we serve. It is possible to serve in many ways. A career in massage can be a path of service or just a job. Purpose and service have nothing to do with the task. Picking up trash is as much a service as being a doctor. Cleaning houses, cutting hair, building houses, and packing cartons all can be paths of service. The commitment to support wellness contributes to the greater good.

Control

Control is characterized by the belief that we can influence events by the way we feel, think, and act. This is internal control, not external control. Internal control involves adjusting ourselves to the situation and looking for ways to respond resourcefully. Those who exert external control attempt to control circumstances and people. It is impossible to control the weather, most circumstances, and most people. Relying on external control is a poor coping mechanism.

The eternal wisdom in the saying, "Grant me the serenity to accept the things I cannot change, the courage to change the things I can, and the wisdom to know the difference" speaks to self-concept and internal versus external control.

The saying "If given lemons, make lemonade" speaks to internal control. Finding the humor in life supports internal control. Not all life events have humor, but most have something that can bring a smile if not a laugh. For instance, one day while I was staring out the window grieving the death of a loved one, a chipmunk jumped up on the sill with so many sunflower seeds stuffed in his little cheeks that they were sticking out of his mouth, and he was trying to stuff more in. This is an example of what I like to call a "chuckle blended with the tears."

Challenge

Living each day as a challenge supports wellness. A challenging day is filled with things to learn, skills to practice, tasks to be accomplished, and obstacles to overcome. Beginning each day with the affirmation "I greet the day and all that it holds" may generate an attitude of challenge. Those who see change as a challenge cope much better than those who do not. Using available, resourceful coping mechanisms to cope with change in life allows the individual to welcome changes as leading to personal development.

Poor stress-coping skills in the form of attempted external control and unproductive emotions, such as unresolved anger, suppress our immune systems and predispose us to infection and poor health. The individual's response to stress, not the stress itself, determines the effect on the person's immunity (see Box 15.8). Wellness includes learning more efficient ways to cope with life, such as through counseling and behavior modification programs if needed.

To improve coping skills, pay attention to people who cope well and ask them to share how they manage. Attending seminars and reading books on effective coping, assertiveness, and development of internal control provide additional resources. Professional counseling can be helpful. Remember, we learned the coping mechanisms we currently have, and we can learn even better ways to cope (Proficiency Exercise 15.7).

PROFICIENCY EXERCISE **15.7**

In the space provided, take inventory of yourself to see what coping mechanisms you have. List three effective coping mechanisms and three that are not as effective. Choose one of these ineffective coping mechanisms and develop a plan to change it.

Effective coping mechanisms:

Ineffective coping mechanisms:

Plan to change one ineffective coping mechanism:

THE SPIRIT

SECTION OBJECTIVES

Chapter objective covered in this section:

6. Implement and respect the importance of an individualized spiritual approach to wellness.

Using the information presented in this section, the student will be able to perform the following:

- Identify a personal approach to spirituality.
- Consider the personal meaning of faith, hope, and love.
- Describe the relationship of spirituality to wellness.
- Respect an individual's spiritual path.

Our spirit is the part of us that transcends. Our spiritual selves "know our truth." Spiritual wellness consists of faith, hope, and love.

Faith

Faith is the ability to believe, trust, and know certain things that science cannot prove. It is the strength of wellness and involves the expression of that connecting strength each day through faith in ourselves, our partners, our families, and humanity as a whole. Faith is essential to wellness.

Hope

Hope is the belief, assurance, conviction, and confidence that our future will somehow be okay. It is the belief that the choices we make now will be the most resourceful choices as we create our future. Without hope, no sense of continuity exists. Temple Grandin, an admirable person with autism, said, "I like to hope that even if there is no personal afterlife, some energy impression [of me] is left in the universe. I do not want my thoughts to die with me" (Sacks, 1996) (Proficiency Exercise 15.8).

Love

Love has no concrete explanation. It is a prerequisite for wholeness, and wholeness is necessary for wellness. This is not romantic love; it is bigger, stronger, more empowering, and mightier. It is quiet, gentle, forgiving, and non-judgmental.

PROFICIENCY EXERCISE **15.8**

Complete the following sentence 10 different ways.

I hope:
I hope:
I hope:
I hope:
I hope:
I hope:
I hope:
I hope:
I hope:
I hope:

PROFICIENCY EXERCISE 15.9

During a learning experience, one or two people may emerge who teach us more than we expected to learn. These individuals may be a fellow student, client, teacher, or other school staff person. Often the learning has nothing to do with the courses we are studying. This is a love sharing. Go to those who have shared their love with you and say, "Thank you."

A teenage boy was struggling to put these most important issues into perspective. He came to his mother and said, "I have figured out the meaning of life." Wondering this herself, she asked her son what he had discovered. The son replied, "When I play my music and I feel great and those who listen to me feel great, then I have shared my love, and my power gets bigger and so does theirs. But if I play my music and only I feel great and those who listen feel bad and weak, then I have taken their power, and this is evil. This is the meaning of life." This type of love celebrates the irrepressible process of life. This is the love of wellness (Proficiency Exercise 15.9).

Spiritual health is essential to wellness. Everyone has a unique belief and experience of faith, hope, and love. Just as with all aspects of wellness, these beliefs and behaviors can be resourceful and adaptive or unresourceful and maladaptive. However, unlike the body and mind, for which the information relating to wellness has been researched and somewhat standardized, our spiritual path and inner peace are beyond hard science and concrete suggestions. Spirituality is a sacred journey and place created by each individual and is to be respected. There are some right ways to a healthy body and mind as previously described. There also are healthy expressions of spirituality, but they are much more varied and less concrete. Resourceful spirituality provides us with faith, hope, and love. These elements strengthen us and protect us from becoming faithless, hopeless, and loveless:

- When we nourish faith, we find strength to survive, thrive, and help others.
- When we nourish hope, we can endure, create, and plan for our future.
- When we nourish love, we care, have empathy, support vibrant life in all its forms, and bring respect and strength to support what is right and good.

Faith, hope, and love combined have far more strength than fear, destruction, and hate. The coming together of those who live a life based on faith, hope, and love—regardless of culture, religion, or experience—forms the spiritual strength and inner peace of our present and potential future.

SUMMARY

Wellness encompasses more than the components discussed in this chapter. Wellness is living life in a simple, gentle, respectful way for ourselves, others, and the environment. Wellness is the result of the healing that takes place on multiple levels when we take care of ourselves; this then extends to caring for others and the planet in general. A competent massage professional practices self-care and educates clients about the basic components of wellness. This chapter has addressed methods for managing physical, emotional, and spiritual stress in life.

Foot in the Door

The massage professional needs to walk the talk. To get and keep your foot in the career environment you desire, your feet first need to walk your way through your own wellness journey. Wellness is a process. How do you determine your own body, mind, and spiritual health status? What do you do to maintain and increase your wellness profile? Would you do the same activities you recommend to clients? The broad spectrum of wellness maintenance directly influences your career. If you are not supporting your own wellness, how you provide massage will be affected. Stamina will reduce, fatigue will increase, clear and concise thinking will be influenced, and mood will be altered. Why would a client walk in your door to receive a massage from an unwell massage therapist? Maintaining your wellness will get your foot in the door and keep it there.

It has been said that when half the world is receiving a massage and the other half is giving a massage, we shall have peace. Wellness is peace within and sharing that peace in simple ways. Sharing this peace consistently with respect and compassion can support wellness and, with faith, hope, and love, provide peace for our world.

Learn More on the Web

The Centers for Disease Control, MedlinePlus, and the National Institutes of Health provide health-related information on a variety of health topics including stress management, recommendations for physical activity, and understanding post-traumatic stress disorder. The US Department of Agriculture website has helpful information on nutrition. The National Institutes of Mental Health resources can assist with developing a comprehensive wellness plan. Specific links are provided on the Evolve site.

Evolve

Visit the Evolve website: http://evolve.elsevier.com/Fritz/fundamentals/.

Evolve content designed for massage therapy licensing exam review and comprehension of content beyond the textbook. Evolve content includes:

- Content Updates
- Science and Pathology Animations
- Body Spectrum Coloring Book
- MBLEx exam review multiple choice questions

FOR EACH CHAPTER FIND:

- Answers and rationales for the end-of-chapter multiple-choice questions
- Electronic Workbook and Answer Key
- Chapter multiple choice question Quiz
- Quick Content Review in Question Form and Answers
- Technique Videos when applicable
- Learn More on the Web

REFERENCES

Chaitow L. *The Body/Mind Purification Program*. Fireside; 1991.

Enns A, Eldridge GD, Montgomery C, Gonzalez VM. Perceived stress, coping strategies, and emotional intelligence: a cross-sectional study of university students in helping disciplines. *Nurse Educ Today*. 2018.

García-Moya I, Morgan A. The utility of salutogenesis for guiding health promotion: the case for young people's well-being. *Health Promot Int.* 2016;32(4):723–733.

Gupta RK, Telles S, Singh N, Balkrishna A. Stress and coping strategies: the impact on health. *Yoga Mimamsa.* 2018;50(1):20.

Kennedy AB, Cambron JA, Dexheimer JM, Trilk J, Saunders RP. Advancing health promotion through massage therapy practice: a cross-sectional survey study. *Prev Med Rep.* 2018;11:49–55.

Langeland E, Vaandrager L, Nilsen ABV, Schraner M, Meier Magistretti C. Effectiveness of Interventions to Enhance the Sense of Coherence in the Life Course. In: Mittelmark MB, Bauer GF, Vaandrager L, et al., eds. *The Handbook of Salutogenesis.* 2nd ed. Cham (CH): Springer; January 1, 2022:201–219.

Lasota A, Mróz J. Positive psychology in times of pandemic: time perspective as a moderator of the relationship between resilience and meaning in life. *Int J Environ Res Public Health.* 2021;18(24):13340. doi:10.3390/ijerph182413340. Published 2021 Dec 18.

Manohar PR. Salutogenesis and ayurvedic solutions for coping with stress. *Annals of Ayurvedic Medicine.* 2016;5(3–4).

Mittelmark MB, Bauer GF. The meanings of salutogenesis. In: *The Handbook of Salutogenesis.* Springer International Publishing; 2017:7–13. https://doi.org/10.1007/978-3-319-04600-6_2.

Mittelmark MB, Bauer GF, Vaandrager L, et al., eds. *The Handbook of Salutogenesis.* Springer International Publishing; 2022:651.

Sacks O. *An Anthropologist on Mars: Seven Paradoxical Tales.* Vintage Books; 1996.

Selye H. *The Stress of Life.* 2nd ed. McGraw-Hill; 1978.

Slimmen S, Timmermans O, Mikolajczak-Degrauwe K, Oenema A. How stress-related factors affect mental wellbeing of university students A cross-sectional study to explore the associations between stressors, perceived stress, and mental wellbeing. *PLoS One.* 2022;17(11):e0275925.

Williams R, Ntontis E, Alfadhli K, Drury J, Amlôt R. A social model of secondary stressors in relation to disasters, major incidents and conflict: Implications for practice. *Int J Disaster Risk Reduct.* 2021;63(102436):102436.

MULTIPLE-CHOICE QUESTIONS FOR DISCUSSION AND REVIEW

The answers, with rationales, can be found on the Evolve site. Use these questions to stimulate discussion and dialogue. You must understand the meaning of words in the question and possible answers. Each question provides you with the ability to review terminology, practice critical thinking skills, and improve multiple-choice test-taking skills. Answers and rationales are on the Evolve site. It is just as important to know why the wrong answers are wrong as why the correct answer is correct.

1. During the massage, a client often speaks of problems with their children respecting house rules. This is a ______.
   a. Body issue
   b. Mind issue
   c. Spiritual issue
   d. Core issue

2. A massage therapist becomes a bit aloof if running behind for a scheduled massage session. This is a ______.
   a. Denial measure
   b. Defensive measure
   c. Salutogenesis approach
   d. Lack of purpose

3. Wellness usually involves a simplification of lifestyle to reduce demands. A stressful outcome of this process is often ______.
   a. Endurance
   b. Financial stability
   c. Dealing with loss and letting go
   d. Increased social support

4. The beliefs one has about the ability to comprehend, manage, and find meaning relate to ______.
   a. A sense of coherence
   b. Denial and defense measures
   c. Pathogenesis
   d. Surrender

5. When breathing in the normal relaxed pattern, ______.
   a. The inhale is longer than the exhale
   b. Deep inspiration is accentuated
   c. Accessory muscles only work on exhalation
   d. The exhale is longer than the inhale

6. A client feels fatigued all the time and explains that they do not seem to sleep through the night. Which of the following may improve their situation?
   a. An afternoon cup of coffee
   b. Taking a long nap in the afternoon
   c. Going to bed and watching television
   d. Spending at least 30 minutes outdoors

7. When one feels confident with commitment, control, and challenges in life, one is ______.
   a. Coping well
   b. Using behavior modification
   c. Functioning from an external locus of control
   d. Reliant on defense mechanisms

8. When a massage therapist is sharing information with a client about methods to achieve well-being, this is called ______.
   a. Counseling and coaching
   b. Health promotion and education messages
   c. Referral for diagnosis
   d. Treatment planning and documentation

9. Massage therapy most directly supports compliance with ______.
   a. Dietary change
   b. Meditation and mindfulness
   c. Physical fitness
   d. Emotional expression

10. Which of the following does not involve evidence-informed information?
   a. Cognitive behavioral therapy
   b. Learning resourceful coping
   c. Spiritual practices
   d. Nutritional supplementation

11. Wellness programs usually include methods to improve communication. Which of the following best explains why communication is more difficult to improve than diet?
   a. Diet and nutrition are more concrete and objective than subjective communication.
   b. Diet is much more dependent on others, whereas communication is independent of others.
   c. Stress focuses change on healthful food choices.
   d. Communication skills are highly genetically influenced, but diet is not.

12. When one is considering the wellness components of a balanced body, mind, and spirit, in which of the following intervention areas is massage most effective?
   a. Promoting a sense of coherence
   b. Restoring an appropriate eating and sleep cycle

c. Normalizing breathing mechanisms
d. Promoting belief system changes

13. A client has been relatively inactive. Recently, the client was diagnosed with diabetes and needs to begin an exercise program. Which of the following best describes the client's level of fitness?
a. Deconditioned
b. Endurance
c. Flexibility
d. Aerobic

14. A client has begun a walking exercise program and is walking an hour per day. Which of the following best describes the program?
a. Stretching and flexibility
b. Aerobic continuous training
c. Circuit-interval training
d. Metabolic anaerobic

15. A client had a severe viral infection 4 years ago and continues to have episodes of relapse. The client was recently diagnosed with fibromyalgia. During assessment, the massage professional notices that the client inhales longer than they exhale and that most of the movement during breathing happens in their upper chest. The client's physician has suggested massage as part of a total management program and asks for a treatment plan. Which of the following is the most reasonable expectation in terms of benefit, cost, and compliance?
a. Weekly massage for 3 months
b. Monthly massage for 12 months
c. Weekly massage indefinitely
d. Massage three times a week for 6 months

16. A 27-year-old client is embarking on a weight management program. The program includes a balanced diet with portion control, appropriate use of nutritional supplements, a well-designed exercise program that combines aerobic and weight-bearing activity, and an emotional support group system. The client wonders what massage may have to offer during this major lifestyle change. Which of the following would be the best and most accurate response to this inquiry?
a. Massage can stimulate similar pleasure and satisfaction centers in the brain as food and can help with cravings that may occur. Massage also can support the exercise program by managing any exercise-related soreness.
b. Massage can restructure the fascial tensegrity network and support the release of accumulated fat from the tissues. Massage can alter the metabolism and support exercise.
c. Massage is relaxing and can be used as a reward for progress. It also influences metabolic rate and aerobic capacity, supporting heart health.
d. Massage can be used to stimulate appetite suppression by increasing dopamine and adrenocorticotropic hormone. Massage also influences the thyroid in such a way as to decrease the fat-storing tendency.

17. A massage professional is struggling with balancing a successful massage career with personal responsibilities. One client is demanding. This client is a local television anchor whose schedule is somewhat erratic. The client feels they cannot maintain a confirmed appointment schedule and needs to be able to call at the last minute for a massage. This client has a combination of tension, sinus, and vascular headaches, as well as irritable bowel syndrome. Both conditions are aggravated by stress. The client notices significant relief after a massage. The massage practitioner has tried to refer this client, but they were unhappy with the massage results. Although the client is demanding, they are also generous and will increase the gratuity substantially when they have received special treatment from the massage therapist. Which of the following best describes the complex nature of this relationship?
a. The massage therapist does not wish to create conflict and avoids confronting the client about the demanding behavior.
b. The client is displaying transference to the point that the professional relationship is compromised, and the massage professional does not know how to reestablish boundaries.
c. The severity of the client's condition makes it difficult for the massage therapist to refer, and the randomness of the illness makes regular scheduling impossible.
d. The massage therapist finds the irregular appointment schedule disruptive to their personal life and has attempted alternative action, but the client has not been satisfied.

18. A client is in generally good health and enjoys massage. The client is extremely value-conscious and asks the massage professional to explain the benefits of regular massage for a healthy individual to determine the cost versus benefit of regular massage treatment. The client also is seeking to determine the optimal frequency of massage for restorative purposes. The client also wonders about various durations of massage application and about the benefits of 30-, 60-, and 90-minute sessions. Which of the following would be most accurate in response to the client's inquiry?
a. Massage is best used weekly for 90 minutes. The approach would be therapeutic change with aspects of palliative care to address the client's desire for a pleasant experience. The outcome of the regular massage application would be to treat identified conditions as they occur. The benefit is to prevent disease from becoming worse and requiring medical intervention.
b. Massage can be used periodically, changing frequency and duration as needed to address specific concerns. The massage would be targeted to restorative care with specific applications that reverse existing health conditions. The benefit would be to meet relaxation and restorative needs.
c. Massage is best used regularly as a restorative and maintenance system. A frequency of once per week is

ideal for these outcomes. Sessions every 2 weeks are adequate. A duration of 60 minutes is typically sufficient to achieve these benefits. The outcome should be prevention of stress-related symptoms and treatment of mild muscular-skeletal conditions as they occur.
d. Massage benefits are increased with frequency of use. The 30-minute massage three times per week is ideal, with occasional 60-minute massage sessions once per week if time does not permit scheduling of the more frequent application. Benefits include stress management and immune system support. Frequent application for shorter duration allows for a slow and relaxing full-body approach to encourage parasympathetic dominance.

19. During assessment, the massage practitioner identifies that a client is moving their shoulders up and down while breathing. The client also indicates an aching sensation in their lower back. Which muscle is likely to be tender to palpation?
a. Latissimus dorsi
b. Quadratus lumborum
c. Rectus femoris
d. Gluteus medius

20. Which of the following situations would be out of the scope of practice for a massage therapist?
a. A client who is sore after an increase in exercise
b. A client who is incorporating relaxation approaches to support sleep
c. A client who is exploring spiritual disciplines to support coping skills
d. A client who is altering their diet and wants to support digestion

Case Studies

CHAPTER 16

http://evolve.elsevier.com/Fritz/fundamentals/

CHAPTER OBJECTIVES

After completing this chapter, the student will be able to perform the following:

1. Use clinical reasoning to integrate the information from science studies and this text to complete a comprehensive history, assessment, and care/treatment plan.
2. Write comprehensive case studies.
3. Analyze care/treatment plans and offer and justify alternate approaches to care.
4. Choose three of the case studies in this chapter, develop a treatment plan that differs from the one presented, and be able to justify the appropriateness of your approach for the condition.

CHAPTER OUTLINE

This chapter integrates the information from this textbook and your science studies. The recommended textbook for anatomy, physiology, pathology, and kinesiology is *Mosby's Essential Sciences for Therapeutic Massage: Anatomy, Physiology, Biomechanics, and Pathology*, although other texts can be used successfully. Competency in the therapeutic massage practice is reflected both in a solid understanding of the content of your science studies and an ability to apply the information practically for individual clients. Clips on the Evolve site contain three additional video case studies showing the process through pretreatment interviews, assessment, and the massage session.

The following 20 case studies cover the most common outcome goals of clients. These cases cover at least 80% of the common conditions seen by massage professionals in day and destination spas and in wellness, franchise, health, fitness, sports, and medical settings. If you carefully study the process of clinical reasoning exemplified in these cases, you should be able to address almost all other conditions you encounter in your professional practice.

Each case study is presented in the following format:

- Case narrative
- Assessment
- Clinical reasoning
- Treatment plan development

The cases present an integrated approach to goal-oriented and outcome-based individual client care. Each case study attempts to describe real situations with complicating factors in addition to the main issues. For example, seldom can you use massage to enhance athletic performance or manage low back pain without having to consider other factors, such as coexisting conditions, work activities, stress tolerance, medications, and client compliance. The massage work environment is a factor; massage on a cruise ship is different from massage in a rehabilitation center. If the client cannot justify the cost or does not show up for regular appointments, even the best treatment plan is meaningless. Skills and knowledge are also factors. What a massage professional with 2 years' experience and entry-level education is able to accomplish is far different from what a professional with 15 years' experience and ongoing professional development can achieve.

This textbook is designed as an entry-level text, with the assumption that you do not have professional experience. One purpose of these case studies is to model the use of a critical thinking process. As a massage therapy student and soon-to-be graduate, you can use these case studies as patterns for how to develop massage treatment plans even when experience is minimal. If you challenge yourself to study the process of each case study, you will begin the habit of thinking in this fashion. The story form for each case is an effective method for learning. Each case can provide a platform for common situations you may encounter in your professional practice. This can be helpful for you as a new massage therapist, so that you do not feel overwhelmed at the beginning of your professional practice. These case studies provide you with examples that you can follow and modify.

Because clients' situations vary so much, writing massage protocol recommendations for an individual condition is almost impossible. For example, the pathology related to irritable bowel syndrome (IBS) is understood in terms of signs and symptoms; however, the issue becomes how that generic information relates to an individual client who seeks help through massage, especially in light of the multiple influences in a client's life. Consequently, recommendations for massage for IBS are very limited; although the information may help a massage professional begin to think about how best to serve an individual client, this is only the beginning. The treatment plan for massage must address each client's entire set of circumstances, not just a single condition the person may have.

The treatment plans presented here have been developed accordingly. Based on many years of professional experience, the authors believe these case studies represent effective processes that will work for most clients. Each case study has a primary goal, with numerous influences that make clinical reasoning and decision making the only effective ways to evaluate and develop appropriate massage treatment plans.

It may be necessary to research the literature with every new client. If the client has a diagnosed condition, it is important to look up information about that medical condition and any treatment being received for it. For example if a client has been burned (as in one of the case studies), the massage professional must understand the different categories of burns, the types of scar development, the treatments used to support burn healing, the expected changes in the tissue after healing, and other related factors. Another reason for literature research is to educate yourself concerning client activities or how to interact with clients from other cultures, those who participate in various activities such as sport or musical performance, individuals with of a variety of functional and cognitive differences, and those who participate in self-care activities such as yoga, diet, and other forms of bodywork. Although this information is not related to pathology, it does help you establish rapport with clients and broaden your understanding of clients' lifestyles.

This type of research begins during the client interview because they are the best source of knowledge about themselves. The fact-gathering portion of the clinical reasoning process continues during the history taking, assessment process, and literature search. This text and *Mosby's Essential Sciences for Therapeutic Massage: Anatomy, Physiology, Biomechanics, and Pathology* provide information on the most common conditions encountered by massage professionals and serve as important places to begin the research process. Textbooks, medical dictionaries, texts on pharmacology and pathology, and the internet can all be used to gather pertinent information to develop appropriate treatment plans. As you have learned throughout the textbook, the website MedlinePlus is very helpful.

For example, a client might come in for massage to reduce aching caused by playing tennis. The client requests massage that has sufficient depth of pressure and drag to address the second, third, and fourth layers of muscle tissue and to increase the pliability of the connective tissue ground substance. If muscle aching were the only condition detected, those methods would be appropriate. However, this same client is taking an anticoagulant medication because of a heart

Box 16.1 Massage by the Numbers

Recall the four main outcomes for massage:
- Relaxation/well-being
- Stress management
- Pain management
- Functional mobility

Also remember the four main approaches to care:
- Palliative
- Restorative
- Condition management
- Therapeutic change

Mechanical force is generated by two actions:
- Pushing
- Pulling

There are nine primary massage methods used to create mechanical force:
- Static methods/holding
- Compression
- Gliding
- Torsion twisting (kneading)
- Shearing (friction)
- Elongation
- Oscillation
- Percussion
- Movement

Methods are adapted by the following 12 modifiers:
- Pressure
- Point of application (location and broadness of contact)
- Magnitude (intensity)
- Direction
- Drag
- Speed
- Pacing
- Rhythm
- Sequencing and transitioning
- Frequency
- Duration
- Intention for outcome

Adapted methods generate appropriate force to load the body tissue to create the following five stresses to which the physiology must adapt:
- Compression stress
- Tension stress
- Shear stress
- Torsion stress
- Bending stress

condition—suddenly, the entire treatment plan changes. The question now becomes how the massage professional can meet the main goal of the client—reduction of deep muscle aching—without causing bruising or other complications arising from the heart condition and the medication taken to treat it. To further complicate the issue, the client wants only a 30-minute massage. To serve the client competently, the massage professional must understand tennis, the training effects that support tennis playing, performance-connected muscle soreness, anticoagulant medication (how and when it is used, the effects and side effects), the client's heart condition and any therapies besides medication used to treat it, and any other pertinent facts. All this information influences the types of massage applications chosen and assists with the decisions on how deep or superficial, how fast or slow, how rhythmic, or how frequent the massage application should be.

The case studies give examples of ways to meet common but complicated massage client goals in the context of the bigger picture. As you study each case, evaluate it to see whether a variation of the recommended treatment plan might be effective. Also, consider all the other conditions that would benefit from a similar treatment plan. For example, one of the cases discusses a client with asthma; however, a similar massage process would be appropriate for someone with emphysema or chronic bronchitis (Box 16.1).

When you study the cases, follow this sequence:

1. Identify the main goal and all the conditions and complicating factors.
2. Identify the overlapping issues that alter the treatment process or the superimposed cautions for massage application.
3. Brainstorm about what you agree with in the presented treatment plan and what you might do differently.
4. Scrutinize the assessment processes.
5. With the physical assessment information, actually put yourself in the positions described and experience how it feels.
6. Relate those postures and sensations to the goals of the client and the recommendations for massage application.
7. Explore the practice model of the massage therapist including the location, fees, and scheduling.

CASE 1. GENERALIZED STRESS AND ANXIETY WITH BREATHING PATTERN DISORDER SYMPTOMS

NOTE: Generalized stress and anxiety with breathing pattern disorder symptoms is the most common stress condition seen by the massage therapist. The approach suggested could also be a platform for assisting those with Long COVID and other post viral situations. This condition is also common in pain and fatigue syndromes and in post-traumatic stress disorder.

The client is 37 years old. Friends and the client's primary care physician recommended massage to help them deal with stress-induced physical symptoms. Three weeks ago they had a complete physical because of being required to purchase a life insurance policy to cover the mortgage on a new home. The family had outgrown their smaller home with the recent birth of their third child. Although the physical indicated that all signs were within normal parameters, the client's blood pressure was slightly elevated. It was recommended that they see their family doctor, who did not find anything medically out of the norm but who did notice that the client was impatient and irritable. The client told the doctor that they were not sleeping well and were experiencing some heartburn about once a week, occasional constipation, and neck and shoulder stiffness. The client had also gained 10 pounds since their last visit 2 years ago. The doctor felt that stress was the main cause of the problems and suggested that they exercise more often, reduce the caffeine in their diet, and lose some of the extra weight. In addition, therapeutic massage was suggested for the muscle stiffness and for relaxation.

The client arrives at a fitness center for the first visit. They have never had a massage and are visibly nervous and in a hurry. The massage professional introduces himself and explains that the first massage session is primarily an initial assessment process that will take 90 minutes and include a 50-minute massage. The cost of the first session is $85. Each massage session after the initial session will last 60 minutes (50 actual minutes of massage), and the cost will be $65 per session. The client states they understand the arrangement and agrees to the assessment and treatment plan process.

Assessment

Observation

The massage professional observes the way the client moves about the office, how they breathe, and the rate of their speech. It is evident that the client is feeling rushed, because they look at their watch many times during the interview and make it clear they need to be at an appointment by 4 PM. The client's shoulders move up and down during breathing. The inhale-to-exhale ratio indicates that the client routinely inhales longer than exhales, seems to swallow air when talking, and belches a couple of times during the interview. The client chews gum, rolls their shoulders back, and often attempts to stretch their neck to the left. The client also pulls at their right shoulder and neck area with their left hand. Their eyes dart about when talking, the voice is a bit too loud for the environment, and they cannot sit in the chair for longer than a few minutes without fidgeting or getting up and walking around. When they do sit still, their fists are clenched. The client smiles often and jokes about being stressed. Their weight is proportional to height but with weight distribution around the waist. The client is right-handed. The client seems a bit uneasy with the idea of a male therapist providing the massage.

Interview and Goals

The interview process consists of casual conversation supported by a client information form. The client information form and conversation indicate that the client is 37 years old, married, has three children, ages 9, 6, and 8 months, recently moved to the city from a small town, and works as an advertising executive. The client has a family history of maturity-onset diabetes, hypertension, and stroke. They have not had any symptoms other than slightly higher than normal blood pressure. They had one surgery as a child for appendicitis, ran track in high school and college, but have not exercised regularly since then. The client enjoys playing basketball and racquetball but has not found a new group of people with whom to play since moving to the city. They occasionally take aspirin for a headache and Tums for heartburn and do not take any vitamins or herbs. They drink coffee and cola beverages and do not smoke. The client was in a car accident 3 years ago and suffered a mild whiplash-type injury. The client has difficulty falling asleep at night. Their spouse tells them they toss and turn and grind their teeth when asleep. Currently, the client feels tired in the morning and gets only about 5 hours of sleep a night. The baby still wakes up at night, and they get up with the child every other night. When asked about their stress load, the client lists the new job, the large mortgage, and the fact that that they are now concerned about health. The client says they have always been a bit high-strung and discloses they worry a lot. The long hours required at the new job are making their spouse angry because they are not keeping up with tasks at home like before they moved. The client sits at a desk, is on the phone a lot, and must attend and run business meetings twice a week.

To allow the client to become more comfortable with the idea of a male therapist, the benefits of massage are explained in relation to therapeutic goals rather than relaxation and pleasurable sensation. The client's main goals for the massage are to sleep better, be more relaxed and less irritable, lower blood pressure, and reduce the stiffness in the neck and shoulder.

Physical Assessment

Posture

Right shoulder is high and anteriorly rotated. Head is slightly forward, and lumbar curve is slightly flattened. Right leg is moderately externally rotated, and right arm is slightly internally rotated. Left knee is hyperextended.

Gait

Stride and arm swing are shortened on the right, and client rolls to the outside of the left foot during the heel strike and toe-off phase.

Range of Motion

Lateral bending of the neck to the left is reduced to 30 degrees. Rotation is equal on both sides but painful during the last few degrees when rotation is to the right. External rotation of the right arm is limited to 75 degrees and internal rotation of the right hip to 40 degrees. Trunk extension is limited to 15 degrees beyond 0 degrees. Eversion of the left foot is slightly limited. Ribs are resistant to being sprung, more so on the left, indicating rigidity in the thorax.

Palpation

Near Touch

Upper shoulder on the right is warm.

Skin

Skin on the right shoulder, pectoralis bilaterally, lateral ribs, neck, and lumbar region have damp areas that redden when stroked. Skin of upper chest bilaterally, right shoulder, and entire lumbar region is taut. Tissue is restricted inferiorly and diagonally to the left on chest and produces a smaller skinfold in lumbar area on the left.

Superficial Connective Tissue

Neck tissue shows mild edema and a sensation of bogginess, as well as a bind resistance to movement toward the left. Connective tissues of the lumbar area and both of the lateral legs palpate shortened and thick. Surgical scar on the abdomen appears bound to underlying structures when moved.

Vessels and Lymph Nodes

No palpable differences.

Muscles

Lumbar and posterior thorax muscles in the second layer are tight but long. Pectoralis major on the right is short. Occipital base muscles are painful to moderate pressure. Abdominals and gluteus maximus are soft and reduced in tone. Hamstrings are short bilaterally. Gastrocnemius and soleus on the left are dense and short. Deep lateral hip rotators on the right are tight and short. Subscapularis on the right is short, and infraspinatus is tight/taut but long. Anterior serratus palpates bilaterally as tender, with tender points corresponding to damp, red areas on the skin. Pectoralis minor on the right is short. Psoas is short bilaterally. Muscles of mastication are tense and short.

Tendons

Subscapular tendon on the right is tender to moderate pressure.

Deep Fascia

Lumbar dorsal fascia, iliotibial band, and abdominal fascia are thick and have reduced pliability.

Ligaments

No apparent changes.

Joints

No observable changes, but some heat, edema, and pain with moderate palpation pressure are noted in the right glenohumeral joint.

Bones

No apparent changes.

Abdominal Viscera

Abdomen is generally soft. Some rigidity is present in the large intestine at the splenic flexure.

Body Rhythms

Heart rate fluctuates from 65 to 80 beats per minute. Breathing rhythm is fast and uneven and does not appear entrained to heart rhythm. Peripheral circulation is good and even.

Muscle Testing

Strength

Pectoralis muscles and adductor muscles test strong, with inhibition in the gluteus medius, which tests weak. Muscles that retract the scapula are weak. Gluteus maximus bilaterally tests weak.

Neurological Balance

Antagonists to pectoralis and internal shoulder rotators are inhibited. Abdominals and gluteus are inhibited.

Gait

Shoulder and hip flexors on the right are not inhibited in the normal reflex pattern. When arm flexors are activated, hip flexors do not inhibit as they should.

Interpretation and Treatment Plan Development

Clinical Reasoning

What Are the Facts?

The main contributing factors are generalized stress with episodes of anxiety and breathing pattern disorder symptoms (these conditions are discussed in Chapters 5, 6, and 15). To work effectively with a client who has these conditions, the massage professional must research them. The general experience of stress is sympathetic dominance in the autonomic nervous system when fight-or-flight or fear mechanisms are detrimental instead of beneficial. When the energy is rallied for these high activity demands but the body stays still, as with this client, the physiological activity manifests internally, resulting in the symptoms of increased heart rate, high blood pressure, digestive disturbances, and changes in breathing. The muscles also assume either the flight or attack position, but movement does not occur; therefore generalized tension builds. When the respiratory mechanism is functioning with auxiliary breathing muscles, oxygen intake may exceed the physical demand, and sympathetic arousal occurs. A vicious cycle begins, with internal and external stimuli increasing sympathetic arousal, which increases breathing and muscle tension, which in turn increases sympathetic arousal. Anxiety with an increase in vigilance (looking for what is wrong) perpetuates. Mood is altered, and physical symptoms manifest in a strange collection of seemingly unrelated symptoms. Because a breathing pattern disorder is a functional process (i.e., the activity is normal but occurs at inappropriate times), no diagnosable pathological condition is present. The most common and measurable symptom is elevated blood pressure, which fluctuates situationally, unlike with primary hypertension, in which the blood pressure is constantly high. Because physical distress symptoms are present but medical tests indicate nothing wrong, people become frustrated. Management of a breathing pattern disorder requires that the individual make lifestyle changes. However, because of the stress syndrome and sympathetic activation, people often look for causal factors outside themselves and can become irritable and restless. This is a common pattern presented by many clients seeking massage.

For this client, stress is professional, personal, and financial. Time urgency is apparent. The client is generally in good health but has mildly elevated blood pressure that is not being treated medically. There is evidence of sympathetic autonomic nervous system arousal, constipation, heartburn, disrupted sleep, upper chest breathing, and history of high-pressure jobs. The client talks fast and is restless, admits to being irritable, grinds teeth at night, and chews gum during the day. This physiological state is supported by an intake of caffeine. Assessment indicates shortening and tenderness in the auxiliary breathing muscles, with the beginning of second-degree functional stress in both the posture (stability) and phasic (movement) muscles.

What Are the Possibilities in Both Function and Dysfunction and the Massage Intervention Options?

The client seems to display breathing pattern disorder symptoms in response to sustained sympathetic arousal. The client has sufficient postural distortion to interfere with the mechanics of breathing, which would cause the symptoms and perpetuate the increase in sympathetic activity.

The client's activity levels are not in balance with the level of sympathetic nervous system arousal. Increased aerobic exercise with a gentle stretching program would be appropriate.

The heartburn the client experiences could be a symptom of acid reflux disease, gastroesophageal reflux disease (GERD), an inflamed stomach lining (gastritis), hiatal hernia, or peptic ulcer. The client's increased abdominal fat could be a contributing factor. The client consumes a lot of caffeine, which aggravates heartburn. Over-the-counter nonsteroidal antiinflammatory medication can also increase heartburn sensation. In addition, pain in the chest may be mistaken for heartburn when it's really a sign of heart disease. The client is using a calcium carbonate–based antacid.

The client is clearly stressed and has some mild anxiety. Causal factors could be the physical changes in posture resulting from extended sitting and talking on the phone, the decrease in physical activity, and/or the buildup of internal pressure from work and family. If this is primarily a cognitive problem, referral to a psychologist is indicated. If the indication is more physical, massage and exercise would help. It is likely that all elements are involved.

Possibilities

1. The massage intervention can be structured to deal with the postural alterations and the shortening in muscle and connective tissue structures that are causing the breathing dysfunction.
2. Massage would support a moderate exercise program by managing post-exercise muscle soreness.
3. The client should experience some benefit; however, it is likely that some sort of cognitive or psychological intervention is needed. A combination of the two approaches would be most satisfactory.

What Are the Logical Outcomes of Each Possible Intervention?

Massage application should reduce the sympathetic arousal, but the effect would be temporary. Adding exercise and stretching would prolong the effects of massage. The breathing function would improve, and the breathing pattern disorder symptoms should diminish, but these results also would be temporary. The client would need to change stress perception or reduce the stress load for symptom reversal. Massage application could help manage the physical stress response if lifestyle changes are deemed impossible at this time or if counseling is avoided. Massage would have to be given often—twice a week at minimum—to be effective.

Cost and time commitments would be required for all interventions. Massage sessions alone twice a week would require 4 hours of total time commitment (massage and travel time), and the cost would be $130 per week. The financial burden for this client is not a concern for a short-term intervention process, but the time commitment is. If the client seeks counseling, massage could be reduced to once a week. The time would be about the same, but the cost would be higher for the counseling appointments. Some of the cost for counseling would be offset by insurance reimbursement.

What Is the Effect on the People Involved for Each Possible Intervention?

The massage therapist is familiar with dealing with these conditions because the fitness center is affiliated with the local hospital's wellness and prevention program. The physician is favorable. The spouse is a bit resistant because the increase in exercise and massage further reduces the client's time at home. If the client's mood improves, the spouse would be more supportive. The client is willing to increase exercise and try massage but is resistant to any type of counseling.

Decision Making and Treatment Plan Development

Primary Goal: Stress Management
Category of Care: Therapeutic Change

Quantifiable Goals

1. Reduce shortening of breathing muscles by 75%. Reduce postural distortion by 50% and increase range of motion in restricted areas by 75%.
2. Increase connective tissue pliability by reducing bind in short areas by 75%.
3. Reduce edema in shoulder by 90%.
4. Normalize blood pressure to appropriate range (under 120/80 mm Hg).

Qualifiable Goals

1. The distressful stress symptoms will diminish, resulting in improved sleep and reduced irritability at work and at home.
2. The client will have a more relaxed demeanor, resulting in improved relationships at work and home.

The goal is to calm the sympathetic autonomic nervous system and introduce a normal balance between the parasympathetic and sympathetic functions. When this is achieved, the client's sleep should improve as a result of a drop in cortisol levels and tossing and turning should diminish because muscle tension will have lessened. The teeth grinding and need to chew gum during the day should decline, which would reduce the strain in the mastication and neck muscles.

Breathing should move from an upper chest breathing pattern to more normal diaphragmatic breathing, with the inhale phase being shorter than the exhale phase in a ratio of 1:4. As the auxiliary breathing muscles relax, posture improves, and air swallowing declines, the belching and heartburn should improve. The neck and shoulder stiffness should diminish when these muscles are no longer used for breathing. Mood should also improve.

Appointments would be scheduled in the evening so that the client can go home and go to bed.

Treatment Regimen

Therapeutic Change

This is a therapeutic change process in the short term with realistic expectations of a condition management treatment program for the long term.

The client decides to join the lunchtime racquetball league for local businesspeople 3 days a week and will commit to a massage twice a week for 6 weeks and then reevaluate, hoping to reduce the massage frequency to once a week.

A general full-body massage session will be used, with a depth of pressure sufficient to elicit the relaxation response. All massage manipulations will be used except friction and percussion because friction causes pain and percussion is generally a stimulating method. The rhythm will be slow and even, meeting the client's body rhythms and then slowing over the course of the session. The direction of massage will be primarily toward the heart but with changes as necessary to address connective tissue bind. Lymphatic drainage methods will be used on the right shoulder. Muscle energy methods will be used, especially to address the eye and neck reflexes and to lengthen all short muscles identified during the assessment.

Because the major tension is in the neck and shoulders, having the client roll eyes in large circles or roll head in small circles while broad-based compression is applied to the tender areas, especially the occipital base muscles, will help. Kneading and skin rolling with myofascial techniques, coupled with lymphatic drainage, will increase pliability in the areas of thick and short connective tissues. Active trigger points in muscles will be addressed with the least invasive measures possible to reduce the guarding response and pain behaviors because pain increases sympathetic arousal. Positional release will be the primary choice and will be applied to the indicated areas in the serratus anterior and intercostal muscles.

Muscles that are inhibited will be encouraged to function through the use of limited tapotement (i.e., not so much as to arouse the nervous system) at the attachments of these muscles.

Joint movement methods will focus on reducing the internal rotation of the right arm and the external rotation of the right leg. Integrated muscle energy methods will be the primary method used and will combine these patterns so that the muscle imbalances can be treated in sequence. The abdominal massage sequence will ease constipation, but caution is required because of heartburn. Prone and supine positioning will also need to be monitored to identify if it creates a heartburn sensation. Side-lying may be a better option.

Teaching the client simple breathing and relaxation exercises, as described in Chapter 15, is appropriate.

CASE 2. MUSCLE TENSION HEADACHE

A 26-year-old female is in good health except for frequent headaches that radiate pain from the back of her skull around her ears and over her eyes. Migraine and cluster headaches have been ruled out. The diagnosis is muscle tension headaches. Because no medical reason has been found for the headaches, they are assumed to be stress related. They do not follow any cyclic pattern. A relationship to the menstrual cycle has not been indicated.

The client has a temporary job as a server while she finishes college. She spends a lot of time sitting, reading, and working at the computer. She notices increased tension in her neck, shoulders, and lower back when she has to spend a lot of time with her studies. She swims three times a week for exercise and is careful with her diet. She has a moderate intake of caffeine and alcohol, and she smokes. She is not under any medical care.

Because common over-the-counter analgesics such as aspirin and acetaminophen bother her stomach, she is seeking an alternative to manage the pain. She has tried chiropractic care, with limited success, and often experiences a headache right after an adjustment. She has heard that massage can help these types of headaches. A friend referred her, indicating that she would be comfortable with a middle-aged female therapist with a home-based practice. The client has completed an informed consent process and has agreed to treatment.

Assessment

Observation

The client is nearsighted and wears glasses. She repositions her glasses often, and she squints in the bright light. She is polite and soft-spoken. She appears frustrated and tired of the inconvenience of the headaches. She is neatly groomed and organized; she provides a list of all the treatments that have been tried, including a food diary and schedules, in an attempt to identify the cause of the headaches. Her weight is normal for her height. She has long, thick hair that she wears in a ponytail.

Interview and Goals

The client's history reveals that she has had headaches for as long as she can remember. She has a headache severe enough to interfere with daily activities about 10 days out of a month. The headaches last about 12 hours, and the pain is a 7 on a scale of 1 to 10 (1 being slight, 10 being extreme). She does not remember any injury or surgery or any childhood diseases other than the normal ones. She had the headaches during adolescence. She generally ignores the headaches, but they are becoming draining. The family history provides no insight. There is a family history of cancer. She wore braces for 3 years and recently had them removed. She has worn glasses and has had long hair since her early teens. She admits to being a perfectionist.

Her goals for the massage are to reduce the frequency and intensity of the headaches.

Physical Assessment

Posture

No obvious postural asymmetry.

Gait

No obvious gait distortions.

Range of Motion

Slightly limited in all directions in the neck with moderate reduction of capital flexion. Temporomandibular joint (TMJ) opens only to two fingers' width (three is normal).

Palpation

Near Touch

Neck near the occipital base and the lower back are warm.

Skin

All areas are normal except for goose bumps and dampness at the occipital base and lower back. Tissue texture is symmetrical and normal. The examiner is unable to lift a skinfold over the entire length of the spinal column.

Superficial Connective Tissue
Superior and inferior binding of connective tissue is present at the occipital base, sacrum, forehead, and calves.
Vessels and Lymph Nodes
Normal.
Muscles
Tender points are noted in the masseter, frontalis, temporalis, and occipital base muscles. Moderate pressure on these points results in pain that mimics the headaches. Neck extensors are short and tight. Surface muscle tone seems generally high. Calf muscles are tight and short bilaterally.
Tendons
Normal.
Deep Fascia
Fascia from the skull to the sacrum binds. Scalp is tightly bound to the skull.
Ligaments
Normal.
Joints
TMJ palpates tender to mild pressure and has reduced range of motion.
Bones
Normal.
Abdominal Viscera
Normal.
Body Rhythms
Rhythmic but fast.

Muscle Testing

Strength
Normal except that head and neck extensors are overly strong. Head and neck flexors are inhibited.

Neurological Balance
Tonic neck reflexes and eye-righting reflexes are overactive; consequently, limb and back extensors do not inhibit when client looks down toward navel.

Gait
Normal except that head seems to be held stiffly when client walks.

Interpretation and Treatment Plan Development

Clinical Reasoning

What Are the Facts?
Muscle tension headaches are a common and recurring problem for many people. They are benign, although all other causes of headaches need to be ruled out. The headaches occur because muscle and connective tissue exert pressure on the nerves and blood vessels in the face, skull, neck, and shoulders. Trigger point activity that refers pain into the headache pain pattern is common. Individuals who are light sensitive or who have visual problems that result in squinting are prone to muscle tension headaches. Heavy headgear or hair that is heavy or styled tightly against the skull presses on pain-sensitive structures. Stress that causes sympathetic arousal, resulting in the attack posture, is a common contributor to muscle tension headaches. Pain of any type can cause the muscles of the head, neck, and face to tighten and can perpetuate muscle tension headaches; in this way, a vicious circle develops. Headaches often "layer," so that even if a migraine is the primary headache type, the pain of the migraine causes an accompanying muscle tension headache.

Postural strain, such as sitting at a computer or driving, or static positions, such as reading a book, result in muscle tension and pressure on pain-sensitive structures, causing a muscle tension headache. Postural strain that attempts to keep the eyes level affects the righting and ocular pelvic reflexes of the neck, eyes, and trunk. Head, neck, and torso flexors should facilitate and head, neck, and torso extensors inhibit when the eyes and head move down toward the midline of the body; the process should reverse when the eyes and head move up, as in looking at the ceiling. Looking right and rotating right cause the muscles on the right to contract concentrically and the muscles on the left to be inhibited and in eccentric function, and vice versa for the left side.

Upper chest breathing is often a contributing factor, because the auxiliary breathing muscles can cause headaches if they are short or have trigger points.

Low back and lower leg involvement is also common and needs to be addressed in conjunction with the more obvious muscle pattern near the head. Connective tissue bind from the occipital base to the sacrum can fix the head, putting pressure on pain-sensitive structures. Poor air quality and noisy environments with uneven or fluctuating lighting can cause headaches. Smoking often contributes to muscle tension headaches.

A muscle tension headache is usually a functional condition, and no obvious pathological condition can be diagnosed. With the client in this case, no pathological reason has been found for the headaches. However, stress is implicated; the client is a self-admitted perfectionist, which supports the stress diagnosis. Shortening of the fascial connection between the skull, occipital base, and sacrum is present. The muscles of the base of the skull and the face, as well as the muscles of mastication, are tender to moderate pressure and reproduce headache pain. The head and neck extensors are short, as are the calf muscles.

What Are the Possibilities in Both Function and Dysfunction and the Massage Intervention Options?
Eyestrain, the weight and position of the glasses, and the heavy hair in a ponytail all may be contributing causal factors. Eyestrain from extended sitting, coupled with the stress of studying, could be contributing to the low back and calf tension.

The clenched jaw and tight arms and legs are components of the attack posture. This posture is part of the sympathetic response and could be part of the symptoms. The noisy environment of the restaurant where the client works could be making the situation worse. Smoking is also a contributing factor. Muscle tension is probably interfering with circulation. No one significant factor appears to be causing the headache pattern; rather, the cause may be the cumulative effect of many small contributing factors, which would explain the random pattern of occurrence. If stress and strain reach a certain level, the headache occurs, such as when the client wears a tight ponytail, has to read in bright light, smokes more than normal, or is stressed by a tight work schedule or a school paper due. The cumulative effect is a headache.

Possibilities

1. Massage and a gentle flexibility program, such as yoga, would help.
2. The heavy hair, eyestrain, and ill-fitting glasses may be causes, and referral to the client's optometrist is prudent. A shorter or more relaxed hairstyle would reduce the weight and strain on the scalp and the muscles in that area.

What Are the Logical Outcomes of Each Possible Intervention?

Some soft tissue factors make muscle tension headaches likely, and these can be addressed with massage. If the muscle shortening is reduced and the connective tissue bind is normalized (conditions noted in the assessment), more external stress may be required to cause the headaches.

A yoga-type activity would reduce stress, help retrain breathing, stretch short tissues, and introduce pliability to the binding connective tissue structures.

A change in glasses to improve the client's eyesight may diminish a causal factor, as might a different hairstyle.

Cost and time are issues. The client is on a limited budget and very busy. Weekly massage sessions would be the minimum required for measurable results.

What Is the Effect on the People Involved for Each Possible Intervention?

The client does not want to cut her hair but is willing to make her ponytail less tight. She will see the optometrist for a checkup. She is not interested in yoga. She will get massages and seems excited about the possibilities for improvement. She is concerned about finances and can afford only two massage sessions a month.

Decision Making and Treatment Plan Development

Primary Goal: Pain Management

Category of Care: Therapeutic Change/Condition Management

Quantifiable Goals

1. Reduce headache pain by 75%.
2. Reduce frequency and duration of headaches by 50%.

Qualifiable Goal

The headaches will decline in number, reducing interference with the client's daily life activities.

Treatment Regimen

Therapeutic Change/Condition Management

The massage sessions will be standard 60-minute appointments at $60 per session, every other week, with time allocated to teach the client self-massage methods. A 10% fee discount applies if 10 sessions are scheduled and paid with cash or check (not credit card) and applied to the 10th massage fee. The client is informed that the massage session includes 5 minutes before and after the massage for assessment and getting disrobed and redressed after the massage is completed. Full-body relaxation massage, using sufficient depth of pressure to produce a parasympathetic effect, will be the main intervention. The primary methods will be compression, gliding, and kneading.

Areas of connective tissue bind, primarily in the occipital and lumbar areas, will require focused work on the superficial fascia, and all methods used will need to have sufficient drag on the tissue. The short calf muscles will be addressed with muscle energy methods to lengthen the muscles. The trigger point areas that refer into the headache pain pattern will be addressed with positional release methods. Pulsed muscle energy or integrated muscle energy methods will be used for areas more resistant to lengthening. Trigger point areas that do not respond to more conservative methods will be addressed with direct compression and stretching of the local tissue, which will be achieved by loading affected tissue with bending and torsion stress. Massage of the face, scalp, and neck is necessary.

The client will be taught self-positional release on the areas of trigger point activity. She will be shown how to apply muscle energy methods, particularly using the position of the eyes or the head to activate a tensing or inhibition of muscles. The main self-help method demonstrated will be to move the soft tissue area restricted by shortened muscles in the position of the tension and then to roll the eyes in slow circles. With this technique, the muscles will move into a facilitated and inhibited neurological pattern. The area then will be gently stretched as the breath is exhaled.

Breathing exercises, as described in Chapter 15, will also be taught as self-help.

CASE 3. GENERALIZED PAIN SYNDROME: SUBCLINICAL FIBROMYALGIA

The client is a 46-year-old female. She works as an administrative assistant for a demanding boss. She has a random work schedule that often involves working into the evening; however, she enjoys the challenges of her job. She has been divorced for 7 years and has two children, who are both in college. Her finances are stable. She is 25 pounds overweight, does not exercise, and does not smoke. She is susceptible to upper respiratory infections and had a bad case of COVID but was not hospitalized. Her sleep and eating cycles are erratic.

She is experiencing generalized muscle and joint aching. She has had symptoms for 5 years, but this past year has been the most difficult. The pain is not constant and fluctuates in intensity and duration. Bad days are beginning to outnumber good days. Medical testing has not revealed any pathological condition. She has seen a rheumatologist and does not quite fit the profile for fibromyalgia syndrome, although she has many of the symptoms and some of the history. Over-the-counter pain medication upsets her stomach.

The client had a severe bout of flu and pneumonia 8 years ago and COVID during the pandemic. Her last physical was 6 weeks ago. Her thyroid-stimulating hormones were a bit elevated, indicating that there may be a thyroid hormone deficiency. Currently she is not being treated with medication but will be retested in 6 months. She is menopausal but still has an occasional menstrual cycle marked by sporadic, heavy bleeding. She is not undergoing hormone replacement therapy at this time. She has mild stress and urinary incontinence. The excess weight is a concern, as is her bone density. A bone scan indicated some bone loss but not sufficient for a diagnosis of osteoporosis. Her cholesterol level is a bit high but still in the normal range.

Her physician recommended an exercise and weight loss program and referred her to the affiliated fitness center, where she saw a brochure for therapeutic massage. She inquired about massage therapy and found that the massage therapist rents space at the fitness center. She called the massage therapist's number, and during the conversation the massage therapist identified that the client's doctor often referred clients to her. This was comforting, and she made an appointment. When she arrived for the massage session, she was surprised to find that the therapist was quite young, in her mid-20s. The massage therapist assured her that she was dedicated to her career and would work diligently to help the client by using her massage skills. The massage fee is $90 for a 60-minute session including pre- and post-massage activities, and the estimated time for hands-on massage ranges from 45 to 50 minutes. The therapist does not accept gratuities or offer discounts. No insurance is accepted. Payment can be made with cash, check, or credit card.

Assessment

Observation

The client is restless, changes position often, and sighs frequently. Movement in the shoulders is noted during normal relaxed breathing. She is neatly groomed and wears high heels. She has a pleasant, even speaking voice. She provides extensive detail in answering all questions. She asks many questions, looking for specific answers. She looks bloated, with indications of swelling in the extremities. Her fat distribution is in the abdomen, creating the "apple shape," which is an indicator of increased risk of heart disease and diabetes.

Interview and Goals

The client does not drink much water; she usually drinks tea or juice. Her client information form shows a family history of autoimmune problems. She has a sister with multiple sclerosis, and her grandmother had lupus. The client had one vaginal birth, and the other child was born by emergency cesarean delivery because of a breech presentation. She takes a multivitamin but no other medications. She has tried various nonsteroidal antiinflammatory drugs (NSAIDs) for pain, but they did not help. Cymbalta was recommended. This medication is thought to work by correcting an imbalance of serotonin and norepinephrine, two brain chemicals known to influence mood. It belongs to a class of antidepressants called selective serotonin and norepinephrine reuptake inhibitors (SNRIs). This medication is also used to treat peripheral neuropathy. The client used the medication for 3 months but did not experience enough relief to justify some of the side effects that occurred. She also read an article explaining that the medication can increase suicidal tendency, which frightened her. The client has been using cannabinoid products, primarily full spectrum edibles and topical CBD lotions.

She indicates that she is stressed but not overwhelmed. She gets a cold every year in the fall, has intestinal gas, and has chronic pain in her muscles and joints. She is restless more than fatigued. She does not participate in exercise and says that she really hates it. She has always been clumsy. She enjoys singing. On a 1 to 10 pain scale (1 being slight, 10 being extreme), she indicates that her pain is usually a 6 with episodes of 8.

Her goals for the massage are to manage the pain and to relax.

Physical Assessment

Posture

Mild lordosis is present, likely functional from wearing high heels. Protruding abdomen, moderate forward head position, and elevated and winged scapula on the left are noted. Shoulders are bilaterally rounded forward, with both arms internally rotated. Legs are externally rotated, more so on the right. Calves are short, and most of the body weight is carried on the balls of the feet.

Gait

Counterbalancing movement of the arms is awkward and reduced. Hips move up and down instead of in a rotational pattern. Most movement occurs at the hips, and client has a short stride. Weight is carried on the ball of the foot, with little heel strike.

Range of Motion

Client is stiff, and her movements are awkward. External rotation and horizontal abduction of the arms are limited by 25%, and dorsiflexion is reduced by 50% bilaterally. Muscle guarding is apparent during passive range of motion, and the client cannot let the body areas go limp.

Palpation

Near Touch

No unusual areas noted.

Skin

Skin feels dry, and pliability is reduced, with binding; skin will not easily lift in a skinfold throughout the body, more so in the lumbar area. Skin shows a reddening, histamine response with light stroking. The effect is most apparent in fleshy areas and less apparent around the joints.

Superficial Connective Tissue

Generally feels boggy and shows nonpitting edema. Edema is more apparent in the legs, which show slight pitting.

Vessels and Lymph Nodes

Normal.

Muscles

Surface layer muscles generally feel soft and nonresilient. Abdominals and gluteus maximus bilaterally are flaccid and long. Second and third layers of muscles (stabilizers and fixators) are short, but client is intolerant of moderate pressure and tenses the surface muscle layer, making palpation difficult. Client is deconditioned as a result of a sedentary lifestyle. Postural muscles (layer three) in lumbar and cervical regions are short. Calves are short, with connective tissue changes resulting in fibrosis, increased tissue density, and ropiness. Muscles of the forearm are tender to palpation with moderate pressure, probably from computer work.

Tendons

Tender points activated by moderate pressure are common in musculotendinous regions body wide.

Deep Fascia

Occipital and cervical fascia, lumbar dorsal fascia, and plantar fasciae are short and bind in all directions.

Ligaments

Joint structure generally is stiff.

Joints

End-feel of joints is stiff and binding. Client guards all range of motion and cannot relax to allow passive range of motion. Light palpation over sacroiliac (SI) and sternoclavicular joints is surprisingly painful.

Bones

Palpation is normal, but caution is indicated because of loss of bone density.

Abdominal Viscera

Difficult to palpate. Surface of abdomen is lumpy. Deeper palpation is uncomfortable to client.

Body Rhythms

Slightly slow and sluggish. Rhythms seem out of sync with each other. Breathing is labored.

Muscle Testing

Strength

Client resists muscle testing, indicating that it hurts to maintain the testing positions. She attempts to cooperate but feels everything is weak and sore. Calves and pectoralis muscles are too strong, and antagonist muscles, especially anterior tibialis and trapezius, are inhibited.

Neurological Balance and Gait

Unable to perform.

Interpretation and Treatment Plan Development

Clinical Reasoning

What Are the Facts?

A strain on the adaptive capacity of the body can manifest as pain syndromes. Generalized pain syndromes are multicausal, and good medical care is required to rule out serious underlying causes. Once a diagnosis of chronic pain syndrome has been made, pain medication and muscle relaxers often are prescribed; however, these are not very successful for long-term treatment. Symptoms that go undiagnosed are especially difficult to treat. In this case the client has not been diagnosed with fibromyalgia, but she displays many of the symptoms.

Fibromyalgia is a condition characterized by aching and pain in the muscles, tendons, and joints all over the body but especially along the spine. Measurable changes in body chemistry and function occur in some people who have fibromyalgia, and these changes may be responsible for certain symptoms. However, fibromyalgia is not associated with muscle, nerve, or joint injury; inadequate muscle repair; or any serious bodily damage or disease. Also, people who have fibromyalgia are not at greater risk for any other musculoskeletal disease. The underlying pathology appears to be related to central nervous system sensitization where normal sensation is interpreted as pain.

The pain of fibromyalgia usually seems worse when a person is trying to relax and is less noticeable during busy activities or exercise. Other symptoms are often associated with the pain, including sleep disturbance, depression, daytime tiredness and headaches, alternating diarrhea and constipation, numbness and tingling in the hands and feet, feelings of weakness, memory difficulties, and dizziness. People with fibromyalgia have "tender points" on the body. Tender points are specific places on the neck, shoulders, back, hips, arms, and legs. These points hurt when pressure is put on them.

Although anyone can develop the condition, it is most common in middle-aged females. People with rheumatoid arthritis and other autoimmune diseases are particularly likely to develop fibromyalgia. Fibromyalgia may also be associated with depression and anxiety.

The causes of fibromyalgia are unknown, but current research is looking at how different parts of the nervous system may contribute to fibromyalgia pain. A person with fibromyalgia may have other, coexisting chronic pain conditions. Such conditions may include chronic fatigue syndrome, endometriosis, interstitial cystitis (painful bladder syndrome), irritable bowel syndrome, temporomandibular joint dysfunction (TMJ), and vulvodynia (chronic vulvar pain).

Researchers have discovered that people who have fibromyalgia process pain signals differently in the central nervous system. As a result, they react more strongly to touch and pressure, with a heightened sensitivity to pain. Some people with fibromyalgia also experience depression. Scientists believe that the condition may be due to injury, emotional distress, or viruses that change the way the brain perceives pain, but the exact cause is unclear. People with rheumatoid arthritis, lupus, and spinal arthritis may be more likely to have the illness. Researchers are looking at the role of substance P and other neurotransmitters and studying why people with fibromyalgia have increased sensitivity to pain and whether specific genes correlate with higher chances of susceptibility. There are alterations in the endocannabinoid system in in some people with fibromyalgia and studies suggest a positive effect of cannabis in fibromyalgia treatment (Berger et al., 2020; Hershkovich et al., 2022; Cohen-Biton et al., 2022).

The onset of fibromyalgia occurs when the stress in a person's life is prominent. Stress often results in disturbed sleep patterns, a lack of restful sleep, and disruption of the production of chemicals necessary to control or regulate pain. Physical and emotional factors may also contribute to the onset of fibromyalgia. For example, a physical illness (e.g., an infection) can cause changes in body chemistry that lead to pain and sleeplessness.

Studies indicate associations between adult fibromyalgia and exposure to stressors such as physical/sexual/emotional abuse and medical trauma (Giorgi et al., 2022). There is evidence that neuroinflammatory pathways affect neuroplasticity in the central nervous system and trigger the onset of fibromyalgia-related symptoms. COVID-19 illness also results in alterations in inflammatory and anti-inflammatory pathways (Kocyigit et al., 2022). Multisystem inflammatory syndrome (MIS) is a rare but serious condition associated with COVID-19 in which different body parts become inflamed, including the heart, lungs, kidneys, brain, skin, eyes, or gastrointestinal organs.

This case describes a typical history pattern of fibromyalgia, including a bad bout of flu and COVID-19, and the accumulation of internal and external stressors over many years. Cumulative trauma and age-related changes, deconditioning from lack of exercise, and a reduction in hardiness are contributing factors. Hormone changes are common. Irregular sleep and eating patterns disrupt the body's sleep/wake cycle. The pain is usually the aching, somatic type. Often any increase in activity results in increased pain over the next 48 hours. This increases the likelihood that the client will remain inactive, which contributes to the problem.

What Are the Possibilities in Both Function and Dysfunction and the Massage Intervention Options?

The client may be slowly deteriorating toward full-blown fibromyalgia. Thyroid deficiency or menopausal symptoms also may be present. Long COVID and dysregulation in the immune system may also be factors. There could be a past trauma history.

Possibilities

1. General constitutional massage may help, with caution regarding the intensity because the pain can be aggravated by massage that is too aggressive.
2. Lymphatic drainage massage is indicated, and light pressure and rhythmic application are appropriate. The deeper muscles that are short and the connective tissue changes should be addressed once pain tolerance has increased and the client can tolerate deeper pressure.
3. The physician recommended an exercise program. Hydrotherapy, with a focus on alternating hot and cold applications, is supported both for relaxation and for stimulating adaptive capacity. Mineral salt soaks can alleviate some aching. Massage would be needed regularly, at least once a week.
4. Massage therapy may be synergistic with cannabis use.

What Are the Logical Outcomes of Each Possible Intervention?

Exercise and massage may increase the pain symptoms in the short term. However, massage is less likely to cause discomfort if given carefully.

Hydrotherapy application of alternating hot and cold with mineral salt soaks would be well tolerated if introduced gradually.

The effects of edible and topical cannabis products may be enhanced.

The client can schedule the time and has the finances.

What Is the Effect on the People Involved for Each Possible Intervention?

The client is not supportive of exercise, and compliance does not seem likely. She is lonely and indicates that the idea of massage and how it feels is comforting to her. She says she would do hydrotherapy but does not like to be cold.

The massage professional realizes that the client has implicated boundary issues and that this is a long-term professional commitment. Without some exercise, the condition will not improve. The client needs to be encouraged to work with a medical exercise professional to support compliance with an exercise program and for possible referral to a nutritionist because changes in hormone balance can affect nutritional needs. A coordinated and supervised program of cannabis use may be beneficial.

Decision Making and Treatment Plan Development

Primary Goal: Pain Management
Category of Care: Condition Management

Quantifiable Goals

1. Reduce aching pain from a 6 to a 4 on a 1- to 10-point pain scale.
2. Reduce constant aching to intermediate aching with more good days per week (4 good and 3 bad).

Qualifiable Goal

The client will be able to perform daily living and work activities more efficiently and participate in a moderate exercise program without intensifying the current symptoms.

Treatment Regimen

Condition management will be pursued, with moderate applications affecting therapeutic change in a three-stage treatment plan.

Some clear soft tissue dysfunctions must be addressed. The lordosis, forward head, rounded shoulders with internally rotated arms, and immobile pelvis with externally rotated legs strain adaptive mechanisms. This posture puts extreme pressure on the SI joints and neck stabilizers and restricts the mobility of the thorax, resulting in shallow upper chest breathing. The shortened calf muscles and plantar fasciae, the result of wearing high heels for so many years, have body-wide implications. Reduced lymphatic movement, strain caused by maintenance of posture, control of postural sway, and restricted breathing all were indicated in the assessment. All these factors must be addressed, but caution is necessary. This client, although not sick, seems to have reached the end of her adaptive capacity. Therapeutic change must be introduced gradually. Slowing degeneration and managing current symptoms are initially most important. Attempting too many adaptations likely would make matters worse.

The three phases of the treatment plan are as follows:

- *Phase 1:* The first phase will focus on general relaxation and hyperstimulation analgesia for pain control. The duration of the massage will not exceed 45 minutes. The massage will be rhythmic and repetitive, using primarily gliding and kneading, with a pressure and depth that the client identifies as pleasurable. Parasympathetic activation and an increase in serotonin are the goals; therefore the massage will have a compressive quality but will not cause pain. Lymphatic drainage and circulation enhancement are appropriate. Foot massage, which is safe and well tolerated, will have a more intense quality, bordering on "good hurt," in an attempt to encourage endogenous pain-killing chemical activity, as well as hyperstimulation analgesia and counterirritation. Localization of this type of intensity to the feet prevents any other delayed muscle soreness from developing. The client will be encouraged to take hot, relaxing Epsom salt baths and be consistent with the mild water aerobics program, set up by an exercise physiologist, that she has agreed to try. This phase could last 12 weeks.

- *Phase 2:* Massage pressure and depth will increase to address the short muscles and introduce the concept of "good hurt" into the areas that are short and tight in the second and third layers of muscles. Tissue elongation methods will address the areas of connective tissue bind in the superficial fascia. Muscle energy, primarily positional release, will be used on tender points identified by the deeper massage. Foot massage of sufficient pressure and intensity to cause a good hurt will continue. The client should be only mildly sore the next day and only in a couple areas. The exercise program will be supported by a focus on water aerobics and mild training with light weights. Self-help will include a splash of cold water after a warm bath and daily cool water foot soaks. The temperature of the footbaths should be decreased to cold within a 2-week period. This phase could last up to 12 weeks.
- *Phase 3:* The goal now is to introduce small, incremental structural and functional shifts to the postural distortion. The massage quality will increase in depth of pressure and drag to address the connective tissue bind in the deeper postural muscle layers and the underlying muscle tension. The massage will remain relaxing, rhythmic, and pleasurable but will take on the quality of an adjunct to the exercise program. Muscle energy methods, particularly integrated methods, can address body-wide muscle interaction patterns. More aggressive connective tissue methods to restore pliability will be introduced with muscle energy methods and muscle lengthening, but this must be coupled with strengthening of the weakened and inhibited muscle patterns. Trigger point activity, particularly in the muscle belly of concentrically short muscles, can be gradually addressed one area per session. Alternating hot and cold showers, beginning with hot and ending with cold, should replace the baths and soaks. This phase will last 12 to 24 weeks.

The entire process could take 1 year.

If the client does not maintain an exercise program, condition management would be a more appropriate treatment and would level out at the first phase of the long-term plan. After 6 months the less invasive applications described in phase 2 could be introduced to see how the client responds. Without a corresponding exercise program, phase 3 would be too aggressive.

CASE 4. NECK AND SHOULDER PAIN WITH LIMITED RANGE OF MOTION

The client is a 34-year-old truck driver. They are right-handed but drive primarily with their left hand. Three years ago the client took a hard fall while riding their mountain bike. They suffered a mild concussion and remember having a stiff neck for about a month. The client is in good health, active, and exercises regularly. They eat a moderate diet and do not abuse caffeine or alcohol or smoke.

The client is experiencing radiating pain into the left scapula and upper deltoid and down the left arm to the elbow. The pain was sudden in onset, and it has an aching, throbbing quality. The pain grows worse as the day progresses, and it is interfering with their sleep, because they cannot find a comfortable position. They also complain of a stiff neck, especially if turning their head to the right. This has been occurring for about 6 months. The client had an upper respiratory infection and a severe cough a month before the current pain symptoms began. The client was referred to chiropractic care by their medical doctor. The chiropractor has had limited success and suspects muscle involvement. Heat provides temporary relief, and cold makes the condition worse. Aspirin helps, as do muscle relaxers, but medications are not the best long-term solution. The client is single, financially stable, and available for appointments on a regular basis. The massage therapist is an employee of the chiropractor.

Assessment

Observation

Client frequently rubs the left side of their neck, left shoulder, and upper arm in a line pattern that follows the brachial plexus distribution. The client is frustrated with the situation but seems happy in general and jokes about the condition and that it is an excuse to get a massage.

Interview and Goals

Nothing out of the ordinary is seen on the client information form other than the information given in the case. Referral information from the chiropractor indicates generalized soft tissue restriction in the neck and shoulder area. In answering a question, the client says that they were on vacation in Mexico for 3 weeks before getting the cold and cough. The cough lasted for a week, and they used over-the-counter cough suppressants. For years the client has ridden a bike at least three times a week for 10 miles. The head injury from their fall was considered minor and was not treated other than with the initial evaluation. They were told the neck stiffness was normal for this type of injury and would dissipate, which it did. They look over their left shoulder while backing up the truck they drive. The client cannot remember doing anything unusual but woke up with the stiffness in the neck and pain in the shoulder and thinks they "slept funny."

The client's goal is to get a massage for a few weeks, but only wants the neck and shoulder pain addressed. The client understands that full-body massage is necessary to address localized problems successfully but says that nothing else bothers them. They intend to keep seeing the chiropractor.

Physical Assessment

Posture

Basically symmetrical with minor rotation of the head to the left. Right leg is moderately externally rotated. Lumbar curve is flat. Chin juts forward with corresponding head tilting backward and forward head position.

Gait

Head is held stiffly during walking. Arm and leg swing appears normal. Weight is carried on the outside of right foot instead of evenly distributed between both feet.

Range of Motion

Right rotation and lateral flexion of the head are limited by 15%. Internal rotation of the right leg is limited by 10%.

Palpation

Near Touch

Client flinched before the neck area on the left was actually touched. Heat is noted in the area.

Skin

Surface is damp with goose bumps from the base of the head to midarm on the left. When rubbed, the area shows increased reddening and itching from histamine response. Resilience is reduced over the area of skin surfaces that are damp and red. Most superficial connective tissue binds in the caudal and diagonal directions to the right. Bilateral bind is seen on the chest from the superior to midsternal area and to the shoulder.

Superficial Connective Tissue

Skinfolds between the scapulae are uneven, with the left side more restricted. Connective tissue bind in all directions exists in the right lumbar area.

Vessels and Lymph Nodes

Normal.

Muscles

The neck extensors, particularly at the occipital base, and the arm horizontal adductors are short. Scalenes on the left are short, with trigger point activity and typical referred pain patterns into the symptom area. All serratus muscles are taut, with the anterior serratus short (concentric) and the posterior superior and inferior serratus muscles long (eccentric). Eccentric muscles display attachment trigger points, and concentric muscles exhibit muscle belly trigger points. Calf muscles are short.

Tendons

Mild tenderness in response to moderate pressure is seen at the subscapular and pectoralis major arm attachments bilaterally.

Deep Fascia

Mild caudal binding (tissue moves up but binds when moving down) occurs in all superficial fascial regions: thorax, abdomen, lumbar area, iliotibial band, calves, and plantar fasciae.

Ligaments

Normal.

Joints

Functional range-of-motion limitations are seen where short muscles reduce extension, horizontal abduction, and internal rotation. No specific joint problems are identified.

Bones

Normal.

Abdominal Viscera

Normal.

Body Rhythms

Breathing rhythm is fast in relation to other rhythms. Client has a tendency for upper chest breathing.

Muscle Testing

Strength

Muscles identified as short tested overly strong, with an exaggerated contraction response. Client had difficulty applying a gradual increase in pressure against resistance and instead responded by quickly jerking and pushing with full strength. These same muscles would not inhibit when the antagonists were contracted. Weakness was noted in the neck flexors. Movement of the eyes downward did not increase neck flexor strength, as would be expected. Movement of the eyes upward, as in looking overhead, increased flexor weakness and significantly increased tension in the neck extensors. Shoulder and hip firing patterns show synergistic dominance.

Gait

Opposite hip flexor and extensor patterns did not inhibit as expected (when the right hip flexors were activated, the left did not inhibit but maintained strength, and vice versa). Arm and leg patterns also were out of sync, with flexion bilaterally and lack of inhibition regardless of direct activation of antagonist or expected inhibition pattern in gait. The hip flexors on the same side, when activated, would be expected to inhibit the arm flexors (i.e., left inhibits left and right inhibits right), but this did not occur. Arm flexors stayed activated and tested strong regardless of the muscle pattern activated.

Interpretation and Treatment Plan Development

Clinical Reasoning

What Are the Facts?

Neck and shoulder stiffness and pain are among the most common complaints a massage professional will encounter. These can have many causal factors. Postural distortion from a rotated or elevated shoulder girdle is common. This condition is often a compensation pattern that develops in response to postural distortion somewhere else in the body. Because the eyes must be positioned forward and level with the horizontal plane, muscle tone, firing patterns, and joint functions commonly shift in this region. To correct this, the entire body pattern needs to be addressed. A common cause of the problem is eyestrain, especially combined with a static seated position, such as occurs with desk and computer work or extended periods of driving. Distorted sleep patterns, often coupled with nasal congestion, add to the situation. Upper chest breathing, such as is found with breathing pattern disorders, almost always involves neck and shoulder compensation. A forward head position strains the neck and shoulder structure. The brachial plexus and cervical plexus are often impinged, because the space through which these nerves travel is crowded, and any increase in muscle tension, changes in the joint position in the area, shortening of the connective tissue, or increases in fluid may result in pressure on nerves and blood vessels. The scalene and pectoralis minor muscles are often involved. (**Note:** Muscle aching gets worse as the day goes on. Joint pain is worse in the morning, gets better during the day, and then increases as the body fatigues.)

The client is young and generally in good health. They have a history of head trauma, along with occupational and recreational activities that have resulted in postural distortion. The anterior flexors and adductors are shortened, and the posterior extensors are inhibited, long, and locked into an eccentric contraction pattern. The generalized connective tissue binding is consistent with repetitive use and the activities that require static positions. Trigger point referred pain patterns are consistent with the symptoms.

What Are the Possibilities in Both Function and Dysfunction and the Massage Intervention Options?

Repetitive strain should be suspected with the static position of truck driving (i.e., looking left and arm positions that shorten the brachial space). The effects of biking also should be considered, given its static position of arms forward, torso bent forward with back rounded, and head forward and extended at the occipital base. Calf shortening and general fascial shortening, attributable to the client's occupational and recreational activities, may be other factors.

Both biking and driving have the arms bent forward with the trunk flexed. This would disrupt gait reflexes over time.

The client displays the typical muscle patterns of a person who has had an extended cough (serratus involvement). An ongoing adaptive process over the past few years likely has finally caught up with the client, and the coughing bout probably further shortened the muscles that surround the brachial nerve plexus. Soft tissue impingement has likely irritated the brachial plexus on the left.

The head trauma and resulting stiff neck may have caused an adaptive process that has deteriorated, resulting in nerve pain in the symptom area. A trigger point referral pain pattern in the scalenes is implicated.

In situations like this, all the stated possibilities probably are involved in the pattern.

Possibilities

1. Massage intervention would need to reduce trigger point activity in all identified areas and increase the pliability of all binding and short connective tissue structures.
2. Muscle energy methods and massage manipulations to lengthen shortened muscles, plus exercise and stretching activities that balance the repetitive posture of driving and biking, should be introduced.
3. Yoga or a similar gentle flexibility and movement system would be a valid option.

What Are the Logical Outcomes of Each Possible Intervention?

Massage and a gentle stretching program would be effective in reducing symptoms.

What seems like a simple problem is actually quite complex, and effective intervention would take longer than the client indicates they are willing to commit to. Because the situation is likely a cumulative adaptive process, the condition may become worse before it improves.

What Is the Effect on the People Involved for Each Possible Intervention?

The client resists the complexity of the situation, believing it is a localized issue, and does not want long-term intervention.

The client is not interested in yoga but would learn about stretching and incorporate some of the stretches.

Decision Making and Treatment Plan Development

Primary Goal: Functional Mobility

Category of Care: Therapeutic Change/Condition Management

Quantifiable Goals

1. Restore normal resting length to concentrically contracted short muscles.
2. Increase right rotation and lateral flexion of the head by 10%.
3. Increase external rotation of the right leg by 10%.
4. Reverse connective tissue bind.

Qualifiable Goal

The client will be able to use arm and turn head without pain during normal daily work and recreational activities.

Treatment Regimen

Therapeutic Change/Condition Management

The treatment plan will consist of 12 90-minute weekly sessions. Each session will include pre- and post-massage procedures and generalized massage with a superficial fascia elongation drag component, coupled with muscle energy and inhibitory pressure and movement approaches such as pin and stretch, to lengthen the short muscles that are directly contributing to the brachial plexus impingement. This will include the lateral neck flexors on the left and the horizontal arm adductors and internal arm rotators bilaterally. Six weekly sessions will be scheduled, and the results will then be evaluated. Gait reflex and firing patterns will be monitored to identify any improvement. Self-help stretching education will be presented to the client. Information will be provided to the chiropractor on massage intervention methods for long-term chiropractic support.

CASE 5. GENERALIZED LOW BACK PAIN WITH LIMITED RANGE OF MOTION

The female client is 28 years old. She is a cashier and bagger at a large grocery store chain and has been on the job for 1 year. She is 40 pounds overweight, with fat distribution primarily in the breasts and abdomen. She has been experiencing low back pain for a few years. The pain is sporadic but worse during her menstrual period, which is also marked by moderately severe menstrual cramps. Since she started working at the store, the menstrual cramps have grown steadily worse.

A general physical indicated no apparent pathological condition. A physical examination ruled out disk and nerve problems and indicated muscle tension and strain. Her doctor said the probable cause is her excess weight. On her doctor's recommendation, she started a walking program and has been reducing food portions to support gradual weight loss.

The doctor also prescribed muscle relaxants to be taken as needed. Lately the client has been taking the medication daily in the evening. The pain worsens as the day goes on; it is relieved initially when she lies down but becomes worse if she lies or sits still for an extended period. She was referred to a physical therapist who designed a rehabilitation exercise program and recommended massage intervention under the physical therapist's supervision.

The physical therapist employs a massage therapist. With less than 1 year of experience, the massage therapist feels confident to address such conditions since they were a physical therapy aid for the PT.

Assessment

Observation

The client is restless; she is in and out of her chair during the entire interview because she is unable to sit for longer than about 10 minutes before her back begins to hurt. Each time she gets up, she places her hands on her knees and pushes herself up. She places her hands behind her back and rubs the lumbar area frequently. When she stands, she distributes her weight evenly on both feet, locks the knees back, and crosses her arms across her chest. She then paces, putting her hand on her left hip. She sighs, as if movement is labored. She also appears to be retaining fluid. Her face is strained. Her manner is pleasant, but her conversation is peppered with negatives and frustration.

Interview and Goals

The history indicates that the client has worked as a cashier since high school and is currently studying computer science. She either stands at the counter, moving groceries and packing bags, or sits in class or at the computer. She has always been a bit overweight, as have her parents. She has never been active, and the only sports activity she enjoys is bowling. Nothing unusual shows up on the history form other than painful menstrual cramps, use of muscle relaxants, and typical childhood diseases. A sharp pain occurs in her back when she coughs or sneezes. Rolling over in bed is uncomfortable. When asked to place her hands on the pain area, she presses across the lumbar area as she moves the pelvis into anterior and posterior rotation. She also specifically points at the SI joints.

She is single and has a small circle of friends. Her parents and sibling live in the next town. She is in a bowling league in the winter. The client's goals for the massage are to reduce her low back dysfunction substantially and to increase her general well-being.

Physical Assessment

Posture

Moderate lordosis, slight kyphosis, and an increased cervical curve with a forward head and a tendency for hyperextended knees are seen. Posture is bilaterally symmetrical from the anterior and posterior views. Postural distortion is most apparent when client is viewed from the side.

Gait

Client walks stiff legged, with little movement at the SI joints. Contralateral arm swing is minimal.

Range of Motion

Trunk flexion in the lumbar area is restricted, and most forward movement occurs at the hips; it is limited by short hamstrings. Muscle spasm pain limits side bending of the torso to 20 degrees bilaterally. Rotation at the lumbar area is limited to the right.

Palpation

Near Touch

Heat is noted in the lumbar area.

Skin

Damp areas are noted in the lumbar area lateral to the spine near the sides of the body, and the skin is generally tight in the areas where symptoms occur. The fingernails have some horizontal ridges and hangnails. Adherence of the skin with binding is palpated in the lumbar area, more lateral and adjacent to the iliac crest.

Superficial Connective Tissue

Bogginess and a mild tendency for surface edema are noted.

Vessels and Lymph Nodes

Normal.

Muscles

Abdominals and gluteus maximus are long and weak. Neck flexors, latissimus dorsi, psoas, hamstrings, quadratus lumborum, and all calf muscles are short.

Tendons

Musculotendinous junction of the hamstrings is tender at the ischial hamstring attachment and taut at the knee attachment.

Deep Fascia

Lumbar dorsal fascia is short and binding, with influence extending up into the cranial base and along the lateral aspect of the legs and bottoms of both feet. The abdominal fascia is loose, nonelastic, and nonresilient.

Ligaments

Reduced pliability is noted around the SI joint.

Joints

SI joint is restricted bilaterally; the knees are hyperextended. Lumbar vertebrae seem compressed. Symphysis pubis is upslipped on the left with a bilateral anterior pelvic rotation, more so on the right.

Bones

Normal.

Abdominal Viscera

Abdomen is soft with no palpable abnormalities.

Body Rhythms

Fast with mild dysrhythmia.

Muscle Testing

Strength

Difficult to assess because client experiences pain in low back during testing. Abdominals and gluteus maximus are weak, back extensors are too strong, and psoas bilaterally appears weak.

Neurological Balance

Difficult to test because client experiences pain. Generally client seems deconditioned.

Gait

Muscle interaction pattern has shifted from the normal opposite arm/leg flexor/flexor-extensor/extensor facilitation pattern to a same-side arm/leg flexor and arm/leg extensor pattern. As a result, the contralateral arm swing has been lost, and a substantially reduced, same-side arm swing pattern is noted. Gluteus maximus does not fire in the normal sequence. Hamstrings fire first during hip extension.

Interpretation and Treatment Plan Development

Clinical Reasoning

What Are the Facts?

Low back pain in the absence of disk dysfunction is common. Causal factors vary, but common elements exist. Client histories include either standing or sitting in static positions, coupled with upper torso twisting or some sort of trauma, such as a car accident or strain during lifting or pushing. Medication is not effective in the management of low back pain. Some sort of pelvic rotation distortion usually is present, as is an upper body compensation pattern of rotated shoulder girdle, altered head position, or change in the thoracic or cervical spinal curvature. Sternoclavicular joint dysfunction is often seen with SI joint dysfunction.

The three most common causes of low back pain are as follows:

- Muscle/connective tissue shortening with some nerve entrapment.
- Tender/trigger point activity in the psoas, quadratus lumborum, and hamstrings, which causes a more generalized, aching pain with painful spasm on sudden movement or coughing and sneezing. This pattern is aggravated by any type of static position, including prolonged lying down, and often results in restless activity, such as changing positions frequently.
- SI joint dysfunction, which has a more localized pain pattern. The pain normally gets worse as the day progresses and eases when the person lies down.

The three forms are often found in conjunction, which further complicates the issue.

The client in this case fits the profile of combined muscle, connective tissue, and SI joint dysfunction. She does not like exercise and movement, especially because walking is labored and awkward. She stands, twists, and lifts weight with her arms as she bags groceries, which puts strain on her low back. She is overweight, with the "apple type" fat distribution that shifts the center of gravity forward, requiring the back extensors to work harder to maintain an upright posture.

She has menstrual cramping, and the low back pain is worse during menstruation. This makes sense, because psoas tightening is common during menstruation. Stress tends to lower pain tolerance and increase muscle tension. The ridges in her nails and the hangnails indicate both long-term and current stress influences. The physical therapist has instituted a rehabilitation exercise program, and the client is following a walking program. Medication has not been identified as a long-term option.

What Are the Possibilities in Both Function and Dysfunction and the Massage Intervention Options?

The client has common symptoms of general low back pain with SI joint involvement. Her job activities are of a type that can commonly aggravate an existing situation. In her case, the job seems to be aggravating the symptoms, which range from occasional and bearable to constant and distressing. She could likely be helped by mobilization of the SI joint, with recommendations provided to the physical therapist.

Because of the edema, some subclinical kidney dysfunction may be present that would result in low back aching; the patient should be referred for diagnosis of this condition. Menstrual difficulties are part of the history and might be an underlying factor.

Stress levels are increased and are likely contributing to the increase in pain perception. Chronic pain is disempowering emotionally and draining on the neurochemical functions of the body. All the endogenous opioids, such as endorphins and other neurotransmitters and mood-elevating neurochemicals such as serotonin, may be insufficient for the current demands in her life, and the results of this insufficiency are sporadic mood difficulties and increased pain perception. Chronic pain can become a habit, leading to a cycle of fear-based reduction of activity, which then increases deconditioning. Chronic pain is a complex psychosocial and physical situation. Referral to the physician with a recommendation for counseling is prudent. The physical therapist would need to be informed of this recommendation and make the referral.

The client's generally inactive lifestyle has resulted in deconditioning and a predisposition to muscle aching. This, combined with her excess weight and the abdominal fat distribution, is likely a main causal factor.

Possibilities

1. General massage can be provided with a focus on restoring pliability to shortened connective tissue structures and reducing trigger point activity in the short muscles, accompanied by muscle energy methods to lengthen the short muscle groups and restore normal firing patterns.
2. Lymphatic drainage massage is indicated to manage the edema.
3. Targeted foot massage is indicated, especially when combined with full-body massage, because it is well tolerated and the client shows shortening of the plantar fasciae.
4. Vacuum decompression methods (cupping) could help with connective tissue binding and be taught as a self-help method.

5. Stress levels could be managed with massage and some sort of gentle movement activity, such as walking, yoga, or both.
6. Aromatherapy is an option in conjunction with massage and as a self-help measure.
7. Recommendations are indicated for an increased intake of water, fresh fruits, and vegetables. A combined, multidisciplinary approach offers the greatest likelihood of sustained benefit.

What Are the Logical Outcomes of Each Possible Intervention?

Cost is a factor in all massage applications. The massage session fee of $45 per session is a major limiting factor.

Time is limited, as is the client's stamina. Too much intervention would tend to overwhelm her, and compliance would decrease. She is already seeing a physical therapist and walking.

Massage may provide the most benefit, with little energy requirement from the client. Aromatherapy and hydrotherapy are self-maintaining and pleasant and have low cost and time factors.

What Is the Effect on the People Involved for Each Possible Intervention?

The client likes the massage, mineral salt bath, and aromatherapy ideas but is resistant to yoga. The client is intrigued by the cupping and would like to try it. She seems a bit desperate, and the massage therapist will have to monitor boundary issues and maintain a supportive relationship with other caregivers.

Decision Making and Treatment Plan Development

Primary Goal: Pain Management
Secondary Goal: Functional Mobility
Category of Care: Condition Management

Quantifiable Goals

1. Increase mobility of the lumbar region by 75%.
2. Reduce pain-affected days by 50%.
3. Restore normal gait and firing patterns.

Qualifiable Goal

The client will be able to perform work and school activities without limitations caused by low back pain 5 out of 7 days a week. She will experience less fatigue when walking.

Treatment Regimen

Condition management will be pursued, with moderate expectations of therapeutic change.

A 45-minute massage in a 60-minute scheduled session will be provided twice a week for the first 4 weeks or until improvement is noted and indicated by reduced pain perception and an increased range of motion. The frequency then will be reduced to once a week. This may be the maintenance schedule because ongoing massage intervention is probably necessary to maintain a stable condition after physical therapy is complete.

The massage will consist of full-body application with a fluid movement focus and incorporation of vacuum decompression on the areas of connective tissue binding.

The focus is to increase mood-elevating chemicals with a broad-based, firm but not painful, compressive force and rhythmic application. Once the stress levels have dropped, the decreased pliability of shortened connective tissue structures can be addressed with methods that elongate and drag the superficial fascia. Reduction of trigger/tender point activity in the short muscles is indicated, using positional release and direct inhibitory pressure combined with muscle energy methods and lengthening for the short muscle groups.

The client will be referred to an aromatherapist for consultation and recommendation regarding essential oils to be used during the massage and for self-application.

The client will be taught self-help measures, including hydrotherapy consisting of soaking baths, heat on the aching muscles, and cold on the joint pain. The client will be taught self-foot massage and how to use softballs, baseballs, and foam rollers to massage painful areas in her back. She will also be taught how to use suction cupping.

Close contact with the physical therapist will be necessary to achieve effective treatment for the client. The client will also be referred to her physician for recommendations regarding counseling for mood regulation.

CASE 6. ATHLETIC DELAYED-ONSET MUSCLE SORENESS

The client is a 22-year-old rookie cornerback professional football player. It is the second week of training camp, and the weather is hot and humid. The training regimen includes various running and sprinting segments, position-dependent drills, and strengthening and conditioning with a weightlifting program. The team's warm-up includes stretching activities. Maximum performance is required to secure a position on the team, and the competition is fierce. During the past 5 days, the players have been wearing full equipment for the morning practice and pads, helmet, and shorts for the afternoon practice. The training staff has been diligent about keeping all players hydrated, and ice baths are available. The client has been regularly soaking his legs in the ice water tubs.

One afternoon the client reports to the trainer that he aches all over and has cramping in his hamstrings and calves. The leg cramping goes away with increased hydration and ingestion of electrolytes. He has been referred to the team massage therapist for management of delayed-onset muscle soreness. The client does not want the massage during the afternoon break because he is afraid it will affect his afternoon practice; therefore he is requesting evening sessions after team meetings.

Assessment

Observation

The client is emotionally pumped but seems fatigued. His movements are generally a bit stiff. He keeps trying to stretch out while talking. He shows upper chest breathing, he is talking fast, and the exhale is shorter than the inhale. His phasic (movement) muscles appear bulked up.

Interview and Goals

When asked how well he is sleeping, the client reports that he is tossing and turning and cannot get comfortable. He also reports a 5-pound weight gain and an increase in thigh, arm, and chest measurements. His history indicates a grade 2 groin pull on the right during the last year of college. It healed well but the area continues to get stiff. He has to keep the area stretched out or he feels the pulling. He has been playing football since high school. Nothing unusual is disclosed in the history form except a recent tendency for constipation. On a pain scale of 1 to 10, he says it feels like a 12.

His goals for the massage are to reduce the aching and stiff feelings and to enhance his athletic performance. The trainer's goal is management of delayed-onset muscle soreness.

Physical Assessment

Posture

Appropriate for football positional demands.

Gait

Slightly reduced stride on the right.

Range of Motion

Abduction of the right leg is reduced by 10% compared with the left leg and has a binding end-feel. Elbow and knee flexion bilaterally are reduced slightly because of soft tissue approximation (muscle tissue bumping into itself).

Palpation

Near Touch

Client generally is giving off heat.

Skin

Generally taut and damp with axillae, feet, and hand sweating. Binding at clavicles may interfere with lymph flow. Tissue in general feels dense but boggy.

Superficial Connective Tissue

Dense.

Vessels and Lymph Nodes

Difficult to palpate because they seem buried in tissue.

Muscles

Muscle tone is appropriate for training effect. General tone is increased from client's first visit a month ago, indicating a response to training effects during training camp. Gluteus maximus bilaterally is short and tight.

Tendons

General tenderness at musculotendinous junction in the phasic (movement) muscles of the arms and legs.

Deep Fascia

Mild binding during both superior and inferior movement in the sheath that runs from the cranial base to the sacrum and continues down the iliotibial band into the calves. Bind also is noted in the abdominal muscles and the pectoralis fasciae.

Ligaments

Normal.

Joints

Aching increased with traction, indicating a soft tissue problem as a primary causal factor.

Bones

Normal.

Abdominal Viscera

Abdominal muscle development makes palpation difficult; appears normal, with some fullness over the descending colon.

Body Rhythms

Fast upper chest breathing pattern.

Muscle Testing

Strength

All muscles test strong, but excessive synergistic recruitment is evident.

Neurological Balance

Generalized hypersensitivity, evidenced by a fast, jerky contraction pattern and inability to contract muscles slowly.

Gait

Normal, but inhibition pattern for the arms is slow to engage (it takes a few seconds for muscles to let go).

Interpretation and Treatment Plan Development

Clinical Reasoning

What Are the Facts?

Delayed-onset muscle soreness is a complicated response to increased physical and muscular activity demands. It can be local or generalized, depending on the activity. Although the term *delayed-onset muscle soreness* indicates a muscle problem, the situation more likely involves the circulatory, lymph, and autonomic nervous systems and breathing functions. Simple delayed-onset muscle soreness in local areas results when a muscle moves repetitively in eccentric action. This is common in any type of weight-training program intended to bulk up, or create hypertrophy, in muscles. Inflammation occurs and possibly some microtearing of muscle fibers. Inflammatory mediators (primarily histamine), which are released during physical activity, increase capillary permeability; as a result, interstitial fluid accumulates, causing simple edema. The increased fluid pressure in the tissue stimulates pain receptors, making the person feel stiff and achy.

In addition the buildup of metabolic by-products (not lactic acid) from exercise irritates nerve endings. Increased muscle tone can result in pressure on lymphatic vessels, interfering with the normal lymphatic flow, further stressing the lymphatic system. In addition, increased sympathetic arousal, which is part of athletic function, especially in contact sports, increases arterial pressure and blood flow. If the normal expansion in the capillary bed of the muscle is restricted because of increased muscle tension and connective tissue thickening, more plasma flows out of the capillaries, requiring the lymphatic system to handle the increased interstitial fluid volume. When the body is in a sympathetic state, the ground substance of the connective tissue thickens to provide more resistance to impact. This process should reverse itself when arousal diminishes and parasympathetic dominance takes over, but often with athletes the arousal levels do not reverse and the connective tissue remains thicker, placing pressure on pain receptors and contributing to stiffness.

The combination of fluid pressure and connective tissue thickening makes the tissue feel taut and dense. More complex patterns result with sustained sympathetic arousal. Upper chest breathing patterns and a tendency for breathing pattern disorders are common and perpetuate the underlying sympathetic arousal.

Management of this condition requires the reduction of any muscle tension interfering with circulation and lymphatic flow, mechanical drainage of interstitial fluid, support for arterial and venous circulation, reduction of the sympathetic arousal pattern, and an increase in ground substance pliability. The process must be accomplished without adding any inflammation to the tissues. Frictioning and any other methods that would cause tissue damage are contraindicated.

Delayed-onset muscle soreness seen in planned training programs is to be expected. Each sport (in this case, football) position places specific demands on certain movement patterns. It is essential that massage applications support the training effect and not interfere with it. Although symmetry in form is ideal, specific sport demand causes hypertrophy in certain muscle groups, and body-wide compensation occurs during a normal training regimen. This has to be considered during the assessment and the application of massage.

This particular client has symptoms of combined delayed-onset muscle soreness and sustained sympathetic arousal. His breathing is appropriate for training activity but is not reversing during downtime; consequently, his sleep is disturbed, and he is constipated. Tissues are filled with fluid, and thickened ground substance makes the tissue feel dense. Connective tissue binding exists in the back and the groin, especially on the right, and in the chest in the area of the right and left lymphatic ducts. Reduced abdominal movement, resulting from the upper chest breathing and the overdeveloped abdominal muscles (primarily the rectus abdominis), does not support movement of the lymph in the abdominal cavity. The muscle strength, with synergistic recruitment and slow response to inhibition patterns, can be attributed to overtraining and sympathetic arousal.

What Are the Possibilities in Both Function and Dysfunction and the Massage Intervention Options?

The client probably is excited about playing professional football and trying to prove himself in camp. He may have some anxiety about making the team, because competition is fierce for his position. This all contributes to sympathetic arousal. He may be overtraining, especially in the weight room, because he is quickly bulking up.

The training regimen in general is a cause of a delayed-onset muscle soreness pattern and stress. The weight of equipment worn during practice (about 20 pounds) is a new strain on the system and adjusting to it can increase soft tissue soreness. Needing to learn all the plays in the playbook adds stress.

Possibilities

In combination with the athletic trainer's support and proper hydration, massage can be focused to achieve the following:

1. Reduce the sympathetic arousal.
2. Soften the connective tissue ground substance.
3. Support lymphatic flow.

Weight training intensity should be reduced to more appropriate levels as recommended by the strength and conditioning coach.

What Are the Logical Outcomes of Each Possible Intervention?

The massage will likely help but needs to be done in the evening before the client goes to bed. This will make scheduling difficult.

The player must stay hydrated, and increased urine production may awaken him at night, interfering with sleep.

If the massage intervention is too intense, he may be sluggish the next day and his performance will be compromised.

Sleep would improve, which would reduce the recovery time. Reflexes should be more appropriate, and coordination and timing should improve, which supports performance.

What Is the Effect on the People Involved for Each Possible Intervention?

Training personnel referred the client; therefore they are supportive. The position coach does not like rookies "babied" and feels that the client should "tough it out" a bit and not look like a whiner. The player has had massage before and liked it but is worried about anything that could affect his performance. He is also confused about the type of massage he has had previously. The "deep tissue" massage left him sore and sluggish for a couple of days. The massage therapist he saw previously overstretched the groin and made the stiffness worse. He has had some massage sessions that were, in his words, "just not worth the time and money." The massage therapist feels that it is important to deal with the situation but does not enjoy beginning massage at 9:30 PM. They are an experienced massage therapist and have been affiliated with this team for 5 years. The team provides the massage location adjacent to the training room for no fee and during training camp provides food and lodging. The players pay the massage therapist directly for the massage sessions at $75 per hour. The player is likely to respond to the nurturing and to notice a reduction in anxiety. He also needs to be educated about qualities of beneficial massage application.

Decision Making and Treatment Plan Development

Primary Goal: Pain Management
Category of Care: Condition Management/Restorative

Quantifiable Goals

1. Reduce pain sensation to a tolerable 5 (on a scale of 1–10).
2. Ease feelings of stiffness by 50%.
3. Normalize breathing.

Qualifiable Goals

The player will be able to perform at or near optimal levels and will be able to participate in all training activities without excessive soreness.

Treatment Regimen

Condition Management/Restorative

Daily massage will be given for 5 days just before bed for 55 minutes at the $75 fee. The frequency then will be reduced to two times per week. Massage application will be primarily adapted to support fluid movement interspersed with rhythmic, broad-based compression and gliding deep enough to spread muscle fibers in all muscle layers. Application of all methods should not create any inflammation or alter the training effect. The player must not be sore to the touch or movement related to massage application. The focus will be on reducing sympathetic arousal and normalizing muscle tension, reflex patterns, and fluid dynamics in the body. Limited use of superficial fascia elongation in the binding tissue of the back, groin, and chest, along with controlled use of kneading, primarily to rhythmically squeeze the capillary beds and soften the ground substance, is appropriate. Abdominal massage to encourage peristalsis, with a specific focus on the large intestines to move fecal matter, is indicated. Breathing, muscle tone, firing patterns, reflexes, and sleep patterns will be monitored as indicators that the player is responding to massage.

CASE 7. THIRD-TRIMESTER PREGNANCY

The client is 34 years old and in the eighth month of her second pregnancy. She has a 9-year-old son. The pregnancy has progressed normally, and the client has had the usual minor complaints of nausea, swelling in the ankles, low backache, and shoulder and neck pain. She has noticed her breathing becoming more labored in the past 2 weeks. She feels pressure on her bladder, but bowel function is normal. She has been receiving massage on and off during the pregnancy. Now that her posture is changing with the increased size of the baby, she is more uncomfortable and wants to begin a more frequent and regular schedule of massage until the baby is born. She lives in the country, and the weather has been snowy and icy. Because she feels clumsy and is concerned about falling, she has been staying home and would prefer onsite massage sessions.

Assessment

Observation

The client's movement is awkward, and she often places her hands on the lumbar area for support. She breathes with her neck and shoulder muscles and is at times short of breath. The baby has taken up all available abdominal space and is still being carried high in the abdomen.

Interview and Goals

The baby has a normal activity level and has not settled into the head-down position. Nothing on the history form indicates problems with the pregnancy or cautions for massage. The client takes prenatal vitamins but no other medications. Her obstetrician is an osteopath who supports massage. The doctor did some joint manipulation earlier in the pregnancy but would prefer that other methods be used until after the baby's birth.

The client's goals for the massage are to be more comfortable in general, to reduce the edema, to sleep better, and to ease the muscle and joint aching in both her low back and neck. She realizes that the effects of massage are temporary, but at this point, even a few hours of relief would be welcome.

Physical Assessment

Posture

Functional lordosis as a result of the pregnancy.

Gait

Normal contralateral gait pattern is evident, but the increased weight in the front, coupled with the change in the center of gravity, makes movement awkward and labored.

Range of Motion

Forward flexion of the trunk is limited by the pregnancy. Lateral bending is limited in both directions and is linked to the client feeling as if she is losing her balance. Range of motion in the ankles and wrists is mildly limited by the edema. Lateral flexion of the head is reduced to 30 degrees bilaterally.

Palpation

Near Touch
Increased heat is noted in the upper shoulders.
Skin
Skin is generally dry and a bit flaky but shows no abnormal color changes. It is slightly rough, and stretch marks are present in the lower abdomen. Hair is a bit dry, and some has fallen out.
Superficial Connective Tissue
Pliable and resilient.
Vessels and Lymph Nodes
Normal.
Muscles
Neck and shoulder muscles that function as breathing muscles are short, as are the back extensors.
Tendons
Tenderness at abdominal attachments.
Deep Fascia
Normal for this stage of pregnancy; abdominal fascia is stretched.
Ligaments
General laxity, normal for this stage of pregnancy.
Joints
Joint play is increased in all major joints. Symphysis pubis is up-slipped on the right. SI joint is mobile but compressed, as are the lumbar vertebrae. The baby restricts rib movement.
Bones
Normal.
Abdominal Viscera
Unable to palpate.
Body Rhythms
Even and slightly slow. Breathing is labored and occasionally out of sync with the other body rhythms. Pulse points are even in the legs.

Muscle Testing

Not performed.

Interpretation and Treatment Plan Development

Clinical Reasoning

What Are the Facts?

Normal pregnancy is a healthy state, with caution implicated for massage. In the first trimester, the main concern is not to overstress the mother in any way that would interfere with normal development of the baby. Deep abdominal massage is avoided, as are any invasive and painful massage or bodywork approaches.

Consideration is necessary for the hormonal changes that may increase sensitivity to odors or mood changes. Breasts enlarge and are tender, and fatigue is common.

During the second trimester, the hormonal changes result in connective tissue changes, and joint stability may become somewhat loose. The abdomen begins to expand and lying on the stomach is uncomfortable unless support is provided. The body's response to hormonal changes evens out.

In the third trimester, strain is put on the postural muscles, because the center of gravity shifts forward. Pressure from the growing baby compresses the abdominal contents; this interferes with normal diaphragmatic breathing and can increase the urgency or frequency of urination. Nonpitting edema is common in the ankles and wrists. Getting comfortable becomes difficult. Backaches and neck and shoulder aching are common. Backache results from the shift in the center of gravity and from the intraabdominal pressure; neck and shoulder pain arises from the use of accessory muscles for breathing. The breasts continue to change and enlarge, preparing for lactation. All these conditions reverse themselves over time after the baby's birth. Management and comfort care (palliation) are the goals at this stage of pregnancy.

This client shows the normal third-trimester adaptations of the body.

What Are the Possibilities in Both Function and Dysfunction and the Massage Intervention Options?

The SI joint pain and lumbar area aching are likely caused by the functional lordosis and joint laxity. The short shoulder and neck muscles are attributable to the use of accessory breathing muscles. The mild edema in the ankles and wrists is common in the third trimester because of the increased strain on the lymphatic system and because some of the lymph pathways are obstructed by the baby and by postural shifts.

Possibilities

1. Full-body pleasurable massage can provide hyperstimulation analgesia to reduce the aching. It also can lengthen the shortened neck and shoulder muscles and assist in movement of the lymphatics, with caution.
2. Caution is indicated with stretching and joint movement, because hypermobility is noted in the joints. The up-slipped symphysis pubis is consistent with the posture shifts and compression of the SI joints; this condition increases the sensation of pelvic instability.
3. Because the client's obstetrician is an osteopath, referral for manipulation of the SI joints and symphysis pubis could bring short-term relief. This could be continued until the baby has been born and the pelvis stabilizes.

What Are the Logical Outcomes of Each Possible Intervention?

The client wants massage at home; therefore the cost is higher to cover travel and setup time. Her spouse and child can be taught basic massage methods so that they can help during the final weeks of pregnancy.

Positioning on the side will require alteration of some massage applications and can strain the massage practitioner's body mechanics somewhat because the ideal positioning for some areas may not be available. The side-lying position is generally supportive and is effective for body mechanics. Additional bolsters are necessary.

What Is the Effect on the People Involved for Each Possible Intervention?

The massage therapist is a young mother herself and can empathize with the client. Therefore the therapist is supportive of home visits for a short time because the client is a regular and is willing to pay a travel fee.

Decision Making and Treatment Plan Development

Primary Goal: Relaxation
Category of Care: Palliative Care

Quantifiable Goal

Increase comfort levels, as self-reported by the client.

Qualifiable Goals

The client will be supported, her stress will be reduced in the final stages of pregnancy, and she will be prepared for effective delivery.

Treatment Regimen

Palliative Care/Limited Condition Management

Full-body massage sessions will be provided twice a week for 1 hour at an in-home rate of $75 per hour plus a $25 travel and setup fee. The massage position will be altered to side-lying.

Pressure will be broad based and applied to a depth that is comfortable. Broad-based compression will be used for the short muscles of the neck, shoulders, and upper chest while the client moves her head or arm in circles to relax the accessory breathing muscles. Gentle traction of the SI joint and lumbar vertebrae to ease compression will be incorporated into the general massage session. Full-body rhythmic massage will create counterirritation and hyperstimulation analgesia, reducing the perception of discomfort for a short time.

NOTE: For these massages, special attention should be given to atmosphere, such as soft music and lighting, with a parasympathetic focus. Scentless massage lubrication should be used because the client is sensitive to odors. Gentle, soothing, circular stroking of the abdomen can increase the pliability of the stretched skin in the area. Foot massage is comforting and balancing. If the client's breasts are aching, she can be taught a circular gliding massage technique for the breast area.

CASE 8. PREMENSTRUAL SYNDROME

The client is a single 29-year-old female with a 5-year-old child. She has been diagnosed with premenstrual syndrome (PMS). After ovulation she is increasingly irritable and anxious. She experiences general swelling and some bloating. Often, but not always, she gets a migraine headache about a week before her menstrual period. Her weight is within normal range for her height, but she can increase half a clothing size during the menstrual period.

She takes ibuprofen as needed for pain, and she is taking a multivitamin and additional B vitamins. She is weaning herself off coffee by switching to green tea, which also has caffeine but not as much as coffee. On weekends she rides her bike and rollerblades for exercise. She has not changed her diet. She recently joined a PMS support group.

The client has a stable income, but the days off work and the mood fluctuations during her premenstrual period are beginning to disturb her employer. Currently, she is 3 days past ovulation and just beginning to experience symptoms.

Assessment

Observation

The client is clearly distressed about her mood swings, as indicated by her emphatic voice tone and her facial expression. She appears bloated.

Interview and Goals

The history form indicates that the client has migraine headaches and that she uses a barrier method for birth control. She has had one pregnancy. She severely sprained her right ankle 3 years ago. She experiences digestive bloat and low backache just before her period. She appears fatigued, and she says she suffers from sleep difficulties and nervous tension the second half of her menstrual cycle. She falls asleep but wakes up frequently and cannot get back to sleep.

The client is intent on management of the PMS and indicates that her goals for the massage are to focus on and deal with the fluid retention and chemical imbalance that accompany PMS.

Physical Assessment

Posture

Posture is symmetrical, with the shoulders slightly rolled forward. Weight is dispersed to the inside of the right foot, and the right knee is mildly hyperextended.

Gait

Normal except for flat-foot loading, in which the weight is on the inside rather than the outside of the right foot.

Range of Motion

Within normal range except for moderate hypermobility in the right ankle.

Palpation

Near Touch
No perceivable abnormality.

Skin
Oily and smooth with binding noted in the superior (cranial) direction (tissue moves down, binds when moved up) around the right ankle and upper chest.

Superficial Connective Tissue
Evidence of fluid retention, with pitting edema in the ankles.

Vessels and Lymph Nodes
Lymph node areas in the axillae display tenderness to moderate pressure.

Muscles
Point tenderness is present in the right medial gastrocnemius.

Tendons
Right Achilles tendon is slightly short.

Deep Fascia
Sheath between the gastrocnemius and the soleus on the right seems bound together with reduced sliding.

Ligaments
Deltoid ligament on the right ankle is unstable and lax.

Joints
Right ankle is hypermobile and has increased joint play.

Bones
Normal.

Abdominal Viscera
Abdomen is boggy and moderately distended. Lower abdomen is tender to moderate pressure.

Body Rhythms
Breathing is uneven and slow, with no current evidence of upper chest breathing. Cardiac pulses are normal but changeable from 55 to 70 beats per minute without change in activity.

Muscle Testing

Strength

Not performed.

Neurological Balance

Not performed.

Gait

Normal except for the gastrocnemius and the soleus on the right, which do not inhibit appropriately.

Interpretation and Treatment Plan Development

Clinical Reasoning

What Are the Facts?

Premenstrual syndrome is a collection of symptoms that include fluid retention, bloating, headache, backache, changes in balance mechanisms and coordination, food cravings, irritability, anxiety, depression, and decreased ability to concentrate. Females may experience a few or many of the symptoms, and this is changeable from cycle to cycle. All of the causal factors for premenstrual syndrome have yet to be discovered. Imbalances in serotonin and dopamine are evident. The increase in progesterone during the post-ovulation period supports fluid retention. Prostaglandins seem to be a factor in the pain and cramping, and aspirin and other nonsteroidal antiinflammatory drugs are often prescribed because they interfere with prostaglandin synthesis. For some females, the symptoms are severe enough to interfere with their lives. They have a type of PMS called premenstrual dysphoric disorder (PMDD).

Common PMS symptoms include the following:

- Breast swelling and tenderness
- Acne

- Bloating and weight gain
- Pain—headache or joint pain
- Food cravings
- Irritability, mood swings, crying spells, depression

No one knows what causes PMS, but hormonal changes trigger the symptoms. This client shows common premenstrual symptoms, especially bloating, fluid retention, irritability, food cravings, and headache. The symptoms are severe enough to compromise her work situation. She also has mild postural distortion and ankle hypermobility.

What Are the Possibilities in Both Function and Dysfunction and the Massage Intervention Options?

Serotonin imbalance is evidenced by chocolate and carbohydrate cravings and dopamine imbalance by the irritability. Because ibuprofen helps the pain and cramping, prostaglandins are likely involved. The progesterone increase during the postovulation period can contribute to the fluid retention, bloating, and breathing changes. The distress from the symptoms could increase the sympathetic fight-or-flight response, creating a self-perpetuating cycle.

Possibilities

1. Massage would promote fluid and neurochemical balance and reduce sympathetic arousal.
2. Recommendations for meditative movement activity, such as tai chi or yoga.

What Are the Logical Outcomes of Each Possible Intervention?

Massage is cost effective, and the closeness of the massage practitioner's office to the client's workplace makes it convenient. The massage therapist works for a franchise, so multiple massage therapists are available for appointments depending on the client's schedule and symptoms. Massage once a week is appropriate during the preovulatory phase; more frequent sessions should be scheduled during the symptom phase. A tai chi class is available through the PMS support group.

What Is the Effect on the People Involved for Each Possible Intervention?

The client is motivated and indicates compliance with keeping appointments. The support group also recommends tai chi or yoga.

Decision Making and Treatment Plan Development

Primary Goal: Stress Management
Category of Care: Condition Management

Quantifiable Goals

1. Reduce self-reported PMS symptoms by 50%.
2. Reduce by 75% the number of days the client takes off work because of PMS symptoms.

Qualifiable Goal

The client will experience increased well-being and reduced mood swings.

Treatment Regimen

Condition Management

Massage appointments will be made weekly until the symptoms appear and then twice weekly until the symptoms dissipate. One-hour sessions are indicated at the franchise membership fee per session. The sessions will include general massage to reduce sympathetic arousal, with a broad-based compressive force and pressure depth that does not cause any guarding or pain. Sufficient pressure will be necessary to influence serotonin, endocannabinoids, and endorphin function. Improved function of these chemicals should reduce food cravings and pain perception and, it is hoped, level the mood fluctuations. Lymphatic drainage will be used to reduce tissue fluid. Because the pressure of superficial lymphatic drainage is very light (just moving the skin), this will be the last method used during the massage.

The client also displays compensation patterns from the ankle sprain and a rolled shoulder pattern, likely from the biking. Because these areas have no direct effect on premenstrual syndrome management and the client's goals, they will not be addressed specifically during the initial treatment plan massage, although improvement may be noted with general massage application. The ankle compensation patterns may become an issue in future sessions, and the treatment plan can be amended at that time.

CASE 9. REPETITIVE STRAIN/OVERUSE INJURY: BURSITIS

The client is a 48 year old who has been diagnosed with bursitis of the left elbow. They are a manager of a retail center, and most of the day involves phone and computer work. The bursa at the olecranon around the attachment of the triceps has become irritated and inflamed. The client fell and hit the elbow 6 months ago. The bursa was injured but healed with no apparent problems. The client recently began a weight-training program that includes biceps and triceps toning and admits overtraining doing both upper body and lower body exercises every day instead of following an alternate-day pattern.

The client was given a cortisone injection at the inflamed site, is taking naproxen, and has been told to rest the area and maintain range of motion but not to lift weight with the arm. The client expresses concern about losing recently acquired muscle tone and bulking. The client became overweight and deconditioned in their early 40s after being very fit in their 20s and 30s. They are determined to reclaim a fit body. The client is already receiving massage on a weekly basis with the goal of managing stress and the muscle soreness caused by exercise. The client is now specifically focused on reversing the bursitis.

Assessment

Observation

The client is a bit restless and impatient. Frustration is evident in their voice over what seems to be a delay in the training program. The client rubs the sore elbow often.

Interview and Goals

The client is taking a muscle-building supplement that contains various vitamins and amino acids. They slipped on the ice and severely bruised the left elbow. It was speculated that they may have ruptured the bursa at the olecranon. The bursitis is in the acute, possibly subacute, stage. The history indicates a family tendency for cardiovascular problems, primarily arteriosclerosis. The death of a relative prompted the client to begin a diet and exercise program. Their blood pressure is slightly elevated but is not being treated medically, and their doctor expects it will fall into normal range with weight reduction, stress management, and exercise.

Physical Assessment

Posture

Mild anterior rotation of the left shoulder and moderate anterior rotation of the left pelvis are seen. The left elbow is carried in a flexed, loose-packed position.

Gait

Client's stride is short when moving forward on the right leg and counterbalances, with the right arm moving into extension instead of the left arm.

Range of Motion

Pain limits flexion of the left elbow to 100 degrees. External rotation of the left arm is limited to 70 degrees.

Palpation

Near Touch

Area of the bursa in the left arm is warm.

Skin

Skin is damp and slightly red near the bursal inflammation. Goose bumps are seen with light skin stroking over the bursal inflammation, and skin binding at the triceps attachment.

Superficial Connective Tissue

Stiffness at the triceps attachment at the elbow.

Vessels and Lymph Nodes

Normal.

Muscles

Triceps and biceps are short on the left. Quadriceps are long and taut, and hamstrings are short on the right. Muscle mass of biceps seems out of proportion to triceps. Internal rotators of the left arm are short, with inhibition of the external rotators. Gluteus maximus on the left is inhibited and not firing appropriately during hyperextension.

Tendons

Tendons are tender to moderate pressure at the right hamstring attachment at the pelvis and at all attachments of the left triceps.

Deep Fascia

Iliotibial band is binding in all directions on the right leg.

Ligaments

No palpable problems.

Joints

Compression of the left elbow joint does not cause additional pain, but traction does; the problem likely is in the primary soft tissue.

Bones

Normal.

Abdominal Viscera

Normal.

Body Rhythms

Fast, with some indication of sympathetic arousal and upper chest breathing.

Muscle Testing

Strength

Triceps muscle on the left is inhibited, and biceps muscle is too strong; quadriceps muscles are inhibited, and hamstrings are too strong on the right. Left gluteus maximus is weak. Trigger point type activity is found in these same muscle groups, with the tender points in the belly of the short, concentrically contracted muscles and at the attachments of the inhibited, long, eccentrically contracted muscles.

Neurological Balance

Client is unable to increase resistance gradually against pressure; uses maximum force; and movement is abrupt and jerky. Abdominal muscles are not firing appropriately.

Gait

Gait patterns are normal, even though local inhibition and increased tone are noted with individual strength testing of direct antagonist and antagonist patterns, especially knee flexors and extensors.

Interpretation and Treatment Plan Development

Clinical Reasoning

What Are the Facts?

Bursitis is an inflammation of the synovial fluid–filled sacs around joints, tendons, and ligaments. Bursitis develops with impact trauma, sustained compression (it is often found in the knees of carpet layers, carpenters, and others who do a lot of work on their knees), and repetitive strain. Repetitive movement causes both friction and a tendency for shortening of the muscle and connective tissue structures, which further increases the tendency for rubbing, causing inflammation. Bursitis can also occur if the position of the bones of the joint and ligament alignment changes or if the muscles pull unevenly on the joint structures.

This type of inflammation responds to applications of ice, nonsteroidal antiinflammatory drugs (e.g., aspirin/naproxen), and, if necessary, localized injection of a steroid. The medications, especially aspirin, thins blood. Massage pressure needs to be monitored to prevent bruising during massage. Areas where the steroid was injected must be avoided because the medication exerts its effect on the local tissues, and massage may disperse the steroid. Recently, transdermal patches of antiinflammatory and analgesic drugs have been used successfully instead of injection, but the same cautions exist. The muscle and connective tissue elements around the inflamed bursa are usually short and lengthening and stretching of this soft tissue is necessary. If the problem is localized and not the result of a more general postural shift, local work may help. However, as soon as the body begins to compensate for the condition, full-body effects develop; therefore even localized bursitis is best addressed in the context of full-body massage.

This client shows connective tissue shortening around the olecranon, with both the agonist and antagonist for elbow flexion short and tight on the affected side. A corresponding pattern that does not show symptoms is present in the opposite leg.

What Are the Possibilities in Both Function and Dysfunction and the Massage Intervention Options?

The previous injury may have caused some scar tissue and shortening and thickening of the triceps tendon. The rotational pattern of the shoulder and hip also increases the likelihood of the triceps rubbing at the attachment on the elbow. The short, tight muscles may be changing the joint angle and orientation of the connecting bones, increasing the likelihood of friction at the bursa. The repetitive strain of the weightlifting for the biceps and triceps is partly causal and likely aggravating the tissue changes from the previous injury. The client admits to overtraining and may be training the flexors more than the extensors of the affected elbow, setting up the muscle imbalance. Massage is indicated, and better results would be obtained if the sessions were scheduled for every other day for 2 weeks.

Possibilities

1. Friction and superficial fascia elongation are options in the areas of connective tissue adhesion.
2. Direct pressure combined with muscle energy methods is indicated for the trigger/tender points in the concentrically short muscles.
3. Lengthening and stretching of the short muscles, with stimulation of the eccentric and inhibited muscles, could be effective.

What Are the Logical Outcomes of Each Possible Intervention?

Massage to lengthen the shortened muscles and ease the connective tissue dysfunction would reduce the tendency for rubbing. If eccentrically activated muscles are further inhibited and become longer, the situation can worsen. Connective tissue binding is at the triceps, and further complications of the situation would need to be addressed in combination with muscle stimulation of the triceps and reduction of excessive shortening of the biceps.

Massage directly over the site of the steroid injection is contraindicated for at least 7 more days, which interferes with application of scar tissue management methods in the area. The client is taking aspirin and therefore may bruise with direct application of compression to trigger/tender points. Alternate methods are needed to address the area. The client needs to ice the area frequently.

Because this is a regular client for the self-employed massage therapist, an increase in massage frequency is a time and cost burden for the client. The massage therapist will have to find available scheduling to accommodate the more frequent appointments.

What Is the Effect on the People Involved for Each Possible Intervention?

Because the client is already receiving massage, the additional appointments are acceptable as long as results are readily apparent within a month. The client's expectations are a bit unrealistic. The client resists ice application.

The massage therapist is willing to accommodate the increase in the number of appointments for a short time.

Decision Making and Treatment Plan Development

Primary Goal: Functional Mobility
Category of Care: Therapeutic Change

Quantifiable Goals

1. Restore range of motion of the left elbow and arm to normal.
2. Reverse any compensation caused by postural changes.

Qualifiable Goal

The client will be able to resume work and moderate, appropriate exercise and weight training without causing irritation of the bursa or elbow.

Treatment Regimen

Therapeutic Change/Return to Condition Management

Full-body 60-minute massage sessions will be increased from once a week to three times per week for 1 month. The focus will be on generalized massage to address the compensation patterns in the opposite leg and the rotational pattern of the shoulder and pelvis. Compression, gliding, and kneading will be applied to the short biceps and hamstrings with tense-and-relax and lengthening techniques.

Percussion and pulsed muscle energy methods will be used after general gliding and kneading to stimulate inhibited muscles. Pin and stretch methods will focus on reducing trigger point activity and lengthening short muscles. In 1 week, connective tissue work will begin on the elbow, with elongation methods and drag of tissue in and out of ease and bind. Kneading and skin rolling will be used to soften the ground substance for the first four sessions of connective tissue application. No additional inflammation will be introduced.

After this application, if heat and other indicators of inflammation are reduced in the area, very controlled use of friction and bending and shearing of thickened tissue can begin. This process needs to be monitored carefully to ensure that the bursitis symptoms do not recur. Naproxen should be discontinued before the introduction of therapeutic inflammation, or the methods will not be as effective, because it is the inflammatory process that changes the connective tissue fiber structure. Depth of pressure will elicit a productive therapeutic edge sensation, and all layers of the short tissues need to be addressed, especially synergists and fixators in the deeper muscle layers.

CASE 10. JOINT SPRAIN WITH UNDERLYING HYPERMOBILITY AND LAX LIGAMENT SYNDROME

The client is a 16-year-old female cheerleader. She has been involved in dance and gymnastics since she was 5 years old. The client is generally in good health but has a history of various sprains and strains.

The current injury occurred when her leg became tangled with a fellow cheerleader's leg, resulting in a grade 1 sprain of the lateral collateral ligament of the right knee. The ligaments on the lateral aspect of her right ankle received a second-degree sprain when she landed on the outside of her foot. This same ankle was sprained last year.

Appropriate first aid was administered, and follow-up medical care included external stabilization and passive and active movement without weight bearing to promote healing with pliable scar tissue formation. Antiinflammatory and pain medications were used for the first 3 days and then withdrawn because these medications can slow healing. The client was on crutches for a few days until she could bear weight on her foot. Weight bearing has been allowed for the past 5 days. It has been 10 days since the accident.

The client's mother cleared the massage with her doctor, who supports the intervention to manage some of the compensation from using crutches and to promote healing of the injured area. The client complains of neck, shoulder, and low back stiffness and pain.

Assessment

Observation

The client is limping slightly. Discoloration is present around the ankle but not the knee. The ankle still appears swollen, but the knee looks normal. The client fidgets during the interview. Her mother is concerned but not overbearing, letting the client answer most questions and adding information where pertinent. The right ankle is wrapped with an elastic support.

Interview and Goals

The history notes multiple sprain injuries and a tendency for generalized hypermobility. The client hopes to participate in a cheerleading competition in 2 months. Her mother is more realistic, thinking it will be at least 3 months before the ankle is strong enough for competition. The client complains of being stiff all over. No unusually pertinent information is indicated on the history form.

The client's goals for the massage are to support healing of the injured ankle and knee, reduce the general stiffness, and reverse the compensation from limping and the use of crutches.

Physical Assessment

Posture

Client cannot achieve full weight bearing on the injured leg. Her posture is very good except for a slight lordosis and hyperextension of her knees, which is common in gymnasts.

Gait

Limited by limping, pain, and a sense of instability.

Range of Motion

Client is generally hypermobile, most likely because of training effects from dance, gymnastics, and cheerleading.

Palpation

Near Touch

Heat is detected at the ankle and knee injury sites and in the shoulders.

Skin

Drag and dampness are present in areas of heat. Bruising surrounds the area of ankle injury. Skin is smooth and pliable with no areas of bind noted.

Superficial Connective Tissue

Connective tissue is resilient. Localized swelling remains at lateral right ankle.

Vessels and Lymph Nodes

Normal.

Muscles

Muscles feel elastic but generally shorter in the belly, especially the calves, hamstrings, and adductors. Supraspinatus, upper trapezius, and pectoralis major and minor are short bilaterally, with tenderness in the axillae where the crutches contact. Psoas is short bilaterally. Muscles of the right leg have increased tone, most likely because of normal guarding of the injured joints. Quadratus lumborum/lateral raphe and the gluteal group on the left are tender to moderate pressure. A very tender area near the musculotendinous junction of the lateral head of the right gastrocnemius palpates like a grade 1 muscle tear.

Tendons

Tendons in the muscles of the right leg are tender to moderate pressure.

Deep Fascia

Resilient and pliable.

Ligaments

Generally loose.

Joints

End-feel is not identified until the joint is in hyperextension. Increased joint play is noted in major mobility joints.

Bones

Normal.

Abdominal Viscera

Normal.

Body Rhythms

Normal.

Muscle Testing

Strength and Neurological Balance

Muscles test normal except for those guarding the injured knee and ankle, which is expected. These muscles are displaying increased tone and are not inhibited as expected. Left quadratus lumborum is firing before tensor fasciae latae and gluteus medius.

Gait

Gait is disrupted by limping and crutches. Flexor patterns in the arms are facilitating together instead of following contralateral patterns. Flexors and extensors of the left leg do not inhibit when tested against the arms.

Interpretation and Treatment Plan Development

Clinical Reasoning

What Are the Facts?

Ligament sprains and muscle strains are common injuries and are diagnosed as slight (first degree), moderate (second degree), or severe (third degree). When a joint shows a sprain (i.e., rupture of some or all of the ligament fibers), there is usually accompanying muscle strain with the possibility of muscle fiber tears. It is important not to stretch muscle tears in the acute phase. Protective spasm (guarding) is intense and painful in first- and second-degree tears. If a total breach of a muscle or tendon has occurred, the person may feel very little pain. First- and second-degree injuries are more painful and have a greater tendency for swelling than a third-degree injury. When a joint is sprained, strain in the muscles that are stretched during the injury is common. Spasm around the tear (tiny microtears to more severe tears) acts to approximate (bring torn fibers together to support healing), protect, and guard the area. In general, all the muscles that surround the joint increase in tone to stabilize and reduce movement. This should dissipate as the injury heals but can become chronic, limiting range of motion of the area. Ligaments begin repair immediately, and the inflammatory response is an important part of this process. Some inflammatory mediators are vasodilators, which help blood reach ligaments. This is important, because ligaments do not have a good blood supply. Muscle tears heal much easier because of the high vascular component of the tissue. It takes 3 to 6 months or longer for a grade 2 sprain to heal fully. Repeated injury contributes to ligament laxity and joint instability.

Sprains are common in people with joint hypermobility. The hypermobility can occur in only one joint (typically associated with recurring injury) or can be more general, appearing in most joints of the body. Some disorders (e.g., Marfan syndrome) are characterized by lax connective tissue. Ehlers-Danlos syndrome consists of a group of connective tissue disorders that can be inherited and vary both in how they affect the body and in their genetic causes. They are generally characterized by joint hypermobility (joints that stretch farther than normal), skin hyperextensibility (skin that can be stretched farther than normal), and tissue fragility.

Most ligament laxity is functional, such as an increased range of motion required in many sports or dance activities. Once the plastic range of a ligament has been increased, it does not return to the previous range but remains long and lax. Joint play is increased, and instability results.

The client fits this profile. She will likely remain hypermobile, with increased compensating muscle tone to provide stability. This situation leads to general stiffness, especially if activity is reduced. Depending on the degree of laxity, the client may find that stretching does not reduce muscle tightness because joint end-feel and longitudinal tensile loading do not occur until the joint is hyperextended or reaches an anatomical barrier.

What Are the Possibilities in Both Function and Dysfunction and the Massage Intervention Options?

The client's gait changes seem to arise from the use of crutches. Because the injury is recent and the crutches are no longer used, gait dysfunction should easily reverse with massage and general activity.

The low back pain may stem from a dermatome distribution referring from the knee combined with postural changes from limping and the use of crutches. The tendency for low back pain may exist because the client's psoas muscles are short.

Possibilities

1. Massage can support the healing process in the acute, subacute, and final healing stages by increasing circulation to the area, maintaining normal and appropriate muscle tone, and supporting mobile scar formation.
2. Referral for diagnosis of the suspected muscle tear is recommended.
3. Referral to a physical therapist or exercise physiologist for a sequential strengthening program for the vulnerable joints is indicated.

What Are the Logical Outcomes of Each Possible Intervention?

Massage intervention would need to be long term to meet the client's goals, with an incremental treatment plan for the current acute and subacute healing stages.

Cost and time are factors, and the mother or father needs to be with the client because she is a minor.

A strengthening program with the goal of decreasing joint laxity should reduce excessive flexibility but will also increase the sensation of stiffness. This concept is in direct opposition to what the client has been taught and practicing for years.

What Is the Effect on the People Involved for Each Possible Intervention?

The client has unrealistic healing expectations and likely will be frustrated with a 6-month intervention plan. She may be confused and resistant to the strengthening program because it makes her body feel different. She has not had massage before and is somewhat hesitant. The massage therapist is a recent graduate of massage school. This client's goals and expectations are somewhat overwhelming. Fortunately she is employed in an independent group massage practice where more experienced massage therapists can be consulted. The massage clinic owner and lead therapist felt that the client would be most comfortable with someone younger and who has an athletic performance background, and the chosen massage therapist played volleyball in high school.

Decision Making and Treatment Plan Development

Primary Goal: Functional Mobility

Category of Care: Condition Management/Therapeutic Change

Quantifiable Goals

1. Reduce generalized stiffness by 75%.
2. Reverse compensation caused by the use of crutches.
3. Support circulation and scar formation in injured areas.

Qualifiable Goals

The client will be able to resume normal daily activities, but not sports activities, within 2 weeks. She will be able to resume full use of the area in 6 months.

Treatment Regimen

Condition Management/Therapeutic Change

Condition management consists of two phases. Therapeutic change is targeted for phase 3.

1. *Phase 1: Acute phase (current).* One-hour massage will be provided three times for the first week. Full-body massage will be used to support circulation and reverse the muscle tension in the shoulders and chest caused by the use of crutches. Specific application of gliding will be used along the sprained ligament and associated strained tendons in the fiber direction of the muscle and toward the injury to help align the scar tissue. Lymphatic drainage in the swollen areas will support healing. Passive range of motion with rocking and gentle shaking to all adjacent joints will encourage mobility and healing in the injured areas.
2. *Phase 2: Subacute phase.* Ice applications will be valuable for 1 or 2 weeks to support pain management. Massage applications will be provided for full-body sessions twice a week for 6 weeks and then reduced in frequency to once a week for 3 months if healing is progressing well. Very gentle gliding across the fiber configuration of the tissue will support mobile scar formation. The intensity of gliding and cross-fiber friction on the injured tissues will gradually increase as healing continues. General increase of tone in the muscles that are guarding will be addressed with muscle energy methods, lengthening, and broad-based compression. Kneading can restore the pliability of the connective tissue ground substance. The area of the gastrocnemius that may have been torn will be treated with caution. No deep pressure will be used, but localized stroking across the grain of the muscle can support mobile scar formation. Because self-stretching is not effective without moving into hyperextension patterns, the client's muscle tissue can be manually elongated during massage. This is accomplished with compression and kneading that introduce bending and torsion stress into the soft tissue between the joints and moving across the tissue fiber direction instead of longitudinally from attachment to attachment. The psoas muscles can be lengthened with muscle energy methods.
3. *Phase 3: Therapeutic change.* Six months of weekly full-body massage will be provided. Once the injury heals, the underlying hypermobility can be addressed. Systematic frictioning can be applied to lax ligaments to introduce therapeutic inflammation and encourage increased connective tissue fiber formation. This will be applied to the injured lateral collateral ligament and lateral ankle ligaments, as well as the rest of the connective tissue stabilizing units of the ankle and knee. This massage application needs to be done in small increments, and the area should not be excessively painful the next day. Pain to the touch with moderate pressure is appropriate, but pain should not occur with movement. This is a painful intervention and needs to be done frequently. It is appropriate to teach a family member to perform the technique. Antiinflammatory drugs should not be used, nor should ice be applied to the area, because the goal is creation of controlled inflammation to encourage collagen formation. Full-body massage with direct tissue elongation should continue. At the end of the 6-month period, the frequency of massage intervention could be reduced to a maintenance schedule of every other week. The client will be encouraged to maintain a strengthening program and to reduce exaggerated joint movements to support restabilization of the joints.

CASE 11. OSTEOARTHRITIS AND ARTHROSIS

The client is a 67-year-old man with osteoarthritis and arthrosis in both knees. He is a sales manager, financially stable, and has a flexible schedule. He has always been active and has a history of participating in high school and college sports. He ran track and played basketball. During that time, he had various minor to moderate injuries, including knee trauma. In his words, "I would just tough it out and play anyway." To compound the problem, he was in a car accident when he was 36 and broke his left ankle. He also spent 12 years in the U.S. Marine Corps as a sergeant.

Currently he enjoys golf and racquetball. He does not want to use a golf cart because he enjoys walking, and he needs the exercise because of a cardiac condition. He plays racquetball for 1 hour on Tuesdays and Saturdays but really suffers from knee pain between those times. His condition is worst at his early morning Sunday golf game. Initially, he is very stiff, which interferes with his golf swing, but he warms up as time goes on.

He uses topical capsicum cream and takes aspirin for the arthritis and for the cardiac condition. He is currently 20 pounds over what his doctors would like him to weigh. The extra weight bothers his knees. He thinks that he has gained some weight because the knee pain has slowed him down.

The left knee is more painful than the right. In the future he may try viscosupplements, which are intraarticular injections of hyaluronic acid. Or he may elect to undergo joint resurfacing or replacement surgery, but for now he is exploring any methods that will allow him to remain active.

He has never had massage and has the support of his physicians. Admittedly, he is skeptical about massage. He says he is not one to be "fussed over" and just wants the job done.

Assessment

Observation

The client is tall, 6 feet 4 inches. He has long legs, a short torso, broad shoulders, and a bit of a potbelly. His center of gravity is high, which places strain on the knees. He carries himself like a Marine. He is loud and gruff but seems kind underneath the facade. He seems a bit nervous about massage therapy. Because the massage therapist is male, there are additional misconceptions about massage that will need to be addressed. His shoulders move when he breathes.

Interview and Goals

The client says he aches all over but that he has lived hard and should expect to be creaky. The joint pain is worse in the morning, gets better as he moves around, and then gets worse again. He has had various and numerous joint injuries and soft tissue trauma. Four years ago his blood pressure rose, and he had angioplasty to unclog two coronary arteries. He takes aspirin to keep his blood thin and to manage the arthritis. He says that he does not seem to bruise easily. He was taking blood pressure medication but did not like the sexual side effects and insisted he go off it. The doctor agreed if the client could keep his blood pressure down with diet and exercise. He has done a good job of this. Nothing else of concern is indicated on the history form. He quit smoking 10 years ago. He used to drink heavily but now drinks only a glass or two of red wine two to three times a week. His sleep is restless because his knees ache. Heat application helps.

The client's goal for the massage is management of his knee pain.

Physical Assessment

Posture

Overall, the client has decent postural symmetry. Cervical curve is flat. Left foot is a bit flat. Ribs are held tight and rigid.

Gait

Client walks stiffly with reduced knee flexion and extension.

Range of Motion

Range of motion in most jointed areas is in the acceptable range for mild daily activities but stiff with resistance during any exercise. The left ankle is moderately restricted in eversion and inversion.

Palpation

Near Touch

Heat is noted at the knees and between the scapulae.

Skin

Rough and binding almost everywhere, with edema at the knees; there is evidence of many traumas (i.e., various scars in many body areas).

Superficial Connective Tissue

Reduced pliability body wide—almost an armor-like feel, with edema (not effusion which is fluid in the joint capsule) at the knees.

Vessels and Lymph Nodes

Seem normal, but ability to palpate is restricted by tissue density.

Muscles

Well-developed but dense and inflexible. Trigger point type activity is evident in quadriceps and gluteals. Muscles that surround the knees have increased tone and isometric contraction in both antagonist and agonist patterns. These muscles obviously are attempting to guard the knee joints.

Tendons

Tender to moderate pressure around the knees and scapular attachments.

Deep Fascia

Thick and inflexible.

Ligaments

Mild laxity at injured ankle and knees.

Joints

Most are within the normal range of motion, but crepitus is common, as is a tendency for leathery or hard end-feel. Knees hurt with compression and traction. Most other joints show resistance to traction, indicating binding. Client indicates that most joints are stiff but not painful. Most of the pain is in the knees.

Bones

Increased bony development around the area of the ankle break. Bump noted in the right clavicle (client forgot breaking it falling out of a tree when a child).

Abdominal Viscera

Difficult to palpate because of internal abdominal fat distribution.

Body Rhythms

Strong and fast. Client breathes with his chest but does not necessarily display breathing pattern disorder symptoms other than talking loudly and mild evidence of sympathetic arousal. Pulses are even.

Muscle Testing

Strength

Client pushes hard against resistance and finds it difficult to use 50% effort. No areas of weakness are noted. Client was unable to isolate a muscle pattern and continually recruited and contracted muscles in areas other than the test area during assessment.

Neurological Balance

Antagonist balance at knees is lost. All muscles around the joint have a tendency for isometric contraction with uneven pull on the knee joint. Synergistic dominance is noted with knee firing patterns.

Gait

Leg muscles do not inhibit as they should against arm activation. Eye reflex patterns do not inhibit movement (phasic) muscles when appropriate. Hip extension and abduction firing patterns are activating in unison instead of in normal sequence.

Interpretation and Treatment Plan Development

Clinical Reasoning

What Are the Facts?

Osteoarthritis and arthrosis are common and have several causes. A genetic tendency to develop this condition is one factor. The most common cause is wear and tear on the joint structure, in addition to past trauma and increased weight. The pain is caused by irritation of the synovial membrane and joint capsule and by muscle contraction, which attempts to guard the area. Osteoarthritis has no cure, but it can be managed to improve the quality of life. Joint replacement surgery is the last option. Advances in technology have greatly improved the outcomes of this surgery, and alternative procedures such as joint resurfacing are more available.

Muscle guarding involves shortening of muscle groups to protect an area. This type of muscle guarding is very different from muscle spasms and cramps, which are spontaneous, painful muscle contractions caused by certain mechanisms in the brain. It usually occurs in all the muscles that cross the joint. Because flexors, adductors, and internal rotators have more mass, when tone increases, the pull is greater from these muscles than from the extensors, abductors, and external rotators. The bone fit at the joint can be pulled out of alignment, creating further irritation in the joint capsule. Also, muscles that cross the joint pull the joint space together. This, coupled with weight bearing at the hips, knees, and ankles, reduces the joint space and increases the potential for rubbing of the bony structures, which then increases inflammation, swelling, and pain. Some increase in synovial fluid in the capsule can be beneficial because an increase in hydrostatic pressure can separate the bone surfaces, easing the rubbing. Arthritic joints often are unstable and have a lax ligament structure. Because the client's knees are affected (closed kinetic chain—hip/knee/ankle), disruption of the knees affects the hips and ankles.

Management includes easing mechanical strain on the knee joint by normalizing the muscle tone without reducing stability and resourceful muscle guarding. Corresponding muscle shortening and weakening in the hips and ankles also must be addressed. Lymphatic drainage–type methods work well if the fluid is outside the capsule. Edema can increase stiffness and reduce range of motion. Sometimes needle aspiration is necessary if excess fluid builds up inside the capsule. If the cartilage is so damaged that it cannot secrete synovial fluid, injections of a viscous material can provide some relief.

Correcting any posture deviation that contributes to the joint irritation may be possible in younger clients, but in older clients, especially after age 75, this becomes more difficult. Pain management is supported with counterirritation and hyperstimulation analgesia applications, a reduction in sympathetic arousal, and an increase in the pain-modulating chemicals in the system. The joints must be kept moving or the condition worsens. Massage that incorporates passive and active joint movement supports pain management, allowing the client to move with less pain. Joint tractioning can offer temporary relief. Application of hot and cold hydrotherapy to manage pain and encourage circulation is appropriate. Cold can be applied after activity, and heat can be used to warm up before activity or as a counterirritation at night to promote sleep.

This client's history and posture give strong indications of the development of osteoarthritis and arthrosis. His body type (long legs with upper body mass) strains the knees in general. In addition, he has used his body hard for a long time.

What Are the Possibilities in Both Function and Dysfunction and the Massage Intervention Options?

The client is still relatively young and in good health. He is motivated to change, as indicated by his previous diet and exercise alterations. The knee joints and left ankle are likely damaged beyond regeneration.

Possibilities

Massage can be beneficial for management of pain, stiffness, and muscle pain related to guarding of the painful joint. Also, deterioration may be slowed, prolonging the time before replacement surgery is required. Generally, increasing tissue pliability and circulation, combined with management of sympathetic arousal, could help this client. Short-term symptomatic pain relief or pain reduction is a reasonable expectation, but the massage effects will wear off, and an ongoing appointment schedule is needed.

1. Racquetball may not be the best activity because the constant running in different directions in short bursts and the starting and stopping are hard on the knees. Swimming could be an option.
2. Gradual introduction of a conservative flexibility program would help.

What Are the Logical Outcomes of Each Possible Intervention?

The recreation center where the client plays racquetball has a swimming pool; therefore access is convenient. A senior yoga class is also available at the recreation center, as is massage. Cost and scheduling are not primary concerns.

Massage has a good likelihood of successful management of conditions if the client has regular appointments and realizes that this is a long-term care program. Cardiac medication may alter the amount of pressure tolerated by the client. Regular reports should be sent to his doctor.

What Is the Effect on the People Involved for Each Possible Intervention?

Swimming does not meet the client's desire for competition. He may try anyway but will not commit. Yoga does not thrill the client, but he is willing to try it if the class is not full of "old fogies." He is willing to play less racquetball and more golf but says golf does not make him sweat like racquetball does, and he needs something to make him sweat. He is a bit put off by the massage therapist being male and in his late 20s. The massage therapist is self-employed and rents space within the fitness center. He is highly recommended by other center members, which helps. The massage therapist is professionally dressed and respectful. He informs the client that the approach he uses is to assess the tissue and then provide intervention as indicated based on outcome goals. The massage area is clinical in appearance. These elements help the client be more receptive.

Patience is necessary for everyone. The progress from the massage will most likely be slow, and the effectiveness wears off. The massage therapist needs to realize that under the gruffness is likely an individual who is afraid and vulnerable. Awareness of and respect for boundary issues are necessary to keep the client empowered.

Decision Making and Treatment Plan Development

Primary Goal: Pain Management
Category of Care: Condition Management

Quantifiable Goal

Reduce the sensation of stiffness and pain by 50% as long as regular appointments are scheduled.

Qualifiable Goal

The client will be able to participate in moderate, low-impact sports exercise activities without being hindered by arthritic pain and joint stiffness.

Treatment Regimen

Condition Management

A long-term massage program is required with an initial schedule of twice a week right after racquetball. This will reduce some of the strain on the client's knees from racquetball. Because of the client's size and the complex application of massage, 90-minute massage sessions are needed. The cost is $100 per session. The appointment schedule will be reduced to weekly as soon as improvement is noted and the client's condition stabilizes.

Full-body massage with multiple goals is needed. The dense and binding connective tissue structure noticed body-wide will need to be systematically but slowly addressed. The focus is on increasing the pliability of the ground substance to reduce muscle density and fascial shortening and maintain more flexibility of the body. Effective methods could be superficial fascia elongation using increased drag in multiple directions (ease and bind, direct and indirect). Active tissue release uses a broad-based application of compression with the forearm, and possibly the knee and foot, against the tissue to compress the soft tissue and carry it away from the bone, with the client actively moving the adjacent joint. Side-lying positioning for the legs and working on a floor mat would facilitate this type of application. Because of frequent movement integration, the client will wear loose exercise shorts during the massage.

The client will likely require varying degrees of pressure and depth of application. The sensation should be at the therapeutic edge sufficient to trigger the release of endorphins, endocannabinoids, and serotonin but not enough to elicit guarding or bracing. Caution for bruising is indicated because of his use of aspirin. Gliding with drag can elongate the soft tissue. Until the client's muscle tone normalizes, use of active resistance for muscle energy methods may be counterproductive. Kneading can load tissue with shear, bending, and torsion stress to increase ground substance viscosity, especially around all the scars.

The knees can be a primary focus after muscle tone and tissue density normalize a bit. The trigger point activity can be addressed, specifically in the quadriceps and gastrocnemius that refer pain to the knees. Traction of the knees can temporarily separate joint surfaces. Surface edema can be moved with lymphatic drainage.

Application of ice and heat between massage sessions will be encouraged. The client can also use one of the many counterirritant ointments and gels that contain menthol as the primary cooling ingredient.

CASE 12. NERVE IMPINGEMENT SYNDROME

The client is a 34-year-old female. She has been a cosmetologist for 12 years and maintains a busy practice. The client has been a business owner for the past 4 years and has two employees. The business specializes in hair weaving and various types of braiding.

She has been experiencing right arm and wrist pain for the past 2 years. She was diagnosed with carpal tunnel syndrome (median nerve impingement), but surgery is not recommended until more conservative interventions have been exhausted. There are also indications of brachial plexus impingement from a minor whiplash injury 3 years ago. Another contributing factor is the client's use of birth control pills.

She is experiencing the typical symptoms of pain in the wrist and hand with numbness in the thumb and first two fingers. The muscles in the hand show no signs of atrophy. Her right arm feels heavy, and she has aching and numbness from her upper arm down into the right scapular area. Tapping the wrist makes the hand tingle and reaching for the floor with the right hand and lateral flexing of the head to the left increases the symptoms. She wakes up at night with her arm feeling numb. Heat applications help. She also takes an over-the-counter pain medication, Aleve (naproxen).

Assessment

Observation

The client's height and weight appear to be normal. She seems a bit swollen. She is a pleasant, energetic, and accommodating person. She draws a distinct line pattern of pain down her arm and hand and across the shoulder under the scapula.

Interview and Goals

The client information form does not indicate any contributing factors other than stress and fatigue from long working hours. She uses birth control pills. The client is "not complaining" because she has worked so hard for her business success. She rates her pain a 7 on a 1 to 10 scale. She indicates that she begins her day at a pain level of 3 and that the pain worsens as the day progresses. She can tolerate the pain in the morning but finds that by the afternoon, her capability is adversely affected.

The client's goal for the massage is to reduce arm pain.

Physical Assessment

Posture

Right shoulder is high and anteriorly rotated. Right arm is internally rotated. Head is tilted to the right.

Gait

Arm swing is short on the right.

Range of Motion

External rotation is limited to 60 degrees. Client resists lateral flexion of the head to the left because it feels tight and makes the arm ache.

Palpation

Near Touch

Anterior triangle of the neck on the right is warm.

Skin

Dampness is noted in the upper right shoulder region, which corresponds with an area of heat. Skin is smooth and resilient. Tissue binds around the right wrist and up into the forearm.

Superficial Connective Tissue
Generally boggy.
Vessels and Lymph Nodes
Normal.
Muscles
Scalenes on the right are short, and scalenes on the left are inhibited and long. Sternocleidomastoid is short and fibrotic on the left, right rhomboids are inhibited and long, anterior serratus is short on the right, right subscapularis is short, and pectoralis minor is short on the right. Wrist flexors are bilaterally short, with trigger/tender point referral activity in the flexor pollicis longus, pronator teres, brachioradialis, and supraspinatus on the right.
Tendons
Tender at insertion of right flexor digitorum group bilaterally. Subscapular tendon on the right is tender to moderate pressure.
Deep Fascia
Palmar fasciae bilaterally are short. Retinaculum on the right is short, with reduced pliability compared with the left hand.
Ligaments
Retinaculum at the right wrist is thick.
Joints
Normal.
Bones
Normal.
Abdominal Viscera
Normal.
Body Rhythms
Normal.

Muscle Testing

Strength
Short muscles with trigger point activity test strong but cannot sustain the resistance because of an increase in symptoms.

Neurological Balance
Normal.

Gait
Muscles in the right arm are not inhibiting appropriately, as indicated in the gait testing protocol.

Interpretation and Treatment Plan Development

Clinical Reasoning

What Are the Facts?
Nerve impingement (entrapment) syndromes are a common cause of nociception. The distribution of pain sensation depends on the nerve impinged. Impinged cervical plexus nerves usually refer sensations up into the head. Brachial plexus nerve impingement refers into the shoulder and down the arm. Lumbar plexus impingement refers into the gluteals and groin or down the side of the leg to the knee. Sciatic nerve pain radiates down the back of the leg. The pain of individual nerve impingement, such as the median nerve in carpal tunnel syndrome, follows the distribution of the nerve. Trigger point–referred pain patterns can follow similar distribution patterns and are a common component of nerve-type pain. The person usually has a history of trauma or repetitive strain resulting in muscle guarding. Fluid retention in vulnerable areas, such as the wrist, can be causal. This can happen with pregnancy or the use of birth control pills. Often the condition has multiple causal factors. Soft tissue impingement of nerves is the easiest of these types of syndromes to manage, and surgery should be avoided if possible because scar tissue formation after the surgery can cause future problems. If surgery is performed, scar development needs to be managed in the acute, subacute, and remodeling stages. Bony impingement usually requires referral to a chiropractor, an osteopath, a physical therapist, or, in extreme cases, a surgeon. Tight muscles, both concentric and isometric (short) and eccentric (long and taut), can press on nerves. Connective tissue shortening and densification are common causes of impingement. Females are somewhat more vulnerable to impingement syndromes such as carpal tunnel syndrome.

This client has multiple causal factors. Her job and increased demands for her service are increasing the amount of repetitive strain in the affected area. The whiplash injury can predispose the scalenes and other muscles of the neck and shoulder girdle to shortening. She is also retaining fluid, likely from the birth control pills.

What Are the Possibilities in Both Function and Dysfunction and the Massage Intervention Options?
The client is likely experiencing brachial plexus impingement, in addition to trigger point activity that is referring into the wrist area. Edema at the wrists is adding to the impingement. The connective tissue at the carpal tunnel is also thick.
Possibilities

1. Massage intervention would need to address each area: short muscles; trigger points in the belly of the muscles; short, dense connective tissue; and edema.
2. Spot work is possible but usually unsuccessful because areas of compensation, although not currently noticed, are likely developing. The client indicates that she is stressed; therefore full-body massage is most beneficial.
3. The client would benefit from a moderate exercise and flexibility program.

What Are the Logical Outcomes of Each Possible Intervention?
Massage is likely to reduce symptoms and prevent the condition from getting worse. It at least would slow the deterioration. Long-term care is probable.

Time is the biggest issue. Also, repetitive strain injury benefits from rest, which the client cannot easily do because of work demands. Early morning weekday appointments are available, and this is the best time for the client.

Because the massage therapist is an employee of the pain clinic the client has chosen for treatment, the clinic may be able to receive some reimbursement from the client's insurance company for the acute care. Insurance probably will not pay for maintenance massage care.

What Is the Effect on the People Involved for Each Possible Intervention?

The client is compliant but unwilling to reduce her work schedule. She says she will begin a regular stretching program, but compliance seems unlikely because of time constraints.

Decision Making and Treatment Plan Development

Primary Goal: Pain Management
Category of Care: Therapeutic Change/Condition Management

Quantifiable Goal

Reduce pain to a 3 on a 1 to 10 pain scale without pain increasing throughout the workday.

Qualifiable Goal

The client will be able to work a 40-hour week without limiting pain.

Treatment Regimen

Therapeutic Change/Condition Management

A 45-minute massage with a lymphatic drainage component will be given twice a week. Methods to increase natural pain-modulating mechanisms and to support the parasympathetic process for stress management are appropriate.

Acute phase treatment will proceed as follows:

- Short muscles will be addressed with general massage and muscle energy and lengthening methods. All layers of muscles will be worked because synergists and fixators are involved. Inhibited antagonists will be stimulated.
- Trigger point activity that refers symptoms in short muscles will be addressed with positional release or integrated muscle energy methods and lengthening. The results will be evaluated before connective tissue methods are introduced.
- The client will be taught self-help methods. Pulsed muscle energy and lengthening for short muscles and positional release for more active referring points will be demonstrated. This phase could take 6 weeks.

After the acute phase, connective tissue methods will be introduced to restore pliability to the dense fascial areas of the right forearm and wrist. Careful use of friction to create therapeutic inflammation is necessary. Monitoring will ensure that the methods do not aggravate the symptoms.

The client will be observed for posture improvement and the development of symptoms in the areas of compensation, such as the low back. Should such symptoms develop, she will be reassessed for muscle length imbalance and connective tissue shortening. Also, trigger points that refer to areas experiencing symptoms will be identified and treated.

When the client's condition is stable, appointments will be reduced to a maintenance schedule of once a week.

CASE 13. GENERAL RELAXATION

The client is a 44-year-old man who is on a vacation cruise. He has a high-stress job and has been having problems in a personal relationship. He will be on the cruise for 2 weeks and would like to schedule four massage sessions, two each week. Although he knows he has numerous minor musculoskeletal issues, he is not interested in addressing any of them. His goal is relaxation and well-being. He has no contraindications for relaxation massage outcomes.

Assessment

Observation

The client appears fatigued and frazzled. His weight appears normal for his height, and he looks moderately physically fit.

Interview and Goals

The client does not report anything on the client information form that would indicate contraindications. He states he is stressed and occasionally experiences tension headaches. He takes no medication, although he takes a daily general multivitamin.

He wants general massage with firm pressure that does not hurt. He does not want to participate; in fact, he hopes to fall asleep.

When asked to describe how he wants to feel and his goal for the massage, he replies that he wants to feel loose, sleepy, and calm.

Physical Assessment

Note: The client did not want to participate in an extensive physical assessment process. Assessment information is gathered during general observation and the first massage.

Posture

Slight forward head position and hyperextended knees when standing in symmetrical stance.

Gait

Somewhat rigid.

Range of Motion

Within normal range.

Palpation

Near Touch
Skin is warm; client has a slight sunburn.
Skin
Skin is normal. Binding is seen in the lumbar and occipital base areas. Client has extensive body hair.
Superficial Connective Tissue
Fibrotic at iliotibial band bilaterally.
Vessels and Lymph Nodes
Normal.
Muscles
Muscle tissue is dense. Hamstrings are short, and abdominals are long and weak.
Tendons
Normal.
Deep Fascia
Plantar and lumbar fasciae are short.
Ligaments
Normal.
Joints
Knee flexion bilaterally is limited by 10 degrees.
Bones
Normal.

Abdominal Viscera
Normal.
Body Rhythms
Upper chest breathing pattern.

Muscle Testing

Not performed.

Interpretation and Treatment Plan Development

Clinical Reasoning

What Are the Facts?

This case falls into the category of palliative care. The focus is on relaxation in a vacation environment, but similar treatment plans would be indicated for individuals having surgery (before and after the procedure), acute care, and care of the terminally ill.

Relaxation and pleasurable sensation are important functions of therapeutic massage. Massage is used to balance autonomic nervous system functions, usually providing reduced sympathetic arousal and increased parasympathetic activity. Relaxation can mean different things to different people. For most clients, relaxation is an experience of parasympathetic dominance. It is important to determine what the client means by "being relaxed." Asking questions that help the client clarify their interpretation of the relaxation experience can provide information on what the physiological outcomes should be.

Soft, rhythmic music and indirect lighting can be helpful in achieving a parasympathetic result. Aromatherapy is an advanced intervention requiring specialized training, but simple, safe application of some common essential oils may be calming. Various applications of heat are also comforting. A warm rice or seed bag or hot water bottle at the feet or behind the neck may be pleasurable. Because the massage is being provided on the cruise ship and in a spa environment, a signature essential oil blend for relaxation and hot packs is available. The spa environment is pleasurable and relaxing. The massage therapist is paid hourly as an employee and receives all gratuities earned.

What Are the Possibilities in Both Function and Dysfunction and the Massage Intervention Options?

The client has numerous areas of short and long muscles actively coupled with connective tissue dysfunction but addressing these areas would not meet the client's goal. The upper chest breathing pattern could be addressed because that should result in a calming effect.

Possibilities

1. The massage practitioner can offer the client a selection of aromas and music, and he could pick the ones he prefers.
2. Warm compresses can be placed over the client's eyes, and a warm pack can be provided for his feet. An alternative would be a warm footbath before the massage.

What Are the Logical Outcomes of Each Possible Intervention?

Because of his sunburn, the client may not want the hot water application.

He may be allergic to the volatile oils in the essential oils.

The massage environment must be quiet. The massage professional must limit conversation so the client can fall asleep if he wishes.

What Is the Effect on the People Involved for Each Possible Intervention?

The massage professional must remain focused on the client's goal and not address the other soft tissue issues identified. The massage professional must be quiet and limit conversation to the necessities of identification of caution, contraindication, and comfort.

Decision Making and Treatment Plan Development

Primary Goal: Relaxation
Category of Care: Palliative Care

Quantifiable Goal

Induce the relaxation response and support parasympathetic dominance, indicated by slowing of breathing and what the client experiences and reports.

Qualifiable Goal

The client will feel relaxed, sleepy, and calm.

Treatment Regimen

Palliative Care

A full-body massage with firm nonpainful pressure will be given using gliding, kneading, compression, and rocking for 90 minutes, with a rhythmic approach used to match the music selected by the client. The pressure level will be moderate to firm but will not elicit discomfort. Sufficient nonirritating lubricant will be used to prevent pulling of the body hair or irritation of the sunburn. The client will be offered a warm, damp towel to remove the lubricant after the massage. The massage professional can do this for the client as a way of gently waking him up after the massage. A massage focused on the feet, hands, head, and face sends the most signals into the central nervous system for relaxation. Attention to the thorax, shoulders, neck, and midback muscles provides inhibition and lengthening of the auxiliary breathing muscles to support relaxed breathing. The client will be positioned in the prone and supine positions. To avoid lumbar hyperextension in the prone position, a pillow will be placed under the abdomen between the pubic bone and umbilicus. The essential oil scent selected will be placed in a diffuser or mist bottle to prevent any skin irritation. The massage practitioner will stay focused and calm, intent on creating a quiet space with empathy and compassion, no expectations, and no interruptions for the client.

CASE 14. SLEEP DISTURBANCE

The client is a 52-year-old female. She is married and has three children, two grown and one in high school. She is satisfied with her personal and professional life most of the time. Currently, she works part time as a nurse but is considering returning to school to advance her career options.

The client is menopausal; she had a hysterectomy when she was 46, but she still has her ovaries. She is taking a low-dose hormone replacement (estradiol) and uses a topical progesterone cream. The estrogen and progesterone, plus nutritional supplementation, have controlled her hot flashes. However, she is still moody and restless, and she is experiencing sleep problems. She is also mildly hypertensive but is not taking medication. She is 15 pounds over her ideal weight. She is active; she plays golf and tennis and bowls. She also hosts a quilting club at her home twice a month. For the past 6 months she has been on a very low-fat diet and has lost 12 pounds. She loves coffee, and she quit smoking 9 years ago.

She has minor aching in her knee joints and is generally stiff in the morning but loosens up with a hot shower and some stretching. She has had an occasional massage while on vacation but has never had massage that focused on a specific outcome goal. She became aware of the benefits of massage in a book she was reading about managing menopause. She and her friends have been discussing methods to address menopausal symptoms and general life changes for this stage of life.

Assessment

Observation

The client's appearance is appropriate for her age. She has some wrinkling, which is explained by the smoking and by the greater susceptibility of Caucasian skin to sun damage. Because she colors her hair, the color and texture will not provide reliable information on stress response. She is a bit overweight, with fat distribution in the lower abdominal area, which is typical for menopause. The fat helps convert body chemicals to estrogen-like substances, replacing the estrogen production of the ovaries. The fat appears to be between the abdominal wall and the skin, which is of much less concern than fat distribution in the abdominal cavity, which is an indication of stress and increased cortisol secretion, prediabetes, and implications for cardiovascular problems. Her mood seems even, although she is a bit intense in her conversation. She yawns and sniffs frequently, which may indicate a tendency for breathing pattern disorder.

Interview and Goals

The client information form indicates that she uses reading glasses; has minor sinus congestion, especially in the fall; and has urge incontinence, which causes a need to urinate frequently, including at night. She tends to bloat and has aching knees and generalized morning stiffness previously mentioned. She has had three pregnancies and a hysterectomy. She has mild hypertension and is fatigued from lack of sustained sleep. When questioned, she reports that just as she is falling asleep, she has to get up to urinate. Then she has difficulty falling asleep again. During the night she either wakes up and then feels the urge to use the restroom or bladder pressure wakes her up. She feels as if she is up and down all night. In an attempt to reduce bladder frequency, she has restricted her fluid intake. She is also having some vivid dreams with the themes of running, looking for things, or trying to find people in a crowd.

She is undergoing hormone replacement therapy and takes a multivitamin supplement for menopausal females that includes some herbs, particularly black cohosh, ginkgo biloba, and extra vitamin E. She also takes a calcium/magnesium with vitamin D supplement. She had her appendix and tonsils removed when she was a child. She is involved with various sports for leisure and exercise, and quilting is her hobby.

Her main goal for the massage is to sleep better. After an explanation of how massage can effect mood-regulating neurochemicals, stiffness, and joint aching, she also became interested in addressing those goals. However, she is mainly concerned about her sleep quality and will base her evaluation of the effectiveness of the massage on this outcome. She indicates that a friend referred her for massage.

Physical Assessment

Posture

Generally symmetrical, but the shoulders are held a bit high and bilaterally rotate forward; so slight at this time that no compensation pattern is noted in any other body area.

Gait

Normal.

Range of Motion

Knees are restricted in flexion, and range of motion is reduced by 10%. External rotation of both shoulders results in a minor reduction in scapular mobility.

Palpation

Near Touch

Slightly increased heat in the upper thorax.

Skin

Surface texture is dry; hair is brittle; nails are well formed, but cuticles are dry and cracked. Elasticity is reduced in upper thorax around clavicles and at sacrum and on the bottoms of the feet. Skin is somewhat tight against the subcutaneous layer and does not lift easily.

Superficial Connective Tissue

Generally reduced pliability, with indications of minor dehydration (pinched skinfold holds its shape longer than normal).

Vessels and Lymph Nodes

Normal.

Muscles

No obvious neuromuscular issues or trigger/tender point activity.

Tendons

Normal.

Deep Fascia

Short and binding.

Ligaments

Slightly dense.

Joints

Minor stiffness with soft but binding (leathery) end-feel. Knees are moderately painful with both compression and traction.

Bones

Normal with reservations; family history indicates possible tendency for osteoporosis.

Abdominal Viscera

Moderate bloat.

Body Rhythms
Breathing is a bit irregular and has an upper chest quality. Heart rate has moments of increased rhythm. Pulses are even bilaterally.

Muscle Testing

Strength
Normal.

Neurological Balance
Normal.

Gait
Normal.

Interpretation and Treatment Plan Development

Clinical Reasoning

What Are the Facts?
The client is menopausal and has typical manifestations of that stage of life; she is taking measures to manage the uncomfortable mood and circulatory changes. She has a family history of osteoporosis and cancer, and she has a history of smoking.

Menopause is a normal process that begins as a female's hormonal patterns change and ovarian production and menstruation cease. Changes in urinary and sleep patterns are common. The urinary stress and urge incontinence can be related to changes in membranes in the urinary tract in response to reduced estrogen levels. Sleep changes are related to urinary urge, hot flashes, low levels of progesterone, and changes in serotonin level in relation to the estrogen level.

Breathing function is mechanically altered with the connective tissue changes, causing an upper chest breathing pattern; this results in oxygen levels in the blood that support sympathetic nervous system arousal.

Connective tissue changes and dry skin indicate mild dehydration and insufficient dietary fat intake. Evidence of osteoarthritis is present in the client's knees (pain on compression), and soft tissue involvement is noted (pain on traction).

What Are the Possibilities in Both Function and Dysfunction and the Massage Intervention Options?
The client may be predisposing herself to connective tissue changes by restricting water and appropriate healthy fat intake. She is doing this because of the weight gain and urinary urge. The reduction in estrogens may have altered the serotonin balance; this affects the production of melatonin, which controls aspects of the sleep cycle. Also, the bladder urgency is disturbing her sleep.

Breathing changes may increase the tendency for sympathetic dominance with increased cortisol levels; these higher levels would interfere with deep sleep and contribute to the types of dreams the client is having.

Possibilities

1. A general full-body massage is indicated, with firm but not painful pressure to encourage parasympathetic dominance and to support mood-regulating neurochemicals for mood and sleep. This massage approach, coupled with a drag quality to increase the pliability of the superficial connective tissue, should address the client's major and minor concerns, including the knee pain. The mechanics of breathing also must be addressed, but the major anatomical reason for upper chest breathing seems to be connective tissue binding with sympathetic arousal.
2. She should be referred to her doctor for the urinary urgency. However, reducing cortisol levels and supporting deep sleep should help with the nighttime urgency.
3. A slow gentle stretching program with a meditative quality is desirable.
4. A consultation with a nutritionist with experience in menopausal changes would help.

What Are the Logical Outcomes of Each Possible Intervention?
The massage should manage the conditions of concern. Regular ongoing appointments are required, and this creates a time and cost burden for the client. Referral to the doctor is necessary to rule out more serious reasons for the urinary problem.

Increasing fluid may temporarily aggravate the urinary stress. The stretching program may temporarily increase stiffness if the client is too aggressive, but moderate stretching would help maintain relaxation, joint mobility, and connective tissue pliability.

The client is self-seeking massage, and this type of client often is the most compliant in terms of keeping appointments and following through with self-help education.

What Is the Effect on the People Involved for Each Possible Intervention?
The massage professional needs to be committed to a regular appointment schedule. She is building her client base from part time to full time and has recently rented a small office space.

Some emotional undertones to the client's case—especially the restlessness, wanting to return to school, and tension with her daughter—may surface during the sessions. The massage professional must maintain appropriate boundaries and make the appropriate referrals. The client likely does not realize the emotional nature of the situation and may be confused if these issues surface. Redirection to the massage process and referral will help.

Decision Making and Treatment Plan Development

Primary Goal: Stress Management

Category of Care: Condition Management/Therapeutic Change

Quantifiable Goals

1. Improve sleep quality, as self-reported by client.
2. Balance mood and physical stress levels, as self-reported by client.
3. Reverse upper chest breathing pattern, as measured by therapist.

Qualifiable Goal

The client will be less fatigued and stiff, which will allow her to perform her desired daily exercise activities.

Treatment Regimen

Condition Management/Therapeutic Change

Weekly 1-hour massage sessions will be provided on an open-ended, ongoing basis. The cost will be $80, and every 10th massage will be complimentary. The client will come to the massage therapist's private office and knows that mobile massage at the client's home is available for $125 for the first massage and $80 for each additional hourlong massage session done on site.

The massage methods used will include gliding with moderate to firm but not painful pressure to increase the levels of mood-regulating neurochemicals and to reduce sympathetic arousal. Gliding also will be done with sufficient drag to cause connective tissue creep in binding areas and to increase viscosity in areas that show reduced pliability. Kneading will also be done, with localized use of skin rolling at the thorax and sacrum to increase connective tissue pliability and glide. Rhythmic rocking to the client's selected soft, slow music will encourage parasympathetic dominance. The range of motion of the knees and shoulders will be normalized with muscle energy methods and lengthening. Binding connective tissue will be addressed with bending and torsion stress applied with compression and kneading to load the tissues.

The client will be taught breathing exercises as presented in Chapter 15. The information in Chapter 15 will also be used to teach her methods of maintaining a supportive sleep cycle.

She will be referred to her physician and nutritionist for diagnosis of the bladder urgency and information for her specific needs.

She will be referred to a gentle flexibility program, such as yoga, to address the connective tissue stiffness and to support sleep and relaxation.

CASE 15. CIRCULATION IMPAIRMENT

The client is 57 years old with type 2 diabetes mellitus. The client is non–insulin dependent at this point and is taking an oral hypoglycemic medication that stimulates the secretion of insulin. The client is 40 pounds overweight, and part of their diabetic management is weight loss. They have lost 25 pounds but have not lost any weight in 3 months.

Their exercise is closely monitored to minimize blood sugar fluctuations. The client walks and uses a rowing machine. The client has begun to notice some impaired circulation in their legs and some burning in their feet. The client reports that they have developed minor symptoms of vascular insufficiency and diabetic neuropathy, a common complication of diabetes. The client's doctors are exploring all options to manage the condition.

The nurse on the diabetic management team has recommended massage for stress management. The client is willing to try anything that can help, and because the massage therapist is affiliated with the medical team, the client feels confident that the nurse who is responsible for the management of their program will supervise the process.

The client is in a long-term relationship and has a good support system.

Assessment

The medical team provided the following information:

The client is 57 years old with moderate type 2 diabetes mellitus. They are being treated with glipizide, diet, exercise, and education in diabetes and stress management. Renal function is good. Recent developments include vascular impairment and diabetic neuropathy in the feet. The massage prescription is for stress reduction with secondary support for peripheral circulation. The frequency and duration are two times per week for 1 hour per session.

Note: This case study is an example of the way a massage therapist responds to a massage prescription. The goals for the massage are determined by the physician. The assessment that follows is done to determine how best to meet those goals and achieve the treatment plan provided.

Observation

The client is visibly nervous and fidgety and prefers to stand to complete the intake process. They wring their hands often and regularly sigh deeply. The client's excess weight is carried in the abdomen and gluteal area.

Interview and Goals

The client reports never having received a massage. The client is ticklish and is concerned about removing clothing. They were in a car accident 10 years ago and had a whiplash injury and a concussion. The client experiences aching after exercise. Other than diabetes, they are in good health. The client works as a maintenance supervisor and troubleshooter for a local manufacturing firm. Alcohol and smoking are no longer part of their lifestyle. The client is determined to do whatever it takes to manage the diabetes since their mother died of complications of the same disease.

The client understands that the goal for the massage is to support relaxation and stress management, which will help regulate insulin levels. Additional outcomes would be to support peripheral circulation and reduce the numbing and prickling sensation in their feet caused by the neuropathy.

Physical Assessment

Posture

Moderate lumbar lordosis and forward head position.

Gait

Clumsy, with a flat-foot landing rather than the normal heel strike–toe off pattern.

Range of Motion

Trunk flexion is inhibited by the abdominal fat mass. Plantar flexion and dorsiflexion are decreased by 20% bilaterally.

Palpation

Near Touch

No noticeable difference.

Skin
Normal except for a bluish cast in the feet. Lower extremities are cool. Binding is present in the lumbar area and at the base of the neck. Palpable fat layer is present under the skin, with excessive accumulation in the abdomen and gluteals.
Superficial Connective Tissue
Bind in the lumbar area, thorax, and calves.
Vessels and Lymph Nodes
Lymph circulation appears normal, but pulses are weaker in the feet, and vessels seem constricted.
Muscles
Somewhat decreased in tone overall, with evidence of exercise-related increased muscle tone in the legs and arms but not in the abdomen or gluteal region.
Tendons
Right Achilles tendon is nonpliable.
Deep Fascia
Binding in the lumbar and anterior thoracic sheaths and nonresilience in the abdomen. Plantar fasciae are short bilaterally.
Ligaments
Normal.
Joints
No evidence of arthritis or pain on compression or traction. Lumbar curve is exaggerated. Knees and feet ache.
Bones
Normal.
Abdominal Viscera
Difficult to palpate because of internal and external fat distribution.
Body Rhythms
Slow, uneven breathing rate.
Muscle Testing
Not performed.

Interpretation and Treatment Plan Development

Clinical Reasoning

What Are the Facts?

Metabolic syndrome is not a disease in itself. Instead, it is a group of risk factors—high blood pressure, high blood sugar, unhealthy cholesterol levels, and abdominal fat. Most of the disorders associated with metabolic syndrome have no symptoms, although a large waist circumference is a visible sign. Metabolic syndrome is primarily caused by obesity and inactivity. Metabolic syndrome is linked to a condition called insulin resistance.

Diabetes is caused by impaired release of insulin by the pancreas, by inadequate or abnormal insulin receptors on the cells, or by destruction of insulin before it can become active. Type 2 diabetes is a maturity-onset form often found in adults who are overweight, especially if a family history of the disease is a factor. Diabetes symptoms include increased thirst and appetite. The high blood glucose levels have detrimental effects on most body systems; these effects include impaired eyesight, neuropathy, impaired circulation, a tendency for thrombosis and emboli, and diminished resistance to infection. Wounds heal slowly, and kidney function is strained. The individual is also susceptible to atherosclerosis. All this must be considered when massage is applied.

The client in this case has impaired peripheral circulation and neuropathy in the lower legs. Kidney function is normal. The client has no history of blood clots. They are taking medication that has common side effects of diarrhea, dizziness, fatigue, headache, heartburn, loss of appetite, upset stomach, sun sensitivity, vomiting, and weakness. Serious side effects of medication that require referral include blood disorders, breathing difficulties, dark urine, itching, jaundice, light-colored stools, low blood sugar, muscle cramps, rash, sore throat, fever, tightening in the hands and feet, and unusual bleeding or bruising. The massage practitioner needs to pay particular attention to dizziness, weakness, breathing, jaundice, itching, and symptoms of low blood sugar (besides dizziness and weakness, these include pallor, a rapid heart rate, and excessive sweating). Diabetic clients should always have their medications with them, and fruit juice or another quick-acting carbohydrate should be available. Muscle cramps, rash, and bruising also need to be considered. Cautions and accommodations are necessary. The skin can become thin and fragile in areas of impaired circulation.

This client is also anxious, indicating sympathetic dominance. They are ticklish and uncertain about removing clothing. The client is overweight, has bothersome knees, and experiences muscle aches after exercise. The client was in a car accident that injured their neck. Assessment identified fascial shortening in the feet, lumbar area, and thorax.

What Are the Possibilities in Both Function and Dysfunction and the Massage Intervention Options?

The possibilities for intervention are limited by the treatment plan provided by the physician. The physician has ordered relaxation massage and support for peripheral circulation with a schedule of biweekly 1-hour sessions.

Of more concern is how to follow the treatment plan when the client is ticklish and nervous about taking clothes off. The client could be introduced to massage through use of a seated massage format over the clothing until more comfortable and then be transferred to more traditional massage on the table with draping.

What Are the Logical Outcomes of Each Possible Intervention?

The chair massage over clothing would address the issue of the client not wanting to remove clothing. However, this type of massage may not provide enough relaxation response to support the goals of the physician. Also, addressing the problem of impaired circulation in the legs would be more difficult.

Tickling can be managed by using more pressure. Because the client's skin is in good shape and has no history of thrombosis or embolism, broad-based compression would be a good method.

What Is the Effect on the People Involved for Each Possible Intervention?

The client would be more comfortable with the chair massage initially, and over time move from the chair to the table. Once they realize massage can be enjoyable and without tickling, they should relax.

Decision Making and Treatment Plan Development

Primary Goal: Stress Management/Pain Management
Category of Care: Condition Management

Quantifiable Goals

As determined by the physician.

Qualifiable Goals

As determined by the physician.

Treatment Regimen

In accordance with treatment orders, the client will be given a 45-minute massage twice a week. The fees will be billed through the physician's office. Massage intervention will begin in the chair, with education provided about the effects of massage. Demonstration of the type of massage used to prevent tickling will be included, and draping methods will also be demonstrated.

While the client is using the seated position, the main focus of the massage will be to reduce sympathetic dominance and support normal breathing. Compression will be applied over the clothing, with shaking and rhythmic rocking of the arms and wrists and passive and active range of motion of the neck.

Once the client's apprehension about getting on the table and taking off clothing has eased, a general full-body massage will be used to promote parasympathetic dominance. The connective tissue shortening will be addressed with fascia elongation methods, always with an awareness of skin fragility. With the increase in connective tissue pliability, circulation and breathing should improve. The short, tight calf muscles will be addressed with slow gliding strokes, accompanied by monitoring for bruising. The calf muscle must have sufficient contractile capacity to promote circulation.

Circulation in the lower extremities will be encouraged with general full-body massage, with compression over the arteries moving proximal to distal. Caution will be used so that any evidence of thrombosis can be detected. The side-lying position will be used for the massage to support comfort due to the large abdomen.

Addressing any areas of discomfort related to past injury or causes other than the diabetes will be cleared with the physician before the treatment plan is altered.

Recommendations to the physician will include massage application to reduce post-exercise aching, which will support compliance with the exercise program; alteration of the exercise program to include some resistance exercises targeting the gluteal and abdominal areas; and normalization of the posture to support optimum energy expenditure. Evidence of an altered upper chest breathing pattern also is seen; because this perpetuates sympathetic arousal, it would be beneficial to address the problem by having the client participate in a breathing retraining program.

CASE 16. FATIGUE CAUSED BY CANCER TREATMENT

The client is a 46-year-old female with early-detected stage 1 breast cancer. The cancer was detected by mammography 12 months ago. She had a lumpectomy and radiation therapy. The outcome looks good. She is currently undergoing treatment with tamoxifen. All medical test results, including those from thyroid and bone density tests, are within normal parameters.

Two years ago the client married for the first time. She managed a bank branch for many years but retired from that job and is seeking a more meaningful career. She loves restoring antiques and hopes to pursue this as both a hobby and a moneymaking enterprise. Although money is a concern for her, she is willing to commit both time and resources to those things that increase the quality of her life. She heard about massage at a support group meeting and was intrigued by studies showing that massage supports immune function and helps with anxiety and depression that can accompany the diagnosis and treatment of cancer.

Her main concern is fatigue. After a year of focusing on treatment, she wants to get on with her life, but the fatigue suppresses her motivation. She experienced fatigue during radiation treatment but expected to resume her normal energy level once treatment was over. In addition to the benefits mentioned in the studies, she hopes that massage will help her regain her energy. Her doctor is supportive of massage but wants to speak to the massage therapist before sessions begin to review the proposed treatment plan.

Assessment

Observation

The client is soft spoken but direct and does not avoid eye contact or difficult topics. Her body motions seem slow, and she appears tired. Her body fat is evenly distributed.

Interview and Goals

Information from the client history form indicates a slight family history of breast cancer but not in her immediate family. She has always been a bit overweight. She had her first menstrual period at 10 years of age, and she still has regular menstrual periods. She has taken birth control pills on and off for years. Birth control is not an issue at this point because her husband has had a vasectomy. She gets an occasional headache but nothing significant. She has had normal childhood illnesses. She feels as if she is not sleeping deeply.

Her goal for the massage is an improved energy level.

Physical Assessment

Posture

Concave upper chest and bilaterally internally rotated arms. Slight kyphosis. Jutting chin with slight forward head position. Flattened lumbar curve with bilateral posterior pelvic rotation. Left knee is hyperextended.

Gait

Weight is carried on the heels, with shortened stride and arm swing.

Range of Motion

Capital and cervical flexion combined allow only 10 degrees of motion. External rotation of arms is limited to 75 degrees. Abduction and extension of shoulders are limited to 20 degrees. Trunk extension at lumbar region is limited to 15 degrees. Hip extension is limited to 20 degrees and dorsiflexion to 15 degrees.

Palpation

Near Touch

Hot and cold distribution seem uneven and erratic.

Skin

Skin is dry and shows obvious effects of radiation in treatment area. Two large moles are present on left shoulder. Bind is present in the thorax between the scapulae and in the lumbar area. Bind also is noted in the hamstrings and calves. Connective tissue seems dense in the lumbar area and hamstrings but thin in the thorax and abdomen.

Superficial Connective Tissue

Scar tissue at the surgical site is pliable, with a small area of bind near the axilla.

Vessels and Lymph Nodes

Normal, although caution is indicated in the left axilla adjacent to the treatment area.

Muscles

Occipital base, arm external rotators and adductors, and hamstring muscles are short. Gluteal group and abdominals are weak and almost flaccid. Calves are short.

Tendons

Pain reported on palpation of the subscapular tendon bilaterally. Achilles tendons are short.

Deep Fascia

Nonpliable and short in the cervical and lumbar areas and in the plantar fasciae. Abdominal fascia is nonresilient.

Ligaments

Normal.

Joints

Minor pain with direct compression over the sacroiliac (SI) joints. Joints of the foot seem immobile.

Bones

Probable fragility over the radiation site.

Abdominal Viscera

Abdomen is soft and has no detectable masses or abnormalities.

Body Rhythms

Uneven and erratic; client feels out of sync with herself. Rhythms fluctuate often.

Muscle Testing

Strength

General muscle strength is fair, with excessive tone in calves and occipital base muscles.

Neurological Balance

Normal.

Gait

Normal contralateral pattern but labored. Gluteus maximus does not fire effectively.

Interpretation and Treatment Plan Development

Clinical Reasoning

What Are the Facts?

The client has received successful treatment for breast cancer. The causes of breast cancer are not fully known. However, health and medical researchers have identified a number of risk factors that increase the chances of getting breast cancer. Risk factors are not necessarily causes of breast cancer, but they are associated with an increased risk of developing the disease. It is important to note that some females have many risk factors but do not develop breast cancer, whereas other females have few or no risk factors but do get the disease. Being a female is the number one risk factor for breast cancer. (**Note:** Males also get breast cancer.) For this reason, it is important to perform regular breast self-examinations, have clinical breast examinations, and have recommended mammograms to detect any problems at an early stage. Massage therapists need to understand the risk factors for cancer in general and in this case for breast cancer specifically.

Factors that can be controlled include the following:

- Having more than one alcoholic drink per day
- Taking birth control pills for 5 years or longer (slightly increases the risk of breast cancer)
- Not getting regular exercise
- Currently using or having recently used some forms of hormone replacement therapy for 10 years or longer (may slightly increase the risk of breast cancer)
- Being overweight or gaining weight as an adult
- Being exposed to large amounts of radiation (e.g., having frequent spinal x-rays during scoliosis treatment)

Factors that cannot be controlled include the following:

- Aging
- Having a mother, daughter, or sister who has had breast cancer
- Having the mutated breast cancer gene *BRCA-1* or *BRCA-2*
- Previously having had breast cancer
- Being young (under 12 years of age) at the time of the first menstrual period, starting menopause later than usual (over 55 years of age), never being pregnant, or having the first child after 30 years of age

Breast cancer can recur at any time, but many recurrences happen within the first 2 years after diagnosis.

Breast cancer may recur locally within the breast or chest area, in areas adjacent to the breast (underarm lymph nodes), or at distant locations (metastatic type). The most common sites for metastatic breast cancer are the lungs, liver, bones, and brain.

This client is 1 year post-diagnosis and has multiple risk factors for cancer development. She is currently taking tamoxifen. The most common side effect of the medication is hot flashes similar to those experienced during menopause. Tamoxifen may induce menopause in a female who is close to menopause; however, it rarely does in young females. Other common side effects are vaginal dryness, irregular periods, fatigue, and weight gain.

The surgical procedure used for breast cancer depends on the stage of the disease, the type of tumor, the person's age and general health, preference, and the physician's recommendation. Surgery is a form of local treatment for breast cancer, as opposed to systemic treatment that involves the entire body, such as chemotherapy. Studies have shown that most females with early-stage disease (stage 1 or stage 2) who are treated with breast conservation measures (procedures that preserve the breast) and irradiation have the same survival rate as females treated with mastectomy.

This client had a lumpectomy, which is appropriate treatment for her stage of cancer, and underwent radiation therapy. Radiation therapy uses high-energy x-rays to destroy cancer cells in the treated area (local treatment). It is most often used with breast-conserving surgery but may also be recommended after a mastectomy for females who have four or more lymph nodes that test positive for cancer cells. The purpose is to destroy any cancer cells that may be left after breast surgery. Radiation therapy may also be used palliatively to relieve symptoms, shrink tumors, and reduce pressure, bleeding, pain, or other symptoms of advanced cancer.

Cancer cells grow and divide rapidly, and they are sensitive to the effects of radiation. Normal cells grow and divide less rapidly and recover more fully from the effects of radiation. The side effects of radiation are the result of temporary damage to the normal cells. It is important to remember that the side effects of radiation are directly related to the dose and the area treated. Common side effects include the following:

- *Local skin reactions:* Itching, redness, or dryness and scaling of the skin. The degree of skin reaction is individualized. Skin irritation continues for approximately 2 weeks after the end of treatment. Healing then begins.
- *Fatigue:* This resolves gradually after treatment.

The client in this case also has a stage 2 postural distortion; this indicates functional stress that is causing a nonoptimal movement pattern characterized by fatigue with moderate activity.

What Are the Possibilities in Both Function and Dysfunction and the Massage Intervention Options?

The main goal for the massage is management of fatigue, which could be residual from the radiation treatment and the stress of the past year. The medication could also cause fatigue or an interrupted sleep pattern. Another factor contributing to the fatigue might be the postural changes making movement labored and tiring, especially so because the client began a moderate exercise program.

Possibilities

1. Massage could act as a stress management method, supporting effective sleep patterns and restoring a more normal movement pattern. This massage approach would be a general constitutional approach with a specific but cautious focus on the postural distortion.
2. The short muscles and connective tissue could be addressed with various massage, muscle energy, lengthening, and stretching methods.

What Are the Logical Outcomes of Each Possible Intervention?

The general massage, focused on quieting the stress response and supporting sleep and well-being, would help with the cancer recovery process in general but would not specifically address the postural changes that may be contributing to the fatigue.

A more aggressive massage approach to increase range of motion and make movement easier may be too aggressive this soon after cancer treatment.

What Is the Effect on the People Involved for Each Possible Intervention?

The doctor supports a more moderate approach that begins with the general massage and introduces the shift in muscle tension and posture gradually.

The client wants to address the problem more aggressively.

The massage therapist agrees with the slower, more cautious approach recommended by the doctor.

Decision Making and Treatment Plan Development

Primary Goal: Stress Management
Category of Care: Condition Management

Quantifiable Goal

Increase restorative sleep by 80% as reported by client.

Qualifiable Goal

The client will be able to participate in reasonable daily activities without fatigue.

Treatment Regimen

Condition Management

One-hour massage sessions (45–50 minutes hands on) will be given on a weekly basis at the massage office for $75 per session.

The main approach is a general full-body massage with sufficient pleasurable pressure to quiet the autonomic nervous system. The application will feel comfortably intense but not painful. The main methods will include variations in depth, drag, direction, speed, and rhythm of gliding strokes. Caution needs to be observed over the irradiated site, where a decrease in pressure is appropriate. Rhythmic rocking and gentle shaking of the joints of the extremities will support relaxation and may increase range of motion. The two moles will be watched for changes, and any changes in the breast or axillae will be referred immediately. Moving the skin and superficial fascia in both indirect and direct patterns of ease and bind can be used over the areas of connective tissue changes. Caution is required over the irradiated skin because of sensitivity and likely skin changes arising from the treatment.

The massage application will be intentional, mindful, rhythmic, and relaxing. Music of the client's choice that is soothing can be used. Once the client shows positive, sustained results from the methods described, positional release and pulsed muscle energy methods and lengthening can be introduced to address the postural distortion. Because the client is taking yoga classes, some postural change should occur that massage can support. Aggressive connective tissue work and invasive methods that introduce any sort of inflammation will be avoided. Any major change in the treatment plan will be approved by the physician.

CASE 17. BREATHING DISORDER: ASTHMA

The client is a 14-year-old male. His parents are exploring support care to help him manage his asthma. The client has been managing his asthma since he was 6 years old. Asthmatic triggers include smoke, perfumes, dust allergy, and exercise. The client has just entered high school and wants to be involved in sports. He shows a talent for golf and is frustrated when his breathing problems interfere with his game.

The client uses a combined medication program that includes Singulair and Ventolin HFA. He does well on the medication, and side effects are minimal. When using the inhaler, he occasionally gets a headache or stomachache, experiences a racing heart, and feels agitated.

Massage therapy was suggested to help with stress and relaxation of breathing muscles. The young man is not so sure about massage therapy. He does not want to take off his clothes, and he does not want his parents in the room watching. He thinks he is doing fine with the medications, but there are indications that he has been overusing his inhaler. The medical team would like him to try relaxation methods before they adjust his medication. The referral by the medical team is for a massage therapist who is a relative of one of the nurses. She is comfortable with adolescents, has golfers as clients, and is in private practice with an office near the client's home.

Assessment

Observation

The client slouches in the chair and looks disgusted. He fidgets. The parents are a bit overpowering and do not let the client speak for himself.

The use of auxiliary breathing muscles is evident. The client is a bit short for his age but appears normal in adolescent development. He is right-handed.

Interview and Goals

In addition to asthma, the client information form indicates headaches and a digestive disturbance (nausea) related to the medication he is taking. The client broke his left collarbone 5 years ago. He has typical adolescent stress and difficulty falling asleep. He is allergic to dust, and his asthma is triggered by sensitivity to scent and smoke. He has some acne on his back, chest, and face. He takes a multivitamin daily.

He does not want to talk about massage for the asthma, but as a goal he is interested in a sports massage application for enhancing his golf game.

Physical Assessment

Posture

Slight kyphosis (common in asthma). Slight anterior rotation and elevation of the left shoulder with a lateral head tilt to the left.

Gait

Normal; arm swing is a bit short bilaterally.

Range of Motion

Arm extension and external rotation are slightly limited bilaterally, more so on the left.

Palpation

Palpation examination was limited because client would not take off his clothes.

Near Touch

Normal.

Skin

Normal (as identified on the arm). Bruise is noted on the right forearm.

Superficial Connective Tissue

Unable to assess.

Vessels and Lymph Nodes

Unable to assess.

Muscles

Breathing muscles are short, tight, and tender to moderate palpation. Tender points in the intercostals and anterior serratus are sensitive to pressure. Trigger point activity is evident in the sternocleidomastoid muscles.

Tendons

Subscapularis and supraspinatus tendons bilaterally are tender to moderate pressure. Muscle attachments at the occipital base are tender to moderate pressure.

Deep Fascia

Short in the cervical area; unable to assess other areas.

Ligaments

Appear normal.

Joints

Acromial clavicular and sternal clavicular joints on the left are tender to compressive force. Facet joints of the upper ribs are fixed and rigid.

Bones

Healing of broken clavicle noted.

Abdominal Viscera

Unable to assess.

Body Rhythms

Breathing is strained, particularly the exhale phase; strain was exaggerated when parents were speaking for client.

Muscle Testing

Strength

Left arm extensors are weak. Rhomboids are weak. Pectoralis major is overly strong and would not inhibit.

Neurological Balance

Reactive muscle twitching occurs with light touch on neck and chest. Shoulder muscles misfire.

Gait

Left arm extensors do not hold when facilitated by the left hip flexors.

Interpretation and Treatment Plan Development

Clinical Reasoning

What Are the Facts?

Asthma is a lung disease that affects 12 million to 15 million Americans, including approximately 10% to 12% of children under age 18. Asthma is a disease of the bronchial tubes characterized by tightening of these airways. It is one of the chronic obstructive pulmonary diseases (others are chronic bronchitis and emphysema). Common symptoms include shortness of breath, coughing, wheezing, and tightening in the chest.

When a person breathes, air is taken into the body through the nose and then passes through the windpipe into the bronchial tubes. At the end of the tubes are tiny air sacs, called *alveoli*, which deliver oxygen to the blood. These air sacs also collect unusable carbon dioxide, which is exhaled from the body. During normal breathing, the bands of muscle that surround the airways are relaxed, and air moves freely. In people with asthma, allergy-causing substances and environmental triggers, such as smoke and scents, cause the bands of muscle surrounding the airways to tighten, and air cannot move freely. Less air causes a person to feel short of breath. Air moving through tightened airways causes a whistling sound known as *wheezing*.

Asthma can be controlled but not cured. It is not commonly fatal, but it can become life-threatening if it is not treated or controlled. Medications are used to prevent and control asthma symptoms, to reduce the number and severity of asthma episodes, and to improve airflow.

Asthma is treated with two kinds of medicines: quick-relief medicines to stop asthma symptoms and long-term control medicines to prevent symptoms. Inhaled corticosteroids are the preferred medicines for long-term control of asthma. One common side effect from inhaled corticosteroids is a mouth infection called *thrush*.

In rare cases, leukotriene modifiers, such as Singulair (montelukast), can have serious psychological side effects such as agitation, aggression, hallucinations, depression, and suicidal thinking.

The client is not interested in massage for the asthma but will discuss massage for his golf game. The restriction in arm mobility and the rotated and elevated shoulder are implicated as disturbing the golf swing.

What Are the Possibilities in Both Function and Dysfunction and the Massage Intervention Options?

The client has compensated for labored breathing since he was 6 years old. This has likely resulted in the postural shift and muscle tenderness identified during the assessment.

Playing golf may be straining the compensation patterns, making his breathing seem more labored. However, golf is a good sport choice because the activity can be controlled and calming, as long as performance remains relaxed and competition stays within reason.

Possibilities

1. A gentle stretching program may be as beneficial as massage and may be more comfortable for the client. Adolescents commonly are very body aware and will assert their need for privacy and independence. The client may be embarrassed about the acne.
2. The initial suggestion for the massage would be for the client to experience a massage over the clothing in a seated position in the massage chair. Because he is a minor, the parents must be present for supervision; however, this could be accomplished by leaving the treatment room door open and having the parents seated just outside the door. Massage could then progress to a mat and still be done over the clothing.
3. Massage on a weekly basis has shown benefit for those with asthma. As the client becomes more comfortable, additional methods could be used. The palpation assessment could be completed when the client becomes tolerant of his skin being touched.

What Are the Logical Outcomes of Each Possible Intervention?

Medication side effects of headache and gastrointestinal distress could be reduced by the massage.

Medication influence on the sympathetic autonomic nervous system may reduce the parasympathetic influence of the massage, reducing benefits.

A stretching program may not address the shortening in the auxiliary breathing muscles that are most affected by the asthma.

What Is the Effect on the People Involved for Each Possible Intervention?

The client will accept massage better if he notices improvement in his golf game. If concrete benefits are seen, his compliance should increase.

The massage professional is uncomfortable talking the client into massage but confident that a focus on golf improvement would also benefit the asthma. Further, the massage professional is uncomfortable with the overbearing parents and would have to establish appropriate working boundaries that respect the client's and the parents' rights.

The client is resistant. The parents are frustrated.

The medical team is very supportive.

Decision Making and Treatment Plan Development

Primary Goal: Stress Management
Secondary Goal: Functional Mobility
Category of Care: Condition Management

Quantifiable Goal

To manage the side effects of medications and reduce sympathetic dominance.

Qualifiable Goal

The client should be able to improve sports performance.

Treatment Regimen

Condition Management

A series of 10 weekly, 60-minute sessions of massage that begin in the chair over the clothing and focus on respiratory function and golf swing mechanics will be provided. The massage therapist provides a package of 10 massage sessions for $550 paid in advance or $65 per session. Broad-based compression, shaking, rocking, percussion, vibration, joint movement (both active and passive), and various forms of muscle energy methods will be used to effectively lengthen short areas in both muscles and connective tissue. Positional release can be used on the tender points identified during assessment and can be taught to the client. Initially the focus will be on the upper body and arms, but gradually it will be extended to a more full-body approach if the client becomes willing.

Referral will be made to a flexibility program, an option that may be more comfortable for the client, allowing him to choose which intervention feels most beneficial. The methods suggested for the massage sessions could be demonstrated on one of the parents so that the client can observe and become more comfortable with the process.

One of the parents must be present during the massage and can observe quietly from the open door during the session. All questions will be addressed before or after the session. During the session interaction will be between the client and massage practitioner unless the client indicates otherwise.

The client and parents will monitor the effects of massage on both the asthma and the golf game and will report to the massage practitioner each session.

The golf pro where the client practices has indicated a willingness to work with helping people understand the benefits of massage and a flexibility program for good golf play. A referral for a meeting with the golf pro is appropriate.

A report will be sent monthly to the client's doctor.

CASE 18. SEASONAL AFFECTIVE DISORDER

The client is a 32-year-old female. She is married and has two children, 6 and 9 years old. She is a teacher but has chosen to stay home while her children are young. She has been diagnosed with a form of depression called *seasonal affective disorder* (SAD). She experiences moderate symptoms, including an increased appetite and a carbohydrate craving, and she gains about 20 pounds every winter. She loses some of the weight in the summer, but over the years she has become overweight. She wants to be alone and has lost all interest in sex. She is fatigued, she says she feels as if she weighs 1000 pounds, and she cannot get enough sleep. She does not want to do anything but manages to drag herself through the day to meet major responsibilities. She has a hard time remembering details and is impatient with unexpected demands on her time. Her muscles ache, and she continually has a dull headache.

She is taking bupropion, which improves mood by boosting brain levels of three different chemical messengers: dopamine, serotonin, and norepinephrine. She has recently begun using light therapy. Both seem to help.

She is interested in complementary methods, especially aromatherapy and homeopathy. She has also read that massage can positively affect depression. She loves massage and has treated herself when on vacation. A holistic health center with a massage clinic just opened in her hometown, and the rates are affordable with a package plan. Her doctor is supportive, especially if massage will help her be more compliant with an outdoor walking program.

Assessment

Observation

The client appears fatigued and has circles under her eyes. She carries excess weight in her hips. She wants to sit down immediately when she enters the office. When she gets up from the chair, she seemingly exerts extraordinary effort. Her demeanor is pleasant but seems forced. She does not offer information but does respond to questions.

Interview and Goals

The client history form indicates that she has headaches, wears contact lenses, has bouts of diarrhea, uses birth control pills, and has some abdominal bloating when she eats ice cream (likely a dairy sensitivity). Muscle aching is described as all over the body, with more stiffness than pain. She has had two pregnancies and one miscarriage. There is a history of heart problems on her father's side of the family. She is fatigued and depressed and has periods of anxiety. Even though she sleeps more than 10 hours a day she does not feel rested in the morning. She has been attempting to lose weight with a low-fat diet. She fell down some stairs a few years ago. She was shaken up and had a slight concussion but was fine in a few days.

The client's goals for the massage are to reduce her depressive symptoms and to support her efforts at relaxation and exercise.

Physical Assessment

Posture

Generally bilaterally symmetrical with no obvious postural distortions.

Gait

Slow and labored with reduced arm swing.

Range of Motion

Within normal range but guarded at the end range.

Palpation

Near Touch

Normal.

Skin

Normal but dry. Hair is dry. Fingers have hangnails.

Superficial Connective Tissue

Very slight bogginess.

Vessels and Lymph Nodes

Normal.

Muscles

Normal; no obvious tender areas or shortened muscles.

Tendons

Normal.

Deep Fascia
Mild bind in the plantar fasciae.
Ligaments
Normal.
Joints
End-feel is normal and soft, but client guards and stiffens before physiological end range of joint movement is reached.
Bones
Normal.
Abdominal Viscera
Soft with evidence of gas.
Body Rhythms
Breathing is slow, with an even inhale-to-exhale ratio and some sighing. Heart rate is within normal range, but pulses are hard to feel.

Muscle Testing

Strength

Muscles test strong, but client exerts extraordinary effort during assessment.

Neurological Balance

Client does not want to sustain pressure against resistance. She says she is tired. Gluteus maximus firing is off. Synergistic dominance is evident.

Gait

Shoulder and hip flexors on the opposite side inhibit instead of facilitate, whereas on the same side, they facilitate. Normal gaiting reflexes appear to be reversed. When client looks down, extensors twitch and flexors and adductors are inhibited rather than facilitated. When client looks up over her head, flexors and adductors inhibit as appropriate.

Interpretation and Treatment Plan Development

Clinical Reasoning

What Are the Facts?

Temporary depression is a normal reaction to loss, life's struggles, or injured self-esteem. However, feelings of sadness that become hopeless and intense, last for long periods, and prevent a person from participating in everyday life are not normal. A mental illness left untreated can worsen, lasting for years and causing untold suffering, and can possibly even lead to suicide. It is important for massage professionals to recognize the signs of depression and refer appropriately (Box 16.2).

Seasonal depression (SAD) is a depression that occurs each year at the same time, usually starting in the fall or winter and ending in the spring or early summer. It is more than just "the winter blues" or "cabin fever." A rare form of SAD known as *summer depression* begins in late spring or early summer and ends in the fall.

People who suffer from SAD have many of the common signs of depression: sadness, irritability, loss of interest in their usual activities, withdrawal from social activities, and an inability to concentrate (Box 16.3). Symptoms of winter SAD differ from symptoms of summer SAD (Box 16.4).

Box 16.2 Signs and Symptoms of Depression

- Sadness (lingering)
- Loss of energy
- Feelings of hopelessness or worthlessness
- Loss of enjoyment of things that were once pleasurable
- Difficulty concentrating
- Uncontrollable crying
- Difficulty making decisions
- Irritability
- Increased need for sleep
- Insomnia or excessive sleep
- Unexplained aches and pains
- Stomachache and digestive problems
- Decreased sex drive
- Sexual problems
- Headache
- Change in appetite, causing weight loss or gain
- Thoughts of death or suicide
- Attempt at suicide

Box 16.3 Common Symptoms of Seasonal Affective Disorder (SAD)

Anxiety: Tension, inability to tolerate stress, phobias.
Social problems: Irritability, loss of pleasure in being with others and a desire to avoid contact, which could even turn into unwillingness to leave the home or bed.
Loss of libido: Decreased interest in sex.
Sleep problems: Tendency to sleep for longer periods; sleep is restless and less satisfying.
Mood swings: In the spring, when SAD lifts, some sufferers experience a dramatic swing in mood and a short period of hypomania, a sudden surge of energy and enthusiasm that brings problems of its own.
Menstrual difficulties: During the winter, premenstrual tension may be worse than in other seasons, causing irritability, sleep problems, appetite changes, and a low energy level.
Hopelessness: Feelings of desperation, which sometimes lead to overdependence on relationships, work, or home.
Excessive eating and drinking: Carbohydrates, alcohol, and coffee.
Increased sensitivity to pain: Headaches, muscle and joint pain.
Other physical ailments: Constipation, diarrhea, heart palpitations.

In the United States 4% to 6% of the population suffers from SAD, and 10% to 20% may suffer from a milder form of winter blues. Three-fourths of sufferers are females, most of whom are in their 20s, 30, or 40s. Although SAD is most common during these ages, it also can occur in children and adolescents. Older adults are less likely to experience SAD. The illness is more commonly seen in people who live at high latitudes (geographical locations farther north or south of the equator), where seasonal changes are more extreme.

To achieve effectiveness and to prevent a relapse of depression, medications generally are prescribed for 6 to 12 months for people treated for first-time depression. These medications usually must be taken regularly for at least 4 to 8 weeks before their full benefit takes effect.

The client in this case is taking bupropion. Bupropion may have the following side effects:

- Drowsiness

Box 16.4 Symptoms of Winter SAD and Summer SAD

Symptoms of Winter SAD

The symptoms of winter SAD include the seasonal occurrence of the following:
- Fatigue
- Increased need for sleep
- Decreased levels of energy
- Weight gain
- Increased appetite
- Difficulty concentrating
- Increased desire to be alone

Symptoms of Summer SAD

The symptoms of summer SAD include the seasonal occurrence of the following:
- Weight loss
- Trouble sleeping
- Decreased appetite
- Agitation
- Restlessness
- Anxiety

- Anxiety
- Excitement
- Difficulty falling asleep or staying asleep
- Dry mouth
- Dizziness
- Headache
- Nausea
- Vomiting
- Stomach pain
- Uncontrollable shaking of a part of the body
- Loss of appetite
- Weight loss
- Constipation
- Excessive sweating
- Ringing in the ears
- Changes in sense of taste
- Frequent urination
- Sore throat

Some side effects can be serious and referral is necessary:
- Seizures
- Confusion
- Hallucinating (seeing things or hearing voices that do not exist)
- Irrational fears
- Muscle or joint pain
- Rapid, pounding, or irregular heartbeat
- Fever
- Rash or blisters
- Itching
- Hives
- Swelling of the face, throat, tongue, lips, eyes, hands, feet, ankles, or lower legs
- Hoarseness
- Difficulty breathing or swallowing

In addition to the depression, the client's gait reflex patterns are disrupted. Also, she is restricting her fat intake.

What Are the Possibilities in Both Function and Dysfunction and the Massage Intervention Options?

The client might not have enough fat in her diet. There is evidence of lactose intolerance with the gas and bloating. Referral to her doctor with a recommendation that she see a nutritionist would be wise.

The client's fall could have disrupted her normal gait patterns. Although not causal to the SAD, walking reflexes have become nonoptimal, requiring increased energy expenditure, which contributes to the fatigue. Working to reestablish a normal gait may help. Wobble board and large gym ball activities could support massage. If improvement is not noted with general intervention, referral to an exercise physiologist would be indicated.

Although medication seems to help, some of the symptoms indicate side effects of the medication, and referral back to the physician for reevaluation of the medication and dosage would be prudent.

Possibilities

1. General constitutional massage has been shown to help those with various types of depression. Massage with sufficient pressure seems to affect the serotonin and dopamine levels, and both neurotransmitters are implicated in SAD. Other neurochemicals influenced by massage may be oxytocin and endocannabinoids.
2. The normal gait reflex patterns can be stimulated with massage, which may make walking less fatiguing.
3. The client could be referred to an aromatherapist but not until approval is obtained from her physician.

What Are the Logical Outcomes of Each Possible Intervention?

Referral to the physician for further evaluation seems a cautious and prudent choice to clarify the client's symptom pattern. This does involve time and cost factors, as do referrals to other professionals. Introducing too many interventions at one time can cause confusion as to what is having beneficial or detrimental effects.

Working with the gait reflexes is a simple and safe intervention during the massage, but the consequences of the fall could be more complicated. A specialist, such as an exercise physiologist, could provide specific protocols for retraining the walking pattern.

General nonspecific massage is likely to provide short-term observable benefits but might not be sustaining if underlying factors exist needing determination. The cost for massage is reasonable, and the location is convenient.

Gym balls and wobble boards are easy to locate and inexpensive. The wobble board requires another person to spot during use to prevent falling. The exercise gym ball is safe to use alone.

What Is the Effect on the People Involved for Each Possible Intervention?

The client likes massage and is interested in aromatherapy. She is open to returning to her physician for further evaluation. The physician is supportive of massage but not of homeopathy. The physician does not know enough about essential oils and so defers to the massage therapist for a recommendation.

The massage therapist feels confident providing the massage but believes some unidentified factors need to be resolved.

Decision Making and Treatment Plan Development

Primary Goal: Stress Management
Secondary Goal: Functional Mobility
Category of Care: Condition Management

Quantifiable Goals

1. Improve gait by 50%.
2. Support the body's natural defenses against depression.

Qualifiable Goal

The client will be able to exercise without pain and fatigue.

Treatment Regimen

The client will be referred back to her physician with the proposed treatment plan for massage and the following recommendations:

- The client may benefit from a nutritional evaluation. Medication side effects concur with the symptoms described on the client history form, and reevaluation of the medication type or dosage may be indicated. The medication dose should be monitored because massage does influence neurochemicals. Gait seems disrupted, and further evaluation from a physical therapist or exercise physiologist may be beneficial. Referral to the aromatherapist is recommended because the client has expressed an interest in this complementary method.
- The client will schedule weekly 60-minute massage sessions, and the schedule will be increased to twice a week if her symptoms worsen. The massage will be a general full-body approach with sufficient pressure for the client to feel the intensity of the session but with no pain or guarding. A general intervention to improve gait patterns will include having the client roll her eyes in large, slow circles while the legs and arms are massaged. After six sessions of the general massage, pulsed muscle energy methods for the arm and opposite leg flexors will be introduced to encourage normal facilitation patterns.
- The client could benefit from a daily session of bouncing and stretching on a large exercise gym ball.

CASE 19. SPORTS PERFORMANCE ENHANCEMENT

The client is a 22-year-old college student studying exercise science and athletic training. They are a competitive marathon runner. Four years ago, the client lost their left leg below the knee in an automobile accident. The client has rehabilitated successfully and has been fitted with both a running prosthesis and a prosthesis for general use.

The client is currently training for a marathon. As an amateur athlete, the client coordinates their own training program and works with a running coach. The client had a first-degree ankle sprain 2 years ago, experiences generalized cramping if overtrains, had one experience of shin splints, and occasionally gets side stitches. These symptoms improve when they drink enough water or sports drinks and properly warm up and cool down.

The client is a student of the sport and is constantly studying the effects of diet and training protocols to enhance performance. They are interested in incorporating massage into the program to support recovery and flexibility and to reduce the potential for injury. Finances are secure resulting from an insurance settlement from the accident. The client has determined they can afford $150 per month for massage and wants the maximum benefit from the investment.

Assessment

Observation

The client is slim, muscular, and fit. There is little evidence of the amputation. The client does not attempt to conceal the prosthesis and speaks freely about the accident and is more concerned about total body performance than the loss of the leg.

Interview and Goals

The client information form indicates minor muscle pain related to training and mild episodes of phantom pain, usually in response to an increase in training. The pain is managed with rest, massage of the stump, and stretching. Right leg symptoms and injuries include calf tightness, shin splints 8 months prior, and an ankle sprain 2 years prior.

The client has occasional fatigue and restless sleep if they overtrain or experience phantom pain. The client is currently being treated for athlete's foot. The client takes performance-based supplements in a well-balanced formula.

The client's goal for massage is support for a training regimen to enhance performance and help prevent injury.

Physical Assessment

Posture

Symmetrical, except for highly developed thigh muscles, with increased development on the left and a slightly elevated iliac crest on the left.

Gait

Normal with the prosthesis except for increased arm swing on the right. They received extensive rehabilitation to support normal gait after the amputation.

Range of Motion

Normal.

Palpation

Near Touch

Nothing abnormal.

Skin

Damp areas are noted at the amputation site and on the medial calf on the right. There are no areas of inflammation, abrasion, or skin irritation from the prosthesis. Skin is smooth and resilient. Small area of bind is noted just under the right clavicle.

Superficial Connective Tissue

Small bind and increased tissue density in the legs.

Vessels and Lymph Nodes

Normal.

Muscles

Normal with hypertrophy in the legs. Decreased pliability with slight increase in density and shortening of the hamstrings. Tenderness and pain radiate to three areas on the stump, two in the vastus lateralis and one in the vastus medialis.

Tendons

Normal except for some shortening in the right Achilles tendon.

Deep Fascia

Plantar fascia is slightly short on the right.

Ligaments

Normal.

Joints

No evidence of inappropriate end-feel or bind. Slight decrease in dorsiflexion on the right.

Bones

Normal.

Abdominal Viscera

Normal.

Body Rhythms

Normal.

Muscle Testing

Strength

Normal.

Neurological Balance

Normal.

Gait

Higher degrees of facilitation between extensors and flexors on the right arm and left leg seem an appropriate compensation for amputation.

Interpretation and Treatment Plan Development

Clinical Reasoning

What Are the Facts?

An understanding of the basic physical concepts involved in exercise and training protocols is important to a massage professional who works with athletes in conditioning, performance enhancement, and injury rehabilitation. To increase a sustainable power output, the athlete must follow a carefully designed training program that will improve the individual's ability to (1) produce metabolic energy by both aerobic and anaerobic means, (2) sustain aerobic energy production at high levels before lactic acid accumulates excessively in the blood, (3) recruit more of the efficient slow-twitch muscle fibers in muscle groups used in competition, and (4) become more skillful by recruiting fewer nonessential muscle fibers during competition. Careful attention to maintaining a sufficient intake of fluids and carbohydrates before, during, and after strenuous competition and training sessions is also important (see Chapter 15).

Shin splints (medial tibial stress syndrome), side stitches, plantar fasciitis, muscle cramps, muscle strains, dehydration, and hyponatremia (diluted blood sodium levels) can quickly make running a painful experience. This client is experiencing shin splints, one of the most common running injuries. This is an inflammation of tendons along the inside of the shinbone. Shin splints result when too much stress is put on tired calf muscles, as occurs with running on hard surfaces. Changing surfaces (from hard to soft) also tends to aggravate the calf muscles. The symptoms of shin splints include aching, throbbing, or tenderness of the shin. Pain is felt when the inflamed area is pressed. The best preventive measure is proper warm-up before a run to help develop flexibility, which is a key factor in avoiding shin splints.

What Are the Possibilities in Both Function and Dysfunction and the Massage Intervention Options?

The client is in good physical condition, with minor changes that seem appropriate compensation for amputation and use of the prosthesis.

Trigger point activity in the leg with the amputation may be causing the phantom pain. An aggressive training program may be contributing to fatigue and muscle aching.

Possibilities

1. Massage is indicated for support of sports training programs. It can facilitate fluid exchange in the muscles, manage symptoms of delayed-onset muscle soreness, and maintain appropriate pliability in soft tissue structures.
2. Massage can help reduce sensation referral in the client's left leg, support restful sleep, and encourage well-being.

What Are the Logical Outcomes of Each Possible Intervention?

The client has specific and realistic expectations for massage and goals that are achievable.

The client has determined that funds are available for massage, but the frequency of massage needed to achieve the desired results might exceed available funds. Massage two times per week would be optimal, with more frequent intervention during intensive training periods. The client's finances support one massage per week.

The massage therapist is aware of the time commitment required to effectively serve a client with these goals.

What Is the Effect on the People Involved for Each Possible Intervention?

All parties involved are supportive of massage, and the massage therapist is qualified to work with this level of athletic performance.

The massage therapist is willing to commit to the time necessary to support this athlete but is concerned about feeling taken advantage of because fee reductions may be required. The client is very independent and a bit demanding but realistic and understanding of the massage therapist's concerns.

Decision Making and Treatment Plan Development

Primary Goal: Pain Management
Secondary Goals: Stress Management and Functional Mobility
Category of Care: Restorative/Condition Management

Quantifiable Goals

1. Reduce episodes of phantom pain by 50%.
2. Reduce post-exercise aches by 50%.
3. Increase sleep effectiveness to support recovery time.

Qualifiable Goal

The client will be able to participate in a training program with minimal discomfort.

Treatment Regimen

Restorative Care/Condition Management

The massage therapist is an instructor at a massage school. The client will receive a 1-hour massage once a week for $150 per month and will allow students to observe and participate in the sessions as part of a sports massage internship program. The athlete will also receive massage sessions at the school student clinic and be supported at various preliminary events by the students.

The massage will be a performance-based, full-body application and will be structured to meet the daily needs of the training regimen. Ongoing contact with the coach is requested. The massage will support rather than seek to change compensation patterns in gait in response to the amputation, because overall posture and performance are good.

Referred pain will be addressed with a variety of methods, and the results will be monitored to see if the phantom pain episodes decrease. The massage will be scheduled in the evening when possible so the client can go to bed afterward. Sleep will be supported through encouragement of parasympathetic activation.

Appropriate methods that affect the neuromuscular/connective tissue and fluid dynamics of the body will be chosen for each session. The client requires various levels of pressure, from light pressure for lymphatic drainage to firm and focused pressure to address the muscles of stabilization in the layer closest to the bone. Care will be taken not to increase inflammation in any area.

CASE 20. SCAR TISSUE MANAGEMENT

The client is a 28-year-old computer technician who works 50 hours per week. They are in good health, active in a variety of outdoor activities, and concerned about maintaining their quality of life.

Six years ago, while burning leaves, the client was burned on their chest. They had first- and second-degree burns, in addition to small areas of third-degree burns. The client was fortunate to be treated in a major burn center and received the best of care. The scarring was managed very well. Only one area had to be grafted, and the donor site was on their thigh; scarring is also present in that area.

Although the areas with a first-degree burn healed with no scarring, the areas with a second-degree burn did scar, with what are called *hypertrophic scars.* The client feels as if these scars are causing tightness across their chest and finds the sensation a nuisance.

The client has had massage a few times before and found that it lessened the tightness in their chest for a short time. The client has read about various forms of connective tissue-focused massage and the effect on scars. In the context of general massage, they would like to explore the possibility of using massage to make them more comfortable and for general stress management. Because the client just received a raise, they haves $100 per month to spend for massage care.

Assessment

Observation

The client is of average height and weight, is fit, and walks with an energetic flair. They are talkative and like to tell jokes. The client is left-handed. They sit calmly during the interview and fill out the necessary paperwork without difficulty.

Interview and Goals

The client information form indicates that the client has some numbness in the burn area. They had various childhood injuries, such as a broken wrist and sprained ankles, but cannot remember just when it all happened. None of the injuries bother them. The burn has been their most serious injury. The client was anxious for a time after the incident and had some nightmares, which has passed. The surgeries underwent were for skin grafts on the third-degree burn areas and for removal of skin from the donor site. The client does not take medication or vitamins and their diet is adequate for an unmarried person who lives with two friends. The client indicates they drink alcohol, use cannabis, and party on the weekends.

The client's goals for massage are general stress management and reduction of stiffness in the burn scars.

Physical Assessment

Posture

Symmetrical, with evidence of slight concavity of the chest. Knees are slightly hyperextended.

Gait

Normal.

Range of Motion

Horizontal abduction of the arms is restricted to 80 degrees. Shoulder flexion on the left is restricted to 130 degrees.

Palpation

Near Touch

No observable problems.

Skin
Skin on the chest has areas of flat scars and areas of scar development that are somewhat rough and raised, with identifiable bands of scar tissue. Areas of pigment change are noted in the scarred region. Skin on the chest and between the scapulae on the back is binding. Skinfold cannot be lifted on burn scars. Skinfold can be lifted on the back with difficulty, and it is uncomfortable for the client.
Superficial Connective Tissue
Moderate stiffness in scarred regions on both the chest and donor area.
Vessels and Lymph Nodes
There is concern over pressure on the vessels in the chest and at the clavicle. There is no evidence of edema.
Muscles
Quadriceps are short, and rhomboids are long.
Tendons
Normal.
Deep Fascia
Pliability of the lumbar dorsal fascia and iliotibial bands is reduced.
Ligaments
Normal.
Joints
Horizontal abduction of the shoulder is limited by soft tissue bind. Sternoclavicular joint on the left is restricted.
Bones
Bone changes in the right wrist indicate healing of a bone break.
Abdominal Viscera
Normal.
Body Rhythms
Full expansion of the thorax is somewhat restricted during deep inhalation. Body rhythm is even, and pulses are in the normal range.

Muscle Testing

Strength
Left arm flexors show weak to moderate resistance.

Neurological Balance
Normal.

Gait
Normal.

Interpretation and Treatment Plan Development

Clinical Reasoning

What Are the Facts?
The client appears to have a restricted sternoclavicular joint on the left; referral to a chiropractor or osteopath is indicated. Treatment for this condition should correct the weak muscles of arm flexion.

Mild to moderate connective tissue binding is present, causing a concavity in the chest and reduction of horizontal abduction of the shoulders. The area corresponds with the burn scars. Corresponding areas of connective tissue bind are noted between the scapulae. The muscles in this area are also tight and long.

The short quadriceps muscles correspond with the hyperextension of the knees.

Burn scars are evident, with reduced tissue pliability and some adhesion.

A burn that causes blisters is a second-degree burn. Typically, this type of burn is characterized as superficial or deep. A superficial second-degree burn involves only the most superficial dermis. It manifests as blistering or sloughing of overlying skin, causing a red, painful wound. Typically, the burn blanches but shows good capillary refill. Hairs cannot be pulled out easily. Healing occurs within 14 days, usually without scarring and without requiring surgical intervention. A deep second-degree burn involves more of the dermis. It may manifest as blisters or a wound with a white or deep red base. Sensation is usually diminished, and healing takes longer than 14 days. Hypertrophic scarring occurs when the healing phase lasts longer than 2 weeks. Debriding and grafting, therefore, are recommended by 2 to 3 weeks.

Studies have shown that stretching the connective tissue with sufficient force creates an elastic response in scar tissue. The most common causes of contractures are scarring and lack of use because of immobilization or inactivity. Severe contracture in this client is not evident, but scar shortening is.

Scar tissue from burns and grafts can be sensitive, and work needs to proceed with caution to ensure that the area is not damaged by the tissue stretching.

What Are the Possibilities in Both Function and Dysfunction and the Massage Intervention Options?
The connective tissue shortening of the burn scars on the chest is probably binding and restricting both upper chest motion and range of motion of the arm.
Possibilities
1. Massage that exerts a drag on the skin and superficial fascia could increase pliability and sliding in the area.
2. General massage on a weekly basis could support stress management, relaxation, and an active lifestyle.

What Are the Logical Outcomes of Each Possible Intervention?
Massage is indicated for the stated goals, but the finances allocated are insufficient to support massage on a weekly basis to address goals.

What Is the Effect on the People Involved for Each Possible Intervention?
The client and massage professional are both supportive of massage and the realistic outcome of the goals, but the finances are difficult. The client has to reassess priorities in terms of where they spend money. They are willing to invest some of the weekend partying money to cover the cost of massage on a weekly basis if they see enough value. The client is willing to commit to a 3-month, 12-session trial period.

Decision Making and Treatment Plan Development

Primary Goal: Stress Management
Secondary Goal: Functional Mobility
Category of Care: Condition Management

Quantifiable Goals

1. Reduce stress symptoms by 75% as reported by the client.
2. Increase connective tissue pliability in burn scars by 30%.

Qualifiable Goal

The client should be able to perform work and daily activities with minor tension on the scar tissue and be less irritated by the tissue changes in the burn scars.

Treatment Regimen

Condition Management

Weekly massage will be provided at $65 per hour session. The massage will consist of elongation techniques with sufficient drag to increase pliability of the scar tissue in the burn and donor areas. Caution will be needed to ensure that the intensity of the work is sufficient to address the connective tissue binding but does not damage the tissue in the area. The connective tissue work will be done before the general massage session, because generating a pulling sensation is likely to feel intense and somewhat uncomfortable. The pressure used will exert force in the horizontal plane to stretch the area of the scars. Methods to introduce tensile and shear stress into the tissue will be used first, and then bend and torque will be added as the tissue becomes more pliable. The intensity of the work will progress slowly. Since the accident is a trauma experience, awareness of trauma informed care is needed.

When the skin and superficial fascia can be lifted, skin-rolling methods will be introduced. The client will not have to endure this work for longer than 10 minutes, and frequent breaks will be included. Because mild inflammation will be introduced into the area, lymphatic drainage will be used to support movement of any restricted lymphatic flow away from the burned area. General massage will be given, with methods used as needed to address range of motion and stress management; these methods will be determined at each massage session. Pressure levels will need to be sufficient to encourage relaxation and stress management goals. The massage rhythm, speed, and duration will address the shift from the stress response to parasympathetic dominance. The massage will be rhythmic with sufficient pressure exerted to address the deeper layers of soft tissue without causing pain or guarding.

Foot in the Door

This final chapter provides examples of 20 common scenarios you may encounter as a massage professional. If you expect to convince employers or potential clients that you are a competent massage therapist, you will need to be able to function as described in the case studies. When you study and practice and if you are taking your education seriously, these skills will get your foot in the door. Ultimately, it is your responsibility to be excellent.

Remember, the cases presented in this chapter reflect entry-level education as presented in this textbook. That means that you still need lots of experience and more education, especially self-teaching.

Each client you work with will be a teacher. When you are attempting to get your foot in the door as a new massage therapy graduate, admit that you are a beginner. However, make sure to communicate your commitment to excellence and passion for massage. You have the foundation to build on if you have been a committed and excellent student. If you have a weakness in your career foundation because you did not devote your energy and time to your massage education, then fix it. Read your books, watch video clips on Evolve, and practice giving massages. Ask (and if necessary pay) for help. Your efforts will get your foot in the door for a massage career, and your skills will keep you there.

SUMMARY

Each of the case studies in this chapter should challenge the student to continue to develop clinical reasoning skills and perfect assessment and technical therapeutic massage skills (Proficiency Exercise 16.1). More important, each case study told a story about a person who was seeking assistance. Remember, the most proficient application of massage is not competent practice—compassion, respect, and desire for the highest good of the client must first be the motivating intent of the massage. Each client you serve has the potential to be a great teacher if you are willing to learn. Knowledge needs experience to support your development as a therapeutic massage professional. Congratulations on your accumulation of knowledge as presented in this text. Our hope is that each one who has learned from this text persists with the accumulation of knowledge and experience to serve and be served in this humble and important profession.

PROFICIENCY EXERCISE 16.1

Create a case of your own following the format used in this chapter.

Evolve

Visit the Evolve website: http://evolve.elsevier.com/Fritz/fundamentals/.

Evolve content designed for massage therapy licensing exam review and comprehension of content beyond the textbook. Evolve content includes:

- Content Updates
- Science and Pathology Animations
- Body Spectrum Coloring Book
- MBLEx exam review multiple choice questions

FOR EACH CHAPTER FIND:

- Answers and rationales for the end-of-chapter multiple choice questions
- Electronic workbook and answer key
- Chapter multiple-choice question quiz
- Quick Content Review in question form and answers
- Technique videos when applicable
- Learn more on the Web

REFERENCES

Berger AA, Keefe J, Winnick A, Gilbert E, Eskander JP, Yazdi C, Kaye AD, Viswanath O, Urits I. Cannabis and cannabidiol (CBD) for the treatment of fibromyalgia. *Best Practice & Research Clinical Anaesthesiology*. 2020;34(3):617–631.

Cohen-Biton L, Buskila D, Nissanholtz-Gannot R. Review of fibromyalgia (FM) syndrome treatments. *International Journal of Environmental Research and Public Health*. 2022;19(19):12106.

Giorgi V, Sirotti S, Romano ME, Marotto D, Ablin JN, Salaffi F, Sarzi-Puttini P. Fibromyalgia: one year in review 2022. *Clin Exp Rheumatol*. 2022;40(6):1065–1072. doi: 10.55563/clinexprheumatol/if9gk2. Epub 2022 Jun 22. PMID: 35748720.

Hershkovich O, Hayun Y, Oscar N, Shtein A, Lotan R. The role of cannabis in treatment-resistant fibromyalgia women. *Pain Practice*. 2022.

Kocyigit BF, Akyol A. The relationship between COVID-19 and fibromyalgia syndrome: prevalence, pandemic effects, symptom mechanisms, and COVID-19 vaccines. *Clinical Rheumatology*. 2022:1–8.

MULTIPLE-CHOICE QUESTIONS FOR DISCUSSION AND REVIEW

The answers, with rationales, can be found on the Evolve site. Use these questions to stimulate discussion and dialogue. You must understand the meaning of the words in the question and possible answers. Each question provides you with the opportunity to review terminology, practice critical thinking skills, and improve multiple choice test-taking skills. Answers and rationales are on the Evolve site. It is just as important to know why the wrong answers are wrong as why the correct answer is correct.

Clinical reasoning and synthesis

1. A massage professional is relocating the massage practice from a city to a rural area. The population is primarily farm workers and factory workers who commute to a nearby city. After interviewing some of the residents from the town, the massage professional discovers that low back pain and fatigue are chief complaints and that the average income is $40,000 per year. Which combination of methods and marketing would be the best to build the new business quickly?

a. General massage with energetic specialization provided in the client's home at a cost of $95 per session. Newspaper advertising used.
b. General massage with myofascial and trigger point specialization in a one-person office. Massage rate set at $60 for a 1-hour massage, with an introductory offer of a free 30-minute massage when a package deal of five massage sessions is purchased for $250.
c. A multi-person office providing space for three full-time massage practitioners and two part-time practitioners, with each practitioner having a particular specialty. Massage fees set at $55 per session. A radio campaign with $5 coupon offered.
d. Subleasing a room in the local cosmetology business and providing general massage for relaxation. Fees set at $65 per session. Advertising done by word of mouth and free 15-minute chair massages on Saturdays.

2. A massage professional has experienced a substantial client base increase the past 3 months because of skills in soft tissue mobilization with massage. They book 25 clients per week and have a waiting list of 15 clients wishing to get appointments. They have attempted to squeeze in an additional four or five clients by extending evening appointments. The fee is $70 for a 1-hour massage. The business nets $900 per week and the massage therapist would like to increase net income by $100 per week. During the last month, they have experienced fatigue and mild shoulder pain, which concerns them. One of the reasons they became a massage professional was to be able to work independently without personnel problems. Which of the following would be the best suggestion from a mentor?

a. Raise prices by $5 per session, limit schedule to 25 sessions a week, and review application of body mechanics.
b. Increase client load by three clients, and switch from general massage to energetic methods.
c. Raise prices by $15 and reduce client load to 20 clients.
d. Hire a massage practitioner and increase client load by 15 clients.

3. A client seeks massage to support parasympathetic dominance and reduce a tendency toward high blood pressure. The client responds best to applications of broad-based very firm compression or deep slow gliding strokes. Skin mobility and flexibility are good, as is range of motion. The client prefers to be nonparticipative during the massage. The client prefers weekly appointments in the evening. The massage professional has been working with this client for 3 months, and although the client is pleased with the work, the massage professional is exhausted after the session. What is the most likely cause?

a. The client is emotionally draining, and the therapist has issues with countertransference.
b. The massage professional finds the sessions complex and interactive, and the constant challenge is fatiguing.
c. The nonparticipation by the client is unrealistic in terms of client goals, requiring the massage professional to work too hard.
d. The client's needs are basic and nonchallenging, and the therapist uses poor body mechanics to maintain the pressure and repetitive nature of the massage.

4. A client is seeking reimbursement for massage fees from their insurance company. They were injured in a car accident, and the massage is primarily palliative. The client has requested a summary report from the massage therapist describing the massage care received over the past 6 months. Where will the massage professional obtain the data to write this report?

a. Treatment plan
b. Client history
c. Informed consent
d. Session documentation

5. A client requested a relaxation massage. The client then complained that the massage felt uncomfortable and that the skin on their back was warm and itching. Post-procedure assessment indicated a histamine response midthorax in the area between T6 and T12. Which of the following components of massage was incorrect in relation to the client's goals?
   a. Direction
   b. Drag
   c. Duration
   d. Rhythm
6. A massage professional is experiencing shoulder pain and has the sensation of tingling and numbness in the arms. They can identify various tender focal points in the trapezius and scalenes when palpating the area. The massage practice has doubled from 10 clients per week to 20 clients per week, and although the massage therapist enjoys the increased income and is pleased now to have a full-time practice, they feel pressured to perform. Instead of relaxing at the end of the day, the massage therapist feels anxious, restless, and fatigued. They also recognize they are breathing more shallowly and yawning often. Which of the following would be the best intervention?
   a. Reduce the number of massage clients to 10 sessions per week and take a monthlong sabbatical.
   b. Reduce the number of massage clients to 15 sessions per week and see their physician for antianxiety medication.
   c. Have a peer check body mechanics to look for overuse of shoulder muscles and speak to their mentor about managing business pressures.
   d. Raise rates so that 10 clients provide the same income as 20 clients.
7. A massage professional recently relocated the business to work in partnership with a mental health professional who refers patients for stress management. The massage practitioner is now required to write monthly reports on client progress and meet with the psychologist. The clients are progressing, and the massage professional and the psychologist can observe the changes, but the reports provided are vague and confusing to the psychologist. Which of the following is the most likely cause?
   a. Use of too many abbreviations in the narrative report
   b. Lack of preassessment and post-assessment in relation to quantitative and qualitative goals
   c. Ineffective informed consent procedures
   d. Subtle physiological changes that cannot be measured
8. A massage professional has been working with a college football player to increase endurance and reduce his tendency toward muscle strains. The massage professional uses a combination of methods to influence muscle tone and resting length, connective tissue pliability, and fluid dynamics, particularly blood exchange in the capillary beds on the lower legs. The massage professional recently has taken a class on muscle energy methods and has been using them to lengthen the muscles of the athlete's legs. The athlete feels looser, but his performance has decreased, and the coach and athletic trainer are not pleased. They feel that something with the massage may be the cause. Which of the following would support the coach and athletic trainer's position?
   a. The training effect on the leg muscles has been disrupted by the introduction of the muscle energy methods.
   b. The massage has caused increased inflammation in the tissues.
   c. The client is fatigued after participating in the muscle energy methods.
   d. The massage professional has not performed the methods correctly.
9. A student of massage is preparing to take final examinations. They have been informed that the exam is comprehensive, timed, and multiple choice. The student has been diligent in their studies and practicum and feels confident to begin working on clients once they graduate. The student feels nervous about remembering all the details studied, especially scientific terminology and clinical reasoning methods. They want to be alert while taking the examination but not anxious. Which of the following would be good advice for this student?
   a. Cram study just before the exam to make sure of all the terminology.
   b. Drink coffee while studying to keep awake, but not before the exam.
   c. Breathe deeply with long inhale and short exhale patterns to decrease anxiety.
   d. Get a massage the day before the exam, sleep well, and remember to exhale slowly while taking the exam.
10. A massage practitioner is preparing to work with a client who has been referred by a peer who is moving to another state. The client is a 54-year-old person who has had successful treatment for breast cancer. The massage practitioner is concerned about meeting the expectations of the client because she was with the referring practitioner for many years. Which of the following areas of professional practice are the most important considerations for the massage practitioner when working with this new client?
    a. Caution for age and hormone dysfunction, professional boundaries, and treatment plan development
    b. Rapport, comprehensive assessment, and alteration of massage application for possible areas of fragile bone structure
    c. Contraindications for cancer treatment, the client's sex, and ongoing mentor-driven rapport issues
    d. Charting, physician referral, and deep tissue massage over scar tissue in the cancer treatment area
11. A massage therapist has just completed a needs assessment for a client who is 37 years old, who is pregnant with her first child, and who has diabetes. This is a complex case because of the client's relatively advanced age for a first pregnancy as well as the complications that diabetes can present. The client is in her first trimester. She has had some nausea and increased fatigue. At this point the pregnancy is progressing normally, and the

diabetes is controlled with diet, exercise, and medication. She has had massage in the past and wants to resume receiving massage during the pregnancy to manage stress and promote sleep. She disclosed during the history that she is anxious about the potential complications of her pregnancy and wants to do whatever is possible to have a normal delivery and healthy baby. Which of the following treatment plans is most appropriate based on this information?

a. The massage should be short and should be done frequently. The pressure would vary depending on the body area being addressed. Fluid movement methods should be avoided.
b. The massage application specifically should target lymphatic drainage. Deep pressure should be avoided. The massage would occur weekly.
c. The massage should target parasympathetic dominance and local muscle aching as it presents. Aggressive stretching should be avoided. Fluid movement methods would be used as needed.
d. The massage application should be scheduled as needed and typically in the evening. The massage should be general and avoid any use of trigger point application or acupressure to avoid the potential for miscarriage.

12. A client often travels for business and uses carry-on baggage that consists of one piece of luggage and one computer briefcase. Both are packed tight and are heavy. The computer case fits on top of the luggage, and the client pulls it around the airport. The client has a slight short-term memory problem and becomes a bit anxious when checking in and going through security. The client becomes somewhat confused during this process and is afraid of misplacing an item such as the boarding pass or photo identification. This client often receives massage while traveling. Which of the following would be the most logical outcome goals requested by this client, and what treatment plan would best achieve these goals?
    a. Stress management and relief from fatigue. Massage would be targeted to generate sympathetic dominance and sleep enhancement.
    b. Stress management and muscle aching in arm and shoulders. Massage would be targeted to generate parasympathetic dominance and decrease muscle tension in the shoulder girdle muscles.
    c. Breathing restrictions and low back pain. Massage would be targeted to reverse breathing pattern disorder and related sleep disturbances.
    d. Headache and relaxation. Massage would be targeted to shift vascular circulation and increase parasympathetic dominance.
13. A young father is taking an active role in caring for his infant daughter. The baby is occasionally fussy, and the dad would like to increase his skills in soothing his baby. He occasionally gets a massage to manage tension headache. While receiving a massage, the father asks the massage practitioner if there is anything that massage can do to calm the baby. Which of the following responses is most appropriate for this inquiry?
    a. The massage practitioner suggests that the father bring the baby in for a few sessions and that they will teach him how to calm the baby with massage methods of compression and range of motion.
    b. The massage practitioner suggests that the baby receive massage when the baby is fussy and that they will be able to use energy-based modalities and hydrotherapy applications to calm the baby.
    c. The massage practitioner indicates they can teach the father a rhythmic breathing technique, and once he perfects the method, if he does it while holding the baby, the baby will relax.
    d. The massage practitioner suggests that the father take a class in infant massage or that they would be willing to give him a few lessons with the baby. Rhythmic massage using a moderate and pain-free depth of pressure has been shown to be calming for infants.
14. A recreational softball player has begun to receive massage for management of fluid retention because of hormone fluctuations. They have responded well to general lymphatic drainage methods as part of the full-body massage application. The client reports that their performance while playing ball has improved and that the improvement coincides with the time frame when they started to get regular massage. They ask the massage therapist for an explanation as to why massage targeted to reducing generalized edema has improved athletic performance. Which of the following is the most logical response?
    a. General massage nonspecifically addresses various aspects of tissue pliability, muscle length–tension relationships, and range of motion. The lymphatic drainage application within a general massage supports restorative mechanisms that encourage recovery.
    b. The correlation is likely a coincidence and not directly related. Only sports-specific massage should increase athletic performance, and the massage practitioner is not trained in sports massage.
    c. The relationship of the massage application to an increase in athletic performance specifically involves increased arterial circulation following the lymphatic drainage method. Increase in circulation supports muscle strength but not recovery after exercise.
    d. The client sleeps longer and therefore is less fatigued. Being more energetic tends to support the movement strategies required to play ball. Lymphatic drainage also has a secondary effect of restoring gait reflexes and normalizing firing patterns involved in muscle activation sequences.
15. A massage therapist is finding it increasingly difficult to work with another massage practitioner who shares the massage area. The co-worker does not maintain the environment in a safe and sanitary way in the opinion of the massage therapist; however, the supervisor does not think that the concerns are serious and will not intervene in the con-

flict. In addition, scheduling conflicts are increasing because both want to work more hours and the client base is available to support an expanded appointment schedule. The conflict is escalating, and either something must be done about the problem or the massage therapist will leave the job. The supervisor does not want this to happen. The owner of the business likes the work of both massage therapists and has tasked the supervisor to solve the problem and will support the solution so long as it can be justified. Which of the following has the most potential to solve the problem?

a. The two massage professionals should be brought together for a problem-solving session using collaboration and should come to agreement about the care of the shared environment and scheduling. A checklist would be developed, and each worker would have to complete the tasks on the checklist at the end of each work period.
b. Each massage practitioner should be provided individual space to maintain as they see fit so long as the safety and sanitation requirements of management are met. Space is available in the facility that can be remodeled at a reasonable cost as long as it also can continue to provide long-term storage of supplies.
c. A cleaning service can be employed to maintain the environment, and the two therapists can continue to share space. The therapist with the most clients will be allowed first scheduling options but must have the schedule approved each week.
d. The conflict between the two professionals has escalated to the point that they will not be able to work together regardless of the solution offered. A decision will have to be made by the owner about which massage professional to ask to leave.

16. A day spa owner is looking to increase business and intends to expand the massage offerings. The business recently has added stone massage and is looking to add more modalities. A massage professional suggests that the spa combine stone massage with aromatherapy and sound vibration to cause a harmonic resonance effect during the session. The owner's policy is to offer only services that can be justified. Can the massage application suggested be reasonably justified, and what would be the most accurate explanation?

a. No. This combination of methods would not be synergistic and actually would negate the effects of modalities being combined.
b. Yes. Research validates that the methods used in this combination enhance each other and support entrainment.
c. Yes. Each method had a logical mechanism of benefit, and these physiological mechanisms appear to be synergistic if not actually validated by research.
d. No. There is no such thing as harmonic resonance, and sound is not caused by vibration, so the explanation is not valid.

17. A massage therapist is looking at various career options. The therapist has completed an entry-level educational program and has passed the licensing exam for therapeutic massage. Now the therapist wants to continue their education with advanced training. The therapist enjoys science studies and problem solving. The therapist likes to work independently but appreciates the expertise of other professionals for peer support and mentoring. The therapist is 32 years old and has a 10-year-old child and reliable child care except for weekends. The therapist has a grandparent in long-term care and feels a strong connection with elder adults. Which of the following career tracks would best support the needs of this person and why?

a. Massage in the medical environment, primarily hospice, because the therapist can determine the hours and work independently yet still be around other professionals. The terminally ill population would satisfy the client's need for a connection with elder adults.
b. Fitness massage targeted to cardiac rehabilitation in a fitness center that works cooperatively with a medical center and a senior citizen assisted-living complex. The flexibility of the environment allows for scheduling, professional interaction, and work with the senior population.
c. Work in a spa setting in a vacation area that serves the retired population. The clients would be elder adults, and the flexibility of the spa environment allows for independent practice and interaction with other professionals.
d. Independent practice in a private office with a varied population but offering senior discounts. This environment offers the most scheduling flexibility. The business location is within walking distance of a long-term care facility and would allow residents to walk to the office for massage appointments.

18. A client is being treated for a chronic low back condition related to soft tissue dysfunction. The client also has diabetes and generalized anxiety. The client believes that massage will help, but during the interview with the massage therapist, the client has difficulty identifying outcome goals for the massage. The client asks the massage therapist for assistance and wants the therapist to explain what the massage would entail for each of the major conditions and what the therapist thinks would be a reasonable set of goals and why. Which of the following is most accurate for responding to this client?

a. Massage can provide symptom relief and symptom management of low back pain of soft tissue origin. Many of the same methods used for low back treatment also are used to normalize breathing. Normal breathing function may help ease the anxiety. The suggested treatment plan is massage to address soft tissue dysfunction in the thorax as it relates to low back pain and to observe for changes in breathing function.
b. Massage for stress management, especially increasing sympathetic dominance, has been shown to be helpful in a diabetic treatment process. The same massage application would reduce anxiety but would not treat the low back dysfunction effectively, although generalized pain management would be possible. The suggested treatment plan is to address diabetic conditions with components of pain management.
c. The low back pain can be addressed mechanically with soft tissue methods, but no other outcomes are reasonable. In addition, the diabetes presents contra-

indications that would limit the ability of the massage therapist to use some of the most effective massage applications for the low back condition. Taking this into consideration, the massage therapist only feels comfortable recommending a general massage application targeted at pain management.

d. The anxiety disorder is likely the underlying cause of the low back condition, and the increased production of serotonin by the adrenal glands is contributing to the diabetes. Massage potentially could reverse both anxiety and low back disorder and substantially improve the diabetic condition. The massage treatment plan would involve breathing retraining, myofascial release, and acupressure to rebalance the energy mechanism in the body, thus improving homeostasis.

19. A massage practitioner is changing from a sport and fitness career path for massage to a spa/wellness center environment massage career. The therapist has a solid fundamental educational background in the science, theory, and practice of therapeutic massage and the science studies that support that practice. Much of the therapist's anatomy studies involved kinesiology and biomechanics with an emphasis in movement. In previous educational endeavors, the therapist had begun an exercise science program and completed most of the science studies, so the therapist is naturally strong in that area. As the exercise science education progressed, the therapist realized a desire for a more eclectic career and felt massage could provide more options. The spa/wellness center at which the therapist will be working targets skin care, general wellbeing, and various combinations of massage and hydrotherapy. A variety of yoga and meditation classes are offered. Which of the following best describes the additional science and methods the massage therapist would need to study to increase their skill for this career change?

a. It would be helpful to increase study of the integument and the effects of skin care products. Knowledge of the physiological effects and application of hydrotherapy would also be beneficial. The study of essential oils also is indicated. Further study of the effects of environment design and client care in a service industry would support career development.

b. It would be important to study Asian massage methods and thermotherapy and to become a cosmetologist to be cross trained in skin care. Communication skills necessary for human services and negotiation and mediation are also important. Increased scientific study on mental health benefits would be useful.

c. Additional scientific studies on the effects of aging and nutrition would be helpful. Esoteric study involving energy-based modalities is also necessary, especially in the area of meditation and mindfulness. Continuing education classes should target connective tissue methods and shiatsu. Business management and human resources studies would enhance marketing skills.

d. A comprehensive study of the circulatory system would prepare the therapist for using lymphatic drainage to treat various skin and pathological conditions. The methods studied would include various ancillary practices such as paraffin treatment, waxing, and debridement. Hot stone massage proficiency is necessary as well. Communication skills for sales would be beneficial.

20. A student is preparing to take final exams to graduate from massage training and then take the state licensing exam. The student is overwhelmed with what to memorize, what to analyze, and in general how to study. Which of the following is the best recommendation for success in passing the various exams?

a. Purchase various study guides, and make sure to know the answers to the questions presented in the guides. Memorize the attachments of all the muscles, but it is less important to know the functions.

b. Concentrate on theory and practice content and spend a lot less time on the science studies. Use flash cards for clinical reasoning activities.

c. Read the textbooks used to develop the exams, and then memorize the terminology. Once this is done, use checklists to eliminate the irrelevant information, and concentrate on definitions and factual recall.

d. Reread the textbooks and concentrate on understanding the content. Study the glossaries to perfect language skills. Write test questions, developing plausible wrong answers and right answers.

Activity

Write at least three more multiple choice questions. Develop plausible wrong answers and be sure the correct answer is clearly correct. Then write a rationale for each question. The more questions you write, the better you will understand the material. Exchange questions with classmates or discuss the issues in class. The questions from all the learners can be combined to create a review quiz.

APPENDIX A

Pathology and Indications and Contraindications to Massage

Indications are determined by evidence provided by research and expert consensus when research is not available. Indications for massage are reviewed in Chapter 6. Determining contraindications is more difficult. When intelligent decision making and experience are coupled with appropriate adaptation, the result is very few contraindications, and most conditions fall into the caution category. However, because this is an entry-level textbook, it is assumed that the reader does not have experience and is still learning the process of critical thinking. Therefore, the recommendations in this appendix are conservative. Because each situation is different, making recommendations on when to give a massage and when not to give one is difficult. Each individual situation must be evaluated to determine whether massage is indicated or contraindicated. The existence of contraindications does not always mean that therapeutic massage is inappropriate. What most contraindications require is caution, which may call for modification of the massage treatment and, in some cases, supervision by and cooperation with the health and medical care team. The clinical reasoning model is a valuable tool for making decisions about contraindications. Specific conditions, symptoms, indications, and contraindications for massage follow. Use a medical dictionary to look up unfamiliar terms.

ABSOLUTE CONTRAINDICATIONS (CI) TO MASSAGE

The following are absolute contraindications (CI) to massage (i.e., massage treatment should not be given or massage is postponed until the condition resolves).

General

1. Acute-stage pneumonia
2. Advanced kidney failure (modified treatment may be possible with medical consent)
3. Advanced respiratory failure (modified treatment may be possible with medical consent)
4. Diabetes with complications (e.g., gangrene, advanced heart or kidney disease, very high or unstable blood pressure)
5. Eclampsia-toxemia in pregnancy
6. Hemophilia
7. Hemorrhage
8. Liver failure (modified treatment may be possible with medical consent)
9. Post-cerebrovascular accident (CVA, stroke), condition not yet stabilized
10. Post-myocardial infarction (MI, heart attack), condition not yet stabilized
11. Severe atherosclerosis
12. Severe hypertension (if unstable)
13. Shock (all types)
14. Significant fever (higher than 101°F [38.3°C])
15. Some acute conditions that require first aid or medical attention:
    - Anaphylaxis
    - Appendicitis
    - CVA
    - Diabetic coma, insulin shock
    - Epileptic seizure
    - MI
    - Pneumothorax, atelectasis
    - Severe asthma attack, status asthmaticus
    - Syncope (fainting)
    - Systemic contagious/infectious condition

Local (Regional): Avoid or Modify Massage in the Indicated Area

1. Acute flare-up of inflammatory arthritis (e.g., rheumatoid arthritis, systemic lupus erythematosus, ankylosing spondylitis, Reiter's syndrome); may be general CI, depending on case
2. Acute neuritis
3. Aneurysms deemed life threatening (e.g., of the abdominal aorta); may be general CI, depending on location
4. Ectopic pregnancy
5. Esophageal varicosities (varices)
6. Frostbite
7. Local contagious condition
8. Local irritable skin condition
9. Malignancy (especially if judged unstable)
10. Open wound or sore
11. Phlebitis, phlebothrombosis, arteritis; may be general CI if located in a major circulatory channel
12. Recent burn
13. Sepsis
14. Temporal arteritis
15. Twenty-four to 48 hours after antiinflammatory treatment (target tissue and immediate vicinity)
16. Undiagnosed lump

CAUTIONARY CONDITIONS

The following cautionary conditions require an awareness of the possibility of adverse effects from massage therapy. Substantial treatment adaptation may be appropriate. Medical consultation often is needed.

1. Any condition of spasticity or rigidity
2. Asthma
3. Cancer (including finding appropriate relationships to other current treatments)
4. Chronic congestive heart failure
5. Chronic kidney disease
6. Client taking antiinflammatory drugs, muscle relaxants, anticoagulants, analgesics, or any other medications that alter sensation, muscle tone, standard reflex reactions, cardiovascular function, kidney or liver function, or personality
7. Coma (may be absolute CI, depending on cause)
8. Diagnosed atherosclerosis
9. Drug withdrawal
10. Emphysema
11. Epilepsy
12. Hypertension
13. Immunosuppressed client
14. Inflammatory arthritides
15. Major or abdominal surgery
16. Moderately severe or juvenile-onset diabetes
17. Multiple sclerosis
18. Osteoporosis, osteomalacia
19. Pregnancy and labor
20. Post-CVA
21. Post-MI
22. Recent head injury

Local (Regional)

Cautionary Conditions

1. Acute disk herniation
2. Aneurysm (may be general CI, depending on location)
3. Any acute inflammatory condition
4. Any antiinflammatory treatment site
5. Any chronic or long-standing superficial thrombosis
6. Buerger's disease (may be general CI if unstable)
7. Chronic abdominal or digestive disease
8. Chronic arthritic conditions
9. Chronic diarrhea
10. Contusion
11. Endometriosis
12. Flaccid paralysis or paresis
13. Fracture (while casted and immediately after cast removal)
14. Hernia
15. Joint instability or hypermobility
16. Kidney infection, stones
17. Mastitis
18. Minor surgery
19. Pelvic inflammatory disease
20. Pitting edema
21. Portal hypertension
22. Prolonged constipation
23. Recent abortion/vaginal birth
24. Trigeminal neuralgia

Other Important Considerations

1. Massage therapists are expected to know how and when to consult with physicians and other health and medical care professionals.
2. Most emotional or psychiatric conditions affect massage treatment. Individual decisions must be made according to case circumstances and, in many instances, medical advice. Medications may be a factor.
3. The client may be allergic to certain massage oils and creams or to cleansers or disinfectants used on sheets and tables. Be aware of potential nut allergies when choosing lubricants.
4. The presence of pins, staples, or artificial joints may alter treatment indications.
5. The massage therapist should be aware of the role of common chronic conditions that affect public health (e.g., cardiovascular disease, cancer, diabetes, substance abuse, chronic mental diseases). The local health department can provide additional information on public mental health services, environmental hazards, occupational health, or various health care organizations available in the community.

Disease/Condition	Indications/Contraindications for Massage Therapy
Aneurysm An aneurysm is a weakening and bulging of the wall of a blood vessel, usually an artery. Aneurysms occur most often in the abdominal aorta and the brain.	Treatment is contraindicated. Refer client immediately to a physician. This is a medical emergency.

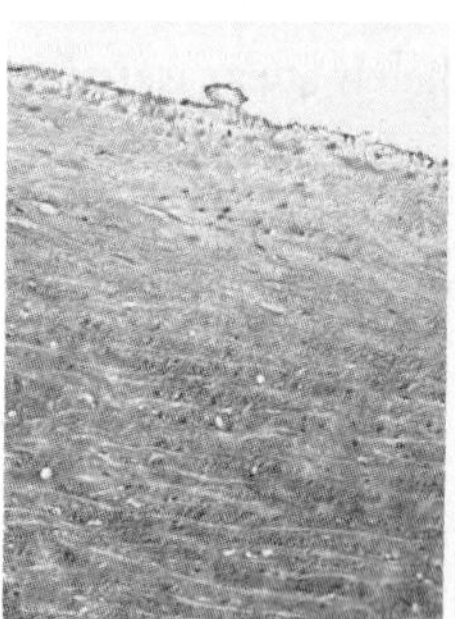
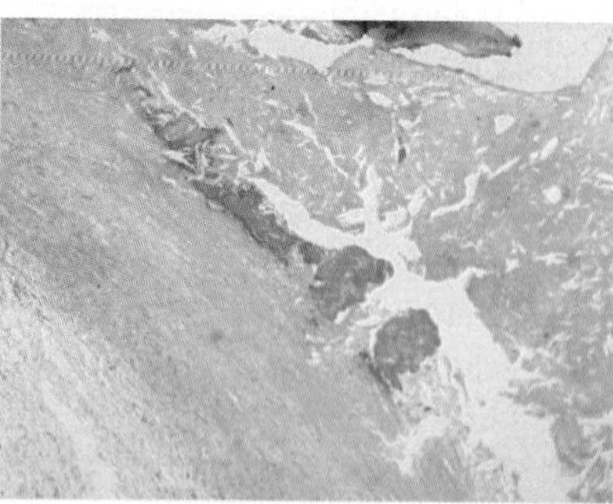

Micrographs of aneurysms. (From Tsang VT, et al: Interruption of the aorta with multilobulated arch aneurysms, *J Thorac Cardio Surg* 133[4]:1092–1093, 2007.)

Disease/Condition	Indications/Contraindications for Massage Therapy
Asthma Acute asthma is spasmodic constriction of the smooth muscle in the bronchial tubes. This is sometimes called an asthmatic attack. Chronic asthmas involve inflammation in the bronchial tubes along with excessive mucus production.	Massage is indicated for clients with asthmas as long as they are not having an asthmatic attack. Between episodes, massage can be beneficial for general stress management and relief of tension in muscles.
Atherosclerosis This is a condition in which arteries become inelastic because of the development of plaques. Because of the inelasticity, atherosclerosis is also called hardening of the arteries. Plaque buildup in the walls of the arteries that supply the heart is referred to as coronary artery disease (CAD). If enough plaque builds up, blood flow can become obstructed, leading to a heart attack or stroke. Because the plaque has a rough surface, thrombosis (formation of a clot in an unbroken blood vessel) can occur. The clot can obstruct blood flow in the area in which it develops, or it can break off and become an embolus.	Mild atherosclerosis is an indication for massage as part of a total treatment program. Advanced atherosclerosis may be a contraindication for massage. A palliative approach might be indicated depending on the medical treatment being provided.

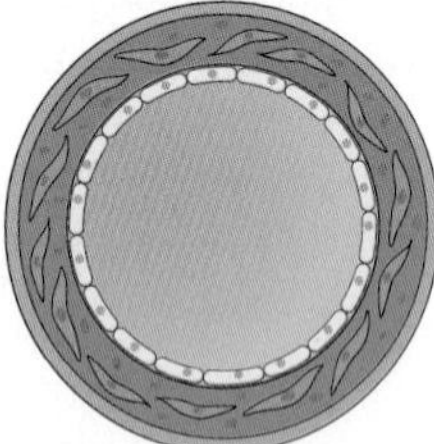

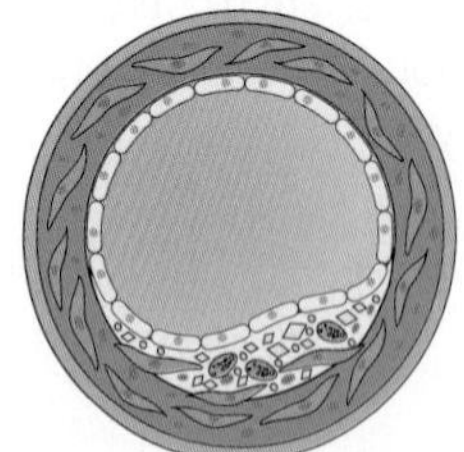

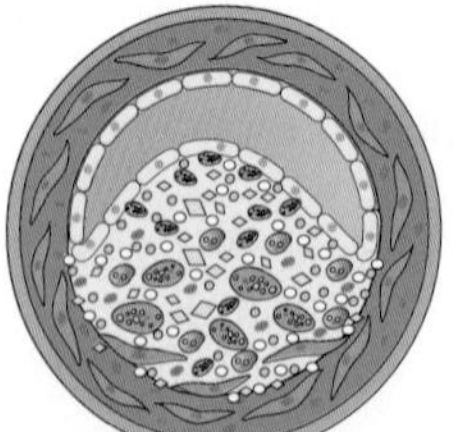

Atherosclerosis. (From Frazier MS, Drzymkowski JW: *Essentials of human diseases and conditions,* ed 4, St. Louis, 2008, Saunders/Elsevier.)

Disease/Condition	Indications/Contraindications for Massage Therapy
Bell Palsy This palsy causes partial or total paralysis of the facial muscles on one side as the result of inflammation or injury to the seventh cranial nerve. 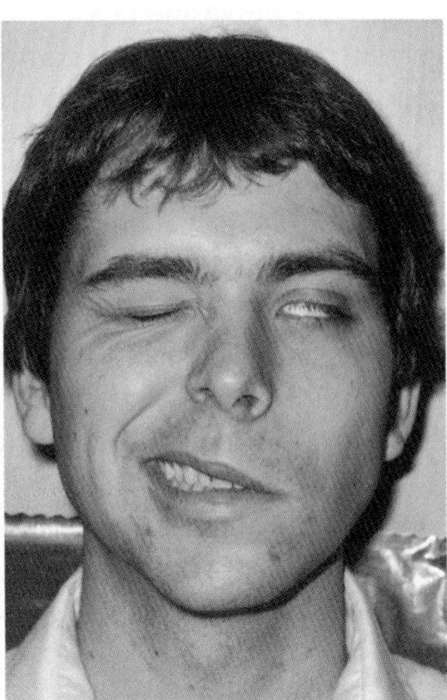 Bell palsy. (From Neville BW et al: *Oral and maxillofacial pathology,* ed 3, St. Louis, 2009, Saunders/Elsevier. Courtesy of Dr. Bruce Brehm.)	Massage approaches can reduce stress. The practitioner must gauge the intensity and duration of any massage application so as not to overtax an already stressed client, aggravating the condition. Shorter, more frequent treatments may be indicated.
Breathing Pattern Disorder This disorder is complex and involves altered breathing patterns. It is associated with stress and anxiety.	Therapeutic massage approaches and moderate application of movement therapies (such as tai chi, yoga, and aerobic exercise) assist with normalizing breathing patterns and altering mood, feelings, and behavior.
Bursitis This is inflammation of the bursae, especially those located between the bony prominences and a muscle or tendon, such as in the shoulder, elbow, hip, and knee. It usually results from trauma and repetitive use. Bursitis commonly occurs in subacromial, olecranon, prepatellar, trochanteric, and retrocalcaneal areas.	Therapeutic massage can help manage pain and support an increase in range of motion. However, massage directly over the bursae is contraindicated.
Cancer *Dysplasia* is the term for a change in normal body cells. Some of these abnormal cells can develop into cancerous cells. Some types of abnormal cells grow slowly and can be treated easily; other types are aggressive and invasive malignancies that can spread to other parts of the body. Common types of cancer include lung cancer, breast cancer, colorectal cancer, leukemia, bone cancer, melanoma (malignant skin cancer), prostate cancer, and stomach cancer. It is important to be able to recognize skin changes that could be related to skin cancer. Common types include basal cell carcinoma, squamous cell carcinoma, and malignant melanoma.	If the cancer is detected and successfully treated before metastasis, the client can receive any type of massage therapy. However, massage for clients with malignancies under active treatment is considered a caution. Additional training is recommended. The massage approach is palliative. It is recommended that the massage therapist work closely with the health care team. The practitioner must adjust treatments for any radiation therapy, chemotherapy, or surgical procedures the client is undergoing. As with most chronic illness and pain, therapeutic massage offers the client palliative or comfort care and may be helpful in reducing stress stemming from the cancer and cancer treatments that the client is receiving. Sometimes clients with colorectal cancer have colostomies. If so, the practitioner needs to adjust treatments to accommodate the colostomy bag. Report any skin changes to the client that may indicate potential for skin cancer. Refer.

Disease/Condition	Indications/Contraindications for Massage Therapy
Carpal Tunnel Syndrome This syndrome results from irritation of the meridian nerve as it passes under the transverse carpal ligament into the wrist. Symptoms include pain, numbness, tingling, and weakness in the part of the hand innervated by the median nerve, namely the thumb, the first and second fingers, half the third finger, and the palm of the hand proximal to these digits.	Various forms of massage application can reduce muscle spasms, lengthen shortened muscles, and soften and stretch connective tissue, restoring a more normal space around the nerve and possibly alleviating impingement. When massage is combined with other appropriate methods, surgery may not be necessary. If surgery is performed, the practitioner must manage adhesions appropriately and keep soft tissues surrounding the healing surgical area supple to prevent reentrapment of the nerve. Before doing any work near the site of a recent incision in the acute healing phase, the client should obtain the approval from the client's physician. In general, work close to the surgical area can begin after the stitches have been removed and all inflammation is gone. As healing progresses, soft-tissue methods can be used to address the forming scar more directly. Direct work on a new scar usually is safe 8 to 12 weeks into the healing period.

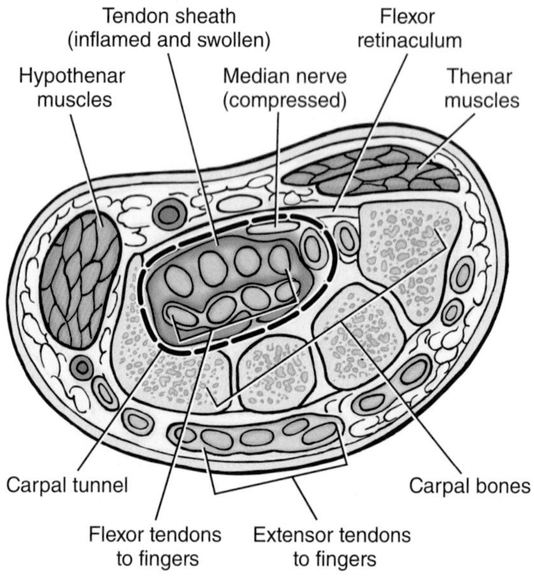

Cross-section of wrist affected by carpal tunnel syndrome.

Contusion A muscle bruise results from trauma to the muscles and involves local internal bleeding and inflammation.	Direct work over the area of injury is contraindicated regionally until all signs of inflammation have dissipated.

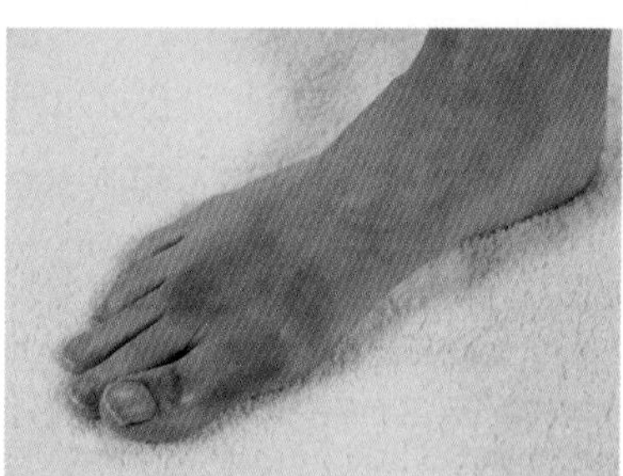

Contusion. (From Fritz S: *Mosby's fundamentals of therapeutic massage,* ed 5, St. Louis, 2013, Mosby/Elsevier.)

Coronary Artery Disease
See Atherosclerosis.

Disease/Condition	Indications/Contraindications for Massage Therapy
Decubitus Ulcer Also called *bed sores* or *pressure ulcers,* decubitus ulcers are caused by impaired blood circulation to the skin. The impairment is due to pressure of the body against a surface, such as a bed, cast, or wheelchair. The impaired blood flow leads to necrosis (tissue death) and a subsequent high risk of infection.	Massage can be beneficial in preventing the development of decubitus ulcers. Once the tissue has been damaged, however, the risk of infection is high, so massage is regionally contraindicated. However, massaging around the edges of the affected area may stimulate blood flow to assist in healing.

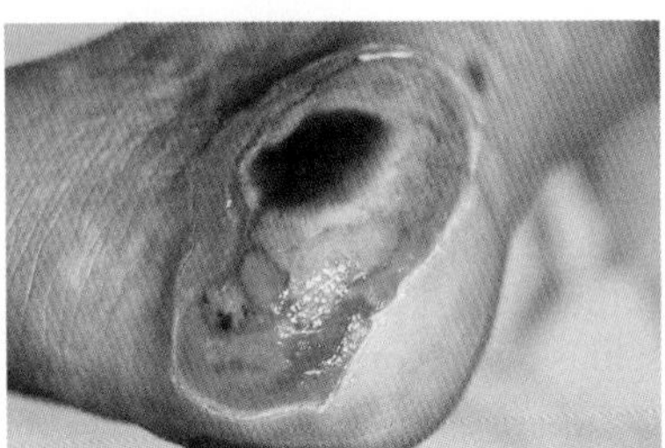

Pressure ulcer, showing tissue necrosis. (From Potter PA, Perry AG: *Fundamentals of nursing,* ed 7, St. Louis, 2009, Mosby/Elsevier.)

Disease/Condition	Indications/Contraindications for Massage Therapy
Diabetes Mellitus This disease results from the pancreas not producing any insulin called *type I* or *type II* where insulin secretion is inadequate to normalize blood sugar levels. Signs and symptoms associated with diabetes mellitus include frequent urination, excessive thirst, increased appetite, fatigue, weight loss, and nausea. Signs and symptoms associated with insulin shock include dizziness, confusion, weakness, and tremors.	Massage for clients who have diabetes should be a supportive part of an overall treatment program. Impaired blood circulation, especially in the extremities, and neuropathy often accompany diabetes mellitus. The massage therapist should refer the client for immediate medical care if any tissue changes are noted. In pain management of diabetic neuropathy, gentle massage techniques can prove beneficial for short-term reduction of pain symptoms.

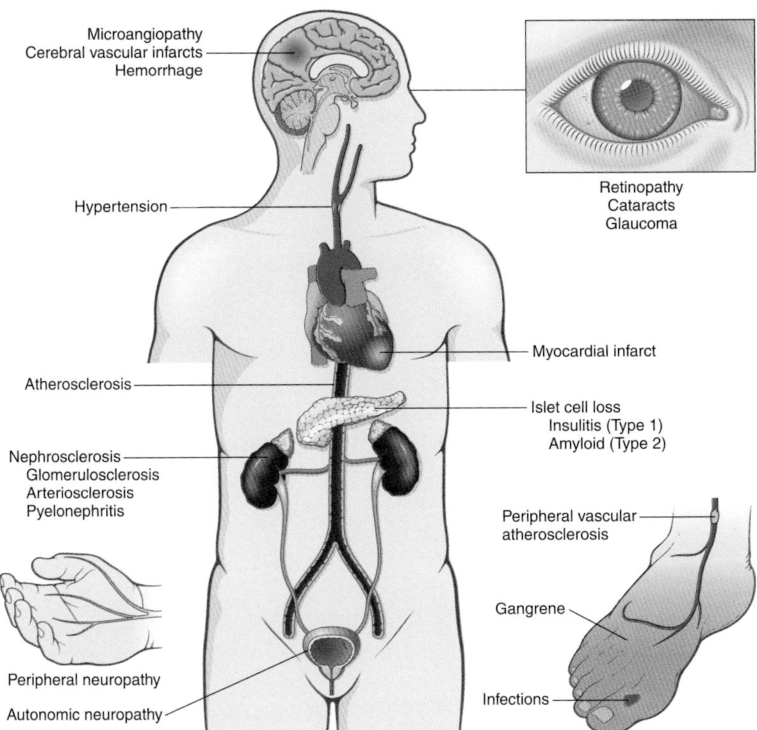

Complications of diabetes mellitus. (From Kumar V, Abbas AK, Aster JC: *Robbins and Cotran pathologic basis of disease,* ed 9, Philadelphia, 2015, Saunders/Elsevier.)

Disease/Condition	Indications/Contraindications for Massage Therapy
Dislocation Dislocation is displacement of the bones of a joint; a subluxation is a partial dislocation.	Massage and bodywork are contraindicated locally over a trauma area until healing is complete. Massage methods are beneficial in supporting the rest of the body during the healing process, especially in managing compensation patterns caused by immobilizing the area. Massage and other forms of bodywork can also help manage secondary muscle tension.
Diverticular Disease Diverticula are small, saclike outpouchings of the intestinal wall in weak areas of the colon. Diverticulosis is the development of these pouches. Diverticulitis is inflammation caused by infection of these pouches. Abdominal pain or referred back pain may indicate gastrointestinal disorders, including diverticular disease.	Clients should be referred to their physicians for proper diagnosis. If the client has been diagnosed with diverticulosis, deep abdominal massage is contraindicated. If the client has been diagnosed with diverticulitis, massage is contraindicated in the acute phase.

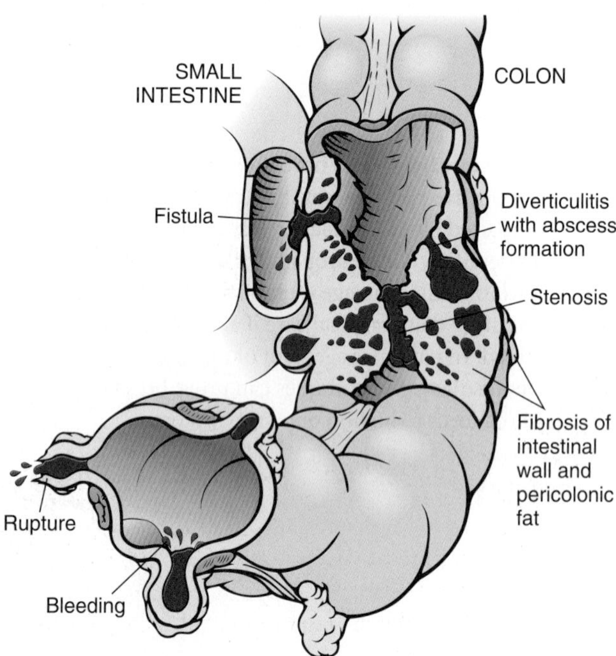

Diverticulosis of the colon. Complications include bleeding, abscess formation, perforation and rupture, fistula formation with adjacent structures, and fibrosis extending into the pericolonic fat. (From Damjanov I: *Pathology for the health professions,* ed 3, St. Louis, 2006, Saunders.)

Disease/Condition	Indications/Contraindications for Massage Therapy
Dupuytren's Contracture This disorder results from the shrinking and thickening of the palmar fascia. The contracture pulls on the tendons of the ring finger and occasionally the little finger, causing them to be permanently flexed.	Local massage is contraindicated if it increases symptoms.

Disease/Condition	Indications/Contraindications for Massage Therapy

Edema

In this condition, excessive fluid accumulates within the interstitial spaces. Edema can be caused by electrolyte or protein imbalances or obstruction in the cardiovascular or lymphatic systems. With pitting, edema tissues do not immediately spring back after being touched.

Massage is contraindicated for most types of edema from unknown cause. Referral is indicated. However, edema resulting from subacute soft-tissue injury, standing for long periods of time, or short-term immobility can be alleviated by massage, as long as there is no other factor contraindicating treatment application.

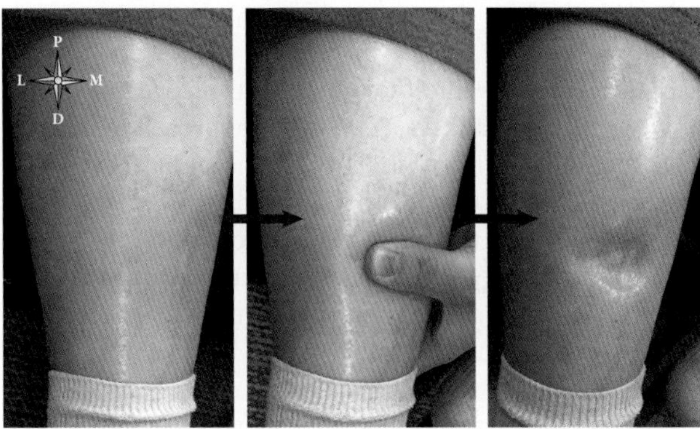

Pitting edema. Note the thumb-shaped depression that does not rapidly refill after an examiner has exerted pressure on the right anterior leg (shin). (From Patton KT, Thompson T, Williamson P: *Anatomy & physiology*, ed 11, St. Louis, 2022, Elsevier.)

Fibromyalgia

This syndrome causes symptoms of widespread pain or aching, persistent fatigue, generalized morning stiffness, nonrestorative sleep, and multiple tender points.

General massage approaches seem to work best to help reduce pain and restore sleep patterns. The client should avoid any form of therapy that causes therapeutic inflammation, including intense exercise and stretching programs, until healing mechanisms in the body are functioning. If tender points have been injected with antiinflammatory medications, anesthetics, or other substances, the practitioner should not massage over these areas.

Gallbladder Disease (Cholelithiasis)

The disease almost always results from a gallstone composed of bile salts or cholesterol lodged in the cystic duct. Abdominal pain or referred back pain may indicate one of several gastrointestinal disorders.

In such cases, referral is necessary for proper diagnosis.

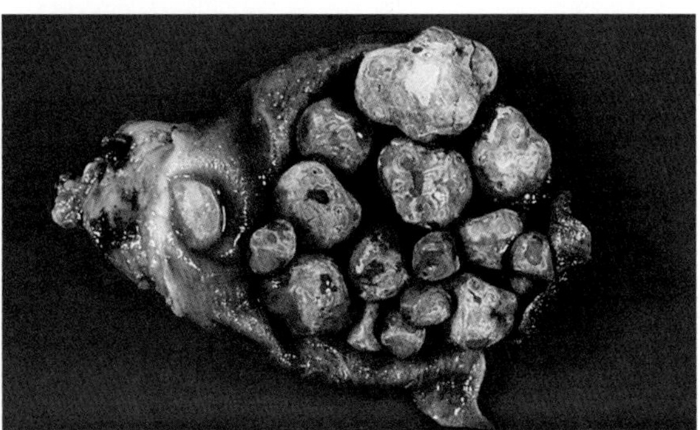

Gallstones. (From Thompson JM, Wilson SF: *Health assessments for nursing practice,* St. Louis, 1996, Mosby.)

Disease/Condition	Indications/Contraindications for Massage Therapy
Headache Pain occurs in the forehead, eyes, jaw, temples, scalp, skull, occiput, or neck. Types of headaches include tension headache, sinus headache, migraine headache, cluster headache, chemical headache, traction, and inflammatory headaches.	Massage therapy is effective in treating muscle tension headache but much less so with migraine or cluster headaches. However, massage can relieve secondary muscle tension headache caused by the pain of the primary headache. Because headache is often stress induced, stress management in all forms usually is indicated for chronic headaches.
Heart Attack A heart attack, also known as a *myocardial infarction,* is permanent damage to the myocardium caused by obstructed blood flow through the coronary arteries to the tissues.	Massage is contraindicated for clients recovering from recent heart attacks. A palliative approach to massage might be indicated for stress management. Once clients have completely recovered, the practitioner may develop treatment plans according to the client's vitality. Comprehensive stress management programs, including therapeutic massage, can help manage heart conditions.
Hepatitis Hepatitis is an inflammation of the liver. It is usually, but not always, caused by viral infection. Acute hepatitis is contraindicated for massage.	Massage for clients with chronic hepatitis requires additional training to manage the contagious nature of the condition. The practitioner must develop treatment plans according to the client's vitality.
Herniated Disk Herniated disk occurs when the fibrocartilage surrounding the intervertebral disk ruptures, releasing the nucleus pulposus. 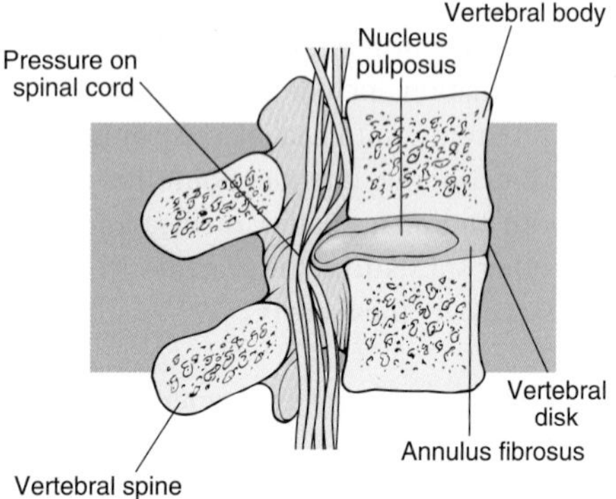 Lateral view of a herniated disk, showing pressure on the spinal cord. (From Frazier MS, Drzymkowski JW: *Essentials of human diseases and conditions,* ed 4, St. Louis, 2008, Saunders/Elsevier.)	Aggressive regional massage, stretching, and joint movement are contraindicated until the acute phase has resolved. However, various forms of massage are important in the management of the muscle spasm and pain surrounding the area of the herniated disk. The muscle spasms serve the stabilizing and protective function of guarding. Without some protective spasm, the nerve could be damaged further; however, too much muscle spasm increases the discomfort. The therapeutic treatment goals should be to reduce pain and excessive tension and restore moderate mobility while allowing the resourceful compensation produced by the muscle tension pattern.
Hypertension This is the medical term for high blood pressure.	For borderline or mild hypertension, massage may be beneficial for managing stress and well-being. However, if the hypertension is due to more serious conditions in the body, massage may be contraindicated. Hypertension that results from other cardiovascular diseases may be contraindicated for massage, but the gentle resting of hands on the body and light massage might be indicated.

Disease/Condition

Indications/Contraindications for Massage Therapy

Irritable Bowel Syndrome

Irritable bowel syndrome (IBS) is also called *spastic colon* or *irritable colon.*

Most chronic gastrointestinal diseases, including IBS, have a strong correlation to stress. Comprehensive stress management programs, including therapeutic massage, can help manage these conditions.

Joint Injuries

Joint injuries are harm or damage related to the bones, ligaments, tendons, cartilage, or any other components that make up the joint. Acute joint injuries include sprains, strains, fractures, and dislocations. Chronic joint injuries include repetitive strain, degeneration, and inflammatory conditions. Pain and swelling of joint injury can be overcome with the judicious and short-term use of pain medication, antiinflammatory medications, and appropriate rehabilitation exercise.

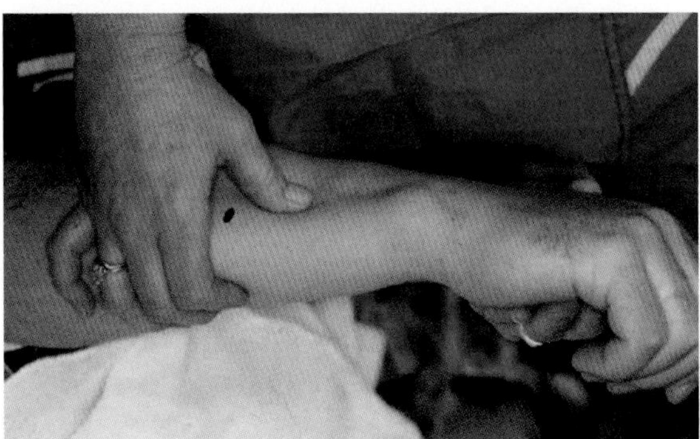

Joint injury. (From Marcotte AL, Osterman AL: Longitudinal radioulnar dissociation: identification and treatment of acute and chronic injuries, *Hand Clinics* 23(2):195–208, 2007.)

Massage is often effective after the acute phase (2 to 3 days post injury). The application of ice, along with rehabilitation exercise, is beneficial. However, ice is contraindicated for some conditions and therefore should be used with caution. Management and rehabilitation of joint problems is a long-term process that often requires a multidisciplinary approach. Although direct work over an area that is actively healing is contraindicated unless supervised by the client's health care team, massage and other forms of soft-tissue work, coupled with movement therapies, can manage compensatory patterns that develop because of casting and other forms of immobilization. Massage application for related chronic joint injury is typically focused on pain management and mobility management.

Kidney Failure

See Renal Failure.

Meningitis

Meningitis is a bacterial or viral infection in the meninges, mainly in the subarachnoid fluid.

Because unusual or unexplained stiff neck is a symptom of encephalitis, clients with this condition should be immediately referred to their physicians for diagnosis. Infectious processes are contraindicated for massage.

Multiple Sclerosis

This involves the destruction of myelin sheaths around sensory and motor neurons in the central nervous system.

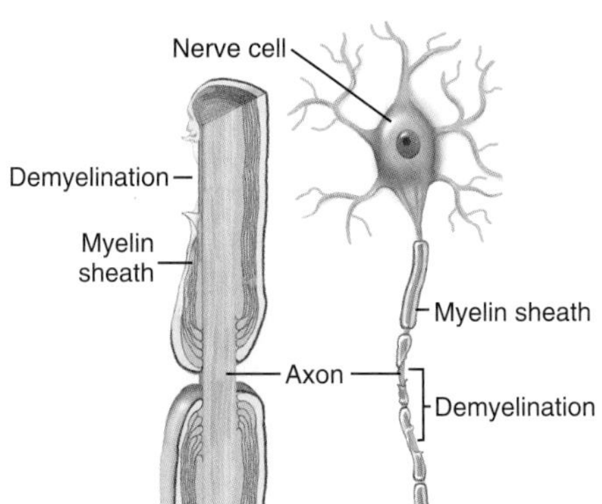

Nerve sheath demyelination seen in multiple sclerosis. (From Shiland BJ: *Mastering healthcare terminology,* ed 3, St. Louis, 2010, Mosby/Elsevier.)

Massage can be an effective part of a comprehensive long-term care program. Stress management also is an important component of an overall care program for any chronic disease. Massage and other forms of bodywork can help manage secondary muscle tension caused by the alteration of posture and the use of equipment, such as wheelchairs, braces, and crutches. Treatments should be developed according to the client's vitality.

Disease/Condition

Indications/Contraindications for Massage Therapy

Muscle Spasms (Entrapment) and Shortening

Muscle spasms are involuntary contractions of skeletal muscle. They are considered to be low-intensity, long-lasting contractions. However, their contractions may compress nerves traveling through them. This is referred to as entrapment. Examples of entrapments include thoracic outlet syndrome and piriformis syndrome.

Various forms of massage are important in the management of muscle spasms and pain. The muscle spasms may serve the stabilizing and protective function of guarding. Without some protective spasm, the nerve could be damaged further; however, too much muscle spasm increases the discomfort. The therapeutic treatment goals should be to reduce pain and excessive tension and restore moderate mobility while allowing the resourceful compensation produced by the muscle tension pattern. Because of the joint structures involved, therapeutic massage should be incorporated into a total treatment program.

Muscle Strain

Strain is an injury to skeletal muscles from overexertion or trauma and can range from mild to severe.

Direct work over the area of injury is contraindicated regionally until all signs of inflammation have dissipated. The therapeutic treatment goals should be to reduce pain and excessive tension caused by compensating postural distortions.

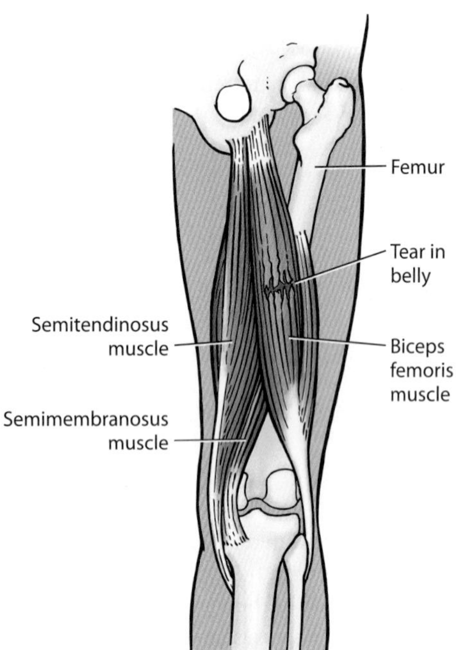

Muscle strain. (From Fritz S: *Mosby's fundamentals of therapeutic massage,* ed 5, St. Louis, 2013, Mosby/Elsevier.)

Neuropathy

Neuropathy is the inflammation or degeneration of the peripheral nerves. Nerve pain is difficult to manage and does not respond well to analgesics.

Massage may provide short-term pain relief by causing changes in neurotransmitter levels and stimulation of alternate nerve pathways, resulting in hyperstimulation analgesia and counterirritation. Any therapy that increases mood-elevating and pain-modulating mechanisms makes coping with nerve pain easier for short periods.

Disease/Condition	Indications/Contraindications for Massage Therapy
Osgood-Schlatter Disease This disease occurs when the tibial tubercle becomes inflamed or separates from the tibia because of irritation caused by the patellar tendon pulling on the tubercle during periods of rapid growth or overuse of the quadriceps.	Regional massage may be contraindicated if inflammation or necrosis is present. Methods that relax and lengthen the muscle and soften the connective tissue are appropriate.

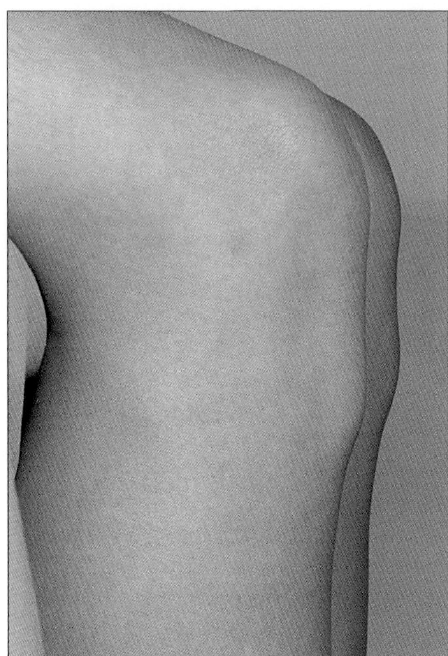

Osgood-Schlatter disease. (From Hochberg MC, et al: *Rheumatology,* ed 4, Edinburgh, 2008, Mosby.)

Disease/Condition	Indications/Contraindications for Massage Therapy
Osteoarthritis/Osteoarthrosis A degenerative joint disease, *osteoarthritis* is the breakdown of joints caused by normal wear and tear. Once the inflammatory response ceases, the condition is called *osteoarthrosis.*	Because the progression and flare-ups of the disease are often stress related, the generalized gentle stress reduction methods provided by massage therapy may be beneficial in long-term management of the condition. The practitioner should avoid friction techniques or any other forms of bodywork that cause inflammation. General pain management methods are helpful. Maintaining pliable soft tissue in the area helps maintain function.
Osteogenesis Imperfecta This group of hereditary disorders appears in newborns and young children. The bones are deformed and fragile as a result of demineralization and defective formation of connective tissue. If skeletal problems create or are part of a permanent condition, supportive care is required.	Massage methods are helpful in the management of compensatory muscle spasms and connective tissue changes. Any type of compressive force or joint movement methods are contraindicated for a fragile skeletal structure, regardless of the cause, unless carefully supervised by the appropriate medical professionals. Light, superficial methods (such as resting the hands on the body, which is used in some forms of touch systems) might be indicated, again with supervision.

Disease/Condition	Indications/Contraindications for Massage Therapy
Osteomyelitis Osteomyelitis is infection in the bone that most commonly affects children and adults older than age 50.	Because this is an infectious disease, massage is contraindicated until the infection is adequately treated.

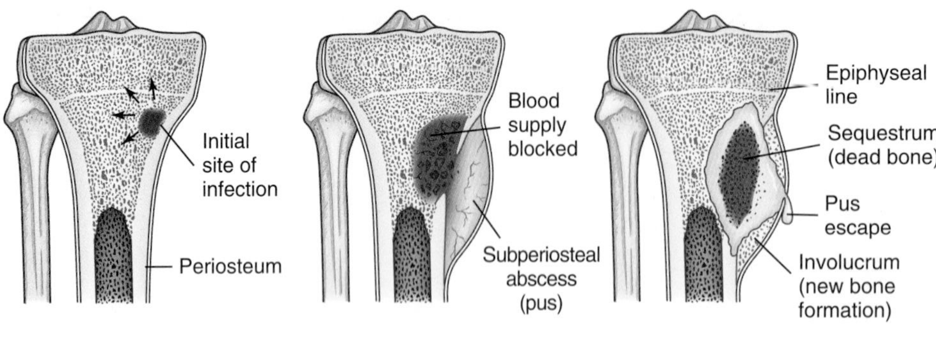

Osteomyelitis. The bacteria reach the metaphysic through the nutrient artery. Bacterial growth results in bone destruction and formation of an abscess. From the abscess cavity, the pus spreads. The pus destroys the bone and sequesters parts of it in the abscess cavity. Reactive new bone is formed around the focus of inflammation. (From Huether SE, McCance KL: *Understanding pathophysiology,* ed 5, 2012, St. Louis, Mosby/Elsevier.)

Disease/Condition	Indications/Contraindications for Massage Therapy
Osteonecrosis (Ischemic Necrosis) Osteonecrosis is the death of a segment of bone, usually caused by insufficient blood flow to the area.	Necrosis usually is a localized condition that requires regional avoidance of the involved bone area. Because massage provides the generalized effect of enhanced local circulation, massaging around the edges of the affected area may be beneficial.
Osteoporosis This disorder is caused by loss of bone mass and density as a result of endocrine imbalances and poor calcium metabolism. The bones become depleted of calcium, other minerals, and protein.	A fragile skeletal structure, regardless of the cause, is a caution for any type of compressive force or joint movement methods. The severity of the condition will determine alterations needed in massage application. Light, superficial methods (such as gentle resting of the hands, which is used in some forms of touch systems) might be indicated.
Paget's Disease (Osteitis Deformans) This is a chronic disorder in which healthy bone is quickly reabsorbed and replaced with fibrous connective tissue that never completely calcifies.	A fragile skeletal structure, regardless of the cause, is a caution for any type of compressive force or joint movement methods. Light, superficial methods might be indicated.

Disease/Condition	Indications/Contraindications for Massage Therapy
Parkinson's Disease In this disease, neurons that release the neurotransmitter dopamine in the brain degenerate, thus slowing or stopping its release.	Because massage has been shown to increase dopamine activity, its use is indicated for managing Parkinson's disease and tremor. In addition, massage therapy and other forms of soft-tissue manipulation may help manage secondary muscle tension.

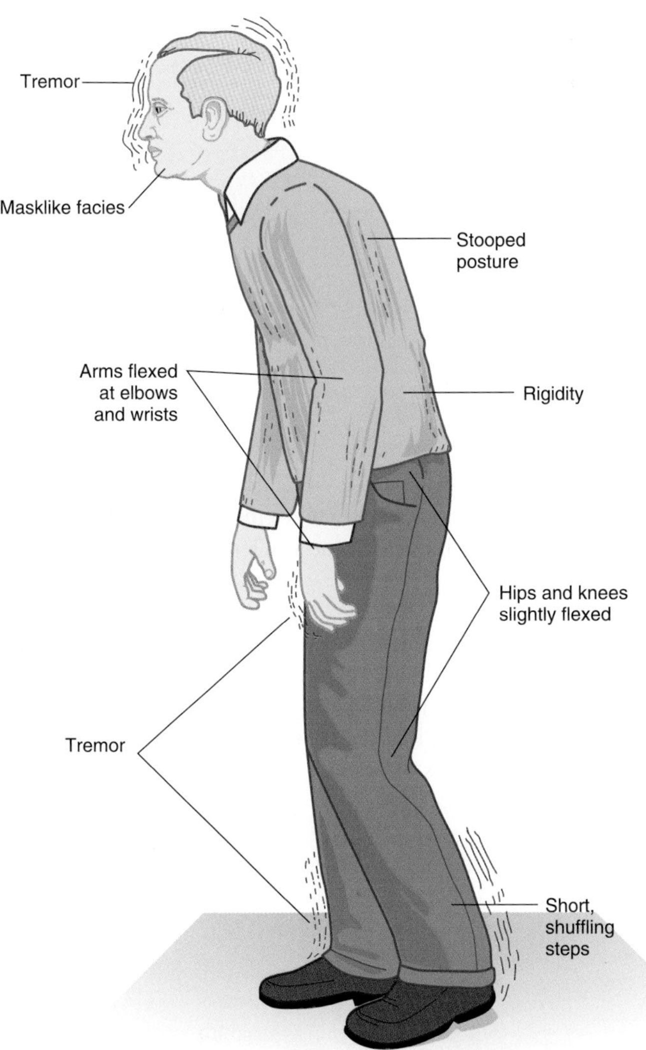

Signs and symptoms of Parkinson's disease. (From Hopper T: *Mosby's pharmacy technician: principles and practice,* ed 3, St. Louis, 2012, Saunders/Elsevier.)

Disease/Condition	Indications/Contraindications for Massage Therapy
Peptic Ulcer A gastric or duodenal ulcer affects the lining of the esophagus, stomach, or duodenum. Ulcers result from tissue damage that never heals because of constant irritation or because healing mechanisms are impeded. 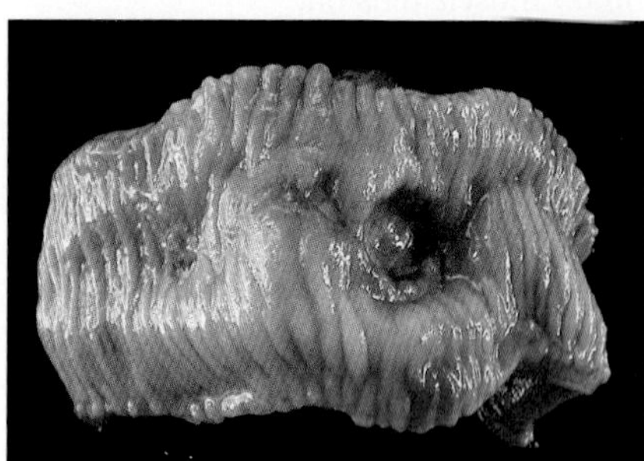 Peptic ulcer. (From Kumar V, Abbas AK, Aster JC: *Robbins and Cotran pathologic basis of disease,* ed 8, Philadelphia, 2010, Saunders/Elsevier.)	Deep abdominal massage is contraindicated for clients with peptic ulcers. Most chronic gastrointestinal diseases have a strong correlation to stress. Comprehensive stress management programs, including therapeutic massage methods, are often effective in managing stress.
Piriformis Syndrome In this syndrome, a hypertonic piriformis muscle compresses the sciatic nerve passing through it, resulting in sciatica-like symptoms.	Massage methods help relieve muscle entrapment of the nerve by reducing tone and lengthening the muscles.
Plantar Fasciitis The condition results from repeated microscopic injury to the plantar fascia and surrounding myofascial structures. Acute-phase plantar fasciitis responds to rest, nonpainful movement, and ice for pain control. 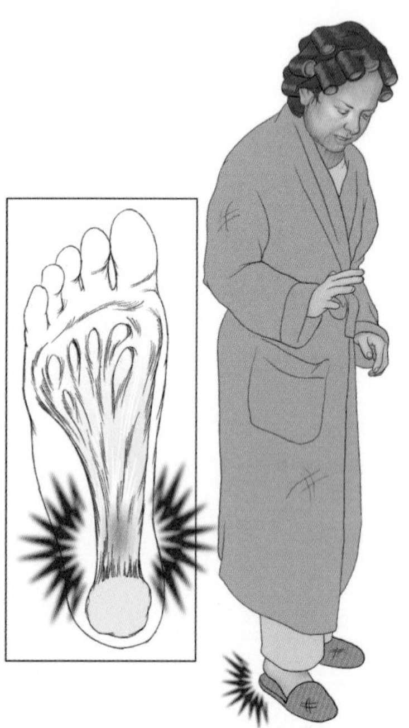 Plantar fasciitis. (From Waldman S: *Atlas of common pain syndromes,* Philadelphia, 2002, Saunders.)	After the inflammation has diminished, soft-tissue methods that address the connective tissue of the plantar fascia and gentle stretching are beneficial. Techniques that release muscular tension in the deep calf muscles can reduce strain on the plantar fascia.

Disease/Condition	Indications/Contraindications for Massage Therapy
Preeclampsia Also termed *pregnancy-induced hypertension* or *toxemia,* the condition is a complication of pregnancy characterized by increasing hypertension, protein in the urine, and edema.	Massage is contraindicated. This is a medical emergency.
Renal Failure Also known as *kidney failure,* this disorder involves the inability of the kidneys to function normally. It may be acute or chronic, and it can be life threatening.	Massage therapy is contraindicated for both acute and end-stage chronic renal failure. Palliative massage methods are appropriate.
Rheumatoid Arthritis This crippling condition is characterized by swelling of the joints in the hands, feet, and other parts of the body as a result of inflammation and overgrowth of the synovial membranes and other joint tissues.	Because the progression and flare-ups of the disease are often stress related, generalized gentle stress reduction massage may be beneficial in long-term management of the condition, especially when part of a total care program. The practitioner should avoid friction techniques or any other forms of bodywork that cause inflammation.

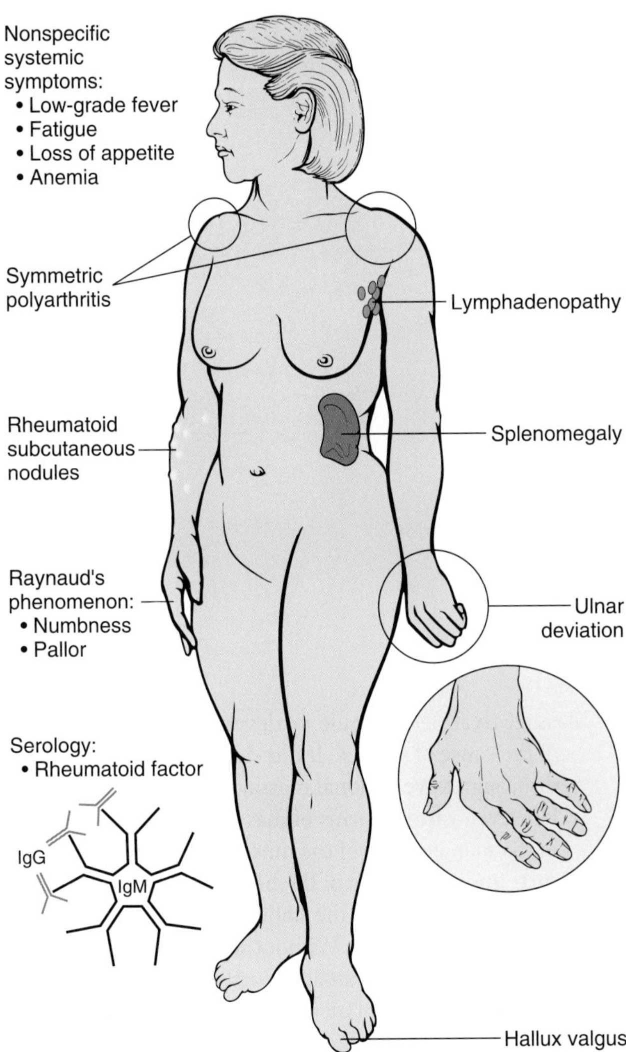

Signs and symptoms of rheumatoid arthritis. *IgG,* Immunoglobulin G; *IgM,* immunoglobulin M. (From Damjanov I: *Pathology for the health professions,* ed 4, St. Louis, 2012, Saunders/Elsevier.)

Disease/Condition	Indications/Contraindications for Massage Therapy
Rotator Cuff Tear Tears often are caused by repeated impingement, overuse, or other conditions that weaken the rotator cuff and eventually cause partial or complete tears.	Massage techniques applied to acute myofascial tears are contraindicated. However, massage therapy may be indicated in the rehabilitative process and as part of a supervised treatment protocol. Massage may be able to help manage and improve compensatory patterns.
Schizophrenia Schizophrenia is the most common mental disorder and includes a large group of psychotic disorders characterized by gross distortion of reality; disturbances of language and communication; withdrawal from social interaction; and disorganization and fragmentation of thought, perception, and emotional reaction.	Therapeutic massage may be supportive in a multidisciplinary approach to treatment, because such methods influence neurotransmitters. However, supervision by the client's health provider is recommended.

Positive symptoms
Hallucinations
Delusions
Disorganized speech
Bizarre behavior

Negative symptoms
Blunted affect
Poverty of thought (alogia)
Loss of motivation (avolition)
Inability to express pleasure or joy (anhedonia)

Cognitive symptoms
Inattention, easily distracted
Impaired memory
Poor problem-solving skills
Poor decision-making skills
Illogical thinking
Impaired judgment

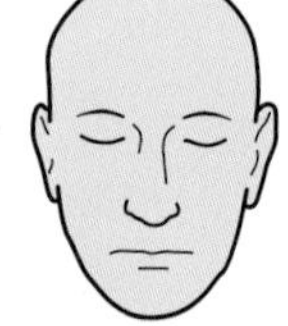

Co-occurring problem
Anxiety
Depression
Substance abuse
Suicidality

All symptoms alter the individual's
Ability to work
Interpersonal relationships
Self-care abilities
Social functioning
Quality of life

Signs and symptoms of schizophrenia. (From DeWit SC: *Medical-surgical nursing: concepts and practice,* St. Louis, 2009, Saunders/Elsevier.)

Sciatica

This is inflammation of the sciatic nerve. It originates in the low back or hip and radiates down the leg.

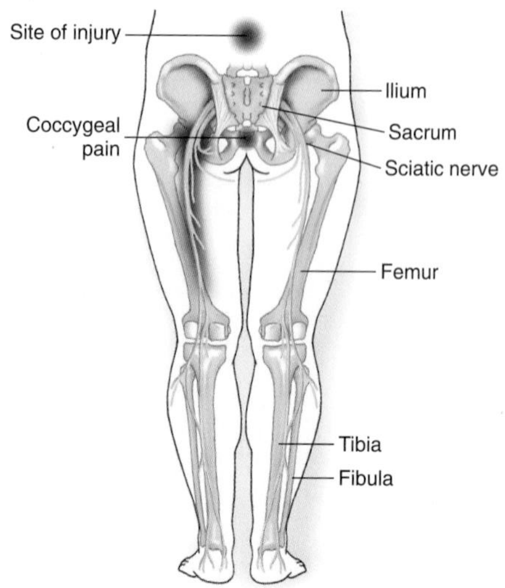

Sciatica. (From Shiland BJ: *Mastering healthcare terminology,* ed 3, St. Louis, 2010, Mosby/Elsevier.)

Massage treatments should be developed on the basis of the cause of sciatica. If it is caused by a herniated disk, aggressive regional massage is contraindicated. However, various forms of massage are important in the management of the muscle spasm and pain surrounding the area of the herniated disk. The muscle spasms serve the stabilizing and protective function of guarding. Without some protective spasm, the nerve could be damaged further; however, too much muscle spasm increases the discomfort. If the cause is piriformis syndrome, then regional massage is indicated. Whether the cause of sciatica is a herniated disk or piriformis syndrome, the therapeutic treatment goals should be to reduce pain and excessive tension and restore moderate mobility while allowing the resourceful compensation produced by the muscle tension pattern.

Disease/Condition	Indications/Contraindications for Massage Therapy
Shingles This is a painful outbreak of the herpes zoster virus along sensory neurons. Herpes zoster is the same virus that causes chickenpox. After an episode of chickenpox, the virus retreats to the dorsal root ganglia, where the immune system usually keeps it in check. Sometimes, however, the virus is able to overcome the immune system, and shingles result. Blisters form along the peripheral nerves associated with the dorsal root ganglia that house the virus. 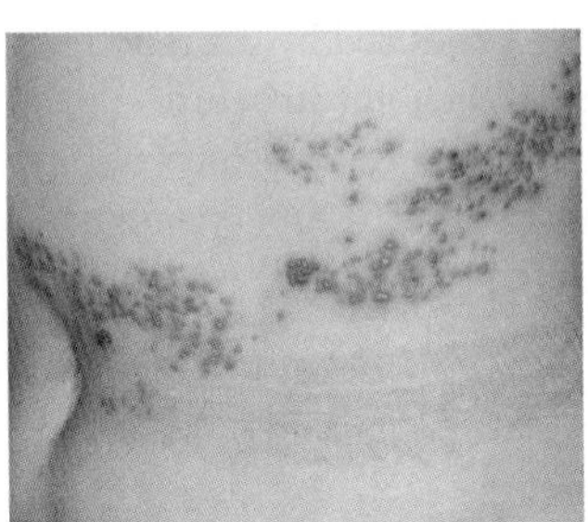 Shingles. (From Habif T: *Clinical dermatology,* ed 4, St. Louis, 2004, Mosby.)	Because shingles is so painful and contagious, massage is locally contraindicated in the acute stages. After the blisters have healed and the pain has gone away, massage is indicated.
Spinal Cord Injury Spinal cord injury involves damage to the spinal cord. The damage usually results from trauma, but can also result from tumors or bony growths in the spinal canal. Loss of motor function in the lower extremities is paraplegia; loss of motor function in both the upper and lower extremities is quadriplegia. 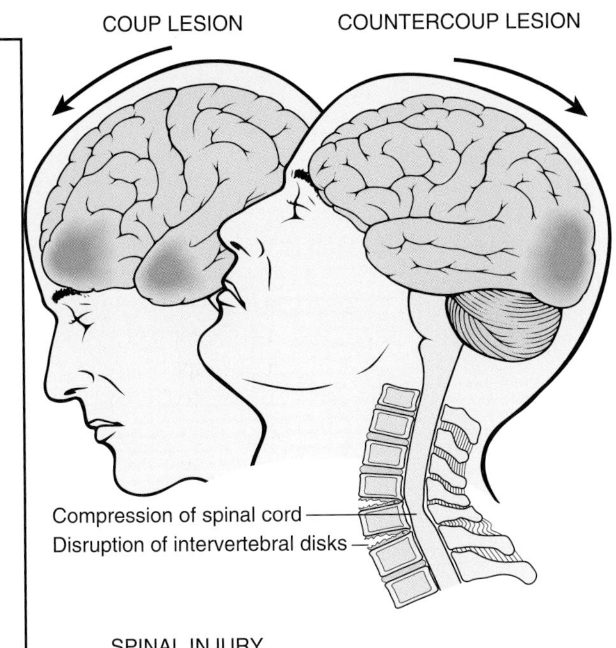 Spinal cord trauma. A coup lesion of the brain occurs at the site of impact, whereas a countercoup lesion is diametrically opposite to the coup lesion. The spinal cord lesion depicted here is caused by hyperextension. (From Damjanov I: *Pathology for the health professions,* ed 4, St. Louis, 2012, Saunders/Elsevier.)	Massage is an effective part of a comprehensive, supervised rehabilitation and long-term care program. Massage and other forms of bodywork can help manage secondary muscle tension resulting from the alteration of posture and the use of equipment, such as wheelchairs, braces, and crutches. Specifically focused massage may help manage difficulties with bowel paralysis. Because massage increases local blood flow, it can help prevent or manage decubitus ulcers.

Disease/Condition	Indications/Contraindications for Massage Therapy

Spondylolisthesis

In this condition, a vertebra becomes displaced anteriorly. It can occur almost anywhere on the spine, but it happens most often in the lower spine.

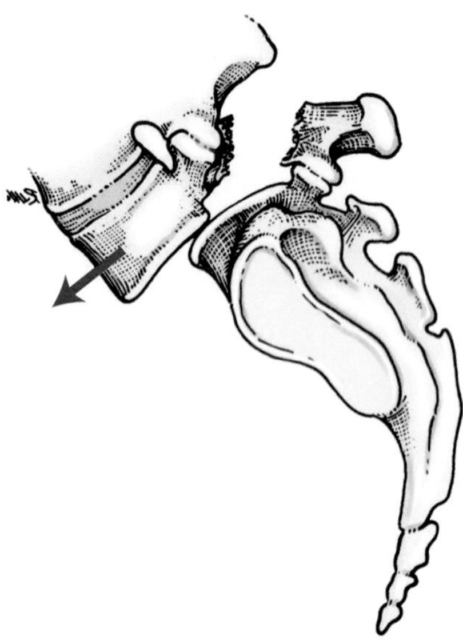

Spondylolisthesis. (In Neumann DA: Kinesiology of the musculoskeletal system: foundations for physical rehabilitation, ed 2, St. Louis, 2010, Mosby/Elsevier.)

Various forms of massage are important in the management of muscle spasm and pain in the accompanying backache. The muscle spasms serve the stabilizing and protective function of guarding. Without some protective spasm, the nerve could be damaged further; however, too much muscle spasm increases the discomfort. The therapeutic treatment goals should be to reduce pain and excessive tension and restore moderate mobility while allowing the resourceful compensation produced by the muscle tension pattern. Because of the joint structures involved, therapeutic massage should be incorporated into a total treatment program with supervision by the appropriate health care professional.

Stress

Stress can be defined as any substantial change in routine or any activity that forces the body to adapt. Stress places demands on physical, mental, and emotional resources. Research has shown that as stresses accumulate, especially if the stress is long term, the individual becomes increasingly susceptible to physical illness, mental and emotional problems, and accidents. In generalized stress conditions, the hypothalamus acts on the anterior pituitary gland to cause the release of adrenocorticotropic hormone (ACTH), which stimulates the adrenal cortex to secrete glucocorticoid. In addition, the sympathetic division of the autonomic nervous system (ANS) is stimulated by the adrenal medulla, resulting in the release of epinephrine and norepinephrine to assist the body in responding to the stressful stimulus. During periods of prolonged stress, glucocorticosteroids (cortisol) may have harmful side effects, including a diminished immune response, altered blood glucose levels, altered protein and fat metabolism, and decreased resistance to stress. Increased activity in the sympathetic ANS can cause symptoms such as chest pain, headache, high blood pressure, muscle aches, forgetfulness, and mood swings.

Massage therapy is indicated for generalized stress management. It is important to rule out any underlying pathology that could be causing the stress-like symptoms. Breathing issues may be related to stress symptoms.

Disease/Condition	Indications/Contraindications for Massage Therapy

Stroke

Stroke is sudden loss of neurological function caused by a vascular injury to the brain. The interrupted blood supply causes brain tissue to die. Stroke is a medical emergency requiring immediate referral.

Once the client is recovering, massage can be an effective part of a supervised comprehensive care program. Massage and other forms of bodywork can help manage secondary muscle tension resulting from the alteration of posture and the use of equipment, such as wheelchairs, braces, and crutches.

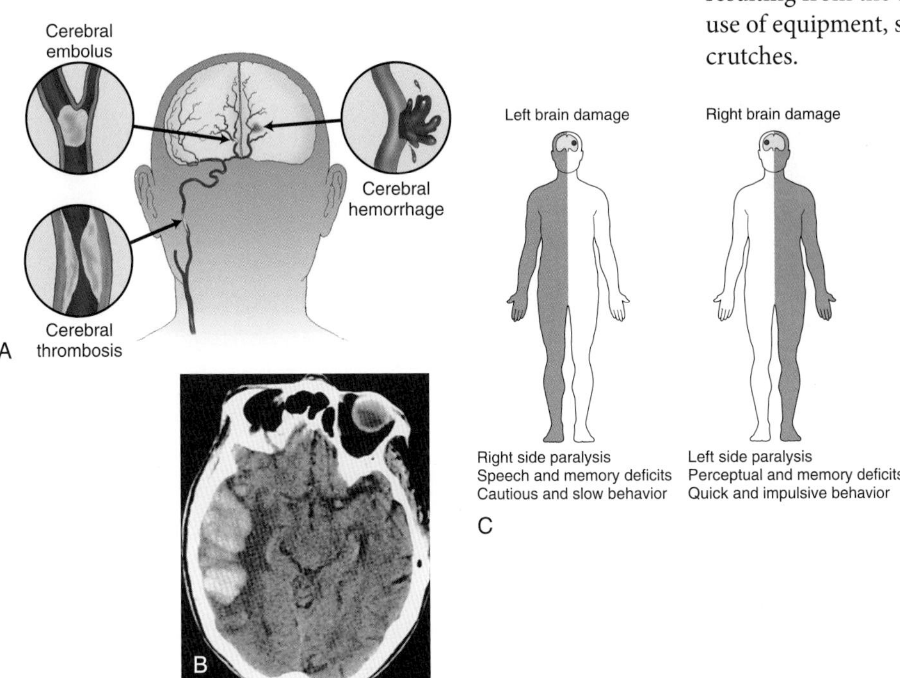

Cerebrovascular accident (CVA). (A) Events causing stroke. (B) Magnetic resonance imaging (MRI) scan showing a hemorrhagic stroke in the right cerebrum. (C) Areas of the body affected by CVA. (A and C, From Shiland BJ: *Mastering healthcare terminology,* ed 3, St. Louis, 2010, Mosby/Elsevier. B, From Black J: *Medical-surgical nursing,* ed 8, St. Louis, 2009, Saunders/Elsevier.)

Tendinitis/Tenosynovitis

Tendinitis is inflammation of a tendon; *tenosynovitis* is inflammation of a tendon sheath.

Any massage methods that increase the inflammatory response are contraindicated. In the acute phase, the use of ice and gentle movement are indicated. Chronic conditions may benefit from methods that improve sliding of the connective tissue structures, relieving the irritation that caused the inflammation in the area.

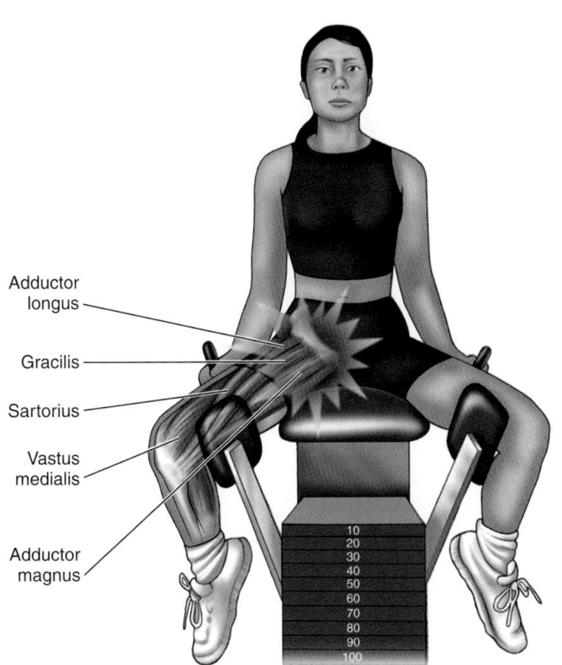

Tendinitis/tenosynovitis. (From Waldman S: *Atlas of uncommon pain syndromes,* ed 2, Philadelphia, 2008, Saunders/Elsevier.)

Disease/Condition	Indications/Contraindications for Massage Therapy

Thoracic Outlet Syndrome

This syndrome occurs when the brachial plexus and blood supply of the arm become entrapped, resulting in shooting pains, weakness, and numbness.

Massage methods help relieve the muscle entrapment of nerves by altering tone and lengthening the muscles.

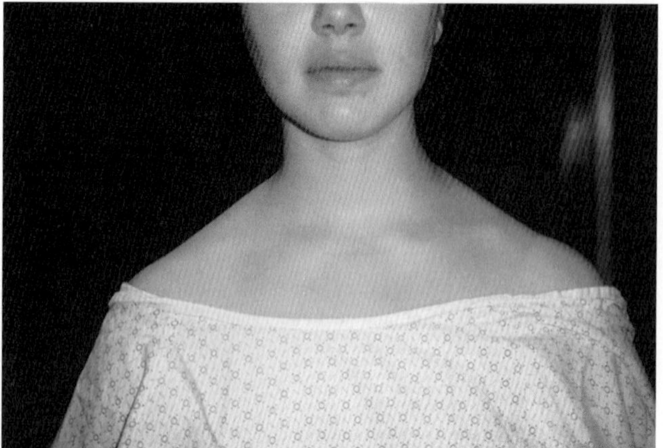

Thoracic outlet syndrome. (From Lederman RJ: Peripheral neuropathies in instrumental musicians, *Phys Med Rehab North Am* 17(4):761–779, 2006.)

Thrombosis

A thrombus is a blood clot. The process of forming a clot in an unbroken blood vessel is called *thrombosis.* A blood clot, bubble of air, fat from broken bones, or a piece of debris transported by the bloodstream is called an *embolus.* When an embolus becomes lodged in a blood vessel smaller in diameter than it is, this situation is called an *embolism.* For example, an embolus that becomes lodged in the lungs is called a *pulmonary embolism.* The major danger of thrombosis and embolisms is that they block vital blood flow to tissues. A common place for thrombosis is in the lower extremities because gravity impedes venous return. This is called a *deep venous thrombosis (DVT),* and it may cause inflammation in the tissues.

Massage therapy is contraindicated regionally and possibly generally because of the pain associated with thrombosis and because massage can further damage debilitated tissues. Clients who are prone to thrombosis take anticoagulant medications, such as heparin or warfarin. These medications make the client more susceptible to bruising, so lighter pressure is indicated during massage, and, of course, the area in which the thrombus is located should be avoided.

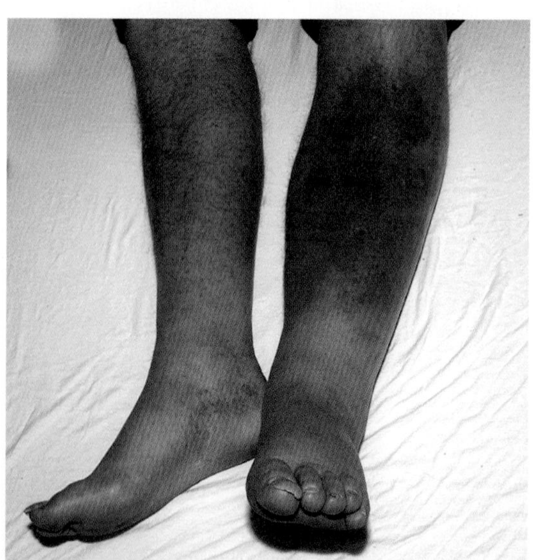

Thrombosis. (From Noble S: Other problems in palliative care, *Medicine* 36(2):100–104, 2008.)

Disease/Condition	Indications/Contraindications for Massage Therapy
Torticollis Also called wry neck, this condition involves a spasm or shortening of one of the sternocleidomastoid muscles. 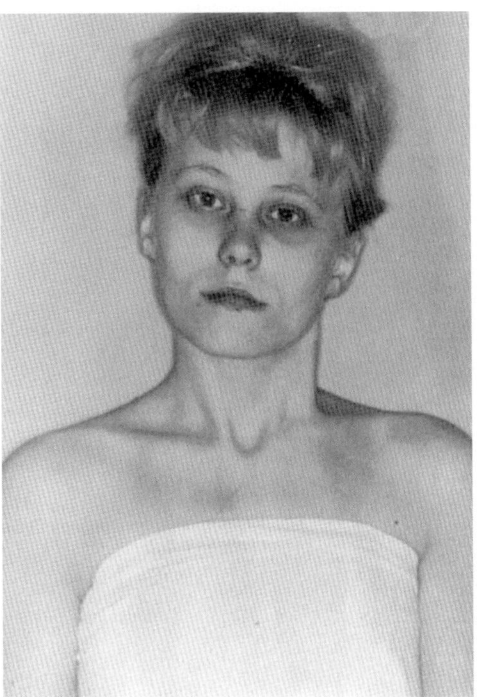 Torticollis in an 18-year-old girl. (From Tachdjian MO: *Pediatric orthopedics,* Philadelphia, 1972, Saunders, p. 68.)	Management of torticollis with massage therapy involves reducing tone in the neck muscles, stretching the contracted muscles, and improving range of motion. Pressure on the blood vessels and nerves deep to the sternocleidomastoid should be avoided.
Vertigo Vertigo is the sensation that the body or environment is spinning or swaying.	Movement therapies can help or aggravate vertigo; therefore, the practitioner must take care to design an individual therapeutic program on the basis of the client's history. Massage methods can deal effectively with muscle tension and diminish anxiety and nausea, but the benefit is temporary because the symptoms return with a recurrence of vertigo.
Whiplash Whiplash is an injury to the soft tissues of the neck caused by sudden hyperextension or flexion (or both) of the neck.	Massage treatment during the acute phase is contraindicated unless closely supervised by a physician or other qualified health care professional. Massage methods are valuable as part of rehabilitation in the subacute phase and can help restore function if the condition is chronic. Extension injury is more severe and requires more carefully applied massage techniques.

SKIN PATHOLOGY: COMMON SKIN DISORDERS

The following photos depict commonly encountered skin disorders. Please note that skin problems may result from various causes, such as parasitic infestations; fungal, bacterial, or viral infections; reactions to substances encountered externally or taken internally; or new growths. Many skin manifestations have no known cause, and others are hereditary.

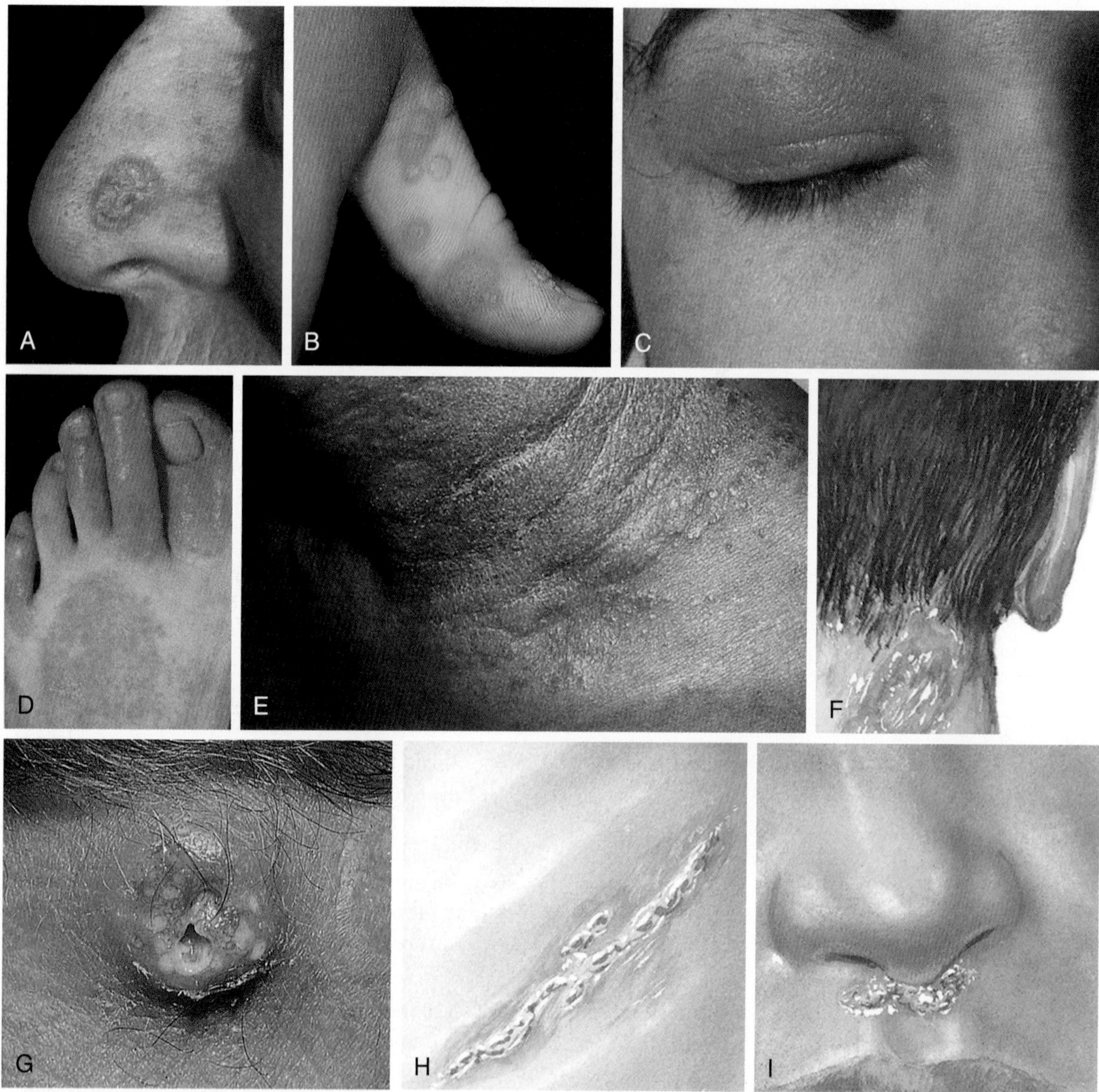

(A) Basal cell carcinoma. From Habif TP: *Clinical dermatology: a color guide to diagnosis and therapy,* ed 3, St. Louis, 1996, Mosby. (B) Common warts. From Habif TP: *Clinical dermatology,* ed 2, St. Louis, 2005, Mosby. (C) Contact dermatitis. Reprinted with permission from the American Academy of Dermatology, ©2011, all rights reserved. (D) Contact dermatitis from shoes. Reprinted with permission from the American Academy of Dermatology, ©2011, all rights reserved. (E) Contact dermatitis from application of Lanacane. From Zitelli BJ, Davis HW: *Atlas of pediatric physical diagnosis,* ed 5, Philadelphia, 2007, Mosby. (F) Dermatitis. From Bork K, Brauninger W: *Skin diseases in clinical practice,* ed 2, Philadelphia, 1998, WB Saunders. (G) Furuncle (boil). From Jaime A. Tschen, MD, Department of Dermatology, Baylor College of Medicine, Houston. (H) Herpes zoster (shingles). From Bork K, Brauninger W: *Skin diseases in clinical practice,* ed 2, Philadelphia, 1998, WB Saunders. (I) Impetigo contagiosa. From Bork K, Brauninger W: *Skin diseases in clinical practice,* ed 2, Philadelphia, 1998, WB Saunders.

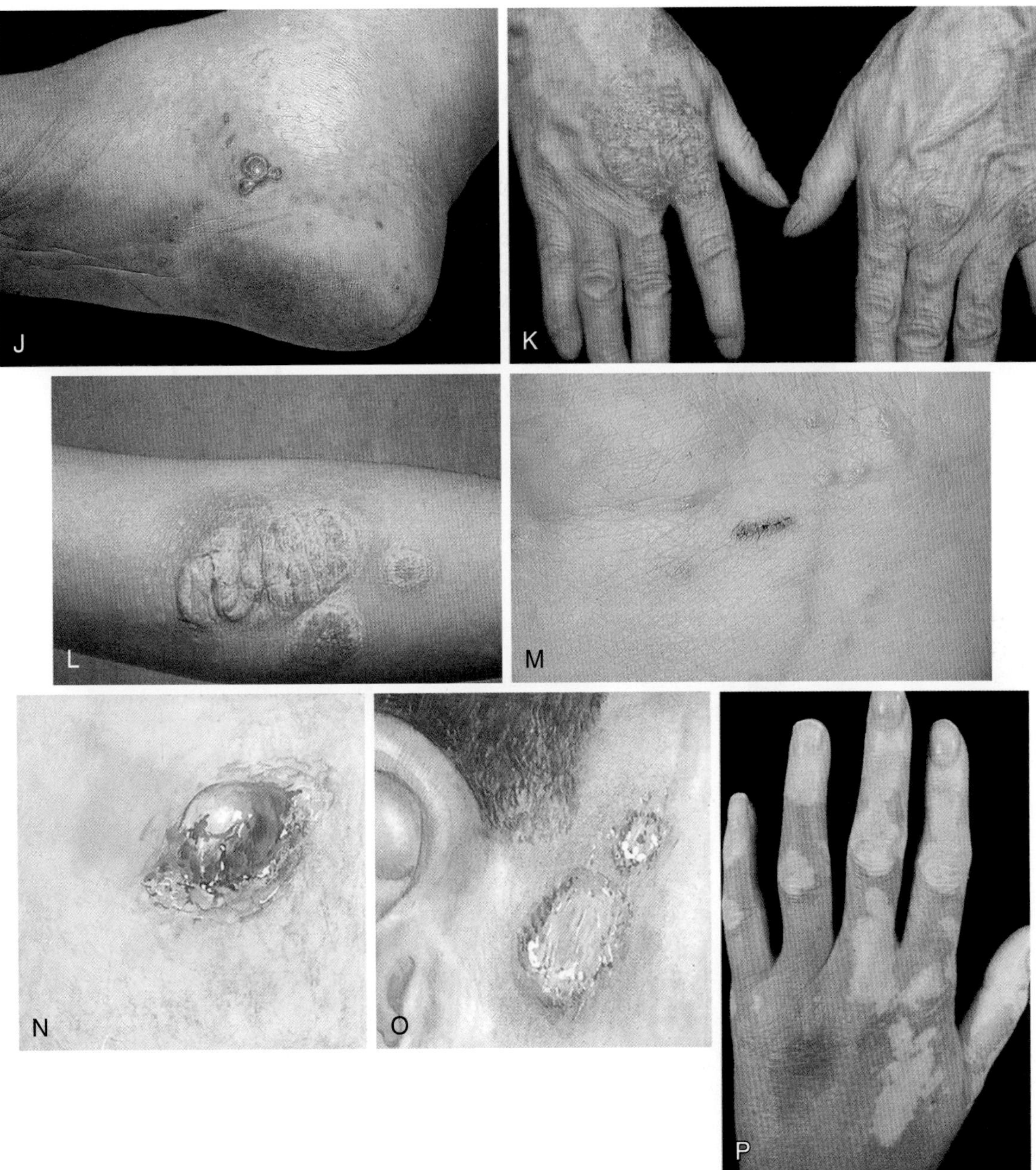

(J) Kaposi's sarcoma. From Habif TP: *Clinical dermatology: a color guide to diagnosis and therapy,* ed 3, St. Louis, 1996, Mosby. (K) Nummular eczema. Reprinted with permission from the American Academy of Dermatology, ©2011, all rights reserved. (L) Psoriasis. Reprinted with permission from the American Academy of Dermatology, ©2011, all rights reserved. (M) Scabies. From Habif TP: *Clinical dermatology,* ed 2, St. Louis, 2005, Mosby. (N) Squamous cell carcinoma. From Bork K, Brauninger W: *Skin diseases in clinical practice,* ed 2, Philadelphia, 1998, WB Saunders. (O) Tinea corporis (ringworm). From Bork K, Brauninger W: *Skin diseases in clinical practice,* ed 2, Philadelphia, 1998, WB Saunders. (P) Vitiligo. Reprinted with permission from the American Academy of Dermatology, ©2011, all rights reserved.

APPENDIX

B Muscle Quick Reference Guide

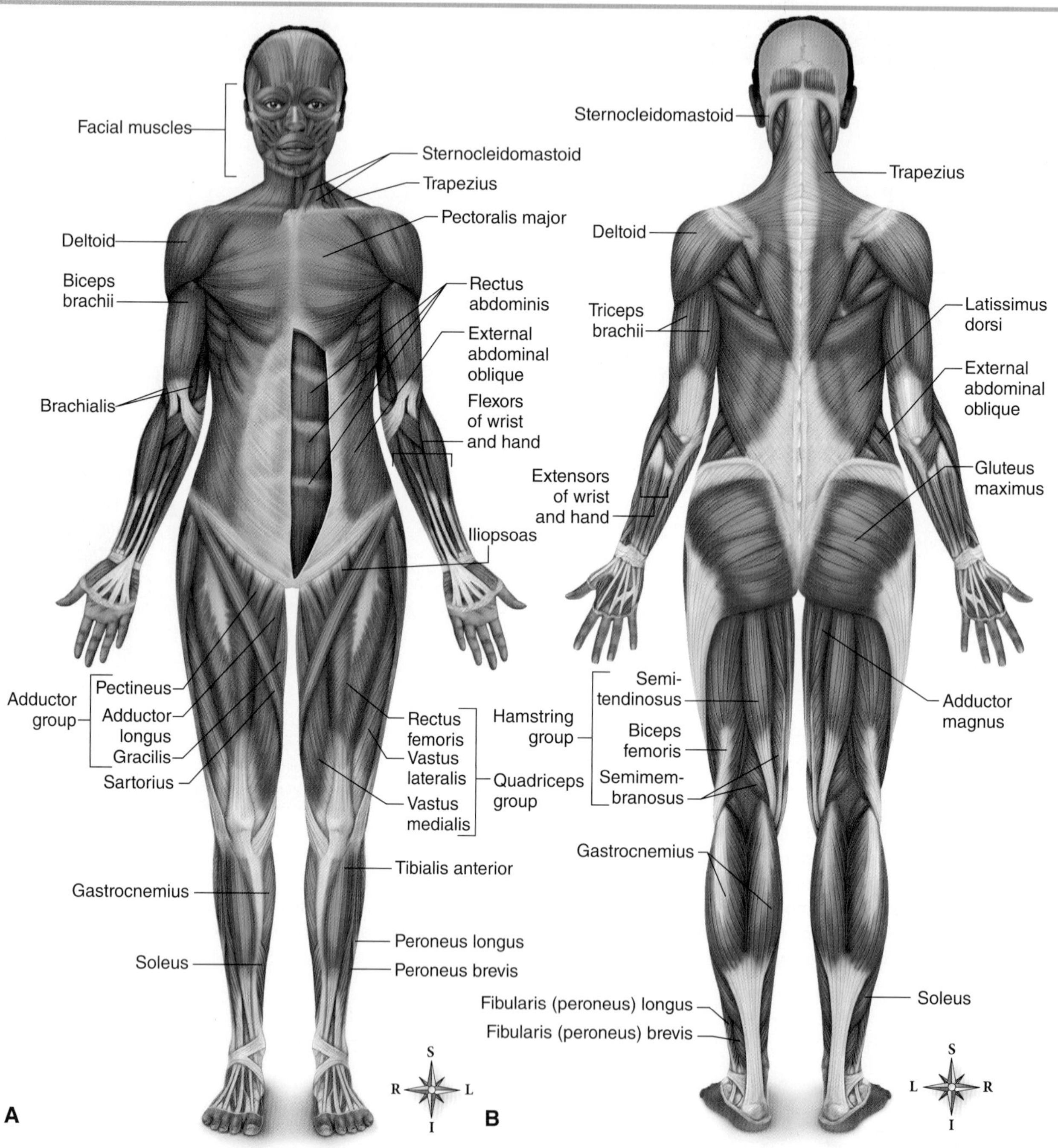

Overview of muscles of the body. A, Anterior view. B, Posterior view. Both views show an adult typical female. (From Patton KT, et al: *The human body in health & disease*, ed 8, St. Louis, 2024, Elsevier.)

Muscle shape and fiber direction can indicate function.

- Muscles shaped like cylinders with vertical fibers typically function on the sagittal plane are movers and sometimes stabilizers (as well as flexors and extensors), and are located on the front and back of the body.

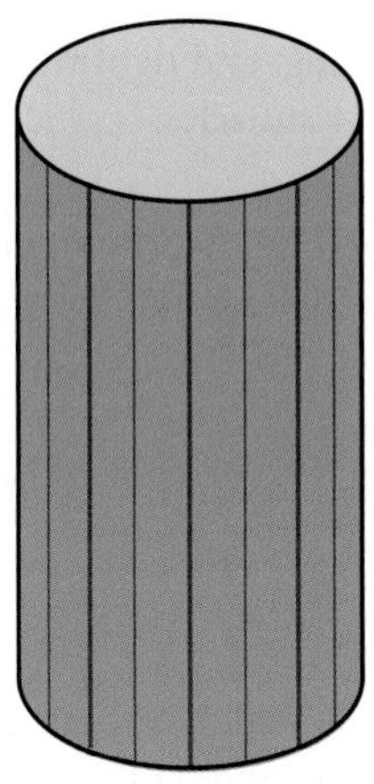

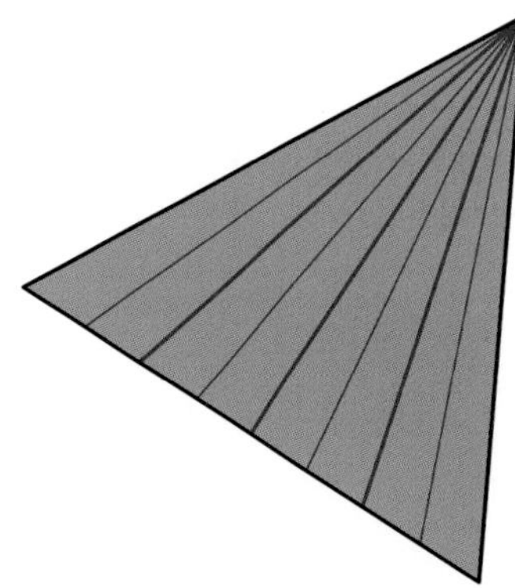

- Muscles shaped like triangles with diagonal fiber direction typically function in the frontal plane and are stabilizers and sometimes movers, as well as abductors and adductors. These muscles are located on the lateral or medial side of the body,

- Muscles shaped like rectangles with horizontal fiber direction function in the transverse plane are stabilizers and rarely movers, but can produce internal and external rotation.

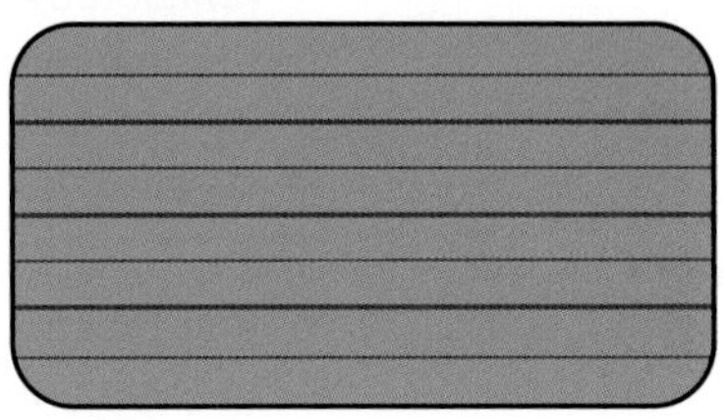

MUSCLE APPENDIX

This chart is an abbreviated, simplified description of the main muscles and referred pain patterns encountered during massage application. Regardless of the exact etiology of the trigger point hypothesis, the concept of clinically observable referred pain patterns remains a helpful concept for assessment.

Muscle Name	Function/Action	Trigger Point Referred Pain Pattern*
Muscles of the Face and Head		
Muscles of Facial Expression		
	Move scalp forward and backward; assist in raising the eyebrows and wrinkling the forehead; draw the eyebrows downward and medially; and create transverse wrinkles over the bridge of the nose.	Galea aponeurotica, muscles over the eyebrows, eyes, ears, nose, and scalp above the ears.
Auricular (ear) muscles	Move the ear.	None identified.
Eye muscles	Open and close the eyelids; provide intrinsic movement of the eyeball.	Superior orbital area above the eyelid.
Muscles that move the mouth	Move lips; aid in mastication; force air out between the lips; and compress the cheek against the teeth.	
Muscles of mastication (chewing)	Move the mouth; close the jaw; provide side-to-side movement and biting; and elevate the mandible.	Near and in the zygomatic arch; anterior, medial, and posterior along the inferior aspect of the muscles near the tendinous junction at the coronoid process of the mandible; temporal region, eyebrow, upper teeth, cheek, and temporomandibular joint; back of the throat, into the ear; upper and lower jaw, the ear, and the eyebrow.

Muscle Name	Function/Action	Trigger Point Referred Pain Pattern*
Muscles of the Neck		
Posterior Triangle of the Neck		
Longus colli and longus capitis	Bend the neck forward (flexion); oblique portion bends neck laterally; inferior portion rotates neck to the opposite side; control acceleration of cervical extension, lateral extension, and contralateral rotation; and provide dynamic stabilization of the cervical spine.	These muscles are difficult to palpate, and thus no specific trigger point locations have been identified. However, the pain from the trigger points in the muscles presents as a sore throat, difficulty swallowing, and tightness in the posterior neck muscles.
Scalene Group		
Anterior scalene	Bends the cervical portion of the vertebral column forward (flexion) and laterally; also rotates to the opposite side and assists in elevation of the first rib, thus functioning as an accessory muscle of respiration; checks (decelerates) cervical lateral flexion and rotation; and stabilizes the cervical spine.	Pectoral region, rhomboid region, and the entire length of the arm into the hand.
Middle scalene	Acting from above, helps raise the first rib, thus functioning as an accessory muscle of respiration; acting from below, bends the cervical part of the vertebral column to the same side; assists flexion of the neck; checks (decelerates) cervical lateral flexion and rotation; and stabilizes the cervical spine.	Pectoral region, rhomboid region, and the entire length of the arm into the hand.
Posterior scalene	When the second rib is fixed, bends the lower end of the cervical portion of the vertebral column to the same side (lateral flexion); when the upper attachment is fixed, helps elevate the second rib, thus functioning as an accessory muscle of respiration; checks (decelerates) cervical lateral flexion and rotation; and stabilizes the cervical spine.	Pectoral region, rhomboid region, and the entire length of the arm into the hand.
Sternocleidomastoid	Assists in flexing the cervical portion of the vertebral column forward, elevating the thorax, and extending the head at the atlantooccipital joint; stabilizes the head; and resists forceful backward movement of the head, tilts the head, rotates the head, and simultaneously acts to control rotation.	Several trigger points are located in the entire length of both divisions of the muscle: head and face, particularly the occipital region, ear, and forehead. Autonomic nervous system phenomena and proprioceptive disturbances are common.
Deep Posterior Cervical Muscles		
Splenius capitis and splenius cervicis	Extend head and neck, draw head dorsally and laterally and rotate head to the same side; check and control cervical flexion and contralateral rotation; and stabilize the cervical spine.	Belly of the muscles closer to the head; to the top of the skull (the pain often feels as though it is inside the head), to the eye, and into the shoulder.

Muscle Name	Function/Action	Trigger Point Referred Pain Pattern*
Erector Spinae Group		
Spinalis thoracis, cervicis, and capitis Longissimus thoracis, cervicis, and capitis Iliocostalis lumborum, thoracis, and cervicis	Extend, rotate, and laterally flex the vertebral column and head; assist with anterior tilt elevation and rotation of the pelvis and spinal stabilization; control and decelerate vertebral flexor rotation and lateral flexion; and stabilize the lumbar spine primarily.	Scapular, lumbar, abdominal, and gluteal areas; bandlike headache into the eyes; stiff neck.
Oblique Muscles, Transversospinalis Group		
Semispinalis thoracis, cervicis, and capitis Multifidus Rotatores Intertransversarii lumborum, thoracis, and cervicis Interspinales	This group of muscles extends the motion segments of the back; rotates the thoracic, cervical, and lumbar vertebral joints; and stabilizes the vertebral column.	Scapular, lumbar, abdominal, and gluteal areas; bandlike headache into the eyes; stiff neck.
Suboccipital Muscles		
Suboccipital muscles Rectus capitis posterior major and minor Obliquus capitis superior and inferior	As a group, these muscles extend and rotate the head in small, precise movements. More often these muscles isometrically function as stabilizers of the head and provide proprioceptive input about head position. These muscles are also important postural muscles and are neural reporting stations on balance and proprioceptive monitors of cervical spine and neck position.	Belly of the muscle, located with deep palpation at the base of the skull, around the ear on the same side; sensation of compressed junction of skull and neck; bandlike headache.
Muscles of the Torso		
Muscles of the Thorax and Posterior Abdominal Wall		
Diaphragm	Participates in respiration; during inspiration (breathing in), diaphragmatic contractions increase the capacity of the thoracic cavity; controls expiration as the diaphragm relaxes; and during breath holding, assists in stabilizing the lumbar and pelvic floor.	None identified.
Serratus posterior superior	Assists in lifting the ribs during inspiration.	Under the scapula near the insertion of the muscle on the ribs and under the upper portion of the scapula.
Serratus posterior inferior	Depresses last four ribs (9 to 12). Some studies disagree that this is the function, finding no electromyographic activity of this muscle during respiration. Seems to act as a stabilizer during forced expirations such as coughing.	Nagging ache in the area of the muscle.
External intercostal muscles	Elevate ribs and draw adjacent ribs together; lift ribs, increasing the volume of the thoracic cavity—ipsilateral torso rotation; and stabilize the thorax.	The intercostal muscles can develop trigger points, which are located by palpating the muscles between the ribs. Pain spans the intercostal segment, especially noticed with deep breathing or rotational movement.

Muscle Name	Function/Action	Trigger Point Referred Pain Pattern*
Internal intercostal muscles	Depress ribs and draw adjacent ribs together, decreasing volume of thoracic cavity—ipsilateral torso rotation; stabilize the thorax.	The intercostal muscles can develop trigger points, which are located by palpating the muscles between the ribs. Pain spans the intercostal segment, especially noticed with deep breathing or rotational movement.
Innermost intercostal muscles	The muscles of this small group attach to the internal aspects of two adjoining ribs. They are believed to act with the internal intercostal muscles.	The intercostal muscles can develop trigger points, which are located by palpating the muscles between the ribs. Pain spans the intercostal segment, especially noticed with deep breathing or rotational movement.
Transversus thoracis	Draws anterior portion of the ribs caudally (reduces thoracic cavity); stabilizes the rib cage.	None identified.
Quadratus lumborum	Draws last rib downward; flexes lumbar vertebral column laterally to the same side; acts to elevate and anteriorly tilt the pelvis; acting bilaterally, extends the lumbar spine and assists forced exhalation, as when coughing; restrains and checks lateral flexion; and assists normal inhalation by stabilizing the diaphragm and the 12th rib and stabilizing the lumbar area.	Gluteal and groin area, sacroiliac joint and greater trochanter: These points are implicated in most low back pain. The dual function of lumbar stabilization (isometric function) and respiration (concentric function) can cause severe pain in the low back with a cough or sneeze if these trigger points are active. Low back pain often is related more to maintenance of posture than trigger point activity; therefore, a common finding is corresponding pain patterns in the muscles that laterally flex the head and neck, such as the scalene muscles.
Psoas major and psoas minor	With proximal attachment fixed, flex the hip joint by flexing the femur on the pelvis; may assist in lateral rotation of the hip joint; acting bilaterally, flex the hip joint by flexing the trunk on the pelvis; can assist extension of the lumbar spine, increasing lumbar lordosis; acting unilaterally, may assist in lateral flexion of the trunk toward the same side; restrain and check trunk and hip extension and contralateral flexion of the trunk; control tendency of lordosis; and stabilize the lumbar spine and help maintain upright posture.	Entire lumbar area into the superior gluteal region; front of the thigh; menstrual aching; can mimic appendicitis. Shortening is a major cause of low back pain. If tension or trigger point activity is located at insertion, pain can mimic a groin pull. Because of postural reflexes, muscles that flex the head and neck are facilitated with psoas activation. A common correlation exists between neck pain and stiffness and psoas pain and low back stiffness. Massage often must address both areas in sequence to be effective.
Iliacus	Flexes the hip joint; may assist in lateral rotation and abduction of the hip joint; with insertion fixed and acting bilaterally flexes the hip joint by flexing the trunk on the femur; tilts pelvis forward (anterior) when legs are fixed; decelerates hip extension; and stabilizes the pelvis.	Inner border of the ilium behind the anterior superior iliac spine.

Muscle Name	Function/Action	Trigger Point Referred Pain Pattern*
Muscles of the Anterior Abdominal Wall		
Transversus abdominis	Constricts and compresses the abdomen, increasing intraabdominal pressure, and supports the abdominal viscera; assists in forced expiration.	Pain located throughout the area but concentrated more in the external circle of the abdominal wall rather than toward the middle near the umbilicus.
Internal abdominal oblique	Compresses the abdominal cavity (some isometric abdominis activity); assists with posterior tilt of the pelvis; flexes the vertebral column, bringing the costal cartilage toward the pubis; laterally bends and ipsilaterally rotates the vertebral column (brings the shoulder of the opposite side forward); and restrains trunk extension.	Pain located throughout the area but concentrated more in the external circle of the abdominal wall rather than toward the middle near the umbilicus.
External abdominal oblique	Compresses the abdominal cavity (some isometric activity); assists in forced expiration; with both sides acting, flexes the vertebral column, bringing the pubis toward the xiphoid process of sternum; laterally bends and brings the shoulder of the same side forward; and restrains trunk extension.	Pain located throughout the area but concentrated more in the external circle of the abdominal wall rather than toward the middle near the umbilicus.
Rectus abdominis	Flexes the vertebral column, bringing the sternum toward the pelvis; compresses the abdominal cavity; assists with posterior tilt of the pelvis (some isometric activity); assists in forced expiration; and restrains trunk extension.	Trigger points often found in the rectus abdominis just below the umbilicus on either side of the linea alba and near the attachment on the ribs. Pain is referred in local area or to groin.
Muscles of Scapular Stabilization		
Trapezius	Upper trapezius elevates and rotates scapula and the shoulder and, with the shoulder fixed, can assist in drawing the head backward and laterally to tilt the chin; the middle portion adducts (retracts) the scapula, draws back the acromion process; lower fibers depress the scapula; the entire muscle, acting bilaterally, assists extension of the cervical and thoracic spine; upper trapezius restrains and controls flexion, lateral flexion, and rotation of the neck and head. Middle trapezius controls and restrains scapular abduction (protraction). Lower trapezius restrains scapular elevation and rotates the scapula. Trapezius stabilizes the scapula and cervical spine.	Neck behind the ear and to the temple; subscapular area; acromial pain.
Rhomboid major and rhomboid minor	Adduct (retract) and elevate the scapula and also rotate it downward so that the glenoid cavity faces down toward the feet; restrain protraction and upward rotation of the scapula; stabilize the scapula.	At the attachment point near the scapular border; scapular region.

Muscle Name	Function/Action	Trigger Point Referred Pain Pattern*
Levator scapulae	Raises the scapula and draws it medially; with the scapula fixed, performs lateral flexion and rotates the neck to the same side; bilaterally extends the neck; restrains and controls head and neck flexion, scapular depression, and lateral flexion of the cervical spine; and stabilizes cervical/scapular function.	Belly of the muscle just as it begins the rotation and at the attachment near the scapula; angle of the neck and along the vertebral border of the scapula; stiff neck in rotation.
Pectoralis minor	Assists in drawing the scapula forward (protraction) around the chest wall; rotates the scapula to depress the point of the shoulder; assists in forced inspiration; restrains scapular retraction; and stabilizes the scapula during movement.	Near the attachment at the coracoid process and at the belly of the muscle; may mimic angina with pain in front of the chest from the shoulder and down the ulnar side of the arm into the fingers.
Serratus anterior	Abducts (protracts) the scapula; rotates the scapula so that the glenoid cavity faces cranially (toward the head); raises the ribs with the scapula fixed and therefore is an accessory muscle of respiration; controls scapular retraction; and holds the medial border of the scapula firmly against the thorax and prevents winging of the scapula.	Along the midaxillary line near the ribs; side and back of the chest and down the ulnar aspect of the arm into the hand; may result in shortness of breath and pain during inhalation.
Muscles of the Musculotendinous (Rotator) Cuff		
Supraspinatus	Abducts the arm; restrains adduction of the arm; and acts to stabilize the humeral head in the glenoid cavity during movements of the shoulder joint.	Shoulder, deltoid, and down the arm to the elbow, often experienced as a dull ache.
Infraspinatus	Provides lateral or external rotation of the arm at the shoulder; restrains and controls internal (medial) rotation of the arm at the shoulder; and acts to stabilize the humeral head in the glenoid cavity during movements of the shoulder joint.	Deep into the shoulder and deltoid area, down the arm, suboccipital area, medial border of the scapula, with limits reaching behind back.
Teres minor	Provides adduction and lateral (external) rotation of the arm; restrains internal (medial) rotation of the arm; and acts to stabilize the humeral head in the glenoid cavity during movements of the shoulder joint.	Posterior deltoid region. Client often experiences limited range of motion when reaching behind the back, such as putting hands in back pocket of pants.
Subscapularis	Rotates humerus medially (internal rotation) and draws it forward and down when the arm is raised; restrains lateral (external) rotation of the arm; and stabilizes the humeral head in the glenoid cavity during movement of the shoulder.	Access is through the axilla near the attachment at the humerus and in the belly of the muscle. Pain in posterior deltoid, scapular region, triceps area, and into the wrist often is mistaken for bursitis because pain often refers to insertion at shoulder.

Muscle Name	Function/Action	Trigger Point Referred Pain Pattern*
Muscles of the Shoulder Joint		
Deltoid	Provides flexion and extension and medial and lateral rotation of the arm and abduction of the arm. Anterior deltoid restrains and controls extension and external rotation of the arm. Middle deltoid restrains arm adduction. Posterior deltoid restrains flexion and internal rotators and horizontal adduction of the arm. Deltoid stabilizes glenohumeral joint during arm movement.	Deltoid region and down the lateral side of the arm.
Pectoralis major	With proximal attachment (origin) fixed, adducts and draws the humerus forward (flexion) and horizontally and medially (internally) rotates it; with insertion fixed and arm abducted, assists in elevating the thorax (as in forced inspiration); controls arm extension, horizontal abduction, and external rotation; and stabilizes the shoulder during overhead activity.	Chest and breast and down the ulnar aspect of the arm to the fourth and fifth fingers.
Subclavius	Draws the clavicle forward and down; stabilizes the clavicle.	Chest and breast and down the radial aspect of the arm to the fourth and fifth fingers.
Latissimus dorsi	With proximal attachment (origin) fixed, medially or internally rotates, adducts, and extends the humerus; depresses the shoulder girdle and assists in lateral flexion of the trunk; with insertion fixed, assists in tilting the pelvis anteriorly and laterally; acting bilaterally, assists in hyperextending the spine and tilting the pelvis anteriorly; controls abduction, flexion, and external (lateral) rotation of the humerus; and stabilizes the lumbar and pelvic area by maintaining tension on the thoracolumbar fascia.	Posterior axillary area just as the muscle begins to twist around the teres major; belly of the muscle near the rib attachments; just below the scapula and into the ulnar side of the arm; anterior deltoid region and abdominal oblique area.
Teres major	Medial or internal rotation, adduction, and extension of the arm; upward rotation of the scapula; controls and restrains flexion, abduction, and external rotation of the arm; and stabilizes the glenohumeral joint.	Near the musculotendinous junction at both attachments; posterior deltoid region and down the dorsal portion of the arm.
Coracobrachialis	Flexion and adduction of the humerus; controls extension and abduction of the scapula; stabilizes the shoulder.	Front of shoulder, posterior aspect of the arm down the triceps and dorsal forearm in the hand.

Muscle Name	Function/Action	Trigger Point Referred Pain Pattern*
Muscles of the Elbow and Radioulnar Joints		
Biceps brachii	Provides flexion of the humerus. The long head may assist with abduction if the humerus is laterally rotated. The short head assists arm adduction. With proximal attachment (origin) fixed, flexes the forearm toward the humerus and supinates the forearm; with insertion fixed, flexes the elbow joint, moving the humerus toward the forearm, as in a pull-up or chin-up; restrains and controls elbow extension and extension of the humerus; stabilizes the humerus at the shoulder and the elbow joint during full extension; and stabilizes the elbow when flexed and holding a weight.	Front of the shoulder at the anterior deltoid region and into the scapular region; also into the antecubital space or the front of the elbow.
Brachialis	Flexes the elbow joint; restrains and controls elbow extension; stabilizes the elbow in full extension and fixed flexion.	Primarily to the thumb, with some pain in the anterior deltoid area and at the elbow.
Brachioradialis	Flexes the elbow joint after brachialis and biceps initiate movement; assists in pronation and supination of the forearm to midposition; restrains and controls elbow extension; and stabilizes the elbow in full extension and fixed flexion.	Wrist and base of the thumb in the web space between the thumb and index finger and to the lateral epicondyle at the elbow.
Pronator teres	Pronates the forearm; assists in flexing the elbow joint; controls supination of the forearm; and stabilizes the elbow joint and radioulnar joint.	Radial side of the forearm into the wrist and thumb. Pain may mimic carpal tunnel syndrome.
Supinator	Supinates the forearm; assists with flexion of the forearm at the elbow when the hand is held halfway between supination and pronation; restrains and controls pronation of the forearm; and stabilizes the elbow and radioulnar joint.	Lateral epicondyle and dorsal aspect of the arm (pain mimics tennis elbow); near the radius in the antecubital space; thumb area.
Pronator quadratus	Provides pronation of the forearm; restrains and controls supination of the forearm.	Belly of muscle; active supination.
Triceps brachii	Extension of the forearm; in addition, the long head adducts and assists in extension of the humerus; restrains elbow flexion and arm abduction and flexion; stabilizes the elbow in extension and fixed flexion to allow carrying weight in the hands; and assists in stabilizing the glenohumeral joint.	Length of posterior arm.
Anconeus (elbow)	Assists the triceps in extension of the elbow joint; balances elbow flexion; and stabilizes the joint capsule of the elbow.	Elbow at lateral epicondyle.

Muscle Name	Function/Action	Trigger Point Referred Pain Pattern*
Muscles of the Wrist and Hand Joints		
Anterior Flexor Group: Superficial Layer		
Flexor carpi radialis	Flexes and abducts the wrist (radial deviation); may assist in pronation of the forearm and flexion of the elbow; restrains and controls extension and adduction of the wrist; and stabilizes the wrist.	Into the wrist and fingers; occasionally into the elbow.
Palmaris longus	Flexes the wrist; may assist in flexion of the elbow and pronation of the forearm; restrains wrist extension; and tenses the palmar fascia.	Into the wrist and fingers; occasionally into the elbow.
Flexor carpi ulnaris	Flexes and adducts (ulnar deviation) the wrist; may assist in elbow flexion; controls and restrains wrist extension and abduction; and stabilizes the wrist.	Into the wrist and fingers; occasionally into the elbow.
Flexor digitorum superficialis	Flexes the proximal interphalangeal joints of the second through fifth digits; assists in flexion of the wrist; restrains and controls finger extension; stabilizes wrist and hand joints; flexes the metacarpophalangeal joints; flexes the forearm at the elbow.	Into the wrist and fingers; occasionally into the elbow.
Flexor digitorum profundus	Flexes the distal interphalangeal joints of the second through fifth digits; assists in flexion of the proximal interphalangeal and metacarpophalangeal joints; assists in adduction of the index, ring, and little fingers and in flexion of the wrist; restrains and controls extension of the fingers; and stabilizes the fingers.	Into the wrist and fingers; occasionally into the elbow.
Flexor pollicis longus	Flexes interphalangeal joint of the thumb; assists in flexion of the metacarpophalangeal and carpometacarpal joints; restrains thumb; and stabilizes the thumb.	Thumb.
Posterior Extensor Group: Superficial Layer		
Extensor carpi radialis longus	Extends and adducts (ulnar deviation) the wrist; may assist in flexion of the elbow and pronation and supination of the forearm; restrains and controls wrist flexion and abduction; and stabilizes the wrist.	From the lateral epicondyle at the elbow down the dorsum of the forearm to various parts of the hand, especially to the web of the thumb and elbow joint.
Extensor carpi radialis brevis	Extends the wrist and assists in abduction (radial deviation) of the wrist and weak flexion of the forearm; restrains and controls wrist flexion and adduction; and stabilizes the wrist.	From the lateral epicondyle at the elbow down the dorsum of the forearm to various parts of the hand, especially to the web of the thumb.
Extensor digitorum	Extends the metacarpophalangeal joints; extends the interphalangeal joint of the second through fifth digits (with the lumbricales and interossei); assists in extension of the wrist; restrains and controls wrist and finger flexion; and stabilizes the wrist.	From the lateral epicondyle at the elbow down the dorsum of the forearm to various parts of the hand, especially to the web of the thumb.

Muscle Name	Function/Action	Trigger Point Referred Pain Pattern*
Extensor digiti minimi	Extends the metacarpophalangeal and (with the interosseous and lumbrical muscles) the interphalangeal joints of the little finger; assists in abduction of the little finger; controls and restrains flexion and adduction of the little finger; and stabilizes the joints of the little finger.	From the lateral epicondyle at the elbow down the dorsum of the forearm to various parts of the hand, especially to the web of the thumb.
Extensor carpi ulnaris	Extends and adducts (ulnar deviation) the wrist; controls wrist flexion and abduction; and stabilizes the wrist.	From the lateral epicondyle at the elbow down the dorsum of the forearm to various parts of the hand, especially to the web of the thumb.
Extensor pollicis brevis	Extends and abducts the carpometacarpal joint of the thumb; extends the metacarpophalangeal joint; assists in abduction (radial deviation) of the wrist; restrains flexion of the thumb and adduction of the wrist; and stabilizes the thumb.	From the lateral epicondyle at the elbow down the dorsum of the forearm to various parts of the hand, especially to the web of the thumb.
Posterior Extensor Group: Deep Layer		
Abductor pollicis longus	Abducts and extends the carpometacarpal joint of the thumb; abducts (radial deviation) and assists in wrist flexion and supination of the forearm; controls thumb adduction; and stabilizes the thumb and wrist.	To the web of the thumb.
Extensor pollicis longus	Extends the interphalangeal joint and assists in extension of the metacarpophalangeal and carpometacarpal joints of the thumb; assists in abduction (radial deviation) and extension of the wrist; restrains thumb and wrist flexion; and stabilizes the thumb and wrist.	To the web of the thumb.
Extensor indicis	Extends the metacarpophalangeal joint and (with the lumbrical and interosseous muscles) extends the interphalangeal joints of the index finger; may assist in adduction of the index finger and supination of the forearm; restrains, stabilizes, and controls flexion of the index finger; and extends the hand at the wrist.	Dorsum of the forearm to various parts of the hand.
Intrinsic Muscles of the Hand		
Thenar Eminence Muscles		
Opponens pollicis	Abducts at the carpometacarpal joint of the thumb; flexes at the carpometacarpal joint; aids in opposition of the thumb to each of the other digits; controls and restrains adduction of the thumb; and stabilizes the thumb.	Into the thumb and the wrist.
Abductor pollicis brevis	Abducts and aids in opposition of the thumb; controls and restrains adduction of the thumb; and stabilizes the thumb.	Into the thumb and the wrist.

Muscle Name	Function/Action	Trigger Point Referred Pain Pattern*
Flexor pollicis brevis	Flexes the proximal phalanx of the thumb; assists in opposition of the thumb; restrains and controls extension of the thumb; and stabilizes the thumb.	Into the thumb and the wrist.
Hypothenar Muscles		
Opponens digiti minimi	Provides flexion and slight rotation of the carpometacarpal joint of the little finger; helps cup the palm of the hand; and stabilizes the little finger.	Little finger and wrist.
Abductor digiti minimi manus	Abducts the metacarpophalangeal joint of the little finger; controls and restrains adduction and flexion of the little finger; and stabilizes the little finger.	Little finger and wrist.
Flexor digiti minimi (brevis manus)	Flexes the metacarpophalangeal joint of the little finger; assists in opposition of the little finger to the thumb; controls extension of the little finger; and stabilizes the little finger.	Little finger and wrist.
Deep Muscles of the Hand		
Adductor pollicis	Adducts the thumb and aids in opposition; restrains thumb abduction; and stabilizes the thumb.	Thumb.
Palmar interossei	Adducts the index, ring, and little fingers toward the middle digit; assists in restraining abduction of the fingers; and stabilizes the hand.	Into the associated finger.
Dorsal interossei manus	Abducts the index, middle, and ring fingers from the midline of the hand.	Into the associated finger.
Lumbricales manus	Extends the interphalangeal joints and simultaneously flexes the metacarpophalangeal joint of the second through fifth digits.	Into the associated finger.
Muscles of the Gluteal Region		
Gluteus maximus	Extends and laterally rotates the hip joint; upper fibers assist abduction of the hip; lower fibers assist in adduction of the hip joint; with femur fixed, assists in extension of the trunk and posterior tilt of the pelvis; the gluteus maximus is active primarily during strenuous activity, such as running, jumping, and climbing stairs; restrains and controls hip and trunk flexion and medial rotation and abduction/adduction of the hip. These muscles are important postural muscles that help maintain the upright posture, stabilize the pelvis, and provide tension to the iliotibial tract to keep the fascial band taut.	Regionally into the gluteal area, especially to the ischial tuberosity, the tip of the greater trochanter, and the sacrum.

Muscle Name	Function/Action	Trigger Point Referred Pain Pattern*
Gluteus medius	Abducts the hip joint; anterior fibers medially rotate and assist in flexion of the hip joint and anterior tilt of the pelvis; posterior fibers laterally rotate and assist in extension of the hip joint and posterior tilt of the pelvis; restrains adduction, medial/lateral rotation and flexion/extension of the hip; and stabilizes the pelvis when a person is standing on one foot.	Along the musculotendinous junction at the iliac crest; low back, posterior crest of the ilium to the sacrum, and to the posterior and lateral areas of the buttock into the upper thigh.
Gluteus minimus	Abducts the hip joint; anterior fibers medially rotate and assist in flexion of the hip joint and anterior tilt of the pelvis; posterior fibers laterally rotate and assist in extension of the hip joint and posterior tilt of the pelvis; restrains adduction, medial/lateral rotation and flexion/extension of the hip; and stabilizes the pelvis when a person is standing on one foot.	Lower lateral buttock and down the lateral to posterior aspect of the thigh, knee, and leg to the ankle.
Tensor fasciae latae	Flexes, medially rotates, and abducts the hip joint; assists in anterior pelvic tilt; extends the knee; restrains hip extension and lateral rotation; tenses the iliotibial tract, counterbalancing the backward pull of the gluteus maximus on the iliotibial tract; and stabilizes the pelvis and knee.	Localized in the hip and down the lateral side of the leg to the knee.
Deep Lateral Rotators		
Piriformis Obturator internus and obturator externus Gemellus superior and gemellus inferior	Provide lateral rotation and abduction of the hip joint when the thigh is flexed; restrain medial rotation and adduction of the hip; and stabilize the hip joint.	The belly of each muscle can house trigger points. Sacroiliac region, entire buttock, and down the posterior thigh to just above the knee.
Quadratus femoris	Laterally rotates the hip joint and adducts the thigh; restrains internal rotation and abduction of the hip joint; and stabilizes the hip joint.	The main trigger points are near the attachments and the insertion. Tension in this muscle may cause deep hip and groin pain.
Muscles of the Posterior Thigh		
Semimembranosus	Flexes the knee and medially rotates the knee joint when the knee is semiflexed; moves the medial meniscus posteriorly during knee flexion; extends and assists in medial rotation and adduction of the hip joint; posteriorly tilts the pelvis; restrains and controls knee extension and lateral rotation; assists in controlling flexion and lateral rotation of the hip; and stabilizes the knee and hip complex.	Several areas in the belly of each muscle and at the musculotendinous junction closer to the knee; ischial tuberosity, back of the knee, and the entire posterior leg to midcalf.

Muscle Name	Function/Action	Trigger Point Referred Pain Pattern*
Semitendinosus	Flexes the knee and medially rotates the knee joint when the knee is semiflexed; extends and assists in medial rotation and adduction of the hip joint; restrains and controls knee extension and lateral rotation; assists in controlling flexion and lateral rotation of the hip; and stabilizes the knee and hip complex.	Several areas in the belly of each muscle and at the musculotendinous junction closer to the knee; ischial tuberosity, back of the knee, and the entire posterior leg to midcalf.
Biceps femoris	Flexes and laterally rotates the knee joint when the knee is semiflexed; long head also extends and assists in lateral rotation of the hip joint and posteriorly tilts the pelvis; restrains and controls knee extension and medial rotation; also restrains hip flexion and medial rotation; and stabilizes the hip and knee complex.	Several areas in the belly of each muscle and at the musculotendinous junction closer to the knee; ischial tuberosity, back of the knee, and the entire posterior leg to midcalf.
Muscles of the Medial Thigh		
Pectineus	Adducts, flexes, and assists in medial rotation of the hip joint and anterior tilt of the pelvis; restrains abduction, extension, and lateral rotation of hip; and stabilizes the hip.	Deep in the groin into the medial thigh and downward to the knee and shin. Pain may mimic hamstring tension.
Adductor brevis	Adducts and assists in flexing the hip joint anteriorly and tilts the pelvis; restrains and controls abduction and extension of the hip; and stabilizes the hip and trunk in the standing position.	Deep in the groin into the medial thigh and downward to the knee and shin. Pain may mimic hamstring tension.
Adductor longus	Adducts and assists in flexing the hip joint and anteriorly tilts the pelvis; restrains and controls abduction and extension of the hip; and stabilizes the hip and trunk in the standing position.	Deep in the groin into the medial thigh and downward to the knee and shin. Pain may mimic hamstring tension.
Adductor magnus	Adducts the hip joint and posteriorly tilts the pelvis; upper portion medially rotates and flexes, whereas the lower portion extends the hip joint; restrains and controls hip abduction; and stabilizes the trunk, pelvis, and hip.	Deep in the groin into the medial thigh and downward to the knee and shin. Pain may mimic hamstring tension.
Gracilis	Adducts and flexes the hip joint; assists with anterior tilt of the pelvis; flexes the knee and medially rotates the knee joint when the knee is semiflexed; controls and restrains hip abduction and extension and knee extension and lateral rotation; and assists in controlling and stabilizing the valgus angulation of the knee and stabilizing the pelvic and knee complex.	Deep in the groin into the medial thigh and downward to the knee and shin. Pain may mimic hamstring tension.

Muscle Name	Function/Action	Trigger Point Referred Pain Pattern*
Muscles of the Anterior Thigh		
Sartorius	Flexes, laterally rotates, and abducts the hip joint; also weakly flexes the torso toward the pelvis when the leg is fixed and anteriorly and laterally tilts the pelvis; flexes and assists in medial rotation of the knee joint; controls and restrains extension, medial rotation, and adduction of the hip and assists in restraining trunk extension; at the knee, restrains and controls extension and lateral rotation of the knee; and stabilizes the knee and hip complex.	Into the hip and medial knee.
Quadriceps Femoris Group		
Rectus femoris	Extends the knee joint; flexes the hip joint; anteriorly tilts the pelvis; restrains and controls knee flexion and hip extension; and stabilizes the knee and hip complex.	Into the hip and knee.
Vastus lateralis	Extends the knee joint and exerts a lateral pull on the patella; controls and restrains knee flexion and medial pull of patella; and stabilizes iliotibial tract and knee.	Into the hip and lateral knee.
Vastus medialis	Extends the leg and draws the patella medially, particularly the lower oblique aspect of the muscle (vastus medialis oblique) with attachment into the adductor magnus; controls and restrains knee flexion and lateral movement of patella; and stabilizes the knee and patella.	Entire anterior thigh, with concentration at the knee.
Vastus intermedius	Extends the knee joint; restrains and controls knee flexion; and stabilizes the knee and patella.	Into the knee.
Muscles of the Anterior and Lateral Leg		
Anterior Muscles		
Tibialis anterior	Provides dorsiflexion of the ankle joint; assists in inversion and adduction of the foot. *Note:* Combined action of inversion and adduction results in supination. Restrains and controls plantar flexion and eversion of the foot. Stabilizes the ankle.	Down the leg to the ankle and into the toes.
Extensor digitorum longus	Extends the phalanges of the second through fifth digits; assists in dorsiflexion of the ankle joint and eversion and abduction of the foot; restrains and controls flexion of the toes, plantar flexion, and inversion of the ankle and foot; and stabilizes the ankle and foot.	Down the leg to the ankle and into the toes.

Muscle Name	Function/Action	Trigger Point Referred Pain Pattern*
Extensor hallucis longus	Extends the metatarsophalangeal joint of the great toe; also assists in inverting and adducting (supination) the foot and dorsiflexing the ankle joint; restrains and controls flexion of the great toes, eversion of the foot, and plantar flexion of the ankle; and stabilizes the great toe and assists in stabilizing the ankle.	Down the leg to the ankle and into the toes.
Fibularis (peroneus) tertius	Dorsiflexes the ankle joint; everts and abducts (pronates) the foot; assists in controlling and restraining plantar flexion of the ankle and inversion of the foot; and assists in stabilizing the ankle.	Down the leg to the ankle.
Lateral Muscles		
Fibularis (peroneus) longus and fibularis (peroneus) brevis	Everts and abducts (pronates) the foot; assists in plantar flexion of the ankle joint; restrains and controls dorsiflexion of the ankle and inversion of the foot; and stabilizes the ankle.	To the lateral malleolus and the heel.
Posterior Leg Muscles		
Popliteus	Assists in restraining knee extension; stabilizes the knee.	To the back of the knee.
Tibialis posterior	Inverts the foot; assists in plantar flexion of the ankle joint; restrains and controls eversion of the foot and dorsiflexion of the ankle; and stabilizes the ankle.	Down the posterior leg to the heel and the sole of the foot into the plantar surface of the toes; can be a factor in knee pain and restricted mobility of the knee and ankle.
Flexor digitorum longus	Flexes the joints of the second through fifth digits; assists in plantar flexion of the ankle joint and inversion and adduction (supination) of the foot; restrains and controls extension of the toes; assists in controlling dorsiflexion of the ankle and eversion of the foot; and stabilizes the ankle and toes.	Down the posterior leg to the heel and the sole of the foot into the plantar surface of the toes; can be a factor in knee pain and restricted mobility of the knee and ankle.
Flexor hallucis longus	Flexes the joints of the great toe; provides plantar flexion of the ankle joint and inverts the foot; restrains extension of the great toe and assists in controlling dorsiflexion of the ankle and eversion of the foot; and stabilizes the great toe, ankle, and foot.	Down the posterior leg to the heel and the sole of the foot into the plantar surface of the great toe.
Plantaris	Provides plantar flexion of the ankle joint; assists in flexion of the knee joint; restrains dorsiflexion of the ankle and assists in controlling extension of the knee; and assists in stabilizing the ankle/knee complex.	Can be a factor in knee pain and restricted mobility of the knee and ankle.
Soleus	Provides plantar flexion of the ankle joint and assists inversion of the foot at the ankle; restrains and controls dorsiflexion and eversion of the ankle; and stabilizes the leg over the foot and ankle.	Down the posterior leg to the heel and the sole of the foot into the plantar surface of the toes; can restrict mobility of the ankle.

Muscle Name	Function/Action	Trigger Point Referred Pain Pattern*
Gastrocnemius	Provides plantar flexion of the ankle joint; assists in flexion of the knee joint and inversion of the foot; restrains and controls dorsiflexion of the ankle and extension of the knee; stabilizes the knee and ankle complex and is involved in maintaining balance in static standing.	Down the posterior leg to the heel and the sole of the foot into the plantar surface of the toes; can be a factor in knee pain and restricted mobility of the knee and ankle.
Muscles of the Foot		
Dorsal Aspect		
Extensor digitorum brevis	Extends the interphalangeal and metatarsophalangeal joints of the second through fourth toes.	The entire foot with areas concentrated at the toes, the ball of the foot, and the heel.
Plantar Aspect: Superficial Layer		
Abductor hallucis	Abducts and assists in flexion of the metatarsophalangeal joint of the great toe.	The entire foot with areas concentrated at the large toe, the ball of the foot, and the heel.
Flexor digitorum brevis	Flexes the proximal interphalangeal joints and assists in flexion of the metatarsophalangeal joints of the second through fifth toes.	The entire foot with areas concentrated at the toes, the ball of the foot, and the heel.
Abductor digiti minimi pedis	Abducts and assists in flexing the metatarsophalangeal joint of the fifth toe.	The entire foot with areas concentrated at the small toe.
Plantar Aspect: Second Layer		
Quadratus plantae	Modifies the line of pull of the flexor digitorum longus and assists in flexion of the second through the fifth digits.	The entire foot.
Lumbricales pedis	These muscles flex the metatarsophalangeal joints and extend the interphalangeal joints of the second through the fifth digits.	Several areas concentrated in the belly of each muscle; the entire foot with areas concentrated at the large toe, the ball of the foot, and the heel.
Plantar Aspect: Third Layer		
Flexor hallucis brevis	Flexes the metatarsophalangeal joint of the great toe.	The entire foot with areas concentrated at the large toe.
Adductor hallucis	Adducts and assists in flexion of the metatarsophalangeal joint of the great toe.	The entire foot with areas concentrated at the large toe.
Flexor digiti minimi pedis	Flexes the metatarsophalangeal joint of the fifth toe.	The entire foot with areas concentrated at the little toe.
Plantar ASPECT: Fourth Layer		
Plantar interossei	These muscles adduct the third, fourth, and fifth toes toward an axis through the second toe; assist in flexion of the metatarsophalangeal joints of the third through fifth toes.	Trigger points seem to follow the bellies of the muscles.
Dorsal interossei pedis	These muscles abduct the second, third, and fourth toes from a longitudinal axis through the second toe; also assist in flexion of the metatarsophalangeal joints of the second through the fourth digits and extension of interphalangeal joints of the second through fourth digits.	Trigger points seem to follow the bellies of the muscles.

*The most common location of trigger points is in the belly of the muscles or at the attachments.

APPENDIX C

Recognizing Human Trafficking Victims

Human trafficking is a growing issue. It is important that you are informed enough to recognize when a person is potentially in danger.

This appendix was compiled from content taken directly from the following three resources:

Homeland Security, *Indicators of Human Trafficking*, https://www.dhs.gov/blue-campaign/indicators-human-trafficking

US Department of Health & Human Services, *What is Human Trafficking*, https://www.dhs.gov/blue-campaign/what-human-trafficking

US Department of Health & Human Services, *Fact Sheet: Human Trafficking*, https://www.acf.hhs.gov/otip/fact-sheet/resource/fshumantrafficking. Fact Sheet: Human Trafficking | The Administration for Children and Families (hhs.gov)

Human trafficking is a form of modern slavery. It occurs when a trafficker exploits an individual with force, fraud, or coercion to make them perform commercial sex or work. In addition to being a violent crime, human trafficking is a public health concern that impacts individuals, families, and entire communities across generations. Prevention requires training and a response from communities, social service providers, health care providers, and other first responders.

There are two types of trafficking:

Labor Trafficking—Individuals are compelled to work or provide services by force, fraud, or coercion.

Sex Trafficking—Adults are compelled to engage in commercial sex by force, fraud, or coercion. Minors are compelled to perform a commercial sex act regardless of the presence of force, fraud, or coercion.

The legal definition of human trafficking describes three facets of the crime: an action, a means, and a purpose. For example, if an individual is recruited by fraudulent means for the purpose of forced labor, that individual has experienced trafficking.

Traffickers use force, fraud, or coercion to lure their victims and force them into labor or commercial sexual exploitation. They look for people who are susceptible for a variety of reasons, including psychological or emotional vulnerability, economic hardship, lack of a social safety net, natural disasters, or political instability. The trauma caused by the traffickers can be so great that many may not identify themselves as victims or ask for help, even in highly public settings.

Many myths and misconceptions exist. Recognizing key indicators of human trafficking is the first step in identifying victims and can help save a life. Not all indicators listed are present in every human trafficking situation, and the presence or absence of any of the indicators is not necessarily proof of human trafficking.

INDICATORS OF HUMAN TRAFFICKING

Recognizing key indicators of human trafficking is the first step in identifying victims and can help save a life. Here are some common indicators to help recognize human trafficking:

- Does the person appear disconnected from family, friends, community organizations, or houses of worship?
- Has a child stopped attending school?
- Has the person had a sudden or dramatic change in behavior?
- Is a juvenile engaged in commercial sex acts?
- Is the person disoriented or confused, or showing signs of mental or physical abuse?
- Does the person have bruises in various stages of healing?
- Is the person fearful, timid, or submissive?
- Does the person show signs of having been denied food, water, sleep, or medical care?
- Is the person often in the company of someone to whom they defer? Or someone who seems to be in control of the situation, e.g., where they go or to whom they talk?
- Does the person appear to be coached on what to say?
- Is the person living in unsuitable conditions?
- Does the person lack personal possessions and appear not to have a stable living situation?
- Does the person have freedom of movement? Can the person freely leave where they live? Are there unreasonable security measures?
- Not all indicators listed above are present in every human trafficking situation, and the presence or absence of any of the indicators is not necessarily proof of human trafficking

RESOURCES

National Human Trafficking Hotline | 1-888-373-7888
https://humantraffickinghotline.org/

Homeland Security Blue Campaign
https://www.dhs.gov/blue-campaign
www.dhs.gov/blue-campaign/infographic

United Nations Office on Drugs and Crime
https://www.unodc.org/unodc/en/human-trafficking/what-is-human-trafficking.html

USA.gov (search "human trafficking")
https://www.usa.gov/

Human Trafficking/Involuntary Servitude | FBI
www.fbi.gov/investigate/civil-rights/human-trafficking
Human Trafficking | ICE
www.ice.gov/features/human-trafficking
Fact Sheet: Human Trafficking | Office on Trafficking in ...
www.acf.hhs.gov/otip/resource/fshumantrafficking
Trafficking in Persons Report 2022
https://www.state.gov/reports/2022-trafficking-in-persons-report/
Human Trafficking |womenshealth.gov
www.womenshealth.gov/relationships-and-safety/other-types/human-trafficking
Human Trafficking | US Customs and Border Protection
www.cbp.gov/border-security/human-trafficking
Human Trafficking | US Department of Transportation
www.transportation.gov/stophumantrafficking
Human Trafficking | Department of Justice
www.justice.gov/humantrafficking
National Strategy To Combat Human Trafficking 2019–2024: Canada
https://www.publicsafety.gc.ca/cnt/rsrcs/pblctns/2019-ntnl-strtgy-hmnn-trffc/index-en.aspx
US Department of Health and Human Services, HHS.gov
https://www.hhs.gov/
Free online courses
SOAR to Health and Wellness Training
https://www.acf.hhs.gov/otip/training/soar-health-and-wellness-training/soar-online
https://www.train.org/main/search?type=course&query=SOAR

Glossary

A

abbreviation A shortened form of a word or phrase.

absolute risk The chance a person will develop a specific disease or potential injury over a specified period.

abuse Exploitation, misuse, mistreatment, molestation, or neglect.

acquired immunodeficiency syndrome (AIDS) A disease of the immune system caused by the human immunodeficiency virus (HIV).

active assisted movement Movement of a joint in which both the client and the therapist produce the motion.

active joint movement Movement of a joint through its range of motion by the client.

active listening Clarifying a feeling attached to a message but not adding to or changing the message.

active range of motion Movement of a joint by the client without any type of assistance from the massage practitioner.

active resistive movement Movement of a joint by the client against resistance provided by the therapist.

acupressure Methods used to tone or sedate acupuncture points without the use of needles.

acupuncture Stimulation of certain points with needles inserted along the meridians (channels) and *Ah shi* ("ouch") points outside the meridians.

acupuncture point An Asian term for a specific point that correlates with a neurological motor point.

acute A term that describes a condition in which the signs and symptoms develop quickly, last a short time, and then disappear.

acute illness A short-term illness that resolves by means of the normal healing process and, if necessary, supportive medical care.

acute injury Indication that damage to the body has occurred such as a fracture, wound, sprain, burn, or contusion.

acute pain A symptom of a disease condition or a temporary aspect of medical treatment. Acute pain acts as a warning signal because it can activate the sympathetic nervous system. It is usually temporary, has a sudden onset, and is easily localized. The client frequently can describe the pain, which often subsides without treatment.

adaptation A response to a sensory stimulation in which nerve signaling is reduced or stops.

adaptive capacity Ability to respond to stress based on hardiness and current stress load.

aerobic exercise An exercise program focused on increasing fitness and endurance.

allied health A division of medicine in which the professional receives training in a specific area of medicine to serve as support for the physician.

altruistic love and kindness The assertion of a common humanity in which other people are worthy of attention and affirmation for no utilitarian reasons but rather for their own sake.

anatomical barriers Anatomical structures determined by the shape and fit of the bones at the joint.

anatomical tools Palms, forearms, fingertips, or knuckles used to apply force to soft tissue.

antagonism The process by which massage produces the opposite effect.

antagonistic When massage produces the opposite effect sought.

antagonists The muscles that oppose the movement of the prime movers.

anxiety A feeling of uneasiness, usually connected with an increase in sympathetic arousal responses.

applied kinesiology Methods of evaluation and bodywork that use a specialized type of muscle testing and various forms of massage and bodywork for corrective procedures.

approach A way of thinking and problem solving during massage.

approximation The technique of pushing muscle fibers together in the belly of the muscle.

aromatherapy A healing discipline involving the use of essential oils.

art Craft, skill, technique, and talent.

arterial circulation Movement of oxygenated blood under pressure from the heart to the body through the arteries.

arthrokinematic movement An accessory movement that occurs as a result of inherent laxity or joint play that exists in each joint. The joint play allows the ends of the bones to slide, roll, or spin smoothly on one another. These essential movements occur passively with movement of the joint and are not under voluntary control.

aseptic technique A procedure that kills or disables pathogens on surfaces to prevent transmission.

Asian approaches Methods of bodywork that have developed from ancient roots of Asian medicine theories and principles.

aspirational ethics Ethical behavior motivated by a professional's desire to provide the highest possible benefit and welfare for the client.

assessment Collection and interpretation of information provided by the client, their family and friends, the massage practitioner, and any referring medical professionals.

asymmetric stance The position in which the body weight is shifted from one foot to the other while standing.

asymmetric standing Standing with one foot in front of the other; the most efficient standing position.

athlete A person who participates in sports as an amateur or a professional. Athletes require precise use of their bodies.

attention The direction of awareness to any object, sense, or thought for the sake of gaining clarity.

autonomy the ability to practice massage therapy independently.

autonomic nervous system The body system that regulates involuntary body functions using the sympathetic fight–flight–fear response and the restorative parasympathetic relaxation response. The sympathetic and parasympathetic systems work together to maintain homeostasis through a feedback loop system.

autoregulation The control of homeostasis through alteration of tissue or function.

Ayurveda A system of health and medicine that grew from East Indian roots.

B

bacteria Primitive cells that have no nuclei. Bacteria cause disease by secreting toxic substances that damage human tissues, by becoming parasites inside human cells, or by forming colonies in the body that disrupt normal function.

balance The ability to maintain the body's center of gravity within the base of support.

bartering The exchange of massage services for other goods or services without using money.

beating A form of heavy percussive load (tapotement) involving use of the fist.

bending Bending loads produce tensile and compressive stresses. Think about bending a wire with both hands; you are actually creating compressive stress on one side and tensile stress on the other.

benign tumor A tumor that remains localized within the tissue from which it arose and does not undergo malignant changes. Benign tumors usually grow slowly.

best practice A technique or methodology that through experience and research has proven to reliably lead to a desired result.

bias The assumption that a theory is true or false without evidence one way or another; bias can occur in the planning, data collection, analysis, and publication phases of research. It can also present as prejudice in favor of or against one thing, person, or group compared with another, usually in a way considered to be unfair.

biologically plausible A hypothesis and the relationship that it proposes are in harmony with existing scientific information.

biomechanics Body motions and the muscular forces used to complete tasks.

biopsychosocial model of medicine An approach to medicine that recognizes that biological, psychological, and social factors all play a significant role in human functioning.

body mechanics Use of the body in an efficient and biomechanically correct way.

body–mind The interaction between thought and physiology that is connected to the limbic system, the hypothalamic influence on the autonomic nervous system, and the endocrine system.

body–mind–spirit The three primary layers that are interrelated, interacting, and integrated to constitute a healthy, balanced, and unified human being.

body segment The area of the body between joints that provides movement during walking and balance.

body supports Pillows, folded blankets, foam forms, or commercial products that help contour the flat surface of a massage table or mat.

bodywork A term that encompasses all the various forms of massage, movement, and other touch therapies.

boundary Personal space that exists within an arm's length perimeter. Personal emotional space is designated by morals, values, and experience.

burnout A condition that occurs when a person uses up energy faster than it can be restored.

breathing pattern disorders A complex set of behaviors that lead to overbreathing in the absence of a pathological condition. These disorders are considered a functional syndrome because all its parts work effectively and the condition is therefore not caused by a specific pathological condition.

C

care/treatment plan A plan used to achieve therapeutic goals by outlining the agreed-upon objectives; the frequency, duration, and number of visits; progress measurements; the date of reassessment; and massage methods to be used.

career A chosen pursuit; a life's work.

categories of force load The five types of loads that can act on soft tissue are tension, compression, shear, bending, and torsion. These five loads fall into two categories: simple loads and combined loads.

caution A condition that requires the massage therapist to adapt the massage process so that the client's safety is maintained.

center of gravity The average position of an object's weight distribution.

centering The ability to pay attention to a specific area of focus.

certification A voluntary credentialing process that usually requires education and testing; tests are administered either privately or by government regulatory bodies.

chakra Energy fields or centers of consciousness within the body.

challenge Living each day knowing that it is filled with things to learn, skills to practice, tasks to accomplish, and obstacles to overcome.

charting A systematic form of documentation.

chemical effects The effects of massage produced by the release of chemical substances in the body. These substances may be released locally from the massaged tissue or they may be hormones released into the general circulation.

chronic A term to describe a disease that develops slowly and lasts for a long time (sometimes for life).

chronic illness A disease, injury, or syndrome that shows minor change or slow progression.

chronic pain Pain that persists or recurs for indefinite periods, usually for longer than 6 months. It frequently has an insidious onset, and the character and quality of the pain change over time. Chronic pain frequently involves deep somatic and visceral structures. It usually is diffuse and poorly localized.

circulation The flow of blood through the vessels of the body.

circulatory A term that describes systems that depend on the pumping action of the skeletal muscle (i.e., the arterial, venous, lymphatic, respiratory, and cerebrospinal fluid circulatory systems).

client A recipient of service, be it from a wellness or health care professional, regardless of their health status. All patients are clients, but not all clients are patients.

client information form A document used to obtain information from the client about health, preexisting conditions, and expectations for the massage.

client outcome The results desired from the massage and the massage therapist.

client–practitioner agreement and policy statement A detailed written explanation of all rules, expectations, and procedures for the massage.

client records All information related to the client.

clinical massage A massage therapy practice involving extensive use of assessment and specific focused techniques and applications with the intention of achieving clinical treatment or functional outcomes and remediation of symptoms.

clinical reasoning A form of critical thinking that targets a specific therapeutic practice.

coalition A group formed for a particular purpose.

code of ethics An agreed-on set of behaviors developed to promote high standards of practice.

cognition Conscious awareness and perception, reasoning, judgment, intuition, and memory.

comfort barrier The first point of resistance short of the client's perceiving any discomfort at the physiological or pathological barrier.

commitment The ability and willingness to be involved in what is happening around us so as to have a purpose for being.

communicable disease A disease caused by pathogens that are easily spread; a contagious disease.

compensation The process of counterbalancing a defect in body structure or function.

complementary, alternative, integrative medicine (CAIM) A group of diverse medical and health care systems, practices, and products that are not generally considered part of conventional medicine.

compression The force or method used to apply pressure into the body to spread tissue against underlying structures. Also, the exertion of inappropriate pressure on nerves by hard tissue (e.g., bone).

compressive stress The result of two pushing forces, directly opposing each other, that squeeze or press an object.

concentric isotonic contraction The application of a counterforce by the massage therapist while allowing the client to move, which brings the origin and insertion of the target muscle together against the pressure.

condition management The use of massage methods to support clients who are unable to undergo a therapeutic change but who wish to function as effectively as possible under a set of circumstances.

confidentiality Respect for the privacy of information.

conflict An expressed struggle between at least two interdependent parties who perceive incompatible goals, scarce resources, or interference from the other party in achieving their goals.

connective tissue The most abundant tissue type in the body; it provides support, structure, space, and stabilization and is involved in scar formation.

contamination The process by which an object or area becomes unclean.

contraindication Any condition that renders a particular treatment improper or undesirable.

control The belief that a person can influence events by the way the individual feels, thinks, and acts.

Coronavirus A group of related RNA viruses that cause diseases such as the SARS-CoV-2 virus.

cortisol A stress hormone produced by the adrenal glands that is released during long-term stress. An elevated level indicates increased sympathetic arousal.

counterirritation Superficial stimulation that relieves a deeper sensation by stimulating different sensory signals.

counterpressure Force applied to an area that is designed to match exactly (isometric contraction) or partly (isotonic contraction) the effort or force produced by the muscles of that area.

countertransference The personalization of the professional relationship by the therapist in which the practitioner is unable to separate the therapeutic relationship from personal feelings and expectations for the client.

cream A type of lubricant that is in a semisolid or solid state.

credential A designation earned by completing a process that verifies a certain level of expertise in a given skill.

cross-directional stretching Tissue stretching that pulls and twists connective tissue against its fiber direction.

cryotherapy Therapeutic use of ice.

cultural appropriation The unacknowledged or inappropriate adoption of the customs, practices, or ideas of one people or society by members of another.

cultural competency A set of congruent behaviors, attitudes, and policies that come together in a system or agency or among professionals that enables effective work in cross-cultural situations.

cultural humility A lifelong commitment to self-evaluation and self-critique of the power imbalances in the client and massage therapist's therapeutic relationship related to cultural diversity.

culture The arts, beliefs, customs, institutions, and all other products of human work and thought created by a specific group of people at a particular time.

cupping The type of tapotement that involves the use of a cupped hand; it often is used over the thorax. Also a form of vacuum/suction-assisted massage.

cutaneous sensory receptors Sensory nerves in the skin.

D

database All the information available that contributes to the therapeutic interaction.

decisions Thought-out responses based on principles, information, and complexities of the situation. Decision making requires a person to consider the facts, possibilities, logical consequences of cause and effect (pros and cons), and possible impact on others.

deep inspiration The movement of air into the body by hard breathing to meet an increased demand for oxygen. Any muscles that can pull the ribs up are called into action.

deep tissue The tissue beneath the superficial structures being treated.

deep tissue work A generic term commonly used to describe a variety of techniques to address specific deep tissues and structures, regardless of the force or pressure exerted or the level of discomfort or pain experienced during or after the application.

defensive climate An atmosphere characteristic of competition that inhibits the mutual trust required for effective conflict management.

defensive measures The means through which the body defends itself against stressors (e.g., production of antibodies and white blood cells or through behavioral or emotional means).

denial The ability to retreat and to ignore stressors.

depression A condition characterized by a decrease in vital functional activity and by mood disturbances of exaggerated emptiness, hopelessness, and melancholy or of high energy with no purpose or outcome.

depth of pressure Compressive stress that can be light, moderate, deep, or varied.

dermatome The cutaneous (skin) distribution of spinal nerve sensation.

diagnosis The process of identifying the disease or syndrome a person is believed to have.

dilemma Difficulty making a decision when there may be multiple ways to address a situation.

direction The flow of massage strokes from the center of the body outward (centrifugal) or from the extremities inward toward the center of the body (centripetal). Direction can be circular motions; it can flow from origin to insertion of the muscle, following the muscle fibers; or it can flow transverse to the tissue fibers.

direction of ease The position the body assumes with postural changes and muscle shortening or weakening, depending on how it has balanced against gravity.

disability An umbrella term for impairments, activity limitations, and participation restrictions, denoting the negative aspects of the interaction between an individual (with a health condition) and that individual's contextual factors (environmental and personal factors).

discipline An area of study involving particular concepts, a specific vocabulary, and so on.

disclosure Acknowledging and informing the client of any situation that interferes with or affects the professional relationship.

disinfection The process through which pathogens are destroyed.

dissociation A state of detachment, discontentedness, separation, or isolation.

diversity The ways in which people differ that make one individual or group different from another.

documentation The process of creating and maintaining client records.

dopamine A neurochemical that influences motor activity involving movement (especially learned fine movement, such as handwriting), conscious selective selection (what to pay attention to), mood (in terms of inspiration), possibility, intuition, joy, and enthusiasm. If the dopamine level is low, the opposite effects are seen, such as lack of motor control, clumsiness, inability to decide what to address, and boredom.

drag The amount of pull (stretch) on the tissue (tensile stress).

drape Fabric used to cover the client and keep the individual warm during the massage.

draping The procedures of covering and uncovering areas of the body and turning the client during the massage.

draping material Coverings that provide the client with privacy and warmth. The most commonly used coverings are standard bed linens because they are large enough to cover the entire body and are easy to use for most draping procedures.

dual role Overlap in the scope of practice, with one professional providing support in more than one area of expertise.

duration The length of time a method lasts or stays in the same location.

dysfunction An in-between state in which one is "not healthy" but also "not sick" (i.e., experiencing disease).

E

eccentric isotonic contraction Application of a counterforce while the client moves the jointed area, which allows the origin and insertion of the muscle to separate. The muscle lengthens against the pressure.

effleurage (gliding stroke) Horizontal strokes applied with the fingers, hand, or forearm that usually follow the fiber direction of the underlying muscle, fascial planes, or dermatome pattern.

electrical-chemical functions Physiological functions of the body that rely on or produce body energy; often called *chi*, *prana*, or meridian energy.

electromyography (EMG) Used to evaluate and record the electrical activity of skeletal muscles.

elongation methods Pulling or pushing tissues to lengthen them.

empathy The ability to identify with the feelings and experience of another.

employee A person who works for another for a wage.

end-feel The perception of the joint at the limit of its range of motion. The end-feel is either soft or hard (see joint end-feel).

endangerment site Any area of the body where nerves and blood vessels surface close to the skin and are not well protected by muscle or connective tissue; therefore deep, sustained pressure into these areas could damage these vessels and nerves. The kidney area is included because the kidneys are loosely suspended in fat and connective tissue, and heavy pounding is contraindicated in that area.

endocannabinoids A group of neuromodulatory chemicals involved in a variety of physiological processes including appetite, pain sensation, mood, memory, motor coordination, blood pressure regulation, and combating cancer.

endogenous Made in the body.

endurance A measure of fitness. The ability to work for prolonged periods and the ability to resist fatigue.

energy The capacity to carry out a particular action, whether it be moving the limbs or thinking.

energetic approaches Methods of bodywork that involve subtle body responses.

enkephalins, endorphins, and dynorphins Neurochemicals that elevate mood, modulate pain, and support satiety by reducing hunger and cravings.

entrainment The coordination of movements or their synchronization to a rhythm.

entrapment Pathological pressure placed on a nerve or vessel by soft tissue.

environmental contact Contact with pathogens found in the environment in food, water, and soil and on various surfaces.

epinephrine (adrenaline) A neurochemical that activates arousal mechanisms in the body; the activation, arousal, alertness, and alarm chemical of the fight-or-flight response and all sympathetic arousal functions and behaviors.

equity The fair treatment of all.

ergonomics The study of the design of equipment, the working environment, and the workload with the goal of reducing musculoskeletal stress on the body.

essential oils Distilled extracts from aromatic plants.

essential touch Vital, fundamental, and primary touch that is crucial to well-being.

ethical behavior Right and good conduct that is based on moral and cultural standards as defined by the society in which we live.

ethical decision making The application of ethical principles and professional skills to determine appropriate behavior and resolve ethical dilemmas.

ethics The science or study of morals, values, or principles, including ideals of autonomy, beneficence, and justice; principles of right and good conduct.

evidence-based practice The use of current best evidence in making decisions about the care of patients.

evidence-informed practices The best available research, plausible suppositions, expert opinion consensus, and practice knowledge based on clinical experience to guide professional practice.

evidence-informed decision making A continuous interactive process involving the explicit, conscientious, and judicious consideration of the best available evidence to provide care.

exemption A situation in which a professional is not required to comply with an existing law because of educational or professional standing.

experiment A method of testing a hypothesis.

external forces Forces that create loads on soft tissue by pushing or pulling on the body in a variety of ways. A belt around your waist is creating an external compressive load. Gravity is an external force. Massage is an external force.

external sensory information Stimulation from an origin exterior to the surface of the skin that is detected by the body.

F

facilitation The state of a nerve in which it is stimulated but not to the point of threshold; the point at which it transmits a nerve signal.

fascial sheath A flat sheet of connective tissue used for separation, stability, and muscular attachment points.

feedback A method of autoregulation to maintain internal homeostasis that interlinks body functions; a non-invasive, continual exchange of information between the client and the professional.

felt sense An internal somatic knowing that is difficult to express using words.

fitness A general term used to describe the ability to perform physical work.

focus/centering The ability to focus the mind by screening out sensation. Also called mindfulness.

force Something that internally or externally causes the movement of the body to change or soft-tissue structures to deform. In physics, a force is any external effort that causes an object to undergo a certain change concerning its movement, direction, or shape.

forced expiration The movement of air out of the body, produced by activating muscles that can pull down the ribs and muscles that can compress the abdomen, forcing the diaphragm upward.

forced inspiration The movement of air into the body that occurs when an individual is working very hard and needs a great deal of oxygen. This involves not only the muscles of quiet and deep inspiration but also the muscles that stabilize or elevate the shoulder girdle to elevate the ribs directly or indirectly.

form/style A particular procedure used to do massage and bodywork.

franchise A business contract through which an individual (the franchisee) purchases the rights to sell or market the products or services (or both) of a large group that has developed a brand (the franchisor).

frequency The number of times a method repeats itself in a time period.

friction Specific circular or transverse movements that do not glide on the skin and that are focused on the underlying tissue. Friction is a force that acts in an opposite direction to movement and holds back the movement of a sliding object.

fungi A group of simple parasitic organisms that are similar to plants but that have no chlorophyll (green pigment). Most pathogenic fungi live on tissue on or near the skin or mucous membranes.

G

gait A walking pattern.

gate control theory A term that refers to a hypothetical gating mechanism that functions at the level of the spinal cord; a "gate" through which pain impulses reach the lateral spinothalamic system. Painful impulses are transmitted by large-diameter and small-diameter nerve fibers. Stimulation of large-diameter fibers prevents the small-diameter fibers from transmitting signals. Stimulating large-diameter fibers (through rubbing or massaging) helps suppress the sensation of pain, especially if the pain is sharp.

gender identity A social construct framework for how people perceive themselves. Gender identity can be consistent with, or different from, the sex assigned at birth.

general adaptation syndrome The process that calls into play the three stages of the body's response to stress: the alarm reaction, the resistance reaction, and the exhaustion reaction.

general contraindications Factors that require a physician's evaluation to rule out serious underlying conditions before any massage is indicated. If the physician recommends massage, the physician must help develop a comprehensive treatment plan.

gestures The way a client touches the body while explaining a problem. These movements may indicate whether they are experiencing a muscle problem, a joint problem, or a visceral problem.

goals Desired outcomes.

Golgi tendon receptors Receptors in the tendons that sense tension.

growth hormone A hormone that promotes cell division; in adults, it is implicated in the repair and regeneration of tissue.

guarding Contraction of muscles in a splinting action, surrounding an injured area.

gua sha Treatment in which the skin is scraped to produce light petechiae.

H

hacking A type of tapotement in which the surface of the body is alternately struck with quick, snapping movements.

hard skills Specific teachable abilities that can be measured.

hardening A method of teaching the body to deal more effectively with stress; sometimes called toughening.

hardiness The physical and mental ability to withstand external stressors.

healing The restoration of well-being.

health Optimal functioning with freedom from disease or abnormal processes.

heart rate variability A physiological phenomenon in which the interval between heartbeats varies.

heavy pressure A compressive force that extends to the bone under the tissue.

hepatitis A viral inflammatory process and infection of the liver.

histamine A chemical produced by the body that dilates the blood vessels.

history Information from the client about past and present medical conditions and patterns of symptoms.

homeostasis The dynamic equilibrium of the internal environment of the body through processes of feedback and regulation.

hormone A messenger chemical in the bloodstream.

hospice A philosophy and practice for end-of-life care.

human immunodeficiency virus (HIV) The virus responsible for AIDS.

hydrotherapy The use of various types of water applications and temperatures for therapy.

hygiene Practices and conditions that promote health and prevent disease.

hyperstimulation analgesia The process of diminishing the perception of a sensation by stimulating large-diameter nerve fibers. Some methods used are application of ice or heat, counterirritation, acupressure, acupuncture, rocking, music, and repetitive massage strokes.

hyperventilation Deep or rapid breathing in excess of physical demands.

hypothesis The starting point of research; it is based on the statement "If *this* happens, then *that* will happen."

I

impingement syndromes Conditions involving pathological pressure on nerves and vessels, the two types of which are compression and entrapment.

implement A tool, utensil, or other piece of equipment used for a particular purpose to augment massage application.

implicit bias A form of bias that occurs automatically and unintentionally and affects judgments, decisions, and behaviors.

inclusion Creating environments in which any individual or group is equally welcomed, respected, supported, and valued.

indication A therapeutic application that promotes health or assists in a healing process.

inflammatory response A normal mechanism characterized by pain, heat, redness, and swelling that usually speeds up recovery from an infection or injury.

informed consent The client's authorization for any service from a professional based on adequate information provided by the professional. Obtaining informed consent is a consumer protection process that requires that clients have knowledge of what will occur and that their participation is voluntary; they also must be competent to give consent. Informed consent is an educational procedure that allows clients to make knowledgeable decisions about whether they want to receive a massage.

inhibition A decrease in or the cessation of a response or function.

initial treatment plan A plan that states therapeutic goals, the duration of the sessions, the number of appointments necessary to meet the agreed goals, costs, the general classification of intervention to be used, and the objective progress measurement to be used to identify attainment of goals.

insertion The muscle attachment point that is closest to the moving joint.

instrument assisted soft tissue manipulation (IASTM) Use of tools to provide a specialized form of massage/scraping of the soft tissues.

integrated approaches Combined methods of various forms of massage and bodywork styles.

integration The process of remembering an event while being able to remain in the present moment, with an awareness of the difference between then and now, to bring some sort of resolution to the event.

integrative medicine The combination of different types of treatments to emphasize care in a wider context of body–mind–spirit interconnectedness and the importance of supporting wellness in addition to treating pathological conditions.

interoception The body's ability to identify and process internal actions of the organs and systems inside the body. Perception of sensations from inside the body including physical sensations related to internal organ function such as heartbeat, respiration, satiety, as well as activity in the autonomic nervous system related to emotions.

intercompetition massage A massage provided during an athletic event.

internal forces Forces that create loads on soft tissue, such as when misaligned joints or poor body mechanics cause soft tissue to shorten, tighten, lengthen, and/or weaken, a process which may load surrounding tissue. One example is a tight muscle or tendon that could compress a nerve running close by, causing pain or dysfunction. Increased pressure in the stomach from overeating is also an example of an internal force.

intimacy A tender, familiar, and understanding experience between beings.

intuition Knowing something by using subconscious information.

isometric contraction A contraction in which the effort of the muscle or group of muscles is exactly matched by a counterpressure such that no movement occurs, only effort.

isotonic contraction A contraction in which the effort of the target muscle or group of muscles is partly matched by counterpressure, allowing a degree of resisted movement.

J

job An activity performed regularly for payment.

joint end-feel The sensation felt when a normal joint is taken to its physiological limit (see end-feel).

joint kinesthetic receptors Receptors in the capsules of joints that respond to pressure and to the acceleration and deceleration of joint movement. The two main types of joint kinesthetic receptors are type II cutaneous mechanoreceptors and Pacinian (lamellated) corpuscles.

joint movement The movement of the joint through its normal range of motion.

joint play The inherent laxity present in a joint.

jurisprudence The theory and practice of the law.

jurisprudence exam A test taken to demonstrate knowledge of a specific piece of legislation such as a massage therapy law.

K

kinesiology The science of the study of movement and the active and passive structures involved, including bones, joints, muscle tissues, and all associated connective tissues.

kinetic chain The process by which each individual joint movement pattern functions as part of an interconnected aspect of the neurological coordination pattern of muscle movement.

L

language Made of socially shared rules that involve sounds, symbols, definitions, and ability to create new words and grammar.

latent trigger point A trigger point that exists but does not refer pain actively. Latent trigger points can influence muscle activation patterns, which can result in poorer muscle coordination and balance, restrict movement, cause muscle weakness, and contribute to the sensation of stiffness.

law A scientific statement that is true uniformly for a whole class of natural occurrences.

leadership The act of influencing others for good, rousing others to action, and inspiring them to become the best they can be as a group works together toward a common goal.

legend drug Any medication that requires a prescription.

lengthening The process in which the muscle assumes a normal resting length by means of the neuromuscular mechanism.

leverage Leaning with the body weight to provide pressure.

license A type of credential required by law; licenses are used to regulate the practice of a profession to protect the public's health, safety, and welfare.

longitudinal stretching A stretch applied along the fiber direction of the connective tissues and muscles.

lubricant A substance that reduces friction on the skin during massage movements.

lymph system A specialized component of the circulatory system that is responsible for waste disposal and immune response.

lymphatic drainage A specific type of massage that enhances lymphatic flow.

M

malignant tumor The type of tumor (cancer) that tends to spread to other regions of the body.

mandatory ethics Ethical behavior that is motivated only by compliance with the law.

manipulation Skillful use of the hands in a therapeutic manner. Massage manipulations focus on the soft tissues of the body and are not to be confused with joint manipulation using a high-velocity thrust.

manual lymphatic drainage Methods of bodywork that influence lymphatic movement.

marketing The advertising and other promotional activities required to sell a product or service.

massage A patterned and purposeful soft-tissue manipulation accomplished by the use of digits, hands, forearms, elbows, knees, or feet, with or without the use of emollients, liniments, heat and cold, hand-held tools or other external apparatus, for the intent of therapeutic change.

massage chair A specially designed chair that allows the client to sit comfortably during the massage.

massage environment An area or location where a massage is given.

massage equipment Tables, mats, chairs, and other incidental supplies and implements used during the massage.

massage mat A cushioned surface that is placed on the floor.

massage routine The step-by-step sequence and protocol used to give a massage.

massage table A specially designed table that allows massage to be conducted with the client lying down.

massage therapist Another term for a massage practitioner; it may also refer to a massage technologist, massage technician, masseur, masseuse, myotherapist, massotherapist, bodyworker, bodywork therapist, somatic therapist, or any derivation of these terms.

massage therapy Consists of massage application as well as non-hands-on components including health promotion and educational messages regarding self-care and health maintenance. Therapy, as well as the outcomes of its practice, can be influenced by therapeutic relationships and communication, the therapist's education, skill level, and experience, and the therapeutic setting. The scientific art and system of the assessment and manual application of certain techniques to the superficial soft tissue of skin, muscles, tendons, ligaments, and fascia, and the structures that lie within the superficial tissue. The hand, foot, knee, arm, elbow, and forearm are used for the systematic external application of external mechanical force using static touch, gliding (effleurage), friction, vibration, percussion, kneading (pétrissage), elongation and stretching, compression, or passive and active joint movements within the normal physiological range of motion. Massage includes adjunctive external applications of water, heat, and cold for the purposes of establishing and maintaining good physical condition and health by normalizing and improving muscle tone, promoting relaxation, stimulating circulation, and producing therapeutic effects on the respiratory and nervous systems as well as the subtle interactions between all body systems.

massage therapy practice A client-centered framework for providing massage therapy through a process of assessment and evaluation, plan of care, treatment, reassessment and reevaluation, health messages, document, and closure in an effort to improve health or well-being. Massage therapy practice is influenced by scope of practice and professional standards.

MCE An acute injury care method meaning Move safely, Compression, and Elevation.

MEAT An acute injury care method meaning Movement, Exercise, Analgesics, and Therapy.

mechanical effects These occur when various types of mechanical force (tension, bending, shear, torsion, and compression) are applied directly to the body, directly affecting the soft tissue through techniques that normalize the connective tissue or move body fluid and intestinal contents.

mechanical methods Techniques that directly affect the soft tissue by normalizing the connective tissue or moving body fluids and intestinal contents.

mechanical response A response based on a structural change in the tissue. The tissue change is caused directly by application of a technique.

mechanical touch Touch applied with the intent of achieving a specific anatomical or physiological outcome.

medical massage A synonym for clinical massage; massage provided in a medical environment.

medications Substances prescribed to stimulate or inhibit a body process or replace a chemical in the body.

mental impairment Any mental or psychological disorder, such as mental retardation, developmental disabilities, organic brain syndrome, emotional or mental illness, and specific learning disabilities.

mentoring Career support provided by a more experienced practitioner.

meridian A nerve tract in the tissue, located in the fascial grooves, along which energy flows.

meta-analysis A high-quality analysis of several similar experiments or studies to test the pooled data for statistical significance.

metastasis The migration of cancer cells.

methicillin-resistant *Staphylococcus aureus* (MRSA) A potentially dangerous type of bacteria that is resistant to certain antibiotics and may cause skin and other infections.

mindfulness Focusing awareness on the present moment.

mobilization The process of making a fixed part movable or releasing stored substances, as in restoring motion to a joint, freeing an organ, or making substances held in reserve in the body available.

modality A method of application or employment of any physical agents or devices. The term is commonly misused to describe forms of massage (e.g., NMT, myofascial, or Swedish).

moderate pressure Compressive pressure that extends to the muscle layer but does not press the tissue against the underlying bone.

motivation The internal drive that provides the energy to do what is necessary to accomplish a goal.

motor point The point at which a motor nerve enters the muscle it innervates and causes the muscle to twitch if stimulated.

movement cure A term used in the 19th and early 20th centuries for a system of exercise and massage manipulations focused on treating a variety of ailments.

multiple isotonic contractions Movements of the joint and associated muscles by the client through a full range of motion against partial resistance applied by the massage therapist.

muscle energy techniques Neuromuscular facilitation, specific use of active contraction in individual muscles or groups of muscles to initiate a relaxation response, and activation of the proprioceptors to facilitate muscle tone, relaxation, and stretching.

muscle spindles Structures primarily located in the belly of the muscle that respond to both sudden and prolonged stretches.

muscle testing procedures Assessment processes that use muscle contraction as a test element. Strength testing is done to determine whether a muscle responds with sufficient strength to perform the required body functions. Neurological muscle testing is designed to determine whether the neurological interaction of the muscles is working smoothly.

muscle tone The nervous system's control of how long or short a muscle is by regulating the degree of muscle fiber contraction. It also refers to determination of the shape and location of a muscle and the density and pliability of all fluid, fibers, and connective tissue of the muscle.

musculotendinous junction The point at which muscle fibers end and the connective tissue continues to form the tendon; a major site of injury.

myofascial approaches Styles of bodywork that affect the connective tissues, often referred to as deep tissue massage, soft tissue manipulation, or myofascial release.

myofascial release A system of bodywork that affects body's connective tissue through various methods that elongate and alter the plastic component and ground matrix of the connective tissue.

N

National Provider Identifier (NPI) A unique 10-digit identification number assigned to covered health care providers.

nerve impingement Pressure against a nerve by skin, fascia, muscles, ligaments, or joints.

neurodiversity The range of differences in individual brain function and behavioral traits, regarded as part of normal variation in the human population.

neurological muscle testing Testing designed to determine whether neurological interaction of the muscles proceeds smoothly.

neuromatrix theory of pain Pain is part of a multisystem response to a perceived threat. There are many inputs to the brain that can trigger the pain neuromatrix, including movement, thought, emotion, touch, memory, fear, and sight. These stimuli can trigger a pain response due to a perceived threat.

neuromuscular mechanism The interplay and reflex connection between sensory and motor neurons and muscle function.

neuromuscular reeducation Therapeutic exercise techniques used to develop and restore balance, movement, coordination, kinesthetic sense, posture, proprioception, muscular tone, and activity through activation of both nerves and muscles.

neuromuscular therapy An umbrella term encompassing a variety of treatment approaches, many of which can be used to address trigger points.

neurotransmitter A messenger chemical in the synapse of the nerve.

nomenclature A system of names.

norepinephrine (noradrenaline) A neurochemical that functions in a manner similar to epinephrine but is more concentrated in the brain.

norovirus A highly contagious virus commonly spread through food or water that has been contaminated during preparation, by touching contaminated surfaces, or through contact with an infected person. Infection can cause sudden onset of severe vomiting and diarrhea.

O

occupation A productive or creative activity that serves as a regular source of livelihood.

oil A type of liquid lubricant.

open-ended question A question that cannot be answered with a simple, one-word response.

opportunistic invasion An infection caused by potentially pathogenic organisms that are found on the skin and mucous membranes of nearly everyone. These organisms do not cause disease until they have the opportunity (e.g., with impaired immunity).

origin The attachment point of a muscle at the fixed point during movement.

orthopedic tests Assessments of bone, joint, ligament, and tendon injuries.

oscillation Any effect that varies in a back-and-forth or reciprocating manner.

osteokinematic movements The movements of flexion, extension, abduction, adduction, and rotation, also known as physiological movements.

overload principle A stressor affecting an organism that is greater than one regularly encountered during everyday life.

oxytocin A hormone that is implicated in pair or couple bonding, parental bonding, feelings of attachment, and care taking, along with its more commonly known functions in pregnancy, delivery, and lactation.

P

pain and fatigue syndromes Multicausal and often chronic nonproductive patterns that interfere with well-being, activities of daily living, and productivity.

pain–spasm–pain cycle Steady contraction of muscles, which causes ischemia and stimulates pain receptors in muscles. The pain, in turn, initiates more spasms.

palliative care Care intended to relieve or reduce the intensity of uncomfortable symptoms that cannot effect a cure.

palpation Assessment through touch.

panic An intense, sudden, and overwhelming fear or feeling of anxiety that produces terror and immediate physiological change resulting in immobility or senseless, hysterical behavior.

parasympathetic autonomic nervous system The restorative part of the autonomic nervous system. The parasympathetic response often is called the relaxation response.

passive joint movement Movement of a joint by the massage practitioner without the assistance of the client.

passive range of motion Movement of a joint in which the therapist, not the client, effects the motion.

pathogenic animals Large, multicellular organisms sometimes called metazoa. Most metazoa are worms that feed off human tissue or cause other disease processes.

pathological barrier An adaptation of the physiological barrier that allows the protective function to limit—rather than support—optimal functioning.

pathology The study of disease.

patient The recipient of care.

patterns The product of the replication of structures and functions that entwine and influence each other.

payroll taxes Taxes that employees and employers must pay based on wages and tips earned and salaries paid to employees.

peak performance Maximum conditioning and functioning in a particular action.

peer support Interaction among those involved in the same pursuit. Regular interaction with other massage practitioners creates an environment in which both technical information and dilemmas and interpersonal dilemmas can be sorted out.

people-first language Way of communicating that puts the person first, not their disability. This "person-first language" puts the focus on individuals, not their functional limitations.

percussion Springy blows to the body at a fast rate to create rhythmic compression of the tissue.

person-to-person contact The transmission of pathogens from one person to another through contact or often by airborne transmission.

personal protective equipment (PPE) Specialized clothing or equipment worn for protection against infectious materials.

pétrissage (kneading) Rhythmic rolling, lifting, squeezing, and wringing of soft tissue.

pharmacology The science of drugs; includes the development of drugs, understanding of their mechanisms of action, and description of their conditions of use.

phasic muscles Muscles that move the body.

physical agents Tools or materials used in the application of therapeutic modalities consisting of energy and materials applied to the client or patient to assist in achievement of therapeutic goals.

physical assessment Evaluation of body balance, efficient function, basic symmetry, range of motion, and ability to function.

physical disability/impairment Any physiological disorder, condition, cosmetic disfigurement, or anatomical loss that affects one or more of the following body systems: neurological, musculoskeletal, special sense organ, respiratory (including speech organs), cardiovascular, reproductive, digestive, genitourinary, hemic and lymphatic, skin, and endocrine. Extremes in size and extensive burns also may be considered physical impairments.

physiological barriers The result of limits to range of motion imposed by protective nerve and sensory functions that support optimum performance.

piezoelectricity The production of an electrical current by application of pressure to certain crystals (e.g., mica, quartz, Rochelle salt) or to connective tissue.

placebo effect Improvement in a patient's disease or condition even if the treatment is not specifically validated.

polarity A holistic health practice that encompasses some of the theory base of Asian medicine and Ayurveda. Polarity is an eclectic, multifaceted system.

POLICE A modern/modified first-aid method of treating musculoskeletal injuries.

positional release A method of moving the body into the direction of ease (the way the body wants to move out of the position causes the pain); the proprioception is taken into a state of safety and may stop signaling for protective spasming.

positioning Placing the body in such a way that specific joints or muscles are isolated.

post-event massage Massage provided after an athletic event.

post-isometric relaxation (PIR) The state that occurs after isometric contraction of a muscle; it results from the activity of minute neural reporting stations called the Golgi tendon bodies.

post-traumatic stress disorder A disorder characterized by episodes of flashback memory, state-dependent memory, somatization, anxiety, irritability, sleep disturbance, concentration difficulties, times of melancholy or depression, grief, fear, worry, anger, and avoidance behavior.

postural muscles Muscles that support the body against gravity.

power differential The difference in knowledge and skills between the client and the professional; it exists because one is placed in the position of controlling the situation.

practices Skills, techniques, and strategies a practitioner can use.

prefix A word element placed at the beginning of a root word to change the meaning of the word.

premassage activity Any activity included in massage preparation, including setting up the massage room, obtaining supplies, and determining the temperature of the room.

prescription An oral or written direction or order for dispensing and administering a health care intervention.

pressure The amount of force applied into the tissue, which is used to indicate magnitude during massage; light pressure indicates small magnitude and deep pressure indicates increased magnitude.

PRICE first aid A treatment regimen for an injury that includes protection, rest, ice, compression, and elevation.

prime movers Muscles responsible for movement.

principle A basic truth or rule of conduct.

profession An occupation that requires training and specialized study.

professional A person who practices a particular profession.

professional autonomy Having the authority to make decisions and the freedom to act in accordance with one's professional knowledge base.

professional touch Skilled touch delivered to achieve a specific outcome, after which the recipient reimburses the professional for services rendered.

professionalism Adherence to professional status, methods, standards, and character.

progress (or session) notes The use of a charting process to record each massage with the client.

prone Lying in a face-down position.

proprioceptive neuromuscular facilitation (PNF) A specific application of muscle energy type techniques that uses strong contraction combined with stretching and muscular pattern retraining.
proprioceptors Sensory receptors that detect joint and muscle activity.
protozoa One-celled organisms that are larger than bacteria able to infest human fluids and cause disease by parasitizing (living off) or directly destroying cells.
pulsed muscle energy Procedures that involve engaging the comfort barrier and using minute, resisted contractions (usually 20 in 10 seconds), which introduces mechanical pumping in addition to post-isometric relaxation or reciprocal inhibition.

Q

qualifiable A term that describes goals measured by criteria determined by the practitioner that indicate when the goal is achieved.
quantifiable A term that describes the measurement of goals by objective criteria (e.g., time, frequency, 1–10 scale) that can demonstrate an increase or decrease in ability to perform an activity, or an increase or a decrease in a sensation, such as relaxation or pain.
quiet expiration Movement of air out of the body through passive action. This occurs through relaxation of the external intercostals and the elastic recoil of the thoracic wall and tissue of the lungs and bronchi; gravity pulls the rib cage down from its elevated position.
quiet inspiration Movement of air into the body while resting or sitting quietly. The diaphragm and external intercostals are the prime movers.

R

range of motion The measurable movement of a joint.
rapport The development of a relationship based on mutual trust and harmony.
reciprocal inhibition (RI) An effect that occurs when a muscle contracts, obliging its antagonist to relax to allow normal movement.
reciprocity The exchange of privileges between governing bodies.
recovery massage Massage structured primarily for the uninjured athlete who wants to recover from a strenuous workout or competition.
reenactment Reliving an event as though it were happening at the moment.
referral Sending a client to a health care professional for specific diagnosis and treatment of a disease.
referred pain Pain felt in an area other than the source of the pain.
reflective listening The ability to restate information in a way that indicates the listener has received and understood the message.
reflex An involuntary response to a stimulus. Reflexes are specific, predictable, adaptive, and purposeful. Reflexive methods work by stimulating the nervous system (sensory neurons), and tissue changes occur in response to the body's adaptation to the neural stimulation.
reflexive effects When various mechanical forces are introduced into body tissues during massage with the intent to stimulate the nervous system, the endocrine system, and the chemicals of the body.
reflexive methods Massage techniques that stimulate the nervous system, the endocrine system, and the chemicals of the body.
reflexology A massage system concentrated primarily on the feet and hands.
refractory period The period after a muscle contraction during which the muscle is unable to contract again.
regional contraindications Contraindications that relate to a specific area of the body.
rehabilitation massage Massage used for severe injury or as part of post-surgical intervention.
relative risk The chance of occurrence expressed in comparative terms by describing the outcome rate for people exposed to the factor in question and compared with the outcome rate for those not exposed to the factor.
remedial massage Massage used for more severe injuries or as part of a post-surgical intervention plan.
research literacy The knowledge and understanding of scientific concepts and processes required for personal and professional decision making.
resilience The capacity to recover quickly from difficulties; toughness.
resourceful compensation Adjustments made by the body to manage a permanent or chronic dysfunction.
resting position The first stroke of the massage; the simple laying on of hands. Also called holding.
restorative care Care that focuses on the restoration or maintenance of physical function.
rhythm The regularity of the application of a technique. If the method is applied at regular intervals, it is considered even or rhythmic. If it is choppy or irregular, it is considered uneven or not rhythmic.
right of refusal The right of either the client or the professional to stop the massage session.
risk management The identification, evaluation, and prioritization of precautionary steps to reduce/curbing the risk.
rocking Rhythmic movement of the body.
root word The part of a word that provides its fundamental meaning.

S

safe touch Secure, respectful, considerate, sensitive, responsive, sympathetic, understanding, supportive, and empathetic contact.
salutogenesis An approach focusing on factors that support human health and well-being rather than on factors that cause disease (pathogenesis).
sanitation The formulation and application of measures to promote and establish conditions favorable to health, and public health in particular.
science The intellectual process of understanding through observation, measurement, accumulation of data, and analysis of findings.
scientific method A means of objectively researching a concept to determine whether it is valid.
scope of practice The knowledge base and practice parameters of a profession.
self-employed Working for oneself rather than another person.
self-employment tax The contribution toward Social Security and Medicare paid by self-employed individuals.
sequencing Refers both to the sequence of strokes (the order in which strokes are applied to a particular body area) and to the overall sequence of the massage (the order in which body areas are massaged).
serotonin The neurochemical that regulates mood in terms of appropriate emotions, attention to thoughts, calming, quieting, and comforting effects; it also subdues irritability and regulates drive states.

service An action performed for another person that results in a specific outcome.

severe acute respiratory syndrome (SARS) A respiratory illness marked by symptoms such as headache, fever, aches, and, commonly, pneumonia.

sexual misconduct Any behavior that is sexually oriented in the professional setting.

shaking A technique in which the body area is grasped and shaken in a quick, loose movement, sometimes classified as rhythmic mobilization.

shear Shear stress is two forces acting parallel to each other but in opposite directions so that one part of the tissue is moved or displaced relative to another part. Shear causes two objects to slide over one another.

shiatsu An acupressure- and meridian-focused bodywork system originated in Japan.

side-lying The position in which the client is lying on their side.

signs Objective abnormalities that can be seen or measured by someone other than the patient.

skin rolling A form of pétrissage that lifts the skin.

slapping A form of tapotement for which a flat hand is used.

SOAP notes A problem-oriented method of medical record keeping; the acronym SOAP stands for subjective, objective, assessment (analysis), and plan.

soft skills Related to social and emotional intelligence.

soft tissue The skin, fascia, muscles, tendons, joint capsules, and ligaments of the body.

soft-tissue deformation Soft tissue that has changed shape. A deformation occurs when internal forces in the material oppose the applied force.

somatic A term that means pertaining to the body and the framework of the body.

somatic dysfunction Impaired or altered function of related components of the somatic (body framework) system: skeletal, arthrodial, and myofascial structures and related vascular, lymphatic, and neural elements.

somatic pain Pain that arises from stimulation of receptors in the skin (superficial somatic pain) or in skeletal muscles, joints, tendons, and fascia (deep somatic pain).

spa From Latin, meaning "health from water."

special tests Methods used to assess the presence and degree of a client's or patient's condition. These assessments commonly involve specific stressing of particular structures.

speed The rate of application (i.e., fast, slow, varied).

spindle cells Sensory receptors in the belly of the muscle that detect stretch.

stabilization Holding the body in a fixed position during joint movement, lengthening, and stretching.

standard precautions Procedures developed by the Centers for Disease Control and Prevention (CDC) to prevent the spread of contagious diseases.

standards of care Treatment guidelines developed by the profession for a given condition, which identify the appropriate treatment based on scientific evidence and clinical experience.

standards of practice The principles that form specific guidelines to direct professional ethical practice and quality care, including a structure for evaluating the quality of care. Standards of practice are an attempt to define the parameters of quality care.

start-up costs The initial expenses involved in starting a business.

state-dependent memory The encoding and storing of a memory based on the effects of the autonomic nervous system and the resulting chemical levels of the body. This memory is retrievable only during a similar physiological experience in the body.

static methods Massage applications that do not use movement.

sterilization A process that destroys all microorganisms.

stimulation Excitation that activates the sensory nerves.

strain/counterstrain The use of tender points to guide the positioning of the body into a space in which the muscle tension can release on its own.

strength testing Testing intended to determine whether a muscle is responding with sufficient strength to perform required body functions. Strength testing determines a muscle's force of contraction.

stress Any substantial change in routine or any activity that forces the body to adapt.

stressors Any internal perceptions or external stimuli that demand a change in the body.

stretching Mechanical tension applied to lengthen the myofascial unit (muscles and fascia); two types are longitudinal stretching and cross-directional stretching.

stroke A technique of therapeutic massage applied with a movement on the surface of the body, which may be superficial or deep.

structural and postural integration approaches Methods of bodywork derived from biomechanics, postural alignment, and the importance of the connective tissue structures.

subtle energies Weak electrical fields that surround and run through the body.

suffering An overall impairment of a person's quality of life.

suffix A word element placed at the end of a root word to change the meaning of the word.

superficial fascia The connective tissue layer just under the skin.

superficial pressure Pressure that remains on the skin.

supervision Support from more experienced professionals.

supine The position in which the client is lying face up.

supportive climate A collaborative environment that leads to mutual trust and to an atmosphere conducive to managing differences.

symmetric stance The position in which body weight is distributed equally between the feet.

sympathetic autonomic nervous system The energy-using part of the autonomic nervous system, the division in which the fight-or-flight response is activated.

symptoms Subjective abnormalities that are not objectively detectable and can only be felt by the patient.

syndrome A group of signs and symptoms that usually arise from a common cause.

synergistic The interaction of medication and massage to stimulate the same process or effects.

system A group of interacting elements that function as a complex whole.

systemic massage Massage structured to primarily affect a particular body system. This approach usually is used for lymphatic and circulation enhancement massage.

systematic review A review summarizing the results of carefully designed health care studies that provides a high level of evidence regarding the effectiveness of health care interventions.

T

tactical athletes Personnel in law enforcement, military, and rescue professions who require unique physical training strategies aimed at optimizing occupational physical performance.

tapotement Springy blows to the body at a fast rate to create rhythmic compression of the tissue; also called percussion.

tapping A type of percussion that uses the fingertips.

target muscle The muscle or groups of muscles on which the response of the methods is specifically focused.

taxpayer identification number (TIN) An identification number used by the Internal Revenue Service (IRS) in the administration of tax laws.

taxonomy The science of classification according to a predetermined system.

techniques Methods of therapeutic massage that provide sensory stimulation or mechanical change of the soft tissue of the body.

tendon organs Structures found in the tendon and musculotendinous junction that respond to tension at the tendon. Articular (joint) ligaments contain receptors that are similar to tendon organs and adjust reflex inhibition of the adjacent muscle when excessive strain is placed on the joints.

tensegrity An architectural principle, developed in 1948 by R. Buckminster Fuller that underlies the structure of the geodesic dome. A tensegrity system is characterized by a continuous tensional network (in the body, tendons, ligaments, and fascial structures) connected by a discontinuous set of compressive elements, or struts (bones).

tension Tension stress (or tensile stress) occurs when two forces pull on an object in opposite directions so as to stretch it, make it longer and thinner, and try to pull it apart.

terminology Language specific to a specialized field of knowledge.

Thai massage A combination of elements from yoga, shiatsu, and acupressure that work with the energy pathways of the body and therapy points located along these lines.

therapeutic applications Healing or curative powers.

therapeutic change Beneficial change produced by a bodywork process that results in a modification of physical form or function that can affect a client's physical, mental, or spiritual state.

therapeutic edge The combination of pressure, drag, and duration that is most beneficial and most satisfying to clients.

therapeutic relationship The interpersonal structure and professional boundaries between professionals and the clients they serve. Also called therapeutic alliance.

thermotherapy The application of heat and cold, often used for rehabilitation purposes.

tissue load Forces load tissues. Tissue loads create stress in tissues, and tissues exposed to force are considered to be loaded. The change in shape of tissue in response to the load is called the strain.

tonic vibration reflex Reflex that tones a muscle with stimulation through vibration methods at the tendon.

torsion Torsional loading, which is usually called torsion, is when forces cause a twist about its longitudinal axis.

touch Contact with no movement.

touch technique The basis of soft tissue forms of bodywork methods.

toughening/hardening The reaction to repeated exposure to stimuli that elicit arousal responses.

traction Gentle pull on the joint capsule to increase the joint space.

training stimulus threshold The stimulus that elicits a training response.

transference The personalization of the professional relationship by the client.

transition Smooth, enjoyable movement from one type of technique to another, or the efficient progression of skills, such as the change from undraping a body area to the introduction of the therapist's hands onto the client's body.

transmission-based precautions Additional precautions beyond Standard Precautions needed to prevent transmission of specific infectious agents and are based on the likely routes of transmission including Contact Precautions, Droplet Precautions, and Airborne Precautions.

transverse friction A specific rehabilitation technique application of a concentrated, therapeutic movement that moves the tissue against its grain over only a very small area.

Trauma-Informed Care (TIC) An approach in the human service field that assumes an individual is more likely than not to have a history of trauma.

trauma Physical injury caused by violent or disruptive action, toxic substances, or psychic injury resulting from a severe long- or short-term emotional shock.

trigger point An area of local nerve facilitation; pressure on the trigger point results in hypertonicity of a muscle bundle and referred pain patterns.

tuberculosis (TB) A bacterial infection that usually affects the lungs but may invade other body systems.

V

vacuum manual therapy Use of negative pressure to create a suctioning effect, lifting tissue. Cupping is one form of this therapy.

vibration Fine or coarse tremulous movement that creates reflexive responses.

viruses Microorganisms that invade cells and insert their genetic code into the host cell's genetic code. Viruses use the host cell's nutrients and organelles to produce more virus particles.

vocation A career or occupation regarded as worthy and requiring great dedication.

W

well-being The presence of positive emotions and moods (e.g., contentment, happiness), the absence of negative emotions (e.g., depression, anxiety), as well as satisfaction with life, fulfillment, and positive functioning.

wellness The efficient balance of body, mind, and spirit, all working in harmony to provide quality of life.

Y

yang The portion of the whole realm of function of the body, mind, and spirit in Eastern thought that corresponds with sympathetic autonomic nervous system functions.

yin The portion of the whole realm of function of the body, mind, and spirit in Eastern thought that corresponds with parasympathetic autonomic nervous system functions.

Index

Note: Page numbers followed by "*f*" indicate figures, "*t*" indicate tables, and "*b*" indicate boxes.

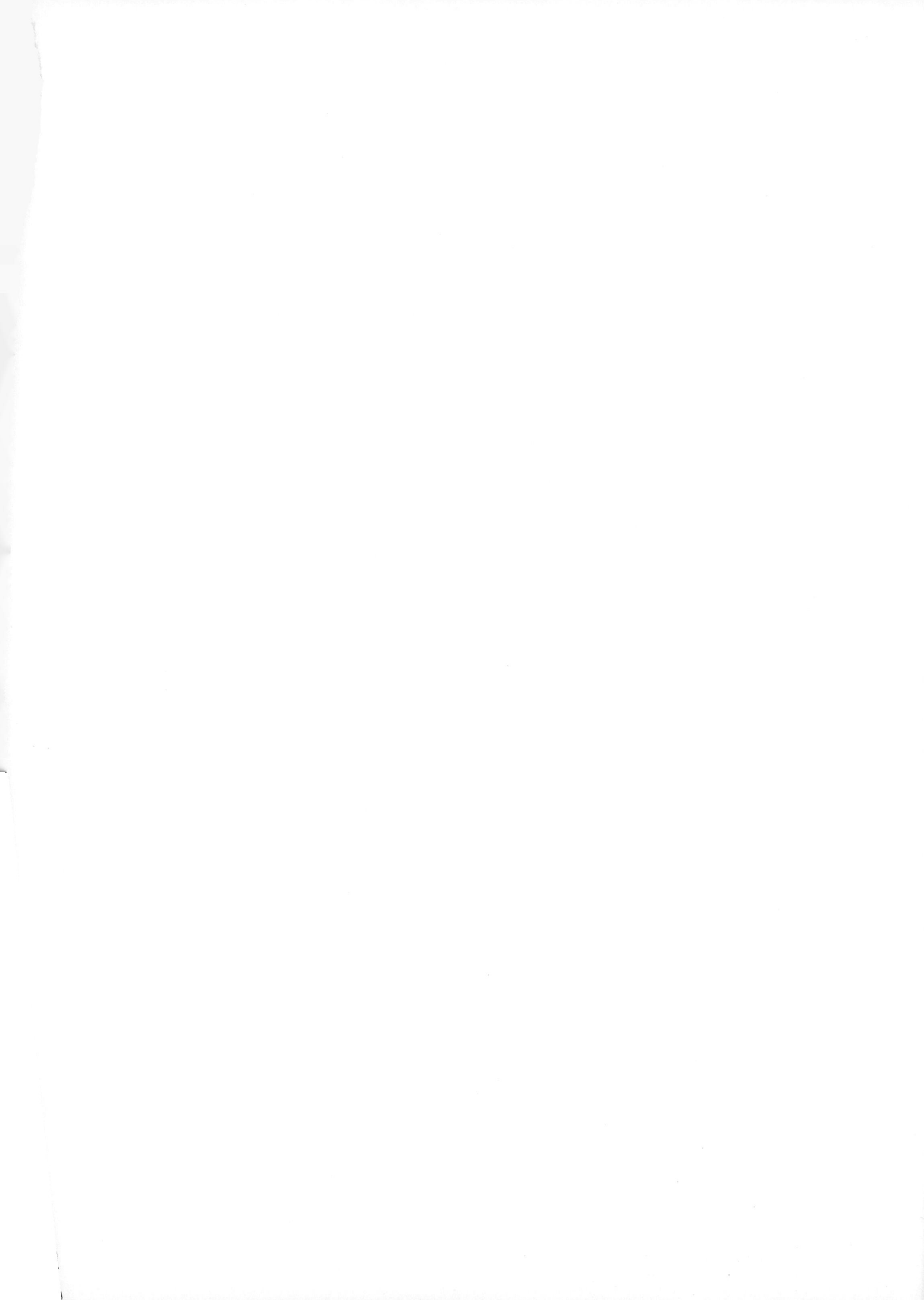